"The best women's health reference book I've ever seen."

—Julianne Moore

"This flawlessly updated edition does justice to the legacy of *Our Bodies, Ourselves,* which has been synonymous with women's empowerment for the past forty years. Incredibly detailed, empowering, and enriched by the extremely diverse opinions and positions of its collaborators, this should be on the bookshelves of women young and old worldwide!"

—Nancy Redd, author of *Body Drama* and *Diet Drama*

"The new edition of *Our Bodies, Ourselves* offers a relatable voice to help make the very confusing reality of health and sexuality as a girl easier to navigate. In a world that doesn't always offer girls such honesty, the new edition of *OBOS* makes me optimistic about the awareness and attitude of this generation of women and girls. My brain was fist pumping the whole way through."

—Tavi Gevinson, thestylerookie.com and editor in chief of *Rookie* magazine

"This revamped edition of *Our Bodies, Ourselves* shows just how far we've come in the women's health movement. The level of inclusiveness of my community—those of us who are queer, trans, or gender nonconforming—is remarkable. If this had been the edition that my mom gave me as a preteen, my life and coming-of-age would have been so different and much less confusing. It also artfully lays out the reality of women's health as a political issue—one that goes way beyond simply understanding how our bodies work. The fortieth-anniversary edition proves that education is a radical act and that sharing our struggles, triumphs, and stories can ultimately change the world."

—Miriam Zoila Pérez, editor, Feministing.com; founder, Radicaldoula.com; and recipient of the Barbara Seaman Award for Activism in Women's Health

"*OBOS* is the most important resource on women's health ever written by and for women. It teaches every woman how to take charge of her own body and helps us all become well-informed health care consumers."

—Loretta Ross, founder and the National Coordinator of the SisterSong Women of Color Reproductive Health Collective

"This is truly the bible on women's health! It has been completely revised and updated for a new generation of women who will need its guidance more than ever as they attempt to take control of their health."

—Susan Love, M.D., author of *Dr. Susan Love's Breast Book* and *Dr. Susan Love's Menopause and Hormone Book* and coauthor of *Live a Little!*

"If only every little girl were born with a copy of *Our Bodies, Ourselves* in her hands, we would raise a society filled with healthy, confident women. And if women could have only one book on their shelves, let it be this classic tome filled to the brim with practical and empowering information."

—Toni Weschler, M.P.H., author of *Taking Charge of Your Fertility*

OTHER MAJOR BOOKS BY MEMBERS OF THE BOSTON WOMEN'S HEALTH BOOK COLLECTIVE

Our Bodies, Ourselves: Menopause

Our Bodies, Ourselves: Pregnancy and Birth

Changing Bodies, Changing Lives

Ourselves and Our Children

The New Ourselves, Growing Older

OUR BODIES, OURSELVES

The Boston Women's Health Book Collective

A TOUCHSTONE BOOK
Published by Simon & Schuster
New York   London   Toronto   Sydney   New Delhi

This publication contains the opinions and ideas of its author. It is intended to provide helpful and informative material on the subjects addressed in the publication. It is sold with the understanding that the author and publisher are not engaged in rendering medical, health, or any other kind of personal professional services in the book. Readers should consult their medical, health, or other competent professional before making medical decisions.

The author and publisher specifically disclaim all responsibility for any liability, loss, or risk, personal or otherwise, which is incurred as a consequence, directly or indirectly, of the use and application of any of the contents of this book.

TOUCHSTONE
Rockefeller Center
1230 Avenue of the Americas
New York, NY 10020

This Touchstone Edition October 2011

TOUCHSTONE and colophon are registered trademarks of Simon & Schuster, Inc.

For information regarding special discounts for bulk purchases, please contact Simon & Schuster Special Sales at 1-800-456-6798 or business@simonandschuster.com.

Designed by Katy Riegel

Manufactured in the United States of America

10   9   8   7   6   5   4   3   2

Library of Congress Cataloging-in-Publication Data

Our bodies, ourselves / The Boston Women's Health Book
Collective.—40th anniversary ed.
    p. cm.
"A Touchstone book."
Includes bibliographical references and index.
  1. Women—Health and hygiene.   2. Women—Diseases.   3. Women—Psychology.
I. Boston Women's Health Book Collective.

RA778.N49   2011
613'.04244—dc23   2011022749

ISBN 978-1-4391-9066-1
ISBN 978-1-4391-8734-0 (ebook)

In loving memory of our close colleagues and women's health advocates Esther Rome, Pamela Morgan, Helen Rodriguez-Trias, Mary Howell, Jose Barzelatto, Allan Rosenfield, Rachel Fruchter, Barbara Seaman, Rita Arditti, Pat Cody, and Rosetta Reitz

■ ACKNOWLEDGMENTS

Producing a book of this size and scope is an enormous undertaking, one that would not be possible without the help and support of many people. We have been fortunate not only to have received input from more than three hundred contributors but also to have worked with some of the most insightful and dedicated women and men involved in the fields of women's health, reproductive justice, and social activism. This ninth edition of *Our Bodies, Ourselves* reflects the great magnitude of their efforts.

Contributors include nationally recognized experts and women of all ages and backgrounds who shared their stories and reviewed, revised, and rewrote each chapter. We are enormously grateful to all of them for donating their expertise and wisdom, and for collaborating to provide the most accurate, up-to-date, and reliable information about women's reproductive health and sexuality. The contributors are listed individually by chapter in the authorship and acknowledgments section, starting on page 869; short biographical statements begin on page 877.

Special mention is due to Susan Blank, Joan Ditzion, Marjorie Greenfield, Mara Kardas-Nelson, Heidi Moore, Lin Nelson, Marcie Richardson, Gary Richwald, Ellen Shaffer, Jocelyn Sims, Evelina Sterling, Kirsten Thompson, and Susan Yanow—each of whom took on the lion's share of writing and revising at least one chapter and participated in many rounds of discussion and editing.

The women who served alongside us on the *Our Bodies, Ourselves* editorial team are an invincible group. BWHBC founder Wendy Sanford dedicated the better part of the past eighteen months to this project, shepherding multiple chapters from the earliest stages of reaching out to contributors to writing and shaping final drafts. We are most grateful for her patience and nuance with words. OBOS Executive Director Judy Norsigian and nurse-midwife Amy Romano also oversaw numerous chapters, improving each one with great insight and hands-on knowledge. Ayesha Chatterjee, assistant program manager for the OBOS Global Initiative, worked passionately to include the stories and perspectives of women's groups around the world who have adapted *Our Bodies, Ourselves* into their own languages and for their own cultures. As anyone who has worked on a large project knows, success rests on the details, and so we are indebted to June Tsang, OBOS program assistant, for her careful attention to every task, including integrating edits and organizing graphics, permissions, and contributors' bios.

The entire editorial team has been inspired by and feels deep gratitude for the extraordinary involvement of those who have contributed over the years to *Our Bodies, Ourselves*. Particular recognition is due the founders of the Boston Women's Health Book Collective as well as to the organization's staff, volunteer board members, and interns, all of whom are listed on pages 873–74. Their early and ongoing efforts and passion have made a true difference in women's lives.

Kiki Zeldes, Senior Editor
Christine Cupaiuolo, Managing Editor

■■■■■■■■■■■■■■■■■■■■■ CONTENTS

We are delighted to present *Our Bodies, Ourselves*—an in-depth look at women's sexuality and reproductive health, from the first gynecological exam to sexual health in our later years.

Since its first newsprint edition published in the early 1970s, *Our Bodies, Ourselves* (OBOS) has enabled women to learn about their bodies, gain insight from the experiences of other women, and consider how best to achieve political and cultural changes that would improve women's lives. This completely revised and updated ninth edition, released on OBOS's fortieth anniversary, covers topics ranging from sexual anatomy, body image, and gender identity to pregnancy and birth, perimenopause/ menopause, and navigating the health-care system.

This edition reflects the perspective and voices of a wide range of women, and their stories are told through new formats. At our invitation, more than three dozen women of all ages and identities participated in a monthlong online conversation about sexuality and relationships; we found their honesty and forthrightness so compelling that the conversation itself became the foundation of a new "Relationships" chapter.

Other new voices include women's organizations around the world that have created their own resources adapted from *Our Bodies, Ourselves*. Throughout the book, you will meet members of the Our Bodies Ourselves

Global Network and read about their work on issues such as abortion, infertility, HIV education and prevention, and social activism. From distributing posters via canoes in rural Nigeria to setting up interactive websites in Israel and Turkey and reshaping health policy in Nepal and Armenia, their efforts exemplify movement building and the power of voices raised in action.

This edition focuses on the core health issues—reproductive health and sexuality—that first brought the Boston Women's Health Book Collective together. Some topics added over the years—such as nutrition, emotional health, and medical conditions that disproportionately or differently affect women—have been omitted this time, in part because information is now more readily available elsewhere. This has given us room to expand on issues such as reproductive rights, violence against women, and environmental health, which not only are centrally related to women's sexual health and well-being but also are areas where, despite decades of advocacy and activism, women still face enormous challenges and obstacles that prevent them from leading safe and healthy lives.

Our Bodies, Ourselves is both a text dedicated to factual information grounded in the best available evidence and a resource about health-care inequities and the work of those dedicated to ending social injustices. The many contributors to this book did not always agree on how to analyze the social, economic, and political forces that affect women's health or how to characterize a medical controversy. When a conclusion remains uncertain, we have shared their questions and concerns so readers can make their own decisions in the absence of the kind of evidence we ultimately hope will be available. Our website (ourbodiesourselves.org) contains additional content, references, and useful links on women's health topics not covered in this book.

As always, we recognize how the personal is often political and thus underscore when individual solutions are not possible or not lasting. Throughout the book, women who have joined with others to bring about change share their stories. The combination of practical information with political critique and women's lived experiences has long been the hallmark of *Our Bodies, Ourselves* and is one of the reasons the book has remained one of the most enduring

OUR BODIES OURSELVES GLOBAL INITIATIVE

Ever since *Our Bodies, Ourselves* became a best seller in the United States, it has inspired women in other countries to adapt it—in part or as a whole—to their unique cultural needs. Through the Our Bodies Ourselves Global Initiative, we support more than twenty-two women's organizations as they develop materials based on *Our Bodies, Ourselves* and use their resources in wide-scale outreach to advance the health and human rights of women and girls in their countries. Although the earliest projects were located primarily in Europe, we have since collaborated with organizations across Africa, South and Southeast Asia, the Middle East, Latin America, and Europe to bring culturally meaningful and reliable information to communities where it is most needed. As a result of our partnerships, resources based on the book are now available in more than twenty-five languages and in print, digital, and other socially interactive formats. You will read about our partners in the "In Translation" sidebars and we invite you to visit ourbodiesourselves.org/programs/ network to learn more.

legacies of the women's movements that grew out of the late 1960s and early 1970s.

Much has changed in the United States since the first edition, when abortion was illegal, birth control was not widely available, and the few available texts on women's health and sexuality—almost all written by men—discounted women's experiences and perspectives. Today, information is abundant, but it is still difficult to find reliable information that encompasses the diversity of women's experiences and teases apart the conflicts of interest inherent in many issues that affect women's health. Far too often, corporate and pharmaceutical interests influence medical research, information, and care, and contribute to the unnecessary medicalization of women's bodies and lives. This not only wastes money and poses avoidable risks but also can discourage women from questioning the assumptions underlying the care they receive and from valuing and sharing their own insights and experiences. The need for a book like *Our Bodies, Ourselves* remains as strong as ever.

Changing the medical system, organizing for better care, and altering the larger social, political, and economic forces that limit women's lives require creative and concerted efforts over a long period of time. We believe that enhancing reproductive health and sexual pleasure can play a significant positive role in all our lives and strengthen us as we work toward sustaining a vision of a world that will better nurture all women, men, and children. We encourage you to explore this book with curiosity and vision.

OBOS *Editorial Team: Kiki Zeldes, Christine Cupaiuolo, Wendy Sanford, Judy Norsigian, Amy Romano, June Tsang, and Ayesha Chatterjee Spring 2011*

Bodies and Identities

CHAPTER 1

Learning about our sexual anatomy and observing and exploring our bodies are good ways to become more comfortable with ourselves and our sexuality. These are also good ways to learn what is normal for each of us and to become aware of changes and potential problems. Understanding the way our sexual and reproductive systems work, how they interact with other body functions, and how they are influenced by our lifestyle, environment, and general well-being can help us enhance sexual pleasure, reduce the risk of some health problems, and make informed reproductive decisions.

We are often far less familiar with the appearance and function of our sexual and reproductive organs than we are with other parts of our bodies. This chapter aims to change this.

The first part discusses female sexual anatomy, including reproductive and sexual organs both inside and outside the body.* It names the body parts and explains where they are and what they do.

The second part of the chapter covers menstruation and fertility awareness. It explains how the menstrual cycle works; the commonalities, differences, and variations in women's cycles; and the physical and emotional changes some women experience. It also addresses how reproduction occurs.

SEXUAL AND REPRODUCTIVE ORGANS: ANATOMY (STRUCTURE) AND PHYSIOLOGY (FUNCTION)

The following descriptions will be much clearer if you look at your genitals with a hand mirror while you read the text and look at the diagrams. Make sure you have enough time and privacy to feel relaxed. Try squatting on the floor and putting the mirror between your feet. If you are uncomfortable in that position, sit as far forward on the edge of a chair as you comfortably can, separate your legs, and put the mirror between them. If you're having a hard time seeing, try aiming a flashlight at your genitals or at the mirror.

The appearance, shape, and size of genitals vary from person to person as much as the shape and size of other body parts. There is a wide range of what is considered normal. By observing your own body, you will learn what is normal for you.

First, you will see your vulva—all the female external organs you can see outside your body. The vulva includes the mons pubis (Latin for "pubic mound"), labia majora (outer lips), labia minora (inner lips), clitoris, and the external openings of the urethra and vagina. People often confuse the vulva with the vagina. The vagina, also known as the birth canal, is on the inside of your body. Only the opening of the vagina (introitus) can be seen from the outside.

Unless you shave or wax around your vulva, the most obvious feature you will see is the pubic hair, the first wisps of which are one of the early signs of puberty. After menopause, the hair thins out. Pubic hair covers the soft fatty tissue called the mons (also mons veneris, mound of Venus, or mons pubis).† The mons lies over the pubic symphysis. This is the joint of the pubic bones, which are part of the pelvis, or hip girdle. You can feel the pubic bones beneath the mons pubis.

As you spread your legs, you can see in the mirror that the hair continues between your legs and probably around your anus. The anus is the outside opening of the rectum (the end of the large intestine, or colon).

The fatty tissue of the mons pubis also continues between your legs to form two labia majora, the outer lips of the vulva. You can feel that the hair-covered labia majora are also fatty, like the mons. The size and appearance of the labia majora differ considerably among women. In some, the skin of the outer lips is darker. The labia majora surround the labia minora (the inner lips of the vulva). The labia minora are hairless and very sensitive to touch.

As you gently spread apart the inner lips, you can see that they protect a delicate area between them. This is the vestibule. Look more closely at it. Starting from the front, right below the mons you will see the inner lips joining to form a soft fold of skin, or hood, over and cover-

---

* This chapter describes female sexual anatomy, but some of us who identify as women do not have this anatomy. Some of us have parts of both male and female anatomy, and some with female anatomy identify as men or as neither sex. For more information, see "Disorders of Sexual Development," p. 14, and Chapter 4, "Gender Identity and Sexual Orientation."

† The formal medical term is given in parentheses if it is different from the English or more familiar term.

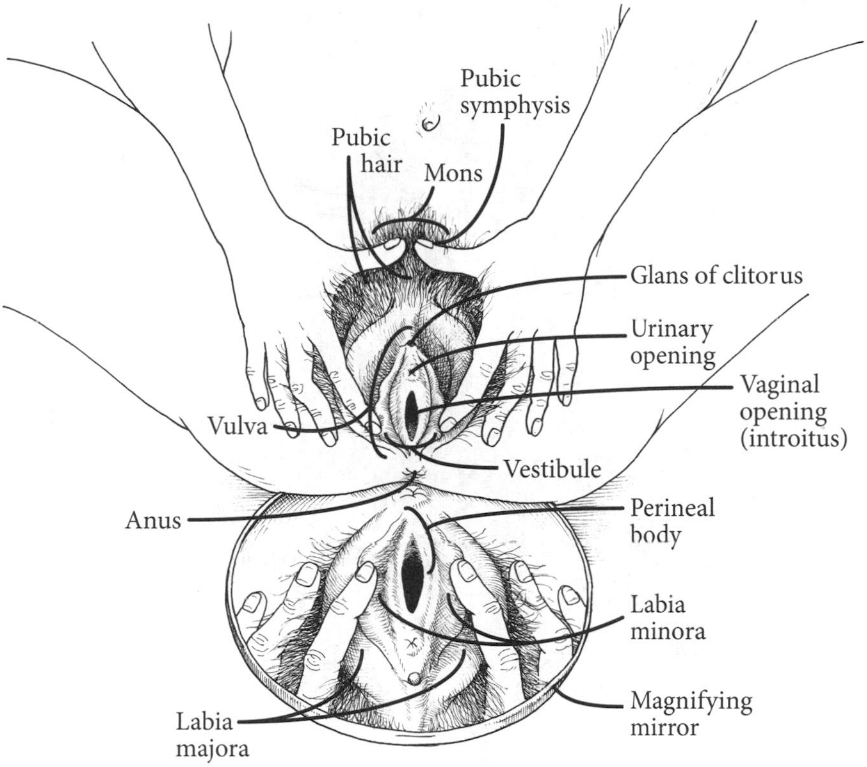
Pubic symphysis
Pubic hair
Mons
Glans of clitorus
Urinary opening
Vaginal opening (introitus)
Vulva
Vestibule
Anus
Perineal body
Labia minora
Magnifying mirror
Labia majora

THE VULVA

ing the glans, or tip of the clitoris. Gently pull up the hood to see the glans. The glans is the spot most sensitive to sexual stimulation. Many people confuse the glans with the entire clitoris, but it is simply the most visible part. Let the hood slide back, and extending from the hood up to the pubic symphysis, you can now feel a hardish, rubbery, movable rod right under the skin. It is sometimes sexually stimulating when touched. This is the body or shaft of the clitoris. It is connected to the bone by a suspensory ligament. You cannot feel this ligament or the next few organs described, but they are all important in sexual arousal and orgasm.

At the point where you no longer feel the shaft of the clitoris, it divides into two parts, spreading out wishbone fashion but at a much wider angle, to form the crura (singular: crus), the two anchoring wing tips of erectile tissue that attach to the pelvic bones. The crura of the clitoris are about 3 inches long. Starting from where the shaft and crura meet, and continuing down along the sides of the vestibule, are two bundles of erectile tissue called the bulbs of the vestibule.

The bulbs, along with the whole clitoris (glans, shaft, crura), become firm and filled with blood during sexual arousal, as do the walls of the vagina. Both the crura of the clitoris and the bulbs of the vestibule are covered in muscle tissue. This muscle helps to create tension and fullness during arousal and contracts during orgasm, playing an important role in the invol-

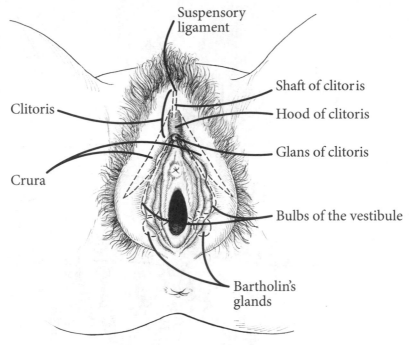

Suspensory ligament

Shaft of clitoris

Clitoris

Hood of clitoris

Glans of clitoris

Crura

Bulbs of the vestibule

Bartholin's glands

DETAILS OF THE CLITORIS

(Dotted lines indicate areas inside the body.)

untary spasms felt at that time. The clitoris and vestibular bulbs are the only organs in the body solely for sexual sensation and arousal.

The clitoris is similar in origin and function to the penis. All female and male organs, including sexual and reproductive organs, are developed from the same embryonic tissue. In fact, female and male fetuses are identical during the first six weeks of development. The glans of the clitoris corresponds to the glans of the penis, and the labia majora correspond to the scrotum.

In some cultures, there is a practice of female genital cutting—removing a girl's clitoris and sometimes even sewing the labia together. For more information, see "Female Genital Cutting," p. 793.

The Bartholin's glands are two small rounded bodies on either side of the vaginal opening near the bottom of the vestibule. They secrete a small amount of fluid during arousal. Usually you cannot see or feel them.

If you keep the inner lips spread and pull the hood of the clitoris back again, you will notice that the inner lips attach to the underside of the clitoris. Right below this attachment you will see a small dot or slit. This is the urinary opening, the outer opening of the urethra, a short (about an inch and a half), thin tube leading to your bladder. Below the opening of the urethra is the vaginal opening (introitus).

Around the vaginal opening you may be able to see the remains of the hymen, also known as the vaginal corona. This is a thin membrane just inside the vaginal opening, partially blocking the opening but almost never covering it completely. Vaginal coronas come in widely varying

VAGINAL CORONA (OR WHAT YOU MAY KNOW AS THE HYMEN)*

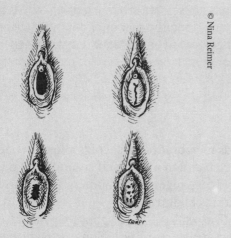

© Nina Reimer

The vaginal corona—generally known as the hymen but renamed by a Swedish sexual rights group in an attempt to dispel many of the myths surrounding hymens—is made up of thin, elastic folds of mucous membrane located just inside the entrance to the vagina. The vaginal corona has no known function; it is probably a remnant of fetal development.

Many people wrongly believe that the vaginal corona is a thick membrane that entirely covers a woman's vaginal opening and ruptures when you have intercourse or any kind of insertive vaginal sex the first time. The myth goes like this: If a bride doesn't bleed from a ruptured hymen on her wedding night, this means that she has had sex and isn't a "virgin." This is not true.

* Content is adapted from *The Vaginal Corona*, a booklet created by the Swedish Association for Sexuality Education, rfsu.se/en/Engelska/Sex-and-Politics/Hymen-renamed-vaginal-corona.

The mucous membrane that makes up the vaginal corona may be tightly or more loosely folded. It may be slightly pink, almost transparent, but if it is thicker it may look a little paler or whitish. The vaginal corona may resemble the petals of a flower, or it may look like a jigsaw piece or a half-moon. It may be insignificant or even completely absent at birth.

The vaginal corona may tear or thin out during exercise, masturbation, tampon use, or any other form of vaginal penetration. Because of this, no one can look at a woman's vaginal corona and know whether she has had vaginal intercourse, or even whether she has masturbated.

In rare cases, the hymen covers the entire vaginal opening. This is called an imperforate or microperforate hymen. Young women with an imperforate hymen will experience monthly cramping and discomfort without the appearance of menstrual blood. In these cases, the hymen can be surgically opened to release accumulated menstrual fluid and to permit tampon insertion or other forms of vaginal penetration. More commonly, a hymen band may be present across the vaginal opening, allowing menstruation but preventing tampon insertion. If the opening is very small or partially obstructed, minor surgery can correct this.

Since the vaginal corona isn't a brittle membrane, the sensation when you first stretch out the mucous tissue folds—whether you're inserting a tampon, masturbating, or having insertive sex—is a highly individual experience. Some women feel no pain at all, while others,

sizes and shapes. For most women they stretch easily—by a tampon, as well as a finger, a penis, or a dildo. Even after the hymen has been stretched, little folds of tissue remain.

If you're comfortable doing so, slowly put a finger or two inside your vagina. If it hurts or you have trouble, take a deep breath and relax. You may be pushing at an awkward angle, your vagina may be dry, or you may be unconsciously tensing the muscles owing to fear of discomfort. Try shifting positions and using a lubricant such as olive or almond oil (not perfumed body lotion). Notice how the vaginal walls, which were touching each other, spread around your fingers and hug them. Feel the soft folds of mucous membrane. These folds allow the vagina to stretch and to mold itself around what might be inside it: fingers, a tampon, a penis, or a baby during childbirth.

The walls of the vagina may vary from almost dry to very wet. Some women naturally have wetter or drier vaginas. Wetness increases with sexual arousal. How wet your vagina is also changes during different parts of your menstrual cycle and over your lifetime. The vagina is likely to be drier before puberty, during breastfeeding, and after menopause, as well as during that part of the menstrual cycle right before and after the flow. Wetter times occur around ovulation, during pregnancy, and during sexual arousal.

Push gently all around against the walls of the vagina and notice where the walls feel particularly sensitive to touch. For some women this sensitivity occurs only in the area closest to the vaginal opening; in others it occurs in most or all of the vagina. About a third of the way up from the vaginal opening, on the anterior (front) wall of the vagina (the side toward your abdomen), is an area known as the Gräfenberg spot, or G-spot. Many women experience intensely pleasurable sensations when this area is stimulated. There are differences of opinion over whether the G-spot is a distinct anatomical structure or whether the pleasure some women feel when the area is stimulated is due to its closeness to the bulbs of the clitoris. (For more information, see "The G-Spot," p. 159.)

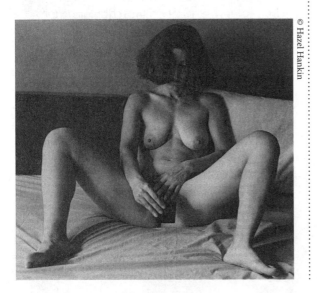

© Hazel Hankin

Now put your finger halfway in and try to grip your finger with your vagina. You are contracting the pelvic floor muscles. These muscles hold the pelvic organs in place and provide support for your other organs all the way up to your diaphragm, which is stretched across the bottom of your rib cage. Some women do Kegel exercises to strengthen the pelvic floor muscles (to learn more, see "How to Do Kegel Exercises," p. 643).

Only a thin wall of mucous membrane and connective tissue separates the vagina from the rectum, so you may be able to feel bumps on the back side of your vagina if you have some stool in the rectum.

Now slide your middle finger as far back into your vagina as you can. Notice that your finger goes in toward the small of your back at an angle, not straight up the middle of your body. If you were standing, your vagina would be at about a 45-degree angle to the floor. With your finger you may be able to just feel the deep end of your vagina. This part of the vagina is called the fornix. (Not everyone can reach this; it may help if you bring your knees and chest closer together so your finger can slide in farther.)

A little before the end of the vagina you can feel your cervix. The cervix feels like a nose with a small dimple in its center. The cervix is the part of the uterus, or womb, that extends into the vagina. It is sensitive to pressure but has no nerve endings on the surface. The uterus changes position, color, and shape during the menstrual cycle as well as during puberty and menopause, so you may feel the cervix in a different place from one day to the next. Some days you can barely reach it. The vagina also lengthens slightly during sexual arousal, carrying the cervix deeper into the body.

The dimple in the cervix is the os, or opening into the uterus. The entrance is very small. Normally, only menstrual fluid leaving the uterus, or seminal fluid entering the uterus, passes

through the cervix. No tampon, finger, or penis can go up through it, although it is capable of expanding enormously for a baby during labor and birth.

CERVIX SELF-EXAM

If you want to see your cervix, find a private, comfortable place with good lighting and gather these supplies: a flashlight, a speculum (a metal or plastic tool used to hold apart the walls of the vagina; see "Where to Buy a Speculum," above), a lubricant such as such as olive or almond oil, and a hand mirror. Wash your hands, then sit back on a couch, a comfortable chair, or the floor, with pillows behind your back for support. Bend your knees and place your feet wide apart.

Familiarize yourself with the speculum. Different styles work slightly differently. All have two bills and a handle. Use the lever to open the bills until the lock clicks. Be sure you figure out how to release the lock before you insert it.

Put some lubricant on the speculum or your vulva. Hold the speculum in a closed position (with the bills together) with the handle pointing upward. Slide it in gently as far as it will comfortably go. If it hurts, stop. Pull it out and try inserting it into the vagina sideways, then turn it. Experiment to see what feels most comfortable for you. Keep in mind that your vagina is angled toward your back, not up toward your head. You can put your finger in your vagina to feel where your cervix is and how to direct the speculum.

Once the speculum is inserted, grasp the handle and squeeze the lever toward the handle to open the bills. Some women find that placing the speculum and finding the cervix take some effort. Breathe deeply and manipulate the speculum gently while looking into the mirror. You will be able to see the folds in the vaginal wall, which may look pink, bulbous, and wet. The cervix looks like a rounded or flattened knob about the size of a quarter. If you don't see it, allow the speculum to gently close and shift the angle of insertion before reopening it, or remove the speculum and reinsert it. Focus the light source on the mirror to help you see better. If you want, a friend or partner can help by holding the flashlight and/or the mirror. If you still can't see your cervix, wait a few days and then try again. The position of the cervix shifts during the menstrual cycle, so it may be easier to see at another time.

When you find your cervix, lock open the bills of the speculum. You will see some cervical and vaginal discharges. Depending on where you are in your menstrual cycle, your cervical fluid may range from pasty-white to a clear and stretchy egg-white texture. The cervix itself may be pink and smooth, or it might be uneven, rough, or splotchy. All of these are normal. If you are pregnant, your cervix might have a bluish tint; if you have reached menopause or are breastfeeding, it may be pale. If you are ovulating, the cervix will appear open with clear stretchy mucus sitting in it. The slit or opening in the center is the os, the opening to your uterus.

You may see small, yellow/white fluid-filled sacs on the cervix that look like little blisters. These are Nabothian cysts and are quite common and do not need any treatment. They are caused by a blockage in the fluid-producing glands of the cervix. Some women have them for years; in other women they come and go. You may also see polyps, pink outgrowths of cervical tissue that dangle on a stalk, looking like a little tongue sticking through the os.

When you are done exploring, unlock and remove the speculum. Some women prefer to remove it after the lock is released but while it's still open; others close the bills first. Clean it afterward with soap and water or rubbing alcohol (isopropyl alcohol) before storing for later use.

Observing the color, size, and shape of your cervix and the changes in your vaginal discharge and cervical fluid during the different stages of your menstrual cycles allows you to learn what is normal for you and can help you recognize when something is wrong. You can do cervical self-exams regularly or during certain phases of your fertility cycle—or maybe just once to check things out.

What's Not Normal

It is normal to have vaginal and cervical fluid, or discharge. However, any of the following found during a self-exam may indicate an infection or another problem.

Recommended Resource: Beautiful Cervix Project (beautifulcervix.com) was founded by a twenty-five-year-old woman who took photos daily for a month to see how her cervix looked throughout the menstrual cycle. The site grew to include photos submitted by women from age twenty to past sixty. There are images of cervixes during pregnancy and after orgasm. You can also view photos of a Pap test in progress.

- Green, gray, or dark yellow discharge
- A significant change in the amount or consistency of discharge
- Any strong odor unusual for you
- Foamy discharge (from gas-producing organisms)

If you find anything that concerns you, see a health-care provider. (For more information, see Chapter 2, "Intro to Sexual Health.")

Internal Organs

The nonpregnant uterus is about the size of a plum. Its thick walls are made of some of the most powerful muscles in the body. It is located between the bladder, which is beneath the abdominal wall, and the rectum, which is near the backbone. The inner walls of the uterus touch each other unless pushed apart by a growing fetus or an abnormal growth. The top of the uterus is called the fundus.

Extending outward and back from each side of the fundus are the two fallopian tubes (also called oviducts; literally, "egg tubes"). They are approximately 4 inches long and look like thin

ram's horns facing backward. The connecting opening from the inside of the uterus to the fallopian tubes is as small as a fine needle. The outer end of each tube is fringed (fimbriated) and funnel shaped. The wide end of the funnel wraps partway around the ovary but does not actually attach to it. The fallopian tubes are held in place by connective tissue.

The ovaries are organs about the size and shape of unshelled almonds, located on either side of and somewhat behind the uterus. They are about 4 or 5 inches below your waist and are held in place by connective tissue. The ovaries have a twofold function: to produce germ cells (eggs) and to produce sex hormones (estrogen, progesterone, testosterone, and many others). The functions of these hormones are only partly understood. The small gap between the ovary and the end of the corresponding tube allows the egg to float freely in the abdominal cavity after it has been released from the ovary. The fingerlike ends (fimbria) of the fallopian tube sweep across the surface of the ovary and wave the egg into the tube after ovulation.

The uterus, fallopian tubes, and ovaries are draped in peritoneum, the thin membrane that lines the inside of the abdominal cavity.

BREASTS

Our breasts make us mammals. Their extraordinary glands produce milk with an incredible capacity to nourish babies' oversize human brains and to fight infection and disease in newborns. Breasts are secondary sex characteristics, which are features that distinguish the sexes but are not directly related to reproduction. Most women think of them as a key component of our sexual selves.

Self-image is often affected by our own and others' reactions to our breasts. Our feelings, both positive and negative, are reinforced by society's obsessive fixation on breasts and the

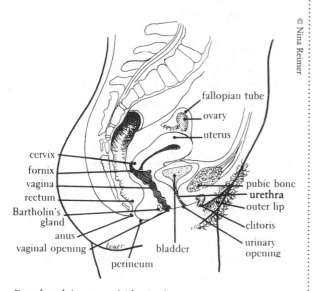

© Nina Reimer

fallopian tube
ovary
uterus

cervix
fornix
vagina
rectum
Bartholin's gland
anus
vaginal opening
perineum
bladder
pubic bone
urethra
outer lip
clitoris
urinary opening

Female pelvic organs (side view)

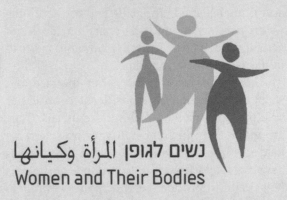

نשים לגופן המרأة וكيانها
Women and Their Bodies

The logo for Women and Their Bodies, OBOS's partner in Israel

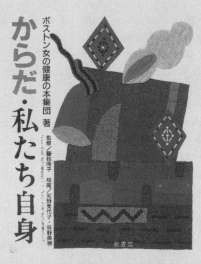

The cover of a Japanese adaptation of *Our Bodies, Ourselves*

Group: Women and Their Bodies

Country: Israel

Resource: Materials based on *Our Bodies, Ourselves* in Arabic and Hebrew

Website: ourbodiesourselves.org/programs/network/foreign

In many cultures, the words and images used to describe female bodies and sexualities are negative, derogatory, and oppressive.

This negative discourse reinforces attitudes that endanger the health of women and girls and silences their voices. It also allows a community to justify or ignore practices that are disempowering and prevent women and girls from fully exercising their rights.

Many of Our Bodies Ourselves' global partners encounter this language prob-

Group: Shokado Women's Bookstore

Country: Japan

Resource: Materials based on *Our Bodies, Ourselves* in Japanese

Website: ourbodiesourselves.org/programs/network/foreign

lem. Here are two examples of women's organizations that effectively changed the tenor in their communities by coining vocabulary that honors women and girls and affirms their sexuality and life experiences.

The Jewish and Arab women who together founded Women and Their Bodies, OBOS's global partner in Israel, note that both cultures prize a woman's ability to bear children, and the end of fertility is often seen as bringing despair. Though this attitude has deep historical and political roots, Women and Their Bodies is concerned about the pressure it places on women to increase the size of their ethnic community by having children. The group is also concerned about social attitudes that affect women who are unable or choose not to have children or are past childbearing age.

Cultural values are often reflected in language. For example, common Hebrew terms for menopause translate to "age of wilting" or being "worn out," and an Arabic term means "years of despair." While developing the Hebrew and Arabic adaptations of *Our Bodies, Ourselves,* Women and Their Bodies was determined to use terms that are respectful and celebratory. With support and help from women in the community, the group ultimately settled on the Hebrew "Emtza Ha'hayim," or "midlife," and the Arabic "San' al Aman," which means "years of security or safety."

In Japanese, words for body parts like vulva, pubic hair, and pubic bone were written using Chinese characters that conveyed "shame" or "shadiness." Shokado Women's Bookstore, OBOS's partner in Japan, revised these negatively nuanced Chinese characters to create neutral or positive terms for the Japanese adaptation of *Our Bodies, Ourselves.*

Since publication, at least one of the terms, "seimo," which translates to "sexual hair," has been integrated into some of the latest Japanese dictionaries. There is also a growing tendency in Japanese society to avoid the Chinese characters that convey "shame" or "shadiness." Instead, the language now increasingly uses neutral characters or "katakana-go"—foreign words turned into Japanese—when talking about male and female bodies. The changes translate into a major improvement, in any language.

way they are used to sell everything from cars to whiskey. This may make it difficult to think about our breasts as functioning parts of our bodies, especially in a culture that heavily markets breast enlargement/augmentation.

Look at your breasts in the mirror or feel them. Like fingerprints, no two breasts are alike, and there is no "perfect" pair. Breasts come in all sizes and shapes: large, small, firm, saggy, lumpy. Your breasts may be slightly different from each other in size or shape. Nipples may lie flat, stick out, or retract (be inverted). The areola (the area surrounding the nipple) may be large or small, darker or lighter, and it usually has little bumps just under the skin. These bumps are the sebaceous glands, which secrete a lubricant that protects the nipple during breastfeeding. Sometimes there are hairs near the edge of the areola. Some women have one breast noticeably bigger than the other. Breast size is not related to the sexual responsiveness of the breast or to the amount of milk you produce after giving birth; small-breasted women are able to breastfeed just fine. Weight gain and loss also affect breast size.

Breasts usually become droopier over the years as skin becomes less elastic and milk glands get smaller. This happens even faster after childbirth (when breastfeeding is completed) and again after menopause, when the milk glands are no longer stimulated to grow.

DISORDERS OF SEXUAL DEVELOPMENT

Disorders of sexual development (or DSDs) are conditions in which a person is born with sex chromosomes, external genitals, or an internal reproductive system that is not clearly male or female. The clitoris may be larger than usual, or the vagina may be small, lack an external opening, or be absent altogether. DSDs are not always visible by looking at the outside genitals; for example, a person may be born with external female genitals but with male chromosomes and internal testes (male reproductive glands) rather than ovaries.

For many years, the term "intersex" has been used by and about people born with genital or reproductive anatomy that is not clearly or exclusively male or female. Recently, concerns about the stigma sometimes associated with the term "intersex," along with advances in treatment and diagnosis, have led to the use of the term "disorders of sexual development" in its place.*

When DSDs are detected in infants, most are surgically assigned a female or male sex at birth, and many discover that their internal organs are different only when they reach puberty. They may not mature physically in the way a typical girl or boy would at that age; for example, those assigned female may not menstruate.

* There is also some controversy over the choice of "disorder" rather than "difference" or "divergence." See, for example, Elizabeth Reis, "Divergence or Disorder? The Politics of Naming Intersex," *Perspectives in Biology and Medicine* 50 (2007): 535-43.

The traditional medical model of treatment for babies born with DSDs, developed in the 1950s, involves using surgery to alter a baby's genitals to look clearly male or female. This practice is based on the assumption that altering the genitals to look as typical as possible and keeping the condition hidden are the only way these babies (and their parents) can avoid emotional trauma and live a "normal" life.

There is growing controversy over the practice of surgically altering babies born with DSD. Often the surgeries themselves create health problems, impair sexual functioning later in life, and contribute to emotional trauma. Angela Moreno, author of the essay "In Amerika They Call Us Hermaphrodites," describes her experience.

When I was twelve, I started to notice that my clitoris (that wonderful location of pleasure for which I had no name but to which I had grown quite attached) had grown more prominent. Exactly one month later, I was admitted to Children's Memorial Hospital in Chicago for surgery. They told me a little bit about the part where they were going to "remove my ovaries" because they suspected cancer or something like that. They didn't mention the part where they were going to slice off my clitoris. All of it. I guess the doctors assumed I was as horrified by my outsized clit as they were, and there was no need to discuss it with me. After a week's recovery in the hospital, we all went home and barely ever spoke of it again. I'm now twenty-four. I've spent the last ten years in a haze of disordered eating and occasional depression. Four months ago, I finally got some of my medical records from Children's Memorial Hospital in Chicago. They are shocking. The surgeon who removed my clitoris summarized the outcome as "tolerated well."[2]

Many people with DSDs and their advocates now believe that cosmetic genital surgery should be performed only when a child or young adult is old enough to make his or her own decisions. Organizations such as the Accord Alliance (accordalliance.org) and the Androgen Insensitivity Syndrome Support Group (aissg.org) are fighting to end the secrecy and shame around DSDs, to develop better approaches to health care, and to create support for healing emotionally from well-meaning but misguided or involuntary medical interventions.

One woman in her twenties talks about the healing this movement brought her.

At the age of eighteen, a workshop on intersex changed my life. I was finally able to get angry at the way I had been treated by doctors, about the assumptions that had been made about me and my body, and about the pressure put on me by doctors that I need to be "fixed." I made the decision that I would keep my body as it is and have finally learned to love and enjoy my sexuality again.

I really believe that the stigma or shame that is used to justify operating on intersex people is a result of this being kept such a secret. The idea that those of us outside the "norm" must conform to the status quo is absurd! If we were all raised with the understanding that not all people are male or female, it would not be so traumatic for those of us outside of the sex binary.

Because breasts react to sex hormones produced by the ovaries, you may notice pronounced changes during the menstrual cycle—your breasts may be bigger and fuller right before you menstruate. This fullness can produce tenderness in some women and can be felt up into the armpit in the part of the breast called the tail. During pregnancy and breastfeeding, breasts often enlarge considerably. They may also swell during sexual arousal. Your breasts may have areas of hardness or softness, different textures, and varying areas of sensitivity.

In girls, around the time the ovaries begin producing estrogen (a year or two before menstrual periods start), the breasts respond by growing. At first, a firm mass develops directly behind the nipple. This is called the bud. As puberty progresses, the ductal tissue in the bud grows out into the fatty tissue, forming branches and lobules to make up the glandular portion of the breast. The fatty and fibrous tissues that support it (stroma) also increase during puberty. Most of this growth happens early, but slower growth continues during the teen years. One breast may develop more quickly than the other, and it's not uncommon for breasts to be different sizes.

With the great increase of sex hormones during adolescence, the milk-producing glands in each breast start to develop and increase in size. During the reproductive years, breast tissue consists of the glandular breast lobules, which are

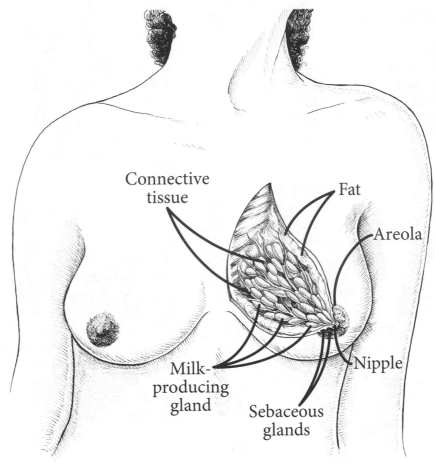

Connective tissue

Fat

Areola

Milk-producing gland

Sebaceous glands

Nipple

Parts of the breast

supported by connective tissue ligaments that anchor breast tissue to the skin and to the connective tissue covering the underlying muscles. Variable amounts of fat fill the spaces between the breast lobules and the supporting ligaments. After menopause, the glandular breast tissue is gradually replaced by fat. The amount of fat in the breast is determined partly by heredity. This fat causes breast size to vary.

Breast Self-Exams

For years, experts advised women to perform monthly breast self examinations (BSEs), believing that doing so would allow women to find potentially cancerous lumps and get diagnosed and treated for breast cancer more quickly. Unfortunately, scientific studies designed to measure the efficacy of BSEs have *not* found that women who perform BSEs are any less likely to die of breast cancer than women who don't perform them. For this reason, many medical guidelines and health organizations no longer recommend monthly BSEs. However, exploring your breasts is a good way to get to know your body and become familiar with what is normal for you.

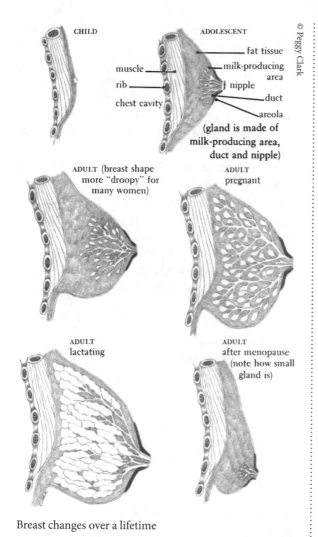

CHILD

ADOLESCENT

fat tissue

muscle

milk-producing area

rib

nipple

chest cavity

duct

areola

(gland is made of milk-producing area, duct and nipple)

ADULT (breast shape more "droopy" for many women)

ADULT pregnant

ADULT lactating

ADULT after menopause (note how small gland is)

Breast changes over a lifetime

STAGES IN THE REPRODUCTIVE LIFE CYCLE

Puberty is the transition from childhood to physical maturity. In women, puberty is characterized by growth of the breasts and pubic and armpit (axillary) hair, and a growth spurt that results in increased height and weight, followed by the end of bone growth. Menstruation starts near the end of puberty, about two years after breast development, on average at about age twelve, though any age from nine to sixteen is normal.

Menstruation continues until age fifty-one on average, but stopping anytime between forty and fifty-five is normal. Menopause technically means the time of the last period, but because periods can be irregular in the last few years, menopause can be identified only retrospectively, after a year of no bleeding. The body changes that occur between the reproductive and postreproductive phases of our lives—a period of time called perimenopause—often take place over as many as fifteen years.

This entire reproductive process is regulated by hormones, chemicals in the bloodstream and in the brain that relay messages from one part of the body to another. The levels of sex hormones are low during childhood, increase tremendously during the reproductive years, and then become lower and differently balanced after menopause.

During the reproductive years, monthly hormonal rhythms determine the timing of ovulation and menstruation. This cycle, the menstrual cycle, regulates our fertility, allowing for the possibility of pregnancy a few days every month. Many women experience signs of this rhythm—changing emotions, changes in breasts, changes in sexual arousal, and even variation in foods we enjoy eating at different times over a month.

MENSTRUATION AND THE REPRODUCTIVE CYCLE

My cycle. My red friend. The curse. Aunt Flo. On the rag. Many different terms—most commonly, my period—are used to describe menstruation. You may have created your own slang, known only to family or friends. This section covers the wide range of experiences with, and feelings about, menstruation.

Menarche (First Period)

The first period may come as a surprise, and negative attitudes from friends or family can color the experience, but most of us find a way to cope and may even look back in humor.

In class, I got up to go to the bathroom. Inside, I noticed that my panties had a funny discharge on them. Then suddenly it hit me: I'd gotten my period! I was so excited and could hardly wait to tell my friends.

The beginning of menstruation is a major marker in the transition from girl to woman. The age of menarche (MEN-are-kee)—when a girl first begins to menstruate—varies, depending on many factors. Some factors are biological; for instance, body fat must be about one quarter of a girl's total weight in order for her to menstruate. Diet, weight, race, environment, and family history also affect when menstruation begins.[3] Women in different countries may have different average ages for entering puberty.

In the United States, the average age of girls' first period has fallen over the last century from around age sixteen to around age twelve, with some girls beginning to develop breasts as early as seven years old. The reasons girls are maturing earlier are not completely clear. Some pediatricians and other medical experts are convinced that childhood exposure to plastics, pesticides, and other environmental endocrine disruptors plays a role. (Endocrine disruptors are chemicals that often act like estrogen and interfere with genetic or hormonal signals, causing changes to the body's finely tuned hormonal system.)

Other possible causes include better nutrition than in the past, obesity, inactivity, premature birth, and formula feeding.[4] A major concern about early puberty in girls is that it increases the odds of developing breast cancer later in life, since longer exposure to sex hormones is a risk factor for breast cancer. Once a girl starts to menstruate, her estrogen levels rise and don't drop off until menopause. All other factors being equal, the more years a woman menstruates, the more years she is exposed to higher levels of estrogen, and the higher her risk of breast cancer.

Some medical conditions affect reproductive development, and not all women have periods. If you haven't seen signs of puberty by age thirteen, or haven't started your period by age sixteen, see a health-care provider.

A twenty-five-year-old woman who does not menstruate says she has discovered how much menstruation is connected with normality in people's minds.

I don't menstruate, and have actually always felt kind of alienated by the way in which female experiences are sometimes centered around menstruation—the idea that menstruating makes someone a "real" woman, for example, or that menstruation is such a quintessential experience that if you haven't menstruated, you don't know what it's like to be a woman.

What Happens During the Menstrual Cycle

As you read this section, you may want to refer back to the drawings and descriptions of sexual anatomy in the first part of this chapter.

The Ovaries and Ovulation

When a girl is born, her ovaries contain about 2 million balls of cells, each with an immature egg in the center. These are called follicles. The ovaries absorb more than half of these follicles during childhood. Of the 400,000 follicles still present at puberty, three hundred to five hundred will eventually develop into mature eggs.

During our reproductive years, follicles develop throughout the cycle, but each month, under the influence of hormones, usually only one follicle develops fully. (Sometimes two or more follicles develop fully, in which case a twin or other multiple pregnancy can result.) Some of the cells in the developing follicle secrete the hormone estrogen. The follicle with the maturing egg inside moves toward the surface of the ovary. At ovulation, the follicle and the ovarian surface open, allowing the tiny egg to float out. About this time, some women feel a twinge or cramp in the lower abdomen or back (called mittelschmerz).

I never knew the word "mittelschmerz" until I was in nursing school. I thought it was such a cool word but was sure I wasn't one of those women who actually experienced it. A year or so later I began tracking all of my fertility signs when I decided to try to get pregnant. I felt a funny cramp on my left side that was a familiar sensation but I had never put two and two together to recognize that it was my body ovulating. I actually exclaimed out loud, "Mittelschmerz!"

A few women experience headaches, stomach pains, or sluggishness at the time of ovulation. Other women feel especially well.

The Egg After Ovulation

After ovulation, the fingerlike ends (fimbria) of the nearby fallopian tube sweep the released egg into the tube's funnel-shaped end. Each tube is lined with microscopic hairlike projections (cilia) that constantly move back and forth. As the egg begins its several-day journey to the uterus, wavelike movements of the muscles in the tube (peristalsis) and the movements of the cilia help it along. If sperm enter the vagina, pass through the cervix, and travel through the uterus into the fallopian tubes, the cilia propel them toward the egg.

If the egg and sperm meet, they may join. (This is conception, or fertilization, when the sperm "fertilizes" the egg.) The fertilized egg then travels the rest of the way along the fallopian tube to the uterus. Whether or not fertilization takes place, the empty follicle that just released the egg from the ovary becomes a corpus luteum (Latin for "yellow body" because of its color). The corpus luteum continues to make estrogen and also begins making progesterone.

If a fertilized egg implants into the uterus, it sends a signal to the ovary to keep making progesterone, which will help sustain a pregnancy by keeping the uterine lining thick and nourishing. If no pregnancy occurs, the corpus luteum is reabsorbed into the ovary after two weeks and the hormone levels drop; this is the trigger that causes menstruation. (See "The Endometrium," p. 20.) The egg disintegrates or flows out with the vaginal secretions.

The Cervix

The kind of mucus or fluid produced by your cervix changes throughout the cycle in response to fluctuations in estrogen and progesterone. While there are general patterns of fluid secretion, each woman's pattern is unique. (See "Fertility Awareness Method," p. 26, for more.)

The cervical fluid is a kind of gatekeeper for the uterus. At ovulation, the cervical fluid becomes slippery and thin, like egg white. It coats the vagina and protects sperm from the vagina's relatively acidic environment. The cervical fluid also nourishes the sperm and changes their structure to prepare them to fertilize an egg. Sperm can live up to five days in midcycle cervical fluid. After ovulation, as progesterone levels increase, cervical fluid thickens into a kind of plug that makes it difficult for sperm to enter the uterus. The vagina gradually becomes drier, too.

If you look at your cervix with a speculum or

feel it with your fingers, you may notice that at about the time of ovulation, the cervix is pulled up high into the vagina. It may also enlarge and soften, and the os (the opening to the uterus) may open a little.

The Endometrium: Lining of the Uterus

The lining of the uterus, called the endometrium, thickens and then thins over the course of a menstrual cycle and thickens considerably during pregnancy. Embedded in this lining are glands that can secrete a fluid that will help nourish a pregnancy until a placenta is formed. In a typical menstrual cycle, estrogen made by the maturing ovarian follicle causes the glands to grow and the endometrium to thicken (partly through an increased blood supply). This thickening of the uterine lining is called the proliferative phase of the menstrual cycle. It can vary in length, generally lasting between six and twenty days. Progesterone, made by the corpus luteum (ruptured follicle) after the egg is released, stimulates the glands in the endometrium to begin secreting their nourishing substance. This is the secretory phase of the cycle and is the only time when a fertilized egg can implant in the lining. In women who have irregular periods, it is the proliferative phase that is variable; for example, a woman with twenty-eight-day cycles ovulates on day fourteen, while a woman with thirty-five-day cycles ovulates on day twenty-one.

If conception does not occur, the corpus luteum produces estrogen and progesterone for about twelve days, with the amount lessening in the last few days. As the estrogen and progesterone levels drop, the tiny arteries bringing blood supply to the endometrium close off. The lining, deprived of nourishment and oxygen, collapses and breaks off starting about fourteen days after ovulation. This is menstruation: the menstrual period or flow.

During menstruation, most of the lining is shed, but the bottom third remains to form a new lining. Then, as a new follicle starts growing and secreting estrogen, the uterine lining thickens, and the cycle begins again.

Menstrual Periods

Women's menstrual cycles vary widely. Counting from the first day of one period to the first day of the next, most cycles last between twenty-three and thirty-six days. For teens the variation can be even broader, from twenty-one to forty-five days. Often we think of periods as occurring once per month (in fact, the word "menstruation" is from the Latin word *mensis*, for "month"). While some women have periods that do occur exactly every month, other women have cycles that are longer or shorter. Some women have consistently regular cycles (bleeding every twenty-eight or thirty-five days, for instance), while other women's cycles vary in length from one cycle to the next. Hormonal contraceptives or breastfeeding may alter the length of our cycles or even stop them altogether. After we have been pregnant—whether we have an abortion, a miscarriage, or give birth—our cycles may change.

Most women's periods last between two and eight days, with four to six days being the average. The flow stops and starts, though this is not always noticeable.

It is possible to have what may appear to be a menstrual period even if you haven't ovulated that month. These are called anovulatory cycles and they are common when menstruation starts and your cycles are getting established. Anovulatory cycles become more common again as menopause approaches.

WHAT MENSTRUAL CYCLES REVEAL ABOUT YOUR HEALTH

Your menstrual cycle provides important information about your sexual and reproductive health. For example, if you suddenly stop getting your periods (but are not pregnant), have much heavier bleeding, or experience very irregular spotting, those symptoms may indicate a gynecological problem.

The menstrual cycle also provides important information about a woman's overall health. Just as blood pressure and heart and respiratory rates are described as "vital signs" key to the diagnosis of potentially serious health conditions, recognizing menstrual patterns may also provide information that leads to the early identification of possible health concerns. Marked changes in menstrual cycles may signal problems with the blood's ability to clot, significant weight change, emotional stress, thyroid disease, autoimmune conditions, hormonal imbalance, diabetes, Cushing's disease, primary ovarian insufficiency (POI), late-onset congenital adrenal hyperplasia (CAH), or even cancer. Menstrual changes can also indicate pregnancy or perimenopause (the years leading up to the final menstrual period). Throughout our reproductive years, when we have medical concerns, the evaluation of the menstrual cycle should be included along with an assessment of our other vital signs.

Menstrual Fluid

The fluid that flows from the vagina during the menstrual period includes much of the uterine lining that has built up during that cycle. In addition to blood (sometimes clotted) and endometrial cells, menstrual fluid contains cervical fluid and vaginal secretions. This mixed content is not obvious, since the blood colors the fluid red or brown. A usual discharge for a menstrual period is about two to five tablespoons, though it often looks like more.

What to Do with the Menstrual Flow

Across time and cultures, women have used and continue to use a variety of products for catching menstrual flow. The choice often comes down to comfort, availability, convenience, and price. You might find the perfect match right away, or you might try different options, looking for more comfort or a better fit.

TAMPONS AND PADS

Many women use commercial tampons or pads (also called sanitary napkins) to catch menstrual blood. These are the products most easily available. Whether you use a product worn outside your body (such as a pad) or a product worn inside your body (such as a tampon) is a personal choice.

COMMON QUESTIONS ABOUT TAMPONS

Will a tampon get lost inside me? No, absolutely not. The vagina is a closed space, and the opening of the cervix is far too small for the tampon to get inside. It is true, though, that a tampon can be forgotten and may slip into a vaginal fold, becoming difficult to find and remove. This can result in a strong odor and brown discharge after a few days. If you have trouble finding the string, you can squat down and reach the tampon with your fingers. For a funny and informative video about this, see "The Lost Tampon" at docgurley.com.

Will tampons make me sick? No. You may have heard that tampons cause toxic shock syndrome (TSS). TSS is a serious but rare condition caused by bacteria. Keeping tampons in longer than eight hours can increase the risk of TSS. If used according to the directions on the package and changed regularly, though, tampons are safe.

If I use a tampon, does that affect my virginity? No again. Virginity generally refers to whether or not someone has had sexual intercourse, not to menstruation or tampons. Tampon use may be one of the factors that play a role in the disintegration of your hymen, but whether you have a visible hymen says nothing about whether you have had sex. For more information on hymens and virginity, see p. 7 and "Virginity," p. 141.

MORE OPTIONS

For many reasons, including comfort, environmental concerns such as a preference for reusable products, and worries about chemical residues, many of us use modified or alternative products to collect menstrual blood. These include all-cotton (sometimes organic) chlorine-free tampons, chlorine-free disposable pads, washable cloth pads, and devices that collect rather than absorb the menstrual fluid. All-cotton and all-organic cotton, chlorine-free tampons are often sold in health food stores and online, and increasingly at some drug and grocery stores. Also, you can make your own cloth pads. There are make-your-own sites online, showing very economical alternatives.

Some women use natural sea sponges that work like tampons. These are also available in health food stores and online. They are reusable and relatively inexpensive. Unfortunately, many pollutants are dumped into oceans and it's possible that sponges may absorb some of these pollutants and cause problems. Therefore, some users boil a sponge for five to ten minutes before using it for the first time and between uses. Doing so, however, shrinks and toughens the sponge and reduces its lifetime.

Some women prefer products that collect rather than absorb the menstrual fluid. The Keeper, the DivaCup, and the Mooncup are three examples of menstrual cups—elongated cups made of rubber or medical-grade silicone that are held in place by suction in the vagina. They can be worn during swimming and other physical activities but not during intercourse or other insertive sex. Some women use a diaphragm or a cervical cap in the same way as a cup. A disposable device called Instead is worn in the upper vagina to collect menstrual flow. The rim softens in response to body temperature and creates a seal to protect against leakage and slipping. (For more information on these products, see youngwomenshealth.org/alternative_menstrual.html.)

It's Your Period—How Do You Own It?

In mainstream Western culture, menstruation is largely taboo. We may hear jokes about it on television, or we may see advertisements for menstrual products, but rarely is menstruation talked about in honest terms. When's the last time you heard menstrual blood even mentioned? Being "fresh" or "clean" is emphasized, and the fact that we menstruate is hidden. Until recently, most menstrual product advertisements tried to be subtle, showing women staying fresh and wearing white while practicing yoga or dancing on the beach. Kotex came out with an ad campaign in 2010 making fun of the genre—to which Kotex readily acknowledged contributing. (Older ads used to include a strange blue liquid representing menstrual blood.) But honesty could go only so far, as none

BLOOD IN THE BOARDROOM

i ask her if she's got a tampon i could use
she says
oh honey, what a hassle for you
sure I do
you know i do
i say
it ain't no hassle, no, it ain't no mess
right now it's the only power
that i possess
these businessmen got the money
they got the instruments of death
but i can make life
i can make breath

—Ani DiFranco,
"Blood in the Boardroom"[5]

of the three major television networks would allow the word "vagina" to be used.

"Fem-care advertising is so sterilized and so removed from what a period is," Elissa Stein, coauthor (with Susan Kim) of *Flow: The Cultural Story of Menstruation*, told the *New York Times*. "You never see a bathroom, you never see a woman using a product. They never show someone having cramps or her face breaking out or tearful—it's always happy, playful, sporty women."[6]

Indeed, we often feel obligated to apologize when discussing menstruation. For many women, there is much more to the menstrual experience than bleeding. Our experiences, both physical and emotional, range widely and sometimes are connected to our religion or culture.

We may have certain traditions around menstruation, passed down through our families—even if the tradition is as simple as what kind of product to use or how best to wash out a bloodstain.

I don't have any bad feelings about it or get upset when I get my period. It's a sign that I'm not pregnant, which makes me happy, because I'm in college right now and I'm not at the stage where I want any kids yet.

Physical and Emotional Changes Through the Menstrual Cycle

The menstrual cycle is governed by hormones that rise and fall in rhythmic patterns. These hormones influence the physical and emotional changes you may experience during your cycles. Some women notice few changes; some experience increased energy and creativity; others experience mood changes (some positive, some negative) and body changes (swollen breasts, for example). Some women have cramps, while others do not. One woman reports happily:

I wasn't the biggest fan of my period, but then I discovered that I have the most incredible orgasms while I'm menstruating!

Premenstrual Changes

Women can have a variety of physical sensations and emotional experiences for several days before menstruation and sometimes during the first few days of menstrual flow. These are caused by the normal hormone fluctuations of the menstrual cycle and are not a sign of a hormone imbalance. Among the more negative changes are mood swings, fatigue, depression, bloating, breast tenderness, and headaches. Sometimes these premenstrual experiences are mild, but sometimes they disrupt our lives significantly.

PREMENSTRUAL MOOD CHANGES AND DEPRESSION

I get upset—sad about simple things—when I get my period.

Some of us experience mood changes before our periods, including some level of depression and emotional irritability. Some of us find that issues that have been with us all along become more pronounced at this time. Others see our moods as authentic expressions of feelings we don't usually feel able, comfortable enough, or secure enough to show. Some women are able to cope with premenstrual mood changes, while others find the intensity of the symptoms and frustrations intolerable.

For some women, certain self-care and nonmedical techniques can help with mood changes. Approaches that have proved useful in a few studies include exercise, calcium, vitamin B6 supplementation (although too much B6 can have serious side effects), and the herb *Vitex agnus-castus* (chasteberry). Approaches that have worked for some women and are still under study include dietary changes such as limiting salt, sugar, caffeine (especially coffee), red meat, and alcohol; massage; reflexology; chiropractic manipulation; biofeedback; yoga; guided imagery; photic stimulation; acupuncture; and bright light therapy.[7]

A small but significant number of women do experience extreme premenstrual depression that interferes with work, social interactions, and general well-being. In these instances, recognition and care are critical. If premenstrual depression interferes noticeably with your daily life (you don't want to get out of bed, you miss work, or you have suicidal thoughts) and nonmedical approaches are not helpful, seek advice from your primary care provider, your ob-gyn, or a mental health professional.

Medical treatments for premenstrual depression include using hormonal contraception continuously, so that there is no menstruation, or taking antidepressant medications called SSRIs. However, there are questions about the effectiveness and safety of SSRIs. (For more information, see "Depression and Other Mental Health Challenges During Pregnancy," p. 389.)

Severe Cramps (Dysmenorrhea)

Women experience many different levels of menstrual-related cramping, from no cramps to severe ones. A particular constellation of symptoms, including cramping and often nausea and diarrhea, may be caused by excess production and release of prostaglandins.[8] (One form of prostaglandins, which are hormonelike chemicals found throughout the body, causes contractions of both the uterine and the intestinal muscles.) With too many prostaglandins, the usually painless rhythmic contractions of the uterus during menstruation become longer and tighter at the tightening phase, keeping oxygen from the muscles. It is this lack of oxygen that we experience as pain. Anticipation often worsens the pain by making us tense up. It's not clear why some women have more uterine prostaglandins than others, but this sort of menstrual cramping is actually a sign of normal hormone cycling and ovulation.

I've always had cramps during my period and sometimes they made me pretty miserable. When my periods returned after I gave birth, my attitude toward cramps changed. Having felt labor contractions, I had an awareness that the cramping was actually just my muscle contracting. I still have moments when menstrual cramps suck (yay for ibuprofen), but I also have moments when I feel them, tune in, breathe, and feel powerful.

There are two types of dysmenorrhea (dis-men-or-EE-yah): primary dysmenorrhea is painful cramping (with or without nausea and diarrhea) not associated with any other pelvic disorder; secondary dysmenorrhea is pain associated with another pelvic problem such as endometriosis, pelvic inflammatory disease, or fibroids. Primary dysmenorrhea is more common and typically starts in the teen years; the pain resolves after a few days of bleeding.

TERMS FOR PREMENSTRUAL CHANGES

The term "PMS," which stands for premenstrual syndrome, is often used with words like "symptoms" and "treatments," as though premenstrual changes are an illness. Some women do experience debilitating discomfort, pain, or mood changes in the days before menstruation. But the label PMS suggests that most women must suffer a "syndrome" each month. This does not reflect the real and significant variation in women's experiences.

Similarly, there is debate about the term and diagnosis "premenstrual dysphoric disorder" (PMDD), which is used to describe a severe form of premenstrual depression. Some critics argue that the term, created by the American Psychiatric Association in 1993, pathologizes menstrual changes by giving women the label of a specific psychiatric "disorder," and reinforces the idea that women are "crazy" once a month and should not be in positions involving great authority or stress.

"When you start calling PMDD—and by extension PMS—a psychiatric disorder, what are you saying about the women of this world?" asks Nada Stotland, a past president of the American Psychiatric Association and professor of psychiatry at Rush Medical College in Chicago. "This reinforces prejudices people already have about women being moody and unreliable." According to Stotland, the majority of women who go to PMS clinics have symptoms that are not, in fact, related to their periods. "Most suffer from depression every day. Others have anxiety and personality disorders. Some are in psychological pain because they are being abused."

Severe premenstrual depression is rare. Pharmaceutical companies whose medications are approved by the FDA for anyone with a PMDD diagnosis sometimes create marketing materials that encourage overuse of this diagnosis. The Bayer pharmaceutical company had to run corrective advertisements to make up for ads that implied that simple irritability and other common premenstrual discomforts were PMDD and should be treated with its birth control pill, Yaz.[9] Its corrective ads explained that PMDD is both rare and severe. In another instance of the possible overuse of a PMDD diagnosis, the European Medicines Evaluation Agency refused to approve drugs for PMDD, raising concerns that women "with less severe premenstrual symptoms might erroneously receive a diagnosis of PMDD resulting in widespread inappropriate short- and long-term use of fluoxitine [Prozac]."[10]

Nonmedical approaches that help some women include Chinese herbs provided by an experienced practitioner of Chinese medicine, applying wet or dry heat over the abdomen, taking omega-3 fatty acids, learning to self-apply acupressure points, and taking ginger supplements.[11] If these methods do not work, consider seeing your health-care provider. Prescription-strength nonsteroidal anti-inflammatory drugs (NSAIDS) such as ibuprofen, birth control pills, other forms of hormonal contraceptives, and the Mirena intrauterine device can diminish severe menstrual cramps for most women.

Very Heavy Periods (Menorrhagia) and/or Irregular Bleeding

You may experience a very heavy period if you did not ovulate during a cycle. This happens to all women occasionally and occurs more often in the teen years, during perimenopause, during times of stress, and after any pregnancy. Heavy periods can also occur if you have fibroids, are using certain IUDs for birth control (the Mirena IUD actually reduces cramps and bleeding), or have an inherited bleeding disorder. The most common inherited bleeding disorder, von Willebrand disease (VWD), affects about 1 to 2 percent of the U.S. population and runs in families. While it is often difficult to diagnose, and there is no cure, VWD can be treated. (For more information, see "Von Willebrand Disease," p. 613.)

Irregular bleeding—off-schedule menstrual flow—can also be caused by recurrently not ovulating, which can be age-related (again, more common in early teens and perimenopause) or from some health problems or severe stress. Bleeding in early pregnancy, which may or may not progress to miscarriage, can sometimes be confused with a menstrual period and can be light or heavy.

If you have heavy periods and/or irregular bleeding, it's a good idea to talk with a healthcare provider, because these can signal serious health problems. (See "What Menstrual Cycles Reveal About Your Health," p. 21.) Keeping a menstrual calendar can help you develop awareness of what a typical flow is for you. (See "Charting Your Menstrual Cycles," below.)

No Periods and Very Light or Skipped Periods

Primary amenorrhea is the condition of never having had a period by the latest age at which menstruation usually starts (sixteen). Secondary amenorrhea is missing periods after having had at least one. Oligomenorrhea is infrequent, erratic periods. Some causes of amenorrhea and oligomenorrhea are pregnancy; menopause; breastfeeding; heavy athletic training; emotional factors; stress; current or recent use of hormonal birth control methods; excessive dieting, anorexia, or starvation; use of some medications, including chemotherapy; obstruction or malformation of the genital tract; hormone imbalance; cysts or tumors; chronic illness; and chromosomal conditions. Sometimes amenorrhea or oligomenorrhea is caused by a combination of several of these factors.

CHARTING YOUR MENSTRUAL CYCLES

Many women find it helpful to keep a menstrual calendar or a special fertility awareness chart. By doing so, we can get to know our bodies, learn what is normal for us, and become advocates for and authorities about our own health. You can use a print or online calendar or diary to chart when you bleed, whether and when you have vaginal secretions, and whether you have a range of physical or emotional experiences (including pain or cramps, heavier or lighter flow, or changes in sexual desire, energy level or mood, breasts, or general physical health). You can find menstrual charts online at the Taking Care of Your Fertility website, tcoyf.com.

Fertility Awareness Method

One way of charting your menstrual cycles is to use the fertility awareness method (FAM).

In addition to being a good tool to assess your gynecological health, FAM is a scientifically validated method of natural birth control and pregnancy achievement. It is based on observing and charting body signs such as changes in the cervical fluid and in the color, size, and shape of the cervix that reflect whether a woman is fertile on any given day.

FAM Is Based on the Following Scientific Principles:

- Your menstrual cycle can basically be divided into three phases: the preovulatory infertile phase, the fertile phase, and the postovulatory infertile phase. You can determine which phase you are in by observing the three primary fertility signs: early morning (waking, or basal body) temperature, cervical fluid, and cervical position.
- The menstrual cycle is under the direct influence of estrogen and progesterone, and the body provides daily signs about the status of these hormones. Estrogen dominates the first part of the cycle; progesterone dominates the latter. Another hormone, called luteinizing hormone (LH), is the catalyst that propels the ovary to release the egg. LH is the hormone measured in ovulation predictor kits.
- Ovulation (the release of an egg) occurs once per cycle. During ovulation, one or more eggs are released. An egg can survive for twelve to twenty-four hours. If a second egg is released in one cycle (as in the case of fraternal twins), it will be released within twenty-four hours of the first.
- The time from a woman's period until ovulation varies, but it is often about two weeks.
- Sperm can live in fertile-quality cervical fluid for up to five days, though typically they live only about two days.

The Primary Fertility Signs

WAKING OR BASAL BODY TEMPERATURE (BBT)
Before ovulation, early morning temperatures typically range from about 97° to 97.5°F (36.11° to 36.38°C), and after ovulation, they usually rise to about 97.6° to 98.6°F (36.44° to 37°C). It's helpful to use a special basal or digital thermometer to get readings that are precise enough to track such small changes. After ovulation, your temperature usually remains elevated until your next period, about two weeks later. But if you become pregnant, it remains high for more than eighteen days.

The important concept to understand is your *pattern* of low and high temperatures. Your temperatures before ovulation fluctuate in a low range, and the temperatures after ovulation fluctuate in a higher range. The trick is to see the whole and not to focus so much on the day-to-day changes. Temperatures typically rise within a day or so after ovulation, indicating that ovulation has already occurred.

A sustained rise in waking temperature almost always indicates that ovulation has occurred. It does not reveal impending ovulation, though, as do the other two fertility signs (cervical fluid and cervical position). After charting a few cycles, if your cycles are consistent, you should be able to see how these three signs interact. It is often believed that most women ovulate at the lowest point of the temperature graph, but this is true for only a minority of women. It's more common for ovulation to occur the day before the temperature rises.

Factors that may disrupt your morning temperature:

- Fever
- Alcohol consumption the night before
- Fewer than three consecutive hours of sleep before taking temperature

USING THE FERTILITY AWARENESS METHOD TO HELP YOU CONCEIVE

By charting your fertility signs every day, you can use the fertility awareness method (FAM) to avoid or to achieve pregnancy. (For more information on using FAM for birth control, see "Fertility Awareness Method and Other Natural Methods," p. 248.) Below is some basic information on using FAM to increase your chances of getting pregnant.* In order to use FAM effectively, you need more information than this book provides. You can take a class or get a book that teaches you specifically how to identify your fertility on a day-to-day basis and provides you with a special FAM chart on which to record. One excellent resource is the book *Taking Charge of Your Fertility* by Toni Weschler.

To use FAM to help you get pregnant, the two most important points to remember are:

1. **Determine whether you are ovulating.** By taking your waking or basal body temperature, you should notice a pattern of low temperatures before ovulation, followed by about twelve to sixteen days of high temperatures. If you don't see an obvious pattern, or if your high temperatures after ovulation last fewer than ten days, consider a medical consultation to make sure that you are ovulating and that the latter phase of your cycle is long enough to sustain a pregnancy.

* Most women don't need to be this scientific in order to get pregnant—with ejaculation or insemination into the vagina every day or two midcycle, most women conceive within six months.

You can also determine whether you are ovulating by using ovulation predictor kits, which test urine for luteinizing hormone (LH). Between twenty-four and forty-eight hours prior to ovulation, women experience a short surge of LH. Ovulation predictor kits measure LH and let you know that ovulation is about to happen.

2. **Have intercourse or inseminate on all days of wet, slippery cervical fluid.** The most fertile day of your cycle will be the last day that you have this slippery cervical fluid. So, for example, if you have wet cervical fluid on Monday, Tuesday, and Wednesday, you should ideally have intercourse or inseminate on each of those days. That Wednesday, though, will be your most fertile day, since it is the closest day to ovulation. (If your partner's sperm count is marginal or low, you should have intercourse or inseminate every other day that you have wet cervical fluid. If the sperm has morphology [shape] problems, every day is better.)

If you conceive, your temperatures following ovulation should remain high, and you won't have a period.

Women are traditionally told to wait a full year before seeking a medical evaluation if they haven't conceived naturally. But you and your partner should both consider doing so after six cycles, if you are timing intercourse or insemination perfectly each cycle according to the steps above and still have not gotten pregnant. If you are over forty, fertility evaluation is recommended after three cycles.

- Eating or drinking before taking an oral temperature
- Taking temperature at a substantially different time than usual
- Heating your body, as with an electric blanket
- Thyroid conditions

CERVICAL FLUID (CF)

Cervical fluid is the secretion produced around ovulation that allows sperm to reach the egg. In essence, fertile cervical fluid functions like seminal fluid: It provides an alkaline medium to protect the sperm in an otherwise acidic vagina. In addition, it provides nourishment for the sperm, acts as a filtering mechanism, and functions as a medium in which to move. Cervical fluid also capacitates the sperm; this process removes the tip of the head, preparing it to fertilize the egg.

After your period and directly under the influence of rising estrogen, your cervical fluid typically starts to become wetter as you approach ovulation. After your period ends, you may have several days of nothing, followed by cervical fluid that evolves from sticky to creamy and finally to clear, slippery, and stretchy (also known as spinnbarkeit), similar to raw egg white. The most noticeable feature of this fertile cervical fluid is its lubricating quality.

After estrogen has peaked and dropped, the cervical fluid abruptly dries, often within a few hours. This is due to the surge of progesterone following ovulation. The absence of wet cervical fluid usually lasts the duration of the cycle.

A trick to help you identify the quality of the cervical fluid at your vaginal opening is to notice what it feels like to run a tissue (or your finger) across your vaginal lips. Does it feel dry? Is it smooth? Does it glide across? When you are dry, the tissue won't pass smoothly across your vaginal lips. But as you approach ovulation, your cervical fluid gets progressively wetter, and the tissue or your finger should glide easily.

As with temperature, certain factors may mask or interfere with cervical fluid:

- Vaginal infection
- Semen (from recent sexual intercourse)
- Arousal fluid
- Spermicides and lubricants
- Antihistamines (which can dry out or decrease fluid)
- Guaifenesin cough medicine (which can increase fluid)

In addition, if you have recently stopped taking birth control pills, you may notice one of two very different patterns: Either you may not produce much cervical fluid at all, or you may tend to have what appears to be continuous creamy cervical fluid for several months.

CERVICAL POSITION

In addition to emitting cervical fluid, your cervix goes through changes throughout your cycle. These changes can sometimes be felt by inserting a clean finger into your vagina (your middle finger is usually easiest, since it's the longest).

The cervix is normally firm, like the tip of your nose, and becomes soft and rather mushy, like your lips, as you approach ovulation. In addition, it is normally fairly low and closed, and rises and opens only in response to the high levels of estrogen around ovulation. The angle of the cervix also changes around ovulation, becoming straighter when estrogen levels are high. (For more on the cervix, see p. 9.)

Secondary Fertility Signs

Secondary fertility signs around ovulation may include pain or achiness near an ovary, increased sexual feelings, and abdominal bloating. Secondary fertility signs do not occur in all women, or in every cycle in individual women. Still, these signs, when apparent, can offer additional information to help identify fertile and infertile phases.

CHAPTER 2 ▪ ▪ ▪ ▪ ▪ ▪ ▪ ▪ ▪ ▪ ▪ ▪ ▪ ▪ ▪ ▪ ▪ ▪ ▪

A woman's body and her sexuality have traditionally been understood and presented as the property and business of everyone but the woman herself. Many of us have been made to feel that knowledge about and care for our bodies—particularly those parts considered primarily sexual—are unnecessary, maybe even inappropriate. Yet learning how to take care of ourselves frees us to feel more comfortable in our bodies and with our sexuality, and enables us to take a more active role in monitoring and maintaining our health.

This chapter covers some steps you can take to protect your sexual and reproductive health, including what you can do for yourself and when to see a health care provider. It also describes what to expect at a gynecological visit and exam and how to advocate for the respectful, compassionate, individualized, and comprehensive care you deserve. Many of the topics addressed briefly in this chapter are covered in more depth in other chapters.

The first chapter in this book, "Our Female Bodies," describes female sexual anatomy in depth. As you read this chapter, you may find it helpful to look back at the drawings, descriptions, and definitions included there.

VULVAR AND VAGINAL SELF-CARE

For the most part, the vulva and vagina need only basic care to stay healthy. Here are some tips to keep your vulva healthy and happy:

- **Lay the groundwork.** Eat well, get adequate sleep, and exercise regularly to help keep all parts of your body healthy.
- **Have smart sex.** Learn the sexual history of your partners and practice safer sex. (See Chapter 10, "Safer Sex"; and Chapter 11, "Sexually Transmitted Infections.")
- **Loosen up.** Thongs can rub back and forth, and tight-fitting pants, spandex, and synthetic underwear can trap heat and moisture and cause irritation. Wear looser clothing and natural-fiber underwear such as cotton. Sleeping without underwear or anything tight allows some air to get to the vulvar area and helps keep the vulvar tissues healthy.
- **Don't douche.** The vagina is a self-cleaning organ, so there is no need to wash inside or douche. In fact, douching can create unhealthy changes in the pH (acidity) and the balance of normal vaginal bacteria.

- **Keep clean.** To help prevent the spread of bacteria that could cause a urinary tract infection, wipe from front to back, reaching from behind, after a bowel movement.
- **Use tampons wisely.** Choose the right absorbency and change tampons every two to eight hours. (See "Common Questions About Tampons," p. 21.)
- **Don't overdo.** To clean your vulva, use just warm water or a gentle, unscented soap applied with your fingers—don't scrub. Avoid lengthy soaks in very hot water, which can dry and irritate the skin.
- **Avoid common irritants.** Skip the scented soaps, body deodorants, and perfumes. These can lead to irritation in some women. If you have sensitive skin, stick to unscented white toilet paper, use a hypoallergenic clothing detergent, and avoid fabric softener/dryer sheets when you dry your underwear or bed sheets.

Vulvas have their own scent, just like other parts of our bodies and the bodies of our sexual

CAN I SHAVE DOWN THERE?

Hair removal is not necessary from a health perspective and in fact can cause irritation and skin infections. If you do opt to trim or remove hair on and around the vulva, proceed cautiously, particularly if your skin is generally sensitive. An electric razor with a pop-up blade is safer and gentler than a regular razor for shaving the bikini line and the mons (the soft tissue over the pubic bone). Avoid hair-removal creams, which can burn the skin. Abrasions and ingrown hairs are common with waxing, so use wax only on the thighs, or see a professional hair remover.

IN TRANSLATION: MY BODY IS MINE

Group: Mavi Kalem

Country: Turkey

Resource: *Bedenlerimiz Biziz* (Our Bodies Are Us), a Turkish adaptation of *Our Bodies, Ourselves*

Websites: bedenimveben.org, mavikalem.org

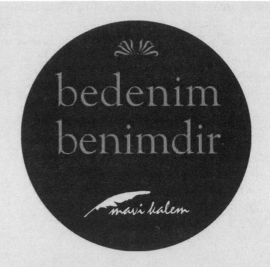

This striking badge, created by Our Bodies Ourselves' partner Mavi Kalem in Turkey, reads, "My Body Is Mine." Distributed by and to young women, along with a pamphlet outlining rights fundamental to health and well-being, it is part of a campaign celebrating sexual and reproductive freedom that has reached nearly twelve thousand women and girls.

According to Mavi Kalem, there are no comprehensive health resources in Turkish. Health information, when available, is shaped by conservative cultural ideas on fertility and childbearing, and focuses on pregnancy, birth control, and sexually transmitted infections. It is difficult to find a resource that analyzes the health and rights of women and girls from their points of view. This forces many to seek information through unofficial channels—friends, older relatives, and mothers—that is not always accurate.

Established in the aftermath of the devastating Marmara earthquake in 1999, Mavi Kalem is committed to the free flow of information and draws on the power of volunteers to drive social and political change. The organization delivers health resources to millions of women, girls, and men, via grassroots workshops, print materials, and discussion groups, both online and in person. Mavi Kalem's website is a unique collaborative and lobbying tool for a growing activist network in the region. The organization also publishes a free monthly women's health magazine, *Zuhre,* which is extremely popular in Turkey and Cyprus.

In the spring of 2011, Mavi Kalem published a Turkish adaptation of *Our Bodies, Ourselves* titled *Bedenlerimiz Biziz.* The book explores the social norms, laws, traditional practices, and religious edicts that make it difficult for Turkish women and girls to exercise their rights. The authors want readers to say, "I read a book and it changed my life."

partners. It's normal for vulvas to smell a little musky or acidic and, during menstruation, to smell somewhat metallic. It's also typical for vulvas to smell different at different times of the menstrual cycle. If a male sexual partner ejaculates inside your vagina, that can alter your scent, too, especially for a day or two after ejaculation. Products that scent or deodorize the vulva or vagina were not designed with our health in mind and play on women's insecurities.

If the scent of your vulva seems particularly strong or unusual, and that change sticks around for more than a few days, it could be a sign of infection. Make an appointment with a health-care provider and, until then, avoid using any commercial vulvar or vaginal treatment or medication not prescribed to you, including over-the-counter yeast infection treatments. If you don't know for sure what the cause is, taking the wrong medication can worsen the irritation and make it difficult to diagnose what if anything is wrong. (See "Vaginal Infections," p. 637.)

GETTING THE SEXUAL AND REPRODUCTIVE HEALTH CARE WE NEED

Throughout our lives there are times when taking care of our reproductive and sexual health involves getting help from health care providers. Many of the chapters in this book, including "Abortion," "Sexually Transmitted Infections," "Birth Control," "Pregnancy and Preparing for Birth," and "Navigating the Health Care System," discuss the types of providers and the specific kinds of care they offer, how to find a provider, how to access care if you don't have health insurance or your insurance doesn't cover the care, and what to expect at a visit.

SEXUAL SELF-CARE

If you experience vaginal, vulvar, or other pain with sexual activity, *stop.* Find out the cause of the pain before resuming. Sex can be painful if you're not fully aroused. Pain can also be caused by a scratch or an abrasion, sexually transmitted infections, and vulvodynia, a chronic pain condition (see p. 187). Sex should be about pleasure, and pleasure is connected to listening to your body and addressing your health needs.

WHEN SHOULD I SEE A PROVIDER?

Most of the time, we visit a provider for our sexual health when a particular need arises: We need birth control or are pregnant or have an unusual vaginal discharge. A gynecological health care visit is also recommended if you have complaints about or issues with your period or any part of your menstrual cycle; if you are experiencing pelvic, vaginal, or rectal pain or discomfort; or if you're experiencing unexplained vaginal bleeding, spotting, or any unusual discharge.

It's also a good idea to have periodic visits once you are sexually active. Since most sexually transmitted infections (STIs) have no noticeable symptoms, it is wise to be screened for STIs before and after you have sex with someone new, if you are sexually active with more than one person, or if you think or know your partner has had sex with someone else. It is recommended that you have a gynecological exam by age twenty-one, even if you are not yet sexually active.

Other reasons to see a provider include:

- You want to start or change prescription contraception.
- You miss three periods or your periods become increasingly heavy or irregular.
- You have unusual genital discharge (which you might notice on your underwear) that lasts for more than a few days or that causes itching or burns or smells bad.
- You have a lump in your breast, or any bumps, sores, swelling, or redness in your genital area.
- You have persistent pelvic or genital pain with menstruation, urination, or sex, or in general, such as when sitting or walking.
- You have unexplained pain in your lower belly or around the pelvic area.
- You have vaginal bleeding that lasts for more than ten days, bleeding at times other than during or around menstrual periods, or flow during periods that becomes unusually heavy or light.
- You are planning to get pregnant.
- You find out you are pregnant.
- You are experiencing a miscarriage.
- You have problems, pain, or discomfort following labor and birth, a miscarriage, or an abortion.

KINDS OF PROVIDERS

Many different types of health care providers offer reproductive and sexual health care to women, including nurse-practitioners, physician assistants, midwives, and doctors such as pediatricians, family practice physicians, and obstetrician/gynecologists (ob-gyns). Some of us obtain care from providers who specialize in women's sexual and reproductive health, while others obtain gynecological care from primary care providers or internists (internal medicine doctors). Different providers have different training, styles, availability, billing practices, and expertise.

SEXUAL HEALTH CARE FOR TEENS

In all fifty states and the District of Columbia, adolescents can seek advice and prescriptions for birth control and medical care for sexually transmitted infections without parental consent or knowledge. In addition, adolescents can consent to HIV counseling and testing in most states. Consent laws for vaccinations and for abortions differ by state. It's important to know, though, that while the visit is confidential, if you use health insurance, the policyholder (usually your parent) will likely receive a notice of services provided from the insurance company.

WHERE TO GET CARE

You can get the get the care you need in a variety of places, including private medical offices and health care clinics. Some clinics provide low-cost or free services. Family planning clinics such as Planned Parenthood that are funded by Title X (a federal funding program overseen by the U.S. Department of Health and Human Services) offer a broad range of related preventive health services, including routine physical exams; education on health promotion and disease prevention; breast and pelvic exams; cervical cancer screening; STI prevention, education, testing, and referrals; and pregnancy diagnosis and counseling. Title X clinics are required by law to see all women, regardless of ability to pay. To find a Title X clinic in your area, visit opaclearinghouse.org/search.

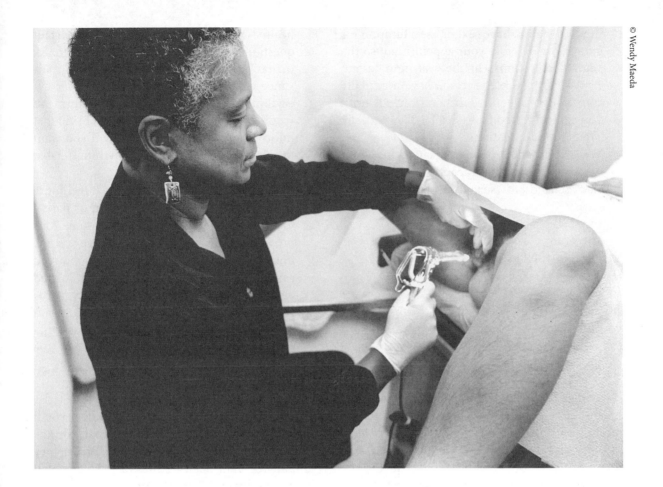

THE GYNECOLOGICAL EXAM

Because many health care visits related to our sexual and reproductive health will include a gynecological exam, this chapter provides an overview of what to expect.

WHAT IS A GYNECOLOGICAL EXAM?

A routine gynecological checkup generally includes an examination of your breasts and a pelvic exam, which includes an external genitals examination, a vaginal exam using a speculum, an internal exam of your uterus and ovaries, and sometimes a rectal examination.

PREPARING FOR A GYNECOLOGICAL EXAM

- **Schedule on a period-free day.** Since menstrual fluid can affect the results of some tests, try to plan your pelvic exam for a day when you won't have your period. Of course, it's not always possible to plan in advance, so if you have your period the day of your exam, call your provider's office or the clinic and ask if you need to reschedule.

- **If you have symptoms, avoid sex and tampons.** If you are having an unusual vaginal discharge or other symptoms that you want evaluated, it's best not to use any medications in your vagina, have sex, or use a tampon for a day or two before your appointment so the vaginal secretions can be seen and tested. And if it's possible that you have a sexually transmitted infection, abstain from sex until you can get tested (see Chapter 11, "Sexually Transmitted Infections").

- **Write it down.** Do you have questions about discharge, pain, contraception, or anything else related to sexual and reproductive health? It can be easy to forget important questions, even when you really want to ask them. Writing down your questions in advance can help you remember to cover everything you need during your appointment. If you chart your menstrual cycles, bring that information with you, especially if you want to ask your provider about anything related to menstruation or fertility.

- **Bring support.** If you think you'd feel more comfortable, ask a friend, partner, or parent to come with you into the exam room. Your provider may ask her or him to leave at some point to ask you personal questions, but you can request the person stay or get invited back quickly. Similarly, if a parent or guardian has come with you to your exam and you want privacy, you have the right to ask that person to leave.

WHEN YOU ARRIVE

When you arrive at the clinic or office, you'll usually be given forms to fill out that ask important questions about your health history and any current health issues or problems you are experiencing. Complete these as fully and honestly as possible, as your answers will help determine your course of care. The information you provide and any test results are confidential.

In the United States, your health information is protected and private according to a law known as HIPAA (hhs.gov/ocr/privacy). You should be notified of the practitioner or clinic's privacy policies in writing, and you will be asked to sign paperwork regarding your privacy, including approving to whom your information can be released and under what conditions. (For more information, see "Rights Regarding Medical Records," p. 677.)

If the reason for your visit includes vaginal pain or irritation, you may be asked to urinate

YOUR RIGHTS AS A HEALTH CARE CONSUMER

No matter where you go for health care, you should be treated without judgment. Conversations about sex should be accurate, clear, complete, and free of prejudice regarding your sexual identity or preferences. If you have questions about contraception or STIs, your questions should be answered directly without comment on whether the provider thinks it's appropriate for you to be having sex. You have the right to make decisions about your body. No one can force you to have a physical exam or undergo any treatment you personally refuse.

Once the exam begins, if for any reason you feel unsafe, or if your provider is being rough, dismissive, or uncooperative, you can end the exam and leave the room; you are never obligated to see an appointment through to the end. Use the word "Stop" to indicate clearly that you don't want to continue. If you say, "Ouch," or are crying, some practitioners may not really notice. Saying "Stop!" loudly and clearly will get their attention and remind them that "no means no," even in the doctor's office.

into a cup so your urine can be analyzed for signs of a urinary tract infection or for a pregnancy test. (Even if you are certain you aren't pregnant, your health care provider may require a pregnancy test before prescribing birth control or inserting an IUD, or as part of a diagnostic workup for a problem like abnormal bleeding or pain.) If you don't need to give a urine sample, use the toilet anyway—gynecological exams are much more comfortable if your bladder is empty.

When you are brought to the exam room, the person doing the initial health assessment—usually a medical assistant, not the provider who will give you the exam—will take some basic measurements, including your height, weight, heart rate, and blood pressure. Then you will be given a gown to wear during the exam and the medical assistant will leave the room so you can undress in private. Sometimes, especially if you are a new patient, your provider may meet with you before you get undressed.

Let someone know if you feel uncomfortable being alone with the provider during the exam. You can ask to have a medical assistant or another attendant in the room. If your provider is a man, many offices do this automatically.

Once you are in the gown, your provider will come in and review your health history (the questions you answered upon arrival) and ask follow-up questions about that history or any current problems or concerns. If you have been doing regular vaginal self-exams (see p. 8) or charting your menstrual cycle (see p. 26), you will be able to tell your health care provider about any changes you have noticed, or simply help her or him understand what is normal for you. If you know anything about the size of speculum that works for you or where your cervix can be found, tell the provider.

Having a gynecological exam is an intimate and invasive experience. But providers who do them over and over again sometimes forget this. If this is your first exam or you have had a nega-tive experience with previous exams or you are feeling very anxious, let your provider know. Ask her or him to go slowly and explain each step as it happen.

Before beginning, your health care provider should wash her or his hands or use antibacterial gel. For the exam itself, your provider will wear gloves.

DURING THE GYNECOLOGICAL EXAM

Many health care providers begin by performing a clinical breast exam. This involves examining your breasts for any possible signs of breast cancer or other breast problems. Usually your provider will begin by visually inspecting your breasts, looking for skin changes or visible lumps. Then your provider will use her or his fingers to feel all parts of your breast, looking for lumps or unusual textures, and check your armpits for swollen lymph nodes.

To begin the pelvic exam, your provider will ask you to lie back on the exam table, move your bottom down to the end of the table, and place your feet in the stirrups, which are metal footrests on either side of the table. Bend your knees and let them relax and fall to each side. Most of us feel vulnerable and exposed in this position, but a good provider will try to make you feel safe. If you feel really uncomfortable, ask if you can sit up more. The exam can be done just as well in this position.

Your provider will first examine your vulva by visually checking to see if your anatomy is healthy. She or he will examine the distribution of your pubic hair, the size and condition of your clitoris, and the architecture of your vulvar lips and opening to the vagina. The provider will look for irritation, discoloration, swelling, bumps, skin lesions, lice, and any unusual vaginal discharge. Sometimes a Q-tip is used to evaluate the entry to the vagina for pain or tenderness.

Next, the provider will begin the pelvic

exam by inserting a metal or plastic speculum in your vagina. Speculums are shaped a bit like duck bills and they come in different sizes and lengths. The speculum will hold the walls of the vagina apart so your provider can examine your vaginal walls and cervix. If your provider is using a metal speculum, she or he may warm it before inserting it. If you are not used to a speculum or what it feels like to have something placed in your vagina, it may be uncomfortable, but it shouldn't be painful. You may feel some pressure in your bladder or around your rectum. Take deep, slow breaths and relax your stomach muscles, your shoulders, the muscles between your legs, and especially your vaginal muscles. A pinching sensation isn't normal. If you are in

WILL A PELVIC EXAM AFFECT MY VIRGINITY?

The short answer is: No. If you were a virgin before your pelvic exam you will be one afterward. Virginity is not a medical or physical condition. Virginity is defined differently by different people, but it most often refers to whether a woman has had penis-in-vagina intercourse. Some people define virginity based on the state of the hymen, a thin, flexible membrane located just inside the entrance to the vagina. But because hymens—also called vaginal coronas—can break and stretch during exercise, masturbation, tampon use, or any form of vaginal penetration, they do not reflect whether a woman has had sex. (For more information, see "Vaginal Corona or What You May Know as the Hymen," p. 7, and "Virginity," p. 141.)

pain, ask your provider to readjust the speculum or use a different size speculum.

Your provider will probably describe the process, step by step. If you want to know more about what's happening, ask. Similarly, if it's easier for you not to hear, ask *not* to be informed every step of the way. Some practitioners keep a hand mirror available. If you want to watch the exam to learn more and to see what your cervix looks like, ask for help in positioning the mirror and light source. If you want to do self-exams in the future (see p. 9), this is a great opportunity to ask questions about how it's done and what to look for.

When the speculum is in place, your pro-

vider will examine your vaginal walls for lesions, inflammation, or unusual discharge and look at your cervix and check for any unusual discharge, signs of infection, discoloration, damage, or growths. A Pap test may be done to check for abnormal cervical cells (see below). Sometimes a smear of vaginal discharge is taken as well, to test for vaginal infections or certain sexually transmitted infections. The speculum will be removed at the end of the pelvic exam.

The Bimanual Exam

After removing the speculum, your provider may insert one or two gloved fingers into your vagina while pressing down on your abdomen with the other hand. This is called a bimanual exam and is done to locate and determine the size, shape, and consistency of the uterus and ovaries. Your provider will feel for any unusual growths or tender areas. Pressure on the uterus is usually painless, but pressure on the ovaries may cause discomfort (like a slightly painful electric shock). The ovaries are difficult to

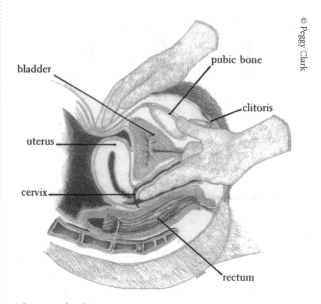

© Peggy Clark

A bimanual pelvic exam

PAP TESTS

A Pap test checks for cervical cell changes that can signal potential health problems, including human papillomavirus (HPV), a common sexually transmitted infection, and cervical cancer. It's done during a pelvic exam using a small spatula or a device that looks like a long Q-tip with a tiny bottle brush on the end. This swabbing may feel unusual or even uncomfortable, like a cramp, light brushing, or scraping sensation.

In 2009, the American College of Obstetrics and Gynecology released new recommendations about Pap tests for women whose risk of cervical cancer is low or average.

- Women should have their first Pap test at age twenty-one.
- Women in their twenties should have a Pap test every two years (assuming prior Pap tests have been normal).
- Women age thirty and older who have had three consecutive normal Pap tests should have a Pap test every three years.
- Women who have had a hysterectomy for noncancerous reasons do not need a Pap test unless they have retained their cervix.
- Women no longer need to have Pap tests after the age of 65.
- Women who have received an HPV vaccine still need to get Pap tests, because the vaccines do not protect against all types of HPV associated with cervical cancer.

If you have had an abnormal Pap result, you should discuss with your clinician how often you should repeat a Pap test, as what is recommended and what you choose to do will depend on your own particular situation. (For more information, see "Cervical Dysplasia and Cervical Cancer," p. 614.)

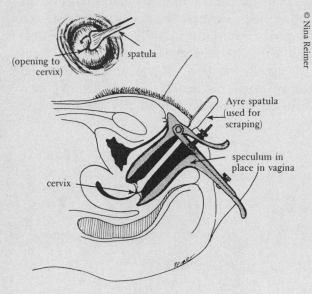

(opening to cervix)

spatula

Ayre spatula (used for scraping)

speculum in place in vagina

cervix

© Nina Reimer

Placement of speculum for a pelvic exam. Spatula scrapes cervix for Pap test (this is usually painless).

find, and sometimes the twinge you feel is the only way the practitioner is aware that he or she is touching them. The bimanual examination is more comfortable and more accurate if you are able to relax your neck, abdomen, and back muscles and keep your arms by your side. Breathing slowly and deeply, exhaling completely, may also help.

The Rectovaginal Exam

Sometimes a rectovaginal exam is part of the pelvic exam. If so, your provider will insert one finger into the rectum and one into the vagina to assess your internal pelvic organs from a different angle. This enables your provider to feel behind the uterus and makes it easier to feel the uterus and ovaries in women who have a tipped (retroverted) uterus. It also helps detect rectal lesions, and tests the tone of the rectal sphincter muscles. Blood in the rectum is sometimes an early sign of colon cancer. A stool test for blood at the time of the rectal exam was used in the past, although a single test at an exam is now considered inadequate compared with a three-day home test or other screening options like colonoscopy.

Some women find the rectovaginal exam unpleasant; others don't mind it. You may feel as if you are having a bowel movement as the practitioner withdraws his or her finger from your rectum. Don't worry—you won't, although sometimes a little stool will leak out. The rectal exam is usually the last part of the exam.

Talking with Your Provider

If you came in for a method of birth control that was not prescribed earlier or was not inserted yet, or for any vaccines, your provider will now address those issues and offer general health advice, either in the exam room or in a private consultation. Findings from your exam will also be discussed.

Many tests, such as Pap and STI tests, do not yield immediate results. If you have had any tests done, your provider should let you know when the results will be ready and how you will be contacted. When you filled out your medical history and office paperwork, you should have been asked whether it's okay for the office to contact you by email or phone. Check this with your provider if you're concerned about who will see or hear the messages.

Hopefully your experience with your provider was positive. But if you don't feel that your concerns were addressed, or if the provider was uncaring or unresponsive to your concerns or questions, ask your friends or family members for recommendations of other providers. Also consider sending an email or a letter to the provider describing your observations and concerns—sometimes clinicians need to be taught by their patients.

Specific Concerns

Some of us have specific physical needs or experiences that can make gynecological exams challenging. Some providers are committed to serving all populations; others are not as educated or sensitive, so the onus can be on us to ask for inclusion or adaptations, understanding that we are entitled to the same care as anyone else.

If you're not certain about a provider's willingness or ability to accommodate you, ask questions when calling to make an appointment, or consider scheduling an appointment to visit the office and meet with the provider in person, prior to an exam. Also contact groups that advocate for your specific needs; some may keep informal or formal lists of recommended health-care providers. Ask for referrals from friends, and look online for reviews.

Sexual Abuse

Many women who have experienced sexual abuse find that pelvic exams, like other kinds of genital contact, can be difficult. You may feel as though you don't have control, and parts of the exam may trigger body memories of sexual abuse and/or assault. You do not have to tell a health-care provider that you have been abused if you don't want to, but disclosing it may help your provider to understand your fears and take extra measures to make you feel comfortable and safe.

If participating more actively in your care would help you to relax, ask the provider to adjust the table or the pillows under your head so that you have a better view of what is going on, or ask to be informed, in advance, of each step in the exam process. Let your provider or staff person know if certain language, or where someone is standing, is potentially triggering for you. If you are being seen after a rape or sexual assault, your provider should use language that accurately reflects your experience and should not use terms like "sex" or "sexual activity" to describe the assault. (For more information, see Chapter 24, "Violence Against Women.")

Disability and Chronic Illness

It's too commonly assumed that sex is not important to those of us with disabilities or chronic illnesses. Your health care provider may not initiate discussions around sexuality, contraception, and sexually transmitted infections unless you bring up those topics. This is where seeing a practitioner who is experienced working with people with disabilities, especially disabilities or illnesses similar to yours, can be especially helpful.

If navigating a medical office or getting ready for an exam or getting up on the exam table will require extra time, call the office or clinic and request a long appointment.

Frustratingly, health care providers sometimes dismiss the physical discomforts of people with disabilities, pain disorders, or chronic illnesses, assuming that any problem is related to our disabilities. Or they talk past us if an interpreter or attendant is present. Our assistants are not surrogates; sensitive health care providers communicate with us directly, maintaining eye contact, and ensuring that our questions are answered.

In any health care situation, you should be treated with respect and patience, particularly if you need assistance with communication. Attention should be paid to your whole health, not just to health issues pertaining to the disability or illness. Adaptation should be provided that meets your needs, and if a provider cannot provide adaptations for whatever reason, a referral should be made to a provider who can. For more information on getting good reproductive and sexual health care if you have a disability, see "Disability Issues" p. 682, and the Women with Disabilities Education Program, womenwithdisabilities.org.

Size

When making your appointment, ask questions to ensure the office understands your needs and will treat you with respect. If you weigh more than 250–300 pounds, let the staff know, as not all providers have tables, scales, gowns, or equipment to accommodate women of size. If a given provider says something can't be done because of size, it usually means that she or he lacks training in providing sexual health care for larger women or has not made the practice accessible.

Both subtle and explicit fat biases are common. Be on the lookout for providers who blame every symptom and problem on your being a woman of size.

Lesbian, Bisexual, or Transgender

I'm so tired of being asked if I want to go on the Pill after I've said I only date women.

Those of us who are lesbian, bisexual, or transgendered may find that our providers make assumptions about us, from whether we're at risk of sexually transmitted diseases to whether we need birth control.

Some staff members or health care providers who do not regularly work with LGBT communities may default to a heterosexual or gender-normative script (meaning they assume that all women are attracted to men and that if you have a vagina, then you identify as a woman). If this happens, remind them who you are and what issues are relevant and appropriate for you. You have the right to be spoken to in the way that you identify your gender, sexual orientation, and/or relationship status. For more information, see Chapter 4, "Gender Identity and Sexual Orientation," and "Homophobia, Transphobia, and Heterosexism," p. 682.

CHAPTER 3 ■ ■ ■ ■ ■ ■ ■ ■ ■ ■ ■ ■ ■ ■ ■ ■ ■

For girls and women, life can often seem like an episode of the reality TV show *America's Next Top Model.* Throughout every phase of our lives, our appearance is judged and critiqued. Our looks are compared with those of our peers, our sisters, the women in the media, or imaginary ideals. No one ever asked if we want to participate in this lifelong competition; being female automatically makes us contestants, subject to constant scrutiny.

Individual experiences also affect how we feel about our bodies. Those of us who have experienced violence or abuse may feel unsafe or unworthy. If we have been ridiculed because of a disability or because of our weight or the color of our skin, we may dislike, mistrust, or even despise our bodies. The response to such hurtful experiences may be to seek what we consider to be a "perfect" body, through excessive dieting or exercising to exhaustion, buying expensive cosmetic products, or surgically changing our appearances—all in the hope that such efforts can shield us from discrimination or lead to success and true love. Sometimes the response is to treat our bodies as if they have little worth—to hurt ourselves, by binge eating or cutting.

Wanting to feel good about our bodies and our appearance is natural. Creating our own style allows us to express ourselves and to reflect our creativity and values. But there are questions most of us wrestle with: How do we nurture a positive body image while we're constantly being judged? How do we deal with pressure to act and look sexier in order to fit in? How do we change a system that marginalizes many of us and that rewards appearances above all else?

While there are many things that divide us as women, dissatisfaction with our looks and our bodies is something too many of us share. This chapter looks at how cultural forces have encouraged us to dislike our bodies and how we each can learn to be more comfortable in our own skin.

THE CRITICISM CONTINUUM

Starting when we're young, we watch older girls and women go through daily transformations, curling or straightening their hair, wearing uncomfortable clothes to achieve the right look, and critiquing their weight. Everywhere we look we see airbrushed models and products to improve our appearance. We internalize the message that as women, we will be defined by our looks and our size, not by our character, smarts, or accomplishments.

The expectations are set even higher now that cosmetic surgery, Botox, and other image-altering options have become normalized in the public consciousness. Not only are we supposed to spend whatever time, money, and effort it takes to look "perfect," but we're supposed to make it look as though perfection comes naturally—no extra effort required.

This pressure extends from when we're very young to well into our older years. Girls just starting school critique themselves and their classmates, wondering who is pretty enough to attract praise and attention, while more older women are developing eating disorders. "I think the degree of despair we are seeing among adult women about their bodies is unrivaled," Margo Maine, coauthor of *The Body Myth: Adult Women and the Pressure to Be Perfect*, told the *New York Times*.[1] At no point, it seems, are we free from being judged or judging ourselves.

The pressures we face have social and financial consequences. Recent studies have shown that thin women earn more on average—about $16,000 a year more, in one study—than their average-size counterparts.[2] Another study found that 57 percent of hiring managers agreed that qualified but unattractive candidates are likely to have a harder time landing a job, and 61 percent of managers (the majority of them men) said it would be an advantage for a woman to wear clothing showing off her figure at work.[3]

Many corporations and medical professionals are all too ready to help us spend our time and money trying to achieve an impossible beauty ideal. The cosmetics, fashion, and diet industries adeptly exploit the message that to be valued, women must do more and spend more to improve their appearance. Through relentless articles and advertisements, the media reinforce the message, playing on our insecurities ("What's He Really Thinking When He Sees You Naked?") or raising new ones ("Top 10 Trouble Spots We Bet You Didn't Notice").

The fantasy that we can completely trans-

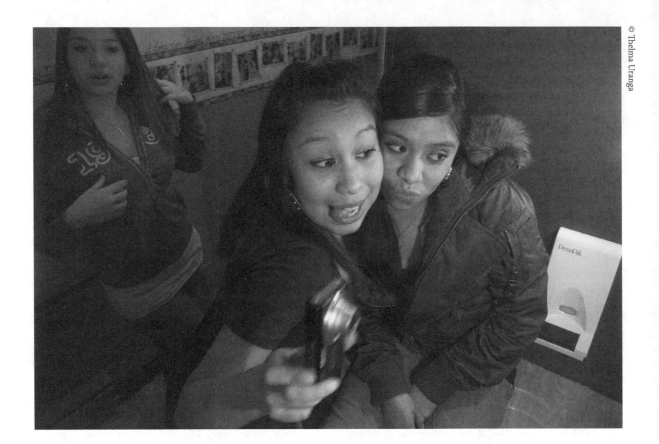

form ourselves often blinds us to the fact that a woman standing 5'4" and weighing 150 pounds will never be able to turn herself into a 5'11", 117-pound supermodel. In fact, even supermodels can't meet supermodel standards unless their images are substantially retouched and Photoshopped. So long as the majority of commercial media aimed at women are supported by advertising revenue from the fashion, beauty, diet, and food industries, there will be no shortage of stories trying to persuade us to do more or try harder.

PERCEPTION AND PERFORMANCE

Messages from commercial media aren't the only ones we internalize; as social media permeate our increasingly digitized lives, the perception and performance of identity are incessant, no longer reserved for when we sit down in front of the TV or pick up a magazine or go to work or head out to a party. From sexting (15 percent of teens twelve to seventeen say they have received sexually suggestive nude or nearly nude photos or videos from someone they know via text[4]) to the updating of Facebook profiles, we are shaping and reshaping our image—or watching others do it—minute by minute. Access to and fluency with digital image-altering tools such as Photoshop have put the power and pressure of commercial media into our own hands.

Many of us have experienced judgment or discrimination from family, friends, and employers based on our appearance. Whether the remarks are subtle or direct, they can leave a lasting impression, as this twenty-three-year-old woman notes: "How do you love yourself when your aunt would feed you boiled zucchini for a week because you were fat?"

The perception of body image for those of us who are lesbian is further complicated. Those of us who choose more masculine markers may feel pressure to be more feminine, but some lesbians experience greater body acceptance; appearance standards within the lesbian community sometimes are less tied to traditional beauty models and allow more room for difference.

Those of us who are transgender experience many of the same pressures that all women face, but the pressures may be enhanced by the desire to present as a woman. As Lucy writes on her blog, *Lovely Lucy: My Life as a Transgender Woman in Academia*:

I've reached the point where I feel like a woman and see myself as a woman but seeing myself as a "man in a dress" hasn't entirely disappeared. When I catch my reflection in the mirror at a certain angle or see a picture of myself, sometimes all I can see are the parts of myself that scream "man!" I know many other trans women have felt the same way.[5]

THE COLOR OF BEAUTY

All too often, the beauty ideal embraced by our culture is a white ideal (and a narrowly defined one at that). As early as the 1850s, skin bleaching and hair straightening were pitched to African Americans as ways to obtain the privileges of white society.[6] Today, women of color around the world apply skin-whitening creams either to lighten or to even their complexions. Some contain mercury, a known toxin that blocks the melanin that gives skin pigmentation.[7]

In the United States, the FDA banned mercury in compounds in most cosmetics, but test-

ing is rarely conducted. In 2010, the *Chicago Tribune* sent fifty skin-lightening creams to a certified lab for testing, most of them bought in Chicago stores and a few ordered online. Six were found to contain amounts of mercury banned by federal law, and of those, five had more than 6,000 parts per million, enough to potentially cause kidney damage over time.[8] The *Tribune* made the full list of products tested available to the public.[9]

Two common active ingredients used in skin-lightening creams are corticosteroids (such as hydrocortisone), which can make the skin more thin and fragile over time and cause excess hair growth and skin rashes and infections, and hydroquinone, which may act as a carcinogen or cancer-causing chemical, although its cancer-causing properties have yet to be proved in humans. Hydroquinone also has been linked with the medical condition ochronosis, which causes the skin to become dark and thick.

Advertisers are now using social media to encourage the virtual whitening of one's skin. The skin care company Vaseline launched a skin-lightening application for Facebook in India, encouraging users to lighten their skin in their profile pictures. According to a representative from the global advertising firm that designed the campaign, the response to the application has been "phenomenal."[10]

The preference for lighter skin is reinforced when a woman of color appears in advertisements or on magazine covers and her skin is digitally lightened. *Elle* magazine came under fire for the dramatic lightening of cover models Aishwarya Rai, a star of Indian cinema, and Oscar-nominated actress Gabourey Sidibe.[11] And though L'Oréal Paris—the world's largest cosmetics maker, whose product line includes skin-whitening creams—denied digitally altering Beyoncé's features or skin tone in a hair color campaign, the singer's skin tone seemed remarkably different.[12]

IN TRANSLATION:
SKIN WHITENING: AT WHAT COST?

Group: Groupe de Recherche sur les Femmes et les Lois au Sénégal (GREFELS)

Country: Senegal

Resource: *Notre Corps, Notre Santé (Our Body, Our Health)*, inspired by *Our Bodies, Ourselves* for French-speaking Africa

Website: grefels.org

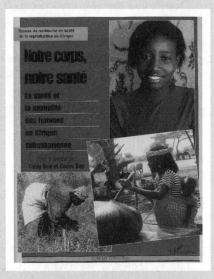

The French edition of *Our Bodies, Ourselves*

The use of cosmetic products to bleach or lighten the skin is a growing issue worldwide, with products heavily marketed in Africa and South Asia, as well as throughout Japan and some Caribbean countries. Lighter skin is not only portrayed as a beauty ideal but also associated with higher economic and social status.

In countries such as Tanzania, the skin-whitening industry is worth millions. Creams cost the equivalent of $4 to $10 each, a huge sum of money in a country where the average daily wage is less than $1. The products are dangerous as well as costly.

Our Bodies Ourselves' partner in Senegal—Groupe de Recherche sur les Femmes et les Lois au Sénégal (GREFELS)—has found that many African women who lighten their skin do so despite being aware of the risks to their health. In the *Our Bodies, Ourselves* for French-speaking Africa, GREFELS explic-itly challenges skin-whitening practices, drawing special attention to possible cancers caused by bleaching.

The authors note in the preface that the book aims to provide African women with knowledge to take care of and appreciate their bodies. "An important part of the book," they write, "is about the representations men and women have about women's bodies, health, and sexuality, about the way women's bodies are used, taken care of, dressed, and/or violated."

While some countries are trying to minimize skin bleaching, specifically by bans on sales, GREFELS believes that a deeper critique of the constellation of factors that influence the health and identity of women and girls in African society is imperative and long overdue.

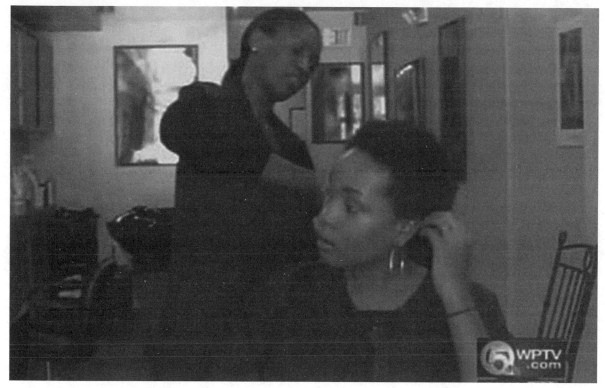

Rochelle Ritchie, a reporter for WPTV NewsChannel 5, goes natural during a special report on black women's hair. (Screen-shot via WPTV.com)

"I LOVE MY NATURAL HAIR"

Hair relaxers, extensions, and wigs marketed to African-American women and others have many potential dangers, from loss of hair to permanent burn damage. Many of the products can contain significant amounts of carcinogens and allergens such as formaldehyde. The choice for many of us to "go natural" would seem to present a simple solution, but it is a testimony to the embedded white beauty ideals that the choice is fraught with anxiety. Relaxed, long hair is considered professional; wearing our hair in braids or cornrows is not. Black women have received fewer promotions and been fired from jobs (or not hired in the first place) for wearing ethnic styles.

When Rochelle Ritchie, a multimedia journalist for WPTV News Channel 5 in West Palm Beach, Florida, did a special report on going natural, she noted that when she started in TV, she was told she needed hair extensions.

So for six years she chemically straightened and artificially lengthened her hair. But she put an end to all that during her report, letting viewers watch as a stylist chopped off Ritchie's damaged hair so she could return to her own natural style. Another woman featured in the piece did the same thing, in part because her six-year-old daughter had developed insecurities about her own natural hair. The daughter was thrilled with her mom's new look—and her own: "I love my natural hair, it's like my mom's, and it's beautiful."[13]

COLORISM, BLACK WOMEN, AND CONTEMPORARY REPRESENTATION

Courtney Young (thethirtymilewoman.word press.com) writes frequently about the intersection of pop culture, gender, and race.

Colorism is a widely understood yet rarely challenged form of discrimination in which the lightness of one's skin tone affords preferential social treatment to one group of people over another. Colorism is so deeply entrenched within the social fabric that there are studies available to prove that lighter-skinned blacks have higher incomes, receive preferential treatment in classroom settings, get hired and promoted at much larger rates within the corporate sphere, more often report the news, and—especially in the case of women—star in more Hollywood films, and even are executed at much lower rates than their darker-skinned counterparts. Though certainly colorism affects men of color, there are particular ways in which it is especially nuanced in the political and social lives of African-American women.

When Michelle Obama took up residence in the White House as first lady in 2009, she brought a new definition of beauty to the world. An extraordinarily accomplished and brilliant woman in her own right, Michelle, to the wide delight of many African-American women, is a dark-skinned woman. Vanessa Williams states, "If a black president represents change, a dark-skinned first lady is straight-up revolutionary. . . . The lingering effects of racism and sexism, coupled with a beauty industrial complex that constantly assaults our senses with images of female beauty that trend toward the lighter end of the racial color wheel, has rendered dark-skinned women nearly invisible in mainstream media."[16]

Issues of colorism and visibility would no doubt be a larger part of the public discussion if that discourse paid more attention to the intersection of race and gender. As it is, the many ways colorism—along with racism and classism—affects women of color are obscured and marginalized. Yet the impacts are felt personally, professionally, and politically.

MORE PRODUCTS, LESS REGULATION

Worldwide sales of fragrances, cosmetics, and toiletries have reached $330 billion per year, with the ten biggest companies accounting for more than half of all sales.[14] The cosmetics and beauty industry spends $2.2 billion on advertising everything from hair dyes to cellulite cream.[15] Although the vast majority of beauty products and magazines are marketed to women, men are no longer exempt from our culture's high expectations. Men's worldwide spending on skin care, hair care, bath and shower products, and deodorant jumped 44 percent between 2004 and 2009.[17] And body-sculpting products such as Spanx that have long been sold to women are now being made for men who want the appearance of a smoother tummy.

Despite its reach, the cosmetics industry is one of the least regulated in the United States—a frightening fact considering that the average

LESBIAN IN/VISIBILITY

Anxieties over hair can be acute for any woman who defies the long and straight ideal. Those of us who cut or shave our hair short, or color or shape our hair in nontraditional ways, especially if we are lesbian or transgender, are more prone to looks from others and even discrimination.

DIS magazine subverts traditional beauty salon imagery with an alternative salon poster featuring hairstyles usually associated with lesbians.[18] "The collection of these creative and varied haircuts brings into stark relief the hyperfeminized options most women encounter at the salon," writes Lisa Wade, assistant professor of sociology at Occidental College.[19]

The poster (available for purchase or free download) is accompanied online by a heady analysis of gender identity and the queer female body in the twenty-first century. It also offers some practical advice for the budget minded:

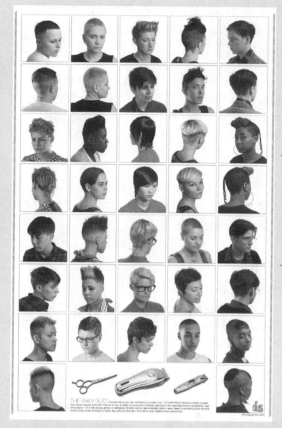

It started with a razor clip, followed by a scissor snip. THE W4W BUZZ features a variety of styles from close-cropped sides with more hair on top, to fades, buzzcuts and undercuts. Because of the seemingly limitless possibilities, age isn't a factor; nor is hair texture, gender, or orientation. Whether you're male or female, trans or sans, these conveniently priced hairstyle solutions are simple and easy-to-meme. Say so long to the salon and hello to your neighborhood barbershop.

woman uses ten beauty products a day.[20] Nearly all of our personal care products are made with at least one and usually several ingredients that have never been assessed for safety by the government or any other publicly accountable institution.[21]

The pursuit of beauty is often fraught with health and safety risks—some that are known and others that we're still discovering. When blood and urine samples from twenty teenage girls from across the country were tested, the samples were found to include an average of thirteen potential hormone-disrupting preservatives, plasticizers, and other cosmetic chemicals.[22] Moreover, carcinogens like formaldehyde and neurotoxins like lead are often found in trace amounts in cosmetics and personal care items.[23] Check out Chapter 25, "Environmental and Occupational Health," for more information.

Indoor tanning is a popular pastime for those seeking the fresh-from-the-beach look, despite studies showing indoor tanning increases the risk of skin cancer.[24] A recent study of college students found that among those who had repeatedly used tanning beds, approximately one-third met an addiction standard, meaning they exhibited dependency the same way others are dependent on alcohol and drugs: They missed class or other activities to tan, felt guilty about tanning too much, and were unable to cut down on indoor tanning time.[25]

FROM LIPSTICK TO LIPOSUCTION, BLUSH TO BOTOX

The quest for beauty and the pressure to conform apply to every body part. Bikini waxing—removing pubic hair that grows outside the swimsuit line—has been replaced by Brazilian bikini waxing, which usually removes every wisp of hair from the genital and anal areas, a painful procedure. As a result of removing all the hair from the pubic region, grown women's bodies more often resemble those of prepubescent girls. And if going bare isn't enough to recapture youth, there's now even genital makeup. My New Pink Button is described by marketers as "a simple to use Genital Cosmetic Colorant that restores the 'Pink' back to a Woman's genitals."[26]

The days when television makeovers consisted of changing one's hair, makeup, and clothes are long gone. Today, participants have their faces and bodies permanently altered through plastic surgery, on national TV, with little discussion of the health and psychological risks. The United States has more plastic surgeons and performs more surgical procedures than any other country—91 percent of which are performed on women.[27]

In 2010, more than 13.1 million cosmetic plastic surgery procedures were performed in the United States. The majority, 11.5 million, are considered minimally invasive. Among these,

A CONVERSATION ABOUT BODY IMAGE AND SELF-ESTEEM

This is an excerpt from an online conversation that developed into the "Relationships" chapter.

Kali: It is painfully easy for us, as women, to find reasons not to like our bodies. Because of my disability, I've had joint problems since I was twelve. Hating my body is something I have struggled with for as long as I can remember. It fails, it breaks, it betrays me. Add to that a few periods of sudden weight gain due to hormonal problems, and let's just say that me liking my body is a very touch-and-go sort of thing.

The thoughts about my body and relationships aren't pretty. "That guy must like me in spite of my appearance." "What is wrong with him? How can he like *this*?" "When he finds out how easily and how often I get injured, he's going to get fed up with this and leave." "I wish I could hide my bulges!"

It may seem odd, but I've found that what helps me with my body issues is creating my own comfort with my body and pushing societal expectations aside. Standing naked in front of a mirror and looking at my body as a statue, with graceful and interesting lines. Finding clothing that actually fit, especially clothing that felt flirty and feminine, or bold and dashing! The less it mattered to me what other people—especially prospective partners—thought, the more confident I was about how other people would perceive my body. It seems utterly paradoxical, and I'm not sure why it works, but it does.

Jordan: It really is frustrating how much perceptions of our bodies play into our perceptions about worthiness for relationships. I've definitely experienced that "I'm so lucky to be with someone who isn't repulsed by me" feeling and I've also had that exploited; people have used me secure in the knowledge that I won't protest because I am afraid of the consequences. And, for the most part, I like my body! I am just aware that the social constructs which surround it make other people think that it is less than acceptable.

Danielle: I want to echo what Kali is saying, about how easy it is to assume someone likes you in spite of something. Just last night, I was talking with my therapist about an ex. I was saying that it was really easy to imagine that the relationship had fallen apart because I'm trans, because transitioning was so hard on both of us, because of my body issues. My therapist asked, "Okay, but what if you'd been together *because* you were trans? Maybe if you weren't transitioning when you were, you never would have been together in the first place."

That had honestly never occurred to me. All women are bombarded with media indicating why our bodies aren't perfect enough. But I'd say trans women (and trans men, to a lesser extent) are additionally laden with messages that our bodies *can't* be attractive. That my very existence is "naturally" repugnant and repulsive.

I'd agree with Kali, too, that finding

things to like about your body is incredibly important. (And clothing that you actually find happiness and comfort with.) Likewise, I think doing something physical is really useful. I feel much better about myself when I'm able to say, "Yeah, I just biked those miles" (or whatever). And exercise endorphins are awesome, even if I don't exercise as often as I'd like.

Cody: Kali, I love what you've written here about creating bodily comfort for yourself and pushing those ugly societal voices out of the way. This has been true and incredible for me as well! I have moments of discomfort in my body, wishing I was smaller or shaped differently, and one of the things that feels best in those moments is to look at my naked body in the mirror and appreciate what I see: broad shoulders, muscle-y arms,

strong thighs. Hips that keep the frame of my body grounded and competent, rough hands.

I have to love this body because it's what I've got, and it's healthier to love my body for what it is than to wish it looked different. If I don't love my body, appreciate my contours, find myself sexy, how can I expect anyone else to feel this way about me? Sometimes I just need to remind myself that I'm hot and perfect and it's an act of bravery and defiance to think such things, in the face of this misogynist culture that wants me to hate myself. Then loving my body becomes political, and so much about me and so much not about anyone else or what they think of my body.

For more from this conversation, check out the "Relationships" chapter.

Botox was by far the most popular (5.4 million), followed by soft-tissue fillers (1.8 million), chemical peel (1.1 million), laser hair removal (938,000), and microdermabrasion (825,000).[28]

Of the more than 1.5 million surgical procedures considered more invasive, breast augmentation (296,000) topped the list, followed by nose reshaping (252,000), eyelid surgery (209,000), liposuction (203,000), and tummy tucks (116,000).[29] No longer treating only the rich, plastic surgeons regularly target working- and middle-class women, some of whom go into deep debt to pay for their surgeries. Job losses during the recession have led more people—both women and men—to consider altering their appearance to look more youthful and, by extension, appealing to employers.

Nearly 210,000 cosmetic plastic surgery procedures were performed on people age thirteen to nineteen in 2009, including almost 35,000 nose reshapings (rhinoplasty) and 8,000 breast augmentations, the most popular types of surgical procedures. Nonsurgical procedures such as Botox injections, which help reduce the visibility of wrinkles, were once reserved for women trying to conceal signs of aging. While Botox is approved by the FDA for children as young as twelve for very specific therapeutic purposes (twitching of the eyelid or crossed eyes, for example),[30] off-label uses are common. Charice Pempengco, a Filipina teenage singing phenom, publicly admitted getting a skin-tightening treatment and Botox injections before her guest appearance on the television show *Glee*; she said she wanted to look "fresh" for the cameras.[31]

ABSOLUTELY SAFE

Absolutely Safe (absolutelysafe.com), a must-see documentary examining breast implant safety, follows the stories of two women, one who wants to have her leaking silicone implants removed and the other looking to have breast augmentation. The viewer meets plastic surgeons who are for and against the surgery, women who have suffered from silicone implants (including the mother of the filmmaker, Carol Ciancutti-Leyva), and members of the FDA committee who determine whether or not to allow silicone back on the market.

"All along the viewer feels powerfully the impact pressures to be beautiful have and have had on American women," says gender studies expert Diana York Blaine. "Breast implants clearly 'solve' the problem while introducing myriad new ones. . . . This film makes starkly clear that the female sense of inadequacy is not an individual phenomenon. Institutionalized sexism affects all of us. Destroying our health seems to be an acceptable solution."

To learn more about health risks, visit breastimplantinfo.org, a project of the National Research Center for Women and Families.

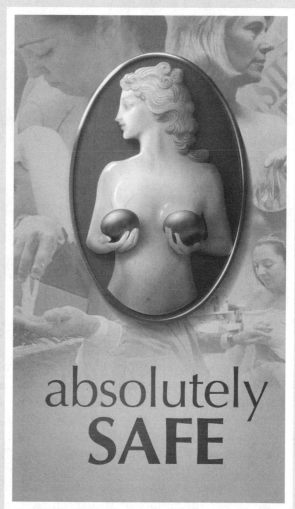

absolutely
SAFE

Special scrutiny is given to new mothers. The media give approval to celebrities who, just weeks after childbirth, flaunt fit figures along with designer diaper bags. The rest of us are expected to follow suit, even if we don't have child care and 24/7 access to a staff of personal trainers and nutritionists (and even if our livelihoods don't depend on appearance). So-called mommy makeovers offer new mothers a package of surgical procedures—breast lift, tummy tuck, and liposuction—to "recover" from what one plastic surgeon calls the "severe physical trauma of pregnancy, child-birth and breast-feeding."[32]

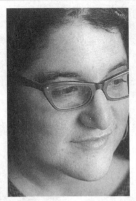

© R.A. McBride

"I LIKE THE WAY MY NOSE MARKS ME"

LISA JERVIS

As an ethnic Jew of a very specific variety –a godless New York City-raised neurotic upper-middle-class girl from a solidly liberal-Democrat family who observed only one Jewish ritual: going out for Chinese food and a movie on Christmas Day –I've had a standing offer for a nose job from adolescence on. "It's not such a big deal," my mom would say. "Doctors do such individual-looking noses these days. It'll look really natural."

It's not too late, you know," she would add in the years after I flat-out refused to let someone break my nose, scrape part of it out, and reposition it into a smaller, less obtrusive shape. "I'll still pay." As if money were the reason I was resisting.

Mainly, I didn't want to be that vain and shallow, and I didn't want scalpels anywhere near my face. But my queasy feelings about plastic surgery aside –the risks, the expense, the frivolity, the blood, the sheer visceral creepiness –I'd have wanted to keep my prominent, bump-adorned honker anyway. Oddly, given how I've felt about my body at various times in my life, I've always been pretty happy with my (dare I say it?) God-given nose.

Of friends my own age who've had nose jobs, most didn't want them but were coerced or shamed into it by older Jewish female relatives: mothers, grandmothers, aunts (an experience I'm eternally grateful my mother spared me). Though in this day and age, the lust for a button nose is more a desire for a typical pretty femininity than for any specific de-ethnicizing, when we scratch the surface of what "prettier" means, we find that we might as well be saying "whiter" or "Gentile."

I like the way my nose marks me. The first time I met another Jewish feminist writer with whom I would end up working, she asked if I was a member of the tribe. I've always appreciated that there's a part of my identity that's instantly recognizable to those who know where to look.

Self-Esteem and Plastic Surgery

It's commonly believed that people who are considered extremely attractive are much happier than everyone else, but research seems to indicate that this isn't true.[33] And, despite the media hype and conventional wisdom that surgery improves self-esteem, there is no research to support that.

If you ask plastic surgery patients how they feel in the months after surgery, many say they feel more self-confident, but when women are asked before surgery how they feel about themselves and then asked the same question a few months or years after surgery, there is no significant difference. They may feel better about the body part that was "fixed," but they don't feel better about themselves. That's because self-esteem is a stable trait for most people, and it doesn't change just because of a change in appearance.[34]

MEDIA DISTORTIONS

The body has become a mere canvas, upon which the digital-age beauty business remasters our image of what is physically possible. But since perfection is ipso facto unattainable, what is really on offer, in the world of beauty as elsewhere, is infinite discontent.[35]

—Ruth Brandon,
Ugly Beauty (Harper, 2011)

Before mass media existed, our ideas of beauty were limited to our own communities. In fact, until the advent of photography in 1839, people were not exposed to real-life images of faces and bodies. Fast-forward to today's digital age and an entirely new landscape in which images inundate us at every turn. Whether we're watching TV, surfing online, or playing video games, idealized young, thin female imagery is everywhere:

I believe that every woman is utterly and completely beautiful. That said, when I find myself faced with produced images of beauty in magazines or billboards, I still can't help but wish I looked like them.

Researchers have found that ongoing exposure to certain ideas can shape and distort our

The continued objectification of women's bodies prompts many of us to objectify ourselves, meaning we internalize the cultural expectations that assert our bodies exist only for the pleasure of others.[36] One woman describes how she defied those expectations during sex:

I worried that he would see a hair here, or a flabby spot there, and be turned off. I noticed that he was never self-conscious about a skin blemish or when he gained a few pounds. So I started copying him and concentrated more on the sexual pleasure I felt. I began enjoying sex a lot more, and he noticed. He said it made him more excited, and the result? A great new circle of passion and sex.

perceptions of reality. How many naked bodies do most of us view on a regular basis in real life—not counting what we see in the media? Very few. But if we're consuming media, especially fashion magazines or pornography, we encounter more naked or seminaked female bodies than we would otherwise. One result of this pervasive imagery is that younger generations are learning what women should look like by viewing what are, more often than not, radically altered and objectified depictions of women in the media. Real women with pubic hair and breasts that aren't perfect round orbs begin to seem unnatural compared with the altered images.

Even if we don't accept the images we see in the media, we are likely to believe that others accept those images and still feel we must alter our bodies to conform to them.[37] Critics say these images are not only promoting a false sense of what our bodies, including our genitals, are supposed to look like, but also affecting our sexual health by encouraging body modifications that can increase the risk of sexually transmitted infections as well as reduce physical sensation and cause other complications.[38]

DESIGNER VAGINAS

Every inch of a woman's body presents a new opportunity for improvement, including our vaginas.[39] Much as with waxing, it's difficult to ignore the obvious link these procedures have to pornography.

Some women have their inner vaginal lips cut and shortened to make them smaller or more symmetrical through a surgery called labiaplasty. The procedure aims to fix labia that are "too large, loose, floppy, bulky, excessive, uneven, redundant, or overpigmented."[40] Others undergo surgical tightening of the vagina, or vaginal rejuvenation, which is touted as increasing women's sexual self-confidence and men's sexual pleasure.[41] This type of surgery has been performed in the United States since the late 1990s, but until recently it was typically performed to treat urinary incontinence in older women. These surgeries often come with major risks, including the possible loss of sensation or pain when aroused.[42] The procedure may even cause some of the same childbirth problems as female genital cutting, including bleeding and tearing in labor.[43]

Although some people believe these procedures will enhance their sexual experiences, no research supports claims of increased sexual satisfaction. Importantly, experts say that perceived sexual enhancement as a result of genital reconstruction may be attributed in part to the psychological reaction to the surgery, rather than to physical changes from the surgery itself. The American Congress of Obstetricians and Gynecologists (ACOG) has stated that these procedures are "not medically indicated, nor is there documentation of their safety and effectiveness." The group also has warned it's deceptive to give the impression that any of these procedures are accepted and routine surgical practices. In addition, ACOG recommends that women considering vaginal procedures be "informed about the lack of data supporting the efficacy of these procedures as well as their potential complications, including infection, altered sensation, dyspareunia [pain], adhesions, and scarring."[44]

Negative comments and pressure from a male partner can influence us to change our bodies, but often the pressure comes from within; we set standards for ourselves that we think we should meet. Los Angeles gynecologist and cosmetic surgeon David Matlock, made famous by the popular television series *Dr. 90210*, has made a career performing and promoting his "Laser Vaginal Rejuvenation" techniques, which he trademarked and refuses to publish. According to Matlock, who claims to have performed more of the surgeries than anyone else in the country, "I can't tell you how many pages and pages of pornographic material woman have brought in

HYMENOPLASTY

Surgical reconstruction of the hymen—more recently referred to as the vaginal corona—is also becoming more popular, particularly among women of Middle Eastern and Hispanic descent. Though the hymen, if there to begin with, can tear, break, or fade away on its own, surgery is done so bleeding will occur during intercourse, a sign in some cultures that the woman is a virgin. See p. 7 for more discussion of the vaginal corona.

to me saying 'I want to look like this.' . . . Even young women will look at loose hanging labia as a sign of aging and want to have it done."[45]

More discussion is needed to reassure women about the wide variation in the appearance of normal genitalia. Comparing pictures of normal and healthy bodies with surgically streamlined ones creates the impression that so-called aberrations are abnormal—when in reality, genital anatomy is as diverse as a person's fingerprints. Furthermore, by promoting a narrow definition of what's normal, female cosmetic genital surgery creates a disincentive for women to deal with cultural and personal forces shaping their body image and sexual identity. "Many women don't realize that the appearance of external genitals varies significantly from woman to woman. As ob-gyns, we know this to be the case from years of experience," said Abbey B. Berenson, M.D., a member of ACOG's Committee on Gynecologic Practice.[46]

The New View Campaign—with the endorsement of dozens of sex educators, doctors, and psychologists from around the world—is demanding new regulations that would require the Federal Trade Commission's consumer protection division to monitor the ads.[47] At a 2008 protest outside the Manhattan Center for Vaginal Surgery in New York City, New View members called for, "More research, less marketing." The group is also calling for a moratorium on the procedures until monitoring and guidelines are in place.[48]

Porn and Profit

As more websites and digital media vie for viewers' attention, it's up to advertisers to take a more compelling, edgier approach. More often than not, that means selling sex—or, more accurately, women's sexuality. (For a roundup of ads that depict the influence of pornography on advertising, visit feministfatale.com.) As the feminist

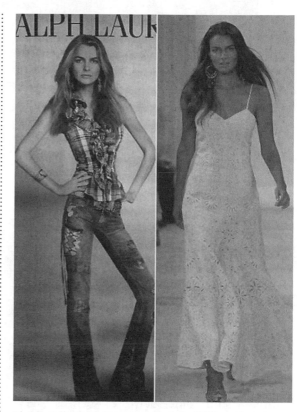

The digitally altered image on the left of Filippa Hamilton, a popular longtime model for Polo Ralph Lauren, caused an uproar in 2009 when it appeared in a department store in Japan. The clothing company eventually apologized for the ad but initiated another controversy soon after by firing Hamilton. "They fired me because they said I was overweight and I couldn't fit in their clothes anymore," Hamilton said.[49]

activist Gail Dines, professor of sociology and women's studies at Wheelock College in Boston, told the New Left Project, "If you just turn on the television, flick through a magazine or look at billboards, you will see that porn has now become a blueprint for how the media represents women's bodies. . . . Today there is almost no soft-core porn on the internet, because most of it has migrated into pop culture."[50]

Male activists have also been part of the movement to reshape attitudes toward body image—especially among men themselves. In

Getting Off: Pornography and the End of Masculinity, Robert Jensen, professor of journalism at the University of Texas, articulates the ways traditional notions of masculinity trap men into a need for dominance in their relationships with both women and other men.

Byron Hurt, filmmaker, antisexist educator and activist, and hip-hop critic, created the award-winning documentaries *I AM A MAN: Black Masculinity in America* and *Hip Hop: Beyond Beats & Rhymes*. In both films, Hurt acknowledges the racism that helped construct black masculinity in America, but he also holds out the possibility of an alternative space in which black men can redefine themselves in opposition to the voices of misogyny, violence, and homophobia.

WHO'S MISSING FROM THIS PICTURE?

Although some older actresses such as Meryl Streep, Annette Bening, and Helen Mirren continue as Hollywood mainstays, the silver screen rarely shows women over forty except in asexual, supporting, or comic roles.[51] Many of the women chosen to portray mothers in the movies are the same age as or younger than men playing their sons. And the older women we do see often look much younger, thanks to careful casting, plastic surgery, and digitally altered images.[52] As a result, those of us who choose to age naturally, without the aid of plastic surgery, meticulous beauty regimes, and restrictive dieting, are sometimes seen as "letting ourselves go."

The media's image of perfection excludes women with visible disabilities. The almost total lack of representation means that the lives of disabled women remain a mystery to many able-bodied people. Disabled women are often portrayed as helpless victims who need protection, or as heroines who have beaten the odds.

Because women with bodies that are disabled, fat, or old are seen as deviating from what is "normal" and desirable, we are often presented as stereotypes rather than as real people. The crotchety old woman, the loudmouthed fat woman, and the desexualized disabled woman with a heart of gold are widespread media clichés. Rarely is our beauty recognized or acknowledged, and we are almost never portrayed as sexual beings:

Living with a physical disability, I have learned from the dominant messages in society that I am not like other women. In fact, for the most part, I'm actually not considered a woman at all.

The percentage of women of color represented in the media has grown, but measures of success are complicated: The inclusion of women of color in some mainstream advertising is often a deliberate tactic to convey how much hipness or attitude a product has.[53] And the body ideal remains the same—skinny and large breasted with long hair—leading some women of color to judge themselves by that norm. One woman notes that as a teenager, she was obsessed with "achieving the 'white girl' look: slim hips, perky breasts, flat stomach. I hated that I didn't look like white models in my magazines."

Mainstream magazines and entertainment media still rarely feature women of color as cover models or lead actors. Consider *Vanity Fair*'s 2010 "Young Hollywood" issue: Nine of the industry's most up-and-coming young female actresses graced the cover—all of them white, thin, and able-bodied.[54]

A young Korean-American woman describes the specific pressure caused by the white beauty ideal:

When I was growing up, everyone in commercials, magazines, and movies had big, beautiful eyes. I wanted bigger eyes, too. Older

AMERICAN ABLE

Media activism takes many forms. The photographer, Holly Norris, and her friend and subject Jes Sachse, who has a rare genetic condition known as Freeman-Sheldon syndrome, created the "American Able" photo series—a marvelous parody of the very specific body type (thin and able-bodied) presented in American Apparel advertising and the media in general.

"This idea of who is beautiful and what's sexy that we see in the media all the time isn't necessarily what beauty is to me or to you," notes Norris.[55]

What began as an assignment for an undergraduate women and popular culture class became part of a group exhibit in May 2010, appearing on more than 270 digital screens throughout the Toronto subway system.

In her statement accompanying the images, Norris says, "Rarely, if ever, are women with disabilities portrayed in anything other than an asexual manner, for 'disabled' bodies are largely perceived as 'undesirable.' In a society where sexuality is created and performed over and over within popular culture, the invisibility of women with disabilities in many ways denies them the right to sexuality, particularly within a public context."

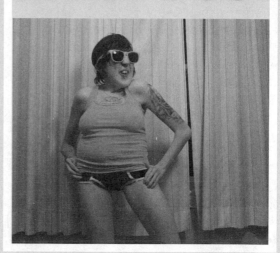

Meet Jes.

© Holly Norris

The series is made all the more compelling by Sachse's obvious joy and boldness. Whether she's wearing a little black dress or little more than tube socks, she owns each shot.

"I look confident in the photos," she said, adding, "I look just how I feel about the work, about the idea, about my body."[56]

Visit hollynorris.ca/americanable for more images from the series. For more on young women's activism around issues of disability and sexuality, see p. 191.

Korean girls suggested using thread or tape to help the double eyelid form. I attempted it, but it never really worked. I just created the illusion with black eyeliner, but I was still really self-conscious about it and struggled with how I looked. I thought I'd get the surgery when I got older, even though my father was against it. Today, I'm thankful I never got it done. There are more Asians in the media now than when I was in high school, which helps. There are people who love the way my eyes look, just like I envied bigger eyes growing up.

MEDIA ACTIVISM

- **If you do not see images of beauty that resemble you, look elsewhere.** Seek out alternative publications, movies, books, and media sites. View mainstream advertising and media images with a critical eye and keep in mind the realities behind them.
- **Examine how your own behavior reflects or supports media tactics.** Would you buy a product if the woman in the advertisement wasn't beautiful? What messages do you internalize?
- **Use your purchasing power.** After popular clothing retailer Abercrombie & Fitch began selling thong underwear for preteen girls, protests and threats of boycotts made it rethink its plans. Refuse to buy products from companies that exploit women and girls in their ad campaigns.
- **Become a media critic.** Blog, tweet, and use Facebook to call out representations of girls and women that are demeaning to all of us.

YOU CAN BE FAT ON TV—IF YOU'LL SUFFER TO LOSE WEIGHT

When larger women are included in popular television shows and movies, they're usually portrayed in relation to weight and their efforts to be thin. Television shows such as *The Biggest Loser* follow the heroic efforts of men and women fighting to lose pounds and gain respect. *The Biggest Loser* draws an estimated 10 million viewers each week. But what does it say about our culture that we applaud these efforts, even if they include dangerous weight-loss techniques,

including self-induced dehydration, severe caloric restriction, and up to six hours a day of strenuous exercise?[57]

At the same time, viewers are clamoring for more diverse and accurate representations on television. Though it was disheartening to see a *Marie Claire* columnist write of the CBS series *Mike & Molly*, "I think I'd be grossed out if I had to watch two characters with rolls and rolls of fat kissing each other . . . because I'd be grossed out if I had to watch them doing anything," the outcry that followed was nothing short of inspiring. Thousands of comments have been left on the post, most of which condemn the snarky critique.[58]

When *Glamour* magazine in 2009 published a nearly nude photo of model Lizzie Miller in a seated position with natural belly rolls, it received an overwhelming amount of positive feedback.[59] The response led to Miller's appearance on *Today*, and the blogosphere buzzed about the surprising inclusion. *Glamour* even dedicated its November 2009 issue to honoring plus-size models and featured a group shot of seven plus-size models in the nude.[60]

But what happens the other eleven months of the year? Despite this welcomed inclusion, women above a size 2 are usually included in fashion magazines and advertisements only in special "real-women" issues or when being directly marketed to—which isn't often enough: Although an estimated 41 percent of U.S. women are larger than a size 14, only 10 percent of retailers cater to them.[61]

Television ads follow the same trend. The clothing chain Lane Bryant stirred controversy over one of its TV ads that featured a plus-size model trying on different lingerie outfits. ABC and Fox initially refused to air it on their popular shows *Dancing with the Stars* and *American Idol*, respectively, claiming it was too "racy." The networks later relented, but only during later portions of the shows. Lane Bryant noted

COMMERCIALIZED CULTURE: THE HISTORY OF WOMEN IN ADVERTISING

Jean Kilbourne (jeankilbourne.com) is an author, speaker, and filmmaker who makes the salient connection between advertising and public health.

"Feminine odor is everyone's problem," proclaims an ad for a feminine hygiene spray. "If your hair isn't beautiful, the rest hardly matters" (an ad for shampoo). "My boyfriend told me he loved me for my mind. I was never so insulted in my life" (cigarettes!).

These ads are some of the earliest in the collection I started in 1968, the year I began studying the image of women in advertising. The examples used in the first version of my documentary film *Killing Us Softly: Advertising's Image of Women* (made in 1979 and remade three times since)[62] seem ludicrous by today's standards. One ad touts a deodorant that is "Made for a woman's extra feelings" (presumably located in her armpits). A woman in a diet ad exults, "I'd probably never be married now if I hadn't lost 49 pounds." (In one audience, a woman shouted out, "The best advertisement for fat I've ever seen.")

It's easy to laugh at these ads and to believe that we've made progress. If only it were true. Certainly we no longer see as many demented housewives pathologically obsessed with cleanliness (these days it's more likely to be antibacterial products), and we see in current ads many more women in the workplace and some (but not enough) men caring for children and even doing domestic chores without screwing them up.

In many ways, however, things have gotten worse. The ideal image of beauty is more tyrannical than ever. Even little children are increasingly sexualized in advertising and throughout the popular culture. Girls get the message very early on that they must be hot and sexy in addition to being flawlessly beautiful and impossibly thin. Women's bodies are still used to sell everything from shampoo to chain saws, and are often dismembered into parts—breasts, legs, buttocks. Sometimes a woman's body morphs into the product, so she becomes the car or the shoe or the bottle of beer. An ad that ran in several upscale women's magazines featured a woman whose pubic hair had been shaved into the Gucci logo. We are encouraged to feel passion for our products rather than our partners.

As advertisers look for new ways to get our attention, they also use ever more graphic depictions of sex and of violence. Ads in the early 1960s, bad as they were, didn't feature women's battered bodies splayed out on the ground or stuffed into automobile trunks.

More important than images in specific ads is the rise in the power and impact of advertising in general. Nearly everything is about marketing these days, from journalism to entertainment to politics. Our entire culture is commercialized in a way unimaginable forty years ago.

I'm afraid there isn't much good news about changes in the world of advertising. But increasingly, people understand that, far from being trivial, advertising is actually a public-health issue that affects us all. In this sense, we *have* come a long way indeed.

that both stations happily ran Victoria's Secret ads during the same time slots, but the stations denied any hypocrisy.[63] After much back-and-forth, the question still remained: Why is the average American woman—who weighs 165 pounds and wears a size 14—so invisible?[64]

TARGETING TWEENS AND TEENS

SELLING INSECURITY

Advertisers understand the buying power of children, tweens, and teens, and aggressively market to them through every available channel. The combination of self-consciousness and spending power makes young people prime targets for corporations. Girls in particular represent an important and powerful revenue source, and savvy marketers make it a point to sell them on the same messages of insecurity they'll hear throughout adulthood, ensuring their lifelong role as consumers.

The beauty industry lures girls when they are young—for instance, by placing variations of the same ads in *Teen Vogue* that it puts in *Vogue*. During adolescence, girls gain an average of twenty-five pounds of body fat, which is necessary for proper development.[65] But in a thin-obsessed culture, it's not surprising that most teenage girls experience body anxiety and go on diets.

A review of twenty-one studies that looked at the media's effect on more than six thousand girls age ten and older found that those who were exposed to the most fashion magazines were more likely to suffer from poor body image.[66] But it's not just fashion magazines. The YWCA in Australia in 2010 sought a PG rating for popular tween magazines *Disney Girl, Barbie,* and *Total Girl*, saying that the publications teach young girls that their bodies need to be improved upon.[67]

Perhaps beyond the direct correlation question lies a simpler question: What kinds of stories are we telling young girls about what it means to be female? What ideals are we encouraging them to meet?

One of the largest marketers to children and tweens is the Walt Disney Corporation, which has crafted a $4 billion empire out of its Disney Princess marketing.[68] In the world of Disney, "Sleeping Beauty" waits to be awoken (and saved) by her prince, "Beauty" falls in love with the man behind "Beast," and Cinderella becomes transformed into a princess thanks to a makeover of hair, makeup, and clothes, despite the efforts of her "ugly" stepsisters. The recurring theme is obvious and simple: Be beautiful and have access to material possessions that help you to be beautiful.[69] (See pp. 119 for a discussion of how relationships are idealized in pop culture and what young adult and adult women remember from Disney stories.)

The real-world contradictions and consequences of Disney's princess marketing became clear when one of Disney's human princesses, fifteen-year-old Miley Cyrus of Hannah Montana fame, posed provocatively for the June 2008 issue of *Vanity Fair* magazine. Cyrus, while initially defending the intentions of the photo shoot, eventually disowned it and claimed, "I never intended for any of this to happen."

In the book *Cinderella Ate My Daughter: Dispatches from the Front Lines of the New Girlie-Girl Culture*, Peggy Orenstein reflects on how Cyrus's ambivalence (whether it was a premediated media stunt or not) reflects how the more the pressure on girls changes, the more it stays the same: "The nineteenth-century Cinderella, Sleeping Beauty and Snow White served as metaphors, symbols of girls' coming of age, awakening to womanhood. The contemporary princesses do as well, and though the end point may be different—marrying the handsome prince has been replaced by cutting a hit single—the narrative arc is equally predictable. In their own way their dilemmas, too, illuminate the ones all girls of their era face, whether publicly or privately, as they grow up to be women—and commodities."[71]

DIY MEDIA

Girls and their allies are taking on the challenges of creating alternative representations of women. In magazines and websites created by, for, and about girls, such as New Moon (newmoon.com) and Teen Voices (teenvoices.com), young women are presenting their own stereotype-busting stories.

Websites such as Shaping Youth (shaping youth.org) and About-Face (about-face.org) are attempting to counter the media's and marketers' influence by providing stories and resources of their own. As girls get older, *Bitch* magazine (bitchmagazine.org) provides a critical and engaging perspective on all aspects of pop culture.

DO I LOOK FAT?

Our self-worth is often tied to the numbers on the bathroom scale. Since mainstream culture tells us that fat women are undesirable to men—and to society in general—many women will do almost anything to be thin.

Yet fat is inextricably linked to the female form; our breasts and hips are, quite simply, made of fat. Women need more body fat than men, and extreme dieting can cause serious health problems; women who are too thin do not menstruate and cannot bear children.

In the United States, one need only call an accomplished woman "fat" to put her in her place. Making women afraid to be fat is a form of social control; we must diet and live in constant terror that we'll gain weight, lest we be ostracized from society.

Conservative radio show host Laura Ingraham dismissed Meghan McCain, an author and pundit (and daughter of Senator John McCain), calling her a "plus-sized model." McCain responded, "What do women think when I speak my mind about politics and I want to have a political discussion about the ideological future of the Republican Party, and the answer is, 'She's fat, she shouldn't have an opinion.' What kind of message are we sending young women?

"It infuriates me," she said. "I'm a political writer on a blog, and all of a sudden I'm too fat to write?"[72]

Current notions about weight are so pathological that even pregnant women struggle to not see themselves as fat. Weight-loss surgery, as well as weight-loss medications and supplements, can pose health risks. In an attempt to shed pounds, nearly half of all women are on a diet on any given day, spending almost $59.7 billion a year on diets[73] that fail the great majority of the time.[74] Researchers have begun to quantify the dangerous increases in stress that accompany dieting, and how dieting has a tendency in the long term to lead to more unhealthy eating habits.[75] Other researchers also found that adolescents who diet put on more weight than those who do not.[76]

Because of the intense focus on body size, our feelings about weight often get tangled up with how we feel about ourselves. "Do I look fat?" is a mantra uttered by many women, yet beneath the surface, it has little to do with weight. Researchers have found that young women often express themselves through what is called "fat talk." In such conversations, we use self-disparaging body talk as a way to bond with peers, with talk about weight substituted for talk about feelings. "I'm so fat" often translates to "I'm depressed," or, "My life is out of control." In return, friends will usually assure the girl that she is thin, thus boosting her self-esteem. Such talk can drive some girls from borderline to full-blown eating disorders.[77]

Because the thin ideal is promoted in the media primarily through images of white women, many believe that women of color do not feel the same pressures to be thin and must not suffer from poor body image. Some studies have suggested that the reason African-American women and girls are shown as generally experiencing higher levels of body confidence than women of other races is in part because studies often neglect to explore attitudes about skin color and hair texture.[78] Other research shows that poor body image and eating disorders do in fact affect women of all races.[79]

African-American and Latino men seem more appreciative of bigger thighs and rounded buttocks, but beyond that, their preference for thin women seems similar to that of white men. My female peers (black, middle aged, and middle class) are all on diets. They're all obsessed with weight and hair length and the importance of those things in getting a man.

Other women who are expected to be naturally thin are sometimes overlooked when they diet excessively. An Asian-American woman talks about the widespread belief that Asian women come in only one size: petite.

Many of my friends weigh less than 100 pounds and keep losing weight, yet nobody calls that anorexia because Asian women are supposed to be tiny. Doctors are subject to these stereotypes, too. At my last physical I weighed 112 pounds; the doctor was shocked, as if I were fat.

WHEN GOOD = SKINNY

Many of us feel stuck between our knowledge of the importance of healthy eating and our desire to accept ourselves. Conversations about feeling fat often revolve around guilt—being "good" and resisting bad-for-you foods, or being "bad" and giving in to temptation. Marketers commonly use "guilt-free" labeling on low-fat or low-carb food, reinforcing this notion, even though the food may not be healthy.

I spent so many years endlessly dieting and trying to be skinny, skinny, skinny. It was so freeing to finally stop and accept my body. As I reach middle age, I know I should eat better, but as soon as I put any restrictions on what I can eat, I feel deprived and instantly crave the very foods that are bad for me.

Though studies show that our well-being and longevity have less to do with weight than health, blatant discrimination against and ridicule of fat people are considered acceptable. In fact, studies in recent years have confirmed a significant increase in discrimination based on

EATING DISORDERS AND HEALTH

Anorexia, bulimia, and binge eating are complicated physical and psychological disorders. Unhealthy nutrition, low weight, and dramatic weight loss and gain can harm major organs and compromise hormonal systems and have a long-term effect on women's health and well-being. Women with eating disorders often suffer from underlying anxiety, depression, obsessive-compulsive disorder, and other psychiatric illnesses. Body size and shape preoccupation, distorted body image, compulsive exercising, and obsessional rituals often linger for years after an acute disorder. The most common fertility-related health problems associated with anorexia are amenorrhea (absence of periods), irregular menstrual cycles, reduced egg quality, ovarian failure, compromised uterine health, and miscarriage.[80]

Primary prevention of eating disorders that involves teaching girls skills for healthy nutrition and body acceptance, leadership and media literacy skills, and a range of coping skills for resisting unhealthy cultural messages can be an early jump start on preventing the long-term reproductive and psychological health issues associated with eating disorders. "Full of Ourselves: A Wellness Program to Advance Girl Power, Health, and Leadership," a program coauthored by Catherine Steiner-Adair and Lisa Sjostrom that promotes body esteem and self-esteem as well as the prevention of eating disorders, is a recommended resource. For more information, visit catherinesteineradair.com/full-of-ourselves.php.

weight.[81] One woman describes how internalizing these attitudes affected her relationships:

In my late teen years, I occasionally engaged in relationships that I didn't particularly want to be in . . . because I felt lucky that somebody would be interested in me in spite of my body. Now I am with a great guy who is attracted to me for many reasons, but partly because of my body.

"Fat" is extremely relative, too—some women consider themselves fat simply because they are larger than most of their peers, or they have suddenly become larger than they were for most of their life. Our national weight obsession is often cast in moral terms, making bias against fat people acceptable. Thin people are assumed to be virtuous, while fat people are considered lazy and lacking self-control.[82] Similarly, larger people are assumed to be unhealthy and unfit. The reality is that some fat people are in excellent health, while some thin people are not.

Tools such as the body mass index (BMI) are unreliable measures of health, as they fail to take into account muscle weight and individual body types. Even medical and insurance tables listing heights and weights do not take into consideration the natural variations in body size.

HEALTHY AT ANY SIZE

While there are clear health risks to being very overweight or obese, the solution most often proposed—for individuals to diet and lose weight—oversimplifies complex realities. We live in a world where highly processed, refined foods are cheap and readily available. The government subsidizes the production of grains including corn and wheat, which are used primarily to make corn sweeteners and refined carbohydrates, but not of healthier foods such as fruits, vegetables, beans, and nuts, thereby creating artificially low prices for the least nutritious options. Processed foods are far more profitable to the food industry, and ads incessantly push fast food, soft drinks, and other high-calorie, low-nutrition products. Dieting and weight loss are a multibillion-dollar industry. Yet this chronic dieting has not slowed the rise in the number of Americans classified as overweight or obese: In 1980, just under half of U.S. adults were overweight; by 2008, this figure had jumped to 68 percent.[83] Dieting is notoriously unsuccessful at producing substantial long-term weight loss: the vast majority of dieters regain the weight they lost, with between one-third and two-thirds regaining more weight than they lost. Body shape is not as changeable as we are led to believe.

Given these realities, an increasing number of health experts are focusing on a model of health called Health at Every Size, which en-

FAT ACCEPTANCE

Society assumes inside every fat person, there is a thin person dying to be set free. But many women are fighting the antifat forces that teach us beauty comes in only one size. For an intro guide to fat acceptance, Kate Harding's FAQ section at (kateharding.net/faq) is a must-read. Harding and Marianne Kirby's book, *Lessons from the Fat-o-sphere*, is a in-depth guide to how to stop judging ourselves and others through distorted body image ideals. For other voices in the movement, check out activists in the blogosphere such as Two Whole Cakes (blog.twowholecakes.com), The Rotund (therotund.com), and Musings of a Fatshionista (musingsofafatshionista.com).

courages women to stop focusing on body size and body weight and instead:

- Accept and respect the natural diversity of body sizes and shapes.
- Eat in a flexible manner that values pleasure and honors internal cues of hunger, satiety, and appetite.
- Find the joy in moving one's body and becoming more physically vital.

For more information and resources, visit Health at Every Size (haescommunity.org).

BUILDING A BETTER BODY IMAGE

It may seem impossible to avoid the persistent images and messages that confront us every day—and inevitable that at least some of the constant chatter will make its way into our heads. But being aware of the way media and advertising distort girls' and women's appearance and cultivate a body-obsessed culture can go a long way in helping to fight their influence.

Progress is also being made politically. Tammy Baldwin (D-WI) and Shelley Moore Capito (R-WV) have introduced the Healthy Media for Youth Act to promote and fund media literacy and youth empowerment programs and support research on the role and impact of depictions of girls and women in the media. It also calls for the establishment of a National Task Force on Girls and Women in the Media.[84] In the wake of an alarming report by the American Psychological Association's Task Force on the Sexualization of Girls,[85] multiple advocacy groups convened the first-ever summit to campaign for change. The SPARK Summit (sparksummit.com), which stands for Sexualization Protest: Action, Resistance, Knowledge, was held in 2010 at Hunter College in New York City. Younger women activists learned about media literacy skills and how to create their own media and build alternative representations. (See p. 818 for more discussion.)

One of the most underdiscussed issues regarding body image and our eating-disordered culture is the loss of joy and authenticity that it engenders. When we become obsessed with our weight and appearance, not only are we unwell physically; we also settle for lives less vivid and fulfilling.

When we are counting calories, overexercising in rote, uninspired ways, and/or spending so much of our mental energy on self-criticism, we forget what we used to *enjoy* doing, such as spending time with friends or pursuing our passions. We also have less time and energy for productive social and political activities that make our communities better places for everyone. It is totally radical for a woman in today's society to heal her relationship with her own body. You can be a model for everyone around you.

Courtney Martin, author of *Perfect Girls, Starving Daughters,* offers these suggestions on how to stop settling for self-hate and reclaim your right to wellness and joy.

- Reconnect with your authentic hungers. What do you feel like eating? When are you hungry? When are you full? All of the wisdom you need lies within, not in the next diet book.
- Move in ways that make you happy rather than getting caught up in strict exercise regimens. The more diverse and joyful your physical activity, the better.
- Don't weigh yourself. Instead ask: How do I feel in my own body right now?
- Interrogate your own self-talk and dispute it when it is either self-hating or judgmental of others' bodies. Invite your biggest fan into your head to counter the criticism. What would your best friend say about the viciousness you just unleashed on your belly?

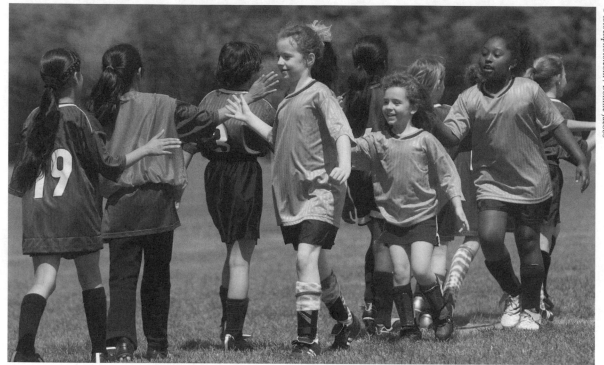

- Change conversations about weight to conversations about well-being.
- Speak up against fat discrimination.
- Ask yourself: When and with whom do I feel happiest and most beautiful? How can I be there, with them, more of the time? Consciously choose your community.
- Put your money where your heart is. Don't buy products from companies that make you feel inadequate, dirty, or insecure in their advertising.
- Get involved in feminism! It offers an empowering lens by which you can understand what you are going through.
- Redefine your notion of what a successful girl or woman looks like. She's not just a high achiever. She's also healthy, resilient, joyful, and full of self-love.
- Make intergenerational friendships that help you see the big picture. Suddenly life may

seem long and the size of your thighs might just prove irrelevant.
- Shift your priorities from achievement and appearance to fulfillment and joy at every opportunity.
- Learn to love the beauty of your own true nature.
- Say it out loud. If you tell a trusted friend or family member about your struggle, you help make it real. This creates accountability.
- Never diet. It is documented that this industry is the gateway to eating disorders.
- Get professional help, if needed, as early as possible. It's critical that you trust your own instincts, not the medical profession's definitions of wellness. Only you know what it's like being inside your own head.

Seeing an individual struggle with body image as part of a larger social and political struggle can be helpful as well. Organizations and movements, such as NOW's Love Your Body campaign, provide a full context for understanding the role of corporations and the media in keeping women dissatisfied with their bodies and offer easily accessible ways to take action on the issue. Check out the presentation on "Sex, Stereotypes and Beauty" at loveyourbody.nowfoundation.org, where you can also find other guides to help develop a critical eye toward beauty standards. Plus, there are tips on everything from staging a mock beauty pageant on a college campus to sounding off to offensive advertisers.

Altering our attitudes and behavior is only a first step in chipping away the prison bars of the beauty culture. In the long run, the only way for any of us to truly break free is to change girls' and women's position in society. As Rose Weitz writes in *Rapunzel's Daughters*, "Only when all girls and women are freed from stereotypical expectations about our natures and abilities will we also be freed from the bonds of the beauty culture."[86]

Fostering this affirmative environment for all of us is ultimately a collective project, where we join forces to educate new generations and transform our present one.

CHAPTER 4 ■ ■ ■ ■ ■ ■ ■ ■ ■ ■ ■ ■ ■ ■ ■ ■ ■ ■ ■

Our attractions and identities are powerful and intimate parts of who we are. More and more, people understand that gender identity and sexual orientation are aspects of life that don't fit neatly into boxes. This chapter addresses these separate yet sometimes intertwined topics that affect our relationships with ourselves, one another, and the world.

CHALLENGING SEX AND GENDER

Sex? Gender? These two words are often used interchangeably, but there are distinct differences. Sex is commonly understood to be based on a person's genitals (clitoris, vagina, penis) and reproductive organs (ovaries, uterus, testicles). These anatomical details are thought to define a person as male or female. If the person's anatomy is not clearly or exclusively male or female, a person is said to have a disorder of sexual development, or DSD (formerly called "intersex").*

Gender is often understood to refer to gender identity, meaning your internal sense of yourself as female, male, or other, regardless of biology. Gender also commonly refers to gender roles or expression, most often to behaviors and physical characteristics considered masculine or feminine in a particular culture at a particular time.

A shortcut way of understanding the difference between gender and sex: Sex is between your legs, gender is between your ears.

GENDER IDENTITY: WHO WE KNOW OURSELVES TO BE

In U.S. culture, gender is believed to follow directly from one's biological sex, so a baby born with a vagina is considered female, called a girl, and expected to grow up to be a woman who acts, dresses, and talks in a manner considered by the culture and her community to be feminine. A baby born with a penis is considered male, called a boy, and expected to grow up to be a man who acts, dresses, and talks in a manner considered to be masculine. In this binary way of thinking, our genitals, not our internal sense of self, are the deciding factor.

Many people challenge the expectation that our biological sex should dictate our physical, emotional, and psychological attributes. What if being a woman isn't about having a vagina (or not having a penis)? What if people don't fit neatly into male/female and masculine/feminine boxes? How we see ourselves and how others perceive us in the galaxy of masculinity, femininity, and the countless points swirling between cannot always be constrained within the two simple categories of man and woman.†

Moving beyond the concept of two fixed gender identities is a new challenge for some of us, and a very personal story for others. Some of us grapple with and analyze our gender; others take it for granted, especially if our gender expression fits society's conventions based on the sex we were assigned at birth.

Where does gender come from? Its source is not entirely understood—and may not be the same for everyone. The formation of gender identity is likely established by hormonal influences in the womb, but it may also be affected by social and cultural factors, including the messages we receive from the media and from our families and communities. Our gender identity and/or gender expression may shift over time.

An increasing number of feminists and other activists are advocating for the expansion or elimination of either-or gender norms, in order to allow for a full range of human behavior and expression. Knowing that gender is separate from sexual anatomy enables us to express ourselves in ways that may conflict with how society dictates we should look and act.

When we live in a world that leaves only the tiniest sliver of room for the least complicated among us, it's difficult to find a place for all our complexities. I am afraid that it pushes us to leave our genders unexplored, and I am pretty sure that it does not allow us to express them in all the ways we would prefer. As it goes with many

---

* See "Disorders of Sexual Development," pp. 14–15, for more on people born with sex chromosomes, external genitals, and/or internal reproductive organs that are not exclusively male or female.

† The idea of a galaxy of gender was expressed in Gordene O. MacKenzie's "50 Billion Galaxies of Gender: Transgendering the Millennium," in Kate More and Stephen Whittle's *Reclaiming Genders: Transsexual Grammars at the Fin de Siècle* (New York: Continuum, 2000).

things, it's easy to be afraid of genders that seem dangerous, unusual, or even merely new.

At the same time, some of us want nothing more than to have our gender identity respected:

As a trans woman, in a couple of my relationships with [non-trans] partners, I felt like I was being objectified—they would often talk about how "cool" it was that I was trans, like I was somehow "above" gender and this super-radical person. They even felt "subversive" for dating me. In reality, I was just being myself, and I am definitely not *outside of gender, and I didn't even really want to be. My gender doesn't make me radical, it just is who I am. I didn't want to be seen as "beyond gender." I just wanted to be seen how I saw myself, which was and is as a woman.*

GENDER IDENTITY: A GLOSSARY

Below are some of the terms most widely used to describe gender identities. Many originated in medical, academic, or activist settings, which might not encompass all perspectives. The terms are fluid, changing meanings over time, and used differently by different communities. A term that pleases one person may offend another. When in doubt, it's best to ask what terms people want used for themselves.

gender identity. How one identifies; a person's innate, deeply felt psychological identification as a woman, man, both, neither, or somewhere in between. Your gender identity may or may not correspond to your external body or sex assigned at birth (the sex listed on your birth certificate).

gender expression. How one looks; the physical manifestation of a person's gender identity, usually expressed through clothing, mannerisms, and chosen names. Your gender expression may

or may not conform to masculine or feminine socially defined behaviors and characteristics.

gender nonconforming. Refers to people whose gender expression is neither clearly feminine nor clearly masculine, or does not conform to mainstream society's expectations of gender roles.

genderqueer. Someone who blurs, rejects, or otherwise transgresses gender norms; also used as a term for someone who rejects the two-gender system. Terms used similarly include gender bender, bi-gender, beyond binary, third gender, gender fluid (moving freely between genders), gender outlaw, pan gender. A twenty-two-year-old woman says:

I identify as genderqueer and very recently have been moving away from also identifying as a woman. I am somewhat androgynous/masculine and I like to mix it up and play around with femininity, to intentionally push myself out of my comfort zone in regards to gender presentation and also to have fun confusing other people. I am very rooted in feminism and come from a long line of feminist ancestors; so while I lately find myself shying away from words like woman and girl and have started using the pronouns they/them/theirs, I also feel very solidly invested in pushing myself and others to expand the definition of the word "woman" to include people like me.

Some genderqueer people don't identify as male or female, and don't consider themselves trans, either, because they're not crossing from one to another but are existing in a third place altogether.

Recently, I have been in the process of informing others of my true gender identity. What I am is androgynous—both man and woman. What my birth sex is, is irrelevant. I'm finding that more and more people are saying things like "What sex is . . . he? . . . she?"—though always to friends, never to my face. I'm finding this very pleasing, although I wish people would say it to me. I do take it as a compliment!

transgender. An umbrella term referring to people whose gender identity and/or gender expression does not fit their sex assigned at birth. Groups often included under the transgender umbrella are transsexuals, genderqueers, people who are androgynous, and people who identify as more than one gender. Drag kings (women who perform as men) and drag queens (men who perform as women) often do so to entertain and may or may not identify as transgender. Similarly, cross-dressers (men who dress as women or women who dress as men) do not usually identify as transgender.

Transgender does not imply a sexual orientation; transgender people may identify as heterosexual, homosexual, bisexual, pansexual, polysexual, or asexual—or consider labels irrelevant or inapplicable. Transgender is sometimes abbreviated as trans or used interchangeably with gender variant.

transsexual. A person who lives and/or identifies as a different sex from the one assigned at birth. In *Whipping Girl: A Transsexual Woman on Sexism and the Scapegoating of Femininity*, the biologist Julia Serano writes that she uses the term to "refer to people who (to varying degrees) struggle with a subconscious understanding or intuition that there is something 'wrong' with the sex they were assigned at birth and/or who feel that they should have been born as or wish they could be the other sex."[1]

For transsexuals, the process of changing gender presentation may range from modifying names and/or use of pronouns to undergoing hormone therapy and possibly surgery to bring one's body more in line with one's gender identity/affirmed gender. Owing to prejudice in some parts of the medical community, high medical costs, and lack of insurance coverage, many transsexuals are unable to afford surgery and instead use clothing, makeup, and mannerisms to live as the preferred gender.

trans. This shortened form could mean transgender or transsexual, and many people use it to mean both.

trans man. A person who was born biologically female and identifies and portrays his gender as male. Sometimes called affirmed male or, simply, male. Also known, especially in medical literature, as female-to-male (FTM) transsexual.

trans woman. A person who was born biologically male and identifies and portrays her gender as female. Sometimes called affirmed female or, simply, female. Also known, especially in medical literature, as male-to-female (MTF) transsexual.

Some people question the use of MTF and FTM:

A lot of trans people have moved away from MTF and FTM, feeling that the terms tend to involve too much emphasis on the "change" part of our identity formation and too little on the "existence" part. That is, once one is defined as MTF or FTM one is left feeling that the transition is what defines our identity, rather than the existence of characteristics or traits of the internal gender, the trans person's so-called true identity.

In other words, how can one be "in transition" from the gender one has always been?

cisgender. Refers to people whose gender identity and presentation fit traditional norms for the sex they were assigned at birth.

cissexual. A person who lives and identifies with the sex assigned at birth. Those who are cisgender/cissexual tend to experience an inner harmony between who they feel they are and how the world sees them. They also enjoy the privilege of having their legal sex and gender identities taken for granted and considered valid in a way that those who are transsexual do not.

Whipping Girl author Julia Serano explains the history and use of cisgender and cissexual—terms that are fairly new and have not been embraced by all gender activists*—on her website, juliaserano.livejournal.com:

As a scientist (where the prefixes "trans" and "cis" are routinely used), this terminology seems fairly obvious in retrospect. "Trans" means "across" or "on the opposite side of," whereas "cis" means "on the same side of." So if someone who was assigned one sex at birth, but comes to identify and live as a member of the other sex, is called a "transsexual" (because they have crossed from one sex to the other), then the someone who lives and identifies as the sex they were assigned at birth is called a "cissexual."

* For more on this topic, see myhusbandbetty.com/2009/09/17/jeez-louise-this-whole-cisgender-thing; pamshouseblend.com/diary/12837/cisgender-and-cissexual-terminology-the-getalonggoalong-moment.

Cisgender and cissexual are neutral terms. Using them avoids singling out those who are transgender as being different or abnormal, and affirms that the spectrum from cis to trans expression is all part of natural variation.

Other gender identity labels. Within queer communities, terms such as butch, femme, and androgynous are used to describe points on a spectrum of masculinity and femininity. Other terms include tranny boys, femme queen, and more. Within straight communities, terms such as girly-girl and tomboy are used to label gender characteristics or expressions. While some people who fit the criteria of these definitions use these terms, others do not.

Regardless of gender identity or sexual orientation, all people have the right to use the term with which they feel most comfortable—and to ask others to respect that choice. It can be painful and awkward when assumptions are made about gender identity based on appearances alone. If you're not sure how a person identifies or what pronoun to use, ask politely. Joanne Herman, author of *Transgender Explained for Those Who Are Not*, explains, "We like your asking much better than if you guess and get it wrong, and we get especially unhappy if you use the pronoun 'it.'"

In addition to he, she, her, and him, some in the transgender community use alternative pronouns such as ze and hir as descriptors. Herman notes that she finds "ze" and "hir" "a bit awkward," but adds that she "felt the same about 'Ms.' at the beginning. Now I'm glad it's the default."[2]

TRANSSEXUAL EXPERIENCE

There is no doubt that from very early on I knew something was wrong. I was a girl, yet my parents named me John Joseph and insisted that I was a boy.

According to the American Psychiatric Association's *Diagnostic and Statistical Manual of Mental Disorders* (DSM), the resource that mental health providers use to diagnose mental illness, transsexuals have a gender identity disorder (GID). Some prefer the term gender dysphoria because it better describes the feeling of being born in a body that doesn't match who you are inside. Others find both terms stigmatizing. In order to have access to the surgeries and/or hormones that some use in order to live successfully in their preferred gender, current medical practice requires a psychiatric diagnosis of GID or gender dysphoria. Insurance coverage, however, is often less available for psychiatric diagnosis.

A revision of the DSM is expected in 2013. Many activists are hard at work seeking to influence the authors to remove the designation of GID as a psychiatric condition.

Many transsexuals who can afford medical care take cross-sex hormones—either estrogen or testosterone, as appropriate to the desired female or male physical expression of gender. Some pursue one or more gender affirmation surgeries (often known by the less-favored older name, sex reassignment surgery). For trans women, surgeries can include feminizing genitoplasty: creation of a neovagina, usually from scrotal tissue (some surgeons use colon tissue); relocation of glans penis to a neoclitoris; and gonadectomy (removal of testes). Surgeries can also include breast augmentation, Adam's apple reduction, and facial feminization surgery. Surgery to alter voice pitch is available, but the results are often disappointing and can result in permanent hoarseness.

For trans men, surgeries can include breast reduction or mastectomy; removal of uterus and ovaries; and phalloplasty, or the technically simpler and therefore less expensive metoidioplasty, both of which involve creating a penis out of the testosterone-augmented clitoris and a scrotum

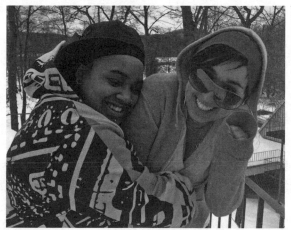

Sasha Alexander and Ana Gordon-Loebl from Pioneering Voices, a Family Diversity Projects exhibit

out of labia majora using skin grafts and testicular prostheses. So far, genital surgery for trans women has been more satisfactory in terms of physical and sexual functioning than that for trans men.

With or without surgery, many transsexuals go through intensive retraining on how to walk and talk and present as their preferred gender.

While cross-sex hormones and surgery can help trans people achieve a better fit between body and identity, these medical interventions are expensive and are not often covered by health insurance (see "Insurance Exclusions," p. 81). Surgery and hormones also carry health risks, require ongoing medical surveillance, and may impair sexual functioning. (See "Side Effects and Risks of Hormone Treatments," p. 80.)

For these and other reasons, many transsexuals manage to live as their preferred gender without pursuing surgery, and some without hormones. Yet in most states, government agencies will not change identifying papers such as a driver's license or birth certificate for someone who has not transitioned medically by means of hormones and surgery. This means that the privileges of full legal transition are frequently

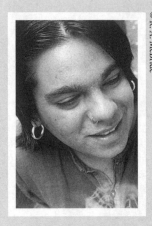
© R. A. McBride

"I CLAIM THE RIGHT TO CHOOSE MY ULTIMATE GENDER"

SUNEEL(A) MUBAYI

I identify as a male-to-female (or male-to-feminine androgynous) transgender or genderqueer person in a male body. I was born and raised as a straight male but started questioning both my gender and sexuality around the age of sixteen for many complex reasons. . . . When I was little, kids in school would make fun of me by calling me "Suneela" to characterize a perceived weak and effeminate nature. I decided to reclaim this, but in a way that would make people think and not assume my gender when they look at my name (Suneel is a boy's name in Hindi). It gives me an androgynous quality, which I like.

Often I'm plagued by self-doubt—am I doing this just to attract attention? I answered it myself when I expressed these doubts to my friend Erica (thank god for her) and she asked me the most fundamental question of all: What does being a woman mean to you? To me, being a woman means having an identity that is feminine but without any preconceived notions, ideas, or mind-sets about what a woman is or what a woman should be—in any sense, be it in terms of looks, actions, habits, social roles, or anything else. Everybody feels like there is some kind of "ideal" man and "ideal" woman. Well, I reject that. I am a woman with no conditions and no strings attached. And no presumptions, either. You may find me rather androgynous, deviant, and gender-bending. I like to dress up, be pierced, and be effeminate or girly.

Yes, I am all those things, or rather, I possess all those qualities. But I claim the right to choose my ultimate gender beyond my traits, looks, qualities, and features, even if it is different from the sexual organs I possess. And whether that's feminine or hermaphrodite or my desired blend of masculine and feminine is my choice. You can love it, be okay with it, be uncomfortable with it, be revolted by it, or leave it. But it's my choice. Being a woman means being a woman.

TRANS BODIES, TRANS SELVES

The upcoming book *Trans Bodies, Trans Selves* promises to be a comprehensive resource for transgender and other gender-variant people. Editor Laura Erickson-Schroth says:

As a medical student I realized that my gender-variant patients and their families were having a hard time finding reliable and comprehensive information about their health and their communities. Inspired by my second-wave feminist mother's battered copy of Our Bodies, Ourselves, *I set out to gather a group of authors and volunteers who could create the same kind of comprehensive community resource, by and for transgender people, that had been created by the Boston Women's Health Book Collective.*

Trans Bodies, Trans Selves will cover health, legal issues, cultural and social questions, history, theory, and more. It will promote trans-positive, feminist, and genderqueer advocacy and be a place for transgender people, partners and families, students, professors, guidance counselors, and others to look for up-to-date information on transgender life. For more information, see transbodies.com.

out of financial reach. As one trans woman says:

Given that the legal determination of gender rides almost solely on a medical chassis, the uneven access to medical help experienced by trans people living with poverty and frequently by trans people of color means that many less-privileged trans folk have a very difficult time attaining legal recognition of our target gender.

Given the extremely high level of antitrans violence, the lack of a legally acceptable ID in one's chosen gender can be a critical missing safety factor.

With or without medical assistance, being able to live as our true selves can mark the end of years of dissonance and inner anguish. Joanne Herman writes about having felt "the wrong primary sex hormone coursing through my body."

I felt like a car running on the wrong kind of gas. I did not fully understand how wrong it was until I replaced testosterone with estrogen when I transitioned genders in 2002. I now have an amazing sense of well-being and harmony that I never knew before. Now my body just hums.[3]

A trans man says:

From the moment I realized I was transsexual, everything changed. Although I'm now legally and "aesthetically" male, I was raised and socialized female, and no amount of hormones or surgery can ever erase that. Nor should it. I have no interest in denying my past, for the years I lived as a woman make me a better man today. . . . I am a strong, proud, transsexual man; I love my life and my body (and am now more inclined to take good care of it); I have a wonderful wife and family; and I am working hard to make the world a better place for those who share my experience.

Becoming the gender you always identified with may seem to others like a radical, gender-transgressing act, but in many ways it is more like coming home.

TRANSSEXUAL HEALTH ISSUES

Few prospective, large-scale studies exist regarding transsexual health. However, the Dutch endocrinologist Louis Gooren, founder of a groundbreaking trans clinic at the Free University Medical Center in Amsterdam, has reported on a thirty-year follow-up of more than three thousand patients.[4] His good news: The trans people seen by the clinic were not at any more risk of early death than cissexual (non-trans)

men and women. Although presumably the trans men and trans women at the Dutch clinic faced some of the health issues touched on in the paragraphs below, they ultimately suffered from the ills of their affirmed gender: heart disease was common in trans men, as in natal men, probably influenced by increased abdominal/visceral fat and high levels of cholesterol and triglycerides. The trans women tended to gain excess weight and were more likely to develop metabolic syndrome, a group of risk factors (including high blood pressure, high cholesterol, and insulin resistance) that occur together and increase the risk for coronary artery disease, stroke, and type 2 diabetes.[5]

What follow are a number of health issues for trans men and trans women in the United States.

Side Effects and Risks of Hormone Treatments

Cross-sex hormone therapy is central to gender affirmation treatment for many if not most transsexuals. At the same time, hormone therapy presents risks. The large randomized, controlled Women's Health Initiative studied certain forms of reproductive hormone therapy in postmenopausal women and demonstrated elevated risks of stroke, blood clots, and breast cancer. (See Chapter 20, "Perimenopause and Menopause," for more information.) Trans women who have not had their testes removed must take high levels of estrogen to suppress testosterone; this increases their risk of thromboembolic disease—the development of blood clots—and calls for close and regular health monitoring. Speaking of his study of three thousand patients, Dr. Louis Gooren highlighted one particular estrogen: "Use of the female hormone ethinyl estradiol [a component of the contraceptive pill but used by trans women in higher dosages] was associated with an increased rate of cardiovascular death and stroke. This was not the case in former users, i.e., those who once took ethinyl estradiol but now take another type of estrogen."[6] For trans men, methyltestosterone taken orally in high doses can cause liver damage. Taking cross-sex hormones, therefore, can create special health issues for transsexual people.[7]

The Endocrine Society (endo-society.org) has published an online listing of medical conditions that can be exacerbated by cross-sex hormone therapy.[8] "Endocrine Treatment of Transsexual Persons: An Endocrine Society Clinical Practice Guideline" is a thorough, evidence-based 2009 guideline with risk factors and recommended protocols.[9] The book *Fenway Guide to LGBT Health* (fenwayhealth .org) is another excellent resource. It addresses sexual functioning, observing that feminizing hormone therapy "tends to reduce libido, reduce erectile function, and decrease ejaculation," while testosterone use is known to increase libido.[10]

If you are a trans person taking hormones, it is vital that you have access to medical providers who understand the implications of cross-sex hormone treatment over a lifetime, who will check regularly to identify and treat possible side effects and risks, and who will stay current with future studies that may reveal which forms and applications of the hormones have the fewest risks. Unfortunately, lack of insurance coverage deprives many trans people of this necessary care.

Insurance Exclusions

In general, because transgenderism is currently defined as a psychiatric condition, U.S. health insurance does not cover hormone treatment or gender affirmation surgeries for trans people. These are most often available only to those who can afford to pay out of pocket for medical care.

One of the many health consequences of this inequity is that a trans person who can't access or afford medical hormone treatment may end up seeking cross-sex hormones from friends, on the street, or online without benefit of the careful screening, quality control, appropriate dosages, and ongoing health care that are so important when anyone is taking hormones. A major risk of obtaining cross-sex hormones on the street is needle sharing, which carries a risk of HIV and hepatitis exposure. Testosterone is usually given by injection, so this is an issue for trans men. Trans women who are frustrated by the presence of facial hair or by futile attempts to raise the pitch of their voices may resort to high-dose estrogen injections as well. (Another danger: Oral testosterone preparations available on the street, often taken by bodybuilders, can cause fatal liver damage.)

In 2008, the World Professional Association for Transgender Health (WPATH) issued a public statement encouraging a shift toward viewing these treatments as medically necessary. The WPATH board of directors "urges state health care providers and insurers throughout the world to eliminate transgender or trans-sex exclusions and to provide coverage for transgender patients including the medically prescribed sex reassignment services necessary for their treatment and well-being, and to ensure that their ongoing healthcare (both routine and specialized) is readily accessible."[11]

Dr. Norman Spack, a longtime advocate and health-care practitioner for trans youth and adults, compares the U.S. system with international models: "In the Netherlands and Belgium, national health insurance covers all costs related to evaluation and treatment of transgendered individuals, including children. . . . This discrepancy in coverage across nations raises questions about U.S. health insurance policy decisions."[12]

Health Screenings for Reproductive Organs

Many trans people cannot afford or choose not to have surgery to remove their reproductive organs. Long-term health, therefore, often requires screening of body parts and organs associated with a gender with which you don't identify. Pap tests for trans men are one example. Health providers in the forefront of trans health care have worked out protocols for a sensitive and respectful approach to this crucial screening. The Sherbourne Health Center (checkitoutguys.ca) addresses trans men's need for ongoing Pap tests and offers a tip sheet for health-care providers.[13] The *Fenway Guide* observes that some trans men who cannot tolerate ongoing pelvic exams consider complete hysterectomy.

Breast tissue exams can be an issue for trans men as well. According to the American Cancer Society and Gender.org, there may still be risk of breast cancer even after sexual reassignment surgery such as chest reconstruction, because breast muscle wall tissue remains. Breast tissue cells might be present in the nipple area as well as throughout the chest area.[14]

There have been a very few reports of prostate cancer in trans females, but since estrogen is one of the treatments for prostate cancer, they almost certainly had the condition before beginning cross-sex hormone treatment.

Fertility Issues

Cross-sex hormones reduce fertility, and this reduction may be permanent even if the hormones are discontinued. Some trans women choose to bank sperm before estrogen treatment or surgical removal of the testicles, to preserve the option of having a biologically related child in the future. Trans men who are on testosterone therapy and then discontinue it may continue to ovulate, even though menstrual periods have stopped. Thus there is a re-

duced but not entirely absent pregnancy risk. The ovaries of trans men retain eggs. Although there is a medical procedure that harvests eggs and preserves them through freezing so a trans man could donate eggs to a partner or surrogate, this option is not generally available, and the life span of frozen eggs is limited.[15]

Medical Intervention for Transsexual Teens

Puberty puts transsexual teens at extreme risk, as their bodies develop the secondary sex characteristics—penis growth and facial hair, or breast growth and menses—of a gender that feels strange, unfamiliar, and unwanted. Transsexual teens are at high risk of depression, self-mutilation, alcohol and drug abuse, and suicide in part because it is difficult for people under the age of eighteen to access appropriate medical treatment.[16] In the United States there are only a few pediatric endocrinology or adolescent medicine programs that work with trans teens.

Following a model developed in the Netherlands, the Gender Management Service Clinic at Children's Hospital Boston offers a temporary hormonal treatment to halt puberty for teens who, after careful screening, are diagnosed with gender dysphoria. This fully reversible treatment gives teens an extra two years to decide whether to take the irreversible steps of cross-sex hormone treatment and surgery. Delaying the development of secondary sex characteristics can reduce social ostracism and psychological distress as well as the need later on for surgeries such as breast reduction or facial hair removal. Interviewed in 2010, Dr. Spack said, "We are beginning to see great success. Patients aren't trying to commit suicide, they're bullied less at school, relationships are better, and mammoplastic surgery may not be necessary."[17]

TRANS EDUCATION FOR HEALTH-CARE PROVIDERS

Most medical practitioners have not yet learned how to treat trans people with appropriate understanding and respectful care. Saber, a trans man whose gynecologist feared that he might have ovarian cancer and sent him to a nearby city for an ultrasound, found that despite his home physician's efforts, the health facility was unprepared for him:

I state my name and that I am here for the ultrasound to check my ovaries for possible cancer. She looks at me and says, "But you're a guy." I explain that I am transgender, female-to-male, and that I am pre-op; that I still have all my female parts. She looks at me and then my chart and says again, like perhaps I am just very slow, "You're a guy, you don't have ovaries." I can tell the word transgender has no meaning for her. She says that she will be right back. After waiting at least fifteen minutes, my partner says, "I am going to go see what is taking so long." My partner comes back in and says, "Everyone is gone. The place is empty. It's dark." Appalling as it was, my partner and I still laugh about the absurdity of it all.

Saber, who subsequently joined the Minnesota Transgender Health Coalition, adds:

Until I can have the surgeries I need, I will continue to be seen in the gynecologist's office on a regular schedule so that if I were to get breast cancer, ovarian or uterine cancer it would be detected early. Unfortunately I cannot afford the surgeries, and so am stuck for now. As long as I have some female organs left in my body I will have to go in for gynecological exams looking like a male.[18]

Whether or not you have made legal changes or undergone surgery, you are entitled to the dignity of being referred to by the name and pronoun of your choice. You should be asked, for example, what you prefer to wear during the exam. A young trans person commented:

Whenever I encounter trans-positive sexual health resources I breathe a deep sigh of relief.

I think trans men and trans women need more vocal support and accessibility in clinics and classrooms, as do those of us who don't transition physically, but find ourselves in sexual, social, and health-related situations that are rarely addressed.

For more information on access to the health care system for LGBT people, see "Homophobia, Transphobia, and Heterosexism," p. 682.

SEXUAL ORIENTATION: WHOM WE ARE ATTRACTED TO

SEXUAL ORIENTATION: A GLOSSARY

asexual. Describes someone who does not experience sexual attraction ever, or for a period of time.

bisexual. Describes people who are romantically/sexually attracted to both men and women—sometimes, though not necessarily, at the same time.

gay/homosexual. Describes men who are romantically/sexually attracted to men, and sometimes describes women who are attracted to women. Often used to refer to men exclusively.

lesbian. Refers to women who are romantically/sexually attracted to women. "Same gender loving woman" is sometimes used in the African-American community.

pansexual. Describes someone who is attracted to people across the range of genders. Often used by those who identify as transgender or genderqueer or who are attracted to people who are transgender or genderqueer.

queer. Historically a derogatory term for gays, this word is now used positively by many lesbian, gay, bisexual, and transgender people and allies. It is sometimes used to describe an open, fluid sexual orientation and/or gender identity/expression.

straight/heterosexual. Refers to women who are romantically/sexually attracted to men, and men who are attracted to women.

Some of us have reclaimed historically negative terms, such as queer, fag, and dyke, and use them affirmatively to describe ourselves. This is a political act that attempts to reclaim the power from these slurs. Rejecting labels is another form of resistance:

I don't identify as anything as far as sexuality goes. I was heterosexual for the beginning of high school, then I had a two-year experience with asexuality, and after that I came into a lovely and mixed-up world that resists labels.

Sexual orientation falls along a spectrum. Although people may choose the nearest applicable label, such as lesbian, they may actually have attractions and even relationships that are not in rigid accordance with that label.

CONFUSING SEXUAL ORIENTATION AND GENDER IDENTITY

Many of us confuse gender identity and sexual orientation. Gender identity is about who we are, while sexual orientation is about who attracts us. Being cisgender or transgender does not predict whether a woman will be straight, bisexual, or lesbian.

The confusion of gender identity with sexual orientation gives rise to misleading stereotypes. For example, some people assume that if a woman is a lesbian, she must have a masculine gender expression—in other words, she keeps her hair short, wears no makeup, and dresses like a man. Likewise, we might assume that because a woman appears masculine, she

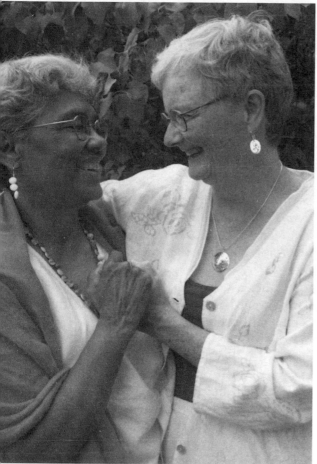

© Ellen Shub

and sexual orientation thus interact dynamically, rather than the latter being static.

When my partner began his gender transition, my lesbian identity had been central to my life and my sense of self for well over a decade, and I didn't know what his transition made me. Some people told me I was "obviously" still a lesbian, but it was just as obvious to others that I was now straight, or bisexual. It wasn't obvious to me at all, and I struggled with it for a long time. Now I've been the partner of a trans man for as long as I was a lesbian, and I've gotten comfortable just not having a name for what I am. I think of myself as part of the family of queers and trans people.

LESBIAN AND BISEXUAL EXPERIENCE

The second decade of the twenty-first century is a promising time for women who have intimate and/or sexual relationships with women. With issues important to the lesbian, gay, bisexual, and transgender communities increasingly in the news, more people all over the country and around the world are recognizing who we are and supporting how we live our lives. The debate over the legal recognition of same-sex marriage has engaged the nation. More and more television shows and movies attempt to portray our lives (albeit not always in the most accurate or satisfying ways). Many people in positions of power and authority—politicians, business owners, and celebrities—are out and proud. Thanks largely to activism from within the LGBTQ community and an increasing emphasis on coming out, many women who love women are living more freely and openly than in generations past.*

must be a lesbian. But being lesbian or bisexual doesn't mean our gender looks or feels a certain way.

The fact that I am femme (that is, traditionally feminine in appearance, with mannerisms perceived as feminine) throws people off; I'm often told I don't "look gay."

Transgender people can identify as straight, lesbian, bisexual, gay, pansexual, or queer. Some who transition gender find that their sexual orientation changes during the process. Gender

---

* Whereas previous editions of *Our Bodies, Ourselves* devoted a separate chapter to women who have intimate romantic/sexual relationships with women, this edition addresses our relationships

BISEXUALITY

Those of us who are attracted to both women and men live out our orientation in many different ways. Some of us date women and men serially, some simultaneously, and some enter relationships with women only or with men only, without acting on other attractions.

Thinking of ourselves as bi may reflect the sense that sexual orientation is a fluid aspect of ourselves that changes over the life span. Sometimes bi is a stopping place in a transition from one orientation to another.

Over time, we may find that a bisexual identity becomes less meaningful in the context of a life partnership with someone. However, for many of us, bisexual identity is lifelong, a proud and essential part of our natures. A woman in a monogamous life partnership may still identify as bi, because this label reflects her inherent capacity for attraction across genders.

I'm a woman who has primarily dated men but has had two short-term relationships with women. I'm in a committed relationship with a man. He is a wonderful, articulate, sensitive feminist whom I hope to marry; and yes, he knows of my past experiences and is open to me having continued relationships with women. . . . My desire for women isn't based on the inadequacies of my current lover but rather a need for some other, some different, some similar thing—all of which I find in women.

Bisexuals are often misunderstood and maligned. Labeled as confused, or not queer enough, people who identify as bi have often been stigmatized. A thirty-five-year-old Latina writes:

I have known I was interested in both sexes since I was six or seven. But, due to the conservative Catholic home I was raised in, my family did not accept same-sex relationships. In my twenties, when I started college, I began to start to explore women, and in my thirties I started to act on it. I love being with another woman; the connection is something I can't put into words. When I talk with my partner about being bi, he thinks it's just a "phase," although I've told him many times that I enjoy being with a woman. So now he prefers not to talk about me being bi. I can feel myself distancing myself from him for not being open to how I feel. When he said, "It's just a phase," it was like he was doubting who I am. It hurt.

In the last few decades, bisexual activists have engaged in ongoing education to dispel common stereotypes, including the idea that bisexual orientation is something that people claim when they are not ready to come out fully as gay or lesbian, or that bisexuals are opportunists who will quickly abandon a same-gender relationship for the greater power and privilege of an opposite-gender connection. We have also continued to contradict the stereotype of bisexuals as inherently promiscuous.

Bi activists have also fought to be included by name in the social, political, and religious organizations that we participate in. In recent years, more and more organizations have changed their names to be inclusive of bisexuals. This has sometimes happened concurrently with those groups working toward greater inclusiveness for and sensitivity to the concerns of people who are transgender. An International Conference on Bisexuality has taken place every few years since 1993, contributing to the growing organization of bi-identified communities nationwide and internationally. There are now active bi organizations in many states and most major cities, and even a bi-specific community center in Boston (biresource.net).

---

with women and with men in a single chapter, "Relationships." As in earlier editions, the experiences and concerns of lesbian and bisexual women appear throughout the book.

- BiNet USA (binetusa.org) maintains listings of all the bisexual organizations and related resources in the United States.
- Bi.org links to bisexual groups and resources around the world.

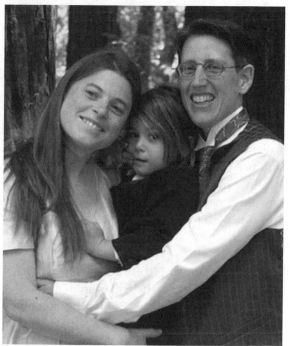

SPECIAL HEALTH ISSUES FOR LESBIAN AND BISEXUAL WOMEN

Lesbian and bisexual women have a few different health concerns from heterosexual women. Research done over the past two decades has revealed a number of factors that can lead to less frequent preventive and diagnostic health care, later treatment, and poorer outcomes for women who have sex with women. More information on the health concerns listed below can be found in the *Fenway Guide to LGBT Health* (fenwayhealth.org).

Cancer Screening

The time interval between Pap tests (for cervical cancer) is almost three times longer for lesbians than for heterosexual women. Cervical cancer screening rates are lower for lesbians compared with heterosexual women, raising concerns that lesbians are not adequately diagnosed or treated.

Stress

Stresses that are associated with long-term concealment of sexual identity and many years of exposure to discrimination can affect health negatively. Some research indicates that lesbian and bisexual women have higher rates of heart disease than heterosexual women, and that people who have experienced discrimination based on sexual orientation or race and ethnicity are more likely to have high blood pressure. Studies also suggest that nondisclosure of sexual orientation can be associated with lower life satisfaction, lower self-esteem, depression and suicide, substance abuse, delay in seeking medical treatment, and increased risk of illness.[19]

Smoking and Alcohol Use

Lesbians are more likely to engage in behaviors such as smoking and drinking alcohol that put them at greater risk for certain cancers.[20]

Smoking

In 1987, the National Lesbian Health Care Survey of the National Gay and Lesbian Health Foundation found that about 30 percent of lesbians smoke, compared with about 23 percent of heterosexual women.[21] More than a decade later, in the Women's Health Initiative, a study of women age fifty to seventy-nine years old, twice as many lesbians reported themselves to be heavy smokers compared with heterosexual women.[22]

Alcohol Use

Research suggests increased rates of problem drinking among lesbians compared with other populations[23] and suggests that substance use among lesbians does not decrease as dramatically with age as it does in the general population.[24] Alcohol use is associated with many health problems, including breast cancer, and can affect choices about safer sex practices, putting a person more at risk for sexually transmitted infections (STIs).

Sexually Transmitted Infections

Contrary to popular belief, women who have sex with women can get sexually transmitted infections. Research shows that many women who have sex with women have current or past sexual relationships with men, and thus have all the traditional risk factors for contracting STIs from men. In addition, STI transmission has been reported in the absence of a history of sexual contact with men: HPV (human papillomavirus) and genital herpes occur among women who have sex with women and report having had no previous sexual contact with men. Lesbians also have a higher incidence of bacterial vaginosis, and women can transmit candidiasis and trichomoniasis to their female partners. Untreated vaginal infections can make a person more susceptible to transmission of HIV and other STIs. For more information, see Chapter 11, "Sexually Transmitted Infections."

Breast Cancer

The primary risk factor for breast cancer is age; other risks include family history, increase in body mass, and not having given birth. Despite the presumption that the latter two factors may put lesbians at higher risk for breast cancer, there is no randomized controlled study that shows an increased risk of breast cancer in lesbian women, and more research is needed.[25]

COMING OUT TO OURSELVES

Coming out is the process of accepting and affirming our sexual orientation or gender identity and deciding how open we will be about it. Before we come out to others, we usually come out to ourselves by acknowledging that we are attracted to people of the same sex, or that we don't identify with gender traits considered appropriate for our sex and/or the sex we were assigned at birth.

Because we grow up in a culture that assumes everyone is heterosexual and that gender always matches sex, becoming aware of and accepting our identity is often a gradual process. Coming out can happen at any age or stage in life. One woman who fought her sexual orientation says:

Coming out of the closet as a lesbian was the hardest thing I ever did. I tried everything to "avoid" being gay. I tried to stay away from women I was attracted to, but finally, after many years, I began to feel much more comfortable with the idea.

Another woman says she couldn't come out until she'd actually had a woman lover, "which was an annoying chicken-egg thing in that not being out made it hard to meet women."

A twenty-nine-year-old woman remembers a similar dynamic that slowed her down:

Part of the reason my girlfriend and I took so long to connect sexually was that when we first met, she thought I was straight. I didn't know how to correct her. As a teenager, when I developed intense crushes on girls and women I knew, I wondered whether I was a lesbian, but discarded that idea because I also had feelings for boys. I

For information and guidance on finding sensitive health care if you are LGBTQ, see "Homophobia, Transphobia, and Heterosexism," p. 682.

thought about identifying as bi but was at a loss about how to back up assertions of that identity with "proof," since I didn't have any experience with either men or women. When I found myself falling for her I felt tremendous anxiety not about how I felt, but about how I could prove to her, without any previous experience with women, that I was sexually interested. I also questioned my own inner certainty that she was who I desired, and that my desire was sexual in nature—a self-doubt I don't think I would have had if the person I was drawn to had been a guy. I don't think I would have thought to myself, "Oh my god, what if I find out I'm just not into guys??"

Some of us come out to ourselves more than once. We may come out as lesbian or bisexual, for example, then later as transgender or transsexual, or vice versa.

The process of questioning our sexual orientation or gender identity can be extremely challenging, but accepting ourselves for who we are is often a relief. After attempting suicide more than once, this woman made a decision:

At the age of forty-five I declared myself female and, in a sane and sober state, worked on matching my body, soul, and spirit into one complete female. It took me five years. Today my body is mine. . . . My birth certificate reads "female."

COMING OUT TO FAMILY, FRIENDS, AND THE WORLD

Letting other people know about our gender identity or sexual orientation can be challenging and life-changing. Each of us must decide individually how much we want to share with our family, friends, and acquaintances.

It took me until I was twenty-seven to decide that I am a lesbian and very proud of it. The coming-out process meant that I gained friends and lost friends. Family made choices to continue their relationships with me or not. Either way, I grew as a woman who loved women. I'm now forty years young and am enjoying being with the woman of my dreams. I cannot fathom what took me so long.

Some of us come out in relative ease and feel our families' embrace:

I'd only realized that there were female-to-males out there about two months before. (All my life, I figured that a lot of girls wanted to be boys, and that male-to-females had so much attention, because who would want to give up being male?) But that day my mother was cooking sauce. We're one of those Italian families, I guess, and I offer to stir . . . Hypnotically, stirring, I start talking, and the next thing I know, I've told her. She wasn't thrilled, and almost four years later, she's still not, but she's my strongest ally in my family. She's just a great mom.

Others find that even liberal family members have trouble accepting the changes:

My dad . . . was big into civil rights in the 1960s (as a white male), marched in Chicago and Washington, etc. But he's had a lot of trouble being okay with my being trans and queer, even though he pretends he doesn't because (I assume)

RESOURCES FOR LGBTQ YOUTH

There are queer and trans teens across the country—we just need to find each other!

It's totally normal to feel confused, depressed, or angry about being different and the negative ways other people often respond to difference. It's important to find peers and adults who can understand and relate. Some schools have gay/straight alliances and promote a Day of Silence (dayofsilence.org) to bring attention to anti-LGBTQ name-calling, bullying, and harassment. Check out the videos at the It Gets Better Project (itgetsbetter .org). You'll hear from people who have been there that life as a LGBTQ person usually improves greatly over time.

Many cities have an LGBTQ center that offers free or sliding-scale counseling, support groups, and social services. Some larger cities have centers specifically for queer or trans youth. Here are some additional resources:

- Gay, Lesbian and Straight Education Network offers support for GLBT teachers and gay/ straight alliances in schools: glsen.org
- GLBT Youth Talkline is a free and confidential hotline offering peer counseling, information, and local resources. The hotline is open Monday– Friday, 5–9 PM PST (1-800-246-7743): glnh.org
- Parents, Families and Friends of Lesbians and Gays is a resource for youth as well as for families. PFLAG has been working hard to become trans-educated and ready to provide support around issues: pflag.org
- Trevor Project is a 24/7 suicide hotline for gay and questioning youth (1-866-488-7386): thetrevorproject.org

it doesn't fit with his worldview of himself as an educated, liberal activist.

One woman warns of feeling pressured to come out:

"More people coming out will relieve the stigma" is something I see a lot. But coming out is dangerous and not possible for a lot of people because of society. For people who can come out and be open, that is great, and I do agree that it helps to diminish stigma, but the burden for fixing problematic social attitudes should not be on the victims of those attitudes!

Another has delayed telling her parents:

I am now a freshman in college and still haven't come out to my parents. A couple of years ago, my father asked me if I was a lesbian. With much hesitation, I answered, "No," because I was scared . . . He said, "Good, because I don't want a fucking faggot for a kid." This statement tore me apart and has delayed my decision to come out to my parents. Most everyone who knows me (including my siblings) knows my orientation. I am currently waiting to tell my parents, for fear that they will kick me out or stop paying for my college.

NATIONAL COMING OUT DAY

Whether you're lesbian, gay, bisexual, transgender, queer, or a straight ally, you can come out for LGBTQ equality on National Coming Out Day (October 11 in the United States, October 12 in England). Many blogs and activists take part online. For more information, visit Human Rights Campaign (hrc.org/ncod).

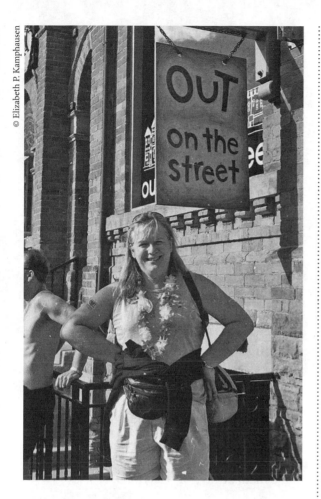

on my appearance. Some people just stared, a few others told me how brave I was, and one person told me that I looked "just like a woman." Another gave me a taste of what it means to be objectified by telling me proudly that I was his very first transsexual.[26]

MULTIPLE IDENTITIES

The experience of living as a lesbian/same gender loving woman varies greatly based on class, gender, race, religion, (dis)ability, and other aspects of our lives. Women of color, for example, are more often judged or rejected by their home communities and at the same time often experience racial discrimination within queer communities.

I was the only openly queer African-American person at my college. When I came out sophomore year, my black friends were supportive yet oftentimes more reserved around me. Many were very religious, and very socially conservative. Others had never met a queer person before. There was always something unspoken between us—Was I still as black as they were? Was my white girlfriend a sign that I had betrayed my race, black men, my friends? Who were these new white queer people that I was now spending time with? Many of my black friends became my closest allies as they learned and grew with me. Those who didn't I lost touch with quickly. But my race will never be separated from my sexual orientation, and vice versa.

The African-American poet and activist Pat Parker wrote in *Movement in Black* about her dream of a society that would embrace her multiple identities:

If I could take all my parts with me when I go somewhere, and not have to say to one of

Some transsexuals have no choice but to come out, because the physical changes are often quite visible. The public nature of the coming-out process can be enormously difficult. The geographer Petra Doan says of her first day back on the job after gender affirmation surgery.

As I entered the building I felt I was entering the eye of a hurricane, at the calm center of a turbulent storm of gendered expectations. As I walked down the hall I could hear conversation in front of me suddenly stop as all eyes turned to look at the latest "freak show." As I passed each office there was a moment of eerie quiet, followed by an uproar as the occupants began commenting

EMPLOYMENT NONDISCRIMINATION

In most places in the United States, it is legal to fire employees because they are trans, lesbian, gay, or bisexual, though some states and municipalities have enacted civil rights protections based on sexual orientation and, in some cases, gender identity and expression. At the national level, the Employment Non-Discrimination Act (ENDA), which would prohibit discrimination against employees on the basis of sexual orientation or gender identity, has been introduced to almost every Congress since 1994 but as of 2011 has yet to pass.[27]

them, "No, you stay home tonight, you won't be welcome, because I'm going to an all-white party where I can be gay, but not Black." Or "I'm going to a Black poetry reading, and half of the poets are antihomosexual," or thousands of situations where something of what I am cannot come with me. The day all the different parts of me can come along, we would have what I would call a revolution.[28]

Many women of color find ways to live openly in both worlds and draw support from an increasing number of queer communities of color.

Some people think that queer and trans are Western concepts and that femme equals looking like Barbie, but that's not how I see it all, as a South Asian queer femme woman. My models for my gender are my grandmother and great-aunties who organized for independence from Britain and [for] labour and women's rights—in short skirts and bobbed hair—in Sri Lanka and Malaysia in the twenties. . . . When I hold my hot-pink "Desi divas against war and racism"

sign at the antiwar rally, I am continuing that tradition.

Lesbian, bisexual, and transgender people with disabilities face additional challenges, including homophobia or transphobia within the disability community. Events organized by able-bodied communities are often not fully accessible or not sensitive to everyone's needs.

I think if I was just queer it might be easy for me to say, well, we just need to end discrimination against queer people, and we just need straight people to see that we are just like them. Whereas, because I'm queer and I have a disability, it's like all of a sudden I'm like, Ya know what? We have this whole bullshit idea of normal that really doesn't apply to anybody. . . . Nobody really fits into that anyway and I especially don't and there is no way I'm going to even if discrimination against queer people ends.[29]

Fat women face size discrimination within both queer and straight communities. People may assume that we're queer because we can't find a man, or that we're asexual.

I am a white, college-educated, twenty-five-year-old queer nonbinary trans person with disabilities living in Northern California. I'm also fat, an advocate for size acceptance. It really is frustrating how much perceptions of our bodies play into our perceptions about worthiness for relationships. I've definitely experienced that "I'm so lucky to be with someone who isn't repulsed by me" feeling, and I've also had that exploited; people have used me, secure in the knowledge that I won't protest because I am afraid of the consequences. And, for the most part, I like my body! I am just aware that the social constructs which surround it make other people think that it is less than acceptable.

BLACK LESBIANS MATTER: AN EXAMINATION OF THE UNIQUE EXPERIENCES, PERSPECTIVES, AND PRIORITIES OF THE BLACK LESBIAN COMMUNITY

In July 2010 the Zuna Institute (zunainstitute.org), a national nonprofit advocacy group for the black lesbian community, released *Black Lesbians Matter*, a national report based on a survey and focus groups with 1,596 black women ages eighteen to seventy.[30] The report gives voice to their most important needs and concerns. Jobs/financial security, health care, and education were the top three concerns, with marriage and mental health coming next.

Highlights of the report include:

- Many women in this survey have had direct experiences with discrimination in areas of employment, with health care providers, and in creating and protecting their families.

- The impacts of invisibility and discrimination have debilitating effects in the lives of black lesbians. These effects are similar to those reported by black Americans who live in poverty.

- Although resilient in the face of extreme obstacles, black lesbians . . . in areas of family, health, visibility, identity, class, and aging suffer disproportionately in comparison to straight whites and blacks, as well as to the broader LGBTQ community.

- Upholding the myth of the "strong black woman" along with the lack of adequate mental health support can lead black lesbians to higher rates of suicide.

- Close to 70 percent of the women surveyed either have children or are planning to have children. The call for visibility, notes the report, is a call to be recognized as a family unit with all the legal rights and privileges granted by law through legally recognized marriages.

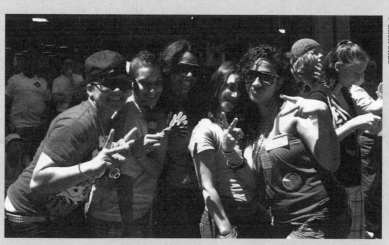

© Ellen Shub

Women celebrating Gay Pride, Boston, 2009.

Some queer spaces are more accepting of fat women:

I'm a queer fat femme of Italian-American and middle-class background. How I experience my sense of self in regard to gender and sexual orientation shifts depending on the context. In straight spaces, I'm likely seen as a straight, fat girl. Since I'm fat, my sexuality is not celebrated or recognized in mainstream society, because fat people are not supposed to be sexual. . . . In queer contexts, however (when other queers perceive my femmeness as queer), I feel quite different. My fat femmeness is celebrated as hot and sexy. I feel motivated to wear clothes that show off my curves, large ass, hips, and breasts.

COUNTERING HOMOPHOBIA, HETEROSEXISM, AND TRANSPHOBIA

Is your school or workplace welcoming to LGBTQ people, or are sexual orientation and gender identity either completely ignored or joked about in cruel and demeaning ways? If you've come out, is your family supportive, or have family members made you feel unwanted unless you "change"?

Some cultures teach us to fear and hate homosexuality and gender variance in others and in ourselves. This hatred hurts all of us, no matter our sexual orientation or gender identity. It turns us against friends and family members, depriving us of important relationships. It causes us to deny attractions or identities that are right for us. And it prevents many from publicly acknowledging friendships with queer or transgender people.

Heterosexism is the assumption—in individuals and in public policy—that heterosexuality is the only normal orientation. A woman whose partner transitioned from female to male reports her mother's response to her new "heterosexual" status:

We are literally the same two people, but after my partner's transition, my mom started sending him birthday cards and inviting him to family events. I thought she'd have a hard time with it, but she was like, "Woo-hoo! Now my daughter has a partner I can actually talk about with my friends!"

Homophobia is fear and hatred of people who are attracted to the same sex:

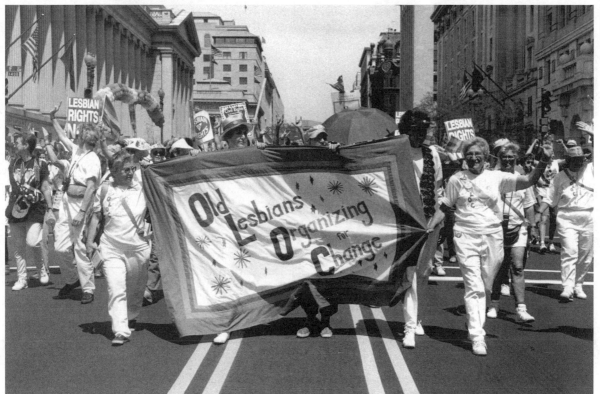

The internalized homophobia—the nagging fears of incompetence, being too different, being unlovable—are still hanging around in my head. But getting up each day . . . each time I do something positive, the homophobia inside me has less power. And each time we do something positive for each other, the homophobia in society has less power.

Transphobia, likewise, is fear and hatred of gender-variant people.

Heterosexism, homophobia, and transphobia lead to laws and practices that deny LGBTQ people legal, religious, and social privileges that heterosexual and cisgender people take for granted. In most places, we are prevented from getting married, filing joint tax returns, and being covered under a partner's health insur-ance (except in companies and cities that allow benefits coverage for domestic partners). We face job and housing discrimination, and the media often ignore or misrepresent us. Essential safer-sex educational materials, when presented in schools, often omit same-sex relationships.

Violence, homelessness, police brutality, chronic underemployment, and poverty dispro-portionately affect transgender people. Many of us who don't easily fit within the two-gender norm find it difficult to attend school, hold jobs, or even go to public restrooms without fear of rejection, harassment, violence, or even arrest.

As a female-bodied genderqueer, I choose to use the women's restroom, but often find myself dealing with unpleasant comments or looks and, on a few occasions, verbal or physical threats/

assaults. As a result, I have avoided using public restrooms, as much as possible, for seventeen years and have now developed urinary tract problems.

It is difficult for trans people to access many services such as rape crisis centers, emergency medical care, homeless shelters, group homes, and domestic violence shelters because these spaces are segregated by sex. Discrimination and harassment in the health-care system mean that we often miss needed medical care. Trans people of color and low-income trans people also are affected by racism and class discrimination that exacerbate the difficulties faced by trans people in general. Transgender and transsexual people also sometimes face discrimination within the queer community:

No one talks about the mental difficulties faced before—and especially after—the transition. Like, for instance, being a (trans) dyke. Like being referred to as "he" in lesbian groups. Like being

banned from places, like the Michigan Womyn's Music Festival.

In many places in the United States and around the world, activists are challenging homophobia and transphobia, and achieving positive change. The Think Before You Speak campaign (thinkb4youspeak.com) raises awareness of the prevalence and consequences of anti-LGBT bias and behavior in America's schools. One goal is to get kids to think twice before saying, "That's so gay." The Policy Institute of the National Gay and Lesbian Task Force (thetaskforce.org) works to advance equality for LGBT people and trains young leaders for the future. The National Black Justice Coalition (nbjc.org) works to eradicate racism and homophobia and advocates for the unique challenges and needs of LGBT African Americans. In schools and colleges, in workplaces, in religious organizations, and in the military, LGBTQ people and our allies are mobilizing for justice while committing the radical act of simply loving each other.

Relationships and Sexuality

■ CHAPTER 5

In preparation for this fortieth-anniversary edition of *Our Bodies, Ourselves,* more than three dozen women, representing a wide range of ages, identities, and experiences, spent several weeks discussing sexual relationships. They asked and answered questions and responded to one another's stories and reflections with encouragement, wisdom, and humor. Their words go back to the book's roots: women discussing their bodies and their lives and learning from the experiences of other women.

Earlier editions of *OBOS* divided the discussion of relationships into two separate chapters—women who love men, and women who love women. In this edition, women of all sexual orientations discuss their lives, from what they enjoy most

MORE ABOUT THE CONVERSATION

In 2010, the *Our Bodies, Ourselves* editorial team posted a call for women to take part in an online conversation. The response was overwhelming; out of hundreds of submissions, thirty-seven participants were selected, ranging in age from eighteen to sixty-three. To learn more about this conversation, visit ourbodiesourselves.org/relationships.

QUESTIONS FOR DISCUSSION

- What are you looking for in a relationship? p. 106
- How do you define—and express—intimacy? p. 109
- What do you enjoy most about being sexual? p. 110
- What role has love played or not played in your relationships? p. 112
- What is it like to be in a relationship when you don't like some or all of your own body? p. 114
- How do media images and portrayals of relationships affect your idea of an "ideal" relationship? p. 119

- How does it affect your relationships when you are with someone whom the world gives more or less power than you have, because of race, income, gender, or disability? p. 124
- What are your experiences in relationships that span racial differences? p. 126
- Have you or your partner discussed having children? If you had differing opinions, how did it affect the relationship? p. 127
- What effect do children have on dating or staying in a relationship? p. 129
- When did you realize that a relationship you intended to stay in was going to be work, and what are some obstacles that can get in the way of relationships? p. 131
- How has sexual abuse and/or physical violence affected your relationships? p. 132
- What has helped the process of healing from sexual or other abuse? p. 135
- How has growing older affected your relationships or what you look for in a relationship? p. 137
- Do you feel affected by relationship time lines? p. 138

about being sexual to their experiences in relationships that span racial and other differences. They also reflect on media images and representations in popular culture that have influenced their views of dating and marriage.

The introductions that follow will tell you a bit about the women you'll meet in this chapter. There's also a list of questions selected from the many subjects they discussed (see above) and a corresponding page number, so you can choose

where you want to start. Throughout the chapter, you'll find statistical snapshots of women's relationships and other related information.

PARTICIPANT BIOS

Alexa: I'm a twenty-two-year-old heterosexual woman, though I've had a few intimate relationships with women in my college years.

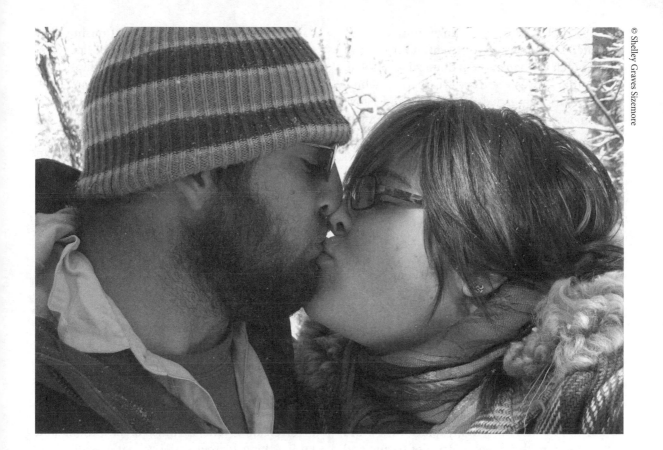

I'm from a working-class family and both of my parents were/are struggling with multiple addictions. I am living a securely middle-class/intellectual/progressive lifestyle. I'm currently living with my monogamous boyfriend of two years.

Ananda: I am sixty-three years old. My relationship with my life partner (married for twelve years) has been nonmonogamous for all of our thirty-two years together. We each have long-term very satisfying other relationships. My main "other" has been part of my life for thirty years; my partner has been in a relationship with a woman who is now also my good friend for fifteen years. Everyone knows about everyone else; there are no secrets. This is a very complex lifestyle and not for everyone; it has been a great challenge and brought much richness to my life.

Astrid: I am forty-seven years old, straight, a Caucasian immigrant from Europe. For six years, I have been a single mom of a daughter; I am twice divorced (once on this side of the Atlantic, once on the other). There has not been much of a dating/sex life in these last years, and it's not only due to the fact that my time is more or less all spent on my daughter and my job. I have also just not really connected with anyone—perhaps I am disillusioned, picky?

Cathryn: I'm sixty years old, was born a hermaphrodite (tetragametic chimera or "true hermaphrodite") and was surgically assigned male at birth. I transitioned as an adult, had surgery to restore my body to close to its original state.

I'm bisexual and have a thirty-four-year-old daughter. I was married for twenty-four years to a very butch woman and I'm physically disabled.

Cecilia: I'm sixty-three years old, white, healthy, happy, married. I love men and I love women, and sex so far has been only with men. My first husband always said he was sure I would cheat on him and if I did, that would be the end of the marriage. His having affairs was all right (old story), and of course it turned out just as he predicted (old story continued). After twenty years, when Love at First Sight came along for me, I didn't hesitate to jump into bed and find out how great sex really could be. When we got engaged, I felt committed and have been since—twelve years.

Cheryl: I am thirty-three years old, African American, heterosexual, a single mother of two sons. I am a trainer of educators in teen pregnancy prevention approaches and programs, which is great work that I feel passionately about and also is reflective of my personal journey as a young mom. My son's father and I ended our relationship when I was in my midtwenties, and I have been on this crazy journey of dating and being in relationships as a single mom.

Chloe: I am a twenty-three-year-old queer transsexual woman. My primary partners are also trans women, though I have dated cissexual women as well.

Cody: I am a twenty-two-year-old white queer kid, looking (somewhat distantly) ahead to a career in nursing. I identify as genderqueer and very recently have been moving away from also identifying as a woman. I am somewhat androgynous/masculine and I like to mix it up and play around with femininity, to intentionally push myself out of my comfort zone in regard to gender presentation. I identify as polyamorous and currently have a primary partner (of four years) and a long-distance date.

Danielle: I'm a twenty-five-year-old pre-operative transsexual lesbian. I'm currently coming out of a long-term relationship that stretched over most of my transition. I'm really interested in nontraditional relationships, how body issues can impact relationships, and how to look toward the future while still focusing on the present in a relationship.

Efia: I'm a thirty-two-year-old black queer woman. Being raised by a father who was an army chaplain/marital counselor and a mother who was a schoolteacher—all in a very loving, nurturing, and religious (and practicing) home—meant that a lot of what I've come to know and own as my sexuality and sexual health was obtained through a little bit of self-discovery and a lot of rebellion.

EJM: I am a heterosexual twenty-four-year-old. I am Korean, growing up half my life in the U.S. and the other half in Korea.

Faith: I'm a twenty-two-year-old single white heterosexual and I was raised by my dad and grandparents. The environment I grew up in was fairly blue-collar, although now I'm privileged to navigate the ivory tower. At school, I'm involved in several feminist organizations and I'm working to revise the sexual assault disciplinary procedures.

Francesca: I am a fifty-year-old never-married black woman. I am the proud mother of a thirty-year-old son. I consider myself an Africana Womanist. I am not currently involved with anyone and have not been for too long! Sexually I am most often attracted to men. I believe for some sexuality can be fluid . . . at least it is for me sometimes.

Gemma: I am a thirty-one-year-old single heterosexual woman. I'm trying to navigate the exciting world of dating while simultaneously wondering if I'm way too picky or way too accommodating. I want very much to become a mom and have recently started to think seriously about how I may do that on my own one day.

Heidi: I am a twenty-six-year-old single

mother with two children. I have been separated two years and will be divorced this month. I would define myself as queer, but to try and put it to more precise words, I seem to move between androgynous and female, and pansexual and asexual. I am currently in an open long-term nonsexual relationship but have been involved in sexual relationships with men and women in the past and probably will be again in the future.

Jaime: I'm straight, white, USA-an, more or less middle class, partnered but unmarried, childless, East Coast, atheist with a mixed Christian heritage, highly (possibly over-) educated, cisgender,* currently mostly able-bodied, twenty-five years old, underemployed, and nonmonogamous. I currently live with a male partner. Thinking of heading back north to find a job soon, which would entail leaving my partner and possibly ending our relationship.

Jordan: I am a white, college-educated twenty-five-year-old asexual queer nonbinary trans person with disabilities. I'm also fat, an advocate for size acceptance, and a practitioner of BDSM.

Judith: I'm not quite twenty-five, white, and cisfemale. I identify somewhere in the queer/lesbian realm. Unfortunately, the political (for me) has yet to translate (fully) to the personal. Although I've been "out" since I was nineteen, I've never been in a relationship, never had sex, never even kissed a girl (or guy, for that matter). I have been on one date (this week, in fact), and am slowly working to sort out the gulf between the sex-positive feminism that informs how I view others' relationships—and the sex-negative and body-negative upbringing that informs my own.

Kali: I'm twenty-six, cisgender, and bisexual.

I'm in a long-term monogamous relationship with a man (coming up on two years). I am white, fat, and disabled. I have a genetic condition called Ehlers-Danlos syndrome, which has caused repeated joint injuries and chronic pain. I'm also a sexual abuse/sexual assault survivor. It has really brought to the fore the need for positive consent instead of passive consent.

Leigh: I am a twenty-eight-year-old queer white woman raised primarily in a single-mother home. My evangelical Christian roots gave me an early commitment to abstinence and virtually no body-positive sex education. Over the years, I have done a lot of intellectual, emotional, and community work to cultivate a new ethic of healthy promiscuity and body positivity. Currently, I tend toward open relationships in which issues such as monogamy, geography, communication, and vocation are negotiated collaboratively.

Lola: I'm a twenty-four-year-old queer, polyamorous, mixed-race, cisgender woman who identifies in my spare time between all those other identities as a "stone femme." Right now I'm pursuing becoming a women's and adult health nurse practitioner to become, more or less, Dr. Queer Medicine Woman.

Lydia: I'm a twenty-nine-year-old cisgender Caucasian woman. I am the daughter of counterculture-leaning parents who home-educated me and my two siblings well into our teens, drawing on free-school/unschool (rather than fundamentalist religious) pedagogies. I am currently enjoying my first-ever sexual relationship after many years of solitary sexual exploration; my girlfriend has been a wonderful, enthusiastic, and encouraging partner.

Madigan: I am a twenty-seven-year-old white, queer, intersex, femme high school dropout. I have worked off and on as a sex worker since the age of eighteen and am currently working as a community organizer. I am very active as an intersex speaker—doing Intersex 101 work

---

* Some women use the word "cisgender" to define themselves, meaning their gender identity is in harmony with their biological sex. For more information, see Chapter 4, "Gender Identity and Sexual Orientation."

with medical professionals, medical students, other academics, and activists.

Mags: I am Latina, thirty-six year old, married bi/les mother of five. I have known I was interested in both sexes since I was six or seven. But, due to the conservative Catholic home I was raised in, my family did not accept same-sex relationships. In my twenties when I started college is when I began to start to explore women and was curious, and my thirties is when I started to act on it. I am out to my husband, who supports my choice in sexuality. I would like to thank all of the people that have been involved in this process because I am now able to discuss openly and candidly with others about my preference and sexuality.

Miriam: I am a twenty-nine-year-old single, heterosexual woman. I had a total abdominal hysterectomy (removal of ovaries, uterus, and cervix) due to ovarian cancer. Surgically induced menopause, its side effects, and surviving gynecologic cancer have greatly affected how I view my sexuality and body, and how I take care of my health.

Nasir: I am a twenty-nine-year-old newlywed and a first-generation American with Nigerian parents. I'm trying to create and maintain a balance in my marriage that will allow it to grow stronger and deeper, taking the best elements of both American and Nigerian cultures, while at the same time making sure I maintain my individuality and uniqueness.

Natasha: I'm fifty-nine; my family background is Ukrainian, Jewish, and Norwegian; and I've been widowed for over seven years from a twenty-five-year partnership/marriage. I have an adopted Latina daughter and two grandchildren.

Nidea: I was raised in a very traditional Dominican household where sex and all women-based conversations were often not spoken about. Overall, I have a very traditional point of view about sex which I apply to myself, and I also have a very liberal point of view which ar-

ticulates itself in my interest in the topic in regard to all women. I am a virgin at twenty-three, single, fascinated and perplexed by sex.

Nina: I am a twenty-five-year-old New Bohemian, which is a fancy way of saying I am unemployed. I am single and I don't bother with labels. As for my relationships, I have allowed myself to be surrounded by some pretty awful people, but each experience has prepared me to make "The List" of attributes I will and will not accept in another person. I stepped up because I was tired of stepping down. I am still waiting for the right person to rise to my level.

Pearl: I am an aging (sixty-two), middle-class, midwestern, white lesbian feminist. My relationship began twenty years ago in a triple that lasted for fourteen of the twenty years we have been together. My partner and I were recently married under the care of our local Quaker meeting. I have spent my career in the disability rights movement. In my outer, public life I am not as wild as I once was, but my private, intimate life is wilder than I could have imagined.

Rebeka: I am an eighteen-year-old African-American/Caucasian bisexual young woman. I am currently a college freshman studying women's studies and psychology. I hope to one day become an ob-gyn or a child psychologist. Although I am bisexual, I have yet to tell my family and friends. I have had one sexual experience with a woman, but other than that I am very new to the whole dating and relationship thing.

Robin: I'm a twenty-year-old genderqueer-identified female-bodied person who is happy and actively sexual in a female body. I am white, middle-class, and able-bodied. I have had sexual relationships with men, women, and transpeople, and am currently in a committed relationship with another genderqueer female-bodied person who has been extremely powerful in opening my mind to the power of consent, body play, and BDSM.

Sloane: I'm thirty-five and have been married to my husband for only two and a half years—still pretty green, but this relationship has been in existence or in the works for just over ten years. I had my first child by cesarean . . . I am still mourning the natural birth we were denied. My husband was laid off and stays home with our child so I am the breadwinner of the family, so to speak.

Sophia: I am an Asian/Hispanic woman in my mid-forties, married to a man of Caucasian descent for twenty years. We have two children. My siblings and I were raised in a very religious household and were heavily indoctrinated in the philosophy that sex before marriage was a sin. I was twenty-two before I had my first sexual experience, with a man who eventually became my husband. I've never told my parents that I had premarital sex. Even now, I can't talk to my mother about anything having to do with sex.

Tasha Maria: I am a heterosexual African-American woman. I am thirty-six years old and I have a seventeen-year-old son. I am single and have never been married, which frightens me because I feel like my time is running out. I never wanted to raise my son alone and wanted to have more children and live what I felt was the American dream.

Victoria: I'm thirty-three, mother to two daughters, married for eight years. When I was in high school and college, I struggled with a lot of shame and fear about my sexuality, and when I was finally able (in my early and midtwenties) to feel confident in my body and my desires, it felt like such an amazing victory. And I really thought I had it all figured out—that I would have great sex for the rest of my life! A few years down the road, I'm realizing that I have an entirely new set of challenges and struggles: changing body, changing relationships, changing desires, crying babies . . .

WHAT (SINGLE) WOMEN WANT

In early 2011, Match.com released findings from the largest and most comprehensive nationally representative study of single men and women.[1] Funded by the dating site, it was conducted in association with the Institute for Evolutionary Studies at Binghamton University and academics from various institutions. Below are some of the key findings.

Marriage, maybe. Seventy-two percent of singles would live with someone in the future without marrying. In the age group twenty-one to thirty-four, 62 percent of single women and men want to marry, 9 percent do not, and 29 percent aren't certain. For singles age thirty-five to forty-four, those numbers drop to: 40 percent of singles want to wed, 19 percent do not, and 42 percent aren't certain.

Independence, definitely. Across every age group, women want more personal space in a committed relationship, as well as more nights out with girlfriends; they are also more likely to want their own bank account and to take vacations on their own.

Older and happier. Singles over sixty-five report the greatest level of happiness over the past twelve months, followed by singles twenty-one to twenty-four years old. Older singles also report being less stressed by being single and, contrary to popular belief, sex is still important to them.

Zoe: I'm a twenty-four-year-old African-American/Puerto Rican heterosexual female. I'm single and childless, and I've never really had any traditional relationships. I would call myself a late bloomer (at least when it comes to having partner sex). I didn't lose my virginity until I was twenty-one and a college senior. Even though I hadn't had sex before then, I've always been incredibly sexual. I've known what sex was from an early age and had a lot of experiences with masturbation beginning around age eight. On the relationship front, I'm a huge commitmentphobe.

PARTICIPANT RESPONSES

WHAT ARE YOU LOOKING FOR IN A RELATIONSHIP?

EJM: I want something that says, "You and your partner are equal human beings and you are sharing a life together." I want a relationship that has mutual respect, equal responsibility, confidence, trust, and sexual compatibility. I want a relationship that allows me to come home and relax without worrying about if I need to fix something in the relationship. I want a relationship that has no violence.

Francesca: What I want in a relationship is patience. It has been many, many years since I have been in a relationship. I have not had sex with a partner in more than twelve years. I am a very sexual being, but I know that since it has been such a long time, I am a bit insecure and need someone who is patient with me to help me navigate back to a place of sexual self-esteem.

Lydia: We've talked, my girlfriend and I, about various types of relationships (open, poly, monogamous) and concluded that both of us are inclined toward monogamy and that's what works for us. After so many years moving solo through life (with amazing friends and family but without anyone to imagine a future with), I am grateful every day to have this person in my life to share (or shelter from) the world with. I love the constancy of having her to wake up with every morning and fall asleep beside every night—and I've kinda surprised myself with how much I enjoy being able to name her as "my girlfriend" and claim that kind of relationship with her, whether I'm talking to friends or colleagues, walking down the street, or writing a check that has both of our names on the top.

Cheryl: I read something once that became a mantra for moments like this in my life: "Love courageously." What that means to me is that love is risky business and scary, but I need to be courageous and do it anyway. When fear shows up, I always play the what-ifs trivia game in my head and sometimes out loud with friends and family. Wisdom always pushes me to consider not just "What if something doesn't work?" but also "What if it does work?"

Ananda: I think that relationships are one of the hardest things we do.

Efia: From a frustrated list I typed into my phone about three weeks ago when I got tired of pining after my last relationship that went horribly wrong:

The Love of My Life . . .
   will be responsible and honest like my father
   will love me unconditionally
   will be beautiful inside and out
   will respect and not hate his mother and father
   will help me when I do and do not ask
   will always have my best interests at heart and in mind
   will bring out the best in me consistently
   will love/cherish my family
   will know how to have healthy disagreements
   will be a grown-up when necessary but a child at heart

will be healthy and encourage me to take care of myself

will be a good father and partner/husband/friend/lover

will have ambition

will love to travel but also like to spend time at home

will be supportive of me

will not be financially irresponsible

will have self-awareness

will *love* music as *much* as or more than I do

Cecilia: I made a list . . . When #1 turned up, I recognized all the traits and went right for it. Then I met a man on a bus. By the time we got off, life had changed. No list, just him.

Heidi: I often feel as though I have been conditioned to want some kind of long-term relationship with a person who I would describe as my soul mate and who will make my life more complete in a way that nothing else can. I don't believe that this fairy-tale relationship exists (for most people), and my opinion sometimes makes me feel like I am disappointing people around me. As a single mother who lives in poverty, I sometimes feel as though I am expected to be in a relationship (especially with a man) if only for financial reasons, like it is selfish of me to get divorced because it is not necessarily what is best for the children regardless of what the relationship was like, and it is even more selfish of me if I then date women, because my children will later be teased because of it.

I have yet to fully process how I think my asexuality fits into this part of my life as far as societal and familial pressures are concerned—as a mom, I am not supposed to be a sexual being, but I am supposed to have additional financial support to provide for my children, such as would be provided by being in a marital relationship.

Cathryn: The one thing I've always hungered for was simply to be cherished; corny, I know. At this point in my life I still want that but am no longer willing to enter a relationship that doesn't leave a lot of room for me, alone. Most of my life I've been the sister/mother confessor to everyone else, the caretaker role, and on some level I want to be both independent and taken care of for a change. I'm drawn to what I call "gentle male energy" but have a lifetime of experiences that leave me to view men as suspect.

Faith: I've been single for a while. I date a lot. I have lots of casual "hookups"—which, generally, only go so far as making out, etc., because I'm personally not a fan of casual sex. Back where I was raised, lots of my high school friends are getting married and having kids—that's what you do once you've graduated from college/high school. At my college, however, the idea of a girl getting pregnant or married is pretty ridiculous; we're all ambitious, young people who want to get their careers in order.

This year, I had sort of an epiphany about the whole thing, which is that I'm not ready for a serious relationship. Ideally, I do one day want to find someone I can share my life with—it seems like a very nice idea. But I have to stop being dissatisfied with myself when it doesn't happen right now.

Natasha: I want a long-term monogamous relationship. At fifty-eight, I don't have time for drama; I want loyalty, a friend with whom I can talk and share my current life and dreams. I want fun, great sex, a witty companion, and someone who shares my values.

Zoe: I want to meet a man I can fall in love with—fully and completely. But not because I think he "completes" me. A man who challenges me to push my boundaries, who nurtures my ambition. A man who has ambition that I can nurture. Someone who will indulge my moods and not be all up in my business 24/7. Someone who understands that I'm already whole and that he's there to nurture that wholeness, to help me grow without welding himself to my side.

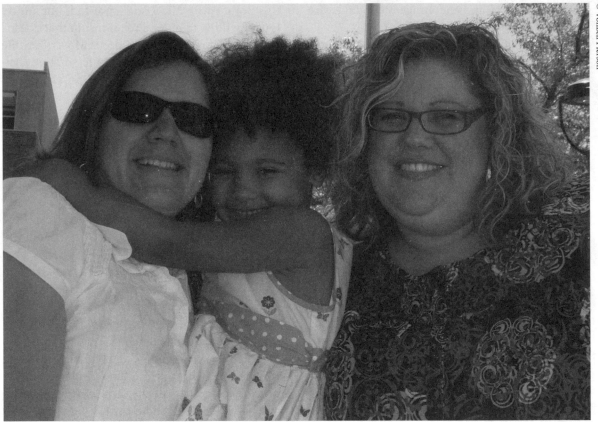

Jaime: I find that when people talk about a successful relationship, they usually mean one that lasts and lasts. Sometimes this is the case even when the relationship is no longer functional or enjoyable—it is successful solely because it still exists. In my book, a successful relationship is one that lasts while it can last and that ends when it needs to end.

Victoria: Over the past few years, I have seen several divorces among my close friends and family, and it's amazing to witness that tipping point when people realize that it is okay to take care of themselves and to place value on their on wholeness and well-being. Particularly because I live in a politically and religiously conservative community, there is a great deal of pressure to "make it work." And some relationships can

be salvaged and can become strong and healthy again. But some can't, and that's okay. It is okay to end those relationships and be alone. It is okay to find strength and comfort and growth in a circle of friends and family. And I love how you're defining that as a success in itself.

Leigh: My current partner of sorts and I have been involved for a year and half and have avoided most of the default terms for describing what was growing between us. At one point, in a conversation with some friends, he stumbled upon the idea of a co-conspirator. This so resonated with who we were becoming in each other's lives and what we both want in a partnered relationship. We are currently in a place of flux due to geographical distance and commitments to projects that energize us but also keep us less directly involved in each other's lives. But through the course of this relationship with him, by experiencing him as a co-conspirator, I can now say that *that* is exactly what I want in a partnership. I want to scheme and dream with someone, undertake projects, work together to build the world we want to live in.

Jordan: Oooh, this resonates with me so much. I definitely think of partners as co-conspirators. (In fact, I think I once posted a personal ad which included the phrase "seeks partner in crime.") I love planning and building things with people (which can be anything from embarking on a papermaking project together to something more personal), and I definitely want to be with someone who shares that and who has a zest for adventure.

Faith: "Co-conspirators" is a really great non-traditional category. I like that it emphasizes the individual agency that each partner has while at the same time giving credit to the mutual impact each has on the creative world building of the other. I, personally, have always desired a partner who will push me to be the best person I can be (and vice versa). In that way, love can transcend more than the two people involved and really impact the larger world.

Ananda: My primary partner and I really are co-conspirators as far as what is next in our lives, what would be fun, what would be different. He is much better than I am at coming up with really new and different things. I look at him askance, hesitant, and then jump in. I am rarely disappointed. The open-spiritedness and the sense of togetherness, in terms of both coziness and intrigue, that the word evokes for me, make it a really great expression of what I want to continue to happen with my partner, even as we age and slow down.

HOW DO YOU DEFINE AND EXPRESS INTIMACY?

Jaime: When I want to express love to a partner without saying it, I put the tip of my nose up against his and wiggle my nose. It's goofy, but it's an intimate gesture for me because it involves being very close, physically, to the other person, and I don't do it to a lot of people. I also express intimacy by telling people secrets. Like the mean rumor someone made up about me from high school that I'd rather forget. Or the abusive relationship I was in and how I can't decide if I want to call it rape.

Madigan: I cannot be sexually or emotionally intimate with someone I don't feel safe with. Physical touch and emotional honesty are two major parts of expressing intimacy with anyone I care about (romantic or otherwise).

Danielle: To truly laugh with someone—not at them or near them, but *with* them—requires a certain amount of intimacy. Because laughter, like any emotional expression, requires the safety to express that joy. The trust that your expression won't be dismissed. The openness and sharing of the moment. It requires an understanding of why the moment is funny, and why the shared experience is important.

Victoria: I think of intimacy as embodied, though not necessarily sexual: These are the friends I hold hands with, give back rubs to, kiss hello and good-bye. And with my partner, when our rhythm is off, when we're struggling to be open in our conversation or we're just disconnected because of our schedules or our priorities, I have to reestablish that connection and intimacy before I want to have sex (whereas he always wants to reestablish connection by having sex). So it's an ongoing conversation in my relationship.

Kali: Intimacy is our inside jokes. It's the way we can be ridiculous and unself-conscious with each other. It's being able to sleep soundly when he's in the same bed with me. It's when a touch can express love, longing, and desire and still be tender. Intimacy is knowing that I can reveal what a geek I am without worrying that he'll be turned off. It's there when we're curled up together in bed, talking.

Nina: Intimacy is all in the details. It's more than sex, and it's more than knowing how to cuddle. It's being able to read your partner's face and know exactly what they are feeling before they tell you. It's knowing the right combination of words to make everything better when their world is falling apart.

Sophia: There are times when my husband and I are in a crowded room full of people and we are feeling a little lost in the crowd. All we have to do is look at each other or lightly touch, and any discomfort with being in a crowd of strangers melts away.

As a nuclear family—as in my husband, children, and I—we are constantly in each other's personal space, but we learn how to accept each other as individuals through mutual trust and respect. We know about and have dealt with all sorts of personal details about each other. I think family intimacy is essential to a child's emotional growth and understanding of personal space and boundaries.

Pearl: Words are difficult to find to describe deep intimacy with a partner. It does involve trust and vulnerability, but those exist within my deep friendships. For me, the intimacy I have with my love/partner is cemented by a knowledge of each other grounded in Spirit. It is that which makes me light up when she comes into the room. It settles me with a connecting look in a large crowd. It is a secret that cannot be known by anyone else. It grows over time, it is still full of surprise, it is not always easy.

Judith: One of the interesting things about intimacy is that—whether it's built slowly or suddenly—it's almost impossible to unravel (completely) once it's there. The relationship it-self may dissolve at some point, but there's still an almost visceral recognition of that person based on an intimacy that existed at one time. I see this with my parents, who divorced in a messy and painful way a few years back, and struggle with the ways they still feel connected, and I see it in my own life as well. There are people I may never be particularly close to again, with whom I nevertheless feel—and expect I will always feel—an intimate bond. That's not always easy, either, but it's important to me. That kind of closeness can transcend a lot.

Cecilia: Intimacy is having no guile, no boundaries. At sixty-three, it is adoring each other's aging bodies: the too-large stomach, the fallen buttocks, the sagging boobs, the small scrapes that take too long to heal, the urgencies, the aches, the relaxation. It is sharing a bathroom and its functions. It is curling up under your lover's armpit and crying for no identifiable reason. It is that glorious morning at the beginning of the relationship when, after luscious sex, you stay in bed for hours telling each other all about your previous lovers. It is knowing when it's time to leave a party because your partner wants to even if you don't. It is being able to talk about your failures and embarrassments. It is being able to say when you're proud of yourself. It is being able to pack each other's suitcases.

WHAT DO YOU ENJOY MOST ABOUT BEING SEXUAL?

Lydia: I love the way sexual activity gives us a nonverbal (or at least partially nonverbal) way of expressing and exploring our connection to each other and the dynamics of our interactions. I feel like the bravery it takes to be in that space of sexual pleasure with another human being (a space that, until now, I have only ever experienced on my own, behind closed doors) is a pretty awesome thing.

Mags: I enjoy making my partner feel things

they may not get from another partner. I think I prefer pleasuring women more than men. I love being able to kiss, touch, lick, and suck on everything that a woman has. I feel like women appreciate the time and effort that the other woman takes in exploring her body and learning different techniques to make her moan.

Heidi: I used to enjoy the feeling of power that I had when I was in charge of a sexual encounter. Knowing that somebody else wanted me in that kind of a way made me feel as though I were special or beautiful or something, I'm not entirely sure what. Now I don't get that feeling anymore. I'm not sure if it is because I can't be bothered, or maybe I'm just jealous of what they are able to feel and I am not.

I do not miss being sexual. I miss intimacy. I miss cuddling at night when I'm falling asleep.

But, for me, there isn't much to enjoy about being sexual right now. Maybe that will change, maybe it won't, but I have to keep working on accepting that this is where I am right now and that it is okay.

Judith: If sexuality is about developing a positive relationship with my body, I enjoy that. If it's about all of my emotionally intimate relationships, across the platonic/romantic spectrum and regardless of how touch is incorporated, I enjoy that. If it's about politics and feminism, and developing agency at the social level so that I can eventually exercise that same agency in my personal life, then, well, there's a lot I enjoy about being sexual.

Danielle: It's been really wonderful, over the course of my transition, to feel more and more "at home" in my own body. To enjoy my own

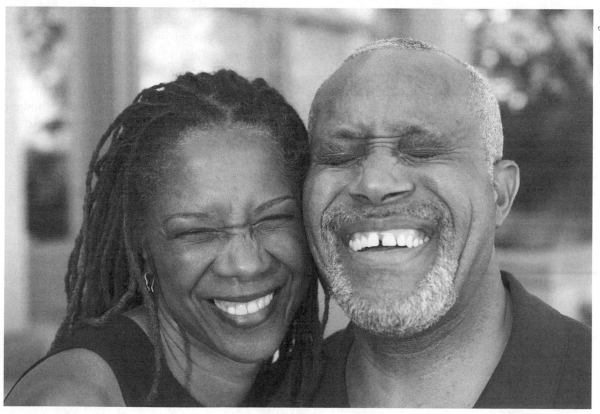

© Big Cheese Photo

breasts (which were a long time coming) or the pleasure of my own smooth skin. I was able to enjoy being sexual before going on hormones or transitioning, but I hadn't realized how *right* things would feel when I felt better about my body, my presentation, and my gender.

Chloe: Totally, Danielle. Prior to transitioning, I had sex fairly often and would say that I liked it but was sort of indifferent. It was fun, sure, but no big deal. After transitioning, things have changed so much. Besides the physical side of things changing (don't know if you had this experience, but for me and lots of other trans women I know, orgasms get harder to have but longer and more, I don't know, whole-body-melty feeling and my skin becomes much more sensitive), just having someone run their hands over my breasts feels "right" in a way I don't really understand, but I never felt that way when I had a flat chest.

I think being (more) comfortable in my body, thanks to hormones and lots of other things, has made sex better for me, and good sex makes me feel better about my body. So it's a nice combo.

Danielle: Yes! I did a whole bunch of journaling recently on my changing experiences with sex over the course of transitioning (not that I'd consider myself "done"), and I think that's a big part of it. Definitely harder to get to, but so much more yummy!

Leigh: Speaking on a raw, visceral level, sex that reaches climax has the incomparable ability to help me focus—to construct, write, create, produce. And I don't mean in a sort of sex-as-muse kind of way, but merely in reference to the clearheaded focus it brings. I masturbated my way through all-nighters reading dense theory and writing papers in grad school. One thing I love about sex with men is how they often fall asleep very quickly after sex and give me space to lie awake mulling over ideas and scheming new projects.

Nina: I did not even *think* to masturbate while I was in graduate school pulling all-nighters. I could have been even greater than I was!

Lydia: I totally use masturbation as a way to focus, ground myself physically, and release non-productive tension. I've never mastered the all-nighter thing, but have used it as a way to wake myself up in the morning. I love morning sex :)

EJM: I think I am the same way. I find my partner always falling asleep quickly, but I find myself being able to focus and my mind becomes more calm, not racing.

Nasir: LOL. It always used to annoy me when men fell asleep. I like the cuddling and the rehashing of what just went down after sex.

Lydia: I don't think falling asleep just after sex is exclusively a male-female thing. Sometimes sex/masturbation helps me fall asleep, sometimes my girlfriend is the one who falls asleep. Sometimes we both do. My girlfriend is less inclined to revisit "what just went down" and create a shared narrative than I am (I'm a compulsive chronicler). It can sometimes be a little lonely. But I think it's more a personality thing than a gender thing.

Ananda: I also masturbated my way through graduate school the second time. I never thought of it as helping me focus but as a way to nurture myself—I was not living with my partner—and to release tension. But, yes, I think you are right, Leigh. Thanks for that thought.

WHAT ROLE HAS LOVE PLAYED OR NOT PLAYED IN YOUR RELATIONSHIPS?

Cody: This question makes me think about "love" versus "in love" and what kinds of relationships we're talking about. Being in love for me is a helpless, head-rushy feeling and requires a lot of trust and intimacy to let myself fall like that. Being in love also has to do with intention, if not commitment: I want the people I'm in love with to be long-term things, and even if it doesn't work out that way, the intention of that needs to be mutual and strong for it to be worth the emotional risk.

I've also had lovers who I haven't really loved at all, but who I've been hot for and enjoyed fucking. I don't think love needs to play any role in sex I'm having, and I don't think that not being in love has impacted the pleasure, intimacy, hotness, or connection of sex for me.

Cecilia: I never could make love with someone I didn't at least think I loved. Note I say "make love." I guess that's key. I don't know if it's because I remained in a fairly conservative segment of society, or because I was brought up in the '50s, or because I'm not hugely sexual, but whatever it is, I have never had sex just because someone was hot and I wanted it. Some version of love has always had to be there. But I really enjoy reminiscing about the few times the sex drive had more to do with it than the love.

Nina: Love in my relationships can be described in a single phrase: *Love the hard way.* In my past relationships I've found that I love too hard without the expectation of reciprocity. I think a lot of my partners did love me in their own little ways. It wasn't until much later that I realized that their subtle love was no match for my unabashed expression of love and devotion.

Ananda: I have learned a lot about myself sexually by having sex with many different men and some women. One of the most amazing sexual experiences I have had in my life was in a threesome with a man and a woman. The orgasm that I had was like falling off a cliff into weightless outer space. If you had asked me forty years ago if I could imagine doing this, I would have said absolutely not. My mother would have been appalled to know. I find these experiences delightful and they have not much at all to do with love but being in the moment.

Francesca: For me sex is better when it is enhanced with love. Yet sex for the sake of sexual need can be good. However, physical closeness,

cuddling, nonsexual intimacy, etc., are always better with love.

Leigh: I really dig the idea of love as action, where demonstration and practice are more important than verbalization and romantic gesture. I don't want to think of love as a solid, assumed foundation, but rather as *praxis*, as the place where ideas/emotions/verbalizations meet practice and action.

Sophia: I can't imagine having the relationship that I have with my husband without being totally in love with him. Our biggest arguments early on were over how to raise our children be-

SNAPSHOT: PERCENTAGE OF WOMEN MARRIED BY AGE GROUP

15-19	1.9 percent
20-34	39.7 percent
35-44	64.3 percent
45-54	64.1 percent
55-64	62.3 percent
65+	40.3 percent[5]

cause of the baggage we carried around about our own childhoods. Within the last decade, we moved four times, a different state each time, while our children were going through elementary, middle, and high schools. Moving and getting adjusted to new jobs, new communities, and new schools during our children's formative years almost tore us apart. The financial, emotional, and day-to-day struggles put our commitment and love to the test to the point where we had to seek therapy. As a very private person, I wanted to solve our problems on our own, but once again, my awesome husband was right about going to see a marriage counselor. It was the best thing we've ever done for our marriage.

The initial passion my husband and I felt for each other has grown into a relationship that is based on fierce devotion and is simultaneously comfortable yet ever-changing. The kind of love, strong emotional connection, I feel for my husband is so powerful now that I can't conceive of feeling the same way about anyone else. Whatever love is, it's what has kept us together.

WHAT IS IT LIKE TO BE IN A RELATIONSHIP WHEN YOU DON'T LIKE SOME OR ALL OF YOUR OWN BODY?

Alexa: I'm currently living with my monogamous boyfriend of two years. As a larger woman (size 18–20, 230 pounds), I occasionally engaged in relationships in my teen years that I didn't particularly want to be in because I felt lucky that somebody would be interested in me in spite of my body. Now I am with a great guy who is attracted to me for many reasons, but partly because of my body.

I recently realized that physical attraction has a lot to do with intimacy, and what I actually resent is that the contemporary media have decided on one type of body that is acceptable to find attractive.

Sophia: I am 5'3" and on average 140 pounds. I've always wished I were thinner and taller. I used to wear loose, shapeless clothes to hide my body. My husband, who is tall and lean, told me that he loved my "curves." I had a hard time believing that he was not just flattering me.

When I got pregnant, I was a little worried about how big I was getting, but my husband just marveled at how my body was changing in response to pregnancy. We had some of our most amazing sex while I was pregnant. After pregnancy, my husband was awestruck by the way my body changed and slowly got back to prepregnancy condition.

I've come to terms with my body. I will never have the body that will allow me to wear whatever I want, but I don't wear baggy clothes anymore. I exercise and eat sensibly for my health, not because I want to get to a certain dress size.

Lydia: For me, the experience of being in a sexual relationship has been incredibly grounding in terms of enjoying my own physicality and the physical presence of others (namely, my girlfriend). I feel like I have permission to really *pay attention* to her body in a way that few settings in our culture offer us: the joy of getting to know, intimately, the shapes and smells and movements of another bodily person. And then the reverse: having someone else become so familiar with my *own* body and take such obvious delight in it.

Victoria: Your description of how your sexuality grounded you in your own physicality really resonates for me. When I started college and started to come into my identity as a feminist, I started to really think about what I'd been taught about sex and my body, and to consciously reject the shame and guilt I'd internalized. I started to masturbate. I read erotica. I had sex for the first time. I talked more openly about sex with other women. And I felt more and more present in my own body, and more and more comfortable with my own sexuality and sexual desire.

Now, at thirty-three, after eight years of marriage and two babies, I feel lost again in my own body. I'm not happy with what I see in the mirror. I'm not happy with my squishy, stretchy belly. I'm not happy with the width of my hips or the jiggle in my thighs. I don't feel the kind of sexual desire that used to make me want to ignore everything else—homework, messy apartment, no food on the shelves—and snuggle up to my partner. And I know, I *know*, I should feel beautiful and proud of carrying babies and embrace the new shape of my body. But it feels really empty when I say those things to myself, or when my partner says them to me.

My two-year-old just peed all over the floor. And I wonder why I don't feel sexy?

Cody: I've just started dating a genderqueer transmasculine person who has had top surgery and takes T [testosterone]. I'm actually surprised to find myself feeling a kind of body discontentment I haven't experienced in a long time. Learning the geographies of my lover's body, hir flat chest and strong arms, small hips and stubbly cheeks, chest hair and defined abs, I'm craving a body like hirs and I can't figure out if it's about gender or about old habits of self-hate. Why do I want to be shaped like that? Is it because I've always struggled with wishing I was smaller and didn't have these wide hips, or is it because I want to transition in the ways that ze has and be read as a boy?

It's a new thing to me, to actually be jealous of a lover's body. I'm hoping I can keep it manifested in sweet affirmations of how hot ze is, in love notes and whispered intimacies, and I can tell hir all the time that ze's a stud. I'm hoping it's not something that makes me sad when we're in bed together, and I feel too big and soft in all the wrong places, and I'm being held by this person whose body is perfect.

Danielle: It was incredibly difficult trying to be in relationships before I transitioned, because someone telling me I was handsome was actually a bad thing. I didn't enjoy being "handsome"; what I really wanted was to be told I was *pretty*.

So finding someone who would tell me that was pretty incredible. And then, as I went on hormones and my body started changing, it was likewise amazing to have someone tell me the changes were making me that much more attractive to her. And having her reassure me about the things I *did* like about my body—smooth skin after shaving, my growing breasts, my hair—was an important part of me finding enjoyment in my own body.

Chloe: Part of the reason having sex with other trans women was important to me early on was that it helped me come to love my own body, too. Seeing them and their body however it was—pre-op, non-op, post-op whatever—as beautiful helped me see my own body as beautiful, too. Part of it was coming to understand how my body worked with new hormones, new feelings, new body parts. Part of it was finally feeling comfortable in my physical body. But part of it was also unlearning cultural stereotypes and socialized messages that make me and other women, trans *or* cis, hate our bodies.

Heidi: My ex-husband was not happy with my body because I have a very small chest. He used to encourage me to get breast implants, which we could not afford. He would watch porn that depicted women with large breasts and make occasional comments that really made me feel self-conscious. I spent a lot of money on specially made push-up bras in an attempt to look as close to his standard as I could. Whenever I was naked around him, I was always very aware of my chest and never entirely comfortable.

Now I try not to care, but I do occasionally feel self-conscious about it. It has become a pet peeve of mine that natural is no longer good enough when it comes to breasts. It also really bothers me that I let him make me feel inadequate (and sometimes still do). He has some extra weight on him, which didn't bother me at all, but I now see it as an example of a double standard in which women's bodies are typically more rigidly scrutinized than men's bodies.

Since having children I haven't been with a partner who does not have experience with a mother who has given birth vaginally, as I am worried about what they would think about the different color and shape that comes with birth. I am also worried about the fact that I don't like to shave, and I have been told that pubic hair is no longer "normal" on women. As much as I like to think that I am happy with my body, and as hard as I try to make that a reality, it really isn't, and it affects many aspects of my life, including my relationships with others.

Victoria: I share your frustration with the idea that natural breasts (and normal pubic hair!) are no longer considered sexy. Honestly, I think someday people are going to look back at breast implants and Botox and bikini waxing and think our culture was completely bizarre.

Cathryn: Pubic hair is totally normal on women—don't buy into that myth. As for the rest, I can relate. I feel much, much better about my body these days, ironically when it's physically broken (multiple back injuries), but there is plenty I would change if I could. But at sixty, just being able to get out of bed in the morning with minimal pain is very nice and serves to put the rest in perspective.

Nidea: There was a point in my life that I hated my body. I didn't fit that saucy Latina image; I was a lost bird that wore oversize clothing. Sexual abuse didn't help my insecurities. I needed to find ways to make myself feel invisible to men and sometimes would even cut myself over it. Family would call me fat, so I was not only dirty but fat, and all I wanted to do was hide under anything I could.

But as I matured, my relationships became a safe haven. Relationships provided a safe and healthy space for me to learn about myself and define and redefine myself. For eight out of the past nine years of my life I had a boyfriend, and I have been single for the past year. I am slowly integrating myself into the single scene, and I am trying to maintain the confidence I built within the security of a relationship—as well as avoid the stereotypes that exist to define and confine me before I can speak for myself.

Zoe: I've always thought that I had a cute face and pretty features, but when I think about my actual body, I start to have doubts. I'm taller than most women, and in heels I'm over six feet. In college, I hung out with a group of girls who were all about 5'2" (if that) and I would always joke that I felt like Gandalf and the Hobbits because I towered over them. To top it off, I'm not a small girl—size 14—so everything about me just felt big.

I don't actually know if I could be with a man I thought was smaller than I am. I would be far too insecure. I've dated a lot of men who are around my size and even that feels strange to me—I tend to feel more comfortable with either larger men or African-American men, who I think are more used to my body type and who I have more in common with culturally. The relationships I've been in that have been most successful have been the ones where my partner reassures me that I'm sexy, attractive, and that he desires me.

Madigan: When I was fifteen it was discovered that I had been born without a uterus or a vagina, a condition known as Mayer-Rokitansky-Küster-Hauser syndrome (MRKH). The diagnosis came after much medical trauma, as I was initially misdiagnosed and put through a painful and unnecessary surgery. I was immediately pressured to have a neovagina created but was too ashamed and shocked to deal with anything at the time. Over the next three years, I hid this secret and was deeply ashamed of my body. I thought if anyone knew, they would reject me or think I was a freak. Being sexual and/or intimate under these circumstances was difficult and painful. I was never able to be sexually present or enjoy myself, as I was always focused on keeping people from penetrating me.

At the age of eighteen, I was in my first long-term relationship with my first love. I decided to be up front about MRKH, and this was a very positive experience for me. A couple of months later, we were attending a queer conference and I stumbled across a workshop on intersex. This workshop completely changed my life. I was finally able to feel the emotions I had stuffed away at fifteen. I was able to get angry at the way I had been treated by doctors, about the assumptions that had been made about me and my body, and about the pressure put on me by doctors that I need to be "fixed"—that even if I wasn't ready at fifteen, I would eventually "have" to have a vagina created. (Lord knows we can't have a woman running around without a vagina!) I also decided that never, ever again would I be sexual with someone who didn't know about my MRKH beforehand. I was terrified of rejection but have never experienced this when I have been honest. I made the decision that I would keep my body as it is and have finally learned to love and enjoy my sexuality again.

Cathryn: Madigan, thank you for telling about how intersexed bodies are just as "normal" as so-called standard bodies. The medical establishment tries to enforce standard bodies on those who may well be comfortable, with some support, in nonstandard intersexed bodies. Bless you.

Miriam: For as long as I can remember, my mother complained about her body. No matter what her size, she always felt she was fat and was very vocal about this. My older sister was always heavy, and her weight was often criticized or discussed at home (and by strangers in public).

Almost every girl I knew complained about her body—about her stretch marks, the size of her hips, her breasts, her thighs. I always kept quiet. I was chubby and felt like if I complained,

As of 2011, Connecticut, Iowa, Massachusetts, New Hampshire, Vermont, New York and the District of Columbia permit same-sex marriages. Maryland, Rhode Island, and New Mexico officially pledge non-discrimination against marriages between same-sex couples from other states.

Other states offer broad protections short of marriage. New Jersey, Hawaii, and Illinois permit civil union, while broad domestic partnership is available in Oregon, Washington, Nevada, and California. Smaller packages of protections for same-sex couples are available in Maryland, Maine, Colorado, and Wisconsin.[7]

The acceptance of same-marriage has also steadily increased, and reflects a remarkably consistent generation gap, with a majority of the millennial generation supporting the right of same-sex couples to marry.

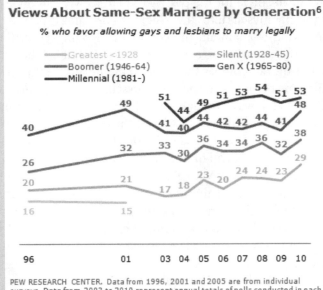

Views About Same-Sex Marriage by Generation[6]

% who favor allowing gays and lesbians to marry legally

Greatest <1928 — Silent (1928-45) — Boomer (1946-64) — Gen X (1965-80) — Millennial (1981-)

PEW RESEARCH CENTER. Data from 1996, 2001 and 2005 are from individual surveys. Data from 2003 to 2010 represent annual totals of polls conducted in each year.

I wouldn't get the reassurance that so many girls were looking for. Or if someone reassured me that I wasn't fat, I would feel like they were lying. And I didn't want to be part of that culture that encourages body snarking, either toward self or toward others.

I don't talk about how I feel about my body. Sometimes I love it, sometimes I hate it. Sometimes I question how someone can be attracted to it, but I know that my insecurities come from myself. I've found that if I fake confidence in my body, I start to feel it. I can be with a lover and not want to be seen naked in the light, but if I pretend I'm comfortable with it I quickly become comfortable. I've decided that I don't want

those moments of not liking my body to affect my relationships.

Faith: I had weight issues when I was in high school. I lost over thirty pounds by the end of it through strict calorie counting and exercise, and have kept it off. However, the feelings of self-loathing from that time period have always stuck with me and my eating is still somewhat disordered because of it.

When I lost my virginity (which was after I'd lost the weight), I remember really not wanting my boyfriend to look at me. I had had so many feelings of shame about my body that it seemed weird to want attention in that kind of way. It didn't dawn on me until later that sex is about appreciating each other's bodies, not to mention truly feeling comfortable in your own. Sex in relationship actually helped me get over a lot of my body issues. I had never been comfortable being naked, even by myself, until someone else had showed me their appreciation for my naked body.

EJM: I grew up with severe eczema. Due to the constant peeling and scars on my body, I have very discolored and uneven skin. In previous relationships, my skin was something unsexy and shameful. I rarely liked the lights on during sex, and if my partner commented on my skin, even the most benign comment, it would put me into a negative thought pattern.

My [current] partner takes an active part in taking care of my skin. When I scratch while I sleep, he will wake up to hold my hand to stop me. On my bad days, he will help me put ointment and creams to ease the pain on my skin. Even this very little gesture has made me feel very comfortable with my skin and showing my skin to him. Because he is a part of my regimen of skin care and prevention, it has been less of a burden. With his help, my skin feels better and it also feels wanted.

HOW DO MEDIA IMAGES AND PORTRAYALS OF RELATIONSHIPS AFFECT YOUR IDEA OF AN "IDEAL" RELATIONSHIP?

Jaime: I see a lot of people in the media like me in some ways. I'm a straight, cis, white women; they are straight, cis, white women. They are mostly thinner and prettier than me, but I'm within a standard deviation of a socially acceptable body. I have these privileges.

My relationships . . . not so much. I can't think of nonmonogamy in mainstream media off the top of my head. And the pop-psychy gender essentialism—yech. I think the closest thing

to the dynamics between my current partner and me are Zoe and Wash from [the TV series] *Firefly* and [the film] *Serenity*. The schlubby husbands and hot but shrewish wives of TV sitcoms we are not. I don't have a TV anymore, and aside from saving money, the dearth of characters and concepts that I can relate to (or even that don't actively piss me off) is a big reason, with my irritation at the lowest common denominator method of portraying women and relationships being prominent.

Danielle: What books/sites have you found useful or more "true" in portraying relationships for you?

Jaime: A lot of feminist blogs are written by women who have relationships more like the kind that I like/have. The main contributors at Pandagon (pandagon.net) and Shakesville (shakespearessister.blogspot.com), for example. They talk about their relationships in the blogs, and it's nice to see a functional open marriage, or just an egalitarian partnership.

I find odds and ends in books that often aren't about the relationships but that include them incidentally. Jasper Fforde's Thursday Next books, with their strong heroine, or just about everything Tamora Pierce has ever written. In nonfiction, there are biographies of people like Jill Ker Conway, Virginia Woolf, and Julia Child, and feminist works on sexuality and women and relationships—*Communion* by bell hooks comes immediately to mind. And queer literature is more likely to portray egalitarian partnerships, so stuff like Alison Bechdel's comics are good for that.

Lydia: I just have to say, love that someone mentioned *Firefly*. And I absolutely adore Zoe and Wash. I agree with you regarding the tiredness of the *Family Guy* or *Everybody Loves Raymond* sitcoms in which a hot and smart woman is somehow inexplicably married to an overgrown man-child. It's so insulting to men, women, straight couples—pretty much anyone who has the gumption to be in a positive, lasting relationship.

Chloe: It's cool that you mention books and the Internet and blogs as media. I think most people were just thinking about TV and pop culture stuff, but it's true, the Internet does offer more options—like you said, if you know where to look, which is a whole other thing. As a trans woman, I've found the Internet crucial to me, especially reading blogs and such. I think that's one of the only places (in media, anyway, not counting people I have met in the "real world") that I saw relationships that at least came close to mirroring my own desires. I hadn't really thought about it that way before reading your post, though. Also, hell yes, *Firefly*! So good.

Jordan: My ideal relationship is never on television. I can't think of a single depiction of a relationship involving a nonbinary trans person on television, let alone someone who *also* has disabilities. As a result of the fact that people like me are basically erased, I think that my perceptions of "ideal" relationships are more pure and self-shaped, if that makes sense. I'm not influenced by relationships I see on-screen, in books, etc., because they are so abstract from who I am that I don't see myself or my relationships at all in them. My ideas about relationships are consequently very much shaped by my own beliefs and thoughts; I must construct my own media because the media pretend that I don't exist.

Rebeka: As a child I did not grow up with a happy family. I never saw what a happy functioning relationship looked like. So as I got older, I watched the Lifetime channel as much as possible. Lifetime is kind of like reading a romance novel. The movies and TV shows they show always have a happy ending: *Touched by an Angel, Walker, Texas Ranger,* and countless fairy-tale movies. Whatever the show, there is always a man and woman who fall in love and are a happy functioning family who live happily ever after.

My mother and brother always make fun of me and say, "She's watching the tampon channel again." I do hope to grow up and have a fairy-tale relationship where we are madly in love with each other and create a beautiful family. I would say that this is the only way I let TV and the media affect me. I am the total opposite of what the media portray and I am very happy with that. I don't need to try and look like what the media portray, because I am far from it. My biggest challenge is just being comfortable with myself and finding someone who likes me for me. Finding a man who isn't affected by the media, now that is the hard part.

Heidi: Children's stories and movies like Disney films introduced me to a heteronormative ideal at a very young age. When I was a young teenager, I started having feelings for some of the girls on my favorite TV shows. I was so ashamed of my feelings toward girls, including my best friend at the time, that I really tried to overcompensate by becoming as boy crazy as possible. I felt normal when I was kissing a boy, even when I was feeling abnormal for not enjoying myself like they do in the movies.

This only got worse in my early twenties. I actually went as far as to get married to a man I knew I didn't love (or even enjoy being with sexually) because I wanted the typical middle-class white-picket-fence life for myself and my children. I thought that I was supposed to get married, that it would make other people happy and provide a "normal" life for my children. That is what I saw throughout the media growing up; rarely were there positive portrayals of a single mother, except for the stories in which she later found a husband.

I am having a similar problem right now. I have not had any interest in dating or having a sexual relationship in about two years. I cannot think of a single television character who is asexual and not considered to be extremely odd in some way. With so much emphasis on sexuality and "hookup culture," asexuality becomes very taboo. I like the fact that women are more than ever free to explore their sexuality, despite the fact that a double standard does still exist between men and women, as does the dichotomy of "good girl" and "bad girl," which is strongly tied to sexuality, but I think there also needs to be a space for women without desires, not because they are "good" or "pure" or abstaining for moral or religious purposes, but simply because they are just not interested in sex, or do not currently feel a strong desire to be involved in sexual relationships.

Sophia: I think the lack of interracial relationships in the media is one of the reasons why my parents were not totally supportive of our relationship when my husband and I started dating. My parents saw very few interracial relationships in their immediate community. They couldn't see how my husband and I could have anything in common. They were afraid that my husband, in the white majority, would take advantage of me, an Asian/Hispanic minority woman. With time, my parents thawed out as they got to know my husband. Now they love him, and they appreciate how thoughtful and sensitive he is to how foreign my parents still feel, even after almost fifty years in the United States, about straying outside their cultural communities.

EJM: I've had the same situation with my parents. I think they are very accepting of my sister-in-law, who is white, and my partner, but I think it is still hard for them to cope with the fact that we are not in the "normal" relationships that they see in their community. I'm really glad to hear how accepting your family is of your husband. It gives me hope that my parents will be able to do the same with my partner and my sister-in-law and see beyond the cultural differences.

Judith: More than shaping my knowledge of the "ideal" relationship, I think media images affect me by severely limiting my sense of what relationship models are possible. Years

after coming out as a lesbian, I still find that if I watch too many sitcoms (with their almost entirely heterosexual pairings), I find myself asking questions about how I'd handle that situation were it to arise with my husband.

It's as if I temporarily forget that the media I'm being fed are not relevant to my own experience. It frustrates me, because I believe in role models; I believe in examining what has worked for others and incorporating the facets that I suspect will work for me. My favorite Disney film, when I was a kid, was *The Little Mermaid*, and yet I was fundamentally uninterested in Eric. I realize now that I selectively identified with Ariel; I connected with her experiences as the youngest daughter, her desire to be somewhere else, and her need to explore, while simultaneously dismissing her love for Eric. For all the problems I see in that film now, it's eye-opening for me to realize that, even as a small child, I had an ability to find my own representation and ignore what failed to speak to me.

These days, I seek out media that represent me, and my understanding of representation has expanded to include more than lesbian relationships. I look for feminist media, queer media, media that emphasize enthusiastic consent, media that do not presume sexuality is easy, media that recognize power dynamics and work to address them creatively. I look for stories in which—to paraphrase *The Celluloid Closet*—the people I most closely relate with are not there to be pitied, feared, or laughed at. In keeping with my days of Disney watching, I still take what resonates with me, in films, books, and television shows, and leave the rest. But I also engage more consciously and actively. I critique the media that don't speak to me, and I create stories and representations of my own to help build a fuller picture.

Chloe: As a trans woman, I have to echo what some folks have already said about the lack of media depictions available to me at all. I had almost nothing to work with from the start. When people talk about trans women in the mainstream media, it's usually to ponder how we could be "crazy" enough to "mutilate" ourselves or something. Our sexuality rarely comes up directly, though it's always there, on the underside. I suspect this is largely because of the ways our decision to transition has long been treated as a sexual fetish or deviancy.

Because of that history, we're thought of as "improperly sexual" no matter what we're doing. It shows up when right-wing propaganda tries to stir up some kind of creepy panic about how we're going to assault other women in the bathroom (because obviously trans women only go into bathrooms for sexual reasons, not just to, you know, pee). I'd say the vast majority of media images of trans women, besides the stupid bathroom stuff, are stories about when trans women (usually young trans women of color) are murdered, and this is often attributed to the stereotype that trans women are all sex workers (and thus, of course, "deserved" it by getting ourselves in dangerous positions). So while trans women's sexuality is not directly talked about in the media, it's usually there, and it's almost always seen as something threatening, immoral, dangerous to both ourselves and non-trans people, something that is perverse or something that gets us killed.

Media portrayals of trans women are getting slightly better, I think, but it brings up a whole other issue—most of what's seen now is of relatively privileged white, middle-class, late-transitioning trans women, like in the movie *Transamerica*. There're still few portrayals of young trans women of color. Or, when we have the occasional positive images like the story of Angel in *Rent*, it's still a tragic story that ends in death. At least it's closer to reality, and at least something is getting out there, I guess.

Kali: What the media say about my relationships now, since I became disabled, is enough to make me both devastated and enraged. The media say that either my partner will leave me, or he is some great self-sacrificing person. There's no room for a relationship where both of us want to be there. Where both of us rely on each other, instead of just me relying on him. The media say that if he stays, it's some kind of amazing act of love, not the more mundane sort of romance that people who are not disabled have. He's not some brave, dramatic rescuer, and I'm not some crippled damsel who needs rescuing. We're just a couple of people in love. That's all. But there's no space in the media for happily ever after for us—either he has to give up his chance at something "better" and live a half life to "save" me (which typically ends in the disabled partner dying), or he has to leave me because my disability is just too miserable for him, and poor disabled me just isn't enough of a woman for him. I try to ignore the media, but I'll admit I have some trouble with the idea that I'm not good enough for him and don't deserve him.

Nina: I am a black woman and I am looking for a partner. Race, color, creed don't really matter, but there are very few positive representations of black women and black women in positive couples. The only representation of the love that I am looking for is in Barack and Michelle Obama. Politics aside, they represent what I want: two educated beautiful black people in love and affectionate with beautiful children. They strive to make a change in the world. You may not agree with their politics, but their love is undeniable.

Rebeka: Nina, I so agree with you. I am a half African/Caucasian-American girl. I am, shall we say, a bigger girl, so I am not portrayed in the media really at all, and if I am, it's not in a very positive way. I am only eighteen, so I am very new to the relationship phase of life. However, I love your Michelle and Barack comment. I hope to one day find love like they have. I just wanted to thank you for being so comfortable being you. I am still coming to terms with myself and sexuality, but it makes me very happy to hear from a strong African-American woman like yourself, who has a strong sense of self. Thank you for being you.

Tasha Maria: I can remember growing up on the South side of Chicago in the late '70s and the images of relationships on television were negative stereotypes of African Americans.

I felt a little better during the '80s when hiphop hit the scene and many of the rappers back then rapped about love. LL Cool J's hit songs "I Need Love" and "Around the Way Girl" were my favorites because he talked about the black women with a lot of respect and love. It also rubbed off on the boys because they wanted to be like LL. We also had *The Cosby Show*, which made me feel like my dream was possible.

After *The Cosby Show* ended and gangsta rap became more popular, a total shift happened, and the African-American woman became a target in the worst way. The images of misogyny filled up the airwaves and the lyrics became more and more disrespectful. The term "baby daddy" was invented in order to explain the increase of unwed mothers.

These images didn't affect just the African-American community but women in general in ways that seem to be irreversible. Even old men like Imus felt the need to describe women as "nappy-headed hos" due to decreasing respect of women.

I turn on many popular television shows and they show interracial relationships usually between an African-American man and a Caucasian woman but rarely do they show a woman like me being loved or respected. Is the African-American woman near extinction? is a common question I have to ask myself from time to time. It has really made me feel sad to hear so many other sisters talk about relationship issues.

HOW DOES IT AFFECT YOUR RELATIONSHIPS WHEN YOU ARE WITH SOMEONE WHOM THE WORLD GIVES MORE OR LESS POWER THAN YOU HAVE, BECAUSE OF RACE, INCOME, GENDER, OR DISABILITY?

Sloane: My husband is a stay-at-home dad for our baby boy, yet many describe his work as "babysitting." When we go to the doctor for well visits, the doctor (male or female) speaks to me and doesn't tend to make eye contact with my husband even though many of the questions are best answered by him. I think it does affect how confident he is in taking care of our son. It is also frustrating for my husband that he spends all day with our son, but our son seems more attached to me because I can breastfeed him and my husband obviously can't (he feeds him breast milk with a bottle while I'm at work).

We went shopping for a used car for me. My husband stayed with our son while I spoke to the salespeople (usually male), who seemed baffled by the scenario. I'm sure all of these little realities filter into how we interact as a couple, but it's difficult to pinpoint how. We have plenty of power struggles, both trying to assert ourselves—even down to deciding how to rearrange the bedroom furniture.

Danielle: A friend and I were discussing a similar situation she's having. Following her maternity leave, she's back at work full-time and he's at home with their baby most of the week. She said it's frustrating for both of them because many of the books of advice are geared for "mommy and baby," so he feels left out and she feels like she's not being a good mother. Likewise, they get frustrated with the way products and information are presented because they don't really apply to their situation. I wanted to let you know you're not the only family who is feeling somewhat lost in how their gender/power/relationship structure "fits."

Astrid: I have dated several men who were older than me and had significant careers—CEO types, full of energy and incredibly self-centered. I have always felt flattered by their attention and have really enjoyed their company. I could always hold my ground in such a relationship and I always knew that my education was not second to theirs. But what I was mostly attracted to was the unfailing (and often unreflected) trust they'd have in their own abilities and qualifications. I think I wanted to be with them because they did what I did not dare to try to achieve myself. Not that I would not have been as qualified, but because I had more doubts about myself and my capabilities. Doubts I certainly had (and still have) because I am a woman.

Madigan: I never got beyond ninth grade in school. I have been heavily involved in social justice activism since I was a teenager and usually have a very different background from most of the people I meet. My current partner is a year older than me and holds both an undergrad and a master's degree. Her family is very well-off and she attended one of the most expensive private schools in the city we both grew up in. We have been together nearly three and a half years now.

We see the world in very different ways and experience financial crises in very different ways. Until I got this well-paying job, I often felt stuck in our relationship for financial reasons and wondered at times if this was part of the reason we were still together. Fortunately, we have a good enough relationship that we have been able to talk about this a lot and have really come a long way as far as this is concerned. Getting a job that raised my income level significantly has leveled the playing field in many ways, but the thought that I could lose this job at any moment never leaves my mind.

Kali: My current boyfriend and I are about equal in education (both have MAs; he's almost done with his PhD; I'm halfway through my JD).

My family is a bit wealthier than his, enough so that I've done much more traveling than he, but that's about all. We're similar in financial situation. The big gap in power in our relationship comes from the fact that he is abled and I am disabled. Well, and the whole female/male disparity.

In general, he's a very progressive guy and both a feminist and disability ally. However, sometimes he doesn't realize things are problematic. I end up shocked that he doesn't get it, and he gets defensive as I try to explain (he says I get condescending). Things like calling a person "blind" when they are really being ignorant (in other words, using disability as a metaphor for bad things). On the other hand, he is very supportive, helping with things that I can't do because of my disability, and has never given me any indication that he thinks less of me for needing his help (on the contrary, he admires my strength and determination to still do what I can do). He always thinks of us as being equals in the relationship. I struggle with that sometimes.

Victoria: My partner dropped out of college the year I graduated from college. He moved in with me while I was in grad school and we got married a year later. And while he has always made significantly more money than me, he always assumes that people look down on him and assume I am smarter and more interesting because I have an MA and work as a professor (adjunct, which basically means temporary and underpaid) while he is a retail manager. It's been a huge issue for us: I feel a tremendous amount of guilt for encouraging him to drop out of college but also some resentment that he wasn't more supportive of my grad school career. He refuses to come to university functions or socialize with my colleagues because he feels out of place. And I've absolutely seen colleagues at the university become awkward and hesitant in conversation with him after asking where

he works, so I understand his hesitation, even though I also find it frustrating.

And unlike many couples, whose power dynamics turn on really recognizable identities, we often have the smoothest, most comfortable interactions with people who don't know us at all and just see us in our role as parents or see our shared interests. It's once people get to know us well enough to know where we work and what our backgrounds are that the awkwardness starts to creep in.

WHAT ARE YOUR EXPERIENCES IN RELATIONSHIPS THAT SPAN RACIAL DIFFERENCES?

Nidea: My last relationship was an interracial one. He was Irish American. We started dating the summer before college and dated through all four years in college. My aunts and uncles would always praise me for catching a great one (yes, like catching a fish or an animal). My parents on the other hand were not as welcoming, questioning why a boy who is white, who has the world in his hands, would want anything to do with a Dominican girl. My father thought I was a "big ho"—the only way a white man would be interested in a Dominican girl had to be sexual—and yet I was still a virgin and wanted to be a virgin until marriage. It just became a huge mess in my mind. How do you keep up with the stereotypes of a Latin woman as either virginal or a "spicy Latina"? There is no room for the gray area.

Zoe: He's a Jewish boy from the Midwest and I'm a black girl (with an adoptive Puerto Rican father and black mother). My mother is really into me dating black men, which is shocking because I so rarely do it. It's also shocking because her husband, my father, is Puerto Rican and a light-skinned one at that. So I don't know where that comes from, but when I think about bringing home a nonblack guy, I freak and wonder how she'll deal with it.

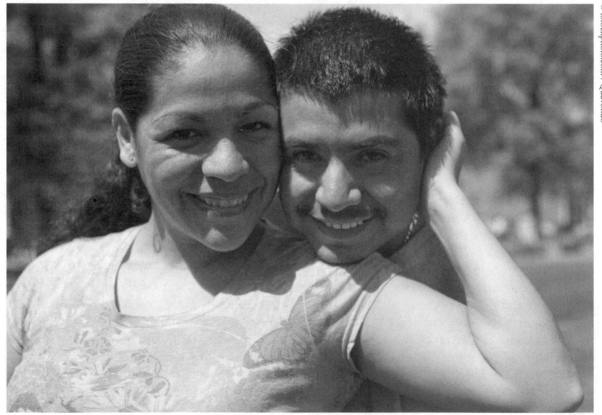

I also hated when I was out with my guy and we'd encounter a group of black men who would give us dirty looks. I always got so scared and superdefensive and tried not to touch him or be affectionate in front of them. I was so afraid that he'd have to "prove his manhood" in front of them and that he would leave me because he'd see how hard it is to love a black girl. It never came to that, ever, but I still fear that when I date white guys. Because I don't think they're used to dealing with things like that.

I will say that I did like that my boy was Jewish, because even though he was white, he still was part of a minority and I felt that connected me to him in a stronger way. Sometimes he'd make little sexual remarks pertaining to me being black—you know, the whole "I like chocolate" type of thing. It's a little bit irritating sometimes, because it's so cheesy, but it never really got on my nerves. Plus, my father will do the same thing on occasion with my mom, so it's not like I never heard that kind of dialogue.

EJM: Although my parents are considered "progressive" in their community in Korea, they still adhere to many traditions. They want me to date a good Christian Korean man and settle down and marry, with very little expectation for my career (this has changed after years of battling).

Their disapproval of my relationships, mostly due to race, became a wedge that broke up many of my relationships, and it was hard for me to respect my parents' wishes and also make my partner happy. My partners were constantly offended that my parents would so openly express their disappointment that I was not dating a Korean. My partners saw it as, my parents *specifically* do not like you because you are white/black/Indian/etc.

My parents also have difficulty coping with different dating cultures. My parents expect my partners to ask for permission to date me, to have a date only once a week, to only meet my siblings and extended family when we are intending to be married. They were constantly baffled by the invitations of my partners' parents during holidays. They would ask me if I intended to get married to my partners, and if not, why would I have any business going to their house on a holiday?

When you have two cultures that do not understand each other, it is definitely an uphill battle. But I found that over the years, my parents have slowly become more accepting of my choices and they are realizing that I cannot be held to *all* of their cultural standards. Dinner with my partner's parents is just dinner and nothing more.

HAVE YOU OR YOUR PARTNER DISCUSSED HAVING CHILDREN? IF YOU HAD DIFFERING OPINIONS, HOW DID IT AFFECT THE RELATIONSHIP?

Ananda: My primary partner is eleven years older than I am. When we first got together I was thirty-one and he was forty-two, with two sons from a previous marriage who were eighteen and twenty. He was done with having kids and had made a definitive decision by having a vasectomy before we met. I had had a baby over a decade before, did not want to be a single mother, so had surrendered her for adoption thinking that I would have a chance to do it right someday. At several points in my thirties, I went through crises about whether to leave this relationship around the baby issue. In the end I stayed. While I don't regret staying—my life has gone in so many incredible directions with his support and partnership—I do regret not having and raising another child.

Victoria: My partner and I always knew we wanted to have children. We both grew up in big families, with birthdays and holidays full of cheerful aunts cooking and uncles talking sports and grandmas and grandpas rocking crying babies and crabby teenagers pretending they didn't want to be there. We've had to unpack a lot of the gender expectations around family and parenting, and we've worked hard to create new patterns and possibilities for our own new little family, but we knew from the beginning that we wanted to do that work.

That said, I don't think parenthood or motherhood is a must-have experience. I don't think it's a necessary rite of passage or path to fulfillment, and I don't think anybody should be pressured by culture or family to undertake this journey if it's not the one you want.

Leigh: The first time the topic of children came up in my current relationship was in the middle of sex. He paused for a minute and asked if I wanted to have children. I thought for half a second and said, "Not really. You?" He said, "Nope. I don't think so." We laughed and continued enjoying ourselves. While that sort of timing could be intense for others, I found it casually thoughtful and spontaneous in the way of just saying whatever thought enters your mind.

We've since had a few conversations about children and if/under what circumstances we might change our minds. Sometimes these arise spontaneously and as a way of talking about the future (something neither of us is generally very inclined toward), and sometimes the conversations arise after a friend or family member expresses excitement at the idea of us making a new person together. I enjoy having the conversations when they arise; they feel very open and lack the pressure that can be present in these conversations as you get older. One of my favorite aspects of our relationship is scheming and dreaming about what we might build together.

Jordan: I am not interested in having children, at all, which seems to be more of an issue as I grow older, as what people used to put down to youthful rebellion is now viewed as socially suspect. I've only had the conversation about

having children once, though, and it was fortunately with someone else who also doesn't want to have children. We talked about the social pressures put upon us and the judgments we encounter, and how relaxing it was to be in a relationship with someone who shared the position of not wanting to have children.

Robin: Even though I'm superyoung (twenty), the topic of children comes up a lot with my partners, less as a serious consideration for current plans, more as a tool for fantasizing/testing the Future. In my current relationship, my partner is especially militant about being anti–child rearing, so I tend to stay away from the topic if at all possible. This affects the relationship in a strange way: While I don't necessarily see myself with this person at an age that I would hope to be taking care of kids (I hope to be an adoptive parent or provide foster care later in life), we are in a more adult relationship and I want to be open about how I truly see myself as an adult. And I find myself in a weird paradox where I don't want to engage in the strange normative narrative of marriage, children, nuclear happiness, and yet I want to acknowledge the part of myself that loves it and has been raised to love it.

Sloane: My husband and I batted the idea of children around for a while. There are enough reasons to have them as there are to not have them. Every other milestone in our relationship seemed to take a while, but when we decided to have a child, we just closed our eyes and jumped. If we'd deliberated on children as long as we did our other decisions, we'd never have a kid.

Aside from having some stability in income and living situation, we didn't deliberate much or have some grand scheme for what the "right" time would be. We figured, okay, let's quit birth control and see how it goes. I was pregnant about two months later. I like how it happened. I enjoyed being pregnant and was happy for the experience of it. It was about as "in the now" as I have ever been. Having my son around is similar to the pregnancy process. I find I'm much more patient than I was before when it comes to how he's developing and moving through stages. We may have another child. That's our leaning, but we'll see how it goes.

Lydia: My girlfriend and I are both approaching thirty, both in graduate school with student loans, looking ahead to another decade-plus of finding our footing financially and in our chosen professions. Right now, we're holding off adopting *pets* until we're sure we can provide for them; providing for children is out of the question for the immediate future.

Still, it's a question we've danced around. My girlfriend is up front about the fact that she doesn't wish to be pregnant or give birth. Ever. She's also pretty clear on her disinclination to be a parent or otherwise care for young children. She hasn't ever told me point-blank that it's a deal breaker in our relationship but is pretty clear about the fact that she doesn't see herself being a parent.

While I can see myself being content and thriving as one half of a couple without children, I think that in the long term I would start to feel impoverished without deeper ties to a multigenerational community.

Cecilia: Having children was a question with my second husband. By then my daughter was in college. So was his daughter, and his son was in high school. We were in our fifties and fabulously in love. Love and babies were what we thought went together, so we thought it would be great to have one. We didn't talk about it much, especially the possible challenges to our families, because we were so sure of our happiness that we trusted all to love. We gave up contraception and made love as we felt like it. It took awhile to realize we were too old. It made me sadder than I ever told him, and it probably made him sadder than he ever told me. When I think now that I could have an eight-year-old in bed down the hall, I wonder what I was thinking!

WHAT EFFECT DO CHILDREN HAVE ON DATING OR STAYING IN A RELATIONSHIP?

Astrid: My daughter's father and I split up when she was three (she is ten now), and he immediately plunged into an intense dating life that led to a continuous string of girlfriends, none of whom lasted for more than a year. My daughter was routinely introduced to them early on—is there anything more endearing and attractive to a new woman than a guy showing off the daughter he dotes on?

I always felt it was my duty to shield my child from a similar experience on my end of things. I have no regrets about setting these priorities—I have never even questioned them. That said, I am finally starting to feel the absence of a grown-up at the dinner table, someone to vent to about how the day has gone. I am forty-seven years old and have spent so many years without a partner that I am not certain I could fit anybody back into my life. But as my daughter gets older, I know I should open up to that possibility again.

Cheryl: I had my sons when I was fifteen and nineteen. Their father was my first boyfriend, and we ended our relationship in my early twenties. I have been dating as a single mom ever since. In my twenties it was much harder to date because most men my age were not comfortable with the idea that I was a mother. They were at a different place in their lives. That was disheartening at times, but along the way I met some great guys who were willing to explore a relationship with me. Of those relationships, my children have only met two men, because until the relationship seems like it may have a long-term future in my life, I don't think it is necessary to involve my children.

I prefer to date men who have children and are active parents, mostly because there tends to be more understanding about the balance of dating and parenting. The man I am currently dating is a single father. Single parenting and dating are difficult at times, and us both having to figure out child care and how to integrate our families into our relationships has presented some real challenges. He is currently deployed to Afghanistan, but we have begun to discuss the future of our relationship and I can foresee that when he gets home we will really have to tackle the blended family challenges.

Heidi: When I was married, I found out that my husband had an affair when I was pregnant with my son. I would think that without children, I would have left right away. I had two children when I found out about it, which was almost a year after their affair had ended. In this case, I think that having kids made me try to make the relationship work. In the end, I found out that he was talking to her again, so I asked him to move out.

I do not date often, but when I do I find it quite difficult. I won't date a person I wouldn't want my children to date someday. And by this I don't mean the exact person—age issues might make that a bit weird—but the type of person. I want to model behaviors that I feel are appropriate for my children, or at least not give them a bad example whenever possible. I have dated people who have invited me to meet their children in the first week, and I find that scary. I don't want people cycling in and out of their lives.

Also, my children are still quite young, and as a student, I do not have a lot of money for things like babysitters. Because of this, it becomes quite difficult to have a life away from them, to meet new people, or to date.

Sloane: My parents had four children and got divorced after thirteen years of marriage. I was in fifth grade when they split. I was—I don't want to say glad—maybe *relieved* that they decided to divorce. They fought a lot and were not well matched.

Now I'm in my own marriage and have to face the question sometimes when things get really bad, when we fight and scream and say horrible things that we don't mean: Should we stay married? Should we raise our son in the midst of this?

A child undeniably and hugely does factor into the equation. I'm very conscientious about what my son is experiencing. I find myself debating, though, about what the bigger picture is. I wonder if being a child of divorce predisposes me to want to cut and run—and will I be modeling that? I wonder if seeing how my husband and I work through our issues will make my son better able to weather his storms. My husband and I love each other. No doubt there. We also need to find a better way to handle conflict. We aren't hopeless, though. We've not been married long, but have been a work in progress for about ten years, and we have improved the way we fight.

I am much more aware of how we fight now that we have a child. How that affects the staying power of our relationship remains to be seen. I guess I won't know the answer until I know it.

Victoria: I have two young daughters, and I really empathize with how it is difficult to be in a relationship with someone who has kids—except that I'm not dating. My partner and I are just trying to figure out how to be parents and also have a relationship with each other as adults like we did before we had children. And some days it all feels very balanced and joyful, and other days it feels like we're on some crappy reality show where you're forced to try and reason with a screaming child and your only help is a pseudospouse the show has chosen for you who doesn't share any of your values.

I cannot imagine trying to establish a relationship with someone new while also trying to parent my girls. It's hard enough to maintain a relationship with a partner I know and love deeply.

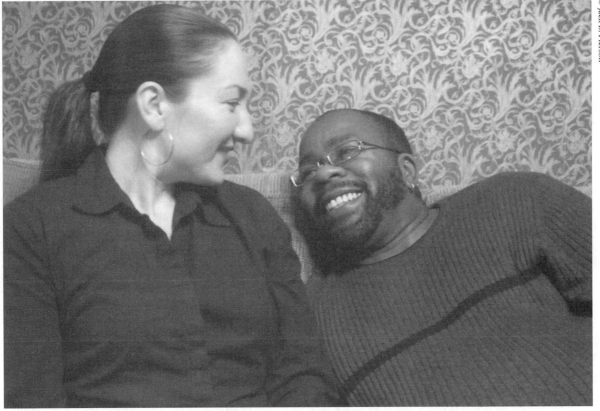

WHEN DID YOU REALIZE THAT
A RELATIONSHIP YOU INTENDED
TO STAY IN WAS GOING TO BE WORK?
WHAT ARE SOME OBSTACLES THAT
CAN GET IN THE WAY OF
RELATIONSHIPS?

Lydia: It's often an exhausting (even if rewarding) experience to remember that my girlfriend does not have the same life experiences and personality that I do, and thus isn't necessarily reading situations the same way I do, or making the same assumptions about what my responses mean. Good communication is so much more than simply speaking up and listening, something I realize now more than ever. It's actually taking the time to break down what

we're saying to each other and what exactly it *means* to both of us.

Sloane: We've just entered a new construction zone with the arrival of our son, now nine months old. I work full-time, my husband is at home taking care of the boy, I'm nursing and have a low libido, I had an unwanted C-section, which has put off our plans of having a second child. It's hard to analyze the situation while in the midst of it, but it's safe to say that I'm realizing again how much work this relationship stuff is.

Ananda: Early on in living with my partner there were the issues of money (especially since I made more money than he did), housekeeping (can be an eternal struggle if you are really opposite on standards of cleanliness or clutter), work (taking too much time and energy), not enough time together or too much time together, and family/children. Over time we have gotten better at not letting these things become obstacles. The first couple of years of my relationship with my primary partner we fought all the time; now we rarely fight and it does not take long to solve or agree to disagree and move on.

Jaime: I approached living with my partner very closely to how I approached living with nonpartner roommates. That is, beforehand we sat down and planned out how housekeeping and cooking would get done, who would contribute what amount of money to household expenses, what activities are and are not permitted in the house, etc. What hurts our relationship is that our standards and methods of housekeeping are not the same, and this is exacerbated by the fact that I am a woman and he is a man. We've been socialized on the matter differently, and then when we see ourselves playing out these stereotypical, harmful gender roles, it adds even more stress to the relationship, aside from the fact that I do more than my share of housekeeping and often ask him to please keep up with his.

This is not to say that I've never lived with messy women; I have, and that is also stressful. The gendered aspect of it really is problematic for us, though, and the fact that we are partners, not just roommates. If we continue to live together, we intend to hire someone to do the cleaning once I have a full-time job and we can afford it. I am totally willing to exchange money for peace in my relationship. I tell you, the next partner I live with must be as tidy as I am. I can't spend my life like this.

Jordan: It really is hard to find people who feel as strongly as I do about a lot of social issues. And it does become a barrier, because I cringe when a partner calls something "crazy" or doesn't understand why something is misogynistic. A big part of becoming more outspoken has also involved being more confident about advocating for myself, and I can't be in relationships with people who don't respect that.

Efia: A single person goes through an infinite number of transitions in life from child to adult, active to inactive, unemployed to employed, nonsexual to sexual, etc. It only makes sense that it's twice as difficult when two or more people decide to combine their experiences, finances, living space, food choices, and whatever else to coexist without undoing everything they've done to become distinct individuals who are trying to establish some identity away from their families or particular upbringing. Once you have a pretty firm grasp on who you are or might be, why in the world would anyone want you to change? Compromise, unconditional love, and acceptance are the hardest things to realize and exercise in relationships, I think.

HOW HAS SEXUAL ABUSE AND/OR PHYSICAL VIOLENCE AFFECTED YOUR RELATIONSHIPS?

Jordan: Cultural acceptance of sexual assault and violence has made it really complicated for me to talk to partners. I fear discussing my rapes with partners because I think, even when my partners are good people, that I will encounter "Why didn't you do this?" "Why didn't you report it?" "Was it really rape?" It means that I can't talk with my partners about why sometimes I freeze up, or shut down, why certain things trigger me, why sometimes I really do not feel like being physically intimate at all. I always feel like I have to hide part of myself in my relationships and as a result it makes it really hard for me to be fully invested on an emotional level because I am constantly performing. And it makes me question how much I can expect a partner to give when I cannot and will not give all of myself.

Astrid: I have been married twice (with a child from my second marriage). I have been beaten by both of my husbands and raped (only once, at least as far as I remember) by my first husband.

I am trying to not let the past experience of physical violence impact my sex life. Much of this abuse I try to simply forget. I have been working with a wonderful, caring therapist ever since my second marriage came to an end, and I am quite confident that I won't fall into the same traps again. Perhaps I am now too cautious and have blocked decent, kind possible partners from my life in the last years—but I'd rather err on the side of caution these days.

It is strange how time can heal. I am forty-seven years old and at least the rape I encountered is more than twenty years in the past. I am convinced there will be more men, more relationships, even some playfulness in my life in the years ahead. The older I get, the more I enjoy sex and the less vulnerable I feel. Perhaps it helps that I have learned to pick better and to say no. Perhaps it is a cheap fix to try to shut out of my mind, as best as I can, those past experiences of violence. But I cannot—I just *cannot*—allow the men who hurt me in the past to take away the pleasure in sex that I am looking forward to in years to come.

Gemma: He was only the second person I ever had sex with. He played rugby with my best guy friend. I wanted to have sex with him. I'd been flirting with him for weeks, and I was excited when it finally seemed to have paid off.

But once we were in my room, it wasn't what I had been hoping for at all. He was really forceful. He held my arms down at my sides; he pushed me onto the bed facedown at one point. I didn't think it was okay to stop him at that point, because I didn't want to seem like I was a prude who couldn't handle a little rough stuff. But I tried to draw the line when he wanted to take off the condom I'd put on him. Unfortunately he didn't listen to me.

I was so confused by it, because it didn't seem to fit a "normal" definition of sexual assault. I couldn't reconcile the fact that I'd said yes to the sex but no to sex without a condom. I didn't realize until two years later that that wasn't okay. I went to a counselor on campus right after it happened and he asked me all these questions about what I was wearing, what I did and said—

things that made me feel like I'd made it happen. (I didn't go back to the counseling center until I was a senior.) At the time I was a resident assistant, and I had a hard time asking for help because it was my job to help other students.

I got into my first serious relationship senior year, after a couple of random hookups that I think I engaged in mostly to prove I was still okay with sex. I told him about it the night we were roughhousing on my bed, and he ended up on top of me. He jokingly said, "What am I gonna do with you now that I have you here?" I felt like I needed to explain why I looked so scared.

It was there all the time for years. I hated being anywhere but on top during sex at first. I hated being in crowds, where it felt like other people's bodies were restricting my movement. It was like a third person in the bed with every partner. Finally, about eight years after it happened, I got sick of that. I can't say I'm over it—you never are—but I made a decision *not* to assume every guy has the potential to be *that* guy, to *not* be nervous and scared, and it has helped. So has talking about it, to friends, partners, and a counselor.

I had an experience just a few months ago that scared me, but for a different reason. I was with a guy who I've known for about seven years. We ended up in bed and it was a little like déjà vu—very forceful, very rough stuff, and not in a way that was sexy or fun at all. I stopped him and made him leave, and he didn't seem to understand that shoving me around and penetrating me so hard that I bled wasn't okay. What scared me about it most was that I knew he'd done it before and would do it again, and maybe with someone who wouldn't feel like she could make him stop. I'm lucky I could. I'm not better than anyone else because I could. I'm really just lucky.

It's there all the time—anytime I hear about a person who's been the victim of sexual assault and hear people asking what she was wearing or why she was walking home alone at night. I make it my business to speak up when I hear that. I don't necessarily tell my own story, but I speak out against victim blaming whenever I hear it, because I'll always remember that counselor who asked me what I was wearing.

Heidi: I have an alarm system that comes with a remote control panic button that I sleep with, which will dial a close friend's number if I push it, because I am still afraid he will make good on his threats to take my daughter.

In a relationship, I have trouble giving up control. Sexually, I cannot let go enough to really enjoy myself, and I am therefore content to abstain from sex. I need to have my own money and I kept my own bank account even when I was married, which I am told is a smart thing to do, but I did it because I did not trust my spouse to pay the bills. I was afraid that I would end up getting evicted yet again. I don't care about little decisions—what movie we watch, where we go for dinner, things like that—but when it comes to big decisions, if I feel as though I was not allowed to make the decision to a large extent, I end up getting extremely nervous.

I also can get triggered rather easily. If a person I am with gets angry or has a behavior that seems aggressive, even if they are playing around, I get very nervous and can have panic attacks. I consider myself to be a very strong person, and I am very vocal in my feminist beliefs and active in the community with antiviolence awareness campaigns, but when something triggers me I can feel so small and insecure again, regardless of how far I have come.

Nidea: I got separated from my parents and I got lost. We always had a safe spot in case that happened, usually in front of the store. I sat there and waited for my parents, a bit frightened because this was the first time it had ever happened to me. I was a little girl who knew no English in this huge store, but someone found me. A man, a bit older than my father, he knew Spanish and somewhat comforted me. As he spoke to me, he would touch me. I didn't understand what he was doing, his hands moving all along my legs and under my skirt. I didn't know what to think; he was saying many nice things to me but at the same time he was touching me. Maybe that was the way in America. No one seemed to notice so I thought maybe it isn't bad. I was in a crowded department store. If it was bad someone would say something, right? By the time my parents came, he wasn't touching me anymore. My parents thanked him, and I got yelled at for getting lost. I got sneakers that day, Patrick Ewing sneakers. Those sneakers always carried those memories attached to them.

Soon after, I met some of my distant cousins. They touched me every single time they visited. In the beginning it was more like a brush against my breasts or my butt. Then they wanted to bathe together, told me it was normal. We were cousins and this was what cousins did in America. It didn't feel bad, but I felt bad, I didn't know why. I wanted it to stop but they would just hurt me; they were older.

One day, my mother had a talk with me. A girl I used to go to school with got raped while waiting for the bus to go to school. My mother then had the sex conversation, what was rape and why it was wrong. The whole purity thing, staying a virgin until you marry, not letting anyone touch you. When you buy something from the store you want it new, right? Not used. I then realized how disgusting I was, how used and violated I had been. I didn't know what to do with myself and just got angry. I would hurt myself; I even attempted suicide. My parents didn't really understand what was going on with me. I was always a quiet child, so I didn't say a word. I just wanted to die.

My boyfriend of four years was willing to understand. I bared my soul and in return he taught me how to love myself, touch myself, and accept myself. But even at times when we were the most intimate with each other, when we wanted to touch each other, I would struggle. I would cry and he just let me. He was sometimes frightened, he didn't know how to deal with it. Sometimes I would be scared of the slightest touch, and to an extent I think it hurt him.

Rebeka: I just want to say thank you for telling this story. A very similar thing happened to me, and to this day I feel disgusted with myself. The whole "it felt good but it was wrong" thing was exactly how I was feeling. I can't have sex out of fear of being touched. Your story gives me hope that I can make it through, and it really helps to know that I am not alone.

Nasir: I too had a cousin who touched me inappropriately a few times one summer. I didn't keep it in, though. I told *everybody* that it was happening, and my mom and aunties dealt with him and the situation quickly. What makes me sad, frustrated, and upset is that the way my cousin was dealt with and the way I was able to say something at age twelve before things really got out of hand is not the norm. I unfortunately know several people who were the victims of rape and sexual assault or abuse who kept it inside for a long time. No one should ever have to deal with that kind of trauma, especially at a young age.

WHAT HAS HELPED THE PROCESS OF HEALING FROM SEXUAL OR OTHER ABUSE?

Nidea: Something that is very difficult but helps so much is to learn how to love yourself for who you are. I really wish I could say definitely when these feelings would go away, but sometimes these feelings come back. But don't let them affect the way you want to live; don't let those who caused you harm be so powerful.

Some of the things that have helped me through this: reading, learning about how other people have coped. Also, music has helped me a lot. I have my feel-good playlist with nothing but positive music: songs by India.Arie, Mary J Blige, and even "Beautiful" by Christina Aguilera.

Natasha: What has helped me heal the most have been my partnership/marriage with my late spouse and my therapist of the last six years. My spouse respected my boundaries, always was concerned about my pleasure, and was happy for me to take the lead.

My current therapist is the first one I could tell everything about the date assaults I survived when I was a young woman, and has supported me in developing my creative gifts in writing, music, and art. I remember taking self-defense and karate classes in my early and late twenties. Both were very important in increasing my self-confidence and facilitating my healing.

Jaime: Time. Feminism. The abuse inflicted upon me was relatively mild, short in duration, and after childhood; it was a partner nonphysically forcing and manipulating me into having sex when I didn't want to or to have kinds of sex I didn't want to. I was eighteen at the time. What I mean to say is that it could have been worse. I didn't recognize it as abuse for a little bit, just as a bad relationship.

With time, it's faded, and I've been able to take it as a learning experience, so that I won't find myself with another partner who does that. And if I should find myself there, I'll recognize it for what it is and GTFO.

I mostly confide in the Internet—the anonymity makes this easier. I'm known as a bit of a strong, stoic woman in real life, so telling most friends and family would make me uncomfortable. I have told a couple of my partners, so that they could avoid doing things that trigger me. The Internet has been the most important resource in my healing. Feminist sites allow me a community, remind me that I'm not at fault, tell

me it gets better, give me vocabularies, and help me process.

EJM: Being open with close friends helps a lot. I did not follow this advice while I was dealing with sexual/emotional abuse while in college. I am a very private person, and I thought that it was best not to burden my close friends with the things that were happening around me. However, I did see a therapist who helped me gain the courage to end the relationship. It was nice to talk to a stranger and hear an outside perspective.

A year later, when I did finally tell my close friends what had happened, instead of being angry at me for not telling them, they gave me hugs. They were thankful that I was able to find the help I needed. It was a huge relief to be able to tell them, and I realized that my life might have been a lot easier if I had their support and love from the beginning.

I continued to meet with a therapist to help me move on from the nightmarish experience I had. It helped me move on from the constant fear that I felt every day and allowed me to accept different relationships in my life. I'm not saying that therapy was the cure-all. I think I still struggle every day with uncertainty of relationships (Will this person suddenly turn on me and terrorize me? Can I cope with having this happen again?), but it helped to find a very patient and caring therapist who matched my needs and personality.

Lola: I was sexually, emotionally, and at times physically abused by a much older boyfriend from age fifteen to seventeen. Jaime said, "Time. Feminism." Yeah, straight up. For me, "time" meant growing old enough to see the teenage me almost as a little sister. I see photos of me back then and think, "Why would anyone want to hurt her? She didn't mean anyone harm." At the same time, with that tiny bit of maturity, I think of telling myself that I couldn't have stopped it or done anything more than I could have at the time. There's a lot of forgiveness there, and peace, that was hard-won.

"Feminism" was definitely the other piece. Being able to connect the personal ("it was just a bad relationship") to the political (violence against women, the overlying tropes of hegemony, power, and consent with older men/younger women) was an enormous relief when I was still unable to give myself the forgiveness I needed and helped me see myself in a larger struggle. It meant not being alone.

Also, I have to say, plain speaking was enormous: just finding the courage to say what happened without using the same tone of voice as you would use at a funeral. Stigma sucks, and for me, at least, I felt released by not acting like it was some big secret. Similarly, I was inspired by an "I was raped" shirt and hope to be strong enough one day to wear one of my own. [The shirts were created in 2008 as part of a rape awareness project.]

HOW HAS GROWING OLDER AFFECTED YOUR RELATIONSHIPS OR WHAT YOU LOOK FOR IN A RELATIONSHIP?

Gemma: I just turned thirty in December, and while I went back and forth between whether or not it was a "big deal," I did make a decision. This was going to be the year, I decided, that I stopped making excuses for guys.

I have had a tendency to give a lot in relationships, to think that I could do something, I could do more, I could try harder to make things work. This is not to say that I shouldn't have to work—I think both people have to—but I definitely have gotten into situations before where, even though I wasn't conscious of it, I was doing way more than my share of the work and really beating myself up when things didn't get better.

I would settle for being the other person's option when he was my priority. And in most cases, *he* would end things with me, and I'd be saying to myself, "Now, why didn't I break that off sooner myself?"

So as I have gotten a little older, I have tried to stop saying, "He probably didn't call because he was busy" or "He probably didn't mean it like that" or "It's no big deal that he forgot I was lactose intolerant even though we've been dating for almost two years" (that actually happened). I think I am doing a better job of valuing myself and being frank about what I want in a partner—and not feeling bad when I have to say no. I am becoming more comfortable with the fact that it is better to be single and look carefully for a good partner than to just have any partner at all.

Francesca: I am approaching forty-nine and have not been in a relationship for more than twenty years. Having never been married, I often now truly wonder if marriage is something I desire. With aging for me comes a sense that I will experience an increased sense of freedom and exploration in this phase of my life. I am now more interested in making intimate connections that have nothing to do with sex before the possibility of sex occurs.

Jordan: I've noticed that as I have grown older, I've gotten a lot less tolerant of, well, to put it frankly, bullshit. When I was younger, I had more of a tendency to be accepting of things that I would find unacceptable now; I would shrink myself to become smaller and less outspoken, for example, and the opinions of the friends of a partner were really important to me. Now I don't really care what people might think of me, and I won't compromise myself. If I have a partner who does or says something I disagree with, I say so, bluntly. I don't stay silent and seethe. And I'm much more choosy about partners in the first place. I don't like to use the word "settle," because it has some bad connotations, but I won't overlook things that I know will become deal breakers later on like I used to do.

I think that this has happened because I've grown into myself much more. I'm perfectly comfortable being alone (as I am now) and prefer it to being in a relationship that doesn't make me happy.

Mags: As I have grown older, I have explored outside the norm. I have been with other women because of a curiosity that I have had since I was younger, but due to the home I was raised in, it was not acceptable to love another person of the same sex. Unfortunately, I do not feel comfortable enough to talk this over with my family because of them being so judgmental and thinking that same-sex relationships are [for] people who are confused or because they were in a bad relationship.

Sophia: Now that my husband and I are approaching our fifties and looking at being empty nesters, we find that we are rediscovering each other in different ways. We don't have the energy or the bodies we had when we were younger. We aren't moving around because of career choices. Our relationship has grown and matured. We are definitely more relaxed with each other and our lives. We enjoy each other's touch and caress, and reach climax or orgasm slower, and sometimes experience it longer. We don't feel as though we have to do everything together as a couple, but we enjoy being a couple. I am glad we are growing old together.

Cecilia: When *Our Bodies, Ourselves* first appeared, I learned to think about my about my body as being sexual. The idea of taking a mirror to see what I looked like "down there" was literally revolutionary. Each year I've gotten older and wiser—and sexier. Now, at sixty-three, I have to begin to think about the next twenty-plus years when the sexy parts of our bodies lose their form. In the past six months I had a startling body change. I lost a lot of weight very fast, and at the same time suffered nearly crippling muscle loss due to a statin drug. My strong, fit, curvy body—one I was proud of—suddenly had loose, wrinkled, empty skin hanging all over it. It was painful to roll over in bed; raising my arms or bending my knees was too uncomfortable to do if I was trying to find physical pleasure.

My husband was wonderful about it, truly concerned about my health and apparently able to get past whatever the visual experience was so that I never felt any hesitation from him about physical intimacy. This month my health has returned; I'm able to exercise, I'm gaining strength, and I think the skin will tighten up to some degree over the next year. But mine will never be a middle-aged body again.

And I have become fascinated by it. Just to get to know it better, I've started taking photographs of my naked self in the mirror—close-ups of the wrinkles, side shots where my chest is nearly flat and my once whistle-inducing ass has disappeared. I don't dislike it, probably because I came into the change with a contented attitude about myself, but it definitely is an adjustment for both my husband and me. My sexuality hasn't diminished, but I think to look at me, one would assume a considerably lower sex drive than I have. My husband says although there is less of me, I feel much the same. I don't quite believe that, but if his senses do, I'm not going to interfere.

I'm also very reassured by this because I can now imagine our physical life as an elderly couple and I can imagine how it will be fulfilling. And what a luxury it is, as I get older, to enjoy the freedom of not feeling I have to work, work, work at everything—just enjoy what I am.

DO YOU FEEL AFFECTED BY RELATIONSHIP TIME LINES?

Nina: I had this idea that I would be married by twenty-five and on my first baby by twenty-eight. I am twenty-five right now and I have been single for the last six years. I used to beat myself up for it, but my mom reminded me of all I have accomplished in my twenty-five years. I feel more equipped now to emotionally handle the kind of relationship I want. I don't think it's an issue of an accepted time line. I think it's up to each individual to determine which time line is good for them.

Faith: As a young person, I feel that when you meet someone who is attracted to you and you are attracted to, you're supposed to instantly act on that physically. This is the feeling I get through dating and talking to friends on college campuses, at any rate. I've always found the whole thing really confusing. For a nontraditional person, I consider myself very traditional when it comes to dating. Mostly, this is just because I like dating. I like the "getting-to-know-you" parts, I like the awkwardness, I like the suspense. However, now it seems more and more like "hanging out" is replacing dating, and there's some sort of sexual expectation that comes with just hanging out in someone's apartment.

Nasir: I agree. There was a sexual time line in my teens and a relationship time line once I hit my midtwenties. The sexual time line to me was more subtle in the sense that you kinda knew where you fit in relation to others your age, but not really, because people lied about how sexually active they were. As for the relationship time line, I feel like I'm way ahead of schedule, being married at twenty-eight. My plan was to start thinking about marriage at thirty, and hopefully be married before thirty-five.

Jaime: My mother is so convinced I'll get married and have kids, though I keep informing her it's not happening. My grandmother (mom's mom) passed last fall, and after the funeral, my mom sorta gave me Grandma's wedding and engagement rings (I'm the oldest granddaughter). That is, she told me that I would get them when I got married. I reminded her it's not happening and suggested that I might have them at some set age if I was then still unmarried. Since then my mom has said I could have the wedding band now and the engagement ring when I get engaged. Which is an improvement.

Lola: As I get older, I also notice that being poly and queer—both identifying as such and being perceived as such—is getting paradoxically both harder and easier. It's getting harder because there is more of a push to get "on the track"—one partner, long term, preferably opposite gendered, engaged in three years, married a year after that, kids within five years after that. It's getting easier for two reasons. First, well, I stand out more. A lot more. In some ways I feel like I'm going to be the last woman standing and I'm afraid that people are going to start yelling louder for me to grow up and get heterosexual and monogamous. Second, and this is more of a positive, I am starting, iota by iota, to figure out who I am, and feel more strength to be that person.

CHAPTER 6 ■

Something I really love about sex is the way it makes me feel alive and at home in my body. . . . It's kind of amazing to realize how much pleasure I can experience in this body.

Sexuality is a state of being, a way of experiencing and giving pleasure to ourselves and others. It has the potential to be a powerful and positive force, deepening our most intimate connections; it also can be a source of great pain. Not everyone has, or wants, sexual feelings. This, too, is part of the range of experiences.

This chapter looks at how sexuality develops through individual desire as well as social and cultural influences. It includes the voices of many women who have shared their diverse experiences around sex and sexuality.

SOCIAL INFLUENCES

What influences sexuality? Nearly everything. Child-rearing practices, government policies, religion, media images, pharmaceutical companies, drug advertisements, violence, and sexual abuse—all these affect how we experience sexuality. Stereotypes based on race, class, gender and gender identity, age, relationship status, disability, and sexual orientation also play a role. Understanding the social and personal influences on our sexuality can help us claim our right to pleasure.

Our sexual desires may reflect social influences and contradictions. For example, a particular sexual act may feel affirming in one situation but degrading in another. You might think someone whistling at you on the street is crude but also enjoy the attention. Or you might fantasize about sexual acts you've been told, or believe, are taboo. It's not uncommon to feel conflicted about what you want sexually. Sometimes it takes time and experience to know what we want and how and when to set boundaries.

GROWING UP

In an ideal world, we would all grow up with adults who talk comfortably and openly about sex and respect our boundaries. If we learn to think of sex as bad and shameful, or if we experience childhood sexual abuse or violence, it may take years of positive experiences later on to heal the relationship with our bodies and sex.

Most of us who experience or are assigned a female gender learn at a young age that we are supposed to make ourselves beautiful and sexy in order to become objects of (boys') desire—but not to enjoy our bodies, not to have desires ourselves. We may come to fear that having desires will automatically lead us into risky sexual behaviors that will, in turn, lead to unwanted

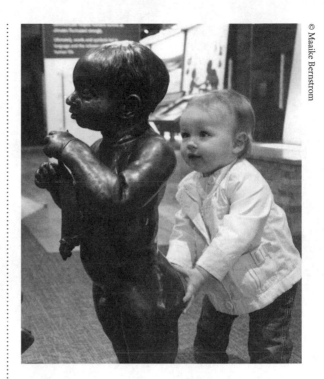

© Maaike Bernstrom

pregnancy, sexually transmitted infections, or sexual assault.

These fears are instilled in us by a culture that sees female sexuality as dangerous and dirty. When we become aware of our desires, we are in a better position to choose whether and how to act on them, and to protect ourselves from risks.

VIRGINITY

The term "virginity" doesn't mean anything, really, but people still use the word like we all know what it means.

Cultural notions of virginity have long shaped sexual attitudes and practices for young women on the verge of exploring sex. A virgin is most commonly considered someone who hasn't had sex—heterosexual intercourse, specifically.

"USES OF THE EROTIC: THE EROTIC AS POWER"

Audre Lorde (1934-1992) was, in her own words, "black, lesbian, mother, warrior, poet." Her powerful essay "Uses of the Erotic: The Erotic as Power" is excerpted here.

The erotic is a resource within each of us that lies in a deeply female and spiritual plane, firmly rooted in the power of our unexpressed or unrecognized feeling. . . .

The erotic functions for me in several ways, and the first is in providing the power which comes from sharing deeply any pursuit with another person. The sharing of joy, whether physical, emotional, psychic, or intellectual, forms a bridge between the sharers which can be the basis for understanding much of what is not shared between them, and lessens the threat of their difference.

Another important way in which the erotic connection functions is the open and fearless underlining of my capacity for joy. In the way my body stretches to music and opens into response, hearkening to its deepest rhythms, so that every level upon which I sense also opens to the erotically satisfying experience, whether it is dancing, building a bookcase, writing a poem, examining an idea.

That self-connection shared is a measure of the joy which I know myself to be capable of feeling, a reminder of my capacity for feeling. And that deep and irreplaceable knowledge of my capacity for joy comes to demand from all of my life that it be lived within the knowledge that such satisfaction is possible, and does not have to be called *marriage,* nor *god,* nor *an afterlife.* . . .

When we begin to live from within outward, in touch with the power of the erotic within ourselves, and allowing that power to inform and illuminate our actions upon the world around us, then we begin to be responsible to ourselves in the deepest sense. For as we begin to recognize our deepest feelings, we begin to give up, of necessity, being satisfied with suffering and self-negation, and with the numbness which so often seems like their only alternative in our society. . . .

In touch with the erotic, I become less willing to accept powerlessness, or those other supplied states of being which are not native to me, such as resignation, despair, self-effacement, depression, self-denial.

And yes, there is a hierarchy. There is a difference between painting a black fence and writing a poem, but only one of quantity. And there is, for me, no difference between writing a good poem and moving into sunlight against the body of a woman I love.[1]

Young women in particular are burdened with conflicting pressures about virginity. On the one hand, popular culture promotes an everyone's-doing-it attitude that can make young women feel something's wrong with them if they're not ready to have sex. On the other, morality messages shame young women into "saving themselves" for marriage.

Jessica Valenti, author of *The Purity Myth: How America's Obsession with Virginity Is Hurting Young Women*, writes about the troubling dynamics of federally funded purity balls (father/daughter dances where girls pledge their virginity to their dads, who promise to protect it until a suitable husband comes along) and abstinence-only programs that compare girls' bodies to wrapped lollipops that become unwanted when used. "While young women are subject to overt sexual messages every day," notes Valenti, "they're simultaneously being taught—by the people who are supposed to care for their personal and moral development, no less—that their only real worth is their virginity and ability to remain 'pure.' "

Also troubling is the messaging about who can attain such purity. The girls most often presented by the abstinence-only movement as examples to idolize are white, are straight, and fit a narrow beauty ideal. "Women of color, low-income women, immigrant women—these are the women who are not seen as worthy of being placed on a pedestal," adds Valenti.

Complicating attitudes further is the pressure to make "the first time" meaningful in every way. A young college student says:

Particularly for girls, there is pressure coming from two opposite ends: the pressure to "lose it" and the pressure to lose it "in the right way." I don't think guys feel that "right way" bit as much.

You may choose to abstain from intercourse and/or other sexual activities for any number of reasons, including just not being ready. You have the right to say no to someone who is pushing you to have sex, and the right to say yes to sex that is pleasurable and responsible:

It's not that I am waiting for marriage, or even for the "right" guy to come along. It isn't that I don't

Recommended Reading: For a fascinating analysis of the cultural construct of virginity, read *Virgin: The Untouched History* by Hanne Blank (Bloomsbury USA, 2007).

like to look sexy and that I don't enjoy flirting or being sexual. It's just that I haven't had sex. I haven't been in the position with a person where I am comfortable and feel safe. For some reason being a virgin in high school is relatively normal, but being a virgin in college seems to have as much of a stigma as being a "slut" does.

If sex were not such a taboo subject, comprehensive sexuality education would not only cover birth control and sexually transmitted infections, but also make room for discussions about pleasure and enthusiastic consent (topics

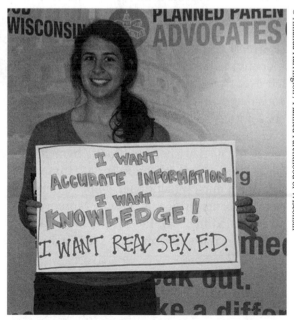

© Amanda Harrington / Planned Parenthood of Wisconsin

The traditional definition of virginity is limiting or even irrelevant for many of us.

As Cara Kulwicki, founder and editor of the curvature.com, notes; "The concept of 'virginity' devalues sexual activity between two partners who cannot engage in penis-in-vagina intercourse, and it devalues female pleasure by focusing on an activity that does not in itself tend to stimulate the clitoris, the most common source of sexual pleasure for women."[2]

that are covered in depth in the next chapter). When women are shamed into always saying no, and men are pressured to always say yes, we all miss out on experiencing our full sexual selves.

Can Anyone Tell?

There is no reliable way for anyone to tell by looking at a woman's genitals whether she has been sexually active. The hymen, more recently referred to as the vaginal corona, a tiny bit of mucous membrane at the opening of the vagina left over from the vagina's development, is often considered an indicator of virginity, but its presence doesn't have any real significance. And not everyone has one.

"Some girls are born without a hymen," says Carol Roye, a nursing professor at Hunter College and a nurse-practitioner, while "others have only a scanty fringe of tissue. Moreover, for all its fabled mystery, the hymen is just a body part."[3] For more information, see "Vaginal Corona," p. 7.

While the hymen can be torn during sex or other physical activity, it doesn't "break." Torn areas can bleed, but it doesn't always happen.

It is also impossible to tell if someone has had sex by how her body looks, how she walks or sits, or by any other means.

STEREOTYPES

Media images and messages often reinforce stereotypes about sexuality. For example, Latina characters on TV shows and in films are often dressed in tight, revealing clothes, while Muslim women are covered head to toe and depicted as repressed. African-American women are often cast as hypersexual when young and asexual when they're older. And media portrayals of African-American men and women in loving relationships are almost entirely absent from popular culture:

What are the young ladies thinking and feeling when the only women who resemble them are shaking their ass in front of the camera for LiL Wayne and Drake? What are the media telling us about African-American women? That we are only good to be video vixens and single.

Racism, which often limits representations of color, exacerbates such stereotypes.

Other stereotypes arise from sexism and general fear of difference. Lesbians are often portrayed as aggressive man-haters; bisexuals as promiscuous, because they refuse to be boxed into an either-or definition of sexual attraction; and trans people as confused, hypersexual, or deceitful. Those of us who express sexuality and sexual desire openly may find ourselves called sluts. Slut shaming is frequently used against young women who are believed to have had sex (even in monogamous relationships) and women who have (or have had) more than one partner. It may also be used as a slur for other reasons:

Those girls, I learned, were nearly every girl—not only the ones who showed interest in sex or had sex . . . but the ones who wore skimpy clothing, read fashion magazines, drank, dated, flirted, or had any investment in finding a partner.

These and other destructive stereotypes influence the ways we do (or don't) assert our desires and the ways we judge ourselves and other women. They affect how others treat us and, when we internalize them and believe them, how we treat ourselves.

In reality, there are enormous differences in sexual experiences and attitudes among women within any racial, cultural, gender, or sexual identity. We can begin to free up the range of sexual values and expression available to *all* of us by approaching one another ready to listen and learn.

BODY IMAGE

We often see ourselves through the eyes of others. Influenced by popular images, we may lose respect for our uniqueness and end up judging ourselves harshly. This can have a negative effect on the ways we express ourselves and the risks we take:

For years I wouldn't make love in a position that exposed my backside to scrutiny, for I had been told it was "too jiggly." Needless to say, this prevented me from being sexually assertive and creative and limited my responses.

We have a good sex life with lots of variety, fantasies, games. The fact that my disability prevents me from bending my leg limits us in some positions, but we just try different ones. Yet . . . I am still struggling with my body. When I am unclothed, I still feel like parts of me are really ugly. I think that when I can finish mourning and cry out my anguish over the disability, then sex will get better for me.

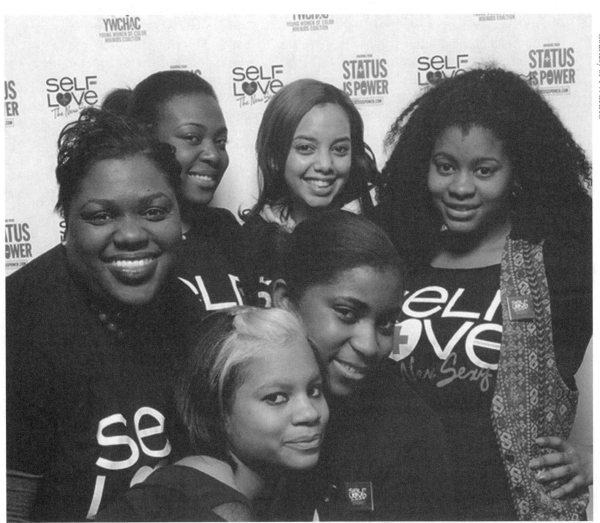

Members of the Young Women of Color HIV/AIDS Coalition at the 2010 Teen Health & Wellness Film Festival in New York City. Learn more at statusispower.com.

Sometimes we find ourselves in the difficult position of trying to help our partners overcome their own negative feelings:

While I love my girlfriend's body without reservation, and think she looks damn sexy in most clothes (not to mention achingly beautiful naked), I know—in part because I've felt that way myself—that when you're feeling lumpish and fat no amount of affirmation from a partner or other friend/family member is going to help drown out those voices in your head. In part this is because we're relentlessly told by media and medical "experts" that not conforming to our culture's physical standards of beauty isn't just unfortunate—it's somehow immoral. I don't have a lot of authority, as just one person (who's blinded by love to boot), to counteract those omnipresent voices of cultural authority that say, "You're bad, you're wrong, you're not beautiful, you're unworthy."

Acceptance that comes from within can be the most satisfying. Getting to where we can block out the damaging messages frees us to love ourselves and our partners more fully:

One of the difficult things about being large is that more often than not other people are the problem, not me. Many times I have felt that people I know wonder at my friendship with my lover. They wonder how a thin person can make love to a large one. The idea, I suppose, is that large women aren't attractive. Nonsense, of course. I enjoy my body immensely when I make love, either to myself or my boyfriend. I never think about my largeness. I simply am it and positively luxuriate in it.

As a woman, and particularly as a trans woman, I sometimes find it difficult to forget all the messages from society and the media about what I'm "supposed to" look like. The possibility that my body can give me pleasure—regardless of whether or not I think I'm thin enough or my breasts are big enough or I'm too tall—is really wonderful.

For further discussion, see Chapter 3, "Body Image"; and "What Is It Like to Be in a Relationship When You Don't Like Some or All of Your Own Body?" p. 114.

POWER

Power differences often play out in sex. Even if you feel equal to a male partner, the culture we live in generally values men more. A female sexual partner may also have more power or status than you because of earning power, level of education, class, race, or other factors. If you are transgender, non-trans lovers may have more respect in society because they operate within the context of a widely accepted gender identity. Though a partner may not acknowledge or even feel that there's a power differential, such privileges can surface in sex, resulting in the following responses:

- You feel you should have sex when your partner wants to, whether you're in the mood or not.
- You feel you should have orgasms to validate your partner.
- You feel you shouldn't ask for what you want, especially if it's different from what your partner is doing.
- You feel you shouldn't use protection if it interferes with your partner's pleasure, even if this leaves you unprotected against sexually transmitted infections.
- If you have a male partner and are sexual without having intercourse, you feel you should help him have an orgasm to relieve his sexual tensions.

"HOW DO YOU FUCK A FAT WOMAN?"

From Kate Harding's essay in Yes Means Yes! Visions of Female Sexual Power and a World Without Rape.

When you are a fat woman in this culture, *everyone*–from journalists you'll never meet to your own mother, sister, and best friend–works together to constantly reinforce the message that you are not good enough to be fucked, let alone loved. . . .

We shouldn't have to devote so much mental energy to the exhausting work of *not hating ourselves*. . . .

Imagine for a minute a world in which fat women don't automatically disqualify themselves from the dating game. A world in which fat women don't believe there's anything intrinsically unattractive about their bodies. A world in which fat women hear that men want only thin women and laugh our asses off, because that is not remotely our experience–our experience is one of loving and fucking and navigating a big damn world in our big damn bodies with grace and optimism and power.

Now try to imagine some halfwit dickhead telling you a rapist would be doing you a favor, in that world . . . imagine a man telling you that you can't leave him, because no one else will ever want your disgusting fat ass.

None of that makes a lick of sense in that world, does it?

It doesn't in this one, either.

Imagine if more of us could believe that.[5]

- If you have a male partner and have intercourse, you feel you should take care of birth control, or you shouldn't use birth control at all if your partner doesn't want you to.

Becoming aware of how externally created dynamics may play out is an important step toward developing respectful and mutually satisfying sexual relationships where consent matters:

[I don't want] a partner who doesn't know that because he's male, his partners don't always tell him when he does things sexually that they'd rather not participate in. After one disastrous relationship with a fellow who was a jerk and didn't have any idea about privilege, I wrote, "Isn't a patriarchal fuckhead" on my list of qualities I desired in future partners.

VIOLENCE AGAINST WOMEN

It is a cruel fact that many women experience or witness abuse—most often from men, but also from women. Childhood sexual abuse, rape, sexual harassment, homophobic or transphobic attacks, battering in our homes—any of these can affect our sexual lives. Even if we don't experience violence directly, the fear of being assaulted, or disturbing news stories or media images, can prevent us from feeling comfortable with sexual partners:

I always feel like I have to hide part of myself in my relationships, and as a result it makes it really hard for me to be fully invested on an emotional level because I am constantly performing. And it makes me question how much I can expect a partner to give when I cannot and will not give all of myself. The actions of rapists do not stop with the rape. They reverberate and echo and

WHEN A PARTNER HAS EXPERIENCED SEXUAL ABUSE

Joan and Allison, together for ten years and married for three, offer their experiences in a relationship in which one partner has experienced sexual abuse

Joan: I am a survivor of physical violence and sexual abuse in my childhood. I attend a support group with other women who are survivors of sexual assault and abuse. Several of the women in the group say they wish they could be a lesbian like me, because it must be easier. All of us were abused by men. I tell them that while my wife does understand some things about my experiences better by virtue of being a woman, it is still difficult for me to avoid triggering my post-traumatic stress disorder and panic attacks during sex. I have friends who talk about monogamy being boring, "vanilla," or oppressive. But I like the stable certainty of monogamy. I don't trust anyone but my wife to touch me intimately.

Allison: Through our relationship, I am also hurt indirectly by the abuse. I want to be very clear that the pain and damage to me are much less severe than that suffered by my wife. She is the one who was abused, and nothing like that has ever happened to me. However, I feel that the perspective of partners of survivors of sexual abuse needs to be represented as well.

When we were first dating, my wife told me she had been abused. I knew that it would be difficult for her to heal, and that this would take a long time. But I wasn't prepared for the fact that some scars are permanent. After ten years of watching her try every medical, mental health, and alternative tactic, I have come to realize that she will never be able to be the person she could have been if she had not been abused. In many ways, she is stronger and more self-aware than a person who has not had to deal with abuse. But she is also anxious, depressed, suffering from post-traumatic stress disorder, and easily frightened during sex. This is in no way her fault. It is something that was done to her, and it pisses me off. I feel helpless because there is nothing I can do to make it better.

I feel that I can never completely relax around my wife, because I have a long mental list of things not to say and places not to touch, so as to avoid triggering anxiety and panic. When we sleep beside each other in bed, there is only one spot, the size of an index card, where I can rest my hand on her body. . . . Sex can be difficult for my wife, and this has been hard on our relationship. She frequently needs to stop during sex. When we are having sex, I always have to hold back to avoid startling her, and because she might want to stop at any moment. This makes it hard for me to get into sex and let my arousal build naturally.

I feel bad for wanting more of her than she has to give. . . . I certainly bring my share of problems to our relationship, too, and she has to deal with them. I'm not doing her a favor; she doesn't owe me anything for my "tolerance." I'm willing to compromise my sexual fulfillment, because in return I get to be married to my caring, funny, intelligent wife, whom I love very much.

continue—what these people did to me is with me for life.

If you have been abused, a sudden touch or gesture from a partner—even one who would never dream of causing harm—can trigger what some call the "sexual alarm system"[6] and cause you to tense up. You may have to show a partner how to disarm the system—for example, by warming up with gentle touching or intimate conversation. It's essential that you go at your own pace and find friends or other supportive people who can help you through this.

More women speak about how they have coped with violence or an abusive relationship, and its effect on later relationships, on pp. 132–137, and in Chapter 24, "Violence Against Women."

RELIGION AND SPIRITUALITY

Many religions have teachings that seek to prohibit certain sexual thoughts and behaviors, especially outside monogamous heterosexual marriage. These attitudes can leave us with negative feelings about our bodies and sexuality. Growing up in a religion in which spiritual goodness is associated with celibacy or the denial of sexual feelings can lead to the idea that sexuality and spirituality are completely split:

All through my teen years, [my] church leaders stressed sexual purity. While I was busy staying sexually pure and modest, I learned absolutely nothing about my body or how I felt sexually. The guilt and shame stopped me in my tracks, and this did not go away when I married. [Recently] I spent a lot of time on a female-oriented sexuality website. After immersing myself in all this female-friendly sexual literature, I finally got in touch with my sexuality and started enjoying sex.

I was raised in a strict Southern Baptist environment in a small town in southern

Arkansas. I knew I was a lesbian at around nine or ten years old. Having repressed my sexuality until I was twenty-eight was very hard. I had no role models to look to, growing up. In my mind, church and being a lesbian just did not go together. Now I know that sex can be a very spiritual, uplifting experience. I wish I experienced it more.

At the same time, some of us have found positive messages about sexuality within organized religion. A woman who attended Roman Catholic schools says:

I was taught that the body was the "temple of the Holy Spirit," and I thought then, as I think now, that having the spirit of God, however we each define God, dwelling within us is . . . beautiful.

Asra Nomani, a journalist who writes frequently about religion and gender issues, has created an Islamic Bill of Rights for Women in the Bedroom that address key issues for women in many religions. It reads in part:

- *Women have an Islamic right to respectful and pleasurable sexual experience.*
- *Women have an Islamic right to make independent decisions about their bodies, including the right to refuse sexual advances.*
- *Women have an Islamic right to make independent decisions about their choice of a partner.*
- *Women have an Islamic right to make independent decisions about contraception and reproduction.*
- *Women have an Islamic right to protection from physical, emotional, and sexual abuse.*[7]

Some of us leave our religions of origin because of the sexual prohibitions. We may choose not to affiliate with a religion at all, or seek out liberal congregations within our own denominations or other denominations that are more sex-affirming.

Reconstructionist and Reform Jewish congregations, Unitarian Universalism, the United Church of Christ, Metropolitan Community Churches, Wicca, and liberal Quakerism (Society of Friends) have a wider acceptance of women's roles and sexuality and may include female clergy and leaders, recognition of same-sex relationships, and comprehensive sex education.

Drawing upon ancient cultures in which women's bodies, sexuality, and fertility were honored as an integral part of nature and life, many women have found wisdom and strength in connecting sexually with a partner and a sense of divine feminine energy. Others have turned to tantra, an Eastern spiritual philosophy, to explore sexual practices that focus on the interconnectedness of life. By investigating sensations of touch and breathing, creating rituals, and paying attention to subtle energies, some women create a sacred connection with partner(s) and higher power(s).

CELIBACY AND ASEXUALITY

CELIBACY

Traditionally, celibacy has meant choosing not to marry. Today, many people use it to mean not having sex with a partner, and sometimes not even masturbating, for a certain period of time. Some people choose celibacy in response to our culture's overemphasis on sex, as a break from feeling the pressure to relate to others sexually all the time.

One woman who grew tired of always having to say yes or no describes her experience with celibacy:

I'm exploring myself as a sexual person, but in a different way. My sensitivity to my body is heightened. I am more aware of what arouses my sensual interests. I am free to be myself. I have more energy for work and friends. My spirituality feels more intense and clear.

In partnered relationships, we may choose celibacy when we want some distance or solitude, or when we just don't want to have sex for a while. This can require careful communication:

I say to my lover, "I don't feel like making love this month, and I may not next month." Now, who does that? Is it okay? Am I allowed? The last thing we were ever taught was that it was okay to try what we want.

Some couples choose celibacy together. It can help couples break out of old sexual patterns, expand sensual/sexual focus beyond genital sex, and make us feel more self-sufficient and independent—all of which can strengthen a relationship.

ASEXUALITY

Asexuality, a lack of interest in sex, is a natural human variation thought to be experienced by about 1 percent of people.[8] It is not the same as a sudden decline in sexual interest or attraction, which may be linked to side effects of certain medications or illness. (For more on variations of desire and the effects of hormones and medications, see p. 182.)

Reporting on her groundbreaking 2008 study based on interviews with 102 asexuals, Susan Scherrer quotes one woman who doesn't feel sexual attraction: "I love the human form and can regard individuals as works of art and find people aesthetically pleasing, but I don't ever want to come into sexual contact with even the most beautiful of people."

Another woman feels sexual attraction but

not the inclination to act on it: "I am sexually attracted to men but have no desire or need to engage in sexual or even non-sexual activity (cuddling, hand-holding, etc.)."

One woman describes her ideal relationship as "the same as a 'normal' relationship, without the sex. We would be best friends, companions, biggest fans of each other, partners in financial, work, and social areas of our lives. I am very physical. I would like to be able to tackle my lover (as in "I love him" not as in "person I am currently having sex with") to the ground, roll around until I pin him, then plant a kiss on his nose, snuggle into the crook of his arm, and talk about some random topic . . . without him getting an erection or entertaining hopes that this will lead to the removal of clothing or a march to the bedroom."[9]

The Asexual Visibility and Education Network, known as AVEN (asexuality.org), offers asexual people a place to connect and learn. The website identifies several aspects of asexuality:

- Unlike celibacy, which is a choice, asexuality is a sexual orientation.
- Asexuality is not a dysfunction, and there is no need to find a "cause" or a "cure."
- Asexual people have the same emotional needs as everybody else and are just as capable of forming intimate relationships.
- Asexuals are generally very different from one another: some experience romantic attraction, some don't. Some experience arousal, some don't.
- Many asexuals talk about having a "romance drive." They need to be intimate with another special person; it's just that the intimacy they desire isn't sexual.
- It may be more difficult to find someone who is willing to enter into a conventional relationship with the knowledge that sex will not be involved, but remember, there are other people with low or no sex drive out there and many people who care more about love and companionship than they do about sex.

CHAPTER 7

SEXUAL PLEASURE

When I'm feeling turned on, either alone or with someone I'm attracted to, my heart beats faster, my face gets red, my eyes are bright. My whole vulva feels wet and full. My breasts hum. When I'm standing up, I feel a rush of weakness in my thighs. When I'm lying down, I may feel like doing a big stretch, arching my back, feeling the sensations go out to my fingers and toes.

When we are aroused by sexual stimulation, from whatever source—fantasies, a certain image or scent, a partner's word or touch—it's common to go through a series of physical, mental, and emotional changes. These changes are often referred to as "sexual response," though it's probably more accurate to refer to sexual responses, plural.

Although there are some commonalities in how women experience arousal, there are also wide variations. Our responses vary not only from person to person but also at different times in our lives and from one sexual experience to the next. There is no one right pattern of sexual response.

This chapter reviews different models of sexual response, followed by a closer look at how we experience sexual pleasure—both with a partner and on our own. Since pleasure is tied to engaging in positive sexual experiences, the voices of women who are at the forefront of building a movement for enthusiastic consent are included here, along with stories from women who have found safe and supportive ways to express their sexual desires. Practical information, including a comprehensive section on lubricants, is also featured.

MODELS OF SEXUAL RESPONSE

You may want to refer to the description of sexual anatomy starting on p. 4 as you read the following information.

Various sex researchers have developed models that attempt to describe women's sexual responses. In the 1960s, William Masters and Virginia Johnson observed and measured women and men engaging in sexual activities in a laboratory setting, and reported their research in *Human Sexual Response* (1966). The Masters and Johnson model outlined four stages of physiological arousal: excitement, plateau, orgasm, and resolution.

It can be helpful to understand the Masters and Johnson model, not because it fits all women or is a standard you should try to follow, but because aspects of it may fit your experience and because so many clinicians still use it. Here's a breakdown of the four stages.

- **Excitement.** During the first stage of arousal, the whole pelvic area may feel full, as erectile tissue in the pelvis, vulva, and clitoris swells with blood, and nerves in that area become more sensitive to stimulation and pressure.[1] In the vagina, this increased blood circulation produces the fluid (transudate) that makes the vaginal walls and inner lips wet—often an early sign of sexual excitement. Women produce different amounts of lubrication; for some, there may not be much lubrication, or it may come later, after sufficient sexual stimulation. Sexual tension affects the whole body as muscles begin to contract. Women may breathe more quickly or experience little shivers. Nipples may become erect and hard, and a flush or rash may appear on the skin.
- **Plateau.** If stimulation continues, one moves into the plateau stage. The responses may continue to intensify as the vagina becomes more sensitive and the glans of the clitoris retracts under the hood.
- **Orgasm.** With enough stimulation of or around the clitoris—and, for some women, pressure on the cervix or other sensitive areas such as the G-spot—a woman may build up to a peak, or orgasm. This is the point at which all the tension suddenly releases in a series of involuntary and pleasurable muscular contractions. Contractions may be felt in the vagina, uterus, and rectum. Many women experience orgasm as a total-body contraction and release.
- **Resolution.** Unless stimulation continues, the resolution stage occurs. During the half hour or more after orgasm, the muscles relax, and the clitoris, vagina, and uterus return to their usual positions (except in the rare disorder known as persistent genital arousal disorder).[2]

Masters and Johnson's work was valuable for women in exploring and asserting the role

INTEGRATION OF BODY, MIND, HEART, AND SPIRIT

Integrating Sexuality and Spirituality (ISIS)—a national survey of close to four thousand women ranging in age from eighteen to eighty-six and representing twenty-two religious faiths—laid the groundwork for sex therapist Gina Ogden's research into what sex means in our lives.

In her books *The Heart and Soul of Sex* and *The Return of Desire*, Ogden offers a different way of looking at sexual responses, based on the ISIS survey. Ogden visualizes a woman's sexual response as multidimensional, including physical, emotional, and spiritual aspects. Her ISIS respondents reported that eroticism is generated in the context of relationship, not only with their partners but also with themselves—body, mind, heart, and spirit. Perhaps most remarkably, sexual satisfaction increased with every decade rather than going downhill

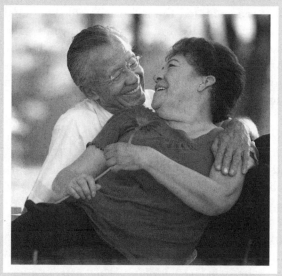

© iStockphoto.com / Aldo Murillo

as it does in the Masters and Johnson model of sex. Yes, those over age fifty were having a better time than the twenty- and thirty-year-olds, reporting that they had been able to move beyond the negative messages of earlier years and embrace the richness of their relationships.[4] Read more at ginaogden.com.

of the clitoris in sexual response. But by focusing their study on people who were very experienced with orgasm during masturbation and intercourse, they reinforced a belief that orgasm and intercourse are necessary to women's sexual response and pleasure. And by offering only one model for human sexual response, Masters and Johnson missed the fact that women who do not orgasm with penetration, for example, also experience pleasure.

In the 1970s, the feminist researcher Shere Hite polled more than three thousand women and discovered that most of them did not experience orgasm through intercourse alone.[3] In the 1970s and 1980s, several researchers and clinicians such as Harold Lief, Helen Singer Kaplan, Bernie Zilbergeld, and Carol Rinkleib Ellison expanded the Masters and Johnson model to include emotional aspects like desire and satisfaction.[5]

In 1997, Beverly Whipple and Karen Brash-McGreer developed a circular model of women's sexual responses, suggesting that if a sexual experience resulted in pleasure and satisfaction, then it could lead to another sexual experience. But if the experience was not pleasurable and satisfying, it might not lead to another sexual experience.[6] In 2001, Rosemary Basson published a nonlinear model of female sexual response that incorporated the importance of emotional intimacy, sexual stimuli, and relationship satisfaction. Basson argues that, contrary to what the linear model suggests, women have many reasons for engaging in sexual activity other than desire.[7]

The best part is the afterglow, when we're both limp and glowing with satisfaction, wrapped around each other. I love the way he knows my body, where to touch, how to touch. The feeling of being so full of him and so full of pleasure that I could explode. The climax of orgasm, whether it's an intense eruption of physical pleasure or an overwhelming emotional sense of being so completely in love with him, brings tears to my eyes.

Despite the limitations of even the revised Masters and Johnson model, psychiatric and medical clinicians, along with pharmaceutical companies, continue to use it to create definitions of sexual health and sexual problems. For instance, a key resource used by U.S. mental health professionals, the *Diagnostic and Statistical Manual of Mental Disorders* (*DSM*), bases its definitions of sexual dysfunction on the Masters and Johnson sexual response cycle. For a critical alternative, see NewViewCampaign.org and the book *A New View of Women's Sexual Problems*, edited by Ellyn Kaschak and Leonore Tiefer, which includes the relational aspects of women's sexuality and allows for a wide range of differences among women's experiences.

Important as sex research can be, there's no need to rely exclusively on experts for accurate information about sexuality. If the models don't fit you, then trust your own experiences. We can obtain powerful data by discussing our experiences with friends or in other groups. In some cases, this information can be enhanced by respectful research that attempts scientifically to record and measure what we experience.

ORGASM

An orgasm can be mild, like a hiccup or a peaceful sigh. It can be a sensuous experience, as the body glows with warmth. Or it can be intensely physical or even ecstatic, causing a loss of everyday awareness. An orgasm can be exclusively physical, or it can include subjective and psychological aspects. Feelings of intimacy can impact orgasms with a partner, and orgasms can enhance intimacy.

An orgasm may feel totally different at different times, depending on whether you are masturbating or with a partner, the type and amount of stimulation, and where you are in your menstrual cycle. Other factors include how you're feeling emotionally and physically; among these are your energy level and degree of excitement.

Masters and Johnson asserted that all female orgasms are physiologically the same (brought about through stimulation of the clitoris, with contractions occurring primarily in the outer

RECOMMENDED FOR YOUR READING PLEASURE

- *I Love Female Orgasm: An Extraordinary Orgasm Guide* by Dorian Solot and Marshall Miller (Da Capo Press, 2007).
- *The Orgasm Answer Guide* by Barry Komisaruk, Beverly Whipple, Sara Nasserzadeh, and Carlos Beyer-Flores (Johns Hopkins University Press, 2010).
- *The Science of Orgasm* by Barry Komisaruk, Carlos Beyer-Flores, and Beverly Whipple (Johns Hopkins University Press, 2006).

third of the vagina). Yet some women describe orgasms that don't fit this model. One orgasm that some women describe as feeling "deep" or "uterine" is brought on by penetration of the vagina. The buildup may involve a prolonged involuntary holding of breath, which is released explosively at orgasm, and there do not seem to be any contractions of the outer third of the vagina.

Women have the potential to respond to sexual arousal throughout the entire body and especially the pelvic region.

Some women find the cervix and uterus crucial to orgasm. Women who have had a total hysterectomy, in which the cervix and the uterus have been removed, may learn to focus on different kinds of sexual stimulation and feelings.

Women with spinal cord injuries who have no feeling in the pelvic area have reported experiencing orgasm and its sensations elsewhere in the body (see "Sex, Disability, and Chronic Disease," p. 189). Women without physical disabilities may also experience such sensations. And some women experience orgasm from thought or imagery alone, without any physical touch.[8]

The Role of the Clitoris

For many women, the clitoris is the organ that is most sensitive to stimulation and plays a central role in elevating feelings of sexual tension. Although it's sometimes called "the joy button," the clitoris is actually much more than a single spot; it is an expansive network of erectile tissues, glands, and nerves. (For more information, see p. 4.)

You or your partner can stimulate your clitoris in many different ways—by rubbing, sucking, stroking, kissing, and using body pressure or a vibrator. Any rubbing or pressure in the mons area or the vaginal lips (even on the lower abdomen and inner thighs) can move the clitoris and may also press it up against the pubic bone.

Some women do not have a full intact clitoris, owing to an accident, sex-reassignment surgery, or a clitoridectomy—surgical removal of the clitoris, which may occur during female genital cutting. For more information, see "Female Genital Gutting," p. 793. Losing the clitoris reduces the capacity for sexual pleasure. If the outer portion of your clitoris has been removed surgically, certain types of touch or movement may be painful, but you may be able to experience pleasure and even orgasm. There still remains the expansive inner network of erectile tissues, glands, muscles, and nerves that contribute to sexual pleasure. And genital surgery does not prevent the ability to fantasize and get turned on by thoughts and feelings.

Once a lover knows my body well enough to be able to get me off fairly easily, it feels so good to relax and relinquish control over what's happening. After, I love feeling sexy and pleased with my body, that it responds to all these fun sensations and I can reliably get release in the way that I crave. For someone who's had a pretty rough relationship with her body over the years, it feels big and important now to be crazy about my body through the way it experiences pleasure.

DID I MISS IT?

Sometimes it can be difficult to know if you've had an orgasm:

The way I've heard about orgasms is there's supposed to be a big release, but that's not the way it works for me. I feel a really intense buildup that feels great, and then suddenly, my clitoris becomes too sensitive to keep stimulating, so I stop. I no longer have a desire to keep going, and I just feel relaxed and tired, in a good way. I always wonder, did I miss the climax? Or was that not really an orgasm?

If arousal occurs without enough stimulation to orgasm, sexual tension subsides eventually without orgasm, though it takes longer, and your genitals and/or uterus may ache. This is the analogue of "blue balls" for men; it has the same cause and will resolve itself. Many women have been convinced (mostly by men) that the male version of this ache is somehow dangerous and deserves immediate relief, while also believing that the female version is of no real consequence because it will go away if you let it.

Some women orgasm once, some twice or more in quick succession. But even though multiple orgasms are possible, this doesn't mean that everyone has them or that you're sexually inadequate if you don't. Partners may expect it, too, yet one orgasm can be plenty, and sexual expression without orgasm can also be pleasurable. Sometimes orgasms (single or multiple) become one more performance pressure or goal:

When I try too hard to have an orgasm, it usually doesn't work and I end up frustrated and bored. For me, it's best if I relax and let it happen if it's going to.

WHAT IF I DON'T COME?

Many women have never had an orgasm or have difficulty experiencing one. Sometimes information or experience are all that's lacking. Some women find it easier to orgasm when the muscles around the outer third of the vagina (pubococcygeus muscles) are strong and well exercised (see "How to Do Kegel Exercises," p. 643) .

Shame about exploring and touching our bodies keeps some of us from learning to bring ourselves to orgasm through masturbation. Sexual, physical, or emotional abuse (past or present) may also impair the ability to orgasm— arousal may restimulate mental and/or physical memories of the abuse, even in a consensual, noncoercive, and trusting relationship.

While some women don't ever experience orgasm, most of us, with exploration and experience, will. If you are distressed by not having orgasms, you can explore how to have one. Experiment with masturbating. Try using a vibrator alone or during sex with a partner. Sex therapists are specifically trained to help women understand the complex blocks to orgasm, which may include physical issues, negative memories, partner dynamics, education, "just say no" cultural messages, and fear of reaching out for what we want. Helpful books and videos are available in the resources section at our bodiesourselves.org.

With a partner, here are some problems that may get in the way of orgasm:

- You don't really want to be having sex with this person right now, or communication about sex is poor.
- You and/or your partner need more sex education in order to understand what's happening during arousal.
- You're too busy thinking about how to do it right, why it doesn't go well or quickly enough, or whether your partner is into it or feeling impatient or tired.
- You're afraid of asking for too much and seeming too demanding.
- You're afraid that if your partner concentrates on *your* pleasure, you'll feel such pressure to orgasm that you won't be able to—and then you don't.
- You're trying to orgasm at the same time as your partner (simultaneous orgasm), which seldom occurs.

- You're angry at, or have unresolved emotional issues or conflicts with, a sexual partner.
- You're angry or scared about something that happened in the past, which may or may not have involved the present partner.
- You're feeling guilt about having sex and cannot really enjoy it.
- You've bought into the assumption that with a male partner, women should have orgasms through intercourse, and it's just not working.
- You've fallen into a pattern of "faking" orgasm to please a partner or to get it over with.

For some women, sexual intercourse may not ever lead to orgasm, even when it feels good. This is perfectly normal. Direct and sometimes prolonged clitoral stimulation both before and during intercourse is often necessary. Intercourse can be about pleasure or connection; it doesn't have to focus on orgasm.

Not being able to have an orgasm with a partner is not by itself a flaw in a relationship, though it can sometimes be a clue that the relationship needs to change in some way. It may also be that you or a partner needs to learn more about your sexual arousal and responses:

Vaginal penetration alone doesn't make me orgasm, and this is true for many women. I need direct clitoral stimulation, and I need it done right. I've only had two partners who have been able to make me orgasm without my assistance at all, out of what I generally count as eleven partners. And even for these two, it took them a good long time to learn how—six months for one and a year for the other—and while both were able to do it via oral sex, only one has been able to do it with his fingers, and then only on occasion. If I'm going to get off during sex, I'm most likely the one who's going to make that happen, and the best way for me to do that is usually with a vibrator.

THE G-SPOT

Some women experience intense sexual pleasure and orgasm when a particular area inside the vagina, approximately one-third to one-half up the front wall, is stimulated. The area was first described by Dr. Ernst Gräfenberg, who published his findings in 1950, and was named the G-spot in his honor.[9] There is debate among researchers about whether the G-spot is a distinct anatomical structure or whether the pleasure some women feel when the area is stimulated is due to its closeness to the bulbs of the clitoris.[10]

If you want to explore whether stimulation of this area is pleasurable for you, set aside a time when you can allow yourself to relax and become aroused. You may want to warm up with other types of stimulation and then use your fingers to explore two to three inches inside the vagina, toward your abdomen. Feel for a rough texture or ridges. It can be helpful to curve your fingers into a "come here" position and explore by massaging and pressing into the area. You may want to experiment with different positions, such as lying on your stomach or squatting. It may be difficult to find, especially if your fingers are especially short and/or your vagina is especially long.

When you first touch this area, it might feel as if you have to pee. That is because the area of the G-spot surrounds the urethra, the tube you urinate through. The sensation may subside after a few seconds of massage. Your G-spot can also be stimulated by a partner's fingers or penis, a dildo, or a G-spot vibrator.

Contrary to popular myth, the G-spot is not a magic button that automatically produces ecstasy when pushed. Yet many find that exploring this area can enhance sexual pleasure.

Female Ejaculation

For some women, sufficient stimulation of the G-spot or the clitoris may lead to ejaculation, the release of fluid from the urethra. Some people doubt the existence of female ejaculation, but from ancient Greek writings to the Hindu *Kama Sutra* to sixteenth-century Japanese artwork, female ejaculation has been described and honored.[11] Sometimes called spraying or squirting, female ejaculation can bring a feeling of powerful release and pleasure:

The sensation when I'm about to squirt is incredibly intense. All my muscles are rigid and I stop breathing and there is nothing I can do to stop what comes next. Then I feel an incredible release as the fluid shoots out of me and my entire body relaxes. It doesn't happen often, and I can't make it happen, but when it does it is pretty wonderful!

Ejaculation can occur with or without an orgasm. Although ejaculate is released through the urethra, it is not clear what the fluid is comprised of. Research indicates that it is chemically different from urine, and some research has found its biochemical elements similar to what is found in male prostate fluid.[12] The amount of ejaculate varies, from about a teaspoon to a gush big enough to create a dinner-plate-sized puddle on the sheets. It looks like watered-down skim milk and the smell and taste may vary during the menstrual cycle.

MASTURBATION

Masturbation—touching yourself sexually—is one way of exploring and enjoying sexual pleasure. It's common for young children to touch and play with their bodies, including their genitals, mostly just because it feels good. The

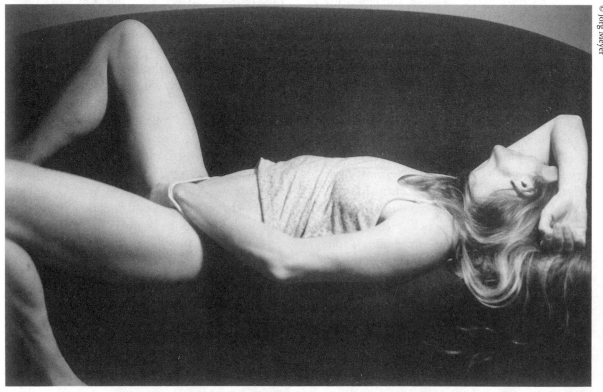

© Jörg Meyer

message that touching ourselves in this way is not okay comes later from parents, schools, and religious institutions, or from the culture around us. Sex-ed classes rarely help, since most don't address masturbation. Back in 1994, during a United Nations conference on AIDS, the then surgeon general Joycelyn Elders was asked whether masturbation should be promoted as a means of preventing young people from engaging in riskier forms of sexual activity. "I think that it is part of human sexuality," she replied, "and perhaps it should be taught." Soon after, Elders lost her job.

Masturbation enables us to explore and experiment with our own bodies and learn what kind of touch feels good. You can discover your own patterns of sexual response without having to think about a partner's needs and opinions. If you want, you can share what you've learned with your partners, by guiding their hands to the places you want touched. It can be freeing to know how to give yourself sensual and sexual pleasure. You become less dependent on others to satisfy you, which can give them freedom, too. Through learning to pleasure yourself, you're more likely to be satisfied with your sexual life overall, and to orgasm more easily—either alone or with a partner:

Masturbating is what I love the most about being sexual. It's powerful. It's sexy. It's a guaranteed good time, and it's a very loving gesture. There is a lot of power and autonomy in putting yourself in charge of your own orgasms.

I think I started to really enjoy being sexual more when I started getting comfortable with masturbating. It wasn't really until I was in college, which seems kind of late now that I think about it. It was really cool to figure out that I could make myself feel certain things and make my own body respond in different ways. Consequently, when I started having sexual

encounters with other people, I could enjoy them more because I felt like I had at least some influence over my own enjoyment.

Female masturbation was something my friends and I in high school never talked about. I knew that women technically could masturbate, but I didn't even know how to go about it when I first started becoming sexual. I hadn't had any luck with self-stimulation, and I didn't have any awareness about what I could do with my body. For a while, this lack of exploration had led me to believe that I was one of those women who would never orgasm. I had never climaxed with my first boyfriend, and I just considered that normal.

I didn't start to pleasure myself until after I started dating my second boyfriend. He was very skilled at oral sex, luckily for me, and sort of showed me what felt good before I even knew what to want/ expect. Without him, I don't know if I would ever have known how to begin touching myself in the right ways. After that, masturbation did become a part of my sexual "routine." And I have to say, sex definitely became better, with all partners, after I'd started. Not only did I know better about what turned me on and got me off, but I became much more comfortable with my body. Being able to experience that kind of sexual pleasure made me feel sexy. It was really kind of an awakening.

After menopause, especially if you're not having sex with a partner, masturbating can help keep vaginal tissues moist. And for women at any age, it is a way of connecting with your body:

Masturbation is my partner. . . . Since I have not been in a sexual or nonsexual relationship for many, many years, this is how I stay tuned to the sexual me.

LEARNING TO MASTURBATE

The first time you try masturbating, you may feel awkward or self-conscious. You may feel as if you do not know how, or give up too soon because you are trying to reproduce what you've seen in the movies or what you've heard from friends. You may feel shy about giving yourself sexual pleasure.

Some suggestions: Find a quiet time when you can be by yourself without interruption and make yourself comfortable. Start by using one or more fingers to touch yourself; add a lubricant or your own saliva if you want more moisture. Experiment with different types of pressure and speed. The clitoris is exquisitely sensitive, and sometimes direct touching or rubbing of the glans (or tip) is painful; indirect or intermittent touching may be more pleasurable.

You can also try crossing your legs and exerting steady and rhythmic pressure on the whole genital area. You can insert something into the vagina—a finger, a cucumber, or a dildo. Other ways to masturbate include rubbing against a pillow, pointing a handheld showerhead at your genital area, or using a vibrator. Sex-positive, woman-owned sex-toy companies are great sources for information as well as products.

At sixteen, like the "good" girl I thought I should be, I gave up masturbation for Lent. Since I defined masturbation only as touching my genitals in a sexual way, in those six weeks I learned that I could have wonderful orgasms through a mixture of fantasy and quietly tensing up and relaxing the muscles around my vagina and vulva. I'm sixty-five now and still enjoying the benefits of what I learned.

I can direct our shower nozzle so the water hits my clitoris in a steady stream. I have a real relationship with that shower! I wouldn't give it up for anything. It's nice when I get up for work and don't have time for sex.

For me, the most pleasurable part is just before orgasm. I feel I am no longer consciously controlling my body. I know there is no way I will not reach orgasm now. I stop trying. I like to savor this rare moment of true letting go!

It's this letting go of control that enables us to have orgasms. If you do not orgasm when you're masturbating, don't worry about it. Just enjoy the sensations:

Masturbating opens me to what is happening in my body and makes me feel good about myself. I like following the impulse of the moment. Sometimes I have many orgasms; sometimes I don't. The greatest source of pleasure is to be able

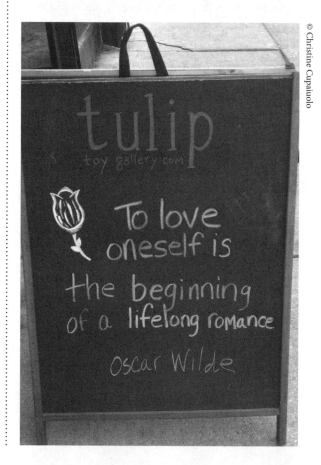

YES MEANS YES

The powerful, candid essays in Yes Means Yes: Visions of Female Sexual Power and a World Without Rape *have transformed the way we think about women's sexuality. Jaclyn Friedman* (Yes Means Yes *co-editor with Jessica Valenti*) *explains the meaning behind the movement:*

You've probably heard the phrase "no means no," and you probably know what it means: if someone says no to any kind of sexual interaction, you must stop. But have you heard the phrase "yes means yes"?

"Yes means yes" is the slogan of a movement to enhance our understanding of sexual consent so that it's clear and works for everyone. The "yes means yes" philosophy is that the only valid sexual consent is enthusiastic consent.

Where "no means no" suggests that, in the absence of your partner clearly objecting, you can do whatever you want, the principle of enthusiastic consent says that you must not do anything that your partner isn't actively excited about (or at least excited to try). And if you can't tell if your partner is enthusiastic, then ask.

There are numerous reasons for this shift. While "no means no" popularized the idea that women's sexual boundaries must be respected (sad to say, a major accomplishment), it's also inadvertently supported the already-pervasive cultural assumption that women only want to say "no" to sex. It also created room for rapists to claim "she didn't say no" as a valid defense if the woman they'd assaulted hadn't verbally protested due to shock, fear, intoxication or any other reason.

Enthusiastic consent clears up this confusion, and in cases of sexual assault puts the onus on the accused to prove the victim was freely consenting, instead of asking the victim to prove she objected strenuously enough. It also challenges the idea that women don't want sex, by assuming that any sexual interaction requires the enthusiasm of all parties involved, regardless of gender.

Like most things, enthusiastic consent is more complicated in practice than it is in principle. Because we still live in a world that punishes women for having too much or the wrong kind of sexual desire, many women feel uncomfortable expressing enthusiasm for sex, even when they very much want a sexual interaction.

Still, enthusiastic consent has the potential to transform the way we think about and engage in sex for the better: by fostering direct, open communication about consent and pleasure, by reinforcing the idea that women can be plenty enthusiastic about sex on their own terms, and by creating a culture in which the only good kind of sex is the kind of sex that's actively good for everyone involved.

Rachel Kramer Bussel, "Beyond Yes or No: Consent as Sexual Process"

Consent is a basic part of the sexual equation. If there's any uncertainty, or if you find that you're using some power to coax someone into sex when they clearly aren't that into it, you need to rethink what you're doing and why you're doing it. . . .

The burden is not on the woman to say no, but on the person pursuing the sexual act to get an active yes.

What does it mean to say to someone, "Fuck me?" Or, to put it a little more delicately, "Touch me?" To tell them exactly how you want to be kissed, licked, petted? Or to tell them just what it is you want to do with them? . . . You're letting your lover—and yourself—know what you're looking for, rather than leaving it up to the imagination. You're giving them explicit instructions and thereby saying "yes" so loudly, they have to hear you. . . .

By embracing a broader concept of consent, we acknowledge that just as "sex" means a lot more than just penis-in-vagina intercourse, "consent" at its best can be about more than just "yes" or "no." It means not taking the "yes" for granted, as well as getting to know the reasons behind the "yes," and those, to me, are what's truly sexy.[13]

Jill Filipovic, "Offensive Feminism"

Sex is about consent and enjoyment . . . Sex isn't about pushing someone to do something they don't want to do. . . . Sex should be entered into joyfully and enthusiastically by both partners; an absence of "no" isn't enough—"yes" should be the baseline requirement. . . . [Women are] sexual actors who should absolutely have the ability to say yes when we want it, just like men, and should feel safe saying no—even if we've been drinking, even if we slept with you before, even if we're wearing tight jeans, even if we're naked in bed with you.[14]

Cara Kulwicki, "Real Sex Education"

[We need] to change the thinking from "sex when someone says no and fights back is wrong" to "sex when someone doesn't openly and enthusiastically want it is wrong." . . . It pains me to think of how different my life would have been if someone had taught me that I was supposed to *want* sexual contact and *say so*; and otherwise it was wrong. I truly thought that fearfully giving up after saying no twenty times counted as consent.[15]

to do whatever feels good to me at that particular time. I rarely have such complete freedom in other aspects of my life.

ENTHUSIASTIC CONSENT

LET'S TALK ABOUT SEX

We all face certain issues in sexual situations, whether it's with a date, a longtime lover, or a spouse: Do I want to be sexually close with this person now? In what ways? What if I don't know—can I say I'm confused? Can I communicate clearly what I want and what I don't want?

Talking about sex can be challenging, whether you're using anatomically correct terms such as vagina, penis, and penetration, or slang terms such as cunt, cock, and fucking. If you find slang degrading, be creative and come up with your own affirming language. Sometimes the vagueness of expressions can lead to miscommunication if both partners are not clear on the meaning. Finding a common language that you're both comfortable with can help.

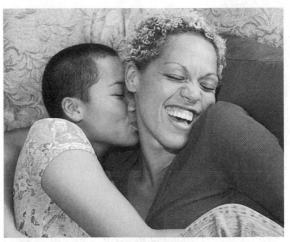
© Thinkstock

I began masturbating at age eleven and engaged sexually with someone else for the first time at fourteen, but I don't think I had really good, enjoyable sex until I incorporated good practices of consent into my sexual interactions with others.

You may want to find a time to talk with your partner(s) when you are *not* having sex and there's no pressure to respond right away. You can practice saying what feels good while exchanging massages, for example, when the atmosphere is less intense. Talking about safer sex, birth control, and sexual techniques or preferences doesn't have to kill the mood. Incorporating these discussions into sexual play can be hot—and can lead to heightened intimacy.

Body language and the sounds we make are also important. Speeding up or slowing down hip movements and placing a firm hand on the shoulder to say, "Let's go slow," are all ways of communicating:

I've liked just saying, "Watch," and showing.

We were both really excited. He began rubbing my clitoris hard, and it hurt. It took me a second to figure out what to do. I was afraid that if

I said something about it, I would spoil the excitement for both of us. Then I realized I could just take his hand and very gently move it up a little higher.

Be aware of the relationship between words and body language. You may be verbally saying yes to some sexual activity, but your body is pulling away or tensing up. Or you may be saying no to going farther sexually while continuing to stimulate yourself or your partner. It's important to communicate what you really want, to stop immediately in the face of any mixed signals from your partner, and to expect your partner always to do the same for you.

Communication is a continuous process. A woman who had found the courage to talk with her partner about their sexual relationship asked in angry frustration, "I told him what I like once, so why doesn't he know now? Did he forget? Doesn't he care?"

He would come almost instantly when we began to make love after marvelous kissing. A little while later, we'd make love again, when I'd be more aroused—aching for him, in fact. I never knew how to alter this pattern, never dared talk about it, and later on found out that he had resented "having" to make love twice.

We had a wildly passionate sex life for a year and a half. When we moved in together, sexuality suddenly became an issue. It turned out our patterns were very different. My lover needs to talk, to feel intimate in conversation, to relax completely before she can feel sexual. I need to touch and to make a physical connection first before I feel relaxed enough to talk intimately. I'd reach out for her as we went into the bedroom, and she'd freeze. We battled it out for months, both feeling terrible, before we figured out what was going on.

Even in the best relationships, asking for what we want may be difficult, and we may feel inhibited about asserting our sexuality openly and proudly. We've been conditioned to think that sex is supposed to come naturally, and talking about it must mean something's wrong. We may hold back from communicating about sex for any number of reasons, including:

- Feeling embarrassed by the words themselves.
- Feeling embarrassed by desires, thinking they might be taboo or a partner will be judgmental.
- After having sex with the same person for years, it feels risky to bring up new insights or desires.

Communicating about sex includes not only talking and negotiating about what both partners want, but also discussing safer sex and, if necessary, birth control. For more information, see Chapters 9–11.

- Communication isn't going well in other areas of the relationship.
- A partner seems defensive and might interpret suggestions as a criticism or a demand.
- Inexperience or confusion over what *you* want at a particular time.

Negotiating how and when it is okay for me to relinquish control over my physical movements— for example, when it's sexy to have my girlfriend restrain me and when it makes me feel slightly panicky—has been a complicated process. I feel bad that I can't give my girlfriend clearer cues about what feels good when, particularly since she tends to retreat pretty quickly when I say, "That didn't feel good this time," to, "Well, then I'll stop doing it altogether." That either-or response comes from (I think) not wanting to do something that I don't like, and not wanting rejection, but there are times when I want a little pain, want a little domination, and I feel bad that I can't give her a clearer sense of when and in what circumstances certain activities feel good and when they don't.

If you do ask for what you want, you may be relieved and gratified to get your desires met. However, if your partner has different preferences, you may have to do some negotiating or look below the surface and figure out the underlying needs. For example, say that you want to spend long hours in bed on a Sunday morning having sex, but your partner wants to get up and go for a run. What are your needs that aren't being met? Do you want more intimacy? Do you need time to unwind? Do you want more sexual attention? What are your partner's needs? Expanding the focus can open up more possibilities of fulfilling both partners' underlying needs.

Learning to talk more comfortably about sex is sometimes easier when you're doing something enjoyable with your partner or with friends. Here are some suggestions:

- Attend a performance of or invite friends over to read aloud from the play *The Vagina Monologues* (events.vday.org).
- Visit a woman-owned sex-toys shop; the employees tend to be knowledgeable, helpful, and nonjudgmental, so don't be embarrassed to ask questions. Or check out sex-toy shops online such as Good Vibrations (goodvibes.com), Babeland (babeland.com), or Eve's Garden (evesgarden.com).

- Host a sex-toys party (like a Tupperware party, but more fun). Look online for woman-owned companies that will put together a party for you and your friends. In some states, laws are in flux about the legality of selling sex toys, so it's best to go through a professional company if you have any worries.[16]

If the problem feels bigger than what you can manage, consider joining or creating a support group. The Self-Help Group Sourcebook (mentalhelp.net/selfhelp) offers tips on how to find or start self-help groups online and in your community. Or look for a certified sex therapist through the American Association of Sexuality Educators, Counselors, and Therapists (aasect.org).

SEX WITH A PARTNER

Sex with a partner allows for endless possibilities: massaging, hugging, licking, kissing, caressing, biting, direct clitoral stimulation, oral sex, vaginal or anal penetration, intercourse, nipple stimulation, fingering or fisting, playing with power and roles, tribadism (rubbing a body part against your partner's genitals), rimming (oral-to-anal stimulation), erotic talk, or sleeping together (really, just sleeping) without sex. We can claim all the dimensions of sexuality that deepen intimacy and pleasure:

During really good, connected sex, I don't worry about things like what faces or noises I'm making, how my body looks or is moving, or how close I am to orgasm. I get caught up in the sensations of pleasure, I notice how my body responds to different kinds of touch, and I can choose either to be 100 percent mentally present or to engage my mind in some kind of delightful fantasy.

In finding out what turns my lover on, exploring her body, tasting her, learning her odors and textures, I am growing to love myself more, too.

I love that moment just before orgasm, when everything in me slows down and homes in on my lover's pleasure, and if I'm achy or tired or sweating it doesn't matter; nothing matters but that moment and the nearing edge of orgasm. I'm a very sexual person and I love getting off too, but for me nothing is truly better than

giving someone else a big, long, breathless orgasm.

We always sleep right up next to each other naked. There's always a lot of touching and feeling, so even though we don't have intercourse that often, I consider us having sex all the time.

Many of us learned that sex with a partner means penetration, with everything else called foreplay. The word "foreplay" can be a problem when it implies that everything that turns us on is merely a step along the way to the big act.

I have orgasms easily during intercourse. Sometimes I love his thrusting deep inside me. Sometimes I don't want the penetration, I want something else. But he feels if we haven't had intercourse, we haven't actually made love.

Some women whose male partners get infrequent erections (owing to age, illness, or other factors) find that their own sexual pleasure actually increases, partly because penis-in-vagina intercourse is no longer the focus of sex. This can be especially true if in the past the woman had intercourse more often than she wanted to, perhaps in order to please a partner.

For some, massages and touching are great for making sexual activity slower and more sensual. Others enjoy sex that is faster and more aggressive. It's all a matter of personal preference, and those preferences can switch or change. It's about what feels good—and right—to you at that moment:

I yearn to feel the crook of her arm under my neck as I sleep. I long to stroke her face and enjoy how good it feels to wake up with her arms around me in the morning. The heat and passion of sex are great, but I think that a gentle

WHEN ONE PERSON WANTS MORE

In an ongoing relationship, there may be times when one partner has a higher level of desire than the other, which can create tension. For some couples, a desire discrepancy may simply be the result of different preferences and bodily rhythms. Communicating clearly, learning about each other's needs, and finding middle ground can help bridge the differences. For other couples, the discrepancy may be due to lack of attraction or to problems in the relationship. Or it could have to do with physical changes. (See Chapter 8, "Sexual Challenges," for more on how illnesses, medications, and hormones can affect desire.)

Many straight women find our partners want sex more often than we do. However, the discrepancy in desire can go the other way, and some women feel constrained by the stereotype that men always want sex and women always want love.

I want sex a lot more often than my husband does. I try not to take it personally when he says no, but sometimes it hurts. I feel rejected. The images on television and in the movies and the jokes that circulate on the Internet always show the man wanting sex more than the woman.

Even if initially your partner or you are not craving physical sex, exploring intimacy with your partner can lead to physical arousal. A sixty-six-year-old

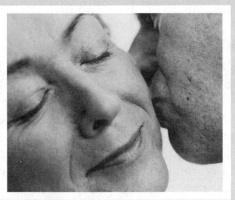

© Antonio Mo / Getty Images

woman who has been with her partner for thirty years writes:

I do feel nostalgic sometimes for the early days when we spent half the day in bed—or out of bed, on the floor, on the sofa, in the shower—having sex. I miss turning to her in the night, thrilled with desire. Fact is, at night we sleep. She and I are busy with work and community, there's not a lot of hot lesbian sexual tension in the movies we see, we have our various aches and pains, and lust rarely takes us over. The good news is that when we haven't had sex in a while, we notice. What works for us then is to set aside a dedicated few hours during which, even if we're not in the mood at the beginning, we find our way to connection with ourselves and each other. With less time, it's mutual masturbation; with more time, it's oral sex. Always it's making love. Getting in the mood, for us, isn't usually about candles and music and sexy pictures, but about time, pure and simple. Time and intention.

caress is more personal. That's what I crave most right now.

SELF-PLEASURING DURING (AND SOMETIMES INSTEAD OF) SEX WITH A PARTNER

Some women get aroused by watching a partner masturbate, or by pleasuring themselves during sex with a partner. It may be something you do without thinking, simply because it feels good to add more stimulation. It can sometimes take time to learn what feels most pleasurable:

When we first started having sex, my husband encouraged me to masturbate because I had so little experience with it. He wanted to learn from my exploration what turned me on. As I got better at it, we often turned each other on by watching each other masturbate, sometimes touching, sometimes just totally into ourselves. It's a beautiful experience. We learned how to give each other orgasms with and without intercourse.

I'm a huge fan of mutual masturbation and would definitely say that it can fall under my personal definition of "sex." I'd even say I often enjoy it more than literal intercourse.

Communicating about masturbation is important, especially if a partner feels left out or threatened. Sometimes it can take a while to get used to the idea that self-pleasuring is something both partners can enjoy:

Neither of us has philosophical problems with the other using masturbation as a way to experience sexual pleasure. But my girlfriend feels bad when I touch myself while we're making love. I had a hard time coming when we first started making love (new context; no longer as private as I was used to, given that someone else was there!), and

she still feels badly about this, even though it certainly wasn't her fault. So I think when I touch myself she feels like she isn't wanted/needed in the room. Whereas I am really turned on by the experience of her being there while I jerk off and experience it as a mutual thing, not something that's better than her or necessarily solitary. So while I don't feel like masturbation is taboo or somehow a betrayal of my partner, I do realize that it can really have a negative effect on a lover's sense of security, and that makes me sad.

One of the ways I know that I'm comfortable with a partner is when I can share the fact that I like masturbation a lot and tend to do it every day. My last real relationship was with a man who knew that I enjoyed masturbation and wasn't threatened by it at all. We would even talk about it and developed our own secret code for when we were doing it. That being said, I think it was different if we were in the same space. While he was fine with me doing my own thing while we were away from each other, the one or two times where I started touching myself while we were fooling around, he'd ask me why I wasn't waiting for him. I think he felt if we were going to be together, we should pleasure each other and not ourselves.

One woman sees it as a team effort:

I think it's hot when I'm comfortable enough to touch myself when a partner is being sexual with me, and I think it's hot when she does the same. I do feel like it opens up a certain vulnerability, though, because it requires some explicit acknowledgment of something you want. . . . It's easy to slip into the mind-set of "I'm touching myself because my partner isn't doing something I want," or "My partner is touching herself because I'm not doing something she wants." But I don't think that has to be true. I think it's possible for someone to simply be comfortable enough

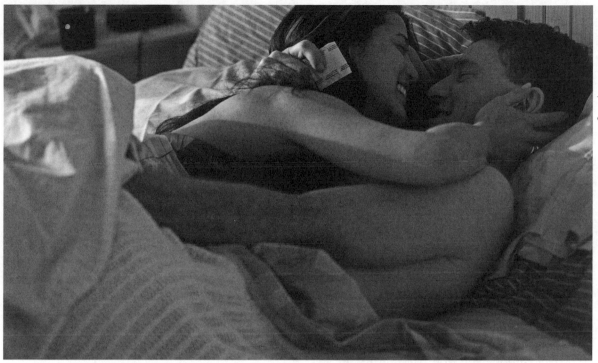

with a partner that her own pleasure becomes a team effort. Which makes things more fun for everyone.

VAGINAL PENETRATION

Women often crave to penetrate or be penetrated during sex, be it by tongue, dildo, penis, or finger(s). Vaginal penetration (which some people prefer to call "insertive sex") can be gentle, playful, intimate, forceful, or passionate. It can be thought of as reciprocal, with one of you enveloping whatever it is the other is using to insert and explore.

I can so clearly remember moving in and around him, and him in me, till it seemed in the whole world there was only us dancing together as we moved together, as we loved together, as we came together. Sometimes at these times I laugh or cry, and they are the same strong emotions coming

from a deep protected part of me that is freer now for loving him.

Penetration can be fantastic for some women, unpleasurable/undesirable for others, or somewhere in between. The key is to communicate to a partner what you want at the time.

If you want your partner to enter you, make sure together that your vagina is wet from vaginal fluid or lubricants. For penetration to give you pleasure, you need to feel sexually excited, your vagina wet and open. Some women may feel ready for penetration immediately; for others it takes more sexual activity, including masturbation. You or your partner can apply water-based lubricants, or even saliva, or use a lubricated condom. Do not use Vaseline or any oils, as these destroy latex condoms, dental dams, and diaphragms.

Certain positions may feel better than others.

WHAT IF IT HURTS?

When you are tense and preoccupied, penetration can hurt. Even if you feel relaxed and sexual, timing is important. If you try penetration before you're fully aroused, your vaginal entrance might be too tight, and you might not be fully lubricated. So don't rush, and don't let yourself be rushed.

As with all sexual activity, if you are sexually inexperienced, frightened, not ready, not in the mood, or angry with your partner, or if your partner is not aware or respectful of your sexual preferences or desires, then penetration can be boring, unpleasant, and even painful. If it doesn't feel good, stop. Play more with external stimulation and wait until you're very aroused, then try again if you want to. Some women experience pain with penetration even when fully aroused. This can be caused by a variety of conditions. (For more information, see "Painful Intercourse/Penetration," p. 185.)

You can sit or lie on your partner, or lie side by side. You can sit up facing each other, with your legs over your partner's legs. Or your partner can enter you from behind and reach around to caress your clitoris, or you can do it, too, in this position.

Pressure at the back of the vagina can be the key to orgasm for some women, but painful for others. If you want deep penetration and pressure on your cervix, choose positions that make these more possible. We are all different shapes and need to find positions that suit us. For those of us with injuries or disabilities, being creative and using pillows for support may increase comfort.

If a man is highly aroused when he begins penetration, he might ejaculate quickly if he moves rapidly back and forth inside you and you move your pelvis against his. If you wish to prolong intercourse, both of you can slow your movements. Experiment with holding your bodies still for a time when he enters you; then begin to move together slowly.

When penetrating a partner's vagina, you can stroke, tap, circle, thrust, and experiment with different rhythms and speeds. Try stimulating her G-spot. You can use a dildo or other sex toy, or put one or more fingers inside and, if you both like, gradually your whole hand (sometimes called fisting). It can feel warm, wet, and wonderful.

Erection-Enhancing Drugs

The increased use of erection-enhancing drugs such as Viagra (sildenafil) has affected the sexual lives of many women who have sexual intercourse with men. Some welcome a male partner's firmer erection and more sustained thrusting; others, for whom penetration isn't necessarily desirable all the time, may find that the drugs contribute to an unwanted focus on intercourse and longer periods before a man reaches orgasm. This is a communication issue as well as a medication issue.

Recommended Reading: For a thoughtful and still timely discussion of Viagra and its effect on relationships, see Abraham Margentaler's *The Viagra Myth: The Surprising Impact on Love and Relationships* (Jossey-Bass, 2003). Meika Loe's *The Rise of Viagra: How the Little Blue Pill Changed Sex in America* (NYU Press, 2004) offers a more academic analysis of the social and cultural effects of Viagra.

ORAL SEX

Sucking or licking a partner's genitals, when done to a woman, is called cunnilingus (slang: going down, eating out) and, when done to a man, is called fellatio (slang: blow job, giving head).

We're really into oral sex, and he's always ready and willing. He'll say, "Do you want to have an orgasm?" And he'll go down on me. It's terrific.

Early on in our relationship (when I was still pretty unsure of how to go about this whole having-sex thing) I made a tentative reference to going down on her and she said (gently) something to the effect of, "Just so you know, I've never been a big fan of oral sex, it doesn't really do much for me." Oh, okay. So I let it drop. But I really, really wanted to taste her, so during lovemaking not long after I kinda kissed my way down to her groin, and then up her thighs, and then (all the while looking for "stop" signals) spread her legs and plunged in . . . five minutes later she had come! "And this," I told her breathlessly, "from a woman who claimed not to like oral sex!" "I didn't until five minutes ago!" she replied. How is that for validation? I really had no idea I was capable of making someone else feel that good, running on instinct like that. It's so incredibly gratifying.

I love oral sex—giving and receiving. When I am giving oral, I get off. It's an incredible feeling. I have had partners who refuse to go down on me because they didn't like it or I didn't shave or whatever. I never didn't give them a blow job because they wouldn't reciprocate. I'm really not willing to make this sacrifice anymore.

At first I was repulsed by the idea of going down on a woman. I thought that we smelled bad, that vaginas were nasty. It was a little pungent and intimidating in the beginning (though less so than

a penis had been!). I soon learned to lose myself in the wonderful textures, tastes, and formations of a woman's genitals.

Like everything in sex, oral sex is good only if we want to be doing it:

Often a guy I'm dating will say, "If you won't have intercourse, just give me a blow job." But if I didn't want him in my vagina, I probably don't want him in my mouth.

Sometimes it's incredibly erotic for me to have his penis moving in my mouth. Since I don't enjoy swallowing his semen, I usually spit it out or let it flow out on the sheets, and that's fine. Sometimes, however, blowing him makes me gag—I don't want his penis filling up my mouth at all. Then we do something else. Or we get in a position where I have more control, like being on top of him with the base of his penis in my hand.

What feels good in oral sex may differ from time to time and from person to person. Hot and cold sensations can be added with ice cubes and edible lotions—you can also try whipped cream, chocolate sauce, or other foods.

ANAL STIMULATION

The anus can be stimulated with a finger, the tongue, the penis, a butt plug, or any smooth, slender object, so long as it has a flared base and can be retrieved easily.

For many people, the anus is a highly sexually sensitive area:

I like having something small in my anus during lovemaking—no pressure or movement, just feeling it there.

Having the area around my anus licked during oral sex is a real turn-on. And anal intercourse when I'm in the mood is incredibly sexy. I love the sensations deep inside me and the thrill of doing something so unusual.

The anus is not as elastic as the vagina, so be gentle. Go slowly, wait until you're relaxed, and use a lubricant (see p. 177). If anal penetration hurts, stop. Don't use numbing lubricants. Suppressing or ignoring pain signals can cause lasting damage.

Anal bacteria can cause serious vaginal infections and cystitis, so if you want your partner's finger or penis or a dildo in your vagina after it has been in your anus, be sure to wash it well first, and use a fresh condom. If you or your partner wants to use a tongue in the anus (sometimes called rimming), using a dental dam with lubrication can protect against getting a stomach infection or a sexually transmitted infection.

Being on the receiving end of anal sex with a man is a very risky activity for HIV transmission. The delicate tissue in the rectum is prone to small tears that make an entryway for the virus. Use a latex or polyurethane barrier (male or female condoms) each time you have anal sex (see Chapter 10, "Safer Sex").

Anal intercourse isn't for everyone:

My husband wants to have anal sex a lot because he likes the tight fit and the exoticness of it. Once it happened. There was lubrication, and everything was right and it felt fine. . . . A few times it's been almost painful and I've stopped it. I wish I liked it better, because I'd love to give him that pleasure, but I have to be honest—I just don't enjoy it.

In our one great try at anal intercourse, I ended up jumping three feet in the air and squealing like a stuck pig. This so terrified him that he completely lost his erection, and we laughed and laughed. I don't think it ever really got in or

anything—somehow we hadn't quite worked out the logistics of it.

FANTASIES

Today as I stretched out before my run, I closed my eyes and imagined my lover's naked body. . . . I could feel her breasts on my face and in my mouth, our bodies reaching out, drawing close, and then wrapped together. The images and feelings sailed me through an hour of strong running.

Most of us have fantasies, sometimes in the form of fleeting images or sometimes as detailed stories. The thoughts and images we carry in our minds can evoke strong physical responses. Many sex researchers assert that the brain is the most important organ of sexual pleasure. Some women experience orgasms from fantasies alone. Sharing fantasies with a partner can be erotic:

We've just started to talk about the fantasies we have during sex. At first it felt somehow disloyal that I've needed fantasies when the other person was such a good lover. Now we figure, the more pleasure, the better.

Fantasies treat us to all kinds of erotic experiences, including situations that seem taboo. Many of us enjoy these stories and images even if we have no interest in acting them out. But if you repeatedly have fantasies that disturb you, you may want to talk about this with a trusted friend or a trained counselor.

Some people say that if you fantasize about sex being forced on you, it means you want to be raped. This is *not* true. Totally unlike actual rape, fantasizing about rape or enacting a rape fantasy is voluntary and does not bring physical pain or violation. For those who grew up learning that "good girls" don't want sex, a fantasy of being forced to have sex may free us of responsibility and can be highly erotic:

In one of my juiciest fantasies, a woman and a man tie me up and make love to me and to each other. There is something extremely erotic in imagining being that powerless. In real life, my lover and I do at times feel totally vulnerable to what the other does or wants. This fantasy lets me play around with the power dynamics that are sometimes so intense between us.

We may distrust fantasies that seem to play into male pornographic images of women as submissive or masochistic, and we may imagine that in a less sexist future, fantasies of dominance would not happen. Yet for some, the fantasy of being dominated is a real and important sexual desire—one that is not necessarily a product of a sexist culture:

One of the biggest struggles I had as a feminist exploring my sexuality in my early twenties was coming to terms with the fact that a lot of my sexual fantasies—at least the ones that lead fastest to climax—have some element of bondage, domination, restraint, coercion. I was really upset by that for a while. Not only am I absolutely against nonconsensual sex on a political, humanitarian level, I also couldn't square my desire to be dominated in sexual fantasy with my extremely strong-willed, bloody-minded personality. In real life, there is nothing that will make me dig in my heels and refuse to cooperate faster than someone telling me I don't have a choice. Yet here I was in my fantasies getting wet and heavy and achingly ready to orgasm when I imagined myself tied down, penetrated, etc., without any option of refusal. In solitary sex, I came to terms with it by realizing that fantasy (over which I have,

ultimately, complete control) is categorically different from reality.

Role-Playing, Sadomasochism (S/M), and Bondage and Discipline (B&D)

There's no limit to acting out situations and fantasies that excite us as long as all parties are consenting and enjoying themselves. We can dress up, and take it off. We can be lusty, vigorous, or needy.

Sometimes when I'm feeling good, I'll create a strip scene for my husband—and for me, since our mirror is strategically placed—and we both get very excited. Now he does it, too, standing in front of the bed, moving his body rhythmically, slowly taking off and throwing down his clothes. I love it. His strength and vulnerability come through at the same time.

In sadomasochistic sex play (S/M) or bondage and discipline (B&D), the playacting is based on fantasy situations of dominance and submission. Partners sometimes act out roles like master/servant, police/citizen, and monarch/subject. BDSM involves one partner agreeing to be vulnerable to the other partner, with boundaries laid out to ensure that lines aren't crossed. Each partner has the ability to stop the activity at any time.

As Stacy May Fowles writes, "By its very nature, BDSM is *constantly* about consent." [17]

Some of us may like spanking or having our hands or feet restrained. We can experiment with activities involving physical pain until the play comes to an end or one partner gives a signal, a prearranged "safe" word or phrase, to stop.

It is important to talk about trust and expectations before being in an S/M or B&D scenario. Safe and consensual BDSM play (sometimes called power-exchange sex) may increase sexual

REFLECTIONS ON BDSM

Kali, who self-identifies as white, fat, and disabled (she has a genetic condition called Ehlers-Danlos syndrome that causes joint injuries and chronic pain), shares her experiences with BDSM.

BDSM has been a sometimes uncomfortable, sometimes ecstatic strain in my life.

My initial reaction was revulsion. I couldn't understand how it could possibly be sexy to be bound or hit. As a fiercely independent, strong (and to be honest, rather prickly) bisexual woman, I could not wrap my head around wanting to submit. But it didn't stay that way.

When I was nineteen, my ex-fiancé and I were having a tickle fight. He, being bigger and stronger, eventually won by pinning my wrists down and straddling my waist. In that position, he kissed me, and suddenly I was on *fire*. Shockingly, passionately aroused. That was a real eye-opener for me.

I later discovered that while I don't like pain much in general (having lived with far too much of it because of my disability), I like being physically overwhelmed, ordered around, blindfolded, tied up, spanked, and lightly whipped. I suppose I fit a stereotype there—type A person in life outside the bedroom, overachiever and so on, but in the bedroom, sometimes I like not having control.

It's tough for me, though, as a survivor of sexual abuse. Pushing boundaries seems to be pretty typical in BDSM, and pushing *my* boundaries is something that must be done with great care. I've had someone take it too far, cause too much pain, push me past my comfort level, and ended up feeling emotionally bruised. I've also had someone gently come right up to the boundaries and, in doing so, make me realize that I craved going just a little farther than I'd thought I would ever want to go.

I have to believe that the person I'm "playing" with will obey the boundaries we negotiated. I have to trust that if I use a safe word, everything will stop. I have to know, at a deep and instinctive level, that they do not want to harm me.

In general, the vulnerability and openness of BDSM have been almost incandescently pleasurable for me. It hits spots that my teenage self could not admit existed.

---

pleasure and open up hidden issues of power present in most human intimacy. Establishing clear expectations is vital to ensuring that a mutual fantasy is satisfying for everyone involved:

S/M, like regular sex, allows people to share an intimate physical experience and an intimate emotional experience, but beyond that, S/M allows my partner and me to share a fantasy life, which is a deep kind of intimacy, very special and unique, that I would not trade for anything.

I think that, as in all things related to a loving, committed relationship, there has to be a great deal of respect and trust involved before there is any room for embarking on uncharted territory. We tried a little S/M after about ten years of marriage, to see what it would feel like, and it was a very valuable experience. It gave us an idea of what our comfort zones were. I don't think we would be able to explore S/M without having total and complete trust and respect for each other.

A twenty-five-year-old queer trans woman with disabilities describes the support she has experienced:

For me, I have found the BDSM community very welcoming and loving, and much more accepting of people like me than the outside community in general. I know that others have had different experiences, but for me my experience there has been primarily very positive and empowering: It has given me autonomy, a greater sense of self, and the ability to connect with lots of lovely people.

ADDED PLEASURE

LUBRICATION

Vaginal lubrication often occurs naturally during sexual excitement and arousal. Women vary in how much lubrication they produce and the amount of lubrication desired for pleasurable sexual activity. Reduced lubrication is very common and can be the result of hormonal changes in a woman's body—during breastfeeding or perimenopause and postmenopause, for instance—or caused by medications such as antihistamines, hormonal forms of birth control, chemotherapy, and medications for ADHD and depression. Also, you may have decreased lubrication if you are dehydrated, or if you're not fully aroused.

Whether you're having vaginal sex with a partner or masturbating on your own, you may want to add lubrication to:

- Decrease painful friction in vagina and/or anus

- Enhance sexual arousal by stimulating the flow of blood to the vulva, which encourages your body to create some of its own lube
- Lubricate the clitoris; this can create more sexual pleasure and an easier route to orgasm
- Change taste during oral sex
- Keep vaginal skin soft and help maintain elasticity of vaginal walls

Lubricants can be purchased online or in person at supermarkets, drugstores, and sex-toy shops.

If you have chronic pain, a lubricant containing lidocaine or benzocaine—numbing agents that can reduce vaginal, oral, or anal pain—may have been prescribed or recommended to you.

When it comes to choosing a lubricant, consider your comfort and safety. Comfort refers to the amount and staying power of the lubricant, which can make a difference in how good the sexual activity feels, and whether the lubricant irritates your genitals. Safety refers to whether the lubricant can be used with latex condoms, the most common type of condom.

If you use latex condoms to protect against pregnancy or sexually transmitted infections, *do not use* any oil-based lubricant, as it can destroy the latex and cause condom failure.

Water-Based Lubricants with Glycerin

The most commonly sold lubricants are water-based with synthetic glycerin, which produces a slightly sweet taste. Most flavored lubricants and warming lubricants contain glycerin. When water-based lubes start to dry, it is best to add water or saliva rather than just adding more lube—the water makes it slippery again.

Types/Products: Astroglide, K-Y Liquid/Jelly, Embrace, FriXion, Wet, Good Head, Revelation, Wet Flavored, ID, Replens, and Liquibeads (suppositories for dry vaginal walls).

Pros: Easy to find, low-cost, safe to use with latex condoms, do not stain fabric.

Cons: Dry out quickly, often sticky or tacky, synthetic glycerin can trigger yeast infections in women who are prone to them, products containing parabens or propylene glycol can irritate sensitive skin.

Water-Based Lubricants
Without Glycerin

If you have recurrent yeast infections, these are the lubricants to use. They can contain vegetable-derived glycerin, which does not trigger yeast infections like the lubes listed above.

Types/Products: Maximus, Ultra Glide, Liquid Silk, Slippery Stuff, O'My, Sensua Organics, Probe, Carrageenan, Glycerin, and paraben free Astroglide.

Pros: Last longer than lubricants with glycerin, can reduce irritation to the genitals, safe with latex condoms, do not stain fabric, usually thicker and provide a cushion, some are more recommended for anal play (Maximus).

Cons: Can have a bitter taste due to the absence of glycerin, usually found only online or at adult stores, those that contain parabens or propylene glycol can irritate the skin.

Silicone Lubricants

These last the longest of all and are especially recommended for women with chronic vaginal dryness or genital pain. Silicone lubricant is different from the silicone used in breast implants and is not considered dangerous; it cannot penetrate through the skin's pores. Most silicone lubricants are hypoallergenic.

Types/Products: Eros, Wet Platinum, ID Millennium, Pink, Gun Oil, Slippery Stuff.

Pros: Safe with latex condoms, stay on underwater, odorless and tasteless, last three times as long as water-based lubricants.

Cons: Expensive, cannot be used with silicone or CyberSkin sex toys, difficult to find (online or adult stores only), must be washed off with soap and water if too much is used.

Oil-Based Lubricants

The following oil-based lubricants can destroy latex condoms, but are safe to use with condoms made from nitrile, polyisoprene, or polyurethane.

Natural Oil-Based Lubricants

These lubricants often can be found in your kitchen. The general rule is that if it's safe for you to eat, it's safe to put on your vulva and inside your vagina. The body can clear out natural oils more easily than petroleum-based lubricants. Certain oils, such as grapeseed and apricot, tend to be thin and therefore better for vaginal intercourse than some of the others.

Types/Products: Vegetable, corn, avocado, peanut, and olive oils; butter; Crisco.

Pros: Great for genital massages, safe for the vagina, safe to eat, good for all forms of sexual play, low-cost, easily accessible.

Cons: Destroy latex condoms, stain fabric.

Other Oil-Based Lubricants

These take longer to clear out of your body than natural oils.

Types/Products: Mineral oil, Vaseline, body lotions, creams such as Stroke 29 or Jack Jelly.

Pros: Great for external masturbation, low-cost, easily accessible.

Cons: Irritate vulva, destroy latex condoms, stain fabric.

SEX TOYS

Sex toys and aids can spice up sexual encounters, make safer sex fun, and be an outlet for creativity. You can try edible body paints or flavored condoms, an egg-shaped electric vibrator or a double dildo, a strap-on harness or a G-spot stimulator.

Sex toys can be bought in person or online. Women-owned boutiques, the first of which opened in the 1970s, often offer feminist, sex-positive information and workshops for women and men.

Don't have time to get a store or can't wait for an online order to arrive? Look around at home: A cucumber dildo or shower nozzle spray can be used for pleasure.

In my early twenties I purchased a couple of vibrators and experimented a little (this was while I was trying to learn how to orgasm), but they didn't really do much for me, and I found anything larger than the silver bullet type of vibrators too uncomfortable to insert and use solo. But the longer lovemaking sessions I have with my partner helped me to relax and play with these toys in new ways. [We] have enjoyed strap-on dildos, lube, and nipple clamps. So being in a relationship has really dramatically improved my opinion of sex toys and deepened my appreciation for the variety of accessories that are out there.

I explored sex toys the summer I was widowed; I was very lonely, crying daily, and needed to comfort myself. I went to our local independent feminist "love store" and, with help from the saleswoman, bought my first vibrator. When it wore out, after some extensive online research I bought some mail-order toys through Good Vibrations and Betty Dodson's website. I wanted to talk with other women about vibrators but couldn't find any women friends who'd discuss them. Nevertheless, I found them great fun to use by myself.

EROTICA

Enjoying erotic entertainment, alone or with a partner, is a way of exploring sexual needs and becoming more comfortable with solitary or shared desires. There is a wide selection of sexually explicit videos, magazines, and books, some created by and for women of all sexual orientations. Online and digital offerings include do-it-yourself videos as well as professionally produced films.

PORNOGRAPHY

Some feminists have sought to make a useful distinction between erotica and pornography, with erotica seen as sexually explicit materials that don't demean or exploit women, and pornography seen as materials that sexualize women's pain or suffering. There's a wide range of feelings about what constitutes erotica, what constitutes pornography, and whether some sexually explicit materials can be harmful to women. Some of us may try to distinguish between hard porn (more graphic/violent) and soft porn (less graphic/more consensual), while some women feel that even soft porn usually promotes male fantasies of sex and thus limits the imagination.

I have an extremely complicated relationship with porn. It's something I started watching early on and I'm comfortable telling people that I watch it. However, when I hear stories like the young girl in Oakland getting gang-raped after a prom, I start to wonder if porn is causing younger people to have an unreal view of what is and isn't acceptable. When it's easy to see a woman have sex with multiple men at one time, they may start to believe that that's every woman's fantasy, when it isn't. I know that when I'm watching porn, it's not what real sex is and I'm comfortable with that. However, I'm not sure everyone is able to separate themselves from that. For a while it got so that I couldn't watch any pornography because

I kept thinking of the message it was sending. However, I'm all for freedom of expression and I get turned on by erotic images. I'm just trying to figure out where to draw the line between my feminist ideals and my sexual proclivities.

I've come to a much more inclusive definition of erotica/porn and realized how valuable it is to have textual and visual stimulation as a way of exploring what turns you on. My girlfriend and I, before we were sexually involved, traded sexually explicit fan fiction (both self-produced and by others) and we've continued to enjoy erotic literature in our relationship.

I really enjoy porn, but only queer/feminist porn. I love Courtney Trouble's work. It's artistic and tasteful. I also love the Crash Pad series. The direction of those is brilliant as well and it's a black lesbian woman who does the directing. That makes me happy.

I reserve the viewing of porn for the times I want to indulge in self-stimulation. I just try to avoid the parts of porn that disgust me—like the excessive spitting on genitalia and close-ups of male ejaculation. It also drives me nuts that women are rarely shown having real orgasms, so I appreciate those that do depict this, since I know it happens in real life. When I find one I like, it's all about the scene for me. If I can imagine what something might feel like to give or receive, or remember a time that I did something similar in my personal experience, it turns me on.

What it comes down to at a personal level is that what some women consider arousing, others may consider unappealing or demeaning. As with fantasies, what you see in erotica/porn may help you explore and enjoy an aspect of your sexual desire without having to act on it.

■■■■■■■■■■■■■■■■■■■■■■ **CHAPTER 8**

For many women, sexual pleasure can be compromised by physical or emotional challenges. The difficulties can be even harder to bear when medical providers find no underlying cause or do not offer suggestions for relief.

This chapter looks at a wide range of issues, including variations of desire and difficulties with arousal, causes of painful penetration that can make sexual intercourse and other forms of insertive sex difficult if not impossible, and the sexual challenges sometimes experienced by women with specific chronic illnesses and disabilities. The chapter also addresses the influence of medications and hormones on physical responses to sex and sexual pleasure.

Stories from women illuminate what has and what hasn't

worked for those of us who wish sex were something that we could enjoy more fully and without hesitation.

VARIATIONS IN DESIRE

Pick up any magazine or read a sex survey, and you're likely to hear how much sexual desire you should have. It's essential to remember that there is no one right amount. Chances are your sex drive fluctuates: Sometimes you want a great deal of sexual activity and can't get it out of your mind, and other times you aren't nearly so interested. Maybe you were sexually quiet for decades and now have strong sexual feelings that make you eager to masturbate, or find a partner, or have sex all the time. Maybe ten years ago you wanted sex every night and now it takes effort, even though you tend to be glad when you do.

A NEW VIEW

Some feminists have questioned the medicalization of sexual desire, seeing it as part of as an effort to legitimize the quest for a moneymaking female Viagra. The feminist researcher Leonore Tiefer and other authors of *A New View of Women's Sexual Problems* (newviewcampaign.org) offer a useful critique. While affirming that certain medications and hormone supplements can help with some sexual problems caused by specific physiological conditions, contributors to *A New View* also identify a range of possible socioeconomic, political, and relationship-based causes for women's sexual concerns.

This fluctuation is true for many of us. Our levels of desire—in terms of both wanting sex and getting aroused—can shift over the years, or from week to week or partner to partner. For some of us, a lack of sexual desire and an inability to get aroused or to orgasm are long-lasting problems that seem unchangeable and cause us distress. Good medical research on the causes of and treatments for these problems is crucial.

I want safe, dependable treatment to be available in case I need it. The rush of sexual desire is too delicious to give up.

How sexual I feel at any given time depends a surprising amount on how much sleep I'm getting, how my partner and I are getting along, whether I'm feeling depressed, what level of antidepressant I'm taking, and a bunch of other even less tangible factors. On those days or months when my desire seems to have dried up, all I seem to be able to tolerate are small, boundaried kisses, and I feel almost smothered if she meets me with a soft-lip, mushy, wet one.

THE QUESTION OF FEMALE SEXUAL DYSFUNCTION AND THE SEARCH FOR A FEMALE VIAGRA

A number of pharmaceutical companies (and medical researchers associated with those companies) have worked over the past two decades to discover medications that enhance women's sexual desire. You may have heard this referred to as the "search for a female Viagra."

This research is crucial for those of us for whom low sexual desire is a result of a physiological problem that might respond to a medical approach. However, we need to be aware that once a product is found, drug companies, in an effort to increase profits, will try to expand the

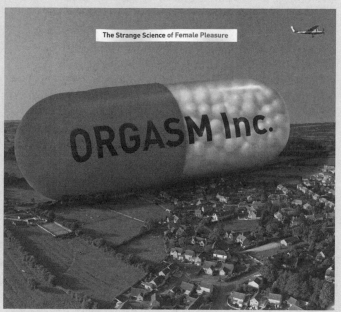

Recommended for Your Viewing Pleasure: In the documentary *Orgasm Inc.*, filmmaker Liz Canner takes viewers behind the scenes of the race to create the first FDA-approved drug for women to treat female sexual dysfunction (FSD). The film takes a sobering yet humorous look inside the pharmaceutical companies and marketing campaigns that are shaping attitudes about the meaning of health, illness, desire, and orgasm. Learn more at orgasminc.com.

The Strange Science of Female Pleasure

market for desire-enhancing medications by encouraging more women to question whether their level of desire is normal.

A particularly problematic aspect of this effort is a new practice of defining all low sexual desire in women as female sexual dysfunction (FSD), a medical disorder deserving treatment. If your levels of desire don't match some cultural norm (if you don't have sex twice a week, for example), you may be encouraged to think that you have a medically significant sexual dysfunction.

It's essential to remember that there is no right amount of sexual desire, just what's right for you. What matters is *your* satisfaction with how much desire *you* feel, not whether your desire is high or low by someone else's standards. Your level of desire is a problem only if it causes you distress. If you're not unhappy with your level of desire, don't let anyone tell you that it's dysfunctional.

For those of us who are unhappy with how we feel, the first step is attending to other factors that can play a role, such as relationship issues or depression. Anxiety and sleep deprivation can also cause low sexual desire. Are you putting in more hours at work, or are you engaged in some other pursuit? You may think something's wrong with your sex drive because you can't even think about wanting sex right now, but your body may be trying to get through the extra level of stress it's been asked to manage. Give yourself time to deal with the stress before concluding that there's something inherently wrong.

If addressing potential underlying causes doesn't help, FSD as a diagnosis can be a welcome validation for those who have wondered what's wrong. Accessible, well-researched, and effective treatments are critical. Online communities and blogs discussing FSD are becoming more common as women seek a balance between the development of necessary medications and an exaggerated medicalization of women's sexuality.

A cultural shift in how we think about desire may be overdue. Traditionally, desire has been understood as a spontaneous motivation to have sex. More recent models point to a nonlinear model of sexual response that incorporates emotional intimacy, sexual stimuli, and relationship satisfaction (see p. 155 for more discussion).

Pharmaceutical companies are in the process of developing other types of medical products to address women's problems with sexual desire and functioning. For a while, they tested some drugs originally created for men, but the results were disappointing. Examples of drugs now sold to men to address erectile dysfunction problems include Viagra (sildenafil), Levitra (vardenafil), and Cialis (tadalafil). Products for women that have been tested in double-blind, placebo-controlled studies include nonprescription remedies such as Zestra (which contains herbal oils)[1] and ArginMax (a dietary supplement), and vibrating apparatuses such as Eros. These are all designed to increase blood flow to the genital areas. Some women have had good results with hormonal supplements such as testosterone, while others have experienced no improvement or even harmful side effects. Research continues to evolve in this area, and it is prudent to investigate the latest data available.

TESTOSTERONE: USES AND CONCERNS

If you mention to your health-care provider that you are experiencing lack of sexual desire, problems with arousal, or difficulty being orgasmic, you may be offered testosterone treatment. Commercially available testosterone supplements were developed for men and have not been approved by the FDA for use by women. (Intrinsa, a testosterone patch for

THE HOPE FOR FLIBANSERIN

In June 2010, a FDA advisory panel recommended *not* to approve the much-anticipated drug flibanserin[2] to treat hypoactive sexual desire disorder (HSDD), which is defined as "low or no sexual interest to the point of distress in otherwise healthy people." The panel found that the drug failed to increase desire and its impact did not justify the risks. Women taking flibanserin had less than one (0.08) additional "sexually satisfying event" (orgasm not required) in a given month compared with women taking a placebo. Possible side effects included dizziness, nausea, and fatigue, particularly with long-term daily use. "For some it may turn out that there is a drug that provides effective treatment," said Amy Allina, program director for the National Women's Health Network. "But this drug is not it."[3]

The German pharmaceutical company Boehringer Ingelheim initially said it would continue its research, but Boehringer later announced it was stopping development of flibanserin.

women made by Procter & Gamble, is available in Europe but has not been approved for U.S. use.) Though doctors can legally prescribe such drugs to women (a practice known as off-label use), they must guess at the right dosage when prescribing products developed for men and/or use a special compounding pharmacy that will mix lower doses for women. Some practitioners will prescribe an ultralow dose of a commercially available testosterone gel for men, such as AndroGel or Testim; specially mixed testosterone cream or gel available from compounding pharmacies; or methyltestosterone capsules to be taken orally (not recommended, however, because of negative effects on lipid levels and the liver).

Measuring women's sexual satisfaction is difficult, so the science supporting the use of testosterone in women is limited. Some women want to try it, especially after exploring non-medical approaches without success. Be sure that you are screened carefully and your baseline blood levels are low in testosterone. Be on the lookout for signs of male hormone excess: Acne, increased facial hair growth, and decreased scalp hair are all indicators that the levels are too high. There are limited long-term safety data on testosterone for women. Testosterone readily changes into estrogen in the breast, so there is a theoretical concern that testosterone supplementation could promote breast cancer.

There are over-the-counter counter topical creams that claim to augment sexual pleasure by increasing blood flow into the genital region, and some practitioners recommend trying them. Avlimil is one example. The instructions say to apply the cream with your finger to the genital area for fifteen minutes—which might explain its effectiveness in aiding arousal.

The only factor consistently linked to sexual desire and satisfaction in studies—more so than testosterone levels—may come as a surprise: exercise. Whether this is due to endorphins, improved mood, or just feeling good about ourselves, exercise is worth a try.

PAINFUL INTERCOURSE/ PENETRATION

Vaginal penetration that you desire typically doesn't hurt, especially if you and your part-

Some women experience not simply a lack of desire, but an aversion to any sexual interactions. Such aversion can arise from deep conflicts about sex, often rooted in past hurts. This may manifest as an extreme, unpleasant sensitivity to touch, or feeling so ticklish that the ticklishness prevents relaxation. Bodies react this way for a reason—they may be protecting us from sexual experiences we can't handle at this point. The American Association of Sexuality Educators, Counselors and Therapists (aasect.org) is a good place to look for help and support.

ner take care that you are receiving sufficient sexual stimulation to be fully aroused. Yet there are times when, even with plenty of arousal and added lubrication, you may experience discomfort or pain. If penetration is at all painful, you owe it to yourself to find out what is causing it and do something about it. A gynecologist can help to determine whether there are physical causes and advise you on treatments. While you are seeking help, you can try alternatives, like masturbating or oral sex with a partner, and anything else that brings pleasure. Open communication between you and your partner(s) makes a difference.

The first few times you have intercourse or experience vaginal penetration, you may feel a small to moderate amount of pain at the entrance to the vagina. There can be some bleeding or no bleeding at all—both are normal. The reasons for the pain are not always clear, but it is typically temporary. An unstretched hymen (vaginal corona) has typically been blamed for this pain at first penetration, but new understandings of the hymen suggest otherwise (see

p. 7). As Hanne Blank, author of *Virgin: The Untouched History*, comments: "If the hymen is substantial, relatively inflexible, and attached around much of the circumference of the vaginal opening, then yes, it's fair to say that the hymen is at issue. But not all hymens meet these criteria, and women without substantial hymens can also experience painful penetration. The truth is that research has not told us with any particular specificity why it is that this discomfort happens, or why it happens for some women (regardless of hymen type) and not others."

The following conditions can contribute to or cause pain during intercourse or other forms of penetration.

Insufficient lubrication. In most women, the wall of the vagina usually responds to arousal by producing a liquid that moistens the vagina and its entrance, making penetration easier. Sometimes there isn't enough lubrication, perhaps because more time is needed for stimulation, or because you may be nervous or tense. Try giving yourself more time to get fully wet.

Insufficient lubrication can also be caused by lowered levels of estrogen, which can make vaginal tissue more fragile and affect the vaginal walls in such a way that less liquid is produced. This affects some women after childbirth (particularly if you're nursing) and women who have to take hormone therapy after breast cancer. Some women also experience this during perimenopause and postmenopause, during which you may need to look for signs other than vaginal wetness to signal arousal (see Chapter 20, "Perimenopause and Menopause," for more discussion). Some women, regardless of their age, simply produce less lubricant. Even if you are not experiencing painful penetration, using a lubricant can dramatically increase sexual comfort, pleasure, and stamina—especially if you use condoms. (The lubricants section on p. 177 has more information on the different types of lube.)

Local infection. Some vaginal infections—like monilia (yeast) or trichomoniasis—can be present in a nonacute, visually unnoticeable form. The friction of a penis, dildo, or finger moving on the vulva or in the vagina might cause the infection to flare up, resulting in stinging and itchiness. A herpes sore on the external genitals can make friction painful.

Local irritation. The vagina might be irritated by a birth control foam, cream, or jelly. First, try a different brand; however, if the irritation persists, it may be in reaction to the spermicide Nonoxynol-9. Alternative spermicides are extremely hard to find, so you may want to consider another birth control method. Though latex allergy is uncommon, some people are sensitive to latex condoms, diaphragms, and gloves. Alternatives include polyurethane condoms, including female condoms. Vaginal deodorant sprays, douches, scented tampons, and all so-called feminine hygiene products can irritate the vagina or vulva, as can body wash, soaps, bubble bath, and laundry detergents.

Tightness in the vaginal entrance. In some situations, size matters—if, for example, a male partner has a large penis and your vagina is small. Keep in mind, though, that a woman's body size is *not* related to size of her vagina. One woman notes that orgasms can help.

I have to be enormously aroused to be able to accommodate a man's penis. It takes multiple orgasms usually, so my partner has to be very patient.

Women's difficulty with penetration is sometimes attributed to vaginismus, believed to be a strong, involuntary tightening of the vaginal muscles, a spasm of the outer third of the vagina. Researchers have not always been able to identify these muscle spasms, writes Debby Herbenick, author of *Because It Feels Good: A Woman's Guide to Sexual Pleasure* and *Satisfaction* and founder of mysexprofes sor.com. "More recently, vaginismus has been described as 'persistent or recurrent difficulties of the woman to allow vaginal entry of a penis, a finger, or any object, despite the woman's expressed wish to do so.'[4] This is an important distinction because it reinforces the point that penetration should be *consensual and wanted*."[5]

Pain deep in the pelvis. Sometimes the thrust of penetration hurts way inside. This pain can be caused by tears and scarring (known as adhesions) in the ligaments that support the uterus (caused by obstetrical mismanagement during childbirth, an improperly performed abortion, pelvic surgery, rape, or excessively rough penetration during sex); infections of the cervix, uterus, and tubes (such as pelvic inflammatory disease—the result of untreated sexually transmitted infection in many women); endometriosis; cysts or tumors on the ovaries; a vagina that has shortened with age; or a tilted pelvis. Penetration in these cases is sometimes less painful if you're on top or lying beside a partner. If penetration consistently causes deep pelvic pain, consider consulting with an experienced gynecological practitioner.

VULVODYNIA

Vulvodynia is a catchall term describing chronic vulvar pain, sometimes without an identifiable cause. It can be extremely difficult and time-consuming to find a practitioner who understands vulvar pain and takes the time to determine why the pain exists and how best to address it. Localized vulvodynia, also known as vestibulodynia (or by an older term, vestibulitis), is marked by a painful burning or sharp sensation in and around the opening to the vagina when there is any kind of penetration.

Pelvic floor physical therapy, hormonal creams, and low-dose tricyclic antidepressants may be helpful in reducing or eliminating the

PELVIC FLOOR PHYSICAL THERAPY

If you have pain with intercourse, your practitioner can refer you to a specialized women's health physical therapist who can evaluate the strength of, endurance of, and any painful trigger points in your pelvic floor muscles. Some women who have developed increased pelvic floor tension find the use of progressive-sized dilators to be effective. These medical-grade dilators may be purchased online or through your health-care provider's office.

pain, which is thought to be caused by an overgrowth of nerve endings; surgery is usually a last resort. For more on vulvodynia, see p. 635. Self-help tips for dealing with chronic pain are available online at the National Vulvodynia Association (nva.org/self_help_tips.html).

I used to enjoy having sex, but around the time I turned thirty, penetration became more and more painful. I saw at least four gynecologists over the next eight years who either suggested that I needed to relax more during sex (grrr) or completely misdiagnosed the pain. Finally, after I talked with a friend about all this, she pointed me toward a gynecologist who specializes in vulvar pain, and he diagnosed it as localized vulvodynia. It was one of the best days of my life—now that I knew what it was, I could start treatment (in my case, estrogen cream and pelvic floor physical therapy worked the best—the pain connection is unclear, but going through the exercises before sex helps). I'm still frustrated by the number of doctors who made me feel it was "all in my head." I've since learned that many women go undiagnosed, which is ridiculous considering how vestibulodynia affects so many aspects of our lives and sexual health.

No matter the underlying cause, when you and your partner are unable to have sex for some time, it can be difficult to start again. Talking with a counselor or sex therapist may be useful. Open communication can sometimes decrease any awkwardness that develops when there's been a physical distance between couples.

EFFECTS OF MEDICATIONS AND HORMONES ON SEXUALITY

MEDICATIONS

Certain medications can affect sexual desire and the likelihood and intensity of orgasms. If you are taking an over-the-counter or prescription drug or herbal supplement and notice a change in your sexual functioning, there may be a connection. For example, antihistamines, which people often take to dry out secretions in the nose, may also cause vaginal dryness. Medications for long-term chronic illnesses and disabilities can affect sexual functioning in a variety of ways (see "Sex With a Disability or Chronic Illness," p. 194, for more information).

Keep a record of the drugs you're taking and note how you're feeling sexually. Some package inserts may identify known sexual effects, but your own record may be the best source of information.

Antidepressants are known to affect sexual functioning. Some SSRI antidepressants (selective serotonin reuptake inhibitors), such as Prozac (fluoxetine), Paxil (paroxetine), and Zoloft (sertraline), as well as SNRI antidepressants (serotonin-norepinephrine reuptake inhibitors) such as Effexor (venlafaxine) and Cymbalta (duloxetine) may reduce sexual desire and the ability to orgasm.

Other antidepressants, such as Wellbutrin (bupropion), have been shown to cause less sexual dysfunction than SSRIs or SNRIs (some women even report an increase in sexual desire). Adjustments in drug dosage sometimes affect sexual side effects.

One woman who takes Prozac says:

When I got in a relationship, I found that some of the sexual side effects are more subtle. I found that while I still experienced desire, it has become really difficult to have an orgasm. And when I do, the quality is different. In the old days, I felt a slow buildup that ended with intense, sudden contractions; now I most often feel a wave of excitement that ebbs and flows but never quite peaks in the same way.

HORMONES

Estrogen, progesterone, and testosterone are hormones that affect a woman's sexual desire and functioning. In terms of sexual desire, the most influential hormone is testosterone, sometimes called the libido or male hormone. In fact, testosterone, like estrogen, is present in both men *and* women, though the proportions differ between the sexes. In women, testosterone is produced through the operation of the adrenals (two small glands near the kidneys) and the ovaries.

Hormonal changes and their effects on sexual desire and functioning are not necessarily a problem. Menstrual and menopausal changes, for example, are a normal part of a woman's development. However, if a hormonal change leads to a drop in desire or sexual pleasure, and you feel dissatisfied with this, you may want to explore other options, such as changing or altering medications or birth control method. Some women who experience vaginal dryness use hormonal supplements, such as estrogen or estrogen/progestin pills and patches, or estrogen cream or rings applied topically in the vagina. (For more about the harms and benefits of hormonal products used for vaginal dryness, see p. 517.)

Many factors affect hormone levels at any given time.

Menstrual cycle. Hormone levels fluctuate throughout our cycles. Many women who menstruate have a peak of sexual desire (libido) before and around ovulation, with a second, less intense peak during menstruation. The lowest level of libido is often prior to menstruation, although there is much variation from this pattern.

Postmenopausal women, and many women using hormonal birth control methods, have less variation in sexual desire.

The Pill and other hormonal birth control methods such as the patch (e.g., Ortho Evra), injectable contraceptives (e.g., Depo-Provera), and the vaginal ring (NuvaRing). Some hormonal birth control methods suppress the usual cyclical nature of hormones and may affect desire and sexual functioning. Some women have more desire, while other women experience less desire, orgasm less easily, and/or experience vaginal dryness. The specific effects of these methods vary greatly among individual women.

Pregnancy. Estrogen and progesterone levels are higher during pregnancy, and blood flow to the genitals increases. These changes, along with other physical and psychological effects of pregnancy, may lead to increased desire for some women. For others, however, fatigue, nausea, pain, fears, or issues with changing body size and self-image may squelch desire.

Nursing. Breastfeeding can suppress ovulation for months after birth, as a result of the high levels of the hormone prolactin and reduced levels of estrogen. Many women report a drop in sexual desire while nursing. Some have no libido at all and become nonorgasmic. This is normal; sexual desire usually returns when the baby is weaned or nursing much less. This normal postpartum variation in desire can be stressful to intimate relationships. For more information, see "Mothers' Health and Well-Being," p. 447.

Perimenopause/menopause. During the years leading up to menopause (which occurs when menstrual periods have stopped for a full year), estrogen levels spike and fall erratically while progesterone levels decline. By one year after the last menstrual period, both progesterone and estrogen are steady at low levels. You may experience less desire and increased vaginal dryness. For some, relief from the fear of pregnancy after you enter postmenopause may allow newfound sexual freedom. (For more, see Chapter 20, "Perimenopause and Menopause.")

Adrenal or ovary removal (oophorectomy). Either of these surgeries may result in a dramatic decrease in sexual interest and frequency of orgasm, in part due to a reduction of testosterone (see more on testosterone above). This is one of many reasons for avoiding unnecessary removal of the ovaries or adrenals (see p. 630).

SEX, DISABILITY, AND CHRONIC DISEASE

Some of us have chronic diseases or disabilities we were born with, such as cystic fibrosis or blindness, or have developed later in life, such as multiple sclerosis or bipolar disorder. Regardless of onset, each of us has the right to fulfillment of sexual desires and to feel good about expressing sexuality. Yet all too often, some people, including health-care providers, assume that teenage girls and women with disabilities are sexless.

GimpGirl Community (GimpGirl.com) aims to bring women with disabilities together in the spirit of support, positivity, and inclusivity. The site includes useful information for women with disabilities and their allies, including a list of recommended gynecologists and clinics with accessible exam chairs or tables. Add your recommendations to help the list grow.

Not only are these attitudes condescending; they can also negatively affect our health and self-esteem. While more is being done to educate the medical community, the pressure is often on us to explain our sexual desires and capabilities and to inform the world around us.

Samantha, who has quadriplegia, says of her relationship with her husband, Michael:

We love each other passionately and often. While the disability does, in reality, affect how we do things and what we are able to do together, it does not define our relationship. Assumptions are always the problem. People can assume, because I'm disabled, that my sexuality, and my ability to enjoy and participate in sex, has been taken away from me. It is fun to be part of an education process aimed at challenging this perception.

Compounding the problem is the fact that having a disability can trigger feelings of alienation or disconnection from our own bodies, causing shame and embarrassment. Reclaiming our bodies for positive sexual experiences may take time and patience, as well as experimentation and support:

I am visually impaired and had to endure multiple medical procedures to prevent blindness or improve my eyesight. Growing up with these challenges often left me feeling like my body was my enemy, so I feel like my sexual development and intimate relationships with others were/ are affected by my heightened insecurities about my body, and I worry about whether or not my significant other would stick around if my vision problems took a turn for the worse.

From dating to the logistics of partner sex, challenges may arise. Lack of knowledge and poorly designed spaces can turn simple issues into huge barriers. We must also decide when and how much to disclose if our disability is not obvious:

I have been surprised at how little most men I have had sex with are bothered by my urostomy [in which urine is collected from the bladder in a small bag attached to the abdomen]. I do tell them before we are in the buff, and it hasn't been too much of an issue. I think they must already accept my disability to some extent before becoming intimate, so perhaps they just see the urostomy as more of the same—part of the disability, which is how I see it.

After my brain injury, I couldn't get spontaneous pictures of people masturbating in public out of my mind and even flirted with the idea of lifting my skirt and doing it myself. These new thoughts were disturbing, and I was afraid to tell my partner, because I worried it would damage our relationship. Then I learned in a support group how a brain injury can change our ability to maintain appropriate sexual boundaries. Eventually, my urges were less frequent, and I became more comfortable with my sexuality.

A great deal of sexual expression involves verbal and nonverbal communication. When one partner is deaf, is hard of hearing, or has a speech disability, we may need to learn new

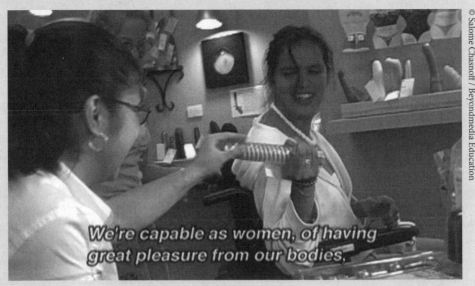

We're capable as women, of having great pleasure from our bodies,

The Empowered Fe Fes visit Early to Bed in the documentary film *Doin' It: Sex, Disability & Videotape.* View the film's trailer at vimeo.com/1474473.

The Empowered Fe Fes, a Chicago-based peer group of young women age thirteen to twenty-four with different disabilities, use video to investigate truths about their lives and their communities and shatter stereotypes about their individual abilities. In the documentary *Doin' It: Sex, Disability & Videotape,* the Fe Fes (slang for female) educate themselves about sex from many angles by talking with activists and scholars. The viewer tags along on a date between a woman with a disability and her able-bodied boyfriend and accompanies the group to a sex toy shop where they learn about feeling comfortable exploring their bodies.

The Fe Fes are sponsored by Access Living (accessliving.org), a disability rights organization. *Doin' It* was created in a media workshop and produced by Beyondmedia Education. A previous year-long workshop that explored growing up as a girl with disabilities led to the creation of the film *Beyond Disability: The Fe Fe Stories.* During that workshop, it came up that only one of the sixteen participants had heard the word clitoris before. This is not uncommon; young people with disabilities are systematically left out of sex education in the schools, the implication being they don't need it. Girls with disabilities are sorely undereducated about sex, and there is a high rate of sexual abuse and domestic violence among girls with disabilities.

The girls' interest in learning more led to the workshop that created *Doin' It: Sex, Disability & Videotape*. The film premiered in 2007 and has been screened in festivals and other venues. It received a best documentary (short) award from the San Francisco Women's Film Festival and an award at Picture This . . . Film Festival in Calgary, Canada. In 2009, Feminist Active Documentary Video Festa in Tokyo translated the video and began distributing the video in Japan.

In the still pictured above, the Fe Fes (Veronica Martinez, left, and Krystal Martinez, right, no relation) are exploring toys at Early to Bed, a feminist sex shop in Chicago. The subtitle in the frame captures the voice-over of Susan Nussbaum, who founded the Empowered Fe Fes with Taina Rodriguez in 1999.

"We're capable as women of having great pleasure from our bodies," says Nussbaum. "And as disabled women, that is something we are often not told about ourselves."

Since the completion of the video, several of the girls who helped produce it have continued to grow as disability activists—challenging the American Medical Association on ethical issues around disabilities, demanding that public officials address access issues, and traveling to the state capital and Washington, D.C., in support of disability rights legislation. To purchase *Doin' It* or other Beyondmedia films on womens' and girls' activism, visit beyondmedia.org.

ways of communicating. Honest and frank discussions about what makes us feel good can be a model for all sexually active people.

I needed to find out if I could actually feel comfortable and communicate to someone who really didn't know me before my accident in order to have sex. At this party, I met a guy, and we eventually had sex. The morning after, I asked him what it was like to be with me, and he answered, "Honestly, at first I was afraid I might hurt you because you are so small, but you talked to me and told me what felt good, and what to do that was good for me, too, so it was great!" In more ways than one, it was great for me as well.

The cultural pressure to be spontaneous with sex can be frustrating if some assistance is needed.

To help maintain independence, a personal-care attendant can help us, or our partner, prepare for sexual activities, though that can be intrusive.

My husband and I are both disabled, so we need a lot of help. We decided that hiring a personal-care attendant was too much of an invasion of our privacy, though. It is very frustrating, but we just don't have intercourse anymore. We have our orgasms through oral sex now, and my husband says we are lucky and that other people would be jealous if they knew.

Certain chronic illnesses and disabilities such as fibromyalgia and some spinal cord injuries have associated pain, so there may be times when we want sexual activity but can't bear to be touched. For some, direct genital stimulation can actually help to block the pain.[6]

Members of the disability community have taught the medical establishment much about sexuality over the years. Research has validated what some of us knew all along—our orgasms are real and can result from genital stimulation or stimulation of other highly eroticized areas. This is true for women with and without spinal cord injury.[7]

The first time I had sex with my boyfriend after I became paralyzed, it was awful. But then, over time, it got better with communication and experience. I was surprised that I could still orgasm after my injury, since no one at the hospital had discussed it with me.

Some disabilities also make us more susceptible to depression by causing changes in brain chemistry and hormone and activity levels, causing us to withdraw from sexual activities. These feelings can be made worse by the medications prescribed. No matter the cause, though, we are not our disability or a bundle of symptoms—a fact that we need to assert and the medical establishment needs to recognize.

Recommended Resources on Sex and Disability: Much writing about sex and disability focuses on male erection issues to the exclusion of women's concerns. These resources are recommended:

- *The Ultimate Guide to Sex and Disability: For All of Us Who Live with Disabilities, Chronic Pain, and Illness* by Miriam Kaufman, Cory Silverberg, and Fran Odette (Cleis Press, 2007).
- *Enabling Romance: A Guide to Love, Sex, and Relationships for People with Disabilities (and the People Who Care About Them)* by Ken Kroll and Erica Levy Klein (No Limits Communications, 2001).
- *A Provider's Guide for the Care of Women with Physical Disabilities and Chronic Medical Conditions* by Suzanne Smeltzer and Nancy Sharts-Hopko (North Carolina Office on Disability and Health, 2005). Though written for providers, this guide gives a clear, comprehensive overview of women's health issues. Available free at fpg.unc.edu/~ncodh/publications.cfm.

Chronic Babe (ChronicBabe.com) was created as an online community for younger women. It includes a help desk, articles, and discussion forums.

SEX WITH A DISABILITY OR CHRONIC ILLNESS

CHRONIC DISEASE OR DISABILITY	EFFECTS ON SEXUALITY	HELPFUL HINTS AND CONSIDERATIONS
Cerebral palsy (CP)	Muscle spasticity, rigidity, and/or weakness may complicate some sexual activity. Knee and hip contractures may cause pain under the pressure of a partner, and spasms may increase with arousal. Some women experience a lack of vaginal lubrication. Menstruation, fertility, and pregnancy are not affected. During delivery, women with severe CP might need a cesarean section.	Sex without vaginal penetration, trying different positions, or propping legs up on pillows may ease spasms. A vibrator or another sex toy can be used for self-pleasure or with another person. Estrogen-containing birth control methods are not advisable for women with restricted mobility. For women taking anticonvulsants, see special precautions below for epilepsy.[8] *A, B, D, E*
Cognitive disabilities (including brain injury, epilepsy, and stroke)	Sexual abilities vary depending upon the location of brain injury (BI). A changed level of interest in sex is possible, as well as decreased vaginal lubrication and difficulty experiencing an orgasm. These reactions are sometimes caused by medications or associated with depression.[9] Irregular periods are common, and it may be difficult to become pregnant. Menopause may also occur earlier. BI and stroke may result in communication, cognitive, and visual-perceptive impairments, as well as loss of sensation, paralysis, and incontinence. Traumatic BI can cause impulsive sexual activity and an inability to read social cues, resulting in frank discussions about sex that others may find socially inappropriate.[10]	If balance, coordination, or strength is an issue, try sexual activities in positions that support the body or require little exertion. Social-skills retraining or working with a neuropsychologist may help to address cognitive or behavioral issues. Estrogen-containing birth control methods and hormone therapy (HT) are not advisable for women with paralysis, stroke, or circulatory disorders. Many antiseizure medications cause a rapid breakdown of hormones in the body, making contraceptives less effective in preventing pregnancy; using a barrier method may be advisable. In a small minority of women with epilepsy, IUD insertion can cause what is known as a reflex seizure.[11] *A, B, C, D, E*
Diabetes and chronic kidney disease	Numerous recent studies have examined the effects of diabetes on women's sexual response, often with varying findings. Some women with diabetes and kidney disease report that orgasms gradually become less frequent and less intense.[12] It is possible that damage to the blood vessels and nerves in the pelvic region impact arousal and orgasm. A lack of vaginal lubrication and recurrent infections can make some sexual activity difficult and painful.[13] Age, depression, and marital status are the most common predictors of sexual difficulties in women with diabetes.[14] Unregulated diabetes and kidney failure may stop menstruation and cause fertility issues. Pregnancy may be complicated for women with all of these conditions and should be closely monitored, including after kidney transplantation.[15]	Using a vibrator enables some women to experience orgasm because the stimulation is more intense. Healthy women with diabetes can generally take the Pill and use other hormonal birth control safely, but women who have hypertension or kidney disease should avoid birth control containing estrogen.[16] It is unclear whether hypertension itself can impair sexual function.[17] It is known that many drugs used to treat hypertension are likely to dampen sexual desire.[18] Topical estrogen cream may be useful for vaginal dryness and pain.[19] Dialysis often brings on heavy and sometimes painful menstruation and may increase sexual desire, though maybe not sexual responsiveness. Kidney transplants usually improve sexual desire, responsiveness, and fertility. *D, E*

CHRONIC DISEASE OR DISABILITY	EFFECTS ON SEXUALITY	HELPFUL HINTS AND CONSIDERATIONS
Heart disease	For those with very serious conditions, including chest pain, palpitations, and shortness of breath, sexual activity may be limited. However, if you can climb two flights of stairs at a brisk pace without inducing symptoms, it's a good sign you're ready to resume sexual activity.[20] (The cardiac responses during step climbing and sex are similar, the average heart rate being 125 beats per minute.) Taking an exercise stress test is the best way to tell if you are physically ready.[21] The fear of inducing symptoms and depression are often primary obstacles to sexual encounters.[22]	Consult a physician to see when and if you can safely begin an exercise regimen. The AMA suggests engaging in sex when rested, waiting one to three hours after eating a full meal to allow time for digestion, and taking prescription medications before sexual activity. Essential hypertension is now being researched as a factor contributing to sexual difficulties.[23] Estrogen-containing methods of birth control pills should not be used, but an IUD is fine, except in women with cardiac valvular disease.[24] **A, D**
Rheumatoid arthritis (RA)	Swollen, painful joints, muscle weakness, and joint contractures may make it difficult to masturbate or to have sex in some positions. Fatigue, stiffness, and joint dysfunction may decrease desire for sex,[25] as can pain and depression.[26] Menstruation, fertility, and pregnancy are usually not affected, but certain antirheumatic drugs may interfere with fertility.[27] Birthing may be complicated if RA is present in the hips and spine. Pregnancy and the use of birth control pills have been linked to symptom improvement and a slight reduction in joint damage.[28]	A vibrator or another sex toy can be used for self-pleasure or with another person. If symptoms respond to heat, plan sexual activities after a hot compress or a hot bath. Experiment with sexual positions and use pillows to avoid pain and for support of affected joints. Estrogen-containing birth control methods are not advisable for those with circulatory problems or restricted mobility. However, for women not at risk for blood clots, these methods and HT might be safely used and may even lessen RA symptoms.[29] **A, B, C, D, F**
Rheumatic diseases (including scleroderma, systemic lupus erythematosus [SLE], Sjögren's syndrome [SS], and systemic sclerosis [SSc])	A decrease in vaginal lubrication is often present, and skin and/or vaginal tightness can make vaginal penetration more painful. SS also causes dry mouth, SLE causes mouth sores, and both SLE and SSc may cause vaginal sores. Delays in becoming pregnant and increased risk of miscarriage have been observed. Consider all methods of birth control with extreme caution if organ complications exist.[30]	Sex without vaginal penetration, and use of a vibrator, topical anesthetic, and vaginal dam, may help to protect fragile skin and sores. Use estrogen cream to help with vaginal pain and atrophy.[31] Women with milder and stable SLE can often safely use estrogen-containing birth control methods[32] and HT without causing a severe flare in symptoms.[33] *Also see RA (above).* **A, B, D, E, F**
Multiple sclerosis (MS)	Depending upon the stage and severity of MS, symptoms will vary and may come and go. Common symptoms include difficulty experiencing orgasm and decreased genital sensitivity, vaginal dryness, muscle weakness, extreme fatigue, pain, and bladder and bowel incontinence.[34] Menstrual and fertility patterns may change; an exacerbation of MS may occur during menstruation, for a few months postpartum, and during perimenopause.[35] Some women report that MS symptoms improve during pregnancy and become stabilized during HRT.[36]	Because sexual difficulties may come and go with other MS symptoms, it helps to be creative. Some medications for spasms and topical anesthetics for pain may be helpful. If balance or fatigue is an issue, use a vibrator or try sexual activities that require less exertion. Some women find that vaginal penetration is painful, but clitoral stimulation feels good. Estrogen-containing birth control methods are not advisable if paralysis or restricted mobility is present. **A, B, D, E, F**

CHRONIC DISEASE OR DISABILITY	EFFECTS ON SEXUALITY	HELPFUL HINTS AND CONSIDERATIONS
Ostomy	Very little has been written about sexual activities and women with ostomies, even today. Surgery often does not impair genital responsivity or fertility. However, some women report pain during vaginal penetration or a lack of vaginal sensations after ileostomy, colostomy, and proctocolectomy surgery.[37]	Use pouch covers and positions that feel comfortable and keep your pouch secured during sexual activity so it does not get in the way or get pulled off. Tablets to neutralize odors may be put inside the pouch. Consider alternatives to the birth control pill, and consult a physician if taking it, because sometimes it is not absorbed completely.[38] *F*
Spinal cord injury (SCI)	Symptoms such as paralysis, loss of sensation, muscle weakness, spasticity, pain, incontinence, and vaginal dryness can all complicate having sex. Changes in the ability to lubricate or feel genital sensations depend on the severity of injury.[39] Orgasms are still possible, regardless of the level or degree of paralysis.[40] They may be similar to those pre-injury or may be more diffuse. Exploration is key to discovering these changes. Areas above the injury may become more sexually exciting.[41] Arousal, self-pleasuring, and sex may increase spasms and the risk of incontinence. Menstruation may stop for several months after SCI, but fertility is not permanently disrupted. Pregnancy increases the risk of developing blood clots, pressure sores, and bladder infections.[42]	Tape down your catheter and move it out of the way so it doesn't get pulled out during sex. Sex without vaginal penetration may help to avoid pain. Taking spasm medication prior to sexual activity may be of assistance. Using a vibrator helps some women experience orgasm. For women with high-level SCI, intense vaginal stimulation (as in childbirth or vigorous and prolonged penetration/vibrator use) can cause automatic dysreflexia (AD), a life-threatening condition.[43] Many women have healthy and painless births, but be on guard for signs of AD and uterine prolapse during labor and delivery.[44] Estrogen-containing birth control methods are not advisable and should not be used if taking antihypertensive medication.[45]
Chronic fatigue syndrome (CFS), fibromyalgia, and myofascial pain syndrome	These chronic conditions cause fatigue, widespread pain, and stiffness that can seriously dampen desire for sex. The possibility of experiencing postexertional fatigue or triggering episodes of pain may make engaging in sexual activities feel too risky.[46] Symptoms usually fluctuate over time and so will their effects on sexuality. Because pain and energy levels change from day to day, patience and creativity are essential.	Pacing yourself and prioritizing where your energy will go—a vital strategy for anyone with these syndromes—may help you have more energy for sex. A vibrator or another sex toy can be useful for hand pain. Experiment with sexual positions and use pillows for support and to reduce pain. Pain is an "antiphrodisiac" and can lead to depression, so symptom management is important.[47] Endorphins released during sexual activity (especially orgasm) may help relieve pain.[48] *A, E*

A. Many medications are directly responsible for negative effects on our sexuality. From dampened sexual desire and decreased vaginal lubrication to delayed or absent orgasm, these difficulties can be very frustrating. These drugs include antihypertensives (diuretics and beta-blockers), antidepressants (selective serotonin reuptake inhibitors, serotonin-norepinephrine reuptake inhibitors, tricyclic and some monoamine oxidase inhibitors), tranquilizers (phenothiazines), spasticity medications, and antiseizure medications (phenytoin [Dilantin]), as well as lithium, risperidone (Risperdal), digoxin, and reserpine (serpasil).[49]

B. The diaphragm may not be recommended if you have poor hand control, recurrent bladder or vaginal infections, or very weak pelvic muscles. If the use of your hands is limited, ask your partner or attendant to help insert the diaphragm. Also, devices are available that make it easier to insert the coil-spring diaphragm, but some hand control is required.

C. The IUD is not a good birth control method for women with a loss of sensation in the pelvic area because of the risk that puncture or pelvic inflammatory disease may go unnoticed.[50] Also, some hand coordination is needed to check the strings every month and make sure the IUD is still in place.

D. Estrogen-containing birth control pills can increase the risk of clotting and cause serious medical problems such as embolism, deep vein thrombosis, and stroke.[51] Newer contraceptive methods such as low-dose oral pills, contraceptive patches, and NuvaRing release less estrogen into the bloodstream than earlier versions of the Pill.[52] Progestin-only methods such as the minipill, Depo-Provera, and implants may be good alternatives because they do not contain estrogen.

Because some birth control medications may interact poorly or be rendered less effective when taken in combination with other drugs, be sure to inform your health-care providers about the medications and dosage you are taking when seeking contraceptive services.

E. A water-soluble lubricant can often be of immense help with a dry vagina or if you feel you have a decreased amount of lubrication.

F. Many women find that ongoing pharmaceutical treatment greatly improves their quality of life by minimizing symptoms. At the same time, safe contraceptive use is mandatory if taking methotrexate (Rheumatrex), cyclophosphamide (Cytoxan), or chlorambucil (Leukeran), since harm to a fetus is likely. These last two medications can also cause permanent infertility, and NSAIDs may cause reversible infertility.[53]

Sexual Health and Reproductive Choices

CHAPTER 9

Our ability to prevent or delay pregnancy is fundamental to our ability to choose how we live our lives. The advent of the Pill and other birth control methods has enabled women around the world to complete our educations, pursue our dreams, and create more egalitarian relationships.

Most of us want contraceptives that are effective and safe, are simple and unobtrusive to use, protect us against sexually transmitted infections—including HIV/AIDS—and can be used before having sex. Unfortunately, the perfect method does not exist. But advances in birth control technology have created more choices than ever before, making it more likely that a woman can find an option that meets her individual needs.

DUAL PROTECTION: PROTECTING YOURSELF FROM PREGNANCY AND SEXUALLY TRANSMITTED INFECTIONS

While birth control methods are highly effective at preventing pregnancy, most methods do not provide protection against sexually transmitted infections.

Dual protection means protecting yourself against unwanted pregnancy and STIs at the same time. You can do this by using condoms every time you have sex. For even better protection against pregnancy, use another birth control method along with condoms. For example, if you are using both the Pill and condoms correctly and consistently, your method is as close to 100 percent effective in preventing pregnancy as you can get without using a permanent method such as sterilization.

Many couples begin by using condoms, but after a period of time, when they feel that they trust each other, they stop using condoms. Unfortunately, trust has little to do with whether a partner is already carrying an STI. If either you or your partner has ever been with another partner, there is a possibility that one of you may be carrying an STI and not know it. For example, half of the people who have chlamydia, the most common STI in the United States, have no symptoms. (For more information, see Chapter 10, "Safer Sex," and Chapter 11, "Sexually Transmitted Infections.")

This chapter provides detailed, accurate, and up-to-date information on each method of birth control. It also addresses questions and concerns that many women share—such as how to choose a method of birth control, how to communicate about birth control with a partner, and barriers that keep us from protecting ourselves.

SOME OBSTACLES TO GETTING BIRTH CONTROL AND USING IT WELL

Shame about sex and negative attitudes toward pleasure and desire prevent people from seeking information about birth control. Laws, medical practices, and public school policies continue to prevent the distribution of accurate information and services—in spite of many studies showing that providing birth control information to teenagers does not make them more likely to have intercourse.

Many of us resist using birth control. Sometimes this is because of shame or fear, or social and political factors, such as poor sex education, a double standard concerning sex, or inequalities between women and men:

- We think that if we are using birth control we can't say no to sex. But using birth control does not mean we always want intercourse: No birth control method all by itself is an affirmative answer to sex. We need to be assertive about our desires and let our partners know that having sex should be a mutual decision, not an obligation.
- We are embarrassed by, ashamed of, or confused about our own sexuality. We cannot admit we might have or are having intercourse, because we feel (or someone told us) it is wrong.
- We are embarrassed by or ashamed of our own bodies or genitals, and feel uncomfortable talking about them in depth and candidly with a health-care provider. Body shame may also keep us from using some

methods that require us to touch our bodies in ways that we feel ashamed of or uncomfortable with.

- We are unrealistically romantic about sex: Sex has to be passionate and spontaneous, and birth control seems too premeditated, clinical, or messy.
- We hesitate to "inconvenience" our partner. This fear of displeasing him can be a measure of the inequality and our lack of control in the relationship.
- We think, It can't happen to me. I won't get pregnant.
- We hesitate to find a health-care provider, who may turn out to be hurried, impersonal, or even hostile. If we are young or unmarried, we may fear moralizing and disapproval. We may be afraid the provider will tell our parents.
- We don't recognize our deep dissatisfaction with the method we are using, so we begin to use it haphazardly.
- We feel tempted to become pregnant just to prove to ourselves that we are fertile, or to try to improve a shaky relationship, and therefore don't use birth control regularly.

WHAT CAN WE DO?

We can learn about the many methods of birth control and teach one another about the available methods. By speaking openly, and by carefully comparing experiences and knowledge, we can guide one another to workable methods and good health-care providers. We can recognize when a provider is not thorough enough and encourage one another to ask for the attention we need. By talking together, we can also gain an understanding of our more subtle resistance to using birth control. We can begin the process of

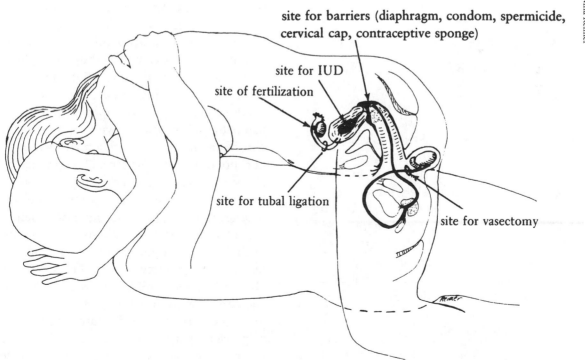

site for barriers (diaphragm, condom, spermicide, cervical cap, contraceptive sponge)

site for IUD

site of fertilization

site for tubal ligation

site for vasectomy

© Nina Reimer

talking with our male partners about birth control, encouraging them to share the responsibility with us. We can join together across state and national boundaries to insist that legislatures, courts, high schools, churches, parents, doctors, research projects, clinics, and drug companies change their practices and attitudes so that we can enjoy our sexuality without becoming pregnant. We can create self-help clinics and other participatory health-care institutions where our need for information, discussion, and support in the complex and personal choice of birth control will be better met. We can use the good clinics that do exist. We can campaign for decent housing, jobs, and child care for all, so that we can choose birth control freely instead of being forced to use it by our circumstances. We can insist that birth control methods be available to

meet the needs of all women, including women of color, women living in poverty, women with disabilities, and women in developing countries. Whatever we choose to do, we can act together.

MEN AND BIRTH CONTROL

At first I was afraid to talk about birth control with my partner. I didn't think he would be interested. As we discussed it, however, I realized that he wanted to prevent unplanned pregnancy just as much as I did. We talked about ways that he could participate in the birth control process, and afterward we both felt more confident in our mutual choices.

Birth control is not just a woman's issue. Men benefit from the use of birth control in many ways, including being able to decide when and if they will father a child and being able to protect themselves and their partners from sexually transmitted infections. When a man leaves the decision about contraception up to the woman, he not only creates an unfair burden for her but also forfeits his ability to prevent an unplanned pregnancy. By failing to take responsibility for contraception, too many men become fathers before they are capable or willing. By sharing decisions about birth control, a man increases the likelihood that his partner will be protected; he also shows that he cares about her and about her future, and that he is a real partner in a sexual relationship, not just a bystander or beneficiary. Having a conversation with your partner about birth control is a good way to learn of his interest in participating in the process, which can also be an opportunity to assess if he is a good choice as a sexual partner.

Our culture and media rarely address male responsibility in the prevention of STIs and unplanned pregnancies. The prevailing societal

---

EMERGENCY CONTRACEPTION

"The condom broke."

"I didn't think we were going to have sex."

"I forgot to take my pill."

"I was raped."

In an ideal world, we would always plan ahead, but the reality is that many of us have found ourselves at risk of a pregnancy that is unwanted. Fortunately, if this happens, we are no longer limited to waiting and worrying. Emergency contraception can be used immediately after unprotected intercourse, or up to five days after. Using emergency contraception greatly decreases the chances of a pregnancy. (For more information, see "Emergency Contraception," p. 251.)

A BRIEF HISTORY: BIRTH CONTROL AND REPRODUCTIVE RIGHTS

Understanding the history of the struggle for birth control and reproductive rights can help us advocate for our rights today.

Over the past 150 years, there have been three significant periods of birth control activism. Each period was followed by a conservative backlash.

- In the 1870s, the first major defense of birth control—called voluntary motherhood—emphasized the dignity of motherhood and women's right to refuse sexual activity. Branding birth control "race suicide," conservative opposition succeeded in criminalizing abortion and categorizing birth control as obscene.
- In the 1930s, Margaret Sanger inspired a resurgence of interest in birth control, fighting to make information and services available to every woman. At the same time, a broad-based feminist movement for legalization of birth control defended the separation of sex from reproduction and supported women's sexual freedom. By midcentury, the "birth control movement" had again died down, and a general conservative trend following World War II put women back into the home and fostered the baby boom.
- By the 1960s, the new rise in feminism had defined birth control as a reproductive right and motherhood as a choice, leading the way to expanded access to contraception and the legalization of abortion. Since then, conservative forces have worked to deny access to reproductive health information and services and to recriminalize abortion. By defining both birth control and abortion as against religious teachings, they have further eroded women's access to reproductive health care.

Conservative forces continue to resist efforts to make safe, reliable birth control and information about birth control freely available to all women, and our rights continue to be at risk. For more information on the fight to keep birth control and abortion safe, legal, and accessible to all women, see "History of Abortion in the United States," p. 337. A good source for news coverage and analysis is RH Reality Check (rhrealitycheck.org).

messages about contraception target women and often ignore the impact that unprotected sex can have on men. Using condoms is the easiest way for men to get involved in the birth control process, but they must be willing to do so. Some men are not interested in using condoms because they have received messages that say it is unmasculine, or they have a preconceived notion that sex is not as good with condoms. These attitudes reveal both a lack of education and a lack of respect for women; they also free men from taking responsibility for their actions.

In addition to buying and using condoms, men can help pay for doctors' visits and drugstore bills; be part of the decision to invest in a long-term, reversible method of contraception; remind us to take the pill each day; help to remove a diaphragm or insert spermicidal foam;

and check to see if supplies are running low. If you and your partner are sure that you will not ever want to have children, or your family is the right size as it is, a vasectomy may be a suitable option (see p. 245). The future holds even more opportunities for men to participate actively in birth control, as several new contraceptive methods for men are currently being developed (see "Emerging Male Contraceptives," p. 247).

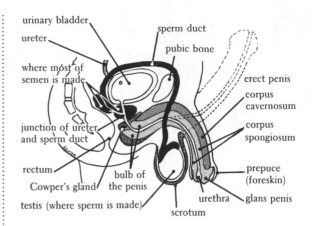

Male pelvic organs (side view)

CHOOSING A METHOD OF BIRTH CONTROL

If you want to use a birth control method other than condoms and spermicides, you need to visit a health care provider. A good health care provider will give you a physical exam, go over your personal and family medical history, and discuss which methods may be a good fit for you. (For advice on how to find a provider or clinic, see "For Teens," p. 207.) If possible, find a health care provider who not only will talk with you but also will listen to what you have to say about your experience with birth control, as finding the best method may involve switching methods or pill brands a few times. If your provider won't work with you, try to find another provider who will. Although health care providers can offer helpful advice about which methods might work best for you, the choice is ultimately yours.

HOW TO DECIDE WHAT'S RIGHT FOR YOU: PERSONAL CONSIDERATIONS

Because there is no one perfect method of birth control that is right for every woman, you need to consider your own needs and priorities. Factors to consider include safety and effectiveness, how much you are willing to risk an unintended pregnancy, how comfortable you are with the potential side effects, how the method is used,

the type of relationship you are in, and the amount of money you can spend. If you have medical problems, chronic illnesses, or disabilities, you may have additional considerations. Insurance coverage or the types of birth control available at a particular provider or family planning center may also determine which methods are available to you.

Below are some questions to think about as you make your decision.

- Am I ready to have or interested in having sexual intercourse at this time in my life or at this point in my relationship?
- Given my lifestyle, what characteristics am I looking for in a method? Can I reliably use a method that I have to remember every day or week, or every time I have intercourse?
- How involved will my partner be in this decision and with the use of the method?
- How safe is this method for me and/or my partner? Do I have any medical or other reasons not to use the method?
- What are the potential side effects and risks of this method? Are these acceptable to me?
- How effective is this method in preventing pregnancy? What would be the consequences in my life if I got pregnant?

If you are a teenager, you may want to wait to start having sex for any number of reasons, or you may just want to hold off on the kinds of sex that present a risk of pregnancy. If you have already made the decision to have vaginal intercourse and don't want to get pregnant, you need to use birth control. Reading this book, talking with your friends and supportive adults, and visiting teen-friendly sexuality websites such as Scarleteen: Sex Ed for the Real World (scarleteen.com) can help you to make healthy choices about if, when, and with whom to have sex, as well as how to protect yourself if you decide to be sexually active.

Have a birth control method picked out and begin using it before the first time you have sexual intercourse. If there is a reproductive health clinic nearby, you can go there and speak with a medical provider. Most family planning clinics, such as Planned Parenthood, provide free or reduced-cost services and supplies. They are also completely confidential. That means no one else will know you have an appointment or are using birth control. You do not need permission from your parents or a guardian to make an appointment or get birth control. If you do not know where there is a clinic near you, you can search for one by zip code or state at Planned Parenthood's website (plannedparenthood.org) or call Planned Parenthood at 1-800-230-PLAN.

No matter what age you are, you can also buy safe and effective methods, such as condoms and spermicides, in most drugstores. Condoms are sometimes given out free in teen centers, clinics, or HIV prevention programs. Whatever method of birth control you choose, use condoms to protect yourself from sexually transmitted infections (STIs). This is especially important because men and women under age twenty-four have the highest rates of chlamydia and gonorrhea.

If you have not been using birth control and have had unprotected intercourse within the past five days, you can use emergency contraception (EC) to prevent pregnancy. For more information, see "Emergency Contraception," p. 251.

- How effective is this method in preventing sexually transmitted infections?
- What are the noncontraceptive benefits to this method? Can it reduce menstrual cramps or help me in another way?
- How much will this method cost? Can I afford it consistently?
- What are my plans for a family? Am I using contraception to delay pregnancy? Am I done with childbearing? Am I choosing never to have children?

EFFECTIVENESS AND SAFETY

Will It Work?
Effectiveness of Birth Control Methods

Though choosing a method involves considering many factors, one of the most important is how well it works to prevent pregnancy.

A method's effectiveness is based on the probability of unintended pregnancy in the first year of use. Effectiveness is usually presented as two numbers: *Perfect use* reflects the effective-

METHODS WOMEN CAN USE WITHOUT PARENTS OR PARTNERS KNOWING

There are times when women need a birth control method that can be used without a partner's knowledge. A recent study of Planned Parenthood clients in Northern California found that nearly one in seven women had a partner who tried to interfere with her efforts to prevent unwanted pregnancy.[1] Birth control sabotage can include hiding birth control pills or flushing them down the toilet, intentionally breaking condoms, and removing contraceptive rings or patches.

There are other times when we don't want people besides our partner to know we are using birth control. For example, if you are a teen, you may be concerned about your parents finding out. If you need to keep your birth control private for any reason, you have some good options.

Totally Invisible: Depo-Provera Shot

This injection of a hormone in your upper arm every three months is one of the most private methods available and is over 99 percent effective if you get your shots at the right time. No one, not even your partner, will know about it unless you decide to tell. It may be challenging to get to the clinic four times a year without someone close to you knowing, but it may also be easier than hiding a pill you have to take every day. (For more information on Depo, see p. 234.)

Only You Know It's There: Implant

This matchstick-size rod is placed just under the skin of your upper arm and is over 99 percent effective. After a nurse or doctor inserts it, you'll have a bandage for a few days and may have some bruising around it. Once it's healed, no one can see that the rod is there. Someone would have to know exactly where to feel your arm to find it. (For more information on the implant, see p. 236.)

Your Partner May Know, but No One Else Will: IUD and Ring

An IUD is a small device that a doctor places in your uterus that provides over 99 percent effective contraception. Partners can sometimes feel the threads that help a doctor remove the device when you're ready. The threads are at your cervix, inside your vagina. (For more information on IUDs, see p. 238.)

The ring, which you can insert yourself, rests near your cervix and releases a small amount of hormone for 92 percent effective contraception. If you're worried about a partner knowing about it or you don't like it there during sex, you can take it out and keep it in a safe, clean place for up to three hours a day. (For more information on the ring, see p. 231.)

ness of the method when it is used exactly as directed, with perfect consistency; *typical use* is the effectiveness of the method when used by real people, who may use the method incorrectly or inconsistently. For example, the birth control pill has a perfect use effectiveness rating of 99.7 percent, which means that if one hundred women use the Pill correctly for a year, fewer than one will become pregnant. In typical use, however—when a woman may forget to take a pill or doesn't get supplies in time—the effectiveness is only about 92 percent, which means that about eight of every one hundred women, or one out of about thirteen women, will become pregnant in one year.* (See "Comparing Birth Control Methods," p. 254.)

How well a method will work for you will be determined by a number of factors:

- The perfect use effectiveness of your chosen method
- How consistently and correctly you use your chosen method
- How often you have intercourse (a woman who has intercourse every day is at greater risk of pregnancy than a woman who has intercourse only occasionally)
- Your age and fertility (younger women are more likely than older women to become pregnant from a single act of intercourse)

To lower your risk of unplanned pregnancy:

- Be sure you have access to your method.
- Be sure you have complete and correct information about the use of your method.
- Use your method consistently and correctly.
- Use two methods together to greatly lower your risk of pregnancy. If one of the two methods is a condom, this also provides protection from sexually transmitted infections.
- Have an emergency method (see p. 251) available for backup if your method fails or if you have unprotected intercourse.
- If your greatest concern is highly effective, long-term, and reversible protection, use a method such as long-acting injections, implants, or an IUD.
- If you are using a barrier or nonmedical method, be aware of your fertile time and avoid intercourse or use extra protection during this time.

---

* Unless otherwise noted, the effectiveness numbers used in this chapter are taken from the Centers for Disease Control and Prevention's U.S. Medical Eligibility Criteria for Contraceptive Use, 2010.

HEALTH CONCERNS: CONTRAINDICATIONS AND SIDE EFFECTS

In general, methods of contraception are safe for healthy reproductive-aged women, although some methods pose health risks for women with particular medical conditions.

When you are considering a particular method, it's important to look at both its contraindications and its side effects. Contraindications are the physical conditions or circumstances that make a method a poor or dangerous choice for a particular woman. For example, it is contraindicated for a woman who is over age thirty-five and smokes to use birth control pills, because they would put her at increased risk of developing a blood clot that could lead to a heart attack or stroke. As another example, having current breast cancer is a contraindication for using any hormonal method. A contraindication means that by using that particular method of birth control you may increase your risk of a serious health problem.

Side effects are the changes that can occur as the result of using a particular medication or device. Side effects can be mild or severe, and can vary greatly from person to person. For example, possible side effects of hormonal methods include changes in bleeding patterns, breast tenderness, and mild headaches. A side effect of some barrier methods may be an increase in urinary tract infections. Some side effects go away completely after a short period of time and some last the whole time you are using the method. Many women experience no side effects at all. For most women, negative experiences with birth control are due to side effects rather than contraindications. In the sections below on individual methods, the subheading "Health Concerns" includes both the method's side effects and the contraindications.

One thing to keep in mind when choosing a method is that brand-new birth control products have not been tested as extensively as those that have been used for decades. The Food and Drug Administration (FDA) approves all methods of birth control, and products that receive FDA approval have undergone up to ten years of rigorous research. However, it can take twenty years or more for some complications to become apparent, especially those that are rare but serious. Drug manufacturers spend a lot of money promoting and marketing new methods, trying to convince you that they are the best. But new, heavily marketed brands are not necessarily any better than older methods, and they may pose risks that are not yet known.

One of the greatest obstacles to women's use of contraception is the fear of possible negative health effects from the use of hormonal methods or the IUD. Some women hear alarming stories that may be based on half-truths, bias, isolated cases, or old information, so it is important to seek out accurate and balanced information before making a birth control decision. It's also important to consider the health risks of being pregnant, which are higher than those of using any form of birth control.

GETTING PREGNANT LATER

You may have heard that using some methods of birth control can affect your ability to become pregnant even after you stop taking the contraceptive.

No method of birth control, except sterilization, permanently interferes with your ability to become pregnant, nor does birth control reduce your ability to have children later in life. In fact, an unintended pregnancy or a sexually transmitted infection can occasionally impact future fertility, so birth control methods, especially those that protect against STIs, may protect your ability to get pregnant in the future.

Some methods may continue to prevent

pregnancy for a short while after you stop taking them. Depo-Provera, for example, may continue to work for some women up to eighteen months after the last injection, though it has no proven long-term effects on fertility. (However, to reliably prevent pregnancy you must get Depo-Provera injections every three months.)

BARRIER METHODS: MALE CONDOM, FEMALE CONDOM, DIAPHRAGM, CERVICAL CAP, SPONGE, SPERMICIDES

Barrier methods prevent pregnancy by blocking sperm from reaching the cervix. They are often used in combination with spermicides. The effectiveness of barrier methods varies a great deal depending on how correctly and consistently they are used. Because they don't enter the bloodstream and are used only intermittently, barrier methods have fewer side effects than other methods. In addition, condoms prevent the spread of sexually transmitted infections, including HIV/AIDS.

MALE CONDOMS (RUBBERS, PROPHYLACTICS)

The condom is typically a latex sheath that fits over the erect penis and prevents sperm from entering a woman's body. It is sold rolled up and stored in a foil or plastic packet. For those who are sexually active, condoms offer the best protection against sexually transmitted infections; only abstinence protects you better. Condoms come in different sizes, colors, and textures.

While most condoms sold are made of latex rubber, some are made from a thin polyurethane (plastic) or polyisoprene material. They, too, protect against STIs; they may also provide more sensation for men who have difficulty

maintaining an erection when using latex condoms; and they can be used by people sensitive to latex. However, they break more often than latex condoms.[2] Natural "skin" condoms (made of lamb membrane) protect against pregnancy but contain pores (microscopic holes) that are large enough to let viruses pass through (but not large enough to let sperm pass through). Therefore, skin condoms do not protect against some STIs, including HIV.

Condoms are a good way for the man to share responsibility for birth control. When you don't know whether you will be having intercourse,

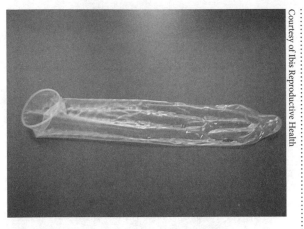

Male condom

condoms can be very convenient. Although some men carry condoms, you should not expect it. Protect yourself by carrying condoms with you. Condoms usually have an expiration date marked EXP on the package. Generally, condoms without spermicide are good for up to five years. Condoms with spermicide last about two years. Keep condoms in a cool and dry place, and throw away condoms past their expiration date. If you are not sure how old a condom is, throw it away and use a new one. Never use condoms that are brittle, sticky, damaged, or discolored. And never reuse a condom.

Effectiveness

Pregnancy Prevention

The contraceptive effectiveness of condoms varies from 85 to 98 percent depending on how well they are used. If used correctly *for every act of intercourse from start to finish*, condoms are 98 percent effective at preventing pregnancy. This means that if a hundred couples use condoms correctly every time they have intercourse for a year, two women will become pregnant. In real life, issues such as not putting the condom on properly, not always using one, or putting it on too late are common, so condoms have a typi-

cal use contraceptive effectiveness of 85 percent. That means that about one in seven women will become pregnant in one year of using condoms.

Some condoms ("spermicidal" or "spermicidally lubricated") contain spermicide, a chemical that kills sperm. The concentration of spermicide is so low in these varieties, however, that they appear to be no more effective at preventing pregnancy than condoms that don't contain spermicide. If you combine using condoms correctly at every act of intercourse with a spermicidal foam, cream, film, or jelly in your vagina, you will have more effective birth control.

Sexually Transmitted Infection (STI) Prevention

The effectiveness of condoms in preventing transmission of STIs—such as HIV, chlamydia, gonorrhea, trichomonas, and hepatitis B—is similar to the effectiveness rate for pregnancy protection, or 80 to 98 percent. Protection from STIs that cause genital sores, such as syphilis, herpes, and chancroid, or from human papillomavirus (HPV)—genital warts—is decreased because the condom may not cover all of the areas that could transmit the infection. Nevertheless, condoms provide the best protection currently available against these infections.

Advantages

- Does not require advance planning, clinic visits, or a prescription.
- Inexpensive and readily available.
- Can be carried easily and discreetly by men and women.
- Best currently available method of protection against STIs, including HIV, and may help prevent cervical cancer (see Chapter 11, "Sexually Transmitted Infections"). By preventing STIs, condoms can protect the ability to get pregnant in the future.
- Allows men to participate in preventing pregnancy and infections.

- May decrease premature ejaculation and prolong intercourse.
- Catches the semen, so nothing drips from the vagina after intercourse.
- No systemic side effects.
- Does not affect menstrual cycles.

Disadvantages
- Requires a brief pause to put on.
- Can reduce sensitivity.
- Some men cannot maintain an erection when using a condom.
- Some men and women can develop an allergy or sensitivity to latex (in this case, condoms made from other materials can be used; see p. 211).

Many of the disadvantages of condoms can be overcome with practice and experience or by switching to a different brand or type of condom.

How to Use
Condom use can be fun for both partners when it is made part of sex. Discuss condom use *before* you have sex. Have more than one condom on hand, in case one is torn or damaged before use or is put on incorrectly, or you have repeat intercourse or change from anal to vaginal sex. Use a condom before the penis comes in contact with your mouth, anus, or vagina, as your partner may discharge a few drops of fluid long before ejaculating. While this pre-ejaculatory fluid is unlikely to cause pregnancy, it may expose you to HIV or other infectious organisms.

1. Carefully open the packet.
2. Unroll the condom a short distance to be sure you are unrolling it in the right direction. If you accidentally put the *outside* of the condom against the head of the penis, discard the condom and open a new one.
3. Squeeze the tip of the condom and unroll it down to the base of the erect penis. The tip will hold the man's sperm. If you do not leave space for the sperm, the condom is more likely to break. If your partner's penis is uncircumcised, pull back the foreskin before putting on the condom.
4. It is important to have enough lubrication. If you do not use a lubricated condom, use a water-based lubricant such as K-Y or Astroglide to prevent tearing or discomfort. If you are using a latex condom, the most common type of condom, never use Vaseline or other oil-based lubricants such as massage oils, suntan lotion, hand cream, or baby oil, as they can weaken the latex. With polyurethane or polyisoprene condoms, any type of lubricant can be used.
5. Soon after ejaculation, the man should carefully withdraw his penis while it is still erect. Hold the condom firmly against the base of the penis to prevent leakage or slipping.
6. Check the condom for visible damage, such as holes or tears, then wrap it in tissue and discard. Do not flush condoms down the toilet; this can cause plumbing problems. Condoms cannot be reused, so use one condom for each time you have sexual intercourse and then throw it away.
7. If the condom breaks, slips off, or was not used, discuss the possibility of pregnancy or infection with your partner. Emergency contraception (EC) can be used after unprotected intercourse to prevent pregnancy (see p. 251).

Health Concerns
The only contraindication for using a condom is if you or your partner has a latex allergy. Severe swelling or difficulty breathing may indicate a

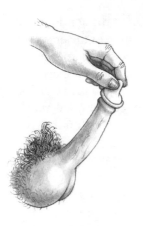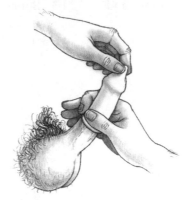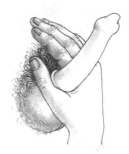

latex allergy; if this happens to you or your partner, see a health-care provider immediately.

Some people develop a mild, local irritation or a rash after using a condom. This may be a reaction to the lubricant, spermicide, or perfumes used on the condom. If this happens to you or your partner, try using a different brand, or a condom without lubrication. If you still have a reaction, try switching to a nonlatex condom; or if you need protection only against pregnancy, you can try natural skin condoms.

Where to Get Condoms

You can find condoms in drugstores, in supermarkets, online, in bathroom vending machines, and on many college campuses. Many family planning clinics, youth organizations, and HIV prevention programs offer condoms for free. The cost in other places varies, depending on the brand and the store, so shop around. Nonlatex condoms are more expensive than latex condoms.

Managing Problems

Some men experience decreased sensitivity with condoms. To enhance sensitivity, try different types of condoms, or add a water-based or silicone lubricant to the outside of the condom, or even a few drops to the inside tip of the condom.

Frequently Asked Questions

- **Can HIV get through a condom?** No. Latex, polyurethane, and polyisoprene condoms, if used correctly, prevent the spread of HIV. Condoms also protect against other STIs. Don't use oil-based lubricants with latex condoms, as they can cause the latex to break down and could allow HIV to pass through. Natural membrane condoms may also allow the HIV virus to pass through.
- **Do condoms make intercourse less enjoyable?** This varies from person to person. Some people dislike them because they can interrupt spontaneity, and some men find they decrease sensitivity. Condoms can also have some positive effects. For instance, both partners may enjoy intercourse more if they don't have to worry about getting pregnant or contracting an STI. Using condoms also may prolong an erection and increase sexual communication.
- **Do condoms fit all men?** Some men believe that condoms are too small or tight for them.

Because heat can cause deterioration, do not store condoms for over a month in a wallet, pocket, or car.

All condoms can stretch to accommodate various sizes. Larger-size condoms are available, although since the condom needs to be snug, most men should use the regular size.

- **Do condoms often break during intercourse?** Condom breakage is relatively rare, but less experienced users may break condoms more often. To prevent breakage, use water- or silicone-based lubricant with latex condoms, and make sure your partner puts the condom on correctly. Condoms are also more likely to break if they are out-of-date, so check the expiration date on the package.
- **Does a person need to use condoms to protect against STIs when having oral or anal sex?** Yes. STIs can pass from person to person during oral, vaginal, and anal sex. Condoms can be used during any of these sex acts to protect against STIs. Anal sex is a particularly high-risk activity, even more so than vaginal intercourse, because the tissue in the rectum tears easily, giving easy access for the virus to enter the person's blood. Using extra lubricant with a strong, preferably latex, condom is recommended. (For more information, see Chapter 10, "Safer Sex.")

THE FC2 FEMALE CONDOM

A female condom is a pouch that is inserted into the vagina before intercourse to prevent pregnancy and reduce the risk of sexually transmitted infections. In the United States today there is only one brand of female condom, the FC2.

The FC2 is a thin sheath made of nitrile polymer with a soft ring at each end. One ring, covered with polyurethane, fits over the cervix and rests behind the pubic bone, acting as an anchor. The larger, open outer ring covers part of the perineum and labia.

Like male condoms, FC2 is available over the counter, without a prescription. Because it is not made of latex, it will not deteriorate when used with oil-based lubricants. It can be inserted before intercourse but should be removed immediately after. The FC2 is prelubricated with a silicone-based lubricant and does not contain spermicide. It does not require precise placement over the cervix. Male and female condoms should *not* be used at the same time, because the added friction between the two condoms could cause them to break. Like the male condom, the FC2 female condom is intended for onetime use.

Effectiveness

FC2 is 95 percent effective in preventing pregnancy when used consistently and correctly. With typical use, it is 79 percent effective.

STI Protection

Although the research on female condoms is not as extensive as that on male condoms, consistent and correct use of the female condom appears to provide a level of protection against STIs, including HIV, similar to that of the male condom.[3]

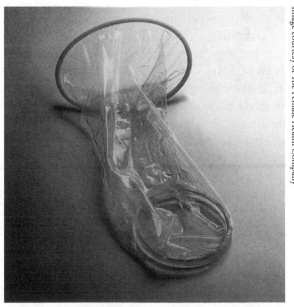

Advantages

- Does not require advance planning, clinic visits, or a prescription.
- Provides protection against STIs, including HIV.
- You don't have to rely on a man to use a condom.
- Provides broader coverage than the male condom, covering the labia, the perineal region, and the base of the penis; this may decrease the chance of passing the viruses that cause genital warts and herpes.
- The outer ring may stimulate the clitoris and make intercourse more enjoyable.
- May help you know your body better.
- No systemic side effects.
- Does not affect menstrual cycles.

Disadvantages

- Not as effective in preventing pregnancy as hormonal methods or a male condom.
- Costs somewhat more than a male condom and may not be as readily available.
- Requires a brief pause to put on.
- Can take practice before insertion becomes easy.
- Some women find that the rings cause discomfort.

How to Use

FC2 use can be fun for both partners when it is made part of sex. Discuss condom use *before* you have sex. Insert FC2 *before* you have any genital contact.

1. Carefully open the packet and find the inner (smaller) ring, which is at the closed end of the condom. Squeeze the inner ring together and push it up into your vagina with your finger. The outer ring stays outside the vagina.
2. When your partner's penis is hard, you will need to guide the penis through the

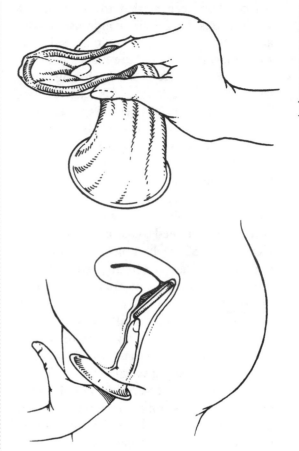

Insertion of FC2 female condom

outer ring, to make sure that the outer ring is not pushed to the side of the vagina. If you find that the outer ring is being pulled into your vagina during intercourse, add extra lubrication inside the condom or to the penis. You can use any kind of lubricant, water- or oil-based, with the FC2.

3. After sex, remove the female condom (if you are lying down, do this before you stand up). Squeeze and twist the outer ring to keep the man's sperm inside the pouch. The condom should come out easily when you pull. After removing the

condom, dispose of it in the trash; do not flush it down the toilet.

Tip: Practice inserting a female condom before you use one during sex.

Where to Get the FC2 Female Condom

You can purchase FC2 female condoms at some retail drugstores, including CVS and Walgreens, HIV/AIDS outreach clinics, family-planning clinics, and sex shops, and on some college campuses. You can also buy them online, including at Amazon.com. A pack of five condoms costs about $12.

For more information on female condoms, visit AVERT (avert.org/female-condom.htm), which works to avert HIV/AIDS worldwide.

Frequently Asked Questions

- **Does the FC2 come in different sizes? Does it have to be fitted?** No, the FC2 does not need to be fitted. It comes in one size that is designed to fit most women.
- **Can the FC2 be used with male condoms?** No. The FC2 should not be used at the same time as male condoms, because the added friction between the two condoms could cause them to fail.
- **Is the FC2 as effective as male condoms?** The FC2 has efficacy similar to male condoms and other barrier methods.
- **Can spermicides or lubricants be used with the FC2?** Yes. It is perfectly safe and effective to use the FC2 with spermicides and all types of lubricants (oil-, silicone-, or water-based).

MICROBICIDES

When used correctly and consistently, male and female condoms offer good protection against pregnancy and STIs. However, some men and women are unwilling to use condoms, and even when a woman wants to use condoms, she may not be able to negotiate their use with her partner.

For these reasons, there is growing interest in additional methods of protection, particularly ones that can be controlled by the woman. Researchers are working to develop microbicides, products that can be applied directly to the vagina to prevent both pregnancy and STIs, including HIV/AIDS. No microbicides are currently available, but they are in development. (For more information, see "Microbicides and PrEP," p. 800.)

DIAPHRAGM

The diaphragm is a dome-shaped, soft rubber cup that fits securely in the vagina to cover the cervix. A spermicide is placed in the cup, facing the cervix, to kill or immobilize sperm and prevent them from entering the uterus and fertilizing an egg. Though diaphragms have no systemic side effects like those of the Pill, they are not as effective in preventing unintended pregnancy. They were once very popular in the United States, but few women use them today.

Effectiveness

The diaphragm has perfect use effectiveness of 94 percent, which means using it every time you have intercourse and adding additional spermicide if you have intercourse again before removal. In typical use the diaphragm is 84 percent effective.

Advantages

- Can be inserted up to six hours before sex and left in for multiple acts of intercourse.
- May help you know your body better.
- Does not affect menstrual cycles.
- Can be used during menstruation to contain flow during intercourse.
- Has minimal side effects.
- Your partner may not know it's there.

Disadvantages

- Does not provide STI/HIV protection.
- Low typical use effectiveness.
- Requires a pelvic exam and fitting at a clinic.
- May not be available at all practices or clinics.
- Needs occasional refitting.
- May increase risk of bladder infections.
- The spermicide used with the diaphragm can be messy.

How to Use

Inserting a Diaphragm

Practice inserting and removing your diaphragm before you have intercourse. It can be awkward at first, but it becomes easy with prac-

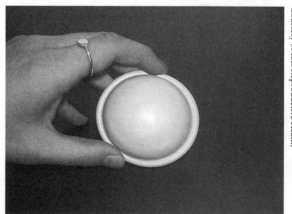

Diaphragm

tice. You can put the diaphragm in any time within six hours before intercourse or vagina-to-penis contact. If more than six hours have passed, either insert an applicator full of spermicide into your vagina, or remove the diaphragm, wash it out, and start again.

1. Put about 1 tablespoon of spermicidal cream or jelly into the shallow cup.
2. Squeeze the diaphragm together by pressing the rim firmly between your thumb and third finger.
3. Squat, sit on the toilet bowl, stand with one foot raised, or lie down with your legs bent.
4. Push the diaphragm up to the upper third of your vagina with the cream or jelly facing up. Your vagina angles toward the small of your back, so it may be more comfortable if you push in this direction.
5. Push the lower rim with your index or middle finger until you feel the diaphragm fit into place. When the diaphragm is in right and fits properly, you should not be able to feel it at all.

Leave the diaphragm in for at least six hours after intercourse. You can leave it in for up to twenty-four hours, but not longer.

Subsequent Intercourse
If you have intercourse again, add more cream or jelly with an applicator. Put it into your vagina, leaving the diaphragm in place at least six hours after the last act of intercourse.

Removal
Choose a comfortable position, slide a finger into your vagina, and hook it under the lower rim of the diaphragm, either between the diaphragm and your vaginal wall or over the rubber dome. Pull the diaphragm forward and down.

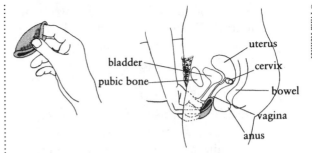

Insertion of diaphragm

Care
Wash the diaphragm with mild soap and warm water, rinse and dry it carefully, and put it into a container (away from light). Do not boil it. To make sure the diaphragm is still effective, check its condition by holding it up to the light or filling it with water to check for holes. Oil-based creams, including some vaginal medications, can damage diaphragms, so avoid contact with those materials.

Get your diaphragm size rechecked after giving birth, after method failure, if you gain or lose more than ten pounds, or after any vaginal surgery. Diaphragms should be replaced every three years.

Where to Get a Diaphragm
Getting a diaphragm requires a fitting by a health-care provider. Because diaphragms are not widely used, you should call ahead to make sure your provider knows how to fit you for a diaphragm and has the proper equipment to do so.

When you have been measured and fitted, practice putting the diaphragm in and taking it out before you leave the practitioner's office, so she or he can tell you whether you are doing it right. (Or go home, practice, and come back in a few days with the diaphragm in place.) Reach in and see what it feels like when it is in correctly, and get help immediately if you have problems, so that when you actually use it, you won't be experimenting. The practitioner should have the diaphragm available right there or will give you a prescription for the proper size.

Health Concerns
Some women cannot use a diaphragm because it can't be made to fit properly. Because diaphragms require manual dexterity, women with physical disabilities like arthritis might not be able to use them effectively without assistance. Women with chronic urinary tract infections or a history of toxic shock syndrome should not use a diaphragm.

Frequently Asked Questions
- **If a woman uses the diaphragm without spermicide, will it work at all?** It might provide some protection, but using a diaphragm without spermicide reduces its effectiveness.
- **Is it okay to leave a diaphragm in all day?** Yes. After intercourse, a diaphragm must be left in for at least six hours to make sure that live sperm do not get past the barrier. Sperm will die in the vagina. After that time, remove and wash the diaphragm.
- **Can a woman use lubricants with a diaphragm?** As with condoms, use only water- or silicone-based lubricants, because oil-based lubricants can damage the latex rubber of the diaphragm. Often, the spermicide itself provides lubrication.

CERVICAL CAP

The cervical cap is a small cup-shaped silicone cap that fits snugly over the cervix (the entrance to the uterus) and is held in place by suction. The cervical cap is used with a spermicidal cream or jelly to immobilize sperm and prevent them from fertilizing an egg.

There is currently one cervical cap available in the United States, called the FemCap. It comes in three sizes and must be fitted by a provider. It has a loop for easy removal.

Effectiveness
For women who have never given birth, the FemCap is 86 percent effective. For women who have given birth, the cap is 71 percent effective.[4] The cap is less effective for women in the first year after pregnancy.

Advantages and Disadvantages
These are the same as for diaphragms; see p. 218.

How to Use
The effectiveness of a cervical cap depends on its fit as well as consistent and correct usage. The FemCap comes in different sizes and needs to be fitted by a medical practitioner, who will show you how to insert the cap. If you have questions, ask your practitioner or go to the website for FemCap (femcap.com). During the first few months of use, there is a higher risk of pregnancy. For better protection during this time, use a condom and check the position of the cap before and after intercourse to make sure it stays in place. If the cap moves during intercourse, consider using emergency contraception (see p. 251).

Inserting or removing a cervical cap is similar to using a diaphragm, but the cap does not fold. When the cap is properly in place, you should feel some resistance when you tug on the removal loop. (See the description of diaphragm insertion and removal, p. 218.)

Care
Care for a cervical cap is similar to a diaphragm (see p. 219). However, using oil-based lubricants will not damage the cap.

Refitting

Giving birth can affect the way a cervical cap fits. Three months after a birth, have your medical provider check its fit.

Health Concerns

The FemCap has the same health concerns as diaphragms; see p. 220.

Side Effects

Some women may experience an allergic reaction to the material of the cervical cap or the spermicide they use. If this happens, consider using another method of contraception.

Where to Get a Cervical Cap

Because most providers are not trained in fitting cervical caps, they are not widely available. However, they are available at many reproductive health clinics and from some other healthcare providers. Call the provider's office before your appointment to find out if the provider can fit a cervical cap.

SPONGE

The contraceptive sponge is a soft disk made of polyurethane that rests against the cervix during sex. The sponge contains the spermicide Nonoxynol-9 to immobilize sperm. It has a loop for easy removal.

Effectiveness

For women who have never given birth, the perfect use effectiveness of the sponge is 91 percent; typical use effectiveness is 84 percent. For women who have given birth, the sponge is significantly less effective: 80 percent with perfect use and 68 percent with typical use.

Advantages and Disadvantages

Although the sponge can be purchased at pharmacies over the counter, the advantages and disadvantage are otherwise the same as for diaphragms; see p. 218.

How to Use

Wet the sponge and insert it into your vagina, dimple side facing the cervix and loop side facing down. It is effective immediately. You can insert it up to twenty-four hours before sex and have intercourse multiple times while it is in place. The sponge must be left in place six hours after sex to be effective, but should not be left in the vagina longer than thirty hours. Throw the sponge away—do not flush—after use.

Health Concerns

The health concerns for sponges are the same as those for diaphragms; see p. 220.

Side Effects

Some women may experience an allergic reaction to the material of the sponge or the spermicide in the sponge.

Where to Get a Sponge

Sponges are available without a prescription at pharmacies and some reproductive health clinics.

SPERMICIDES

Spermicides kill sperm so they cannot fertilize an egg to cause a pregnancy. The chemical Nonoxynol-9 (N-9) is the active ingredient in most spermicides, which are available in different forms: foam, jelly, cream, film, and suppositories. Spermicides are most effective when used consistently and correctly with a barrier method of birth control—a condom, diaphragm, or cervical cap. They give no protection against HIV; in fact, some research indicates that Nonoxynol-9, when used more than once a day, can increase the risk of acquiring HIV.[5] However, spermicides containing N-9 are a safe contraceptive option for women at low risk for HIV/STIs who do not use the product more than once a day. (See "Safety of Nonoxynol-9 When Used for Contraception" p. 223.)

Effectiveness

When used perfectly on their own, the different formulations of spermicides range in effectiveness from about 82 to 85 percent. With typical use, however, they are about 71 percent effective. As with all methods that depend on use with each act of intercourse, a spermicide's effectiveness varies widely depending on how correctly and consistently you use it. Spermicides are most effective when used with a barrier method such as a condom, diaphragm, or cervical cap.

Advantages

- Available without a prescription.
- Lubrication may increase pleasure.

Disadvantages

- Women who use N-9 more than once a day appear to have an increased risk of HIV transmission.
- Low typical use effectiveness.
- Can be messy.
- May make oral sex less pleasant.
- May irritate vulva or vagina and increase risk of urinary tract infection.
- Requires a brief pause.

How to Use

Spermicides can be used alone or with a diaphragm, cervical cap, or condom to reduce the risk of pregnancy. Insert the spermicide within a half hour before intercourse. If it was inserted more than one hour before intercourse, it will have lost much of its effectiveness. Add more spermicide for repeated intercourse. Leave spermicide in your vagina for six hours after the last act of intercourse. Avoid douching in general, but if you must douche, wait at least six hours (douching washes away spermicide).

Types of Spermicides

Foam

Foam comes in a can and is the consistency of shaving cream. It is inserted using an applicator that comes with the can and is effective immediately. Follow the manufacturer's instructions for use.

Creams and Jellies

Creams and jellies are inserted into the vagina with an applicator and take effect immediately.

Vaginal Contraceptive Film (VCF)

VCF comes as paper-thin squares that dissolve over the cervix. After it's inserted, it takes about fifteen minutes for the VCF to become effective. Follow the manufacturer's instructions for use.

Suppositories

Suppositories are inserted into the vagina like a tampon and pushed up toward the cervix. It takes about twenty minutes for the capsule to dissolve and become effective.

Side Effects

You or your partner may experience genital irritation, a rash, or itchiness if either of you is allergic to ingredients in a spermicide. If this happens, you may need to use another method of contraception.

Where to Get Spermicides

Spermicides are available over the counter in any drugstore or can be bought in family-planning clinics or online.

If you become pregnant while using spermicide, the pregnancy will not be affected.

HORMONAL METHODS: PILL, MINIPILL, RING, PATCH, SHOT

Hormonal contraceptives come in many forms—daily pills, weekly patches, monthly rings, and quarterly injections. They work by using hormones similar to the ones our bodies produce to prevent the release of eggs. Combined hormonal contraceptives use both estrogen and progestin. Progestin-only contraceptives do not contain estrogen.

For hormonal methods to work, you have to use them as directed and on schedule. They protect against pregnancy, but not against STIs, including HIV.

HORMONAL METHODS AND MENSTRUAL BLEEDING

Menstrual bleeding—a period—is the result of the interaction of the hormones estrogen and progesterone in our bodies. Estrogen causes the lining of the uterus (the endometrium) to thicken in preparation for pregnancy; progesterone further develops the lining of the uterus and maintains it during pregnancy. If no pregnancy occurs in the cycle, there is a fall in progesterone, and the lining is shed. This lining is what is expelled during menstruation.

Hormonal contraceptives use synthetic hormones to suppress ovulation and prevent pregnancy. Most birth control pills contain some form of estrogen and a synthetic form of progesterone called a progestin. These hormones stabilize the uterine lining and encourage more regular bleeding patterns. Progestin-only methods such as Depo-Provera, implants, and some pills contain no estrogen. They can lead to irregular or absent bleeding.

These changes in bleeding patterns can cause relief or concern. For example, some women worry that not bleeding while using the

pill or another hormonal method causes unshed blood to build up inside the uterus. This is not true. Methods with combined estrogen and a progestin reduce the uterine lining and progestin-only methods prevent the lining of the uterus from building up, so there is nothing to shed. Another concern is spotting between periods or irregular bleeding. Irregular bleeding occurs most frequently in the beginning of method use, when the uterine lining has not completely thinned. This is not harmful, but it can be very annoying.

Skipping Your Period

Some women are now opting to use the Pill, patch, or ring continuously for several months in order to skip periods. Some new brands of pills are packaged to be used this way. If you do not have a brand of pills designed for continuous use, you can skip your periods by using regular monophasic pills this way: Take only active pills in one pack, skip the inactive pills, and go directly to the next packet of active pills. After three months, or when you begin to have spotting, take inactive pills for a week. Then begin using the active pills again. If you use the patch or ring, wear it for the recommended time, remove it, and immediately begin the next patch or ring. Studies show that using the pill continuously is as safe as using it with monthly bleeds.[7] The long-term health effects of using continuous hormonal contraception have not been studied.[8] Many women are happy to skip periods, although some miss the monthly reassurance that pregnancy has not occurred.

WHERE TO GET HORMONAL CONTRACEPTIVES

All hormonal methods—the Pill, patch, ring, minipill, and shot—are available by prescription only. You must see a health-care provider. The clinician will discuss your medical history with you, check your blood pressure, and give you any other medical exam that may be needed. If a hormonal contraceptive is right for you, the clinician will give you a prescription and may be able to give you a starter pack. Pelvic exams are not necessary to begin hormonal contraceptives.

THE PILL—ORAL CONTRACEPTIVES

Combined pills are the most popular type of birth control used in the United States and among the most commonly used methods worldwide. What is commonly referred to as "the Pill" is actually many different brands and several different regimens that may differ from one another in the dosage and type of hormones. Women can choose a regimen in which they bleed every month, every three months, or less frequently than that. You may need to try more than one type of pill before you find one that works well for you and does not cause unacceptable side effects.

Combined pills come in one-month or three-month packs. One pill is taken every day. Most of the pills have a combination of synthetic estrogen and progestin; the remaining pills have no hormones and are called spacer pills, sugar pills, or inactive pills. Bleeding begins during the time you take the inactive pills. The specific types of hormones and the number of active and inactive pills vary by brand.

The original birth control pills had twenty-one days of active pills and seven days of inactive pills. Some newer pills have twenty-four active pills and four inactive pills; this regimen reduces irregular bleeding. Many brands of these pills now have generic versions, which are less expensive than the new, patented varieties. Since the generic pills have been around for longer and are better studied, the risks associated with using them are better understood.

The Pill works by preventing the ovaries from releasing eggs. It also prevents fertilization by causing the cervical fluid to thicken, making it harder for sperm to enter the uterus. The Pill is a very effective method of birth control, although it does not protect against sexually transmitted infections, including HIV/AIDS.

Effectiveness

With perfect use, the Pill is over 99 percent effective. Perfect use means that the woman takes a pill at about the same time every day and never misses a pill. With typical use, the Pill is about 92 percent effective. That means that about one in thirteen women who use the Pill becomes pregnant in the first year of use.

Advantages
- May cause lighter or more regular bleeding.
- May reduce painful periods.
- Does not interrupt spontaneity.
- May reduce incidence of ovarian cysts and fibrocystic breast changes.
- May relieve premenstrual syndrome (PMS).
- Protects against uterine and ovarian cancers.
- Provides some protection against pelvic inflammatory disease.
- Does not require a pelvic exam for use.
- May reduce acne.
- Certain types can be used for emergency contraception (see p. 251 for more information).

Disadvantages
- Does not protect against STIs, including HIV.
- Must be taken as directed; can be difficult to remember.
- Can have unpleasant side effects on mood or libido.
- Raises risk of venous thromboembolism (blood clots in the veins), heart attack, and stroke for some women.
- Requires a prescription, which must be regularly filled.

How to Use
If you begin taking the Pill within five days after your period starts or within five days after an abortion, it is effective immediately. If you begin at any other time, the Pill becomes effective after one week (so use a backup method or avoid intercourse during that week). To lower your risk of STIs, use condoms as well. Combining condom and pill use also increases your protection from pregnancy.

Starting the Pill
A common way to start taking the Pill is to begin on the first day of your period or the day of an abortion. Some women prefer to start on the first Sunday after they begin their period or the first Sunday after an abortion. Starting pills on Sundays has the advantage of usually having your period begin on a Monday or Tuesday, and thus not having periods on weekends.

Some health-care practitioners now recommend the Quick Start method. Following a negative pregnancy test, you take your first pill in the clinic or office. Use a backup form of birth control for one week.

Continuing
Take one pill every day until you finish an entire pack. If you take your pill at the same time you brush your teeth, eat a meal, or perform another daily activity, it may be easier to remember. If you have a mobile phone, you can also set an alarm as a reminder to take your pill. Start a new pack immediately after you finish the old one.

Missed Pills
Missing pills is the most common reason for becoming pregnant while using birth control pills. Missing the first day(s) of a new pack of pills is the most dangerous in terms of decreasing their effectiveness, so make sure to refill your prescription before you run out. If you forget to start a new pack on the right day or if you miss a pill during the cycle, here's what to do.

Late Start
- If you are one or two days late starting the next package, take two pills as soon as you remember and one pill each day after. Use a backup form of birth control for one week.
- If you are three or more days late starting the next package, start with the first pill in the package and use a backup method of birth control until you have taken seven ac-

SAFETY OF THE PILL

The birth control pill is one of the most intensely researched medications in history. Since its development more than fifty years ago, it has been used by millions of women worldwide.

The early pill formulations raised concerns about blood clots, heart attack, and stroke, spurring exhaustive research on oral contraceptives beginning in the 1960s and '70s. Since then, new formulations of the Pill with low-dose hormones have been introduced, and today's pills contain about one-eighth to one-tenth of the estrogen in early pills. Research has concluded that today's birth control pills are safe for most women, and that healthy, nonsmoking women have little if any greater risk of heart attack or stroke than women who do not use the Pill.

Any woman of any age has a tripling of her risk of blood clots while on the Pill, although this risk is still quite small overall. To put the risk in perspective, the risk of a blood clot during pregnancy is double the risk of getting a blood clot while on the Pill. Women with some cardiovascular conditions or some chronic illnesses and women over age thirty-five who smoke should not take the Pill. In rare cases, women who use birth control pills may develop liver tumors. Some evidence suggests that oral contraceptive use slightly increases the risk of getting cervical cancer or breast cancer among women under thirty-five,[9] but these associations are controversial and have not been fully established.

Long-term use of the Pill provides significant noncontraceptive health benefits. Long-term use protects against ovarian and endometrial (uterine) cancers, and research suggests that these protective effects may last up to fifteen years or more after stopping the Pill. Women who take the Pill have lighter, shorter periods (thus reducing the risk of anemia), are less likely to develop ovarian cysts, and have a decreased incidence of pelvic inflammatory disease (PID).

Though the information listed above is based on research on the Pill only, it is reasonable to infer that the same cautions and side effects apply to all methods that contain both estrogen and progestin, such as the patch and the ring.

tive (hormonal) pills in a row. If you had unprotected intercourse during the time you missed pills, consider using emergency contraception (see p. 251). If you have questions, call your health care provider.

Missed Pills During the Cycle
- If you miss one pill, take the missed pill as soon as you remember and take your next pill at your usual time. This may require taking two pills in one day. If you miss your pill by twenty-four hours, take both the one that is late and the one that is due.
- If you miss two pills in a row in the first two weeks of the pack, take two pills on the day you remember and finish the rest of the pack as usual. Use a backup form of birth control for one week.

- If you miss two pills in a row in the third week of the pack, keep taking one pill every day until you have finished the active (hormonal) pills. Then set aside the rest of the pack, including the inactive pills, and start taking a new pack of pills. Use a backup form of birth control for one week.
- If you miss three or more pills in a row in the first two weeks, take one pill as soon as you remember, then keep taking one pill every day. Use a backup method of birth control until you have taken seven active (hormonal) pills.
- If you miss three or more pills in a row in the third week, take one pill as soon as you remember, then keep taking one pill every day until you have finished the active (hormonal) pills. Don't take the inactive pills. Go directly to a new pack and take the whole pack. Use a backup form of birth control for one week.

Missing any of the last, inactive pills of a combined pill package will not raise your risk of pregnancy. Skip the pills you missed and be sure you start your next pack on time. (This is not the case for the minipill; see p. 233.) Know what regimen you are taking and which pills are active and which are inactive.

Missed Periods

Women taking the pill often have shorter and lighter periods. A drop of blood, even if it is brown, during the week you are taking no hormonal pills is counted as a period when you are on the Pill.

If you miss one period and you took all of your pills correctly, and you don't have any signs of pregnancy, the chances of pregnancy are very low. It is not uncommon to miss a period while on the pill. If you miss two periods in a row, it could be either normal or a sign of pregnancy. Take a pregnancy test either at home or with a health-care provider, but keep taking your pills, in case you are not pregnant. If you become pregnant while on the Pill and continue your pregnancy, there is no evidence that the Pill increases the health risks to your baby.

Health Concerns

Contraindications

Women who are over thirty-five and smoke generally should not take the Pill. Women who have any of the following conditions also should not take the Pill.

- Severe hypertension (high blood pressure)
- History of heart attack or stroke
- Clotting disorders or blood clots in the legs or lungs
- Migraine headaches with aura
- Unexplained vaginal bleeding (until diagnosed; then the Pill may be a treatment)
- Current breast cancer
- Known or suspected pregnancy
- Liver disease
- Heart disease
- Major surgery with prolonged immobilization
- Gastric bypass surgery

The Pill is generally not recommended for women who have a history of breast cancer, diabetes with complications, or certain types of gallbladder disease, or who take certain antiseizure medications or rifampin, a tuberculosis medication.

Women who have given birth should wait three weeks before beginning a birth control method that contains estrogen. Women are at high risk for blood clots for several weeks after a pregnancy, and adding a birth control method that contains estrogen increases that risk. Because estrogen can interfere with the quality or quantity of your milk production, women who

HORMONAL BIRTH CONTROL AND MOOD CHANGES

Studies of women using combined hormonal birth control methods have shown that they experience a variety of moods. For some women, birth control improves mood. Most studies of progestin-only birth control, such as Depo-Provera (the shot), an implant, and the Mirena IUD, show on average little or no difference in mood changes. However, there is enormous variability in any individual woman's response to her own hormones and any synthetic hormones she takes. Some women report feeling depressed when using hormonal birth control. Because Depo-Provera initially puts more progestin into the bloodstream than methods that emit a lower, steady dose of progestin, some women find it to have a greater negative effect on both mood and libido (sex drive) than other hormonal methods. For these reasons, it makes sense to pay attention to your body and emotions when using birth control methods that contain hormones.

breastfeed may want to use a different method of birth control. (For more information, see "Suitable Contraceptive Methods to Use While Breastfeeding," p. 251.)

Danger Signs

If you experience any of the following symptoms while taking the Pill, you should call your health-care provider or go to an emergency room immediately.

- Severe leg or arm pain, swelling
- Chest pain or shortness of breath
- Severe headaches
- Eye problems, such as sudden blurred vision

Drug Interactions

Certain medications reduce the effectiveness of the Pill. These include antiseizure medications (phenytoin [Dilantin], phenobarbitol, carbamazepine [Xeloda]), rifampin (a tuberculosis drug), and Saint-John's-wort. If you are taking any medications or herbal remedies, tell the provider who is prescribing the Pill. You may need to add a backup method of birth control.

There have been anecdotal reports of antibiotics interacting with oral contraceptive pills. However, there is no scientific evidence that antibiotics (other than rifampin) interfere with oral contraceptives. Because of the anecdotal reports about this issue, some women choose to use a backup method (such as condoms) while taking antibiotics and oral contraceptive pills.

Getting Pregnant Later

Women who want to become pregnant may stop using the Pill at any time. Pregnancy may occur right away or after several months. The Pill does not affect your long-term fertility.

Side Effects

- Irregular bleeding or spotting
- Nausea
- Breast tenderness
- Spotty darkening of the skin (melasma) (rarely)
- Mild headaches
- Mood changes, including depression or decreased sex drive

Side effects usually go away after two to three cycles of pills. If any side effects are bothersome after two to three cycles, continue taking your pills and call your health-care provider for an appointment. Though these side effects can make you uncomfortable, they are not danger-

WILL BIRTH CONTROL MAKE ME GAIN WEIGHT?*

The Pill (and also the patch and the ring) does not cause weight gain.[10] However, we sometimes *feel* as if we've gained weight after starting birth control. It's hard to know exactly why this happens. It may be because many women start birth control for the first time while transitioning from the teens into the twenties, a time of natural weight gain. If a woman gains weight at this time, it's easy to put the blame the Pill, the patch, or the ring. The truth is each of these methods can be used without an expected weight gain.

One method of birth control, the shot (Depo-Provera), *does* lead to weight gain for some women. A recent study showed that, in the first six months of use, one out of four shot users gained 5 percent or more of her starting weight.[11] (For example, if you were one of these women and weighed 170 pounds when you got your first shot, you would gain nine or more pounds within six months.) The women who gained weight in the first six months were more likely to go on gaining weight while they continued the shot. However, the majority of women (three out of four) didn't gain much weight, averaging 1.4 pounds in the first year of using the shot. The shot might not be the best choice if you already have trouble with your weight, particularly since there are options that provide protection against pregnancy and aren't linked to weight gain (like the implant, an IUD, the ring, the patch, and the Pill).

Long-acting methods that also contain progestins, such as the implant and the hormonal IUD, are not linked to weight gain like the shot.

* Excerpted with permission from SexReally.com.

---

ous. Sometimes a different pill will make a difference. If you feel that you must stop the Pill immediately, be sure to abstain from vaginal intercourse or use another form of contraception. The contraceptive effects of the Pill—as well as the side effects—go away as soon as you stop taking it.

The Pill as Emergency Contraception

Some brands of the Pill can be used for emergency contraception. EC is taken within five days after unprotected intercourse to prevent pregnancy. (For more information, see "Emergency Contraception," p. 251.)

CONTRACEPTIVE PATCH

The contraceptive patch—currently marketed under the name Ortho Evra—is a prescription method of birth control. The patch looks like a square Band-Aid and is applied to the abdomen, buttocks, upper arm, or upper torso. The patch is changed once a week for three weeks, left off for one week, then resumed. The patch works by slowly releasing a combination of estrogen and progestin through the skin. These are the same hormones found in the combined birth control pill and therefore the patch works the same way and has the same side effects (see p. 228).

Effectiveness

The patch is a very effective reversible method of birth control. With perfect use, the patch is about 99 percent effective; with typical use it's about 92 percent. The patch is less reliable in women over 198 pounds, but so few women over this weight participated in studies of the patch that the level of effectiveness cannot be reliably calculated.

The patch works best when it is changed on the same day of the week for three weeks in a row. Pregnancy can happen if an error is made using the patch, especially if

- It becomes loose or stays off for longer than twenty-four hours
- The same patch is used—left on the skin—for longer than one week

If either of these things happens, follow the directions in your package insert, consider taking emergency contraception (see p. 251), and call your health-care provider.

Advantages

These are the same as for the Pill (see p. 225), although some women find the weekly patch more convenient than the daily pill.

Disadvantages

These are the same as for the Pill (see p. 225), except that you have to remember to use a new patch once a week rather than to take a pill every day.

How to Use

Apply the patch within five days of the first day of your period or within five days of an abortion. If you start at another time, use a backup method for seven days. One patch per week is used for three weeks in a row. The day of the week you apply the patch will be the same day you change it a week later. On the fourth week,

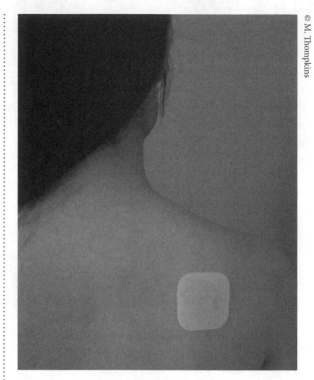

© M. Thompkins

Birth control patch

don't wear a patch, and your menstrual period should start. A new patch is applied seven days after removal to start another month of birth control. It does not matter if you are still bleeding.

The patch can be applied anyplace on the body that is clean and dry except on open sores or on the breasts. Don't put it on after you have applied body lotion. The patch can be worn swimming or in the shower but should be checked afterward. About 2 percent of the time, a patch will completely fall off. If it partially or completely falls off, refer to the instructions.

After giving birth, wait three weeks to apply your first patch. You are at higher risk for blood clots for three weeks after a pregnancy, and adding the patch increases that risk.

Health Concerns

Unlike the Pill, the patch provides a steady amount of estrogen that does not change over the course of a day. However, the average amount of estrogen in the blood of patch users is about 60 percent higher than in users of low-dose pills. There is conflicting evidence on whether this higher baseline of estrogen for patch users has serious health effects; some studies have shown a higher incidence of blood clots in women using the patch, while others have not. Other than this concern, the health risks and contraindications of the patch are the same as those for the combined pill (see p. 227).

Some research studies have shown that breast tenderness, painful periods, and nausea are more common with the patch than the Pill, and that women are more likely to quit using the patch than the combined pill.[12] Another possible side effect unique to the patch is skin irritation, rash, or redness where you apply the patch. Other side effects are the same as for the combined pill.

VAGINAL RING

A vaginal ring is a thin, transparent, flexible ring that you insert into the vagina to prevent pregnancy. The vaginal ring is left in place for three weeks and then removed for one week, providing one month of birth control. It slowly releases into the body estrogen and progestin, which stop ovulation and thicken the cervical fluid, creating a barrier to prevent sperm from fertilizing an egg. The ring does not protect against sexually transmitted infections, including HIV. Currently, the only type of ring available is NuvaRing, although a one-year ring is in development.

Effectiveness

The vaginal ring is over 99 percent effective as birth control when used perfectly. With typical use, the effectiveness is about 92 percent.

Advantages

- Can be worn for twenty-one to thirty days, providing protection from pregnancy one month at a time.
- Private—no visible patches or pill packets.
- Does not need to be fitted for use.
- Otherwise the same as for the Pill (see p. 225), although some women find the monthly ring more convenient than the daily pill.

Disadvantages

- May change vaginal discharge or cause vaginal irritation.
- Otherwise the same as for the Pill (see p. 225), except that you have to remember to use a new ring once a month rather than to take a Pill every day.

How to Use

The vaginal ring must be inserted within the first five days of beginning your period or within five days of an abortion. You may also choose to change the ring on the first day of the month and use the calendar as your guide for when to replace each ring. The ring is effective after seven days during its first use, so use a backup method for the first week. After the first month, it is effective continuously, as long as you don't forget to insert a new ring after the seven-day break. If you started the ring on time, you are protected from pregnancy during the seven-day break.

If you're taking the Pill or using another form of hormonal birth control, you can switch to the ring without losing protection from pregnancy.

Inserting the vaginal ring is much like inserting a tampon or a diaphragm. You can squat, stand with one leg raised on a chair, or lie down. Squeeze the ring between your thumb and index finger or twist it into a figure 8, then gently push it into your vagina. Because the ring is not a barrier method, you don't have to worry about the exact placement. Push the ring far enough in so it feels comfortable. Usually you can't feel it at all.

The ring remains in the vagina for three weeks, though if you prefer to have the ring out during sex, it can be removed for a maximum of three hours in any twenty-four-hour period. Remove it by inserting a finger into your vagina, hooking the side of the ring, and pulling it out. If you have completed the three weeks and are done with the ring, wrap it in its foil pouch and put it in the trash; avoid flushing it down the toilet to prevent hormones from being released into the environment. Your period should start within the next few days. For another month of birth control, insert a new ring seven days after removal of the last one, even if your period has not ended.

New rings should be stored until use in the refrigerator if possible, or at room temperature, but at no more than 77°F, and away from direct sunlight.

If the ring slips out of your vagina and it has been out for less than three hours, you are still protected from pregnancy. Rinse it with cold or lukewarm water (not hot) and reinsert it as soon as possible. If you lose the original ring, insert a new one as soon as possible. If more than three hours have passed, your protection is significantly reduced. You need another method of birth control until the ring has been back in place for seven days in a row. If you had unprotected intercourse when the ring was out for more than three hours, consider using emergency contraception (see p. 251).

Health Concerns

Women with an easily irritated vagina, a dropped uterus, a dropped bladder, rectal prolapse, or severe constipation may not be able to use the vaginal ring. Your health care provider can help you decide.

The hormones found in the ring are similar to those found in the Pill. Women who cannot use the Pill for health reasons also cannot use the ring. The health risks, benefits, drug interactions, and danger signs of the ring are the same as those for the combined pill (see p. 227).

Side Effects

In addition to the side effects described for hormonal contraceptives, ring users may experience some minor side effects, including vaginal discharge or irritation.

MINIPILLS (PROGESTIN-ONLY ORAL CONTRACEPTIVES)

Minipills are progestin-only birth control pills that contain progestin but no estrogen. Minipills come in packs of twenty-eight pills, and one is taken every day. The minipill prevents fertilization by thickening the fluid around the cervix and blocking sperm from entering the uterus. It also affects the transport of the egg through the fallopian tubes. The minipill may also prevent ovulation. It does not protect against sexually transmitted infections, including HIV.

Effectiveness

Minipills are 98–99 percent effective with perfect use and 87–92 percent effective with typical use, slightly less than regular birth control pills. For women who are breastfeeding, they provide almost 100 percent protection from pregnancy and do not affect milk supply.

Advantages

- Contains no estrogen. Since most of the side effects and medical risks of combined pills come from the estrogen, minipills avoid these effects.
- Unlike combined pills, minipills do not reduce the incidence of ovarian cysts; their advantages are otherwise the same as for combined oral contraceptive pills (see p. 225).

Disadvantages

- Does not protect against sexually transmitted infections, including HIV.
- Must be taken every day at the same time; missing one pill can result in pregnancy.
- Increases the risk of functional ovarian cysts (not dangerous).
- May cause irregular bleeding or spotting.
- Requires a prescription, which must be filled by a pharmacy regularly.

How to Use

Minipill packs have no inactive pills. Each pill contains hormones, so it is important to take a pill every day at the same time. Forgetting a minipill or taking it late increases the chance of pregnancy more than missing a combined pill does.

Using a backup method such as condoms or spermicide increases minipill effectiveness. To lower your risk of sexually transmitted infection, use condoms as well.

Starting Minipills

Take the first pill on the first day of your period. Take one pill daily, at the same time of day, even during your period.

After the First Pack

As soon as you finish one pack, begin the next one. Start your next pack even if you are still bleeding or have not started your period. Continue taking one pill every day.

If you have problems with the minipill, call your health-care provider. If you stop taking minipills, you must use another birth control method to avoid pregnancy.

Missed Pills

- If you are three or more hours late taking the pill, take it as soon as you remember. Use a backup method for forty-eight hours.
- If you miss one pill, take the missed pill as soon as you remember, and take the next one at the usual time. This may mean taking two pills in one day. If you miss only one pill and make it up, you probably will not get pregnant. Use a backup method for two weeks.
- If you miss pills for two days, take two pills each day for the next two days. Use a backup method for two weeks. You may have some spotting or bleeding, but if the bleeding is like a period, call your provider.
- If you miss pills for three or more days, use a backup method and call your provider for instructions.

If you missed one or more pills and you had unprotected intercourse, consider using emergency contraception. Progestin-only ECs (called Plan B or Next Choice) are higher doses of the minipill. (See the section on EC, p. 251.)

Getting Pregnant Later

Women who want to become pregnant can stop using minipills at any time. Pregnancy may occur right away or after several months.

Health Concerns

You should not use the minipill if you are already pregnant, have breast cancer or advanced liver disease, have had gastric bypass surgery, or take certain anticonvulsants or rifampin (a tuberculosis drug).

Benefits

Women using progestin-only hormonal contraception have a decreased risk of pelvic inflammatory disease. You may have less menstrual cramping and pain, lighter periods, and less chance of anemia. This method can be used by women who cannot use estrogen.

Side Effects

The most common side effect for women using minipills is irregular bleeding or no bleeding at all. If you do not bleed for sixty days, take a pregnancy test or call your provider, but continue taking your pills. The minipill may also cause mood changes, headaches, and decreased sex drive.

Drug Interactions

Minipills are affected by the same medications as the pill. See "Drug Interactions" (p. 228) for information on which medications can decrease effectiveness.

THREE-MONTH SHOT (DEPO-PROVERA)

Depo-Provera is an injection of the hormone progestin. Depo prevents pregnancy for three months. It is usually given in the arm or buttock. The high level of progestin prevents fertilization by stopping the ovaries from releasing eggs, thickening the cervical fluid, and changing the uterine lining, making it harder for sperm to enter or survive in the uterus. You have to get a new shot every three months. Depo-Provera does not protect against sexually transmitted infections, including HIV.

The fact that Depo is a long-acting method is both its strength and its weakness. For women who like the shot, knowing that they are protected from pregnancy for at least three months is very important. But for those women who have unpleasant side effects such as ongoing bleeding, knowing that these effects may continue for another three or more months can be difficult. After the last shot of Depo-Provera, it can take more than six months for the drug to completely leave the body. If you are considering using Depo, talk to your provider about what your options would be if you experience side effects.

Effectiveness

Depo-Provera is over 99 percent effective as birth control provided you get your next shot at the correct time every three months. Because not all women are able to get the next shot on time, its typical use effectiveness is 97 percent. After the first shot, make an appointment for the next shot.

Advantages

- The most private method of birth control.
- Does not require monthly supplies or attention.
- Effective after twenty-four hours.
- Does not interrupt sexual spontaneity.
- Contains no estrogen. Because most of the side effects and medical risks of combined pills come from the estrogen, Depo avoids these effects and can be used by women who cannot use the combined pill.
- May stop bleeding after continued use.
- May decrease risk for ovarian and uterine cancers.

Disadvantages

- Does not protect against STIs, including HIV.
- Requires regular injections every three months.
- Causes some loss of bone density, most of which is replaced when a woman stops using it, although its long-term effects on bone strength remain unclear.
- May delay ability to get pregnant after method is discontinued.
- Can cause weight gain.
- Possible irregular bleeding or no menstrual bleeding at all (seen as a benefit for some but not others).
- If side effects occur, the hormones cannot be removed. It may take months for periods to get back to normal.

How to Use

You will probably be given your first shot of Depo-Provera during—or within five days after the start of—your period. If there is no chance you are pregnant, it can first be given at any time during the cycle. After twenty-four hours, the shot provides effective birth control for the next thirteen weeks.

Depo can also be started immediately after a birth or during the first seven days after an abortion, including immediately after an abortion.

If you are more than a week late for your shot, use a backup method of birth control for the next two weeks. If your period is over two weeks late and you have had unprotected intercourse during that time, consider taking a pregnancy test before receiving the next dose. Remember that it can take six to nine months for your menstrual cycle to return to normal after you stop Depo-Provera.

If you have heavy or continuous bleeding after your first injection, you can have a second injection as early as four weeks after your first injection; this second injection should stop your bleeding.

If you decide to switch from Depo-Provera to the birth control pill, the vaginal ring, or the contraceptive patch, it is recommended that you start your new method on the date the next injection is due. It is not harmful to start earlier; it just means that you will be double covered to prevent pregnancy. If you decide to switch to an IUD, it can be inserted anytime during the three months following the last injection.

Getting Pregnant Later

If you want to become pregnant, you can stop using Depo-Provera at any time. Depo's contraceptive effect can last an average of four to six months after your last injection, and for some women, it can last up to eighteen months. (However, some women become pregnant immediately after stopping, so don't count on the long-term effect if you do not want to be pregnant.) If you think you might want to become pregnant in the next year, Depo is probably not a good choice for you.

Health Concerns

If you suspect or know you are pregnant, or you have breast cancer, you should not use Depo-Provera.

Depo-Provera is not recommended if you are planning to get pregnant soon. It probably should not be used by women who have multiple risk factors for cardiovascular disease, severe hypertension, history of heart attack or stroke, diabetes, or advanced liver disease.

Risks

Depo-Provera causes some loss of bone density, though its long-term effects on bone strength remain unclear. Recent research indicates that bone density loss is worse for adolescent women or with longer use of Depo-Provera and may not be completely reversible, especially when a woman's diet does not provide enough calcium. For this reason, it's important for women using Depo to exercise regularly and eat calcium-rich foods. If this is difficult for you, you may want to consider switching to a different method of contraception after two years.[13] Some evidence shows that you can help protect your bones by adding a small amount of estrogen if using Depo for more than two years.

If you become pregnant while using Depo-Provera and continue your pregnancy, you may have a slightly increased risk of premature birth.

Benefits

Women using Depo-Provera have a decreased risk of endometrial cancer and pelvic inflammatory disease. You may have less menstrual cramping and pain, fewer periods, and less chance of anemia.

Side Effects

All women who use Depo experience changes in menstrual bleeding. This is not dangerous. Spotting, heavy bleeding, and no bleeding are common side effects. After a year of use, over half of all Depo users stop having periods (amenorrhea); two-thirds stop by the end of the second year. It is not possible to predict who will experience amenorrhea. Many women like not having periods, while others find it unsettling. Irregular bleeding is the most common reason for discontinuing the use of Depo.

Many women who use Depo-Provera gain some weight over time, usually about 1.5 pounds in the first year. One in four Depo-Provera users experiences rapid weight gain, and may gain up to eighteen pounds in the first year.[14] (For more information, see "Will Birth Control Make Me Gain Weight?" page 229.)

Symptoms some women experience during use of Depo-Provera include headaches, nervousness, mood changes, bloating, hot flashes, decreased interest in sex, breast tenderness, acne, hair loss, and backache. After the last shot of Depo-Provera, it can take more than six months for the drug to leave the body. Side effects may linger until the drug is completely gone.

Drug Interactions

No medications have been shown to lower the effectiveness of Depo-Provera.

LONG-LASTING CONTRACEPTIVES: IMPLANTS AND IUDS

Long-acting birth control includes the contraceptive implant and intrauterine devices (IUDs). These methods are highly effective, and because you don't have to take any action for them to work, there is no difference between their perfect and typical use effectiveness. Fewer than one in one hundred women using these methods will become pregnant in a year. Some women find these methods convenient because they require fewer clinic or pharmacy trips. Although they may be expensive up front, depending on your health-care coverage, they can be the most affordable methods over time. They provide highly effective protection against pregnancy but do not protect against STIs, including HIV.

WHERE TO GET LONG-ACTING METHODS

Getting an implant or IUD requires a visit to a doctor or clinic, where a skilled clinician places the contraceptive in a quick, nonsurgical procedure. These birth control methods can last for years but do not have to be used that long. They can be removed at any time, and your fertility returns immediately. Removal, which is also done by a skilled clinician, takes just a few moments.

IMPLANON (CONTRACEPTIVE IMPLANT)

Implanon is a single soft, progestin-filled capsule that is inserted under the skin in a woman's upper arm. It works in the same way as other progestin methods, preventing ovulation and thickening the cervical fluid, thereby preventing sperm from entering the uterus. Implanon offers a safe, long-term, reversible contraceptive option.

Effectiveness

Implanon is over 99 percent effective—as effective as tubal sterilization, but reversible. It lasts up to three years.

Advantages

- One of the most effective reversible birth control methods.
- Can be used privately.
- Does not interrupt spontaneity.
- You don't have to think about contraception for up to three years.

- Can be used by women who are breast-feeding.
- Contains no estrogen. Because most of the side effects and medical risks of combined pills, the patch, and the ring come from the estrogen component, Implanon avoids these effects and can be used by women who cannot use combined pills, the patch, or the ring.
- Provides steady, very low does of progestin.
- Fertility returns quickly once implant is removed.

Disadvantages

- Does not protect against STIs, including HIV.
- Most women experience irregular bleeding and changes to periods.
- Requires a trained medical provider to insert and remove.
- Side effects can last until removal.
- Can cause slight increase in ovarian cysts (not dangerous).
- Rarely, can cause an infection or bruising in the arm immediately after insertion.

How to Use

Implanon is inserted by a health-care provider in a medical office. Implants are usually inserted during or a few days after your period to ensure that you are not pregnant. However, they can be inserted anytime, as long as you are sure you are not pregnant.

Insertion

An insertion usually takes less than five minutes. A local anesthetic is used on the inside of the upper arm, and the Implanon inserter is used to place the device. The inserter is a needle similar in size to needles used to draw blood. The implant is placed just under the skin. Both you and the provider must feel the implant under the skin to confirm that it is in the correct location. Your arm may feel bruised or tender for several days. Implants are effective within twenty-four hours of insertion.

Removal

You can have an implant removed on schedule (after three years) or anytime before then. Local anesthetic is used on the arm, then a small incision is made and the provider pulls out the implant. The typical removal takes less than a minute. The incision made for removal may leave a small scar on your arm. Fertility may return immediately or within a few months.

Health Concerns

Women who suspect or know they are pregnant, or have breast cancer, should not use implants.

Implants are generally not recommended for women who have a history of stroke or breast cancer, severe liver disease, unexplained vaginal bleeding until after it is diagnosed, intolerance to irregular bleeding, or progestin allergies. Cautions and side effects are the same as with other progestin-only contraceptives.

Risks

Irritation, scarring, or infection may occur where the implant is inserted. If your incision area becomes red, swollen, or painful, call your health-care provider.

Benefits

Women using Implanon may have a decreased risk of pelvic inflammatory disease. You may have less menstrual cramping and pain, fewer or lighter periods, and less chance of anemia.

Side Effects

The most common complaint of women using implants is irregular bleeding, which occurs most often during the first months but can last the entire three years the Implanon is in place. Bleeding patterns can be unpredictable, and a small proportion of women have almost continuous spotting. Low-dose oral contraceptives or estrogen taken in addition to using the implant may help regulate cycles.

Some women may experience side effects such as acne, headaches, breast tenderness, and weight gain. A small number of women have reported mood swings, abdominal pain, painful periods, and hair loss. If you have negative side effects that are disrupting your life, you can have your implant removed at any time.

INTRAUTERINE DEVICES (IUDs)

Intrauterine contraceptives (IUDs) are small plastic devices that contain copper or progestin and are placed inside the uterus. A string attached to the IUD extends downward through the cervix into the upper vagina, allowing the IUD to be removed. The IUD is usually not noticeable during intercourse and is effective for up to either five or twelve years depending on the type.

Currently, there are two types of IUDs available in the United States: ParaGard and Mirena. The two IUDs are used similarly but prevent pregnancy by different methods.

The ParaGard, also called the Copper T, has a tiny copper wire wrapped around the plastic body. The ParaGard works primarily by releasing copper ions into the uterine fluid; these ions make sperm unable to swim or fertilize an egg. Periods may be heavier or cramps may be more intense for women using ParaGard. Women who have been on the Pill prior to insertion of ParaGard may find this particularly noticeable because periods on the Pill are generally much lighter with less cramping than without it. The ParaGard is FDA-approved for use for up to ten years and has been shown to be effective for up to twelve years in studies.

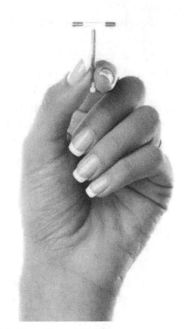

ParaGard IUD, or Copper T 380a

The Mirena IUD works by releasing steady, small amounts of a progestin (levonorgestrel), which prevents ovulation and thickens the cervical fluid. Thicker cervical fluid prevents sperm from advancing from the vagina into the uterus. If sperm do get through, they are less vigorous and less able to fertilize an egg, if present. The progestin in the Mirena decreases menstrual bleeding and cramping for most users. About a third of users will have no period after a year of using the Mirena. The Mirena is approved for use up to five years.

The IUD is now used by more than 160 million women worldwide. It is one of the safest, best tolerated, and most effective methods of contraception available.

Effectiveness

IUDs are over 99 percent effective, as effective as tubal sterilization. That means that for every one hundred women using an IUD, fewer than one will become pregnant in a year.

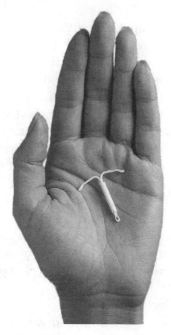

The Mirena IUD, or levonorgestrel-releasing IUD

Advantages

- Immediately effective.
- Private.
- Does not affect spontaneity.
- Does not interfere with breastfeeding.
- You don't have to think about contraception for as long as it is in place.
- Effective for five to twelve years, depending on type.
- ParaGard is nonhormonal.
- Mirena, which is also used as a treatment for heavy bleeding and painful periods, may decrease bleeding and cramping.
- Mirena does not contain estrogen and provides a steady, very low dose of hormone.
- Cheaper than many methods if you use it for more than a year.

Disadvantages

- Does not protect against STIs, including HIV.
- Placement of the device and removal require clinic visits and a pelvic exam.
- Can cause spotting and irregular bleeding in the first three to six months.
- Can be expelled (uncommon).
- ParaGard can cause heavier cramps and bleeding during periods.
- Up-front costs (the IUD and the insertion charge) may be expensive and are not always covered by insurance.
- Perforation of the uterus can occur (very rare).

How to Use

The IUD needs to be inserted by a trained, skilled medical provider. Ask your provider about her or his experience inserting IUDs. Your provider will insert a speculum, clean the cervix with a cotton swab dipped in a cleansing solution, and apply a clamp on the cervix. While pulling slightly on the clamp (to straighten the uterus), the provider will insert a straight instrument about the width of a toothpick to measure the depth of the uterus. The IUD, which is folded inside a narrow tube, is then inserted to the correct depth. During the insertion, the arms of the IUD unfold inside the uterus. Then the provider removes the inserter and clamp, trims the strings, and removes the speculum. The whole insertion process usually takes only a few minutes, and may cause strong cramping or a feeling of light-headedness. Insertion is painful but brief. By the time you finish saying "Ow!" it's over. It is recommended that you take a nonsteroidal pain reliever (such as ibuprofen) before you have an IUD inserted. The cramping should go away in a few minutes or hours.

A good time to insert is during ovulation or menstruation, or just after childbirth or abortion, when the cervix is dilated. However, IUDs can be inserted at any time in a woman's cycle, provided she has no chance of being pregnant

IUD SAFETY CONCERNS

Though the IUD is the second most widely used method of birth control in the world, it has not been popular in the United States. This is largely due to the fact that in the 1970s, one type of IUD, the Dalkon Shield, was found to be unsafe, causing an increase in pelvic infections among users and resulting in the deaths of twenty women. Thousands of women filed lawsuits, and by 1985 the company had declared bankruptcy. Most IUDs were pulled from the market at the time, and the reputation of IUDs was damaged.

The IUDs now available are safer and have not been found to increase the risk of pelvic infections except for a small risk right around the time of insertion if a woman has an undiagnosed STI. Talk to your health-care provider if you are concerned that you might have an STI.

(unless it is within five days of unprotected intercourse and is being used as emergency contraception; see p. 242).

Six weeks after insertion, you may have a return visit with your provider to make sure the IUD is in place and there are no signs of infection. If you experience heavy vaginal bleeding, lower abdominal pain, abnormal discharge, or unexplained fever, you should see your provider as soon as possible. These could be signs of expulsion (the IUD falling out) or infection. Depending on when an IUD was inserted and the skill of the provider, there is a 0.5–7 percent chance of expulsion.

Checking IUD Strings

If you are comfortable putting your fingers into your vagina, you can check to make sure your IUD is in place. Some providers will advise you to check your strings after your first period on the IUD, but it's not a requirement. (If you do check your strings, make sure not to pull on them.) If you have severe pain or cramping lasting more than a few days after the insertion, you may have a partially expelled IUD. If this is the case, you would be able to feel feel the hard plastic of the IUD at the opening of your cervix. If you think your IUD may be partially expelled, abstain from intercourse or use another contraceptive method until you see your provider to determine whether the IUD is still in place.

Missing Periods

Absent periods are common with the Mirena but not with the ParaGard IUD. While pregnancy is extremely unlikely, you should take a pregnancy test if you miss a period while using a ParaGard IUD. If you have a positive pregnancy test or any concerns about your IUD, call your health-care provider.

Health Concerns

You should not use an IUD if you have any of the following conditions:

- Current pelvic infection or STI
- Known or suspected pregnancy
- Had a serious infection within the past three months after giving birth or after having an abortion (puerperal sepsis or postseptic abortion)
- Endometrial cancer or untreated cervical cancer
- Unexplained vaginal bleeding before diagnosis
- Current breast cancer (for Mirena only)
- Wilson's disease or an allergy to copper (ParaGard only)

IUDs are generally not recommended for women who have fibroids that have changed the shape of the uterus, for women who have ovarian cancer or have AIDS and are not clinically well on antiretroviral therapy, or for women who have advanced liver disease. ParaGard is generally not recommended for women who already have heavy bleeding or very painful periods. Women with anemia or severe menstrual cramping and heavy flow can use the Mirena IUD to improve these conditions.

Using an IUD does not increase your risk of STIs or pelvic infection; having unprotected sex without a condom with someone who has an STI does. If you have an STI at the time your IUD is inserted, you are slightly more likely to develop a pelvic infection in the next twenty days. You can be tested for STIs on the day of IUD placement and treated if needed. If you get an STI while you are using an IUD for birth control, you are no more likely to develop a pelvic infection than anyone else who gets an STI. The Mirena actually protects against pelvic infections. You can be treated for STIs or a pelvic infection with the IUD in place.

Risks

Piercing or perforation of the uterine wall is a very rare event that can occur during IUD placement (less than one time in a thousand insertions). In general, a partial perforation of the uterine wall heals quickly, no treatment is required, and your fertility is not affected. Very rarely, it can cause more serious complications. More experienced medical providers have much lower rates of perforation.

Rarely, an IUD may become embedded in the uterine wall. An embedded IUD is still effective, but it can be painful and may need to be removed. There is a risk of surgery and infertility if an IUD becomes embedded, but—to repeat—this situation is very rare.

If you become pregnant while using an IUD, have the IUD removed, whether or not you want to carry the pregnancy to term. An IUD in place increases the risk of miscarriage or premature birth. If the strings are not visible to remove the IUD, it is usually left in place until the end of the pregnancy, or removed at the time of an abortion.

Because the IUD is so effective at preventing pregnancy, women using IUDs are at lower risk of ectopic pregnancy (when a fertilized egg attaches and grows outside the uterus) than women using less effective contraception or no contraception at all. But in the unlikely event that a woman does become pregnant while using an IUD, she is more likely to have an ectopic pregnancy than other women. Ectopic pregnancy can be very dangerous and requires emergency medical attention. (For more information, see "Ectopic Pregnancy," p. 466.)

Benefits

The IUD offers very effective protection from pregnancy without systemic side effects and decreases a woman's risk of getting endometrial cancer. The Mirena IUD decreases menstrual bleeding and cramping, and has recently been approved by the FDA for the treatment of heavy bleeding. Thirty percent of Mirena users stop having menstrual bleeding altogether. Mirena IUDs are also used in the treatment of endometriosis, although they have not been FDA approved for this use.

Side Effects

Longer, heavier, or more painful menstrual periods are the most common complaint of ParaGard IUD users. If you are already borderline anemic, increased menstrual flow may cause anemia. Some women have spotting between periods.

In the first three months of use, prolonged bleeding is also a common complaint with the Mirena. It takes about three months for the lining of the uterus to thin down, and during this time, bleeding can be erratic or heavy at times; it almost always settles down after three to six months. During the first month, 20 percent of users experience bleeding of more than eight days in duration, but by the third month, only 3 percent have prolonged bleeding.

The side effects of the Mirena IUD are similar to those of other progestin-containing methods but are generally less intense, because the effects are more local and the blood levels of progestins are much lower. The Mirena can cause a slight increase in ovarian cysts. These cysts are benign and usually resolve in two to three months. Mirena rarely can cause headaches, acne, mood changes, and a decrease in sex drive.

Getting Pregnant Later

If you want to become pregnant, you can have the IUD removed at any time. You may become pregnant immediately or within a few months.

ParaGard as Emergency Contraception

The ParaGard IUD is very effective for emergency contraception. You can prevent pregnancy after unprotected intercourse by having a ParaGard copper IUD inserted within five days. It is 100 percent effective in preventing pregnancy and can then be left in place as a method of birth control for up to twelve years.[15]

PERMANENT METHODS: FEMALE AND MALE STERILIZATION

There are several options for female sterilization: tubal ligation, Essure, and Adiana. They all work by stopping the egg from traveling to the uterus from the ovary and preventing sperm from reaching the fallopian tube to fertilize an egg.

Female sterilization should be considered permanent and irreversible. Although procedures exist to "untie" the tubes, they typically involve major surgery, cost many thousands of dollars, are not covered by insurance, and work only about half the time. In vitro fertilization, another option for sterilized women, is also costly and carries its own risks. You should consider sterilization only if you are certain you will not want to become pregnant in the future.

TUBAL LIGATION

Tubal ligation, commonly known as "getting your tubes tied," is a surgical sterilization technique that closes the fallopian tubes. In this procedure, fallopian tubes are cut, burned, or blocked with rings, bands, or clips. Tubal ligation is effective immediately. It does not protect against reproductive tract infections or sexually transmitted infections, including HIV.

A tubal ligation can be performed at any time under local or general anesthesia in a clinic, doctor's office, or hospital. Minilaparotomy and laparoscopy are the two most common techniques. Be sure to discuss the risks and benefits of different techniques with your health-care provider before deciding which one to use. If you are having a baby and want a tubal ligation afterward, talk to your doctor about sterilization options at the time of birth.

In a laparoscopy, the abdomen is filled with carbon dioxide gas so that the abdominal wall balloons away from the uterus and tubes. A laparoscope, a small telescopelike instrument, is inserted into a small cut just below the navel. Another instrument is inserted through an incision just above the pubic hairline to cut, sew, or burn the tubes. In a minilaparotomy, the surgeon makes a small incision just above the pubic hair and moves the fallopian tubes toward the incision to cut, sew, or burn the tubes.

After surgery, take two to three days off and

perform only light activities for a week. You may have sex again when you feel comfortable, usually after a week. If you have surgery performed through your vagina, don't put anything into your vagina for two weeks to avoid infection.

ESSURE

Essure is a method of sterilization that does not require surgery or general anesthesia. A small flexible spring is inserted into each fallopian tube. This sterilization technique is considered a major advance over surgical methods because it poses fewer risks of complications. Unlike surgical sterilization, Essure is not effective immediately; it becomes effective three months after the procedure, when an X-ray dye test shows that the tubes are successfully blocked.

The procedure is performed in a doctor's office. The doctor passes a thin, fiber-optic tube attached to a video camera through the cervical canal into the uterus, and inserts a tiny device into each fallopian tube. The devices expand, and over the course of about three months, fibrous tissue grows into them to block the tubes. In the United States, the FDA requires a test three months after Essure insertion to confirm that both fallopian tubes are blocked and the devices are in the right place. Rarely, the devices are found to be in the wrong location or have fallen out before the tubes are blocked.

Essure blocks both fallopian tubes 95 percent of the time. The most common reason for failure is that the doctor is unable to place the device in one or both fallopian tubes. Most women who have the procedure are able to go home about an hour afterward and return to work the next day.

Because Essure is made of the metal nickel, you should let your health care providers know you have been sterilized using the device. Some procedures—such as electrocautery of the lining of the uterus (endometrial ablation)—cannot be done with a metallic object present. Although research to date has shown the method to be very safe, its relative newness (it was introduced in 2002) means some risks may not have been identified yet.

ADIANA

Adiana is a new type of nonsurgical female sterilization that uses a silicon implant about the size of a grain of rice. Because it's nonsurgical like Essure, Adiana carries fewer risks than surgical sterilization. It becomes effective about three months after the insertion procedure, when an X-ray dye test shows that the tubes are successfully blocked.

The insertion is performed in a doctor's office. The doctor passes a thin tube through the cervical canal into the uterus. Radio waves released at the tip of the tube heat a short section of each fallopian tube. The tube is then used to place a tiny silicon implant on the heated spot. Over about three months, fibrous tissue grows into the implant to block the tubes. As with Essure, the FDA requires a test three months after Adiana insertion to confirm that both fallopian tubes are blocked. Research has shown that the method blocks both fallopian tubes 95 percent of the time.

Effectiveness

All surgical sterilization procedures are over 99 percent effective. The nonsurgical procedures are 95 percent successful. Once properly placed, Adiana and Essure take three months to become effective. After the three-month follow-up test shows that the tubes are blocked, Adiana and Essure are more than 99 percent effective.

Advantages
- Permanent birth control.
- Does not interrupt sexual spontaneity.

- Requires no daily attention.
- Cost-effective in the long run.
- Tubal ligation is immediately effective.
- Essure and Adiana are nonsurgical.

Disadvantages

- Does not protect against STIs, including HIV.
- Tubal ligation requires surgery and has risks associated with surgery, such as bleeding, infection, and anesthesia problems.
- Essure and Adiana take three months to become effective.
- More risk than male sterilization.
- Should not be considered reversible.
- Possible regret, especially if done before age thirty or immediately after giving birth.

Health Concerns

Tubal ligation is generally not recommended for women who have had difficulties with previous surgeries.

Adiana and Essure are not recommended for women with fibroids that change the shape of the uterus, women with iodine allergies (because the tests used to confirm blockage may contain iodine), or women who have given birth or had a pelvic infection in the last three months. Adiana is not recommended for women taking medications such as steroids that suppress the immune system. Essure is not recommended for women who are allergic or sensitive to nickel.

Risks

Tubal ligation is abdominal surgery and carries the risks of any surgery, including infection and a reaction to the anesthesia. If you have a high fever, swelling, or pus at the incision or severe abdominal pain or bleeding, call your doctor. You can shower the day after your surgery, but take care not to rub or pull on your incision for at least a week. Rest for a few days before you start all your normal activities again; you should feel fully recovered within a week.

If you had a laparoscopic procedure, your stomach may be swollen from the gas in your abdomen, and you may have back or shoulder pain. This will go away within a few days as your body absorbs the gas.

Following Essure or Adiana placement, serious complications occur in less than 1 percent of women. These can include an injury to the uterus, vasovagal response (slowing of the heart rate and dilation of the blood vessels, resulting in low blood pressure and light-headedness, which can occur during any gynecological procedure), or fluid overload (the absorption of too much water in the body, which can, in rare instances, lead to serious breathing problems or other complications). However, in studies, women with these complications recovered quickly and did not need to stay overnight in the hospital.

Pregnancy is unlikely after a successful sterilization (about one in two hundred women will become pregnant in the first year following sterilization). When a pregnancy does occur, it has a substantial chance of being located in the tube instead of in the uterus (ectopic pregnancy). This can be very dangerous and requires immediate medical attention. Women who have surgery to reverse a tubal ligation and become pregnant also have a higher chance of ectopic pregnancy. Thus, any pregnancy after sterilization (reversed or not) needs to be evaluated with ultrasound to ensure the pregnancy is within the uterus.

Benefits

Female sterilization does not affect a woman's ability to enjoy sex. Usually, hormone levels and a woman's menstrual cycle are not noticeably changed by sterilization. Ovaries continue to release eggs, but the eggs stop in the tubes and are reabsorbed by the body. Some women experience improved sexual pleasure with the end of concerns about becoming pregnant.

Side Effects

Common side effects immediately following Essure and Adiana placement include mild uterine cramping or pain, nausea, and light bleeding. These usually go away within a few days.

After tubal ligation, some women report irregular and painful periods or no periods, midcycle bleeding, or lack of interest in sex. However, a large study of over ten thousand women found that those with surgical sterilization were more likely to have reduced bleeding and less menstrual pain compared with women who had not been sterilized, and no more likely to have midcycle bleeding.[16] A third of the women in the study used a hormonal method of birth control, such as pills or Depo-Provera, before their sterilization procedure, and quitting a hormonal method can lead to cycle irregularity.

Getting Pregnant Later

Female sterilization is considered a permanent method of birth control. Surgery to reverse a tubal ligation is effective only about half the time. Reversal procedures are technically challenging, expensive (over $5,000), and usually not covered by insurance. Another option for achieving a pregnancy after sterilization is in vitro fertilization.

MALE STERILIZATION: VASECTOMY

A vasectomy is a sterilization technique for men. It involves minor surgery to cut the vas deferens, the tube that carries sperm from the testes to the penis. The man still produces semen, but when he ejaculates, there are no sperm in the semen.

Male sterilization is a simpler procedure than surgical female sterilization. It is usually done in a doctor's office or a clinic and takes less than fifteen minutes. The practitioner applies a local anesthetic (such as lidocaine), makes one or two

Sterilization has a long history of abuse. Women with disabilities, poor women, and women of color have been disproportionately targeted for sterilization. Although U.S. federal guidelines now require that special informed consent procedures be followed, the problem of sterilization abuse remains in some places. For more information on the history of sterilization, see "Sterilization Abuse" at the Our Bodies Ourselves website, ourbodiesourselves.org.

small incisions in the scrotum, locates the two vasa deferentia, removes a piece of each, and ties or burns the end. Because sperm are already in the vasa deferentia, men are not sterile immediately. For this reason, it is important to use another method of birth control until the man has a negative sperm count, or for three months after the procedure. Since vasectomy does not protect against sexually transmitted infections, men should also continue to use condoms to protect against STIs.

No-scalpel vasectomy is used increasingly throughout the world. It was developed in China, where it is now the standard technique. In no-scalpel vasectomy, a practitioner uses an instrument to puncture a tiny hole in the scrotum, lifts the vas deferens out through the hole, removes a piece of it, and then ties or burns the end. No-scalpel vasectomy is as effective as the scalpel method but has a lower complication rate.[17]

Vasectomy does not affect a man's sexual function. It leaves the man's genital system basically unchanged. His sexual hormones are unaffected, and there is no noticeable difference in his ejaculate, because sperm make up only a small part of the semen. Even if they know these facts, some men still worry that a vasectomy will affect their sexual performance. Talking with someone who has had a vasectomy can help relieve anxieties.

Vasectomy has become increasingly popular over the past years. Men often choose vasectomy after the failure of another birth control method; when they want to spare their partner from more-invasive surgery (female sterilization); or because they want to have complete control over their fertility.[18] Nearly 13 percent of U.S. married couples use vasectomy as their contraceptive,[19] and in some countries, such as New Zealand, almost half of men over forty have opted for it.[20]

Recent advances allow some vasectomies to be reversed through an expensive microsurgical procedure. However, the longer a man has had his vasectomy, the lower the chance of success. In addition, reversals usually aren't covered by insurance. Pregnancy rates after a vasectomy reversal vary widely; even a skilled surgeon may have only a 30 percent success rate.[21] Vasectomy should be considered permanent.

Effectiveness
Vasectomy is over 99 percent effective and is considered permanent.

Advantages
- Permanent birth control.
- Does not interrupt sexual spontaneity.
- Requires no daily attention.
- Does not affect pleasure.
- Less complicated than female sterilization.

Disadvantages
- Does not protect against STIs, including HIV.
- Not immediately effective.
- Requires minor surgery.
- Rarely, the vas deferens rejoins.
- Should be considered a permanent method; may not be reversible.

NONMEDICAL METHODS: WITHDRAWAL, FAM, LAM, ABSTINENCE

WITHDRAWAL (PULLING OUT)

Withdrawal (coitus interruptus) involves removing the penis from the vagina before ejaculation so that the sperm is deposited outside the vagina and away from the lips of the vagina. It is also called "pulling out" and is often used in combination with other methods such as condoms, fertility awareness, or periodic abstinence. Withdrawal offers no protection against sexually transmitted infections.

When used consistently and correctly, withdrawal is slightly less effective than male condoms at preventing pregnancy. Using the method successfully requires good communication and an experienced partner who knows his body. Your partner must:

- Know when he is going to ejaculate
- Demonstrate that he does not ejaculate very quickly, before he realizes it
- Have the experience and self-control to pull out in time

Effectiveness
Withdrawal is between 73 and 96 percent effective at preventing pregnancy, depending on how perfectly it is done. With typical use, one of about every four women relying on withdrawal alone becomes pregnant during the first year. With perfect use, one of twenty-five women becomes pregnant during the first year.

Advantages
- Withdrawal can be used to prevent pregnancy when no other method is available.
- Using withdrawal in combination with other methods may increase their effectiveness.
- No health risks or side effects.

EMERGING MALE CONTRACEPTIVES

Birth control has traditionally been the responsibility of women, and most methods of contraception work by altering a woman's fertility. Currently the only methods of male contraception are vasectomy and condoms. Vasectomy, while very effective, is permanent, and therefore is not appropriate for those who may wish to have children in the future. Condoms, because they must be used for each act of intercourse, are not widely used among committed couples. There is a critical need for safe, reliable, and reversible birth control methods for men. Despite this need, development of new contraceptives for men has been slow and poorly funded.

However, several new methods of male contraception are in development. China will likely have a hormonal contraceptive for men in the next decade. Although it's often referred to as the "male pill," it will be administered by injection every eight weeks. The majority of men in clinical trials consider the method acceptable.[22]

Also in the next decade, India may have a truly innovative birth control method known as RISUG. It is a compound that renders sperm unable to swim. A small amount is injected into the vas deferens in a ten-minute procedure. Clinical trials show it is highly effective, begins acting almost immediately, and has few side effects. Researchers found that RISUG in animals can be reversed with another injection that flushes it out of the vas deferens; they are now evaluating its reversibility in men.[23]

Although these new contraceptives for men are in advanced stages of research, they will not be available in the United States anytime soon. It will take many years and more large-scale clinical trials for the Food and Drug Administration to thoroughly evaluate them.

For more information on experimental male contraception, see the website of the Male Contraceptive Coalition at male contraceptives.org.

- Promotes communication and responsibility between partners.
- Free.

Disadvantages
- Does not protect against STIs, including HIV.
- Interrupts spontaneity.
- Requires a great deal of self-control, experience, and trust.
- Not for men who ejaculate prematurely or are sexually inexperienced.

How to Use
The man withdraws his penis from the vagina before or when he feels he has reached the point when ejaculation can no longer be stopped or postponed. He ejaculates outside the vagina, being careful that semen does not spill onto his partner's vulva. Men who use withdrawal must be able to know when they are reaching ejaculatory inevitability—the point in sexual excitement when ejaculation can no longer be stopped or postponed.

FERTILITY AWARENESS METHOD (FAM) AND OTHER NATURAL METHODS

FAM

FAM is a scientifically validated method of natural birth control that involves charting fertility signs to determine whether or not you are fertile on any given day. Fertility awareness can also be used to achieve pregnancy or for greater body awareness in general. (For more information, see p. 26.)

FAM as birth control involves some background research, record keeping, and a daily time commitment. It also involves being comfortable touching your own vagina and vaginal fluids. In order to use FAM effectively, you need more information than this book provides. You can learn more about FAM in the book *Taking Charge of Your Fertility* by Toni Weschler or by taking a class (see Recommended Resources).

How FAM Works

By charting your primary fertility signs (waking temperature, cervical fluid, and cervical position), you can determine which phase of the cycle you are currently in. Unlike the obsolete rhythm (or calendar) method, which relies on past cycles to predict future fertility, FAM effectively identifies your fertile phase, the time when ovulation is about to happen, and when it has occurred. You can then use your daily fertility observations to know whether or not you are safe for unprotected intercourse on any given day.

Couples can choose either to abstain or to use another method during the woman's fertile phase. It should be understood, though, that if you choose to have intercourse using another birth control method during your fertile phase, FAM cannot be any more effective than the method itself.

Effectiveness

If FAM is used perfectly by a motivated couple who abstain during the fertile phase, the effectiveness rate is approximately 95–97 percent over the course of a year. It is difficult to know how effective it is with typical use. Various studies show that the effectiveness of natural family planning varies greatly; 75–90 percent per year is commonly reported in the medical literature. Natural methods of contraception are most appropriate for strongly motivated women and couples who can commit to learning the method thoroughly and following the rules consistently.

Advantages

- No health risks or side effects.
- Can increase a woman's awareness and understanding of her gynecological health, hormonal balance, and fertility.
- Promotes communication and responsibility between partners.
- After the cost of initial instruction, costs nothing to practice.

Disadvantages

- To learn it correctly requires taking a class or reading a book, and it usually takes about two cycles to assimilate FAM's basic principles.
- Does not protect against STIs, including HIV.
- Requires considerable commitment, cooperation, and self-control, by both you and your partner.
- Typical failure rate is higher than with other methods.
- Can be challenging to practice while breastfeeding, owing to the unpredictability of ovulation.
- Takes a few minutes a day to take your temperature and chart your fertility signs.

New Technologies

Technologies such as calculators, computer programs, saliva tests, and urine tests are increasingly available to help determine fertility. However, these high-tech methods are more appropriate for women who are trying to achieve pregnancy rather than avoid it. This is because most of these methods do not give you enough warning of impending ovulation to account for the possibility of sperm surviving for up to five days in the uterus and fallopian tubes.

BREASTFEEDING AS BIRTH CONTROL

You should never assume that you are infertile simply because you are breastfeeding. But breastfeeding can prevent ovulation, and thus work as a natural form of child spacing, *if* certain criteria are met. The frequency with which a woman breastfeeds is the primary factor in determining when fertility returns. Breastfeeding every few hours—even if only for a minute or two each time—is most effective at preventing ovulation.

Exclusive or full breastfeeding is not the same as frequent breastfeeding. The amount of time that a baby spends sucking or the amount of milk the infant receives are not factors in the effectiveness of breastfeeding as birth control.

Other factors can influence the return of postpartum fertility, including the use of pacifiers, whether or not food or liquid other than breast milk is given to your baby, or even whether you sleep with your baby. A woman who wishes to practice a form of natural contraception following birth has a couple of options.

Lactational Amenorrhea Method (LAM)
You can use LAM during the first six months if you are exclusively breastfeeding.

This method must be very strictly followed to be effective. Even then, its success is contingent upon such frequent nursing that it is often difficult for women in Western societies to rely

on completely. But the guidelines state that you are not likely to ovulate if you meet all of the following criteria:

- Your menstruation has not returned since childbirth.
- Bottle feeds or regular food supplements are not introduced.
- Your baby is under six months old.

The first criterion of LAM is that you have not resumed periods. If you are breastfeeding, any vaginal bleeding before the fifty-sixth day after birth is almost always anovulatory (meaning no ovulation has taken place) and therefore can be ignored. Any bleeding after the sixty-fifth day should be considered a sign of resumed ovulation.

The second criterion means that you are strictly breastfeeding and not giving your baby any other food or even offering a pacifier. The contraceptive effectiveness of LAM is maintained only if the intervals between night feedings do not exceed about every four hours. So the shorter the intervals between all feedings, and the closer you keep your baby to you, the more likely it is that LAM will be effective. To further increase the effectiveness of LAM, some instructors suggest that you nurse once or twice per hour during the day and several times at night during the baby's first few months.

Fertility Awareness Method (FAM)
This can be used throughout the return of your fertility, as well as afterward. The rules for practicing FAM while breastfeeding differ from those used in other circumstances and are not described in this book. FAM can be used most effectively if a woman can consult with a FAM instructor, whether in person, on the phone, or online. The website Taking Charge of Your Fertility (tcoyf.com) is a good site to learn more. (For more information, see p. 26.)

The basic principle is that the breastfeeding

woman observes her cervical fluid during the day. It typically shows a pattern of either nothing or dry cervical fluid day after day, or a combination of both. These days are considered safe. As soon as a woman's cervical fluid pattern begins to change to a wetter consistency, her body is indicating that she may be preparing to ovulate again. She must consider herself fertile on any days of wet vaginal sensation or wet cervical fluid, as well as three days beyond the last day of wetness.

Nursing once or twice per hour during the day and several times at night during the baby's first few months usually results in unambiguous protection from pregnancy, meaning that you will have "dry cervical fluid" (essentially no wetness) and a dry vaginal sensation. Once you have established this dryness, you can usually nurse less frequently after the first few months and still maintain dryness indicative of protection.

If you have not learned how to use FAM or do not strictly meet the LAM criteria, it is best to use another method of birth control while breastfeeding.

ABSTINENCE

Some of us define abstinence as not having any sexual contact with another person. Others consider ourselves abstinent when we don't have intercourse but engage in sexual practices such as hugging, caressing, touching a partner's genitals, or having nonvaginal sex. This section uses the terms complete abstinence and sex without intercourse (sometimes called "outercourse") to differentiate between these two kinds of abstinence.

Effectiveness
Complete, continuous abstinence is 100 percent effective. However, because many people who plan on being abstinent at some point engage in unprotected intercourse, its typical use effectiveness is far lower.

Sex without intercourse is 100 percent effective if no semen comes in contact with the vulva or vagina.

Advantages
Complete Abstinence
- The most effective form of birth control.
- No physical side effects.
- Protects against STIs.
- Free.

Sex Without Intercourse
- Highly effective form of birth control.
- Free.
- Allows you to experience sexual pleasure with a partner without risking pregnancy.

Disadvantages
Complete Abstinence
- Going without sex for long periods of time is unappealing for many of us.
- If our commitment to abstinence wavers, we may become sexually active without protecting ourselves against pregnancy and STIs.

Sex Without Intercourse
- Slight risk of pregnancy if semen gets close to your vagina (see p. 310).
- Risk of transmitting an STI.

Your Health
Women who abstain completely from intercourse are less likely to

- Get a sexually transmitted infection
- Have an unplanned pregnancy
- Become infertile as a result of an STI
- Develop cervical cancer

Many of us who are abstinent will have intercourse at some time in our lives. If you're considering intercourse, take time to educate yourself about birth control options and safer sex, rather than making a spontaneous decision during a passionate moment.

EMERGENCY CONTRACEPTION

Emergency contraception (EC) is contraception that can be used *after* unprotected intercourse or a birth control failure to prevent pregnancy. EC can be used any time from immediately after unprotected intercourse to up to five days after. Using emergency contraception greatly decreases the chances of a pregnancy. Emergency contraception does not work if you are already pregnant. It does not cause abortion.

There are now four safe and effective methods of emergency contraception available: commercial forms of emergency contraception pills (ECPs), combined birth control pills, progestin-only pills, and IUDs.

In the United States, Plan B, Plan B One-Step, and Next Choice are available without prescription to women and men seventeen years and older. Women age sixteen and under need a prescription. However, in some states, pharmacists are allowed to prescribe ECPs directly to women of any age, eliminating the need for a clinic visit. As of 2011, the following states allow this: Alaska, California, Hawaii, Maine, Massachusetts, New Hampshire, New Mexico, Vermont, and Washington state. The newest commercial ECP, Ella, is available only by prescription regardless of age.

Although some forms of emergency contraception have been used for several decades, most women and many providers still do not know that it is available and effective. If more women knew about and were able to get emergency contraception when needed, many unintended pregnancies and abortions could be prevented.

EMERGENCY CONTRACEPTIVE PILLS (ECPs)

Emergency contraceptive pills (ECPs), also known as "postcoital contraception" or the "morning-after pill," work by changing a woman's hormone levels in the same ways birth control pills and other hormonal methods work. They give the body a short, high burst of synthetic hormones that disrupt natural hormone production needed for ovulation and pregnancy. ECPs prevent pregnancy by inhibiting ovulation or by disrupting egg and sperm transport, fertilization, or implantation. Most women can safely use ECPs even if they cannot use birth control pills as their regular method of birth control. ECPs can be used within five days of unprotected sexual intercourse.

It is not advisable to use ECPs as your only

SUITABLE CONTRACEPTIVE METHODS TO USE WHILE BREASTFEEDING

- Abstinence—complete or outercourse.
- Barrier methods.
- Copper T IUD.
- Mirena IUD.
- Depo-Provera injection.
- Implanon.
- FAM/LAM.
- Minipills (progesterone-only pills).
- Combined hormonal contraceptive methods like the Pill, NuvaRing, and Ortho Evra patch can be used beginning six weeks after giving birth. However, if you are breastfeeding, these methods may diminish the quantity or quality of breast milk.[24] This possible risk may outweigh the benefits of these methods.

protection against pregnancy if you are sexually active or planning to be, because they are not as effective as other contraceptive methods. Using ECPs frequently won't hurt you, but it will get expensive.

The FDA currently approves three types of emergency contraceptive pills: pills that contain only progestin, pills that contain both progestin and estrogen, and pills that contain the antiprogestin ulipristal acetate. (Mifepristone, or RU-486, can also be used for emergency contraception. It has a lower pregnancy rate and fewer side effects than currently available pills[25] but has not been approved for this use in the United States and is very expensive, $350–$650.)

Progestin-only ECPs include Plan B, Plan B One-Step, Next Choice, and the minipill. Progestin-only ECPs are slightly more effective than combination pills and cause few if any side effects.

The second type of ECP uses both estrogen and progestin. Currently, no combination pills are sold specifically as ECPs, but many brands of the daily birth control pill can be used at a higher dose for emergency contraception. To find out which pills you can use and the proper dose for each, call the Emergency Contraception Hotline at 1-800-584-9911 or go to ec.princeton.edu/questions/dose.html. This method often causes nausea and discomfort, but many women believe that the protection is worth it.

The newest ECP, the antiprogestin pill Ella, is more effective than progestin-only pills at preventing pregnancy, but it is more expensive.

Health Concerns

Because ECPs are used for only a short time, most women—including some who have been told by a doctor that they shouldn't take birth control pills—can safely take them. If you have a serious health problem that prevents you

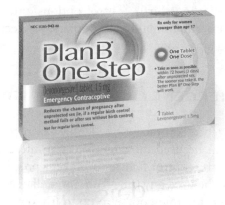

Courtesy of Teva Women's Health, Inc.

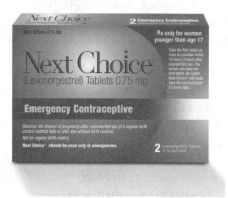

Courtesy of Watson Pharmaceuticals, Inc.

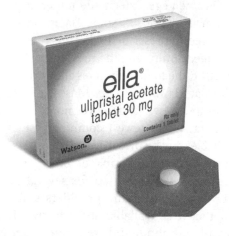

Courtesy of Watson Pharmaceuticals, Inc.

from taking regular birth control pills, consult a health-care provider. Certain medications may interfere with Ella, so discuss any other medications you're taking with your provider.

If you could be pregnant already, it is a good

idea to take a pregnancy test before using emergency contraception. ECPs should not be used by women who are already pregnant—not because the pills are thought to be harmful, but because they are ineffective at terminating established pregnancies. If after taking the pills you become pregnant anyway, there is no evidence of danger to the fetus.

How to Use

Some people call emergency contraceptive pills "morning-after pills." But you do not have to wait until the morning after. You can start the pills right away or up to five days after you have had unprotected intercourse—that is, intercourse during which you did not use birth control or your birth control may have failed. The sooner progestin-only or progestin-plus-estrogen ECPs are started within the five-day (120-hour) window, the more effective they are. Ella, however, is equally effective on all five days after unprotected sex.

Effectiveness

Plan B and Next Choice reduce the chance of pregnancy by 88 to 95 percent. If a hundred women have unprotected intercourse, about eight will become pregnant; if the one hundred women use Plan B, only one will become pregnant. Plan B is 89 percent effective for all women who take the pills within the first three days. Taking the pill within the first twenty-four hours may increase effectiveness to as much as 95 percent.

Combined estrogen and progestin pills are slightly less effective than progestin-only pills. They reduce the chance of pregnancy by 75 percent.

Ella reduces the risk of pregnancy by 98 percent. It is equally effective regardless of which day it is taken.

Side Effects

Progestin-only pills have few or no side effects. Nausea and vomiting are the most common negative effects of taking emergency contraception pills that contain both estrogen and progestin; about half the women who take them feel nauseated, and about 20 percent vomit. For this reason, some practitioners advise taking the pills with food or with an antinausea medication such as an over-the-counter remedy for motion sickness. Other negative effects include breast tenderness, dizziness, abdominal pain, and headaches. Using combination pills for emergency contraception may also change the timing of your next menstrual period: It may begin a few days earlier or a few days later than usual.

The most common side effects of Ella are abdominal pain, cramping, and irregular bleeding. Less common side effects include headache and nausea.

How to Use the IUD as EC

The ParaGard IUD, also known as the Copper T, is very effective at preventing pregnancy if inserted within five days after unprotected intercourse. The IUD works as an emergency contraceptive by rendering sperm unable to swim, changing the unfertilized egg, or preventing the implantation of a fertilized egg. Once inserted into the uterus, ParaGard can be left in place and used as your regular method of birth control for up to twelve years.

Women who cannot use the IUD for birth control (see p. 240) should not use it for emergency contraception, either.

Effectiveness

Using the ParaGard IUD within five days of unprotected intercourse reduces the risk of pregnancy by 100 percent.

COMPARING BIRTH CONTROL METHODS

METHOD	PERFECT USE EFFECTIVENESS: NUMBER OF WOMEN IN 100 WHO WILL BECOME PREGNANT IN ONE YEAR	TYPICAL USE EFFECTIVENESS: NUMBER OF WOMEN IN 100 WHO WILL BECOME PREGNANT IN ONE YEAR	% WOMEN CONTINUING USE AT ONE YEAR	STI PROTECTION	AVERAGE COST*	COST PER YEAR*
No method	85	85		None	Free	Free
Barrier Methods						
Male condom	2	15	53	Good	$0.60–$3 each use	Depends on use
Female condom	5	21	49	Good	$1.50–$3 each use	Depends on use
Diaphragm	6	16	57	None	$100–$200 for method and fitting	$35–$65
Cap (no previous vaginal birth)	–	14	Unknown	None	$100–$200 for method and fitting	$35–$65
Cap (previous vaginal birth)	–	29	Unknown	None		
Sponge (no previous vaginal birth)	9	16	57	None	$0.50–$3 each use	Depends on use
Sponge (previous vaginal birth)	20	32	46	None		
Spermicides	18	29	42	None	$0.50–$4 each use	Depends on use
Hormonal Methods						
Pills (combined/mini)	<1	8	68	None	$10–$55 per month	$120–$700
Patch	<1	8	68	None		
Vaginal ring	<1	9	68	None		
Depo-Provera	<1	3	56	None	$75–$150 per quarter	$300–$550
Long-Acting Methods						
Implanon	<1	<1	84	None	$800 over 3 years	$275
ParaGard	<1	<1	78	None	$650 over 12 years	$55
Mirena	<1	<1	80	None	$900 over 5 years	$180

METHOD	PERFECT USE EFFECTIVENESS: NUMBER OF WOMEN IN 100 WHO WILL BECOME PREGNANT IN ONE YEAR	TYPICAL USE EFFECTIVENESS: NUMBER OF WOMEN IN 100 WHO WILL BECOME PREGNANT IN ONE YEAR	% WOMEN CONTINUING USE AT ONE YEAR	STI PROTECTION	AVERAGE COST*	COST PER YEAR*
Nonmedical Methods						
Withdrawal	4	27	43	None	Free	Free
Fertility awareness	3-5	12-25	51	None	Free after training	Free after training
Permanent Methods						
Tubal ligation	<1	<1	100	None	$1,500–$5,000	Depends on fertile years remaining
Essure	<1	<1		None	$2,500–$5,000	
Adiana	<1	<1		None		
Vasectomy	<1	<1	100	None	$250–$1,000	
Emergency Contraception						
Pills	Not applicable	Not applicable	Not applicable	None	$10–$50 per use	Depends on use
ParaGard	Not applicable	Not applicable	Not applicable	None	$650; can use for 12 years	$55

*Costs for prescription birth control vary dramatically depending on where you live, what health coverage you have, and what type of health care provider you visit. You may be able to get free clinic visits or birth control—ask your provider.

Where to Get Emergency Contraception

Emergency contraception is available at family-planning clinics, health-care providers' offices, and pharmacies. You can ask your provider to write you a prescription in advance so you have it on hand if you need it. The IUD must be inserted by a trained provider.

Frequently Asked Questions

- **What is my risk of pregnancy from unprotected intercourse?** The likelihood of becoming pregnant after a single act of unprotected intercourse depends on where you are in your menstrual cycle and on your body's unique fertility levels.

- **What if I engage in unprotected intercourse but ejaculation does not occur? Is sperm present in pre-ejaculatory fluid?** The chance of pregnancy is probably extremely low. Three small studies found no motile sperm in pre-ejaculatory fluid.[26] (However, HIV *can* be detected in pre-ejaculatory fluid.) If you are worried about the possibility of pregnancy, or if you are not sure whether ejaculation did occur, consider using emergency contraception.

- **When should my next period come after I take emergency contraceptive pills?** After taking ECPs, some women have a period early, and some women have irregular bleed-

Abortion rights opponents oppose EC and claim it is abortion, which ends a pregnancy, rather than contraception, which prevents one. However, EC works either by preventing ovulation or by preventing implantation of a fertilized egg in the uterus. The international medical community agrees that pregnancy begins with implantation, so EC acts before pregnancy even occurs.

ing that is not really a period. The duration of the irregular bleeding is not predictable. You should have another normal period within the next month. If not, you should get a pregnancy test to make sure you're not pregnant.

- **What if I have sex after taking emergency contraceptive pills?** Emergency contraceptive pills do not act as ongoing birth control. They will not protect against pregnancy from unprotected intercourse that occurs after the pills are taken.

- **Is there a limit to the number of times emergency contraceptive pills can be used?** There are no safety concerns with using ECPs repeatedly. However, ECPs are not as effective as many other methods of contraception. EC is also expensive to use repeatedly. You (and your wallet) might benefit from finding an ongoing method of contraception.

For free information about preventing pregnancy after unprotected intercourse and to obtain names and telephone numbers of health care professionals in your area who can provide emergency contraception, call the Emergency Contraception Hotline at 1-800-584-9911 or visit not-2-late.com.

■ ■ ■ ■ ■ ■ ■ ■ ■ ■ ■ ■ ■ ■ ■ ■ ■ **CHAPTER 10**

S ex that we say yes to and actively participate in can be pure pleasure, allowing us to express desire, playfulness, intimacy, vulnerability, and power. Unfortunately sex can also expose us to the risk of pregnancy and to sexually transmitted infections (STIs). In most cases, STIs can be treated. However, some STIs, if left untreated, can cause serious long-term health consequences, including chronic pain, infertility, cancer, and even death.

How do we enjoy pleasure and also protect our health? How can we explore our sexuality and avoid infection and unwanted pregnancy? Many of us know the basic answers, but in the heat of the moment, most of us have, at some point, failed to use the protection that would be in our best interests. Fortunately, we can help ourselves by better preparing for those moments.

This chapter talks about sex-positive ways to protect yourself and your partner(s) from STIs. Please see Chapter 9, "Birth Control," for ways to prevent unwanted pregnancy. For details on the different types of STIs, along with STI diagnosis and treatment, see Chapter 11, "Sexually Transmitted Infections."

WHY PRACTICE SAFER SEX?

Safer sex refers to steps you can take before and during sexual activity that are known to reduce the risk of STIs. The term "safer sex" is used instead of "safe sex" because sex with a partner is never guaranteed to be 100 percent safe.

Many of us have heard of HIV, the virus that causes AIDS, and other STIs such as gonorrhea, chlamydia, HSV (herpes simplex virus), and HPV (genital human papillomavirus, a leading cause of cervical cancer and genital warts). What we may not know is how common they are. While it's hard to know exact numbers, it is estimated that there are approximately 19 million new STI infections in the United States each year, with about half of the new cases occurring in young people age fifteen to twenty-four.[1] Approximately one in four young women between the ages of fourteen and nineteen in the United States is estimated to be infected with one or more of the most common STIs: HPV, chlamydia, herpes, or trichomoniasis.[2]

More than two dozen bacterial, viral, or parasitic infections are known to be transmitted largely or exclusively through sexual contact. Many people do not know that they are infected because they have never been tested and because most STIs have no noticeable symptoms. Bacterial and parasitic infections are commonly treated with antibiotics or other prescription drugs. There is no cure for viral infections; treatment aims to prevent or reduce symptoms. Having an untreated STI can make you more

SAFER-SEX BASICS

Safer sex refers to sexual practices that can reduce or eliminate exposure to STIs, usually by preventing the exchange of blood, semen, or vaginal fluids. Using condoms consistently and correctly is an essential component of safer sex.

vulnerable to a second STI (including HIV), and it may cause the symptoms of a second infection to be more serious or painful.

Some STIs, such as herpes and HPV, and genital ulcer diseases such as syphilis and chancroid (a bacterial infection characterized by painful sores) can be transmitted from contact with skin that is not covered by a condom. The risk is reduced only when the infected area or site of potential exposure is protected.

THE TALK

Whether you are considering sex with someone new or negotiating sexual choices in a long-term partnership, there are key questions to consider: When and how do you talk with your partner(s) about sexually transmitted infections? Which activities have a lower—or higher—risk of STI transmission? How do you decide which protection is best for you—and then follow through on your decisions?

Thinking about these questions and talking through the answers with your sexual partner(s) are the first steps toward enjoying your sexuality while staying safe. It can be good to know that those conversations can be comfortable—and empowering. One twenty-two-year-old says:

TEN MYTHS ABOUT STIs

1. **You can tell by looking if someone has an STI.** There is no way to know for sure who may have HIV or another STI. Many people don't know themselves that they are infected. Many STIs are silent diseases, meaning that they produce few, if any, symptoms.

2. **Being sexually exclusive with one partner will keep me safe.** A monogamous relationship reduces the risk of infection, so long as neither partner came to the relationship with an existing infection. However, many people enter new relationships not knowing if they are infected with an STI, and people don't always tell the truth about their past or present sexual practices. If you are having sex with only one person but that person has other partners, you can be exposed.

3. **If he pulls out before he comes, I can't get infected.** Pre-cum—drops of fluid that the penis discharges during arousal—can contain HIV, other STIs, or even sperm. It's best to use a condom as soon as the penis is erect.

4. **My birth control will protect me from STIs.** Condoms are the only birth control method that offers dual protection against pregnancy and STIs. The pill, hormonal injections and implants, diaphragms, and the IUD do not protect against STIs.

5. **Lesbians don't get STIs.** All women who engage in certain sexual activities are at risk for STIs, though the risk is less for women who have sex only with other women. Some STIs can be trans-mitted between women by genital-to-genital or oral-to-genital contact that involves the exchange of vaginal fluids or by sharing sex toys, and some can be transmitted by skin-to-skin contact.

6. **I have an STI and we've already had sex, so there's no point using protection.** Practicing safer sex is still essential. Your partner may not yet be infected, and even if you share an STI, you could have different types or strains of the same infection that could make the infection worse for both of you. Or your partner could un-knowingly have a different STI, which could speed up the progression of your current infection. You and your partner can pass an infection back and forth if you're not both treated.

7. **I am too young (or too old) to get an STI.** Girls and women of any age who are having sex can contract an STI. Adolescent girls have the highest risk because their cervix cells don't pro-duce as much protective cervical fluid as, and are more susceptible to infec-tion than, the adult cervix. Tears in the vaginal wall, which are more common in postmenopausal women owing to decreased production of natural lubri-cants, can increase susceptibility to bacteria and infections.

8. **STIs happen to other people, not me. Besides, you can't get an STI the first time you have sex.** Anyone engaging in certain sexual activities with someone who has an STI can contract an STI, whether it's the first time or the hundredth.

9. **My partner and I fool around naked and have oral sex, but we haven't gone all the way, so we're not at risk.** Not having anal or vaginal intercourse decreases your risk of getting an STI, but some infections can be spread by oral sex and by skin-to-skin contact. You can contract HPV, for example, if your partner is infected and you rub your genitals together. Herpes is transmitted by genital or oral contact with a developing or existing sore; the virus can also be spread without symptoms.

10. **We shower before sex so we won't spread infections.** Lather up if you want to, and then cover up. Washing the genitals, anal area, and hands before and after sex, and between anal and vaginal or oral contact, is good hygiene and may cut down on urinary tract infections, but washing does not prevent STI transmission. (Douching, by the way, is never a good idea; it may even push infections higher up in the vagina and affect other reproductive organs, and it alters the vaginal flora, making you susceptible to other infections.) After you wash, don't forget to reach for that condom or dental dam.

In the past, I've mostly had sex with people I've flirted with, hooked up with, or had sex with more than one time—that is to say, I haven't had many one-night stands without any flirting or courtship leading up to sex. In these contexts, I've found it easy to have check-ins about STI status before getting too hot and heavy. I've had friends stop sweaty make-out sessions to check in, and had hookups that seemed to be headed toward sex stay as just making out because of explicitly communicated worries about STIs. These have always been comfortable conversations (in my experience) that are about respecting each other and wanting to have fun, and not about shame or stigma.

As someone who's received good sexual education from a young age, I've always thought of STIs as just part of the picture, if you're ever going to have casual hookups. That is to say, I don't get freaked out by folks who have STIs; I expect people in my community (including potential lovers) to have experiences with them, and the best thing I see to do is to keep myself educated and to continue to have open conversations about how to stay safe.

A thirty-two-year-old woman acknowledges that it took awhile to take charge of protecting herself:

I get tested often and, as far as I know, I have not contracted anything, but it horrifies me that I have left my fate in other people's hands too often. At thirty-two, I finally have the fortitude to demand safe sex and verbal communication about any future partner's sexual history, or I will simply not get involved. It just took a little too long to get here.

Agreeing to use protection can help both of you feel more relaxed and intimate. You may find that you are better able to explore and enjoy sex when you are more confident that you will not get (or give) a sexually transmitted infection—and being assertive about safer sex can help you be more expressive about your sexual desires and preferences.

It's best to talk with your partner(s) about STIs before having any kind of sex. It may be hard to do, but it's an important part of protecting your health and that of your partner(s). If possible, start with a casual conversation when you are not being sexual, or try an icebreaker, like, "What kind of condoms do you like best?" or "Have you ever tried flavored condoms?"

Many people find it helps to talk first with friends or health-care providers about how to introduce the topic and which conversational strategies work best. For some, humor is a great way to help pave the way for more serious discussions. If talking about safer sex is extremely difficult, either because you're uncomfortable or because there are safety concerns, see "It's Not That Easy: Challenges to Protecting Ourselves," p. 269.

Here are some suggested questions to ask each other:

- Has either of us, or any of our other/previous partners, ever had an STI? When? What was it? Did it ever come back?
- Have we or any of our other/previous partners ever been tested for an STI or had an abnormal Pap test?
- Have we both obtained preventive sexual health care, including STI screenings?
- How many sex partners have each of us had in the last six months? Were they male, female, or both? What are we doing or have we done with our other partners to make sex safer?
- Are alcohol and other drugs involved when we have sex?
- What do we each usually do to make sex safer?
- What are we going to do right now to prevent infection?
- If we're finding it difficult to talk about these subjects, what can we do to create an environment where it's okay to talk about STIs?

If you think you or your partner may have an infection, it's best to abstain from sexual contact

SAFER SEX AT ANY AGE

According to the "National Survey of Sexual Health and Behavior" released in 2010, only 25 percent of those age fifty and over who were single, had a new sex partner, or had multiple partners within a year said they had used a condom the last time they had sex. Almost 40 percent had never been tested for HIV.[3] Older women are often not tested for STIs, in part because we are not seen as sexual. It's important to let your health care provider know if you are starting a new relationship, if you have more than one sexual partner, or if you think you should be tested for STIs for any reason. You have the right to request STI testing and should not be required to give your reasons for wanting it, if you prefer not to.

until both of you have been tested and treated—and until you both know the potential risks of sexual contact and how best to protect yourselves. In the meantime, enjoy safer activities, such as massage or mutual masturbation. (For more information on screening, testing, and treating STIs, see Chapter 11, "Sexually Transmitted Infections.")

JUST USE IT

The "just do it" message of popular culture suggests that sex should be completely spontaneous. We rarely see couples on television or in movies discuss sexually transmitted infections or reach for the condoms before the lights go out.

Tip: Keep barriers handy. Many of us have had experience with needing protection only to find it wasn't within reach—in which case we're more inclined to do without. At home, keep protection next to your bed or near where you might have sex. Also keep a few condoms or dental dams in your purse or bag; replace them regularly in case the packaging gets damaged

But in the real world, people every day are talking, planning, and taking precautions to protect each other's health. With knowledge and communication today, we can avoid health problems tomorrow—and that makes sex a lot more fun.

I HAD UNSAFE SEX—WHAT SHOULD I DO?

If you've had unprotected sex with someone and you're not sure about the person's history, you should have an STI check before having sex with anyone else. Most STIs are symptom-free, so testing is necessary to rule out infections. It's also a good idea to talk to your health-care provider about STIs that may not show up right away after exposure and get advice on whether you should be retested later.

Some STIs can be prevented even after exposure. If you have unprotected sex with someone who you either know or think might have HIV or hepatitis A or B, you may be able to get medication from your health-care provider that will prevent the infection from developing. It's important to act immediately, if you need to do this. (For more information, see "Decreasing Risk *After* Exposure," p. 286.)

HOW TO PREPARE FOR (ALMOST) EVERY SEX ACTIVITY

Some sexual activities carry a much greater risk of contracting or transmitting an STI. One way to think about it is to imagine a risk ladder, with the lowest-risk behaviors at the bottom and the highest-risk behaviors at the top. The higher you go on the ladder, the more you need to ensure that you have the appropriate tools to help you stay safe. The following sexual activities are rated by how risky they are when performed without protection.

ACTIVITY-SPECIFIC SAFER-SEX RECOMMENDATIONS

High Risk

Anal Intercourse
This is a high-risk activity for STIs, much more so than vaginal intercourse because the tissue lining the rectum is very fragile and, unlike the vagina, the rectum does not self-lubricate. The rectum's lining tears easily, making it is easy for viruses, bacteria, or other germs to get into the bloodstream. For sufficient protection, your partner should use a male or female latex condom with plenty of lubricant. (Female condoms can be adapted for use in the rectum; see below.) Thicker lubricants are suggested for the safest anal sex.

Massaging the anus with a finger or sex toy, or oral-anal sex play, can be a pleasurable prelude to anal (or other) sex, and it may help relax the muscles so that the condom is less likely to break during penetration.

Vaginal Intercourse
The vaginal lining can easily get tiny tears or abrasions that allow HIV and other infections into the bloodstream. Female or male condoms

TOP TEN SAFER-SEX TIPS

1. **BYOC** (bring your own condom). Don't rely on a partner to have condoms, dams, or lube. Always have your own supply, and check the expiration dates before use.

2. **Role-play safer-sex conversations with friends.** Brainstorming strategies for dealing with difficult responses and practicing what to say can help you to be more comfortable and assertive when the time comes to talk about it for real. The best input and advice may come from people who share your experiences and who truly understand your concerns.

3. **Create basic limits and boundaries around safer sex in advance.** Writing them down can help remind you that they're important and nonnegotiable.

4. **Avoid getting so drunk or high** that your judgment may fail you.

5. **Make safer sex part of sex,** rather than something that interrupts sex. For example, put on male or female condoms together.

6. **Don't rush into higher-risk activities.** First take your time with low- or no-risk activities, which can help build trust and communication (and also feel really good).

7. **If you have a history of sexual or other abuse** and feel this interferes with your ability to be safe, seek the help of a therapist, counselor, or support group to assist you in your healing and to help you select partners and sexual settings that make you feel comfortable.

8. **Choose partners who don't put all the responsibility for safer sex on you.** Look for partners who are comfortable putting safety discussions on the table.

9. **Work toward being able to talk more candidly about sex and sexual health with friends and partners.** It's easier to be safe when you don't feel ashamed.

10. **Don't feel bad about yourself if you find this difficult.** Many of us were taught that talking about sex isn't "romantic" or that "nice girls don't." But we can, and we do—and it gets easier with practice.

---

offer the best protection. Use a lubricated latex, nitrile, polyisoprene, or polyurethane condom (not lambskin) with added condom-safe lubricant, if desired. No other method of protection has been conclusively proved to prevent STI transmission (including HIV). (For specific tips on proper condom use and lubricants, see "Condoms 101," p. 266.)

Medium Risk

Oral Sex on a Man

While this is not as risky as vaginal or anal sex, it still carries a risk of transmitting or contracting STIs, especially if you have just had dental work or have open cuts in your mouth. And if you have oral herpes (HSV-1), you can transmit it through unprotected oral sex. For maximum protection, use a condom as soon as the penis is

KNOW YOUR RISK

SEXUAL ACTIVITY (FROM MOST RISKY TO LEAST RISKY)	TOOLS FOR SAFER SEX
High Risk	
Being on the receiving end of anal intercourse	Male or female condom, lubricant
Vaginal intercourse	Male or female condom, lubricant
Medium Risk	
Oral sex on a man	Male condom, lubricant
Oral sex on a woman	Dental dam or other barrier, lubricant
Rimming (licking your partner's anus)	Female condom, dental dam, or plastic wrap
Lower Risk	
Dildos, sex toys	Soap and water, condoms
Deep manual sex (sometimes called fisting) and finger play	Soap and water, latex gloves
Water sports (sex partners urinate on each other)	Soap and water

erect, before any oral contact, since the pre-cum (drops of fluid that the penis discharges during arousal) can contain HIV. Use a new condom each time. If licking plain latex doesn't do it for you, try using a flavored condom.

Oral Sex on a Woman

This carries some risk, especially if the woman has her period or any open sores, like genital shaving cuts. And if you have oral herpes (HSV-1), you can transmit it through unprotected oral sex. For maximum protection, cover your partner's vulva and/or anus with a barrier, such as a dental dam, a cut-open latex glove or condom, or a female condom.

Rimming

Licking your partner's anus carries some risk of STI transmission. For protection, use a female condom inserted rectally or a dental dam.

Low Risk

Dildos, Sex Toys, and Vibrators

Shared toys can transmit some STIs from one partner to another. Wash all toys thoroughly in hot soapy water between use. For extra protection, you can clean a sex toy with 10 percent hydrogen peroxide, or soak it for twenty minutes in a 10 percent bleach solution (one part household bleach, nine parts water). Make sure to rinse all toys with water after cleaning with chemicals. If you're sharing a dildo with a partner or partners and washing is not an option, use a condom on the dildo.

Deep Manual Sex and Finger Play

Deep manual sex (putting a hand or several fingers into the rectum or vagina) is low risk for the person doing the inserting, although it is possible to get an STI if you have sores, cuts, or cracks on your hands or fingers. Deep manual sex carries some risk for the person on the re-

Take extra precautions during sexual activities that may involve blood, which is a very effective transmitter of some STIs. For people with HIV, for example, the highest concentration of HIV is usually found in the blood, with less in the semen and still less in the vaginal secretions. Direct contact with even small amounts of blood, including menstrual blood, can transmit infections, including HIV or infectious hepatitis B and C.

If engaging in bondage or S/M (sadomasochism), negotiate first with your sex partner(s) to limit the chances of blood, semen, or vaginal fluids entering the vagina or coming into contact with irritated or cut skin. If an abrasion or cut does happen, clean it well with running water, cover it with a bandage, and keep it away from body fluids. Clean any S/M gear after use.

ceiving end, because the internal tissue can be easily bruised or worn away. While this may not by itself cause STI transmission, it could put you or your partner at risk of infection if you have unprotected intercourse before healing has occurred. Finger play (playing with the vagina or labia or touching your partner's anus) is less risky.

For protection for deep manual sex, consider using latex gloves. For finger play, you can use finger cots, which cover only a single finger. Change them with each use.

Water Sports
This term refers to sex partners urinating on each other. This is relatively low risk, as long as there is no blood in or mixed with the urine. Men's urine carries a slightly higher risk because urine comes through the same channel—the urethra—as semen, and might pick up a virus or trace bacteria as it leaves the body. Protect your eyes, and avoid any broken skin or cuts. Urine itself is sterile.

Other Less-Risky Activities
Kissing, hugging, massages, hand jobs, and mutual masturbation are all low risk.

Avoid getting your partner's semen or vaginal fluids on your skin if you have small cuts or sores. Also avoid getting semen in your eye during sex play, as STIs can be transmitted this way.

BARRIERS THAT WORK

Male condoms, used on the penis during vaginal and anal intercourse and oral sex, are the most accessible and best-known barrier protection. When used consistently and correctly, male condoms are highly effective in preventing STIs. Most male condoms are made of latex. People with latex allergies can also get good protection from nitrile, polyurethane, and polyisoprene male condoms. Lambskin condoms do *not* provide STI protection. Using a lubricant with a condom can help prevent condom breaks and also prevent tears or abrasions in the vagina.

Female condoms, which are designed to be inserted into a woman's vagina, can also be used for protection. While most women use these vaginally, some also prefer them to male condoms for protection during anal sex. The only female condom currently approved for sale in the United States is the FC2. It can be used for vaginal and anal sex, and for oral sex on a woman. While the research on female condoms is not as extensive as that on male condoms, consistent and correct use of the female

FLUID BONDING

Fluid bonding means sharing body fluids with only one person, and using protection with all others. This reduces risk, though only if you have both been tested beforehand for the full range of STIs. Fluid bonding requires that both partners use protection consistently with other partners and never have unprotected sex with anyone else, not even "just this once." Exposure to several partners, either your own or your partner's partners, increases your chances of getting an STI.

I started having safe(r) sex with everyone but my primary partner about a year and a half ago, and my concerns about STIs changed with that new context. Now I'm obligated to keep not only myself but also my partner STI-free, and I take that very seriously. It has to do with the practicality of being fluid bonded and both STI-free, and also with this pact that we made that's got to do with keeping our relationship primary. Now I don't feel like I can push boundaries at all when it comes to safe sex.

condom appears to provide a level of protection against STIs, including HIV infection, similar to the male condom.[4]

Both male and female condoms offer protection against HIV, gonorrhea, and chlamydia, which are spread through body fluids. Condoms also offer some protection against infections like herpes simplex virus (HSV) and human papillomavirus (HPV) that are spread through skin-to-skin contact. But these infections can still be transmitted by sores or warts that may not be visible and by contact with parts of the genitals not covered by the condom. Because the female condom covers more surface area, it may potentially offer more protection against HPV and herpes than male condoms.

You can get female condoms at some retail drugstores (including CVS and Walgreens), HIV/AIDS outreach clinics, family-planning clinics, and sex shops, and on some college campuses. You can also buy them online, including at Amazon.com. A pack of five condoms costs about $12. If you've used female condoms in the past and found that they were too noisy, you might want to give them another try—they have recently been redesigned, and the material now used is nitrile, which is soft and quiet.

Other barrier methods can be used for mouth-to-vagina or mouth-to-anus contact, or to protect infected areas not covered by a condom. Squares of latex (dams) are available online, in some drugstores, at Planned Parenthood centers, and at sex shops. (For more information, see "Dental Dams and Do-It-Yourself Barriers" below.)

CONDOMS 101

The following guidelines provide basic information on male and female condom and lubricant use for safer sex. (For more information on condom use for birth control, see Chapter 9, "Birth Control.")

- Store condoms in a cool, dry place. Do not use a condom if the packaging is torn or damaged.
- Avoid using a condom that's been in a pocket or the bottom of a purse for a long time, or in a glove compartment or vending machine, where it may have been compromised by heat or otherwise damaged. Never use condoms that are brittle, sticky, or an unusual color.

DENTAL DAMS AND DO-IT-YOURSELF BARRIERS

If you're engaging in mouth-to-vagina or mouth-to-anus contact, you can protect yourself and your partner by using a barrier such as a dental dam. These rubber sheets, also used by dentists, tend to be small and thick, although some sex boutiques carry ones that are larger, thinner, and flavored. A special kind of dam, Sheer Glyde, has been approved by the FDA specifically for safer sex.

Female condoms can also be used for oral sex on a woman. Once the female condom is inserted in the woman's vagina, gently pull the outer ring forward and use the condom as a barrier between your mouth and your partner's vagina and anus. Many women like this because it is already lubricated. You don't need to hold the female condom in place with your hands once it is in, and the ring can also be moved over the clitoris to increase your partner's pleasure.

The following do-it-yourself (or DIY) techniques may have some merit in extreme circumstances. However, there is no guarantee of quality control when you make or use these and you may be increasing the risk of barrier failure.

- You can adapt a male condom to use as a barrier by vertically cutting it with scissors.
- You can also turn a latex glove into a barrier: First, wash out the powder, then cut off the four fingers, and slit it up the side, leaving the thumb intact. Try lubricating the side that touches your partner. Be sure to keep the same side against her vulva, and keep track of which side is which so you don't touch the body fluids you are trying to avoid.

Remember that male and female condoms, dams, and other barriers don't protect you from getting infected in places they don't cover.

- Check the expiration date on each condom before you use it. Generally, condoms without spermicide are good for up to five years; condoms with spermicide last about two years. If you are not sure how old a condom is, throw it away and use a new one.
- Put the condom (male or female) on before any genital, oral, or anal contact occurs. The male condom has to be on the penis when it's erect and before it touches your body, especially the vulva, mouth, or anus. Likewise for a female condom; insert it before any skin-to-skin contact occurs.
- Use a new condom each time you have sex.

Have more than one with you in case you have sex again or if a condom is damaged. If you are having both anal and vaginal intercourse, put on a new condom after anal intercourse and before beginning vaginal intercourse. Or try what this woman suggests and insert female condoms in both the anus and the vagina.

They can be lubed well (inside and out), then inserted—one into the anus and a second one into the vagina. When this is done, the male or other insertive partner can go back and forth freely from anus to vagina as the couple's energies desire without fear of infection.

If you or a partner experiences irritation with latex male condoms, don't despair! The irritation may be due to spermicide (chemicals that kill sperm) on the condom, so try a brand without spermicide. If you experience itching, a rash, or dryness, you might be sensitive to latex. Try using a polyurethane, polyisoprene, or nitrile condom. Sometimes vaginal irritation with condoms can be due to attempting intercourse too soon, before you're aroused enough and the vagina is lubricated.

LUBRICANTS

Lubricants help to prevent condom breaks and also prevent tears or abrasions in the vagina or rectum. They can also make sex more pleasurable for you and your partner. Use only water-soluble lubricants, not oil-based ones, with latex condoms. Oil-based products include Vaseline, baby oil, suntan lotion, massage oils, and some hand creams. These can damage a latex condom within minutes and destroy its protection.

Oil-based lubricants, however, have no effect on nitrile or polyurethane condoms. If you prefer oil-based lubricants, make sure that the condom you are using is made of polyurethane, polyisoprene, or nitrile.

Lubricants can be applied directly to the clitoris, labia, or anus, or inside the vagina. Putting a tiny amount in the tip of a male condom

The birth control chapter has more information on condom use. For detailed instructions on how to use a male condom, see p. 213. For instructions on how to use a female condom, see p. 216.

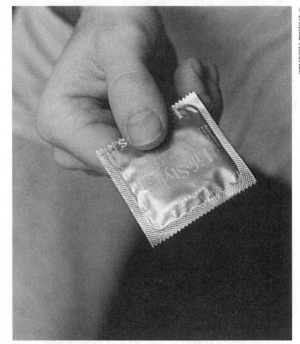

© Donna Alberico

may give the man extra pleasure—which could be a plus in persuading him to use condoms. Be careful to use only a tiny drop, and only in the tip, not the sides, so the condom won't get loose and slip off.

You can use prelubricated male condoms. However, avoid using condoms prelubricated with spermicide, as the main ingredient, Nonoxynol-9 (N-9), can cause vaginal and rectal irritation and increase STI risk. (For more information, see "Safety of Nonoxynol-9 When Used for Contraception," p. 223.) Many condoms are available without added N-9; visit your local pharmacy to find a brand that works for you.

For more information on lubricants, see "Lubrication," p. 177.

IT'S NOT THAT EASY: CHALLENGES TO PROTECTING OURSELVES

Female and male condoms, gloves, and dental dams are known to stop the transmission of STIs, including HIV. Yet many of us don't protect ourselves consistently or effectively. Why?

OUR OWN ATTITUDES

Who, me? . . . I'm not a gay man or an addict . . . I'm too young . . . I can tell who's infected . . . I love him so much—he'd never do anything to hurt me . . . If I bring a condom, he'll think I'm a slut . . . I'm a lesbian, why do I need protection? . . . I'm afraid he'll refuse . . . She's too important to risk losing . . . I can't carry condoms around—my mother would find them . . . He knows I need the drugs, so I can't make trouble . . . I'm not worth protecting . . . He'll get mad . . . Talking about sex is too embarrassing . . . I just can't deal . . .

Many of us have had at least one of these thoughts or conversations in our heads or with friends. Even when we know what's right, it can be incredibly difficult to follow through. It's all too easy to forget that our health—and our partners' health—is *our* responsibility.

A woman who works in HIV prevention says:

It can be particularly awkward when you are in love and don't want to do anything to upset your partner or to imply that you can't trust each other. When love comes into the relationship, condoms often go out the window.

Another woman says it is one thing to talk about being responsible—and much harder to take action in the moment.

It is hard to imagine murmuring into someone's ear at a time of passion, "Would you mind slipping on this condom just in case one of us has an STI?" Yet it seems awkward to bring it up any sooner if it's not clear between us that we want to make love.

Or, to put it more directly:

A condom seems to pour cold water on the romance by saying, "Okay, to be brutally honest, we've both slept with other people." The condom seems like a statement of distrust: "You could give me a disease; you could kill me."

Sometimes, you might be the one resisting safer sex—maybe because you think that a partner will like you more if you agree to sex without condoms. Some of us may feel that using barriers implies we are untrustworthy or "dirty," or that if we suggest using a barrier, a partner may make those kinds of assumptions about us. Others feel that condoms reduce intimacy or closeness.

If you are the resistant partner, check in with yourself and balance what you know about risks to your health or that of a partner with attitudes that discourage using protection.

OVERCOMING OBSTACLES

Other factors may make it more difficult to acquire and consistently use protection.

- **Drug and alcohol use.** Even with the best of intentions, intoxication can compromise judgment and weaken resolve to use protection. If a sex partner is also under the influence of drugs or alcohol, practicing safer sex becomes even less likely.
- **Lack of information.** Unprotected sex is more common when information about STIs and pregnancy risk is not available. You can

obtain solid information from health-care providers at family-planning clinics such as Planned Parenthood. Other sex-positive and comprehensive sources of information can be found in Recommended Resources.

- **Cost and access:** These remain formidable obstacles for many women. Call a health clinic or Planned Parenthood and explain that you'd like to discuss safer-sex options but your resources are limited. Many clinics offer safer-sex supplies free. At the very least, you can almost always get condoms from clinics just by walking in the door, without even having to register as a patient.

WHEN A PARTNER RESISTS SAFER SEX

Look, I know how to protect myself. But it's just not that easy. When I hand him a condom, he says, "What's the matter, baby? Don't you trust me?" What am I supposed to say to that?

For many of us, a partner's resistance to safer sex may be the most challenging obstacle we face.

Some people feel that sex isn't as good with barriers, or that barriers reduce intimacy.

Some men are afraid they won't stay hard with a condom on, even though the base of

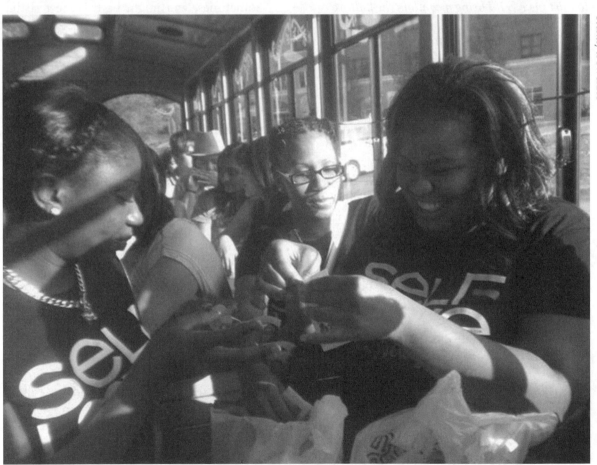

Courtesy of YWCHAC

Young Women of Color HIV/AIDS Coalition prepare to pass out condoms.

male condoms usually helps maintain an erection. Partners who are used to being in charge sexually may resent it when women initiate safer sex. Many sex workers' clients refuse to pay for protected sex, or they pay more for sex without condoms. A lesbian may believe there's no HIV or other STI risk for lesbians. Suggest using protection, and your partners may feel that you're accusing them of sleeping around or of using drugs.

Negotiating safer sex can be especially difficult in abusive or controlling relationships. Talking about safer sex is more risky for some of us; even if we understand that we need to speak up in order to protect our lives and health, it may be almost impossible, or even dangerous, to do so. The choice may be between unsafe sex or violence, abandonment, or homelessness. If your partner reacts to your request to practice safer sex with threats or with physical or emotional violence, see Chapter 24, "Violence Against Women."

Being honest and direct with our sex partners is an excellent goal. But the *most* important thing in the short term is to reduce your risk of pregnancy or of contracting HIV or another STI. If you are not yet at the point where you can insist on safer sex (and your partner is male), here are a few things women have tried.

- With a new partner, say that you always use condoms because they are your preferred method of birth control.
- Say that you are about to get your period—or that you think you may have a minor infection—and want to use something so your partner isn't exposed. Even though it doesn't feel good to make up reasons, it may still be safer than not using anything for protection.
- If you use a female condom, point out that it's your body, your female condom, and your choice to protect your health and the health of your partner.

For more ideas about how to respond if you ever feel pressured to have sex without a condom, visit the American Social Health Association's page on negotiating condom use at ashastd.org/condom/condom_negotiation.cfm.

EMPOWERING OUR SCHOOLS AND COMMUNITIES

Conservative religious groups and political organizations in some parts of the United States have spent considerable energy blocking comprehensive health education in schools and advocating for abstinence-only sex education. Studies have shown that abstinence-only programs are not effective in preventing STIs. A large study of adolescents who pledged to abstain from sex until marriage, for example, found their rates of STI transmission to be similar to those of non-pledgers. The study indicated that even though pledge takers initiated sex later, they were less likely to seek STI testing and less likely to use condoms when they did have sex.[5] Many states also experienced a rise in teenage pregnancy after putting in place abstinence-only curricula and later began to reconsider the approach. For more information on state and federal policies aimed at preventing STIs and teen pregnancies see "Politicizing Reproductive Health," p. 765.)

STI education programs work—if they are supported. School education programs that make condoms available report fewer students having intercourse and a higher level of safer-sex practices among students who are having sex.[6] And studies show that accurate sex information and vaccination against STIs, such as hepatitis B or HPV, do not increase sexual activity among young adults.[7]

We urgently need to keep developing and providing culturally relevant education, prevention, and treatment for everyone, especially young and low-income women who are at high-

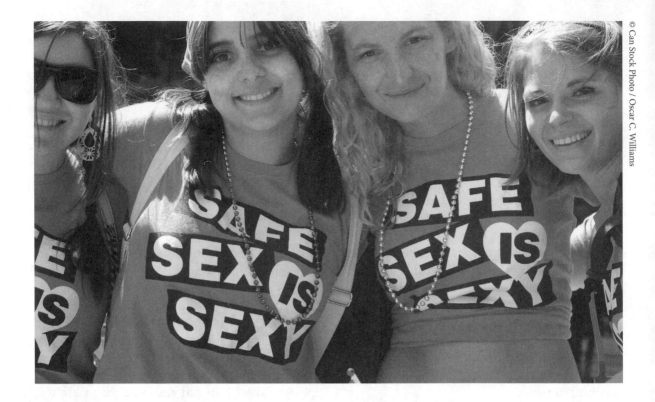

est risk. It's imperative for safer-sex education programs to engage the people they serve in designing and implementing programs. Attitudes about sex are shaped in part by community, economic status, and life experiences. Factual knowledge is essential, but cultural awareness is also necessary in discussing potentially successful strategies for negotiating safer sex.

A Latina from Chicago writes that in lower-income communities in particular, "Sexuality is one area over which men still feel like they have some control in their lives. If the women bring home the safer-sex message, we may become lightning rods for the frustration and anger the men feel as a result of racism, unemployment, and poverty. The educational strategy has to be developed by the community itself."

What works best? The nonprofit organization Advocates for Youth lists the following characteristics of effective sex education, based in part on research by Douglas Kirby and Sue Alford.[8] These are helpful starting points for any group or organization.

- Offer age- and culturally appropriate sexual health information in a safe environment for participants.
- Cooperate with members of the target community, especially young people.
- Assist young people to clarify their individual, family, and community values.
- Assist young people to develop skills in communication, refusal, and negotiation.
- Provide medically accurate information about both abstinence and contraception, including condoms.
- Have clear goals for preventing HIV, other STIs, and/or teen pregnancy.

THE NYC CONDOM AVAILABILITY PROGRAM

In 1971, the New York City Department of Health started distributing free male condoms in the city's STI clinics. In the 1980s, the onset of HIV/AIDS led to the expansion of free male condom distribution to HIV/AIDS service organizations and organizations serving injecting drug users. In 2005, the Health Department launched a condom-ordering website for easier access and bulk orders. Average monthly condom distribution then rose from 250,000 to 1.5 million.

The primary goal of the NYC Condom Availability Program is to increase consistent male and female condom use to reduce HIV, STIs, and unintended pregnancies in New York City. The program makes condoms more widely available, generates conversation and community buy-in around safer sex through participation in community events, and provides valuable education and training regarding safer-sex practices. The program strives not only to increase correct and consistent condom use throughout the city, but also to normalize condom use and accessibility.

On Valentine's Day, 2007, the agency set a national precedent with its NYC Condom campaign, in which a standard, premium lubricated LifeStyles condom was packaged in a chic, Gotham-inspired NYC-branded wrapper. The NYC Condom provides New Yorkers with a uniquely cosmopolitan condom while increasing condom use and awareness. In 2009, the NYC Condom Availability Program distributed more than 41.5 million condoms, and the NYC Condom can now be found at over three thousand locations around the city. Free female condom distribution began in 1998 and nearly 1 million free female condoms were also distributed in 2009. For more information on NYC Condoms, go to nyc.gov/condoms.

- Focus on specific health behaviors related to the goals, with clear messages about these behaviors.
- Address psychosocial risk and protective factors with activities to change each targeted risk and to promote each protective factor.
- Respect community values and respond to community needs.
- Rely on participatory teaching methods, implemented by trained educators and using all the activities as designed.

CHAPTER 11 ■ ■ ■ ■ ■ ■ ■ ■ ■ ■ ■ ■ ■ ■ ■

Every woman has a right to enjoy her sexuality without fear of disease. That means we need to know how to protect ourselves from sexually transmitted infections (STIs), how to find treatment if we get one, and how to avoid spreading an infection without giving up our sex lives.

Sexually transmitted infections range from a temporary bother to life-threatening. If left untreated, some can cause infertility or chronic pelvic pain, or be transmitted during pregnancy or birth to a fetus or newborn baby. Having an STI can make a person more susceptible to other infections, including HIV, the virus that causes AIDS.

You can catch some STIs just by touching or kissing an infected area. But the biggest risk for women is from vaginal or anal intercourse without a condom. You can also catch some infections, like HIV, by sharing needles during drug use.

While it's in our interest to use protection during sexual activity, to get screened for STIs as needed, and to pursue necessary treatments, we don't always know how to do this or make the right decisions or follow the best practices. Most STIs have no visible symptoms, so we are often not aware that we or our sexual partners are infected. And because of lingering negative social attitudes toward sex, even the idea of having a sexually transmitted infection can bring up embarrassment, shame, anger, and fear. The social stigma attached to STIs (how others think about someone with an STI) can make it difficult to use protection or to seek needed care or resources:

My husband told me he'd slept with someone else and might have gotten an STI. I didn't know what to do. . . . I saw an ad yesterday for an STI hotline, and after a lot of hesitation, I called. It was a relief to get information without anyone knowing who I was.

If one person in a supposedly monogamous couple gets an STI, it may be from sexual contact outside the relationship, either recently or in the past. Some infections can be present without symptoms for years and have been acquired before the current relationship. It can help to remember that STIs are a health problem—like any other health problem—and not a sign of wrongdoing.

I was diagnosed six years ago, and then found out my boyfriend at the time had been cheating on me. . . . I was hurt, embarrassed, felt unlovable, disappointed, and angry at myself because I knew I should have been using protection all of the time especially since I knew he had a history of being unfaithful in past relationships. Six years later,

I see my diagnosis as a hidden gift . . . strange, huh? But it forces me to have conversations [with potential partners] about sexual history, my chosen form of protection which is condoms, and [about] readiness to have sex or not.

WHAT ARE STIs?

Sexually transmitted infections (STIs)—also called sexually transmitted diseases (STDs)—are a variety of mostly bacterial and viral infections (diseases) that are passed from one person to another primarily through anal, vaginal, or oral sex.

STIs are among the most commonly reported diseases in the United States today. The most recent national estimates suggest that there are approximately 19 million new cases of

Recommended Reading: For the latest STI information, including screening and treatment guidelines, visit these sites:

- American Social Health Association (ASHA): ashastd.org
- Centers for Disease Control and Prevention National Prevention Information Network: cdcnpin.org/std/

For teens and young people:
- Go Ask Alice!: goaskalice.columbia.edu
- I Wanna Know: iwannaknow.org (ASHA's teen/parent site)
- Scarleteen: scarleteen.com
- Sex, Etc.: sexetc.org
- Teen Clinic: teenclinic.org
- Sexuality and U: sexualityandu.ca/teens/teens

STIs each year, half of them among fifteen- to twenty-four-year-olds.[1] Approximately one in four young women between the ages of fourteen and nineteen in the United States is infected with one or more of the most common STIs.[2]

The STIs most common in the United States are human papillomavirus (HPV), genital herpes, trichomoniasis, chlamydia, gonorrhea, syphilis, hepatitis B, and human immunodeficiency virus (HIV)—the virus that causes AIDS. All of these STIs are covered in detail in this chapter. Other infections that can be transmitted via several different routes, including sex—such as hepatitis A and C, cytomegalovirus (CMV), and molluscum contagiosum—are not addressed here. If you have sexual contact outside the United States or with someone who is from another country and are being checked or tested for STIs, tell your health-care provider.

HOW ARE STIs TRANSMITTED?

STIs can be spread through semen, vaginal fluids, and anal secretions, and through discharge from sores or lesions caused by STIs. HIV and hepatitis B can also be spread by contact with the blood of an infected person. Herpes and HPV are usually spread through skin-to-skin contact with the affected area.

The risk of transmission is greatest during anal and vaginal intercourse, but STIs also can be transmitted by oral sex and, less commonly, by unwashed sex toys. Most STIs can be transmitted from one person to another even when there are no obvious signs of infection, and even several years after a person was infected.

HOW CAN I PROTECT MYSELF FROM STIs?

The only 100 percent sure way to protect against STIs is to abstain from having sex. But you can be sexually active and still greatly reduce your chances of getting an STI. Your risk of infection depends on whether your partner has an STI, what kind of sexual contact you have, and whether you use protection.

Statistically, people who have more than one sex partner are more likely to get an STI. People who have one partner at a time generally have less risk than people who have multiple partners. If you have only one partner, however, you may still be at high risk if your partner has other partners in addition to you.

You can reduce your risk of getting an STI by getting vaccinated against HPV and hepatitis B (see "Vaccinations to Prevent STIs" below) and by following safer sex practices—practices that prevent the exchange of blood, semen, or vaginal fluids. Using condoms consistently and correctly is an essential component of safer sex. (For a thorough discussion of prevention and protection methods, see Chapter 10, "Safer Sex.")

WHAT ARE THE SYMPTOMS OF STIs?

The most common symptom is having no noticeable symptoms and not knowing you have an STI—which is why prevention and screening

VACCINATIONS TO PREVENT STIs

Vaccinations are available to protect against the types of the human papillomavirus (HPV) most likely to cause significant disease and against hepatitis B.

- **HPV.** Two vaccines (brand names Cervarix and Gardasil) protect against the types of HPV that cause most cervical cancers. Gardasil also protects against the types of HPV that cause a majority of genital warts. These vaccines are given in three shots, and it is important to get all three doses to get the complete protection. The vaccines work best for young people who are not yet sexually active and have not been exposed to HPV. Some clinicians also recommend the vaccine for young women under twenty-six, even if sexual activity has already occurred, but others do not, because the vaccine's benefit declines with time since first sexual intercourse. HPV vaccination does not prevent acquiring all HPV types so it is important to continue to get regular Pap tests. (For more information, see "HPV Vaccines," p. 616.)

- **Hepatitis B.** In the United States, most hepatitis B is acquired sexually. The hepatitis B vaccine is recommended for all infants, starting at birth, and children and adolescents younger than nineteen who have not been vaccinated. It's also recommended for adults who have not already been immunized, especially for people whose sex partners have hepatitis B; sexually active adults who are not in a long-term, mutually monogamous relationship; people who share needles, syringes, or other drug-injection equipment; people who have close household contact with someone infected with the virus; and those who work in situations that may put them at risk of hep B exposure. The vaccine is usually given as three or four shots over six months to a year.

Both the HPV and the hepatitis B vaccines can be costly,* especially since they both require multiple shots. Most private health insurance plans cover some or all of this cost. If you are eighteen or under, the National Vaccine for Children (VFC) program will provide this and other vaccines free. If you are over eighteen and don't have insurance or your insurance doesn't cover the vaccinations, check with a local public health department, which may have an immunization branch that provides free or low-cost vaccines. Additionally, Merck, the company that makes Gardasil, has a patient assistance program that may cover the cost of your HPV vaccine. For more information, go to merck.com/merckhelps/vaccines/home.html.

* HPV, 3 shots, $275; hep B, $75-$165.

are important for everyone who is sexually active. Most women with chlamydia or gonorrhea infections don't realize that there is anything wrong unless they are tested or infected partners notify them of exposure.

Some untreated STIs may lead to pelvic inflammatory disease (PID). Painful symptoms can include abdominal pain and fever, at which point the fallopian tubes may be blocked and fertility already permanently damaged. The CDC estimates that untreated STIs cause at least 24,000 women to become infertile each year in the United States.[3]

If STI symptoms occur at all, they can include

- Itching, discharge.
- Unusual smell from the vagina or anus. Take note when the color or smell of your vaginal fluids changes.
- Growths, bumps, blisters, sores, or rashes, often around the genitals or anal area.
- Sharp pain in the lower abdomen.
- Pain or burning while urinating or having sex.
- Bleeding between menstrual cycles.

If you have any of these symptoms, abstain from sex and consult a health-care provider immediately. It might be something other than an STI, but it's still good to get it looked at. Even a garden-variety yeast infection, causing vaginitis, can irritate the lining of the vagina and make you more vulnerable to getting a STI. Get yourself checked and treated.

A few infections may appear as more general symptoms, although these may be transient. People infected with HIV, for example, may experience a set of flulike symptoms such as high fever, sore throat, swollen glands, extreme fatigue, and rash within the first month after becoming infected.

The cancer-causing types of HPV have no noticeable symptoms and are detected only when abnormal cervical cells appear on a Pap test.

CHLAMYDIA AND UNDERSCREENING

Chlamydia is the most commonly reported infectious disease in the United States; more than 1.2 million cases were reported by clinicians and clinical laboratories to the Centers for Disease Control in 2009.[4] But CDC research also indicates that chlamydia—which is fully and easily treatable but can cause chronic pelvic pain and infertility if left untreated—is often undiagnosed; over 2.8 million new cases, more than double the number of reported cases, are estimated to occur each year. The CDC recommends that all women twenty-five and younger who are sexually active be tested for chlamydia at least once a year but estimates that only about 47 percent of young women are actually tested.[5]

For more information on possible symptoms for specific STIs, see "Bacteria- and Parasite-Caused STIs," p. 289, and "Viral STIs," p. 294.

ARE STIs CURABLE?

STIs that are caused by bacteria, protozoa, and other small organisms—such as chlamydia, gonorrhea, syphilis, and trichomoniasis—can be cured with medication. However, curable in this case means that the progression of the infection can be stopped and the organism eliminated; any long-term damage already done to your body, including damage to your fertility, can't be reversed. This is why STIs should be detected and treated as soon as possible.

Genital-area infestations caused by skin parasites such as crabs (lice) and scabies (mites) cause itching and rash and can be passed along through sexual or nonsexual contact (towels, sheets, clothes). Parasites can be cured by using medicated creams and lotions.

Viral STIs—such as genital herpes, some HPV strains, HIV, and hepatitis A, B, and C—can be treated to relieve symptoms or slow infection progression, but medicine will not cure (or eliminate) the infection. Each of these viruses behaves differently. (For information on how to treat specific viruses, see "Viral STIs," p. 294.)

WHAT IS THE CONNECTION BETWEEN HIV AND OTHER STIs?

Any STI can alter healthy tissue and increase vulnerability to other STIs, including HIV. Why does this happen? STIs may cause skin cracks, sores, inflammation, or lesions on the vulva or in the vagina, making it easier for HIV to get into the bloodstream. Also, HIV targets white blood cells, which fight infection. When you have an STI, your body sends more white blood cells into the genital area to deal with it. Unfortunately, this means more target cells for HIV to infect, and this raises the risk of HIV taking hold in the body after exposure.[6]

WHEN SHOULD I GET SCREENED OR TESTED?

Since most STIs have no apparent symptoms, it's a good idea to get screened before you have sex with someone new, if you have more than one partner, or if you think or know your partner has had sex with someone else. (For information on specific STI screening guidelines, see "Screening," p. 284.)

If you think you or your partner(s) has been

TEENS AND TESTING

In all fifty states and the District of Columbia, adolescents can seek testing and medical care for STIs without parental consent or knowledge. In addition, adolescents can consent to HIV counseling and testing in most states. Consent laws for vaccinations differ by state.

STI testing may be provided confidentially, but if the test or treatment is billed to an insurance company, the policy holder (who may be a parent) will be informed of the charges via the explanation of benefits. Therefore, it is crucial that you discuss costs and billing in advance to prevent unwelcome disclosures. Some clinics provide low-cost or free services. (For more information, see "Where to Go for Care," p. 285.)

exposed to an infection, go for testing and possible treatment right away, and encourage your partner(s) to do the same. Remember, you might have an STI and not have any noticeable symptoms. (See "Where to Go for Care," p. 285.)

HOW COMMON ARE STIs?

Most STIs disproportionately affect women, especially young women. Nearly half of all new STI cases occur in people age fifteen to twenty-four,[7] though this age group accounts for only one-quarter of the sexually active population. Adolescents and young adults are at greater risk because they are more likely to have unprotected intercourse and to have short, consecutive relationships, are biologically more susceptible to infection, and face obstacles to getting sexual and reproductive health care.

The reported rates of chlamydia and gonorrhea, for example, are highest among females fifteen to nineteen years old,[8] and many people acquire HPV infection during their adolescent years.

Racial and ethnic minorities face different rates of risk, with African Americans being the most severely affected by STIs. They represent 12 percent of the U.S. population but in 2008–2009 accounted for about 71 percent of reported gonorrhea cases and approximately half of all chlamydia and syphilis cases—48 percent and 52 percent, respectively, according to the CDC's "Sexually Transmitted Disease Surveillance" report, which tracks reported cases of chlamydia, gonorrhea, and syphilis.

The risk is greatest for those living in poor urban communities, where the number of people with STIs is statistically larger. Economic status, racial segregation, disparities in incarceration rates, and limited access to affordable and quality health care are some of the factors that contribute to increased STI rates.[9] (For more information, see "Who Gets Infected?" p. 282.)

BIOLOGICAL FACTORS

In general, women are more at risk than men to contract STIs through heterosexual intercourse, simply by design. Any secretions are in contact with the relatively large surface area of the vaginal walls longer then they are in contact with a penis. Furthermore, the vagina is a warm, moist environment, making it an ideal place for viruses, bacteria, and protozoa to multiply.

Adolescent girls have the highest risk because their cervix cells don't produce as much protective cervical fluid as, and are more susceptible to infection than, the adult cervix.

Infections are possible at any age, however, and women who are no longer menstruating may also be at increased risk. In menopause, the vaginal lining gets thinner and often somewhat drier due to decreased production of natural lubricants. Older women can get small breaks in the skin during vaginal intercourse or other penetrative sex, making them vulnerable to sexually transmitted infections. Many health-care providers wrongly assume that older women don't have or don't want sex anymore and are much less likely to give older women STI prevention messages and screening tests. If you are dating again after a long-standing relationship has ended, tell your health care provider about your new sex partner(s).

Regardless of age, try to find a well-informed health-care provider with whom you can talk freely about your sexual health before you have any problems.

RISK FOR WOMEN WHO HAVE SEX WITH WOMEN

If you have sex exclusively with other women, your chance of getting an STI is lower than that of women who have sex with men. However, women in same-sex relationships can be exposed to and transmit STIs, including HPV, HIV, herpes, and—less likely—chlamydia. The CDC reports that limited data are available on the risk of STIs for women who have sex with women, but risk varies depending on the STI and sexual practice (oral-genital sex; sex involving rubbing genital skin together; vaginal or anal sex using hands, fingers, or penetrative sex toys; and oral-anal sex).[10]

Many women involved with women either have had or will have sex with men, or may have been raped or have engaged in risky behavior, such as sharing needles or sharing sex toys with partners whose STI status is unknown. Defining risk only in terms of sexual identity can be deceptive; our risk for STI depends on what we do sexually, not how we identify ourselves.

For lesbians, coming out to a health care provider may be difficult. It is important in order to make sure appropriate information, tests, and treatment are given for STI symptoms. However, even when you explain your sexual orientation, some providers may still have difficulty fully understanding the needs of women who have sex with women:

Recently, I met with a new gynecologist, and I told her I was sexually active with women. . . . Later, during the exam, she said we wouldn't need to bother with tests for STIs. I was really surprised. She assumed I couldn't get an STI because my partners are women. Fortunately, I knew that wasn't accurate.

For more information on coming out to your provider and finding lesbian- or bi-friendly health care, see "Homophobia, Transphobia, and Heterosexism," p. 682.

IMPACT OF FEMALE GENITAL CUTTING

Women whose genitals have been cut in the practice of female genital cutting (FGC, also referred to as female genital mutilation) have a higher risk of catching an STI from an infected partner because of unhealed ulcers, inflamed vulval membranes, and small sores resulting from intercourse, or having a smaller vaginal opening due to scarring. FGC is also linked with increased rates of pelvic inflammatory disease, among many other complications.[11]

SOCIAL AND CULTURAL FACTORS

On average, women have fewer financial resources than men; we are also more likely to be single parents and primary caregivers for those who are ill. For some of us, lack of money can mean lack of access to prevention and treatment. It can also mean we are too preoccupied with our own day-to-day survival, and that of our family members, to pursue safer-sex materials and/or necessary screening and treatment. In these ways, economic injustice contributes to higher rates of untreated STIs, and thus to a higher risk of transmitting STIs among sex partners within communities where poverty is a significant problem.

In cultures that value passivity and submissiveness in women, it can be difficult for a woman to refuse unwanted sex and/or to negotiate condom use. A male partner may refuse to use protection, even if he is having sex with other women or men on the side. For many women, fear of sexual violence and/or financial dependence on a male partner makes negotiating safer sex undesirable or impossible. (See Chapter 10, "Safer Sex," for tips on negotiating condom use.)

Dr. Susan C. Ball, associate professor of medicine at New York Presbyterian Hospital, points out that "the result of this imbalance in sexual power has led to the infection of countless women around the world and of the babies born to them."[12]

Many cultures discourage women from touching or looking at their genitals, making it more difficult to notice early signs of an STI. We may also be more sensitive to the shame and stigma associated with having an STI and thus delay diagnosis and treatment.

The insensitivity of some medical institutions to women—especially to women of color, poor women, uninsured women, and women who don't speak English—results in many delaying seeking care or testing. Those of us with low incomes and little formal education may find that health-care providers are too quick to suspect that we have an STI, while those of us who seem middle or upper class, or who are married or older, can go through a health visit without the topic coming up at all. Both forms of bias can be damaging.

Cultural, biological, and economic factors

WHO GETS INFECTED? UNDERSTANDING RACIAL DISPARITIES IN STI OCCURRENCE, PREVENTION, AND CARE

Considering the United States' history of racial discrimination and unequal access to health care, and our national discomfort with race and sexuality, it isn't surprising that sexually transmitted infections take their greatest toll in communities of color. Blame is often put on individual behavior, but the numbers are more likely due to underlying social conditions that our country has failed to confront.

In 2009, African Americans, who account for 12 percent of the population, represented 71 percent of gonorrhea infections and approximately half of all chlamydia and syphilis cases. Overall, their rate of chlamydia was more than eight times that among whites. Young African-American women experienced significantly higher rates of chlamydia and gonorrhea than any other group. Other groups also disproportionately affected are young Hispanic men and women age twenty to twenty-four, whose chlamydia and gonorrhea rates are twice that of whites in the same age group. And among American Indians/Alaska Natives, the rate was more than four times that among whites.[13]

The incidence of many STIs—especially HIV—is higher in poor, segregated neighborhoods. These numbers give rise to stereotypes in which women and men from economically disenfranchised communities are portrayed as promiscuous and irresponsible about STI protection.

In fact, researchers have found that women in poor African-American communities who engage in the lowest-risk sexual activities are much more likely to acquire STIs than women in communities with low rates of infection who engage in higher-risk sex.[14] This suggests that the community within which you live and choose your partners has a major impact on how much risk you face.

Why might communities that are hard-hit economically, many of which are communities of color, have higher STI rates?

- Fewer hospitals and treatment centers and lower-performing and less funded schools mean less access to STI education, prevention, and treatment.
- Less money available for safer-sex supplies such as condoms.
- High incarceration rates. Owing to race, class, and educational bias, the U.S. criminal justice system imprisons a disproportionate number of people of color; more than 60 percent of the prison population is composed of racial and ethnic minorities, most of whom are from inner cities.

Some public-health experts have noted two troubling trends with so many African-American and Latino men behind bars:

One is the shift in the patterns of marriage and courtship that result when so many men are removed from a community. The other is an increase in the number of "multiple concurrent sexual partnerships," in which individuals are engaged in sexual relationships with more than one person at a time. In many communities, when one sexual partner is imprisoned, the person left behind chooses another partner. When widespread, this behavior creates an efficient, effective pattern for introducing and maintaining an STD through a network of sexual relationships.

Concurrent sexual partnerships, our research indicates, are a more effective engine for transmitting STDs than sequential partnerships. In the latter case, an infected individual is more likely to be diagnosed before a new partner is infected. In the former, an individual infected by one partner can immediately pass the infection on to another, potentially spreading it quickly through the network. As people move in and out of relationships and in and out of communities, such infections become almost impossible to treat efficiently. Movement in and out of prison aggravates these trends.[15]

Bradley Stoner, chair of the board of directors of the American Social Health Association, says the numbers are an important reminder that STIs are a critical public-health threat. The data on disparities, he says, "show that minority populations continue to bear a disproportionate share of the STD burden. It is time to focus more aggressively on STD prevention and control efforts, and turn our attention towards destigmatizing STD testing and treatment."[16]

Increasing accessibility of STI services is crucial, as is involving the communities themselves in the design and delivery of the services. At the same time, we need to find ways to address the complex economic and racial injustices that contribute to these disparities. One of many groups working toward these goals is SisterLove (sisterlove.org), an Atlanta-based sexual health and reproductive justice organization with a focus on HIV/AIDS.

may combine to increase women's risk of STI transmission. Despite the conventional wisdom that female sex workers are more likely to transmit HIV or another STI to male clients, it is actually more likely—because of women's biological vulnerabilities—to be the other way around. Many male clients resist condom use or offer to pay more for unprotected sex. Some sex workers build on experience, by, for example, inserting a female condom before accepting a client or swiftly slipping on a condom as part of sex play. Indeed, in some communities, sex workers also work as effective safer-sex educators and have helped train other safer-sex educators.

Women's prisons offer another example of the interplay of biological and social factors. When women arrive in prison with an untreated STI, unhealthy living conditions and insufficient medical care can lead to less attentive treatment, more health complications and suffering, and a higher death rate from HIV/AIDS. Some prisoner-initiated groups—including groups in Lexington, KY, Marianna, FL, and Dublin, CA, and in the Washington, DC, Detention Facility and New York's Bedford Hills prison—have worked to bring AIDS support, education, and awareness to prisons. The groundbreaking work of the AIDS Counseling and Education group

NEEDLE DRUG USE

All recreational drugs can impair judgment, and this may make it less likely that someone will practice safer sex. IV drug users also need to consider how to inject safely, as shared needles may be contaminated from a prior user with HIV or other blood-borne infections. A recent CDC study in California noted that in the preceding twelve months, 32 percent of injection drug users had shared works or needles, and 63 percent had had unprotected sex.[17] Needle exchange programs have been successful in helping women reduce the risk of HIV transmission.[18]

In 2007, 16 percent of new HIV cases among U.S. women were due to injection drug use, down from 22 percent in 2002. Although most women with HIV become infected through unprotected intercourse with an infected man, the partner's drug use can be the source of the HIV infection that he passes on.

Injection drug use is particularly common in hard-hit socioeconomic areas where access to quality care and to treatment for addiction is inadequate. Inaccessibility of care can fall especially hard on women, who are more likely to have daily responsibility for children and may thus face extra obstacles to making use of any treatment or rehab options that are available.

(ACE) at Bedford Hills has been documented in the book *Breaking the Walls of Silence: AIDS and Women in a New York State Maximum-Security Prison.*[19] Prison officials have often opposed or disbanded these peer education groups, despite or perhaps because of their success at educating and organizing prisoners, but the ACE group was still going as of late 2010.

Improving women's health experiences with STIs will depend on fundamental social changes that address poverty, racism, and sexism. It is important to make public officials understand that when particular communities are hard-hit by STIs, such factors are at work—not an inherent tendency to sexual infection on the part of any social group.

As the Department of Health and Human Services notes, a key to improving STI prevention and treatment efforts in communities hit hard by racism and economic distress is to involve community members "at all stages in the process of devising and implementing prevention and control strategies."[20] (For tips on creating culturally appropriate sex education programs, see "Empowering Our Schools and Communities," p. 271.)

It is crucial that we take care of ourselves and work to change the systems that make self-care so difficult. Too often, public support is lacking for the tools we need: comprehensive health insurance and health care, drug treatment programs, adequate housing, healthy and affordable food options, and child care. We all have a right to enjoy sex without risking our health, to advocate for ourselves and one another, and to get the medical care we need.

SCREENING, TESTING, AND TREATING STIs

SCREENING

Some screenings, such as Pap tests that look for precancerous cervical changes, are offered to almost all women. Other screening tests are recommended only for pregnant women or at-risk groups, which usually include sexually active adolescents, people with a history of STIs, people with new or multiple sexual partners, people who use condoms inconsistently, and people who use drugs or do sex work.

You can find specific STI screening guidelines at the following websites:

- Centers for Disease Control and Prevention: cdc.gov/std/treatment
- The California STD/HIV Prevention Training Center: stdhivtraining.org/resource.php?id=15

Individual risk depends not only on behavior but also on the prevalence of disease in your community. In urban communities and communities with high rates of poverty, some populations, especially African Americans and, to a lesser extent, Latinos, may be at greater risk, and broader voluntary screening of individuals without symptoms may be warranted.

The Limits of Screening

Sensitive and specific tests are available for chlamydia, gonorrhea, syphilis, HIV, herpes, trichomoniasis, and chancroid. However, no test is perfect, and even the best tests available occasionally produce false negatives and false positives. Sometimes, tests miss the presence of an STI, if the person exposed is still incubating the infection (for HIV, this is also known as the window period), or if the specimen isn't collected or processed properly. There also are some STIs for which there is currently no commercially available lab test (e.g., for *Mycoplasma genitalium*).

Recommended Screening for Pregnant Women

Untreated STIs can reduce your ability to become pregnant and in some instances cause infertility. Because they can increase the likeli-

hood of pregnancy complications and can infect a fetus or infant, early diagnosis is essential.

Pregnant women should be offered screening for HIV, syphilis, hepatitis B, and chlamydia, and possibly gonorrhea. A test for hepatitis C is recommended for women who use or have used injection drugs or received blood products, transfusions, or transplants prior to 1992.[21]

An early prenatal visit is also a good time to check for bacterial vaginosis (BV) and to have a Pap test if it wasn't done during the previous year or two. Some experts recommend that women who have had a premature delivery in the past be screened and treated for bacterial vaginosis at the first prenatal visit.

Infections first acquired during pregnancy are the most likely to be passed to the baby. Chlamydia, gonorrhea, syphilis, trichomoniasis, and BV can be treated and cured with antibiotics during pregnancy. Viral STIs cannot be cured, but antiviral medication may be appropriate for pregnant women with herpes and definitely is for those with HIV.

You may need more testing later on during your pregnancy if you are at risk of exposure (e.g., if you have new sexual partners). (For specific considerations, see the section below on individuals STIs.)

WHERE TO GO FOR CARE

- **Public-health clinics (also called STI or STD clinics).** Government-funded sexually transmitted disease clinics provide services, usually regardless of a person's ability to pay. Clinic staff members are likely to have a lot of expertise in testing, diagnosing, and treating most STIs, and the setting may offer more privacy than your usual provider's office.

  To find the nearest walk-in facility, visit hivtest.org. Enter your zip code and it will produce a list of nearby clinics that perform tests for HIV and other STIs, with detailed

DECREASING RISK
AFTER EXPOSURE

If you think you might have been exposed to HIV or hepatitis A or B, you may be able to obtain treatment immediately, without waiting for tests. Postexposure prophylaxis (PEP) involves taking a short-term antiretroviral treatment to reduce the likelihood of infection after potential exposure.

If you are exposed to HIV through your job or through unprotected sexual activity or shared needles, you can go to an emergency room within seventy-two hours of suspected exposure (the sooner the better) and request this treatment (referred to in nonoccupational cases as nPEP). The drugs used in the twenty-eight-day PEP regimen for HIV can cause serious side effects and are expensive (around $1,000), but they have the potential to prevent HIV infection. Insurance may cover some of the PEP costs.

The earlier PEP is begun, the more likely it is to be effective. If you have not been vaccinated against hepatitis A or B, it is best to seek PEP treatment within twenty-four hours of exposure to hepatitis B[22] and up to two weeks (though as soon as possible) after exposure to hepatitis A.[23] Unvaccinated individuals should receive HAV immune globulin within two weeks of the exposure. People receiving PEP should also get vaccinated.

information about costs and the types of tests offered. You can also call the Centers for Disease Control's national hotline (1-800-227-8922) for clinics in your area.

- **Family-planning and community clinics.** Most family-planning providers (such as Planned Parenthood clinics, local health departments, and other community clinics) also offer affordable and knowledgeable STI counseling, testing, and referral. In the rare cases when they don't, they'll know where you can get them. They are also likely to treat you with particular sensitivity around sex-related issues. Many are low cost and also have sliding-scale fees. To find a clinic near you, go to plannedparenthood.org and enter your zip code.
- **Primary care provider.** Go to your regular health-care provider if you're likely to receive clear, understandable responses to your questions. Family physicians, family nurse-practitioners, and physician assistants are trained to test for and treat STIs.

  However, not all providers have the necessary equipment to do routine STI testing, and they may not know enough about these diseases. Ask whether your treatment follows the most recent CDC treatment guidelines.
- **ER.** If you have been forced into sexual activity and you're afraid you've been exposed to a disease, most emergency rooms can give you preventive treatment for STIs, including HIV. Tell the ER staff if you need emergency treatment after being raped or sexually assaulted. Some ERs also have rape kits to collect evidence and can help you file a police report if you wish to make one. (For more information, see "Rape," p. 700.)

  Unless you really need emergency care, however, the ER isn't the best place to go. Since ERs focus on trauma and life-threatening illnesses, the hospital emergency staff won't be able to give you the time, expertise, and sensitivity you may need to deal with STI issues. Also, test results will likely take longer when performed in the ER.

PREPARING FOR YOUR HEALTH-CARE VISIT

- **Find a health care provider you trust.** Some providers are uncomfortable talking about sex, or may make assumptions about whether we might have an STI or not based on their own cultural biases.

  Though we're often limited by cost or insurance restrictions, try to find a provider who is comfortable discussing sexual health and with whom you are comfortable (public-health and family-planning clinics, listed in the previous section, have staff trained in discussing all sexual issues). Ask for recommendations and look for someone who provides complete and understandable information, encourages and answers questions, and accepts your sexuality and gender identity.

- **Call ahead or look online.** Find out what services are offered and how much you'll have to pay. Tests may involve only a small co-payment, but there may be a fee for the visit.

- **Think ahead about confidentiality.** Everyone is entitled to confidentiality regarding STI medical care and records, and every state has laws guaranteeing minors the right to confidential STI care. However, if you are a minor and have insurance through your parent(s), be aware that your parent, as the insurance policy holder, will receive notification from the insurance company that includes an explanation of the charges or benefits. If this is unacceptable, look for a clinic that provides free or low-cost testing. (See "Where to Go for Care," p. 285.)

- **Self-care.** It's fine to use an ice pack or take over-the-counter pain medicines for genital pain. However, don't put any cream or ointment on a sore, as that could make it more difficult for the test to detect the organism.

If you have trouble urinating, avoid drinking alcohol and eating spicy foods (both of which may irritate your urinary tract) until you have received treatment and the infection has cleared up. In some cases, a hot bath may make the pain less intense.

- **Don't have unprotected sex or douche.** Douching before STI testing can make the test results less accurate and your infection worse. So can unprotected sex.

- **Ask for support.** Some people arrange to bring a friend with them to write down information and offer emotional support. Make sure that anyone who accompanies you is someone whom you trust and with whom you can be honest about anything your provider might ask, including the range of your sexual practices and relationship issues, such as intimate partner violence. If there are things you would like only your provider to know, you may want to go into the appointment alone. Or you can arrange to have a private time with the provider (apart from your support person). Some facilities/providers do not allow another person in the room, even at the patient's request. This is in order to prevent any barrier to the honest exchange of information or potential compromise to patient confidentiality.

AT THE CLINIC OR DOCTOR'S OFFICE

- **Be honest.** It is important for your provider to know if your sex partners include men, women, or both; whether you have had new partners since the last visit; and the sites of exposure. Although some women engage in anal sex, many health care practitioners do not ask about it. Don't wait for your provider to bring up specific sexual practices. Be forthcoming in order to get the most comprehensive and accurate care.

- **Make sure you get all the tests you need.** Although providers may be able to diagnose herpes by sight, for example, lab tests can provide more specific information. Ask exactly which STIs you are being tested for; some have to be diagnosed from symptoms because there's no reliable screening test. (For more information on recommended tests, see "Screening, Testing, and Treating STIs," p. 284.)
- **Ask about vaccinations.** As of 2011, there were two effective vaccines on the market to prevent HPV. One is against the two cancer-linked types of HPV, while the other covers the same high-risk types and, in addition, the two types that usually cause genital warts. It's important for women who receive an HPV vaccine to continue with recommended cervical cancer screening (such as Pap tests). Vaccines are also available against hepatitis A and B infections. (For more information, see "Vaccinations to Prevent STIs," p. 277.)
- **Make sure you understand your diagnosis and what you need to do to get well.** If you've been diagnosed with an STI, it's important that you know what medication you will be taking and for how long; the potential side effects, including drug interactions with hormonal birth control and other medications; how long to wait before resuming sex; and any follow-up tests or treatment required. Don't be embarrassed to ask questions.
- **Don't leave with unanswered questions.** If your provider is too busy to answer questions, ask to speak to someone else. Find out how long it will take for your symptoms to clear up and what you should tell your sex partner(s) and when you can resume sexual activity. If the office will try to reach you later with test results, provide an appropriate phone number or email address where you can be reached, and discuss whether a message may be left for you. Or schedule a date to call or to return for your results. Make it easy for your provider to reach you and treat you if needed.

FOLLOW-UP

- **Call with more questions.** It's hard sometimes to think of everything to ask on the spot. If you have more questions after your visit, call back and ask for the information you need.
- **Take *all* prescribed medication.** Even if you feel better or the symptoms disappear, finish taking the full course of medication. Incomplete treatment can result in drug-resistant strains of the infections growing in your body, and these can cause more complications.
- **Make a plan with your partner.** If you or your partner has a bacterial STI (such as chlamydia, gonorrhea, or syphilis), you and all your partners (and their partners) must be treated, and take all medication as prescribed, before you have sex again. If not, you can keep reinfecting each other. Your partner(s) may not need to see a provider: You may be able to provide antibiotics to your partner(s). Ask your provider if he or she can give you medication that you can give to your partner(s). Also ask how long you need to wait after you and your partner(s) have been treated before resuming sexual activity.
- **Hang in there:** You may feel uncertain about your treatment. Tests are not perfect; sometimes treatments are a burden or they don't work, and that means more medical visits, time, and money. But the alternative—not getting treatment—is worse, because it puts your long-term health, and that of your partner(s), at risk.

- **Reporting requirements:** Health-care providers are required by law to report to the public-health department certain STIs, including, but not limited to, chlamydia, gonorrhea, syphilis, chancroid, and HIV/AIDS.[24] Public-health departments use reported information about STI diagnoses to help identify risk factors for disease, detect and respond to outbreaks, interrupt the spread of infection, and plan prevention programs. Although names are included with case reports, individual information is confidential and by law cannot be disclosed by the health department to anyone else. HIV cases diagnosed by anonymous (as opposed to confidential) testing do not get reported to health departments.

If you are diagnosed with gonorrhea, syphilis, HIV/AIDS, or (sometimes) chlamydia, a public-health official or social worker may ask you for the name(s) of anyone you may have caught the infection from or have given it to. The official or social worker may contact these people, without using your name, to encourage them to seek testing and treatment. You may also choose to contact sex partners yourself. Doing so may save their fertility or even their lives, as well as that of their other or future sex partners.

Partner notification services such as inSPOT (inspot.org) enable users to electronically notify their sex partners that they have been exposed to HIV or other STIs and that they should seek medical care. The site lets people notified to put in their zip code and find a testing location near them.

BACTERIA- AND PARASITE-CAUSED STIs: CHLAMYDIA, GONORRHEA, SYPHILIS, AND TRICHOMONIASIS (TRICH)

Bacterial STIs and trich (caused by a parasite) are spread by sexual activity. They cannot be spread through contact with toilet seats, doorknobs, swimming pools, hot tubs, bathtubs, shared clothing, or eating utensils.

The good news is that these STIs are curable through treatment with antibiotics. Curable, that is, as long as you see a health-care provider, get tested and treated, follow through on all the medication, avoid sexual contact until cured, and make sure that your sexual partner(s) will get testing and treatment as well.

There's bad news, too. Like viral STIs, bacterial STIs often give no warning signs or symptoms. This means you can get infected and infect your sexual partner(s) without knowing it. Serious complications that cause irreversible damage can progress silently before you ever recognize a problem; these complications include pelvic inflammatory disease, infertility and life-threatening ectopic pregnancy. The longer that bacterial STIs go untreated, the more damage they can do. Medication will stop these infections, but it will not repair any permanent damage done before treatment begins.

If you are being treated for a bacterial STI or trich, you'll be at high risk for reinfection unless you avoid sex until you and your sex partner(s) complete successful treatment. Reinfection rates among women diagnosed with and treated for chlamydia and gonorrhea are high, in many cases because their partners do not receive treatment. Having multiple infections increases a woman's risk of serious reproductive health complications, including infertility.

CHLAMYDIA

Chlamydia is caused by the bacterium *Chlamydia trachomatis*. In the United States, about 1.2 million cases of chlamydia were reported in 2009,[25] but chlamydia often goes undetected and undiagnosed; over 2.8 million new cases, more than double the number of reported cases, are estimated to occur each year.

Transmission

Chlamydia can be transmitted during vaginal, anal, or oral sex. If there is infected vaginal fluid on your fingers, or discharge from the penis of an infected man, touching your hand to your eye can also infect your eye. If you have receptive anal intercourse, you can get a chlamydial infection in the rectum. Chlamydia can also be found in the throats of women and men who have had oral sex with an infected partner.

Pregnancy and Childbirth

Chlamydia can be passed from an infected mother to her baby during vaginal childbirth. Chlamydia is a leading cause of early infant pneumonia and conjunctivitis, or pinkeye, in newborns.

Possible Signs and Symptoms

Most women with chlamydia have no apparent symptoms. The bacteria initially infect the cervix and the urethra. Women who have symptoms sometimes have an abnormal vaginal discharge or a burning sensation when urinating. If the infection spreads from the cervix to the fallopian tubes, some women may still have no signs or symptoms; others may have lower abdominal pain, low back pain, nausea, fever, pain during intercourse, or bleeding between menstrual periods. If it spreads to the rectum, chlamydia can cause rectal pain, discharge, or bleeding, or may be present with no symptoms at all.

Men's symptoms include discharge from the penis or a burning sensation when urinating. Men might also have burning and itching around the opening of the penis.

Screening and Diagnosis

Yearly chlamydia testing is recommended for all sexually active women age twenty-five or younger, older women who have a new sex partner or multiple sex partners, and all pregnant women.[26] As chlamydia can be confused with gonorrhea, you may want to get tested for both.

The presence of *Chlamydia trachomatis* can be confirmed by lab tests done using a swab from cervix or vagina or using urine. If you've had receptive anal intercourse, a rectal swab for chlamydia is recommended.

Treatment

Oral antibiotics. Be sure your partner(s) will be treated as well, to avoid reinfection. In some states, a clinician can legally provide antibiotics or a prescription for antibiotics for you to give to your sex partner or partners. Retesting is recommended three months after being diagnosed with chlamydia to detect new infections, which can be due to sex with undiagnosed and untreated sex partners.

Complications

Chlamydia can spread into the uterus or fallopian tubes and cause pelvic inflammatory disease (PID). This happens in about 10–15 percent of women with untreated chlamydia. PID can lead to internal abscesses (pus-filed pockets of infection and inflammation that are hard to cure) and long-lasting, chronic pelvic pain. PID can damage the fallopian tubes enough to cause infertility or increase the risk of ectopic pregnancy.

Chlamydia can also increase the chances of becoming infected with HIV, if you're exposed.

GONORRHEA

Gonorrhea is caused by *Neisseria gonorrhoeae*, a bacterium that can grow and multiply easily in the warm, moist areas of a woman's reproductive tract, including the cervix, uterus, and fallopian tubes. It can also multiply in the urethra (urine canal) in women and men. The bacterium can also grow in the mouth, throat, eyes, and anus.

Gonorrhea is the second most commonly reported infectious disease, with more than 301,000 cases reported to the CDC in 2009,[27] but it's estimated that more than half of all new infections go undiagnosed.[28]

Transmission
Gonorrhea is spread through contact with the penis, vagina, mouth, or anus.

Pregnancy and Childbirth
Gonorrhea can be passed from an infected mother to her baby during childbirth and cause blindness, joint infection, or a life-threatening blood infection.[29] Treatment of gonorrhea as soon as it is detected in pregnant women reduces the risk of transmission during childbirth.

Possible Signs and Symptoms
Most women who are infected with gonorrhea have no noticeable symptoms. If symptoms do appear, they can include increased vaginal discharge, vaginal bleeding between periods, or a painful or burning sensation when urinating. Since these symptoms are nonspecific, they can be mistaken for a bladder or vaginal infection.

Men's symptoms can include a burning sensation during urination or a white, yellow, or green discharge from the penis. Sometimes men with gonorrhea get painful or swollen testicles.

Rectal infection in both men and women can occur without symptoms or may include discharge, anal itching, soreness, bleeding, or painful bowel movements. Infection in the throat may cause a sore throat.

Screening and Diagnosis
It's recommended that clinicians screen all sexually active women, including those who are pregnant, for gonorrhea infection, particularly those at increased risk for infection (that is, if they are young or have other individual or population risk factors).

A urine sample or a swab of your vagina, rectum, throat, or urethra is used to collect bacteria that can be identified in a laboratory for gonorrhea confirmation. The nucleic acid amplification DNA test (NAAT) is the most accurate type of test and is widely available.

Treatment
Antibiotics can successfully cure gonorrhea. However, drug-resistant strains of gonorrhea are increasing in many areas of the world, including the United States, complicating treatment. Because many people with gonorrhea also have chlamydia, antibiotics for both infections are usually given together. In some states, a clinician can legally provide antibiotics for you to give to your sex partner or partners. Retesting is recommended three months after being diagnosed with gonorrhea to detect new infections, which can be due to sex with undiagnosed and untreated sex partners.

Complications
In women, gonorrhea is a common cause of pelvic inflammatory disease (PID; see above, under chlamydia). More rarely, advanced gonorrhea can spread to the blood or joints. The most common symptoms are aching and swelling in the joints (usually in the hands or feet), but gonorrhea can spread, causing skin lesions and infections of the heart, the bones, and the sheaths

that cover the nervous system (meninges). In very rare cases, it can be fatal.

SYPHILIS

Syphilis is caused by the bacterium *Treponema pallidum*. After being greatly reduced in the United States in the twentieth century, syphilis rates have increased. In 2009, reported syphilis cases increased 5 percent over the previous year, for a 39 percent increase since 2006.[30] Most of the increase is in men who have sex with other men.

Transmission
Syphilis is transmitted through direct contact with a syphilis sore. Sores occur mainly on the external genitals, or in the vagina, anus, or rectum. Sores also can occur on the lips and in the mouth.

Transmission of the organism most often occurs during unprotected vaginal, anal, or oral sex. Barrier methods such as the male or female condom or dental dam are important tools to prevent the spread of infection. They do not, however, offer protection from sores outside the area covered by the barrier.

Genital sores caused by syphilis make it easier to transmit and acquire HIV infection. Syphilis-type sores are usually painless and can bleed easily. When they come into contact with oral and rectal mucosa during sex, this contact increases the infectiousness of and susceptibility to HIV. There is an estimated two- to fivefold increased risk of acquiring HIV if you are exposed to HIV when syphilis is present.

Pregnancy and Childbirth
Because syphilis can pass from a woman to her fetus, pregnant women are routinely screened for syphilis. If syphilis treatment is given early in the pregnancy, the fetus probably won't be affected, since syphilis often takes a few months to cause damage to a fetus. Later on, since medication can stop the disease but cannot repair damage already done, a baby may be stillborn or have serious abnormalities at birth.

An infected baby may be born without signs or symptoms of disease. However, if not treated immediately, the baby may become developmentally delayed, have seizures, or die. In most states, prenatal testing is required by law.

Possible Signs and Symptoms
Untreated syphilis typically goes through several stages. Primary syphilis is characterized by a (usually) painless sore, or chancre, at the spot where the bacterium entered the body; the chancre heals on its own, but syphilis remains active if untreated. Individuals with untreated primary syphilis usually develop secondary syphilis, usually at about two to eight weeks after the appearance of the original sore. In secondary syphilis, the bacteria have spread into the bloodstream.

Secondary syphilis is often characterized by a skin rash, which may appear as rough, red, or reddish-brown spots on areas including, but not limited to, the palms of the hands and bottoms of the feet. Lesions may also appear on mucous membranes, and individuals may experience fever, swollen lymph glands, sore throat, patchy hair loss, headaches, weight loss, muscle aches, and fatigue. Rectal infection in both men and women may include discharge, anal itching, soreness, bleeding, or painful bowel movements, but may not have obvious symptoms at all. Infection in the throat can cause a sore throat.

Screening and Diagnosis
Screening is recommended for all pregnant women and anyone at increased risk for syphilis infection, including sex workers, people who exchange sex for drugs, people diagnosed with HIV, carriers of other STIs, and those who have

had contact with someone who has active syphilis.[31] Individuals living in communities with increased levels of syphilis are often offered screening.

Syphilis can be diagnosed based on physical examination findings, microscopic identification of syphilis bacteria, and blood testing. A second test is usually required to confirm the diagnosis.

Treatment

Syphilis is easy to cure in its early stages. A single shot of an antibiotic generally cures a person who has had syphilis for less than a year. Additional doses are needed to treat someone who has had syphilis for longer than a year. Be sure to abstain from sexual contact until the syphilis sore or rash is completely healed or a follow-up test shows that you have been cured.

Complications If Untreated

Symptoms of secondary syphilis resolve with or without treatment, but without treatment the infection can silently progress and cause damage to the body's internal organs, including the brain, nerves, eyes, heart, blood vessels, liver, bones, and joints. This occurs in about 15 percent of cases. By the late stage, this damage can be serious enough to cause paralysis, numbness, gradual blindness, dementia, and death.

TRICHOMONIASIS

Trichomoniasis is the most common curable STI in young, sexually active women. An estimated 7.4 million new cases occur each year in women and men.[32] Trichomoniasis is caused by the single-celled protozoan parasite *Trichomonas vaginalis*. The vagina is the most common site of infection in women (resulting in small open sores on the vaginal wall), and the urethra is the most common site of infection in men.

Transmission

The parasite is transmitted through penis-to-vagina intercourse or vulva-to-vulva contact with an infected partner.

Pregnancy and Childbirth

Pregnant women with trichomoniasis may have babies who are born early or with low birth weight.

Possible Signs and Symptoms

Symptoms may include a frothy yellow-green vaginal discharge with a strong odor. The infection also may cause discomfort during intercourse and urination, as well as irritation and itching of the genital area. In rare cases, lower abdominal pain can occur.

Most men with trichomoniasis do not have apparent symptoms; however, some men may temporarily have an irritation inside the penis, mild discharge, or slight burning after urination or ejaculation. The symptoms may disappear within a few weeks without treatment. However, an infected man, even a man who has never had symptoms or whose symptoms have stopped, can continue to infect or reinfect a partner until he has been successfully treated.

Screening and Diagnosis

Screening for trich is recommended for women with symptoms and as part of a comprehensive STI evaluation. Women with new or multiple sex partners—especially if not using condoms—are also recommended to have a screening test.

Diagnosis can be confirmed by looking at a sample of vaginal discharge or with newer tests that use rapid antigen detection and NAAT methods. The newer tests are more accurate.

Treatment

Trichomoniasis can usually be cured with prescription drugs, either tinidazole, given by mouth in a single dose, or metronidazole (Flagyl), which should not be used by pregnant women in the first trimester. Many women who take metronidazole experience unpleasant effects, such as nausea, headache, diarrhea, metallic taste, joint pain, and numbness of the arms or legs. Avoid alcohol while taking metronidazole, as the combination can make the effects of both worse.

Your partner or partners need to be treated before you have sex with them again so that you do not get reinfected.

Complications If Untreated

Having trichomoniasis increases susceptibility to HIV, and may also increase the chance that an HIV-infected woman will pass HIV to her sex partner(s).

BACTERIAL VAGINOSIS AND YEAST

Vaginal infections can also be caused by bacterial vaginosis (BV), which is possibly sexually transmitted, and yeast, which can be sexually transmitted but most often isn't. (For information on both of these, see pp. 644 and 645.)

VIRAL STIs: HERPES, HPV, HEPATITIS B, AND HIV/AIDS

HERPES

Herpes is a very common infection caused by herpes simplex virus type 1 (HSV-1) or herpes simplex virus type 2 (HSV-2).

Genital herpes can be caused by either virus, while oral herpes (fever blisters or cold sores around the mouth and lips) is almost always caused by HSV-1. Women with frequently recurrent genital herpes (more than two to three outbreaks a year) usually have an HSV-2 infection, while genital herpes due to HSV-1 outbreaks are usually milder and less frequent. More than 60

million people in the United States have genital herpes, about 50 million with HSV-2 and 10 to 20 million with HSV-1.

More than 80 percent of people infected with HSV-2 are unaware that they have genital herpes because they have no symptoms or only mild symptoms that have gone unnoticed or are attributed to other common genital conditions such as vaginitis, painful urination, or hemorrhoids.

Transmission

Herpes is spread by contact of the mouth, genitals, or skin with either developed or developing herpes blisters. Transmission is also possible between outbreaks, when invisible or asymptomatic viral shedding occurs from the original site of infection. Both HSV-1 and HSV-2 are most often spread by people who are asymptomatic, meaning they are not experiencing any signs or symptoms at the time of transmission. Thus, you can get herpes, or give it, without you or your partner knowing there is an infection. The risk of transmission can be reduced if the partner with herpes takes a daily dose of antiviral medication on an ongoing basis, uses condoms, and refrains from sex at the first sign of an outbreak.

When HSV-1 is present around the mouth, it can be transmitted through oral secretions or sores and spread through kissing or sharing toothbrushes, drinking glasses, or eating utensils. If you have sores on your lips or in your mouth, avoid oral sex. Don't kiss anyone—especially not infants, young children, or pregnant women. If you touch the sores with your fingers, wash your hands with soap and hot water, especially before touching your eyes or putting in contact lenses.

HSV-1 infection of the genitals is usually caused by oral-to-genital contact with a person who has HSV-1 infection. It can also be caused by genital-to-genital contact, but this is less common than mouth-to-genital contact.

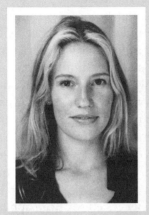

© Ali Price

BREAKING THE NEWS

JENNIFER BAUMGARDNER

When I was twenty-six, I got herpes from a lovely guy on our first real date. At first I held out hope that the searing pain in my vulva, fever, and chills were just signs of a bad urinary tract infection, but a trip to my gynecologist confirmed otherwise. I had HSV-1, more commonly known as oral herpes, but I had it on my genitals. Because of the popularity of oral sex, having this variety was becoming as common as having *genital* herpes on one's genitals.

To be honest, I was initially very depressed after diagnosis. I pored over my Mayo Clinic health book and *Our Bodies, Ourselves* for days, wondering what my future held. The books sort of scared me, actually, because (for good reason) they mention all of the more dangerous possibilities that might come with herpes. For instance, I might have many outbreaks each year, and it appeared likely that I would have to have a C-section if I ever got pregnant. If a lesion infected the baby during delivery, he or she could be made blind. I also felt sort of trapped in the relationship with the carrier –although I really did like him –because I feared telling other lovers or being rejected. As it turned out, I haven't had any other outbreaks in the eight years since diagnosis, and I'm currently seven months pregnant. My doctor says that most women can have vaginal births as long as they aren't having an active recurrence. She's putting me on a drug that suppresses outbreaks (acyclovir) for the last month or so of my pregnancy, as a precaution.

As for telling lovers, I have had three since that guy who gave me my gift of a lifetime. Breaking the news is a little excruciating–and one person was really upset to hear it–but it has never derailed my love life. I went on to have a long relationship with the guy who was so upset, so he eventually got over his fears. The worst thing that happened was that I did give it to someone once. I had no symptoms but must have been shedding the virus, and I have tended not to use condoms after a relationship gets serious and committed. He had one bad outbreak, the initial one, but has never had a problem since.

One thing that helped me to deal with having an STI was to realize that I was part of a mighty big club. Another thing that helped was telling my dad, a doctor in my hometown of Fargo, ND. The first thing he said was, "Hey, it's not going to be a big deal. Herpes is not one of the most serious medical conditions you are likely to have during your lifetime." He was right.

[Update: Jennifer writes that she has had not one, but two, vaginal births without complications.]

Generally, the HSV-2 infection is contracted during penile-vaginal or penile-oral contact, or genital rubbing with someone who has a genital HSV-2 infection. It is very rare to acquire an oral infection with HSV-2 through oral sex with someone who has genital HSV-2.

If you or your partner has a genital herpes outbreak, avoid all contact with active sores or places where sores tend to occur. Do not have intercourse—even with a condom. Wait until seven days after the sore heals. The virus can spread from areas not covered by the condom, and it can be transmitted in sweat or vaginal fluids to places the condom doesn't cover.

Pregnancy and Childbirth

Tell your health-care provider if you have genital herpes flare-ups. Discuss the pros and cons of taking a daily antiviral medication for a month prior to delivery, in order to reduce the risk of transmission to the newborn during vaginal delivery. Pregnant women who don't have herpes should avoid unprotected sex with a partner who has herpes.

Recent research suggests that transmission from partners' oral herpes to the pregnant mother's genitals, and then on to the fetus, accounts for an increasing proportion of newborn herpes cases. Women with primary outbreaks of genital herpes during birth are at highest risk of transmitting it to the newborn. As a result, some clinicians recommend that women not receive oral sex in the last half of pregnancy.

If you have prodromal (early-warning) symptoms such as tingling or aching, or active sores at the time of labor and delivery, a cesarean delivery is usually recommended. After birth, take care not to infect the infant. Don't touch genital or oral herpes sores, and wash your hands thoroughly before touching the baby.

Possible Signs and Symptoms

Most people with genital herpes have no noticeable signs or symptoms. For those with outbreaks during the initial episode, there may be pain at site of the sore(s), painful urination, vaginal discharge, swollen glands, fever, and body aches. Women with severe outbreaks may be unable to pass urine easily. The initial outbreak is usually the most painful and takes the longest time to heal. A health-care provider can give you prescription medication to lessen the severity.

Typically, another herpes episode can appear weeks or months after the first, but it is almost always less severe and shorter than the first outbreak. In the 20 percent of genital herpes infections when signs do occur, they typically appear as one or more blisters on or around the genitals or rectum. The blisters break, leaving tender ulcers (sores) that may take two to four weeks to heal. If you are unaware of typical herpes symptoms, you may attribute the sores to something else, such as a scratch or zipper cut. Genital herpes can also cause nonspecific symptoms such as genital or anal itching, rashes, burning on urination, or achiness—which could lead you to think you have vaginitis, a urinary tract infection, or hemorrhoids.

Recurrences may be triggered by stress or lowered resistance, getting your period, sex, certain foods, and sunburn. These episodes often decrease after the first year, but they can last in some cases for five to ten years or even longer. Some people with repeated genital herpes experience early-warning signs of an upcoming herpes episode: fever, malaise, or unusual sensations like tingling, itching, pain, burning, or pressure at the site of the original infection. The prodrome period can last up to two days and stops when the blisters appear.

LIVING WITH GENITAL HERPES

Herpes is an inconvenience and a pain, but it's something you learn to live with.

You may feel shocked when you first discover you have herpes. You may feel isolated, lonely, and angry, especially toward the person who you think may have infected you. You may become anxious about initiating or staying in long-term relationships or having children.

After the first big episode of herpes, I felt distant from my body. When we began lovemaking again, I had a hard time having orgasms or trusting the rhythm of my responses. I shed some tears over that. I felt my body had been invaded.

Most people find that over time they are able to adjust to and manage the emotional and health aspects of herpes. Learning the facts about the virus and seeking support when needed are important steps.

I contracted HSV-1 in the genital area when I was twenty-three. When I first found out I was infected by my boyfriend, who had a cold sore when he went down on me, I was angry. Why hadn't he known it could be spread by oral sex? Why didn't I know? Then I worried I'd have to stay in the relationship, and I wasn't so sure I wanted to. When we broke up a year later, it was hard at first telling new partners—or knowing when to tell them. I'm now married, and while I worry about infecting my partner, he's never stressed over it. That helps me to relax.

It may be easier to cope with herpes if you are able to talk about it openly and let people close to you know when you're feeling run-down. Identifying what triggers your flare-ups and reducing stress, if you can, may lead to fewer outbreaks.

The National Herpes Resource Center, run by the American Social Health Association (ashastd.org/hrc), provides comprehensive information for people with herpes. You'll also find a list of herpes support groups (called HELP groups) in the United States and Canada; many of these groups also welcome people with HPV infections.

Screening and Diagnosis

While asymptomatic adolescents and adults are not routinely given blood tests for herpes antibodies, the CDC recommends that health-care providers include HSV-2 antibody testing of the blood as part of a comprehensive evaluation for STIs.

If you have lesions, your health-care provider will likely be able to diagnose genital herpes by sight, but clinical diagnosis should be confirmed by laboratory testing. It can be helpful to know which type of herpes you have, as recurrences and virus shedding without symptoms are much less frequent for genital HSV-1 infection.

Treatment

There is no treatment that can cure herpes, and the infection can stay in the body indefinitely.

You can take a course of antiviral medications to treat individual outbreaks, though the medication is not as effective during recurrences as during the initial infection.

If you experience frequent outbreaks, talk to your health-care provider about taking a daily low dose of antiviral medications to help reduce the frequency and duration. This is called suppressive therapy, and daily use can reduce the likelihood that you will you infect your partner(s) and, if you are pregnant, transmit herpes to your baby during birth. It can also reduce the psychological distress associated with herpes outbreaks.

If you are having an outbreak, avoid using over-the-counter creams or ointments, as they can interfere with the healing process. Keep the area clean and as dry as possible and wear comfortable loose clothing that allows the area to get air. Avoid underwear made from synthetic material.

Some people recommend taking a supplement of the amino acid lysine (L-lysine). While some research has suggested that lysine supplements can reduce the frequency of recurrences or reduce healing time, other studies have not found this to be true.

Complications

Genital herpes can cause recurrent painful genital sores, and infection can be especially severe in people with suppressed immune systems. Regardless of severity of symptoms, genital herpes frequently causes psychological distress in people who know they are infected (see "Living with Genital Herpes," above).

HSV-2 infection increases the risk for HIV infection by at least twofold. This is likely because even microscopic ulcerations can provide an entry for HIV. The immune response to HSV-2 can also make HIV-infected individuals more infectious.

HPV (HUMAN PAPILLOMAVIRUS) INCLUDING GENITAL WARTS

Human papillomavirus (HPV) is the most common STI in the United States. The CDC estimates that more than 50 percent of women will become infected sometime in their lifetime, though most will never know it. About 20 million people—men and women—are thought to have an active HPV infection at any given time, with 6 million new cases each year.[33]

There are more than one hundred types of HPV; about thirty of them can be transmitted through sexual contact. Most people who have HPV do not develop any symptoms or health problems from it. HPV infection often goes away without any treatment within two years, as the body's immune system clears the infection on its own. However, because this infection is so common, even those infections that clear on their own cause a large number of genital warts and abnormal Pap tests while the infections exist.

However, some HPV infections persist for many years. Some types of HPV cause warts to appear on or around the genitals and anal area. These genital warts, technically known as condylomata acuminata, are most commonly associated with two HPV types, HPV-6 and HPV-11. Other HPV types can cause cancer of the cervix in women and, less frequently, vaginal, vulvar, anal, and throat cancer, as well as penile cancers in men. The HPV types associated with warts, however, are not generally associated with cancer.

Two types of HPV in particular, types 16 and 18, together cause about 70 percent of cervical cancers. There are about twelve thousand cases of cervical cancer diagnosed in the United States each year, and more than four thousand deaths. There are now two vaccines that can prevent infection with these specific types of HPV. (For more information, see "Vaccinations to Prevent STIs," p. 277.)

Transmission

HPV is spread by skin-to-skin contact (most often genital-to-genital), not through an exchange of bodily fluids.[34] Barrier protection, such as condoms, can reduce the risk of infection, but HPV can be spread by skin contact in places the condom doesn't cover. Even after the warts have been removed, it is possible for the virus to be shed from the area originally infected; this means the infection can be transmitted without either sexual partner being aware of it.

HPV can be contracted from one partner, remain dormant, and then later be unknowingly transmitted to another sexual partner. People do not know they have been infected by HPV unless they see genital warts or have an abnormal Pap test.

Potential Signs and Symptoms

Warts may appear within several weeks after sexual contact with a person who is infected with HPV, or they may take months or years to appear, or they may never appear. Genital warts can cause itching, irritation, and bleeding. Around the anus, where they are more likely to be discovered by touch rather than sight, warts can be mistaken for hemorrhoids.

Some HPV infections cause flat, abnormal growths in the genital area and on the cervix; however, HPV infections of the cervix usually do not cause any symptoms.

Pregnancy and Childbirth

Genital warts may grow during pregnancy or in women with weakened immune systems; they appear cauliflowerlike as they grow. During pregnancy, they can make the vaginal wall less elastic and delivery more difficult, although this rarely occurs.

Screening and Diagnosis

Genital warts can be diagnosed by a visual inspection. Sometimes, ordinary skin tags and moles in the genital area can look like warts. Infrequently, the clinician may need to biopsy the area to determine if there is a wart present.

The most common way of finding out if you have one of the two cancer-associated types of HPV infection is through a Pap test—a small sample of cells is scraped from your cervix and examined in a lab for signs of abnormal cell changes. Pap tests can detect cell changes that may need to be monitored with more frequent exams or, in some cases, treated. (For more information, see "Pap Tests," p. 40.)

For women age thirty and older, a Pap test may be done in combination with an HPV DNA test. Your health-care provider takes a swab of cells from the cervix, just as for the Pap test, and the cells are analyzed in a laboratory. Currently available tests may identify fourteen of the high-risk HPV types associated with cervical cancer, or may focus on just a couple of high-risk types.[35] A negative Pap test and negative HPV test may mean the time before the next Pap test can be extended.

DNA tests currently are approved for use with women over age thirty (for whom HPV is less likely to clear naturally) and as a follow-up test for adult women who have unclear Pap test results. This test is rarely used for women under thirty because HPV exposure is so common and our bodies typically clear the infection without treatment.

Screening for cervical cancer is recommended for women who have been sexually active and who have a cervix. The U.S. Preventive Services Task Force recommends against routine screening of women older than sixty-five if they have had regular normal Pap tests and are not otherwise at increased risk (i.e., have a new sex partner or multiple sex partners).

Tests may take several weeks to complete. If you are infected with HPV, keep in mind that it doesn't mean that you will develop cancer.

Treatment of Warts

Genital warts can be treated by a health-care provider or by oneself. Health-care providers use mild acids (trichloroacetic acid), freezing (cryotherapy), burning with an electrical current (electrocauterization), or lasers. There are three prescription genital wart treatments that can be used at home. These treatments usually require repeated applications from a few weeks to a few months.

In some cases, warts return, so you may need repeated treatment. Talk with your health-care provider to decide which treatment might be best for you.

Complications

Genital warts are seldom dangerous, but they can be uncomfortable and can cause embarrassment with a new sexual partner. Some women report discomfort during sex at the place of infection even after warts have been removed.

HPV is the most common cause of cervical cancer, which affects about twelve thousand women in the United States each year. It can also cause vulvar, vaginal, anal, penile, and throat cancer.

For more information, resources, and support groups, visit the National HPV and Cervical Cancer Prevention Resource Center, created by the American Social Health Association, at ashastd.org.

HEPATITIS B

Hepatitis B is a viral infection that affects the liver. It can range in severity from a mild illness lasting a few weeks to a serious, lifelong illness.

In 1990, routine hepatitis B vaccination of children was implemented; it has dramatically decreased the rates of the disease in the United States, particularly among children. In 2007, there were an estimated 43,000 new infections in the United States, though the official number is much lower.[36]

Hepatitis B can be acute or chronic. Acute hepatitis B virus infection is a short-term illness that occurs within the first six months after someone is exposed to the virus. Most adults will clear the infection on their own, but 10 percent of people who are infected will become carriers who develop long-term health problems, including serious liver damage and liver cancer. There are an estimated 800,000 to 1.4 million people in the United States who have chronic hepatitis B.[37]

The best way to prevent hepatitis B is by getting vaccinated. For more information, see "Vaccinations to Prevent STIs," p. 277.

Transmission

Hepatitis B is fifty to one hundred times more infectious than HIV. It is usually spread by sexual contact through the exchange of bodily fluids such as blood or semen. Among adults in the United States, sexual activity accounts for nearly two-thirds of acute hepatitis B cases.[38]

Infection can spread among drug users who share needles, syringes, and other drug-injection equipment. Individuals can also become infected through direct contact with the blood or open sores of an infected person, by sharing razors or toothbrushes, or through exposure to blood from needles or other sharp instruments used in tattooing and body piercing.

Many people with chronic hepatitis B virus infection do not know they are infected, since they do not feel or look sick. However, they still can spread the virus to others and are at risk of serious health problems themselves.

Pregnancy and Childbirth

Hepatitis B can be passed from mother to baby during pregnancy and childbirth. Most newborns who become infected with hepatitis B virus do not have immediate acute symptoms, but they have up to a 90 percent chance of developing chronic hepatitis B.[39] This can eventually lead to serious health problems, including liver damage, liver cancer, and even death. Maternal screening for hepatitis B and early immunization of the baby right after birth, as well as follow-up immunization for those not vaccinated at birth, can prevent transmission.

Possible Signs and Symptoms

Often people who have hepatitis B have no symptoms. When symptoms do occur, they can include loss of appetite, weakness, muscle pain, headache, fever, dark urine, and yellowing of the whites of the eyes.

Screening and Diagnosis

Pregnant women should be screened at their first prenatal visit. Talk to your health-care provider about screening for hepatitis B infection if you live with a person who has hepatitis B, have had sex with a person who has hepatitis B, are HIV-positive, or use injection drugs.

Blood tests are used to diagnose infection and to determine whether you have antibodies to hepatitis B, which would mean you're not at risk. If you have chronic hepatitis B, your household members and sex partner(s) should be immunized against it.

Treatment

If your hepatitis B infection is acute—meaning it is short-lived and may go away on its own—your health-care provider will likely work with you to reduce any symptoms you experience while your body fights the infection. Follow-up blood tests may be needed to ensure the virus has left your body.

If you've been diagnosed with chronic hepatitis B infection, your health-care provider can suggest which antiviral medication may be most appropriate for you. If your liver has been severely damaged, a liver transplant may be an option.

Complications

Chronic hepatitis B is a serious disease that can result in long-term health problems, including liver damage, liver failure, liver cancer, or even death. People with untreated hepatitis B can become chronic carriers and spread the infection.

HIV/AIDS

HIV is the human immunodeficiency virus, which can lead to acquired immune deficiency syndrome, or AIDS. HIV damages a person's body by destroying specific blood cells, called CD4+ T cells, which are crucial to helping the body fight diseases.

In the United States, women and adolescent girls now account for 27 percent of annual new HIV infections, up from 7 percent in 1985.[40] This translates to more than 278,000 women and adolescent girls living with the infection.[41] Women and girls of color—especially African-American women—are disproportionately affected compared with white women.

The HIV prevalence rate for African-American women (1,122.4 per 100,000) is nearly four times the rate for Hispanic/Latina women (263 per 100,000) and nearly eighteen times the rate for white women (62.7 per 100,000).[42] Approximately one in thirty African-American women will be diagnosed with HIV at some point (as will approximately one in sixteen African-American men).[43] Relatively fewer cases have been diagnosed among Asian, American Indian/Alaska Native, and Native Hawaiian/other Pacific Islander females.

Among women diagnosed with AIDS in the

United States in 2008, 77 percent of African-American women, 75 percent of Hispanic/Latina women, and 65 percent of white women became infected through heterosexual contact.

Transmission

Two conditions must be met for HIV to pass from one person to another.

- The virus must be present in sufficient quantity. Five bodily fluids—blood, pre-ejaculate (pre-cum), semen, vaginal fluid, and breast milk—can carry enough virus to cause infection. Saliva, tears, sweat, urine, feces, and vomit (unless they are mixed with blood) do not ordinarily contain enough virus to cause infection.
- The virus must have a way to get into the bloodstream. HIV can enter a body through the mucous membranes that line the vagina and rectum; directly into the blood from a shared IV-drug or tattoo needle; through the skin via any open cut, wound, or scratch; through the mucous membranes in the eyes and the nose; and through the opening of a man's penis. Oral sex, rimming, fisting, fingering, and deep kissing are considered lower-risk activities for HIV transmission than penis-in-vagina and penis-in-rectum sex, unless blood is involved.

The virus can enter mucous membranes more easily if there are tiny cuts, inflammation, or open sores due to another STI or a vaginal infection. Therefore, your risk of becoming HIV infected or potentially infecting a partner is increased if you or your partner has other STIs that are untreated, or if you have untreated vaginitis or bacterial vaginosis (BV), a condition in which there is an imbalance of bacteria in the vagina.

Practicing safer sex is important even when both partners are HIV-positive. Unprotected sex among HIV+ partners can lead to mixing or exchanging viral strains, so one partner may spread resistant viruses to the other. Protection from other STIs is important as well. Barrier methods such as condoms and dental dams are recommended, as appropriate, for every sexual encounter. If one partner is infected and the other is not, using a barrier method can prevent infection of the uninfected partner. (For more information and guidelines on practices to prevent HIV transmission, see Chapter 10, "Safer Sex.")

HIV can also be transmitted by sharing drug needles with an infected user. If you are considering getting a tattoo or a piercing, make sure that you find out what steps are in place at the facility for sterilizing needles between clients.

Pregnancy and Childbirth

HIV can pass from mother to fetus (this is called vertical transmission) during pregnancy and childbirth. If you want to have a child and think you might have been exposed to HIV, get tested before you become pregnant.

In the early days of the HIV infection, women were often discouraged from becoming pregnant, owing to the 30 percent chance of HIV being transmitted to the child before or during birth and the likelihood that the child would be without a parent in the near future. That is no longer the case in the United States. Early testing, rapid testing at the time of labor and delivery, effective antiretroviral medication, and cesarean sections for women with high viral loads have contributed to reducing the rate of transmission from mother to baby to under 2 percent in the United States and other industrialized nations.[44]

Since HIV can pass to the infant through breast milk, the CDC advises against HIV+ women breastfeeding if they live in the United States or other areas where baby formula is

NEW HIV PREVENTION METHODS IN DEVELOPMENT

There is a desperate need for new prevention methods to halt the spread of HIV/AIDS. New kinds of cervical caps and diaphragms are being tested for effectiveness in HIV prevention, and researchers are trying to develop an effective vaccine.

The Centers for Disease Control and Prevention also are involved in several studies looking at the safety and efficacy of certain HIV medications that could be taken daily by people who are at high risk to try to lower their chances of infection if exposed to HIV. This preventive procedure is known as pre-exposure prophylaxis (or PrEP). Breakthrough research published in late 2010 found PrEP to be effective in a group of 2,500 gay men who took a combination of emtricitabine/tenofovir daily.[45] The men who received the antiretroviral medication, marketed under the name Truvada, experienced 44 percent fewer HIV infections overall than those who were in the placebo (or control) group that did not receive Truvada. Those who took the medicine regularly had much higher levels of protection. Larger studies are under way in the United States and abroad. PrEP has potential to assist efforts to prevent HIV transmission and specifically help women worldwide as a female-controlled prevention method in places or situations where condom use is unavailable or not an option. (For more information on PrEP, see the CDC website at cdc.gov/hiv/prep.)

There is an urgent need for prevention strategies that can be controlled by women, with or without their partners' consent, and microbicides are being developed explicitly for this use. Microbicides are substances that, when inserted in the vagina or rectum, could substantially reduce the risk of getting or transmitting STIs, including HIV. There are no effective microbicides currently on the market, but some are in development. (For more detailed information, see "HIV Prevention Methods," p. 799.)

readily available and can be safely prepared. In areas where there is limited access to formula and to clean water, some experts believe that the benefits to the baby of exclusive breastfeeding outweigh potential risks of HIV transmission.[46] Researchers are currently investigating whether certain types of antiretroviral therapy may help prevent transmission in cases where breastfeeding is necessary.

Women with HIV-positive male partners who want to bear children have several options. Some fertility clinics use special sperm-washing techniques that can remove viral particles, allowing the couple to conceive an HIV-negative baby. Other couples choose to conceive using donor insemination from an HIV-negative donor. If you would like to become pregnant and you have an HIV-positive partner, consult with a fertility expert to learn more.

Possible Signs and Symptoms

People with HIV often experience a flulike illness four to six weeks after the actual time of infection. This illness, recognized as acute HIV infection, corresponds to the seroconversion of the HIV antibody from negative to positive. Symptoms that occur at this time can include fever, swollen glands, rash, sore throat, muscle aches, fatigue, or outbreaks of herpes zoster or aseptic meningitis. The symptoms are often experienced as a bad cold or flu. Once seroconversion has occurred, most patients feel entirely healthy and may have no further symptoms of HIV infection for years. During this period, however, people can transmit the virus to others through unsafe sex or by sharing needles.

Screening and Diagnosis

The Centers for Disease Control advise routine voluntary HIV screening for all persons thirteen to sixty-four years old—adults, adolescents, and pregnant women—as a normal part of medical practice, similar to screening for other treatable conditions, in all health-care settings.

The guidelines indicate that blood tests should be repeated at least annually for everyone likely to be at high risk for HIV, including injection drug users and their sex partners, persons who exchange sex for money or drugs, sex partners of HIV-infected persons, men who have sex with men, and people who have had (or whose sex partners have had) more than one sex partner since their most recent HIV test.

If you are starting a new sexual relationship, it's a good idea for both you and your partner to get tested prior to having sex. If you or a partner has multiple sex partners (or you have reason to think this is the case), consider an annual HIV test. If you are pregnant, the test should be part of your prenatal medical screening. If you go for testing and treatment of another STI, consider including a HIV test.

See "HIV Testing," p. 306, for more information on when and where to get tested. Support groups and counselors are available at some testing sites to help you with testing decisions.

Course of HIV/AIDS

HIV attacks T cells (CD4 lymphocytes), which are central to a healthy immune system. If HIV is untreated, immune function eventually begins to break down. If T cell levels go below 200/mm, symptoms of AIDS start to appear. These include weight loss, fatigue, swollen glands (lumps in the neck, armpits, or groin), and skin rashes. Night sweats, fevers, thrush (an oral yeast infection), headaches, diarrhea, and loss of appetite can also occur.

Opportunistic infections—such as pneumocystis pneumonia (PCP), Kaposi's sarcoma (a cancer-causing virus), cytomegalovirus, esophageal candidiasis, or lymphoma—often occur when the immune system has been severely damaged by HIV.

Women with HIV often have unique complications. Recurrent vaginal yeast infections, chronic pelvic inflammatory disease, frequently recurring or disseminated genital herpes, or progression of human papillomavirus (HPV) infection can occur—and may indicate that HIV infection has progressed to AIDS.

Treatment

Antiretroviral therapies (ART) may allow people to live with HIV for decades, possibly for a normal life span. The goal of ART is to reduce the amount of HIV in the blood to undetectable levels. Achieving this usually allows the T cell levels to rise, sometimes back to normal levels, enabling the body to resist opportunistic infections. ART used to require taking multiple pills in multiple doses, but now it is sometimes as simple as taking one pill once a day. The increasing effectiveness of HIV treatment has dramatically reduced death rates and improved quality of life, and HIV is now often a manageable long-term illness. In addition, people who take their ART very consistently, without missing doses, are far less likely to pass HIV to a partner.[47]

Treatment can be challenging, however.

While many people experience initial side effects of the medications, including nausea or diarrhea, some have long-lasting side effects such as fatigue, bone loss, and fat redistribution. Some of the medications have been associated with diabetes and liver disease, and some may interfere with treatments for other conditions. It is important to make sure your HIV medicines are compatible with other medications you are taking, as well as with birth control pills. Tell your health-care providers all the medications you're taking to ensure you are prescribed the right medications at the right doses.

Taking ART consistently, as prescribed, is crucial. It is important to find a medical regimen that you are able to follow and tolerate. HIV mutates very quickly and can become resistant to an antiviral drug if too many doses are skipped or missed. If you don't take the drugs consistently, you may develop HIV strains that are drug-resistant, and you may not be able to use the drugs later in the course of the illness.

Not every person with HIV needs to be on medication; the decision is influenced by factors such as viral load and CD4 count. Current guidelines recommend antiretroviral therapy for those with T cell counts less than 500/mm.[48] Talk to your health-care provider about how to decide. Everyone who wants ART should have access to it, regardless of gender, socioeconomic or educational status, housing status, or drug use.

To complement the highly effective antiretroviral medications, some people with HIV and AIDS use acupuncture and Chinese herbs, meditation, yoga, massage, and many other holistic approaches to healing.[49] Some people find that these help reduce the side effects of the medications, bolster the immune system, and help cope with the stresses of illness.

Some AIDS service organizations, hospitals, and clinics provide alternative therapies regardless of an individual's ability to pay. The AIDS Care Project of Boston, for example, draws on federal and local public-health funding to offer acupuncture and traditional East Asian medicine at low or no cost in communities where HIV is prevalent.[50] If you have health insurance, some complementary treatments may be covered. (For more information, see "Complementary and Alternative Therapies," p. 674.)

HIV treatments are constantly evolving. For more information, see The National Women's Health Information Center's section on women and HIV/AIDS: womenshealth.gov/hiv/treatment.

How Do I Get Tested?

Testing is available in many hospitals, clinics, test sites, and doctors' offices. Visit hivtest.org (a service of the CDC) for locations near you.

In general, public-health clinics have a lot of experience with HIV testing and treatment, and they often offer post-test counseling, which your doctor or local hospital may not. Your results there will be confidential—that is, while your privacy is protected, the health-care provider knows your results and can follow up quickly. You can also go to an anonymous testing site or pursue a home test (see below).

Confidential test results will become part of your medical record. Testing laboratories are not required to share test results with insurance plans, but you should check your state laws and individual insurance plan. If you file a treatment claim for HIV or AIDS, your insurance company will know you are infected with HIV.

What Kind of HIV Test Should I Take?

- **Conventional HIV antibody test.** This is the most common test and involves drawing blood for the standard serological enzyme-linked immunoassay (EIA) test. These test results typically take about a week. Confirmation of a positive result (Western blot) is always done on the same sample, and a positive test is not reported until the results of the Western blot are known.

  Negative test results are considered accu-rate and definitive, unless a person is in the window period—the four to six weeks between when a person is infected with HIV and when the body has made enough antibodies to be detected by a laboratory test—in which case the test should be repeated three months after known exposure. Commercial tests are available for use with blood or saliva.

- **Rapid tests.** Rapid tests detect HIV antibodies and results can be available in under thirty minutes. They are especially helpful in settings where immediate results are important, such as in jails (where inmates come and go rapidly), in childbirth (to prevent mother-to-child HIV transmission), during outreach, or where it is unlikely that a person will return to get the results, including emergency rooms and STI clinics. Unless you're still in the window period, a negative result is over 99 percent accurate. A rapid test positive result is only preliminary; additional confirmatory testing is required to make the diagnosis of HIV. Emergency rooms across the country are increasingly making rapid testing available, especially when it can be linked with appropriate follow-up for people who do have positive results.

- **Home testing.** Available online and in most pharmacies, home test kits make it possible to collect a blood sample in private. You prick your finger, place a smear of blood on the piece of filter paper provided, and send it to a specified lab. The smear is identifiable only by an identification number. Seven days later, you can call a toll-free number to hear the results. Unfortunately, the quality of home test kits is highly variable. Although many kinds of kits are available online, currently only one—the Home Access HIV-1 Test System (homeaccess.com/HIV_Test.asp)—is approved by the FDA. A drawback of home kits is that they do not include provider counseling or referrals.

- **PCR.** This new type of test looks for HIV in a cell's RNA. This test can help make the diagnosis earlier in the course of infection than an antibody test, but because it is very expensive it isn't widely used.

Coping with the Test Results

If your test result is negative (and you are not in the window period), you may feel relief and gratitude, especially if you have been exposed to HIV. You may also ask, "Why not me?" if you have friends who suffer from the disease.

Finding out that you are negative may give you additional motivation to do what you can to stay negative. Or you may find, as some people do, that once you hear that you are negative, it is difficult to keep practicing safer sex or using clean needles. A support group, counselor, or friend may help you find your balance.

If your test result is positive for HIV, it is important to talk about your status with someone you trust and to give yourself time to take in the diagnosis. Help and guidance are available; to find out more, visit AVERT's section, Learning You Are HIV Positive: avert.org/positive.htm.

Getting the Best Health Care Possible

Finding health care is a crucial step, especially finding a provider experienced in treating HIV infection. So is negotiating whatever insurance or disability benefits might be available to you.

Because there are so many variables in treatment and new treatments are evolving, people with HIV do best when they see a physician who specializes in HIV. This may not be easy in rural areas or in smaller cities where there are fewer cases of HIV. In larger urban areas, there are specialized HIV centers and clinics that address the medical and socioeconomic aspects of the disease. Not everyone who is positive needs to be treated, but it is important to find an HIV specialist you trust so that you can learn where you stand, how to stay healthy, and how to protect your partner(s) from infection.

What follows is what should be the basic, minimal standard of care for all people with HIV or AIDS.

- **Evaluation.** A full physical exam with blood work, including CD4 cell (or T cell) monitoring and viral load testing, will help you plan and assess treatment. T cell monitoring indicates how well your immune system is doing; viral load and genotype testing indicate how much HIV is in your body and whether the virus is resistant to any of the currently available treatments. Other parts of routine care include a thorough review of your medical and medication history; periodic screening for other STIs, hepatitis, and TB exposure; review of vaccination history; referrals to a dentist and an eye doctor; and a referral to a gynecologist to screen for cervical cancer.
- **Vaccinations.** Vaccinations should be brought up to date, especially for pneumonia, hepatitis A and B, tetanus/pertussis, and flu, and possibly HPV. Your health-care provider may also want to discuss and assess your risk for conditions such as tuberculosis, herpes simplex virus, yeast infections, and other opportunistic infections.
- **Treatment.** Treatment should be based on the best available guidelines for the management of HIV and AIDS (see p. 304).
- **Support.** Emotional well-being is important, as are nutritional advice and the assistance of a social worker. Many if not most HIV-specialized care centers can refer you to appropriate support networks if they are not available on-site.

For more information on getting the best health care possible, see Chapter 23, "Navigating the Health Care System."

CHAPTER 12 ■ ■ ■ ■ ■ ■ ■ ■ ■ ■ ■ ■ ■ ■ ■ ■

I thought I was pregnant because I missed my period, but I tried not to think about it. I didn't want to talk to anybody because I was too scared. My mother would never let me forget it, so I didn't want to tell her, and I didn't want to tell any of my friends because I was afraid word would get around school.

Are you worried that you might be pregnant? You're not alone. Almost half of all U.S. women become pregnant without planning to at some point in their lives.

If you think you are pregnant, you may feel joyful and excited about the possibility of becoming a mother. You may also feel shocked, terrified, ashamed, or simply not ready to be a parent.

The first thing to do is to confirm whether you are pregnant. The earlier you know, the more time you'll have to plan. If you are nervous about the results, try to find someone who will provide support when you take the test and as you make your way through the process of finding out about and deciding among your options. You have the right to whatever support and advice you want, as well as the right to make your own decisions.

If you are pregnant, you might know what you want to do immediately, or you might find the decision agonizing. Many of us change our minds once we are faced with the reality of being pregnant, even if we always thought we knew what we would do. Be gentle with yourself. Remember that there is help to guide you through this time, regardless of your circumstances.

FINDING OUT

Any woman who has begun her periods, has not experienced menopause, and has vaginal intercourse with a man can become pregnant. Most unexpected pregnancies occur when the couple is not using birth control or is using birth control inconsistently or incorrectly. However, birth control methods can occasionally fail, even when used correctly. (For more information, see Chapter 9, "Birth Control.")

THE TEST

There are two different kinds of tests you can take to find out if you are pregnant.

- **Home pregnancy tests:** These generally test for human chorionic gonadotropin (hCG), a pregnancy-related hormone that can be found in urine. These tests are very accurate and can be used starting about the time

SIGNS OF PREGNANCY

Early signs of pregnancy vary from woman to woman and even from one pregnancy to the next. Here are some signs many women experience:

- A missed, lighter, or shorter-than-usual menstrual period
- Breast tenderness or enlargement
- Nipple sensitivity
- Frequent urination
- Feeling unusually tired
- Nausea and/or vomiting
- Feeling bloated
- Cramps
- Increased or decreased appetite
- Feeling more emotional than usual

Other causes besides pregnancy can produce these symptoms. Do not assume that you are pregnant until a test confirms it. If you are hoping you're not pregnant and you're sexually active, continue using birth control until you take the test in case it was a false scare.

EMERGENCY CONTRACEPTION

Emergency contraception (EC) is a kind of contraception that can be used up to five days *after* unprotected intercourse or birth control failure. Using EC dramatically decreases your chance of getting pregnant. For more information, see "Emergency Contraception," p. 251.

IS IT POSSIBLE TO BECOME PREGNANT WITHOUT HAVING INTERCOURSE?

It is possible, though very rare, for you to become pregnant without intercourse. Pregnancy is possible if sperm is on a hand that is then put into your vagina; if sperm lands in your vulva, right near the entrance of your vagina; or if clothing or material that is completely saturated with semen is in direct contact with your vagina. However, because sperm ejaculated outside the body survive only minutes to a few hours, getting pregnant without intercourse is highly unlikely.

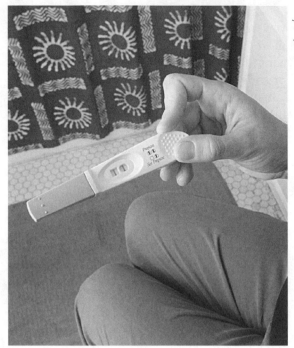

© Lynda J. Banzi

when you would have gotten your period. Most home pregnancy tests work similarly: You either put a test stick into your urine stream while urinating, or you collect urine in a cup and then put the test stick into the cup. After you wait a certain number of minutes, the results window on the stick will show either a line (bold or faint) or no line. A line is a positive test, which means you are pregnant. If the test is negative and it is less than one week past the time when you would have gotten your period, you should take the test again in several days.

You can buy home pregnancy tests at most grocery stores and drugstores. They usually cost between $5 and $15. You don't need to be over a certain age and you don't need a prescription to buy them.

- **Blood test:** Done at a doctor's office or at a health clinic, a blood test identifies if there is hCG in your blood. It can tell if you are pregnant about a week before you would expect to get your period.

FACTS ABOUT UNINTENDED PREGNANCIES

- More than 3 million unintended pregnancies occur every year in the United States.[1]
- About three-fourths of teen pregnancies are unintended.[2]
- Half of unintended pregnancies occur among the 11 percent of women who were not using birth control during the month they became pregnant.[3]
- The majority of unintended pregnancies among women who use birth control result from inconsistent or incorrect use.

SIGH OF RELIEF

If you suspected that you were pregnant but turn out not to be—and you don't want to become pregnant—here are some tips:

- Find a birth control method that is more suited for you. There are continual improvements and new options, and what may not have worked for you in the past could be substantially different now. See Chapter 9, "Birth Control."
- Buy emergency contraception (see p. 251) and keep a package on hand for backup.
- If you are being sexually abused, contact the Rape, Abuse & Incest National Network (rainn.org, 1-800-656-4673), or contact the National Domestic Violence Hotline (the hotline.org, 1-800-799-7233). More resources are available in Chapter 24, "Violence and Abuse."

SIGH OF REGRET

If you are not pregnant but realize that you wish you were, you now have time to prepare. To learn more about taking care of yourself and conceiving a child, see "Trying to Conceive," p. 356.

DECIDING WHAT TO DO

Once you learn that you are pregnant, you will need time to adjust to the news and the vast range of emotions that follow. Even if you are thrilled, you and/or your partner may feel emotionally, physically, spiritually, or economically unprepared to become parents now.

Your next step is to decide whether to continue the pregnancy or to have an abortion. If you decide to carry to term, you may choose to raise the child yourself or have the child raised through closed or open adoption or foster care.

Many of us feel emotionally torn for a long time before we choose the next step. Your body will be going through hormonal changes that affect emotions and feelings. Quiet reflection and talking with close friends or family may help you think through the possibilities.

Yet it is important to make a decision while it is still early in the pregnancy, so that you can either get prenatal care or have an abortion before the twelfth week of pregnancy, the easiest and safest time to have an abortion. Not making a decision will limit your choices.

Trust yourself; you can determine what is best. It is a highly responsible and moral act to clarify the right choice for you. The National Abortion Federation offers a free online guide that can help you decide. "Unsure About Your Pregnancy? A Guide to Making the Right Decision for You" is available in the Publications and Research section at prochoice.org.

FINDING SUPPORT

A partner who is loving and nurturing can offer wonderful support as you face an unexpected pregnancy. But even if you don't have such a person in your life, you deserve and need to be respected during all aspects of pregnancy and decision making.

FAMILY PRESSURE

Most of us have a relative who believes he or she knows what is best for everyone in the family. Some of us also have mothers or other relatives who always welcome a new child in their home, no matter what—and think you should, too. This could be because of religious beliefs, mourning over the loss of another child, or someone's identity as a caretaker. But this is *their* bias, and you are your own person with your own goals and needs.

Others of us have parents who are ashamed of and concerned about the effects of a child on them or their family. In either case, it can be difficult to go against your family's wishes—especially when family members threaten to withdraw support or seem angry with you—but ultimately you're the one who has to make and live with the decision.

A STRONG-WILLED PARTNER

Your partner may have passionate reasons for wanting you to carry to term or to abort, but even the most noble reasons might not reflect what is best for you. And sometimes the reasons are not so noble—for instance, he may fantasize that a child will suddenly turn your tumultuous relationship into a beautiful partnership. Or he may use a child or an abortion as another excuse to control your life.

If these situations are familiar, trust your instincts and seek support elsewhere. This is a vulnerable time for you; make sure to spend time reflecting on what you want, not what others want you to do. If your loved ones have strong opinions about what you should do, you may need to seek support to stand against their opinions or to wait until you have made your decisions before telling them. Sometimes doing what your heart says means going against what others want. Seek help from an objective friend or family member, or a counselor or trusted mentor.

ABORTION

Abortion is safe and legal in the United States, although your financial situation, age (if you are under sixteen), and where you live can make finding a way to get an abortion stressful. The safest, easiest, and most affordable time to get an abortion is within the first three months of pregnancy (calculated from the day of your last period). It can be difficult to get an abortion after

twelve weeks. For more information, see Chapter 13, "Abortion."

I was using the Pill with my long-term boyfriend. After we broke up, we had breakup sex, and the condom broke. One time was all it took! He did not want to be a father. I knew I could financially care for a child, but I did not feel it was moral to have a child who knew her/his father did not want her/him. I also did not feel emotionally secure [enough] to raise a child alone. I had an abortion and felt tremendously relieved.

CARRYING TO TERM

If you decide to carry your pregnancy to term, it is important to find a doctor or midwife who can determine how far along you are and help you get the care you need during pregnancy. For more information, see Chapter 15, "Pregnancy and Preparing for Birth."

I was in a stable, if long-distance, relationship, with a supportive guy who I knew would be behind me no matter what I chose. I spent a week thinking, wondering, agonizing, and writing. At the end, I realized that I wanted to be a parent,

IF I CONTINUE THE PREGNANCY, CAN I STAY IN SCHOOL?

Poverty is the reality for nearly all teen mothers and their children. One huge contributor to poverty is lack of education. One-quarter to one-third of female dropouts say that becoming a parent played a role in their decision to leave school.[4] Additionally, nearly 50 percent of female high school dropouts are unemployed, as opposed to 30 percent of women who earned a high school diploma.[5]

According to Title IX of the Education Amendments of 1972, teenage mothers have the legal right to remain in school, as well as the right to voluntarily enroll in special programs or schools for pregnant and parenting students. Many such programs in the United States assist teen parents by offering counseling, prenatal care, and day care, in addition to providing opportunities to obtain a high school diploma outside a traditional public high school. To find such a program in your area, ask a school guidance counselor or an employee at a local family planning clinic, or inquire at the office of your local school district.

I told my significant other that he could leave now, or he could stay and be a father. I'm glad he decided to stay. I've told my daughter, who is three now, this story many times. It's one of her favorites. I want to make sure she knows that I wasn't forced into having her, that I chose to be her mother.

SINGLE PARENTING

Parenting with the child's father is not always possible or desirable. As more children grow up without a father at home and more women become economically independent, it is increasingly socially acceptable for us to parent on our own. Babies are remarkably resilient and adaptable when they have a consistent, emotionally nurturing caretaker who keeps them comfortable, properly fed, and safe.

FOSTER CARE

If you decide to carry your pregnancy to term but are unsure about whether you'll be able to parent your child, you have several options, including putting your child into foster care and relinquishing the baby through adoption.

Foster care is a temporary situation. Throughout history, shared child rearing in extended families and among friends has helped ensure that as many children as possible have a chance to thrive. Almost a quarter of all children in foster care in 2008 were in relatives' homes.[6] Obtain a lawyer for negotiations for either informal foster care with a friend or family member or the government's formal foster care system. A legal document, even with a family member, will reduce a lot of assumptions and guessing about financial support, regaining custody, visitation, and many other factors.

The goal of foster care should be to provide you time to resolve your problems and make decisions about your parenting ability. Close to half of the children who left foster care in 2008 were in care for less than one year.[7] It is not in a child's best interest to remain in the foster care system for an extended time. Children who spend many years in foster care often end up going from one placement to another. If you have honestly reflected on your circumstances and believe that you will not be able to parent, consider adoption so that the child has the stable home she or he needs.

ADOPTION

I started to take a real long look at my situation and what kind of a parent I would be and what I wanted my child's life to be like. It hit me like a ton of bricks: I was not ready, nor anywhere near ready, to be a mommy. . . . So I did a lot of thinking, a lot of crying, and a lot of soul-searching, and I decided that the best option for me would be to place my child for adoption.

As recently as the 1970s, unwed women who became pregnant were sometimes sent away during pregnancy and coerced to surrender their babies for adoption. The secretive nature of closed adoptions is now considered psychologically unhealthy for both the woman and the child. Today, increasing numbers of birth mothers are choosing open adoptions, which allow birth parents to have some level of ongoing contact with their children. If you choose closed adoption, consider picking an agency that will keep information about you to give to the child and adoptive family if they request it. Also be sure that the agency is willing to help you find out how things are going later on, even if you feel now that you will never want to know.

Adoption can be a difficult choice. If you choose this route, you will be well served by creating a deliberate adoption plan with an adoption counselor and by using a reputable agency. A good agency pays for your legal and counseling services and does not offer you money. It treats you, not the adoptive family, as the client. To find a reputable agency, visit the Child Welfare Information Gateway (childwelfare.gov/adoption) or call 1-888-251-0075 and ask how to contact an adoption specialist in your state. Most states require adoptive families to undergo an evaluation. If your state does not require one, consider what your own requirements for the family would be.

Usually, you, as the birth mother, get to choose the adoptive family from a pool of applicants. If you are not offered this opportunity, you may want to choose another agency. Many agencies require adoptive families to provide yearly updates to the birth mother. It may be possible to write letters to the child and have them placed in a file for her or his future.

There have been many changes in multiracial adoption over the last twenty years. A good agency prioritizes matching the child's background with that of the adoptive parents. If that is not possible, look for a family with connections to a community that shares your values. If you or the birth father is of Native American descent, the Indian Child Welfare Act of 1978 may affect the adoption. (For more information, visit the National Indian Child Welfare Association's website, nicwa.org.)

You can also find an adoptive family through a newspaper ad, an independent adoption facilitator, a medical practitioner, or a lawyer. In such circumstances, you create the adoption plan directly with the adoptive parents and/or their lawyer. Keep in mind that the lawyer will have the clients' best interest at heart, not yours. Whether you choose an agency or a private adoption, it is advisable to have your own lawyer and counselor. An adoption counselor can work with the birth father and both of your families as well.

NOW THAT YOU'VE MADE YOUR CHOICE

Be gentle with yourself. Whatever route you decide to follow, you may grieve for the path you did not take. Grief is normal. It does not mean that you have made the wrong decision but rather means that you are feeling a loss. Reach out to others who have made similar decisions for discussion and support.

CHAPTER 13 ▪ ▪ ▪ ▪ ▪ ▪ ▪ ▪ ▪ ▪ ▪ ▪ ▪ ▪ ▪ ▪ ▪ ▪ ▪

Unless we can freely decide whether to continue a pregnancy, it is impossible for us to control our lives, to enjoy our sexuality, and to participate fully in society.

While there are more contraceptive options now than ever before, no birth control method is 100 percent effective, and access to reproductive health information and services is unevenly distributed, geographically and economically, both in the United States and worldwide. In addition, gender inequality, coercion, and violence mean we are sometimes unable to choose or control when we have sex.

Almost half (49 percent) of all U.S. pregnancies are unintended.[1] No woman should have to remain pregnant or become a mother against her will. Each woman must be able to decide whether or not to continue a pregnancy based on what she believes is best (see Chapter 12, "Unexpected Pregnancy"). Our ability to make these personal decisions should not be restricted by the government, religious institutions, or any individual. Unfortunately, abortion rights opponents in the United States have succeeded in placing many obstacles in the way of women who seek abortions.

WHO HAS ABORTIONS–AND WHY?

Abortion is one of the most common medical procedures in the United States. About one in four pregnancies, excluding miscarriages, end in abortion.[2]

U.S. abortion rates have declined from a high of 29.3 per 1,000 women aged fifteen to forty-four in 1981 to 19.6 per 1,000 women in 2008.[3] Approximately 1.21 million legal abortions were performed in the United States in 2008.[4]

On the basis of current abortion rates, about one in three women in the United States will have an abortion by age forty-five. There are many misconceptions about who has an abortion. The following statistics demonstrate that women who have abortions cannot be put in a single category.[5]

- Women between the ages of twenty and twenty-four obtain 33 percent of all abortions; women ages twenty-five to twenty-nine obtain 24 percent; teenagers obtain 18 percent and women thirty-five and older obtain 11 percent.
- Non-Hispanic white women account for 36 percent of abortions; African-American women, 30 percent; Hispanic women, 25 percent; and women of other races, 9 percent.

- Thirty-seven percent of women obtaining abortions identify as Protestant, and 28 percent identify as Catholic.
- Poor and low-income women account for more than half of all abortions; 42 percent of women obtaining abortions have incomes below the federal poverty level (in 2010, this was $10,830 for a single woman with no children).
- About 61 percent of abortions are obtained by women who have one or more children.

The most common reasons women give for having an abortion include concern for or responsibility to other individuals; inability to afford a(nother) child; interference with work, school, or the ability to care for dependents; difficulties with husbands or partners; and not wanting to be a single parent.[6]

FINDING AN ABORTION PROVIDER

Although abortion has been legal in all states since 1973, accessibility depends on which state you live in, how far away you are from a provider, how much money you have or what your insurance will cover, and how far along you are in your pregnancy. Eighty-seven percent of U.S. counties have no abortion provider.[7]

Most abortions are provided by freestanding clinics. Some specialize in abortion exclusively, while others provide a range of reproductive health care services.

Fewer than 5 percent of abortions are performed in hospitals. Over the past twenty years, the number of hospitals providing abortions has decreased—from 1,405 in 1982 to only 610 in 2008.[8] While only a small number of abortions are performed in hospitals, the impact of the decrease is greatest on women in rural areas, low-

FREQUENTLY ASKED QUESTIONS

Women and the public in general are exposed to a great deal of misinformation about abortion. In some cases, abortion rights opponents have intentionally spread myths. What follows are the facts.

- **Is having an abortion safe?** Having an abortion is safe, and very few women experience complications. Having an abortion poses fewer risks to a woman than going through pregnancy and birth.

- **Will having an abortion affect my ability to get pregnant in the future?** Uncomplicated abortion poses virtually no risk to a woman's future reproductive health, as shown by numerous studies. Very rarely, serious pelvic infection can cause damage to the fallopian tubes, which can increase the risk of ectopic pregnancy or fertility problems. You can decrease this risk by seeking prompt treatment if symptoms of infection occur.

- **Does having an abortion increase my risk of breast cancer?** No. In 2003, the National Cancer Institute convened a workshop of more than a hundred experts from around the world to evaluate the research. These experts concluded that "induced abortion is not associated with an increase in breast cancer risk."[9]

- **Do women who have had an abortion suffer from post-traumatic stress disorder, "post-abortion syndrome" (PAS), or "post-abortion stress syndrome" (PASS)?** No. In spite of claims by abortion rights opponents that women who have abortions are at risk of PAS or PASS, no such syndrome is recognized by any mainstream professional organization.[10] In fact, studies have shown that women most frequently report relief, positive emotions, and decreased stress after an abortion.[11] Some women also feel sadness and loss after an abortion, as well as anger, confusion, shame, and guilt, even when they know they've made the best decision. Abortion is not associated with long-term psychological distress.[12]

income women who depend on hospitals for health care, and women whose health requires hospital services. It also reduces the opportunities for training new health care providers to perform abortions.

The resources below can help you find an abortion provider and/or help with funding an abortion.

- **Planned Parenthood**, plannedparenthood.org, enables you to search by zip code or state for Planned Parenthood clinics that provide abortions, including those that provide abortions after the first trimester. You can also call Planned Parenthood at 1-800-230-PLAN.

- **The National Abortion Federation** (NAF) Hotline provides referrals to member clinics in the United States, Canada, and Mexico City: 1-877-257-0012. For information about abortion and other resources, including financial assistance, call NAF's other hotline

The following list includes some of the questions you may want to ask when you call for an appointment.

Medical Issues

- What abortion methods are available to me? What are the differences in terms of numbers of visits, costs, and restrictions?
- Is there anything about my physical condition or in my medical history that could interfere with my getting an abortion at your facility? Is there an upper weight limit for your abortion care? Will you perform an abortion if I'm HIV-positive?
- What pain relief and other medications are available? What is the difference in cost?
- Will the clinic be responsible for routine follow-up care? For treating complications? What type of backup services are available in case of emergency?
- I need a Pap test or chlamydia testing. Can I get these done when I come in for the abortion?
- Will birth control be available if I want it?

Financial Issues

- How much does the abortion cost? Must the fee be paid all at once? Is everything included, or will there be additional charges? At what point in the pregnancy will the fees increase?
- Will Medicaid or health care insurance cover any of the cost?

- Does your clinic have funds to pay for my abortion?
- Do you know of any other resources that may help with funding?
- If calling Planned Parenthood: Do I qualify for any financial support for the abortion?
- Can you bill my insurance company directly?

State Laws

- Are there age requirements? Do I have to tell my parents, get their consent, and/or bring proof of age? Will my parent or guardian need to visit the clinic? (For more information, see "Parental Consent and Notification Laws Affecting Teens," p. 325.)
- Is there a mandatory waiting period between the counseling and when I can have my abortion? Can I have the counseling over the phone, or do I have to come to the clinic?

Clinical Procedures

- How long should I expect to be at the clinic? Will everything be done in one visit?
- Can I bring someone else with me? Can she or he stay with me throughout the counseling and the procedure? If not, why?
- Will there be a counselor or nurse with me before, during, and after the abortion?
- How will my privacy be protected before, during, and after the procedure? Will my medical records be protected?

- Will there be someone in training performing my abortion?
- Will there be staff people who speak my native language? If not, will an interpreter be provided?
- Can you accommodate any special needs I have (for example, wheelchair accessibility)?
- Will there be protestors? If so, does your clinic have escorts who will accompany me into the clinic? How will I recognize them?
- Do you have counselors who can provide follow-up counseling after the abortion? Do you have names of private therapists you can give me who work with women before and after abortions?

The National Abortion Federation offers free brochures you can download, including "Unsure About Your Pregnancy? A Guide to Making the Right Decision for You" and "Making Your Choice: A Woman's Guide to Medical Abortion." These brochures, which are available in several languages, can be found at the National Abortion Federation (prochoice.org), under Publications.

number: 1-800-772-9100. You can also visit NAF online: prochoice.org.

- **The National Network of Abortion Funds**, fundabortionnow.org, maintains local funds in most states that can provide referrals, offer help with funding, or help identify sources of funding.

When looking for a clinic or provider, watch out for "crisis pregnancy centers," often listed as "abortion alternatives." These centers often draw women in by offering free pregnancy testing or ultrasounds and advertise themselves as counseling and referral agencies. In reality they are run by groups opposed to abortion. They are not staffed by trained health care providers, and they try to dissuade women from having abortions by giving misleading and inaccurate information. For example, they may tell you that the pregnancy is further along than it really is or that abortions are dangerous and cause breast cancer and/or infertility (they don't; see "Frequently Asked Questions," p. 318, for more information). Such centers are often located close to clinics that do provide abortions and have similar names.

Also steer clear of websites that claim to sell pills for abortion. While one type of abortion, medication abortion, uses pills to induce abortion, there are unfortunately many websites that will send fake pills or charge your credit card and send nothing. Contact the resources above to get honest information about medication abortion.

PREPARING FOR YOUR ABORTION

It's natural to feel anxiety and anticipation before your appointment, as you might before any medical procedure. Try to go about your normal activities and get a good night's sleep. It's important to avoid excessive alcohol, street drugs, and strong sleeping pills before the abortion.

Most abortions performed in the clinic are done while you are awake, with drugs that help you relax and ease the pain of cramping. If you are having heavier intravenous (IV) sedation or

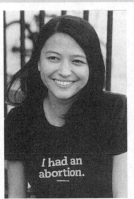
© Ali Price

I had an abortion.

IF I HAD LISTENED

A'YEN TRAN

If I had listened to the subway ads for postabortion trauma counseling or the men at the clinic brandishing rosaries and yelling racist pleas not to "kill your black/Hispanic/Oriental baby," things would be different. I would not hold a degree, and I would not be building a career. My child's father would have been a man who sexually, emotionally, and mentally abused me. Worst of all, my child would not have the financial and emotional support necessary for a healthy life.

When I was nineteen, I got pregnant for the first time. On the recommendation of a friend, I opted for a medical abortion. I was left to go through the process alone, which made the experience difficult. While my side effects were unusually strong, I was grateful and relieved to have been able to have an abortion.

Several years later, in college, I got pregnant again. The pregnancy may have been from a condom breaking or from carelessness in not applying the condom before the first moment of penetration. This time I had a surgical abortion. The doctor was kind and caring, and her assistant held my hand and told me what was happening.

I told my friends that I was having an abortion, and they offered ample emotional support. I didn't feel alienated, because I was part of a vocally pro-choice community. Now I coordinate a group of abortion clinic escorts to deflect the harassment of antichoice protesters.

If I had listened to the antichoice protesters, I would not be able to pursue my life goals. Currently, the World Health Organization conservatively estimates about 47,000 women die every year due to lack of access to safe abortion services. I want to change that. The world I envision is filled with happy, healthy, nourished babies and parents.

general anesthesia, you will probably be advised to avoid food after midnight, though clear liquids may be allowed.

Prepare for variable temperatures in the clinic rooms by dressing in layers. You can bring music, and you may even be able to listen to it during the procedure. Be sure you have documentation that the clinic requires, such as identification and your insurance card or some other means of paying for the abortion.

Even when abortion feels like the right decision, it may still be difficult. You may feel a wide

FUND ABORTION NOW . . . BECAUSE WOMEN'S LIVES MATTER

I realized I was pregnant two months ago, and ever since we've been working to come up with the money needed to terminate the pregnancy. During the day, I locked myself in the bathroom so that my kids wouldn't see me cry. I couldn't even sleep anymore, fearing that it might be too late at this point and feeling "forced" to have a child I don't feel equipped emotionally or financially to care for.

Last Monday, I sold my engagement ring to pay for groceries. That night, I sat up until three in the morning, looking online for someone who could help me pay for an abortion and help me find a clinic. I sent an email to the National Network of Abortion Funds, asking if they could help. The next day, a woman called me back with the names of a bunch of clinics and walked me through a plan to find the money for my abortion. It took a ton of phone calls and a couple of days, but in the end I got help from three different abortion funds around the country. Yesterday I had my abortion, and last night I slept for the first time in weeks.

The National Network of Abortion Funds estimates that each year more than 200,000 women who seek abortions need help paying for the procedure. The Hyde Amendment (1976) prohibiting federal Medicaid coverage of abortion and the lack of abortion providers in many communities make it difficult for many low-income women—including a dispro-

portionate number of women of color and immigrant women—to afford an abortion.

The National Network of Abortion Funds is a network of grassroots groups that work to break down economic barriers to abortion by providing financial assistance to women who cannot afford abortion care. The network is made up of more than a hundred individual abortion funds throughout the United States, Canada, Mexico, and overseas that raise money to help women cover the cost of abortions and related expenses, including travel, food, lodging, and child care. Some also provide counseling and other support services.

The National Network of Abortion Funds supports every woman's ability to make the most profound decisions about her life and her family, regardless of the amount of money in her bank account. Since 1993, the National Network of Abortion Funds has been supporting the work of individual abortion funds through training and resource sharing, and working to change the unfair policies that make abortion inaccessible. For nearly twenty years, the National Network of Abortion Funds has led the fight for repeal of the Hyde Amendment and worked to keep the experiences and lives of women affected by Hyde at the forefront of the conversation about abortion funding.

While abortion funds make abortion accessible for 20,000 low-income women a year, it is only by changing laws like the Hyde Amendment that abortion will be truly accessible to all women. To find out more about local abortion funds or the work of the National Network of Abortion Funds, visit fundabortionnow.org.

range of feelings, from sadness and grief to anticipation and relief. It can be confusing when even though you have decided that having an abortion is best for you, you still feel bad. Journal writing can be helpful, as can talking with a friend, acknowledging your feelings, honoring your decision, and having self-compassion. See "Resources for Support," p. 335, for recommended hotlines and websites.

Think about whether you would like someone to accompany you to the abortion procedure. Some clinics will allow a companion to stay in the room with you during the abortion, and some will not. If having someone with you is important to you, ask the clinic beforehand if it is allowed and seek out a clinic where it is.

WHAT TO EXPECT AT THE CLINIC

Though some private doctors' offices and clinics do not attract protesters, at other clinics there are regular "sidewalk counselors" and demonstrators. If you are concerned, call ahead and ask what you might encounter. Abortion providers are usually well prepared—there may be escorts who will meet you outside and accompany you into the clinic. If you live nearby, you may want to drive by or go to the clinic ahead of time to get familiar with the area. You will want to avoid direct contact with the protesters, even when they get close to you and say things that are mean and hurtful.

Once inside the clinic, you will fill out a medical history form. A health worker will check your vital signs (blood pressure, pulse, and temperature), repeat a urine pregnancy test, and draw blood to check for anemia and the Rh factor.* You may have an ultrasound exam to

PARENTAL CONSENT AND NOTIFICATION LAWS AFFECTING TEENS

If you are under age 18, you may be required to tell or get permission from one or both parents or a guardian before you can get an abortion. As of August 2010, thirty-four states require some parental involvement, while sixteen states and the District of Columbia allow minors to get an abortion without parental notification and/or consent.[13] To find out about the specific laws and policies where you live, visit the Guttmacher Institute at guttmacher.org/statecenter and click on your state.

Most pregnant teens do consult with their parents, either on their own initiative or when encouraged by an abortion provider.[14] The Abortion Care Network offers guidance on how to talk to your parents about your pregnancy at: abortioncarenetwork.org/mom-dad.

However, some teens don't feel safe telling a parent. If you have a parent who is abusive or so strongly opposed to abortion that you fear telling him or her, you have other options. A process called judicial bypass allows minors to seek permission from a judge to get an abortion, rather than from one or two parents. Many abortion clinics can help you negotiate the free and confidential process of obtaining judicial bypass.

---

* Blood is either Rh-positive or Rh-negative. If you are Rh-negative and the fetus is Rh-positive, you may form antibodies against the Rh factor in the fetal blood cells. In a subsequent pregnancy, these antibodies can react against an Rh-positive fetus, causing serious

harm. To prevent you from forming these antibodies, your provider will give you an injection of a blood derivative (one brand name is RhoGAM) within seventy-two hours after the abortion.

confirm how many weeks pregnant you are. The length of a pregnancy is usually counted from the first day of the last normal menstrual period (LMP) and not from the day of conception (fertilization).*

A health worker or clinician will talk to you about your decision to have an abortion and tell you what to expect during and after the procedure. In most clinics, if you are less than nine weeks pregnant, you will be given the choice of an aspiration (surgical) abortion or a medication abortion (see "Abortion Methods," below). The educational session is a time for you to ask questions and express any concerns. The clinic may also offer informational videos or group counseling sessions where you can talk with other women who are having abortions. In some states, staff/health care workers are required to give you materials or information that will try to discourage you from having an abortion. This is not because they want to do so but because certain states require it—a result of antiabortion politics. Once you have the information you need and your questions have been answered, you will be asked to sign consent forms. The next steps in your visit depend on the type of abortion you are having.

Many abortion providers now ask their patients if they would like to see the ultrasound image of their pregnancy during their appointment. Some women find the viewing helpful to their decision-making process. Others do not want to view the image. Either way, you should think about what you want and be sure to let the staff member performing your abortion know what you want.

Most women who have abortions in the United States are highly satisfied with their

care.[15] When you call to make an appointment (and, of course, while you are at your appointment), ask about anything that concerns you. Trust your feelings about the way you are treated on the phone as well as in person. You should not have to defend yourself to anyone; you should feel supported in your decision and how you want your care to be provided.

A staff member at a clinic describes how it can and should be:

At our clinic, counselors are trained to help each woman sort out her feelings. We do not invade anyone's privacy if she tells us that her decision is clear and not coerced, and that she does not want to discuss her reasons or feelings. At the same time, if she needs to talk through what she's feeling, we spend time working through those emotions with her. Women talk with each other, not just with the counselor. We provide very detailed and accurate information about the abortion procedure. A woman can have a friend stay with her during the abortion. When there is a decision to be made, the woman herself is an active participant.

ABORTION METHODS

In the United States, most abortions (88 percent) are performed during the first trimester, meaning through the twelfth week of pregnancy.[16] First-trimester abortions are performed using one of two methods: vacuum aspiration (also called surgical abortion) or medication abortion (also called medical abortion or abortion with pills). In vacuum aspiration, suction is used to remove the pregnancy; in a medication abortion, the pregnancy is interrupted and expelled over the course of a few days using medicines.

In the United States, most second-trimester abortions are done by dilation and evacuation (D&E), which involves dilation of the cervix and

* Though the date of your last menstrual period (LMP) can provide an estimate of how pregnant you are, LMP dating can be inaccurate, particularly for women with irregular menstrual cycles. A clinician will make the final assessment about how advanced the pregnancy is through a pelvic exam or ultrasound.

the use of instruments and suction. Alternatively, women who are more than twenty weeks pregnant may have the option for an induction abortion using medications that cause the pregnancy to be expelled.

Which abortion method is used will depend on how pregnant you are; your medical history, including any medical conditions or drug allergies; the training of the person performing the abortion; the equipment and supplies available; the approaches favored by the local medical community; and your own preferences.

MEDICATION ABORTION

A medication abortion, also called medical abortion or abortion with pills, consists of a two-drug regimen that ends a pregnancy within the first nine weeks of pregnancy. A medication abortion is different from using emergency contraceptive pills (EC, otherwise known as morning-after pills) such as Plan B, which can be taken up to three days after unprotected intercourse to prevent conception, or ella, which can be taken up to five days after unprotected intercourse. (For more information, see "Emergency Contraception," p. 251.)

In the United States, the most common kind of medication abortion involves the drugs mifepristone (also known as Mifeprex, RU-486, or the "abortion pill") and misoprostol. The mifepristone is taken orally at the doctor's office or clinic, and the misoprostol is used later, usually at home. In a few clinics, Methotrexate (an injection) plus misoprostol is used for medication abortion.* Methotrexate is more common in Canada, where women do not yet have access to mifepristone.

Medication abortion with mifepristone/

---

* Most clinics now use mifepristone plus misoprostol because it is more effective than methotrexate. Methotrexate is available in some clinics because it is less expensive than mifepristone.

misoprostol is very safe and about 95 to 98 percent effective. In 2 to 5 percent of cases, women will need a vacuum aspiration to complete the abortion. This may be because the drugs didn't work and the pregnancy continues (about 1 percent of the time) or because of heavy or prolonged bleeding. Since September 2000, when the U.S. Food and Drug Administration approved mifepristone, more than a million women in the United States have safely used mifepristone/misoprostol,[17] and millions more worldwide have used it since it first became available in France in the late 1980s.

Mifepristone works by blocking progesterone, a hormone that is needed to sustain a pregnancy. Without progesterone, the embryo detaches from the uterine lining. Misoprostol, a prostaglandin that is either inserted into the vagina or allowed to dissolve inside your mouth (between your cheeks and gums or under your tongue), causes the cervix to become soft and the uterus to cramp. The embryo is then expelled in what seems like a heavy period.

After taking the mifepristone at the doctor's office or clinic, you may experience bleeding, nausea, or fatigue. Even if you have bleeding, it is very important to take the misoprostol as instructed. Most clinics recommend that you use the misoprostol twenty-four to forty-eight hours after the mifepristone. The waiting time is important and increases the likelihood that the medications will work.

Most women use the misoprostol at home. Cramping and bleeding, possibly heavier than your normal period, will usually begin within a few hours. You can take over-the-counter pain relievers such as aspirin, Tylenol, or ibuprofen for the pain, and many women find that a heating pad or hot water bottle helps relieve the cramping. Other common side effects include nausea, vomiting, diarrhea, fever, chills, or fatigue.

It is normal to have more bleeding than a normal menstrual period and pass blood clots.

EARLY ABORTION OPTIONS*

ABORTION PILL/MEDICATION ABORTION WITH MIFEPRISTONE AND MISOPROSTOL	ASPIRATION ABORTION (SUCTION OR VACUUM ASPIRATION)
How far along in the pregnancy can I be?	
Up to nine weeks from the first day of your last period	Up to twelve to fourteen weeks from the first day of your last period
What will happen?	
The abortion takes place at home.	The abortion takes place in the office.
• *Generally, in the office*, you swallow the abortion pill (mifepristone). Most women feel fine after taking mifepristone. Some women have nausea.	• The actual abortion procedure takes five to ten minutes.
• *At home*, twelve to seventy-two hours later, take the misoprostol bucally (in the cheek) or vaginally, as instructed by your health care provider.	• The doctor puts instruments in your vagina and uterus to remove the pregnancy.
• The abortion starts one to four hours after you take the misoprostol. You have heavy bleeding and cramps for a couple of hours.	• You return to the clinic if you are experiencing problems or if you would like to see a provider (a return visit is not required).
• You check in with your clinic about a week later to be sure the abortion is complete.	
How painful is it?	
You will have mild to very strong cramps off and on during the abortion. Pain pills help.	You will have mild to very strong cramps during the abortion. Pain pills help.
How much will I bleed?	
Heavy bleeding with clots is common during the time you are passing the pregnancy. After that, lighter bleeding may continue off and on for one to two weeks or more.	Most women have light bleeding for one to seven days. Bleeding may continue off and on for a few weeks.
How much does it cost?	
For both types of abortion, the exact cost depends on where you go.	
Can the abortion fail?	
The pills work 95 to 98% of the time. If the pills fail, you must have an aspiration abortion.	It works 99% of the time. If it fails, you must have a repeat aspiration.
Can I still have children afterward?	
Yes. Neither type of abortion lowers your chances of getting pregnant or staying pregnant in the future.	

(continued)

ABORTION PILL/MEDICATION ABORTION WITH MIFEPRISTONE AND MISOPROSTOL	ASPIRATION ABORTION (SUCTION OR VACUUM ASPIRATION)
Is it safe?	
Both pills have been used safely for more than ten years in the United States and over twenty years in Europe. Big problems are rare. Medication abortion carries at least ten times less risk of health complications than continuing a pregnancy.	Aspiration abortion has been done safely for over forty years. Abortion in the first eight weeks is the safest, and problems with any first trimester abortion are rare. Surgical abortion carries at least ten times less risk of health complications than continuing a pregnancy.
What are the advantages?	
• You won't have shots, anesthesia, or instruments in your body • It may feel more natural, like a miscarriage. • It can be done earlier in the pregnancy than an aspiration abortion. • Being at home instead of in an office may be more private. • You can choose to have someone with you, or you can be alone.	• It is over in a few minutes. • You see less bleeding than you would with a medication abortion. • Medical staff members are with you during the abortion. • It can be done later in the pregnancy than a medication abortion.
What are the disadvantages?	
• It takes one to two days to complete the abortion. • It is not the same for all women. • Bleeding can be very heavy and may last longer than with an aspiration abortion. • Cramps can be severe and last longer than with an aspiration abortion. • It cannot be done as late in the first trimester of pregnancy as an aspiration abortion. • It cannot end a tubal pregnancy.	• It is more invasive; instruments are inserted through the vagina and into the uterus. • Anesthetics and pain medicines may cause side effects. • You have less control over the abortion procedure and perhaps over who is with you. • The vacuum aspirator may seem noisy. • It cannot be done as early in pregnancy as a medication abortion. • It cannot end a tubal pregnancy.

* Adapted with permission from the Reproductive Health Access Project, reproductiveaccess.org/fact_sheets/early_abortion_options.htm.

You may also see light pink or whitish wispy tissue, which is the gestational sac. The embryo is less than half a centimeter long at this stage and is often embedded in a blood clot. Severe lower abdominal cramps typically mean that pregnancy tissue is passing out of the uterus. The cramping may occur in waves (see "Controlling Pain and Anxiety," p. 331, for coping techniques). Generally, cramping will subside after the tissue passes (about four hours, but each woman's body is different). The bleeding will gradually decrease over the next few days, and light spotting often continues for one to three weeks.

Though complications are rare, if you have heavy bleeding (enough to soak through two or more thick full-size sanitary pads per hour for two consecutive hours), have sharp abdominal

EXPERIENCES OF WOMEN WHO HAVE HAD A MEDICATION ABORTION

In the United States, the percentage of women who choose the method varies quite a bit from region to region and clinic to clinic. In 2005, 22 percent of women who were less than nine weeks pregnant chose a medication abortion.[18] Nationally it is estimated that medication abortion is used in 10 percent of all abortions.[19] Some of the reasons include a desire to avoid an invasive, surgical procedure; a perception that it is better, easier, or more "natural" ("like a miscarriage"); and a feeling that it is more private. Most important, studies show that the overwhelming majority of women surveyed are satisfied with whatever method they choose.[20]

This was a very personal and private procedure, which enabled me to have some control over this difficult situation. This procedure is not for every woman. The bleeding and cramping last longer [than an aspiration abortion] and are somewhat unpredictable. The hardest thing is the waiting between taking the medication and finishing the abortion. Aspiration would have been faster. However, for me it was better because I'm more private. I was comfortable being in my own home. Even though I did have side effects, this was [an] easier procedure, both emotionally and physically.

pain or pain in your lower back, or have a fever of 100.4°F or higher that lasts for more than four hours, call your provider or the clinic. (For more information, see "Symptoms to Watch for After an Abortion," p. 336.)

Most clinics require a follow-up visit to confirm that the abortion is complete. The clinician will do a physical examination, ultrasound, or blood pregnancy test. Sometimes these services can be managed by phone without having to return to the clinic. If the pregnancy is continuing, you will need to have a vacuum aspiration abortion. If the embryo has stopped growing but some pregnancy tissue still remains in the uterus (sometimes called an incomplete abortion), the clinician may give you more misoprostol, empty the uterus with suction, or simply ask you to return for another visit.

You will likely get your next period within about four to six weeks after using the misoprostol. Some women find that this first period after a medication abortion is heavier or has more clots than normal. A small percentage of women have an episode of extra heavy bleeding about three to five weeks after the misoprostol. (See "Aftercare," p. 334, and "Symptoms to Watch for After an Abortion," p. 336, for general abortion aftercare information and other symptoms that may warrant a call to your provider.)

VACUUM ASPIRATION ABORTION

Although the number of women in the United States choosing medication abortion (abortion with pills) is increasing each year, vacuum aspiration (also called suction abortion or surgical abortion) is the currently the most common method used for first-trimester abortions. In vacuum aspiration abortion, the uterine contents are removed by suction (aspiration), which is applied through a cannula, a thin tube that is inserted into the uterus and connected to a source of suction, either an electric pump or a handheld syringe. (If no electric pump is used, the abortion is a manual vacuum aspiration, or MVA.)

Vacuum aspiration abortion is a safe medical procedure. About 1 in 300 women who have a vacuum abortion in the first twelve weeks of pregnancy experience a complication that requires hospitalization.[21] The risk of death from abortion is always lower than the risk of death involved in carrying a pregnancy to term. However, gestational age—how far along the pregnancy is—is the most important risk factor in death from abortion. For abortions at under eight weeks, the risk of death is less than one in one million, compared with 9 in 100,000 at twenty-one weeks.[22] This is one reason why it is important to obtain an abortion as early as possible.

Before starting the procedure, the clinician will perform a pelvic exam to check the size and position of your uterus. In some clinics, ultrasound may be used either before the procedure, to confirm how far along you are in the pregnancy, or during or after, to ensure that the uterus has been emptied. Be sure to tell your provider if this is your first pelvic exam, and feel free to ask questions. Taking deep, slow breaths and staying as relaxed as possible may make the exam more comfortable.

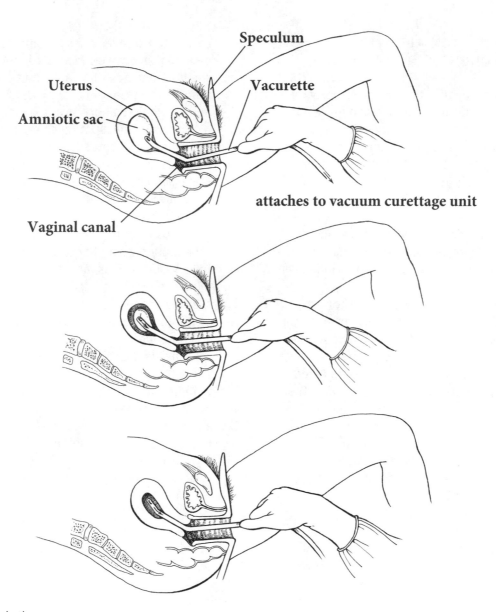

Speculum

Uterus

Vacurette

Amniotic sac

attaches to vacuum curettage unit

Vaginal canal

Vacuum aspiration

Next, the clinician will insert a speculum into your vagina to separate the vaginal walls and bring your cervix into view. Although you may feel pressure, this should not hurt. Ask the clinician to adjust the speculum if it pinches.

After washing the cervix with antiseptic so-

lution, the clinician will place a tenaculum (a long-handled, slender instrument) on the cervix. This instrument allows the clinician to hold the cervix in the proper position during the abortion; you may feel a pinch or a cramp when it is applied. Next, the local anesthetic solution is in-

CONTROLLING PAIN AND ANXIETY

Although it's natural to feel scared or anxious about experiencing pain during any abortion procedure, most women find the cramping tolerable. If you are having a medication abortion at home, you'll want to be somewhere comfortable where you can lie down and be close to a toilet. Use pillows for support, and try to find a comfortable position. A heating pad or hot water bottle may help relieve the cramps, and deep rhythmic breathing, which you can do on your own or with a support person, may help reduce pain and anxiety. Your provider may offer a prescription for pain medication or suggest over-the-counter pain relievers.

Ibuprofen is the generally the most effective painkiller for cramps. You can also use other nonsteroidal anti-inflammatory drugs such as naproxen (Aleve) and diclofenac. Acetaminophen (Tylenol) or aspirin also help, though aspirin may increase the bleeding. Do *not* use mefenamic acid (Dolfenal) or other antispasmodics; misoprostol makes your uterus contract in order to push out the pregnancy, and mefenamic acid or antispasmodics can interfere with the abortion process.

For vacuum aspiration, local anesthesia injected into the cervix helps relieve pain that may occur during dilation (opening) of the cervix. In addition, the clinic may offer medications either orally or through an IV that will help you relax and feel less discomfort and anxiety. These medications, sometimes called moderate intravenous sedation or conscious sedation, are different from general anesthesia and will not cause you to lose consciousness.

Some facilities offer general anesthesia for women who want to be asleep during the abortion. However, because general anesthesia can, in rare cases, cause complications such as breathing problems, uterine atony (failure of the uterine muscles to contract normally), and bleeding, it is usually not used for abortion.

Because each of us experiences and copes with pain in our own way, it's important to talk with your provider about what the clinic offers, the difference in cost, and what will work best for you.

---

jected around the cervix in two or more places. Although many women are apprehensive about this step, injections into the cervix are usually less painful than injections in other parts of the body. You may feel pressure, a pinch, or nothing at all. You may also feel a slight burning sensation as the medicine is injected into the cervix and brief cramping and nausea. Some women also experience ringing in the ears and tingling in the lips or tongue.

Once the cervix is numb, the provider will gradually stretch the opening of the cervix by inserting and removing dilators (tapered rods) of increasing size. You will probably feel pressure and perhaps some cramps on and off. Dilating typically takes less than two minutes.

Next, the cannula—a sterile strawlike tube—is inserted through the cervix into the uterus. The size of the cannula depends on how pregnant you are; it may range from the size of a small drinking straw to that of a large pen (half an inch). The clinician connects the cannula to a handheld vacuum device (manual vacuum aspiration) or an electric vacuum device and then moves the cannula back and forth to draw out the pregnancy tissue. If the clinician uses a vacuum machine (electric vacuum aspiration), you may hear the humming of the machine and a whooshing noise when the cannula is removed. The aspiration by handheld or electric vacuum usually takes only a few minutes.

You'll likely feel some cramping as the uterus contracts and empties. The contractions are important, because they squeeze shut the blood vessels of the uterus. The cramps may range from mild to intense, but they usually lessen immediately after the cannula is removed or within the next several minutes.

After wiping out your vagina and checking for bleeding, the practitioner will remove the speculum. She or he will examine the tissue to be sure the pregnancy has been fully removed. Sometimes women ask to see the pregnancy tissue. If you would like to, let the provider know.

A staff person will make sure you are feeling okay. Then you can move into a more comfortable room to sit or lie down for a while.

I was really nervous about being awake during the abortion, especially because I'm afraid of needles. But the numbing part felt more like pressure than pain, and the cramps were bad for only a few minutes. I held my partner's hand, did some deep breathing, and I couldn't believe how fast it was over.

I experienced some pain with the procedure, but mostly, it was just a series of new sensations. I had never been so aware of my uterus. I spent an hour lying down to recover. I remember being elated—it was over! The only way to describe it was relief!

ABORTION AFTER THE FIRST TRIMESTER

In the United States, about 12 percent of all abortions take place after the first trimester, at thirteen weeks of pregnancy or later, and about 1.4 percent of all abortions take place after twenty-one weeks of pregnancy.[23]

Women have later abortions for a number of reasons: not knowing of a pregnancy or how far along it is; difficulty raising money for an early abortion; indecision about how to handle an unplanned pregnancy; health problems that develop or worsen during pregnancy; or because serious impairments in the fetus are detected.* In one study, 58 percent of women who had a later abortion would have liked to have had the abortion earlier. Nearly 60 percent of women who experienced a delay in obtaining an abortion cite the time it took to make arrangements and raise money.[24]

The cost of abortion rises throughout the second trimester. In addition, these abortions require more time off from work or school and may require longer travel distances to find a provider. Although the health risks of abortion increase with gestational age of the pregnancy, the complication rates are still very low.[25]

The most common method of second-trimester abortion in the United States is dilation and evacuation (D&E), which involves removing the fetal and placental tissue with a combination of suction and instruments. A small number of second-trimester abortions are done by inducing labor with drugs, a procedure called induction abortion.

Many women prefer D&E to induction, because it is quicker and does not require hospi-

---

* To read one woman's story of having a later abortion because of fetal impairments, see "My Late-Term Abortion" at the Our Bodies Ourselves website, ourbodiesourselves.org.

talization or going through the physical and emotional stresses of labor. Some women, however, desire an induction abortion for many of the same reasons women choose medication abortion in the first trimester. Occasionally, women ending wanted pregnancies (because unexpected problems arise) decide to labor with an induction procedure in order to hold the fetus and say good-bye. This may also be possible after some D&E procedures (called intact D&Es).

DILATION AND EVACUATION

Having a dilation and evacuation (D&E) abortion is similar in many ways to having a vacuum aspiration procedure (see p. 328). Because the pregnancy is further along, however, the cervix needs to be opened wider to allow the larger pregnancy tissue to pass, which requires the clinician to soften and dilate the cervix ahead of time. This process of cervical preparation can take anywhere from a few hours in the early second trimester to a day or two for later procedures.

There are two main methods of cervical preparation: osmotic dilators and misoprostol, one of the drugs used in medication abortion. Osmotic dilators are short, thin rods made of seaweed (laminaria) or synthetic material (Dilapan). After inserting a speculum, the clinician places one or more osmotic dilators in the cervical opening. The placement takes only a few minutes. The dilators absorb moisture and expand over the next several hours, gradually stretching the cervix open. You will likely feel pressure or intermittent cramping as your cervix dilates. If you are having a later second-trimester abortion, you may have more osmotic dilators placed on the following day.

Once osmotic dilators are inserted, you should not touch or put fingers into your vagina, rub your belly, or get a massage. The osmotic dilators are removed at the time of the abortion. It's important to keep your appointment to complete the abortion; if you miss your appointment and the osmotic dilators are left in the cervix, you are at increased risk of infection, bleeding, and miscarriage.

The second way of preparing the cervix uses the medication misoprostol, which is a prostaglandin that softens the cervix (for more information about misoprostol, see "Medication Abortion," p. 325). The small misoprostol tablets may be placed between your cheeks and gums, under your tongue, or in the vagina a few hours before your abortion. Follow the recommendations of your clinician. Side effects with the doses used for cervical preparation are uncommon but may include cramping, nausea, mild diarrhea, or chills and/or a fever. Sometimes osmotic dilators and misoprostol are used together, particularly for later abortions or intact D&Es. For later abortions (after about twenty weeks LMP), an injection into the abdomen may be given to ensure fetal demise before the procedure is started.

Your provider may recommend stronger pain medication or sedatives for a D&E than would be necessary for vacuum aspiration, in addition to local anesthesia in the cervix. If necessary, the provider uses dilator instruments to enlarge the cervical opening further. Then the clinician removes the pregnancy (fetal and placental tissue) with vacuum aspiration, forceps, and a curette (a small, spoonlike instrument). This takes a few minutes, and you may feel a tugging sensation and some strong cramping as the uterus empties.

INDUCTION ABORTION

As the name implies, induction abortion involves medications that cause the uterus to contract and expel the pregnancy. After a certain point in pregnancy (usually around twenty-four weeks), a D&E can no longer be performed and the only option is an induction abortion. The experience is similar to labor, although as the fetus is smaller than a full-term baby the process may last a shorter time. Painful contractions can last for several hours or even a day or so. The procedure usually takes place in specialized facilities or hospitals, where the quality of care and degree of personal attention vary. Although a few specialized clinics have dedicated space for induction abortion, most general hospitals don't. Therefore, you may find yourself on a ward with women who are delivering babies. If possible, bring a partner or friend to support you and to help ensure that you get the compassionate treatment you deserve.

Preparation for an induction abortion is much the same as for D&E, except that you may need to plan for an overnight stay in the hospital or hotel located near the clinic. You will have blood tests and an ultrasound exam, and the clinician may use osmotic dilators to prepare your cervix (see p. 333).

Medications to induce abortion can be given in a number of ways. Most commonly, prostaglandin suppositories or misoprostol tablets are inserted into your vagina every few hours. Oxytocin (Pitocin) may be given through an IV line. For later abortions, an injection into the abdomen may be given to ensure fetal demise. Although this may sound scary, the abdomen is numbed before the injection, and you will probably feel only a slight cramp when the needle enters your uterus.

Each woman's experience is different. The contractions will probably feel like mild cramps at first and then become more intense. When the amniotic sac breaks, you will feel a gushing of warm liquid from the vagina. Later, you may experience a lot of pressure in the rectal area as the fetus is expelled. If the placenta does not come out within a few hours, your provider may use suction or a curette to remove it.

For pain, you may be given strong medications, sedatives, or epidural anesthesia (regional anesthesia commonly used in childbirth). Relaxation exercises, deep breathing, and the support of a friend can help make the contractions easier to tolerate. Medications are also available to control common side effects such as nausea, vomiting, and fever. You should be as comfortable as possible during the abortion process, so be sure to ask for more pain medication or support if you need it.

For more information on abortion after the first trimester, see ansirh.org/research/late-abortion.php.

AFTERCARE

After a vacuum aspiration or D&E abortion, you will go to a recovery area to rest. The staff will periodically check your vital signs and bleeding. It is normal to bleed moderately or even to pass small clots; the intensity of the cramping usually lessens during the first half hour. Depending on the procedure, the type of anesthesia you had, and how you are feeling, you may stay in the recovery area from twenty minutes to an hour or more. If you had IV sedation or general anesthesia, you will need someone to drive or accompany you home.

Before you leave, the staff will provide information about what to expect over the next few days and what signs to look for that might indicate a complication (see "Symptoms to Watch for After an Abortion," p. 336). Be sure you know the emergency number to call in case problems arise. You may also receive antibiotics to prevent infection and a medication to help minimize the bleeding (avoid alcohol, as it can increase bleeding). Avoid putting anything into your vagina (no tampons, no sexual intercourse, and no douching) for five days after the abortion, as the cervix is open and there is a greater chance of an infection during this time.

You may also be advised to rest and to avoid heavy lifting and strenuous exercise. Self-care is important, but work, school, and family circumstances may make some of these recommendations unrealistic. In addition, no studies have shown that these activities actually increase the risk of complications after abortion. The best guide is to listen to your body and use common sense.

Because you can get pregnant again shortly after an abortion, even before your first period, it's important to use reliable birth control if you don't want another pregnancy. For more information, see "Starting Birth Control After an Abortion," p. 337.

You may be given a follow-up appointment for two to three weeks after the abortion. At this visit, the clinician will check how you are doing emotionally and physically. Most women feel fine and do not have any problems after an abortion, but it's also normal to feel tired or to have cramps for several days. Bleeding ranges from none at all to a light or moderate flow, which may stop and then start again. Some signs of pregnancy (such as nausea) usually get better in a day or two, while others (such as breast tenderness) may take a week or two.

Emotionally, most women report feeling relief after an abortion, but it is also perfectly normal to have mixed or even negative feelings. The decision to terminate a pregnancy can be sad or stressful. It may be made more upsetting by the stigma against abortion fueled by those who are opposed to abortion rights.

One woman describes such an experience when she became pregnant at age 19:

I knew from the moment I found out that I didn't want to carry the pregnancy to term, but I was overwhelmed by images everywhere telling me that it was "wrong" to consider abortion. . . .

When I searched for information on the Internet, I was bombarded by religious websites with brutal pictures of aborted fetuses. When I tried to go to my friends for help, I was told they were "so excited" and couldn't wait for me to have a baby. My boyfriend kept saying how much he wanted a son. No one asked me what I wanted. I felt robbed of choice, like my body was being controlled by everyone but me.

My dreams of going to college and moving out were over because of one mistake. Finally, some kind of switch went off in my head. I couldn't afford to care what other people thought. I wanted my life back. If that is selfish, then I was willing to be selfish. What kind of mother would I be, anyway? The next day I made an appointment, but it was hard. I cried a lot. But that was two years ago, and I will be graduating from college in a few months. Most importantly, I tell myself every day that I made the right choice, and I know in my heart that I did.

SYMPTOMS TO WATCH FOR AFTER AN ABORTION

Your abortion provider is usually the best source of information or care if problems arise. If you require medical attention and cannot return to your abortion provider for care, ask for the best place to go in your area. You may not have a choice in emergency situations, but try to stay away from Catholic-owned hospitals or practitioners, as they oppose abortion and may not give you the most compassionate and appropriate care. If possible, bring a support person with you. When you receive care at another location, be sure to let the abortion provider know. This helps the clinics track their abortion complications and improve the quality of their services.

Abortion-related complications are rare in the United States, but they do happen. Below is a list of symptoms that may indicate a problem. If you have any of these symptoms or other concerns, get help immediately.

HEAVY BLEEDING

All women bleed during an abortion. In rare cases, some women bleed more than is safe. The best way to tell if you are bleeding too much after an abortion is to keep track of the number of pads you are using and the number and size of any clots. Call your provider if you soak two maxi pads an hour for two hours in a row, if you pass large clots, or if you begin to feel lightheaded.

The main way that your uterus controls bleeding after an abortion is to contract, squeezing the blood vessels shut. Heavy bleeding can occur if your uterus relaxes too much (uterine atony) or if some fetal or placental tissue is left in the uterus (retained tissue or incomplete abortion). Very rarely, excessive bleeding can be due to a uterine injury that occurred during the abortion.

PAIN

Uterine cramping is normal after any kind of abortion, but persistent or severe pelvic pain may indicate a problem. Contact your provider if intense pain persists after you've used a heating pad and taken pain relievers.

The most common cause of severe pain is an infection. Most infections are mild and can be treated at home with antibiotics prescribed by your provider. Postprocedure pain may also be caused by retained fetal or placental tissue (incomplete abortion) or clots (hematometra). If the tissue or clots don't pass on their own, you may need medication or a vacuum aspiration to empty the uterus.

In rare instances, pain may also indicate ectopic pregnancy, when an embryo is implanted outside of the uterus, most commonly in a fallopian tube. A growing pregnancy can stretch and burst the tube, causing severe pain and bleeding in your abdomen. Although ectopic pregnancy is rare, it poses serious health risks and requires immediate medical attention. An ectopic pregnancy is not removed by vacuum aspiration or medication abortion using mifepristone. It is usually treated with methotrexate or surgery. (For more information, see "Ectopic Pregnancy," p. 466.) In very rare cases, severe pain without an accompanying fever can be the sign of a lethal infection caused by the bacterium *Clostridium sordellii*.

FEVER

If you have a sustained fever of 100.4° Fahrenheit or above, you may have an infection. Misoprostol can cause a short-term fever. However, if your temperature remains elevated many hours, or if you have severe pain, call your provider.

CONTINUED SYMPTOMS OF PREGNANCY

Symptoms of pregnancy, such as nausea, bloating, or breast tenderness, typically resolve within a week or two following an abortion. If these symptoms persist, you may still be pregnant and should visit your provider. Taking a home pregnancy test is not useful, because you can continue to test positive for four to six weeks after a complete abortion, due to pregnancy hormones that are still in your body. Also, if you began using a hormonal birth control method (the Pill, patch, or vaginal ring) right after the abortion, know that these can cause pregnancy-like symptoms, particularly during the first few months of use.

STARTING BIRTH CONTROL AFTER AN ABORTION

Your abortion provider can tell you about the different types of contraception available and give you a method or prescription before you leave the clinic, if you so choose. Most contraceptive methods can be started immediately following the abortion—see chart on p. 338.

Condoms are the only method of birth control that also protect against sexually transmitted infections (STIs). To protect yourself from HIV/AIDS and other infections, use condoms even if you are using another form of birth control. For more information on contraception, see Chapter 9, "Birth Control." For more information on preventing STIs, see Chapter 10, "Safer Sex."

HISTORY OF ABORTION IN THE UNITED STATES

Abortion has been used to control fertility in every known society, regardless of its legality. It was practiced legally in the United States until about 1880, by which time most states had banned it except to save the life of the woman. Antiabortion legislation was part of a backlash against the growing movements for suffrage and birth control—an effort to control women and confine them to a traditional childbearing role.[26]

It was also a way for the medical profession to tighten its control over women's health care,[27] as midwives who performed abortions were a threat to the male medical establishment. Finally, with the declining birthrate among whites in the late 1800s, the U.S. government and the eugenics movement were concerned about "race suicide" and wanted white U.S.-born women to reproduce. More than most other medical procedures, the legality of abortion is linked to women's status and political power, as well as to

STARTING BIRTH CONTROL AFTER AN ABORTION

METHOD	WHEN TO START AFTER ASPIRATION, D&E, OR INDUCTION ABORTION	WHEN TO START AFTER MEDICATION ABORTION
Birth control pills, patch, vaginal ring, implant, Depo-Provera	On the day of abortion or within five days after	On the day of misoprostol use or within five days after. With heavy bleeding, you may wish to wait two to three days to use the vaginal ring.
Intrauterine device (IUD)	Immediately after abortion or at a follow-up visit. Expulsion rate may be higher if the IUD is inserted immediately after second-trimester abortion.	At or anytime after a follow-up visit when passage of the pregnancy is confirmed
Diaphragm, cervical cap, spermicides	After a first-trimester abortion, you can be fitted for a diaphragm immediately. You can be fitted for a cap when you resume sexual intercourse. After a second-trimester abortion, wait four weeks to be fitted for diaphragm or cap.	As soon as you resume vaginal intercourse
Condoms	As soon as you resume vaginal intercourse	
Fertility awareness method	Wait three cycles to be sure your normal pattern has resumed, and use a backup method until then.	
Sterilization	Anytime after you have made your decision	

the population and economic objectives of the society.

Even when it was illegal, abortion was widely practiced. The ability of a woman to obtain an abortion at all, let alone one that was safe, depended upon her economic situation, her race, and where she lived. Women with money could often leave the country or find a physician who would perform the procedure for a high fee. Poor women, for the most part, were at the mercy of incompetent practitioners with questionable motives. Often unable to find a provider, poor women and women of color disproportionately turned to dangerous self-abortions, such as inserting knitting needles or coat hangers into the vagina and uterus, douching with dangerous solutions such as lye, or swallowing strong drugs or chemicals. All women were subject to the desperation, shame, and fear created by the criminalization of abortion.

I had an illegal abortion, which led to infection, and I was close to death. I ended up in a legal hospital with a real doctor who managed to pull me through. Thank god the pregnancy was terminated. All this rubbish about guilt feelings is just that. Ask me if I would do it again knowing the risks—YES—absolutely. Thank heaven it's legal now, so women don't have to endure life-threatening situations.

When I was 15 and pregnant, abortion was illegal. I was denied any choice—I had a baby that I gave up for adoption. This experience has been a driving force in my life. I became an ob-gyn; I do abortions because I am totally committed to making sure that other women have the options that I didn't have.

Laws prohibiting abortion took a heavy toll on women's lives and health. Because many deaths were not officially attributed to unsafe, illegal abortion, it's impossible to know the exact number. However, thousands of women a year were treated for health complications due to botched, unsanitary, or self-induced abortions; many died, or were left infertile or with chronic illness and pain.

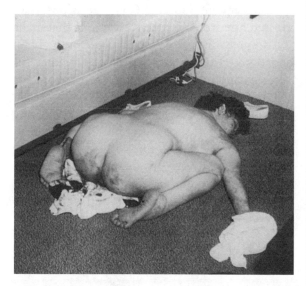

This controversial photograph first came to widespread notice when it appeared in *Ms.* magazine in the early 1970s. It was later included in *The New Our Bodies, Ourselves* as a depiction of an anonymous victim of an illegal abortion. We now know that the photo is of Geraldine Santoro. The story of her life and tragic death from an illegal abortion is told in the documentary film *Leona's Sister Gerri.* (Files of Dr. Milton Halpern, former medical examiner, New York City.)

MAKING ILLEGAL ABORTION SAFER

Before abortion was legalized, some dedicated and well-trained physicians and other medical practitioners risked imprisonment, fines, and loss of their medical licenses to provide abortions.[28] Through word of mouth, women found out how to obtain abortions. By the 1960s, the Clergy Consultation Service on Abortion, a network of concerned pastors and rabbis, and feminist groups had set up referral services to help women find safer illegal abortions.

In Chicago, a group of trained laywomen called the Abortion Counseling Service of the Chicago Women's Liberation Union went even further, creating an underground feminist abortion service. The group, whose code name was Jane, provided safe, inexpensive, and supportive illegal abortions. Over a four-year period, the group provided more than 11,000 first- and second-trimester abortions with a safety record comparable to that of today's legal medical facilities. Laura Kaplan, a former Jane member and the author of *The Story of Jane*, describes the women involved:

We were ordinary women who, working together, accomplished something extraordinary. Our actions, which we saw as potentially transforming for other women, changed us, too. By taking responsibility, we became responsible. Most of us grew stronger, more self-assured, confident in our own abilities. In picking up the tools of our own liberation, in our case medical instruments, we broke a powerful taboo. That act was terrifying, but it was also exhilarating. We ourselves felt exactly the same powerfulness that we wanted other women to feel.[29]

Throughout the world, wherever abortion is illegal and unsafe, committed people take enormous risks to provide safe abortions clandestinely, to treat women who have complications, and to help women find safe providers.

ORGANIZING TO CHANGE THE LAW

In the 1960s, inspired by the civil rights and antiwar movements, women organized a women's liberation movement. They fought, marched, and lobbied to make abortion safe and legal. At speak-outs, women talked publicly for the first time about their illegal abortion experiences. The women's movement, joined by sympathetic allies within the medical profession, made visible the millions of women who were willing to break the law and risk health and life to obtain an abortion. The movement also connected abortion rights to gender equality.

Between 1967 and 1973, about one-third of states reformed (fourteen) or repealed (four) restrictive abortion laws. Changes included allowing women access to abortion in certain circumstances, such as when the pregnancy was the result of rape or incest. In 1970, New York became the first state to legalize abortion on demand through the twenty-fourth week of pregnancy (Hawaii had earlier legalized abortion through twenty weeks, but only for residents of that state). Two other states (Alaska and Washington) followed, and women who could afford it began flocking to the few places where abortions were legal. Feminist networks offered support, loans, and referrals and fought to keep prices down. But for every woman who managed to get to New York, many others with limited financial resources or mobility still sought illegal abortions.

On January 22, 1973, the U.S. Supreme Court struck down all existing criminal abortion laws in the landmark *Roe v. Wade* decision. The court found that a woman's decision to terminate a pregnancy in the first trimester was protected under the "right of privacy . . . founded in the Fourteenth Amendment's concept of personal liberty." The court allowed states to place restrictions in the second trimester to protect a woman's health and in the third trimester to protect a viable fetus. However, the Court held that if a pregnant woman's life or health were endangered, she would not be forced to continue the pregnancy at any stage.

LEGALITY AND ACCESSIBILITY

The positive impact of *Roe v. Wade* on women's health in the United States was enormous. Fatal infections and hemorrhage due to abortion complications mostly became things of the past. However, the court did not secure abortion access for all women. Almost immediately after *Roe* passed, opponents of abortion rights began mobilizing, though it was not a major political issue for the Republican or Democratic parties as it is today.

Though unable to ban abortion outright, abortion rights opponents, through legislation and subsequent Supreme Court decisions, have created hundreds of state restrictions that make it extremely difficult for many women to obtain abortions. These state restrictions, which include excluding abortion from insurance funding, demanding that teens consult with one or both parents, and creating mandatory waiting periods and counseling sessions, have been devastating for the most vulnerable women: young women; women with low incomes, a disproportionate number of whom are women of color; women who live in rural areas; and women who depend on the government for health care.

Some abortion rights opponents go further in their efforts to impede women from having abortions by blocking access to clinics and harassing and intimidating abortion providers, patients and supporters. Operation Rescue gained notoriety in the 1980s for blockading clinic entrances, which provoked tens of thousands of arrests nationwide. Clinics have also been the targets of bombings, arson, anthrax threats, and acid attacks.

The massive protests and invasions of clinics

decreased after Congress passed the Freedom of Access to Clinic Entrances Act (FACE) in 1994, but FACE has not stopped the strategy of harassing individual doctors and their families by picketing their homes, circulating wanted posters with their pictures, publicizing their names online, or participating in direct violent attacks against doctors and clinic staff, including murder. Harassment and violence against providers have led to a sharp decrease in services.

In May 2009, Dr. George Tiller, an abortion provider in Wichita, Kansas, became the latest victim of antiabortion extremists when he was shot and killed in his church. Because Dr. Tiller's clinic was one of only a handful in the United States known to offer later abortions, including third-trimester care for women with serious health conditions or carrying fetuses with anomalies, he had become the most prominent target of antiabortion extremists in the country. His death inspired much reflection and activism around the words he often proclaimed: "Trust women."

A health care provider speaks about the impact of the violence:

The fear of violence has become part of the life of every abortion provider in the country. As doctors, we are being warned not to open big envelopes with no return addresses in case a mail bomb is enclosed. I know colleagues who have had their homes picketed and their children threatened. Some wear bullet-proof vests and have remote starters for their cars. Even going to work and facing the disapproving looks from coworkers— isolation and marginalization from colleagues is part of it.

Many physicians continue to provide abortions, despite the difficulties, because they deeply believe in women's right to choose. Dr. Susan Robinson and Dr. Shelley Sella, two physicians who worked with Dr. Tiller in Wich-

ita, say of their ongoing commitment to providing abortions:

Women have always needed abortions and will always need them. A very few will need abortions late in pregnancy. Rather than empathizing with these women and respecting their difficult decisions, society vilifies them and the providers who care for them. We believe it is a privilege to support women's decisions, to care for them, and to help turn their desperation into relief.

Dr. Tiller believed that kindness, courtesy, justice, love, and respect are the cornerstones of the doctor-patient relationship. He believed that women are capable of struggling with complex ethical problems and arriving at the best decision for themselves and their families. We share this belief. We are proud to continue his legacy.

RESTRICTIONS ON FUNDING

Insurance funding for abortion has been a central battleground. When the Supreme Court decided *Roe v. Wade* in 1973, public and private insurers covered abortion as a surgical procedure. In 1976, Congress passed the Hyde Amendment, which banned federal funding for abortion through Medicaid (a joint state-federal program for low-income people) unless the woman's life was in danger. Though some Medicaid programs use state funds to provide abortion coverage, they cannot access federal funds to do so. Although Hyde has since been altered to include exceptions for pregnancies that are the result of rape and incest, many women who should be eligible for funding are unable to obtain it. A recent study of abortion providers' experiences billing for Medicaid coverage in these circumstances found that less than half of the eligible abortions were reimbursed and one state represented most of these reimbursements, meaning that many states do not comply with the law.[30]

Twenty state Medicaid programs do not fund abortion under any circumstances.[31] When Medicaid is denied, poor women wait on average two to three weeks longer than other women to have an abortion because of difficulties in obtaining the necessary funds.[32] When abortion is delayed, health risks to the woman increase. A later second-trimester abortion is also more expensive than a first-trimester procedure.

Congress has extended the ban on federal funding for abortion to other groups, including military personnel and their dependents, federal employees and their dependents, teenagers participating in the Children's Health Insurance Program, members of the Peace Corps, disabled recipients of Medicare, federal prison inmates, and Native American women.[33]

Some of the restrictions on federal funds are even more stringent than those applicable to poor women eligible for Medicaid. For example, women serving in the military cannot obtain a federally funded abortion even when the pregnancy results from rape or incest. In fact, military doctors and health care facilities cannot provide abortions even if women pay themselves.[34] Women must go to private hospitals and clinics, though these are not available in many regions where women are stationed.

Lack of funding continues to be a significant barrier to abortion for thousands of women each year. It has also continued to be a rallying point for opponents of abortion. In the 2009 debate over health care reform, antiabortion legislators succeeded in passing an amendment to the legislation that expanded restrictions on insurance coverage of abortion, effectively excluding abortion coverage for millions of women. (For more information on how health care reform affects women's reproductive health care choices, see "The Politics of Reproductive Rights," p. 773.

CREATING OBSTACLES TO ACCESS

Abortion rights opponents have persuaded many states and localities to adopt mandatory waiting periods—which require women to wait up to thirty-six hours between receiving state-imposed, often biased information, and being able to have an abortion. These requirements burden women and doctors with extra costs and stress and result in delays in women obtaining care.[35] As the number of abortion providers dwindles, more women must travel longer distances for abortion services, stay overnight and pay for a hotel, take time off from school or work, or arrange for child care.

Until the 1992 case of *Planned Parenthood v. Casey,* the Supreme Court held that these laws were unconstitutional, finding that they did not promote women's health or real choice but were designed to stop abortion and express state disapproval of women who sought them. However, in the *Casey* decision, the Court allowed states to impose "informed consent" and waiting periods. As of 2009, thirty-four states specified the information that women must receive before consenting to abortion and twenty-six states require that women wait between consent counseling and the abortion procedure. As with parental consent, state approaches are diverse.[36]

Biased information laws in some states require that doctors give misleading information to women. For example, some states' written materials claim that abortion may be linked to an increased risk of breast cancer, despite the fact that the National Cancer Institute has concluded that no such link exists.[37] Similarly, some state materials discuss only the negative emotions a woman might experience after an abortion, entirely omitting the relief experienced by many women and ignoring the conclusion of the American Psychological Association that a

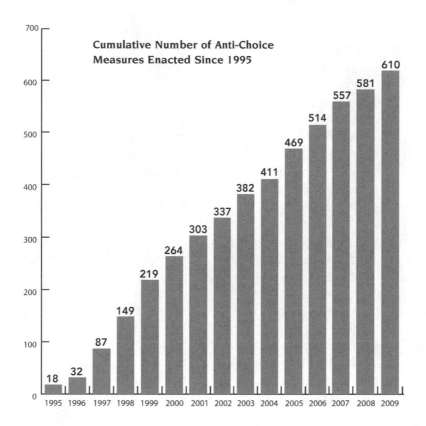

Cumulative Number of Anti-Choice Measures Enacted Since 1995

Who Decides 2010, NARAL Pro-Choice America Foundation

legal first-trimester abortion poses no greater risk of mental health problems to a woman than does carrying a pregnancy to term.[38] The goal of these biased information laws is not to give women information but to discourage abortion as an option.

Parental consent and notification laws also restrict access to abortion for girls and young women under age eighteen. Currently thirty-four states have laws requiring some parental involvement.[39] As a result of these laws, some teens must seek judicial bypass (permission from a judge) or leave their home state and travel to states with less restrictive laws to obtain services.[40]

Another strategy to erode abortion access is Targeted Regulation of Abortion Providers

laws, also known as TRAP laws. These laws, in place in thirty-five states, impose burdensome and medically unnecessary requirements, which are sometimes extremely expensive to implement. For example, some states have passed laws requiring that the offices of physicians who

DO YOU KNOW YOUR STATE'S ABORTION LAWS?

Visit the Guttmacher Institute State Center (guttmacher.org/statecenter/sfaa.html) for a look at the laws and policies that affect your state.

WEAKENING THE CONSTITUTIONAL PROTECTION FOR ABORTION

From 1973 until 1992, the Supreme Court rejected dozens of state efforts to limit access to abortion. With two big exceptions, the Court enforced *Roe v. Wade*'s ruling that until the point of viability, the state could regulate abortion only to protect the health and well-being of women.

The exceptions were the 1979 ruling in *Bellotti v. Baird*, which said that states could insist that a minor obtain parental consent or persuade a judge that she was mature or that abortion without parental notification was in her best interest, and the 1980 ruling in *Harris v. McRae,* which said that payments for medically necessary abortions could be excluded from the otherwise comprehensive Medicaid program.

Abortion rights opponents continued to persuade state and local legislatures to adopt more restrictive laws. In 1992, the *Planned Parenthood v. Casey* decision upheld a highly restrictive Pennsylvania law that included mandatory waiting periods, parental consent, and biased information. Further, the Court abandoned the legal principles of *Roe* and allowed laws designed to limit access to abortion at any stage of pregnancy, so long as the law does not place an "undue burden" on a woman's access to abortion. Though the decision said that spousal consent was an undue burden, in the aftermath of *Casey,* hundreds of restrictions have been passed and not seen to be in violation of the new standard.

Most recently, in the 2007 case *Gonzales v. Carhart,* the Supreme Court upheld the so-called Partial-Birth Abortion Ban Act. The law was passed by Congress and signed by President George W. Bush in 2003. Although there is no medical procedure known as "partial birth," the law has been interpreted as prohibiting doctors from performing an intact D&E (a procedure where there is no instrumentation before the fetus is removed) unless the fetus is no longer alive. The ban has resulted in doctors either choosing a procedure that is less safe for the woman needing a later abortion or ensuring that the fetus is not alive before starting the abortion. The PBA ban opened the door to state restrictions on later abortions.

In her dissent to *Gonzales v. Carhart,* Supreme Court Justice Ruth Bader Ginsburg decried the ruling, saying:

Today's decision is alarming. . . . It tolerates, indeed applauds, federal intervention to ban nationwide a procedure found necessary and proper in certain cases by the American College of Obstetricians and Gynecologists (ACOG). It blurs the line, firmly drawn in Casey, *between previability and postviability abortions. And, for the first time since* Roe, *the Court blesses a prohibition with no exception safeguarding a woman's health.*

provide abortions must meet health facility licensing requirements that are not imposed on other providers of comparable medical procedures. TRAP laws make abortion services more expensive and cumbersome for women, and they force the closure of some clinics. A law passed in 2010 in Virginia will likely cause seventeen of Virginia's twenty-one clinics to either close or spend millions of dollars in unnecessary and costly modifications to their clinics that do not enhance patient safety.

A more recent strategy of abortion rights opponents is to claim that because a fetus feels pain, later abortion should be banned. Several states have passed laws or introduced legislation saying that women must be told that fetuses feel pain or have set limits on how late women can seek abortions. In April 2010, Nebraska passed a law banning abortion after twenty-two weeks LMP (since a woman's last menstrual period) based on the claim that the fetus feels pain at that stage. The Nebraska law grants exceptions after twenty-two weeks LMP only in cases of medical emergency, the pregnant woman's imminent death, or a serious risk of "substantial and irreversible physical impairment of a major bodily function." It excludes the woman's mental health as a reason for abortion.

Though restrictions based on claims of fetal pain are growing in popularity, the best available scientific evidence indicates that a human fetus probably does not have the functional capacity to experience pain until after the beginning of the third trimester of pregnancy and that it is unlikely that pain can be experienced until after birth.[41]

REPRODUCTIVE RIGHTS AND JUSTICE

Abortion rights opponents have created an atmosphere that is stigmatizing, threatening, and too often violent. Sometimes just identifying oneself as prochoice can feel risky. But abortion rights activists continue to fight for reproductive rights and justice—by organizing large national demonstrations, engaging in clinic defense, conducting public education campaigns, and providing support for abortion providers and women who have abortions. See "What You Can Do," above, to take part in this movement.

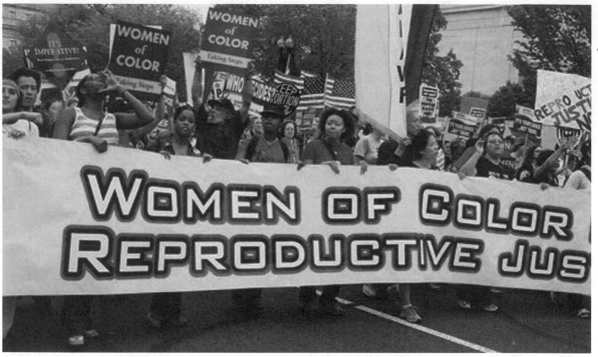

March for Women's Lives in Washington, D.C. (2004)

Over the years, the fight for reproductive rights has evolved into a movement for reproductive justice, organized by women of color and allies. Reproductive justice groups prioritize the rights of the least privileged women and see reproductive freedom as part of the larger fight for human rights and social justice. To learn more and to read voices from the movement, see "Organizing for Change: Reproductive Health and Justice," p. 813.

Childbearing

O ur choices about motherhood have expanded enormously over the past sixty years. In generations past, the
lack of effective birth control, along with rigid societal expectations, meant that almost all women who were fertile had
children. Today, however, access to birth control, legal abortion, reproductive technologies, and adoption make it possible for more of us to control whether, with whom, and when to
have children. In addition, changing laws and social mores
have led to greater acceptance of women who decide not to
have children, as well as of single women, same-sex couples,
and other nontraditional families who seek to conceive or
adopt a child.

For some women, the urge to have a baby is strong and clear:

Sometime when I was eighteen, some specific biological thing started to tick inside me—I think I actually have a memory of feeling it start, or at least of suddenly becoming aware of it. Out of nowhere came this deep hunger to be pregnant, to have a tiny living creature inside me, to experience my body going through the processes of pregnancy and childbirth. I think about being pregnant all the time, and my belly and my chest actually ache when I see pregnant people or small babies.

Others are equally certain that children are not in the future:

I am not interested in having children at all. . . . Fortunately [I am] with someone who also doesn't want to have children. We talk about the social pressures put upon us and the judgments we encounter, and how relaxing it is to be in a relationship with someone who shares the position of not wanting to have children.

And many of us find ourselves, at some point (or points), struggling with ambivalence:

I still debate whether or not I want to have children. Some of the reasons relate to whether or not I really want to dedicate that much of my life to children at the sacrifice of personal pursuits versus whether or not I think I will regret it or feel lonely one day for not making that choice.

Life's realities often interfere with our desires. You may be single and not want to raise a child alone or in love with someone who doesn't want to be a parent. Limited financial or other resources may make it difficult to imagine having and raising a child. You may find yourself pregnant without having consciously made a decision to do so, or you may be infertile or have an illness or disability that prevents conception, pregnancy, or parenthood. Having more control of our fertility can give us the ability and time to think deeply and fully about becoming mothers, but sometimes, for all the consideration we give it, what occurs is the opposite of what we intended.

THINKING ABOUT THE QUESTION

Children can bring joy and complexity into our lives in ways we might not even imagine. As they grow and change, we grow and change along with them. It can be wonderful sharing activities, stories, and places with our children that meant something to us when we were young. Children can challenge and inspire us to make the world a better place, and they give us a way to be part of the continuity of life. Many of us want to nurture and love children of our own and consider having a baby to be one of the richest human experiences.

I loved being pregnant, and our partnership while I was pregnant and when our girls were new babies was amazing: our emotional and sexual intimacy was intense. The feelings of joy and love and hope that I've experienced as a parent are like nothing I could have imagined.

At the same time, being a parent involves exchanging spontaneity and relative control of everyday life for a huge responsibility, complicated schedules, and relative chaos. Juggling your needs and dreams alongside the needs and demands of your child is an ongoing challenge. You may fear bringing children into a troubled world or want to pursue dreams incompatible with child rearing. Being child-free often means more personal freedom and more time, money, and energy to invest in relationships, work, and other interests and passions.

Not having a child has given me time to pursue my love of singing and theater. It allows me to

AGING AND FERTILITY

For various reasons, including access to birth control, more career and educational opportunities, and economic concerns, more women in the United States are delaying childbearing. Today about one in five women has a first child after age thirty-five.[1]

Many women who try to have a baby in their mid- and late thirties or early forties have no problem getting pregnant. Yet fertility does decline as we age, and many other women struggle to get pregnant or are unable to get pregnant or carry a pregnancy to term. This reality can put us in a bind: We may feel unready to have a baby now while also concerned about not being able to become pregnant later. For these reasons, it's important to understand the effect aging has on chances of conceiving and carrying a pregnancy to term.

During any given menstrual cycle, a twenty-five-year-old woman has about a 25 percent chance of becoming pregnant. This percentage begins to drop in the late twenties and decreases more significantly in the mid- and late thirties, until by age forty a woman has about a 5 percent chance of conceiving per cycle.[2]

These statistics sound more alarming than they are, though. A younger woman is *not* five times more likely to conceive than a woman of forty; she is simply more likely to get pregnant in fewer cycles. Over the course of a year, a woman who is between the age of thirty-five and thirty-nine has approximately a 60 percent chance of spontaneously conceiving (with no fertility interventions). The rate jumps to 85 percent after two years.[3]

Age affects our ability not only to conceive but also to carry a pregnancy to term. Chromosomal abnormalities, the cause of more than half of all miscarriages, are more likely as we age. A woman in her twenties has a 12 to 15 percent chance of having a miscarriage each time she becomes pregnant, while a woman in her forties has close to a 50 percent risk of miscarriage.

Statistics provide valuable information on the likelihood of conceiving and/or carrying a pregnancy to term. They cannot, however, predict what will happen for any individual woman. In addition, decisions about when to try to become pregnant, especially as we get older, are often complicated by factors that have little to do with age. Many of us put off having children because we don't feel emotionally or financially ready or because we don't have a partner and don't want to be a single parent. Yet waiting means that we may be unable to get pregnant when we are ready. Recognizing this reality in no way diminishes the importance or value of education, career, or other life choices that lead us to postpone childbearing, but it places front and center how difficult it can be to make decisions and compromises about when to try to get pregnant.

focus on myself, which is important to me because I'm in a helping profession. I can't quite imagine seeing clients all day and then going home and

taking care of kids all night. I do sometimes feel like I'm missing out on something really important, but most of the time I'm happy with my choice. I like having children in my life but not being responsible for them.

Like many of the choices we make, the decision whether to have children is influenced by our families, our communities, our culture, and the society in which we live. It can be difficult to separate our genuine feelings about being a mother from the external pressure most of us feel to have a child:

I debate this question under the shadow of the mainstream media that try to scare women into thinking marriage/children is the most important thing in life. . . . People, especially women, who remain single are seen as failures regardless of how successful and fulfilling the rest of their lives may be.

As we think about whether to parent, many questions arise. Some have straightforward answers. Others are more complicated: Does my job give me financial stability? Do I have a stable household? Is my partner or any other household member abusive in any way? What about alcohol and drugs? Are there family medical problems that might be passed on genetically? Do I have parenting skills, or am I eager to learn them? How will I juggle work and child care? If I am single, how would having a child affect any new intimate relationships? Do I have adequate health care insurance and accessible health care? What will the financial costs be? What kinds of values would I want to encourage in my child, and who could help me do this? What kind of community would I want to raise children in? Would I have support if I or my child develop a disability? Am I ready to prepare a child to deal with difficulties in life, such as racism, sexism, and homophobia? Am I too young? Do I know what I'm doing? Am I too old? What if something happens to me and someone else has to raise my child?

And that's just the start. If you have a partner, talk about the kind and amount of involvement in child rearing you each would want to have. Would one of you stay home with the baby? Would you find child care? If your partner is a man, you may want to be especially conscientious about discussing how he, too, and not just you, will be balancing parenting, work, and other priorities.

Try, too, to evaluate your emotional resources for parenting. Are there caring people around you to help you keep your perspective, your temper, your sense of humor, and your sanity in the midst of the emotional upheaval, changes, and chaos that occur with parenthood? Is there a mother or mother figures you can turn to for advice, support, and resources?

Answering "no" to any of these questions does not mean you should not have children. They are just considerations. Many of us feel that it's impossible ever to feel completely ready to be a parent:

My husband and I batted the idea of children around for a while. There are enough reasons to have them as there are to not have them. Every other milestone in our relationship seemed to take a while, but when we decided to have a child, we just closed our eyes and jumped. If we'd have deliberated on children as long as we did our other decisions, we'd never have a kid!

A NOTE ON LANGUAGE

It's difficult to find a term for having no children. Many people use "child-free." This chapter does also, although the term does not take into account the many ways that children—and commitments to children—may be in our lives even if we are not parents.

INFLUENCES ON YOUR CHOICE

Here are some common challenges, misconceptions, or issues that can influence the decision-making process:

- **Avoiding a conscious decision.** Some women let nature "decide" by not using contraception. Others delay so long that the decision is made by default.
- **Giving in to pressure from family members or peers.** Your parents especially might be eager for you to have children so they can have grandchildren, or your extended family may expect you to have children by a certain age. You may also feel pressure if many or all your friends are becoming parents, possibly making you feel you should do the same.
- **Letting your partner decide for you.** He or she might be eager to have a child or might want you to promise *not* to. You may go along with such a wish if you're afraid your partner will get angry or leave or if you're uncertain and just want the decision to be over. When you're newly in love, you may go along with your partner's wish to have a baby together or to abort a pregnancy and then regret it later. Pay attention to your feelings and seek support outside your relationship if you're having difficulty sticking up for yourself.
- **Thinking your partner will change.** In your eagerness to form a family, you may ignore warning signs that your partner isn't ready for parenthood. It's a mistake to think that negative traits or habits will disappear when your partner becomes a parent or that parenting itself will improve a partner's behavior. In addition, if you or your partner has a drug or alcohol problem, is irresponsible or immature, or is explosive and violent, it is unlikely that he or she will change when the baby arrives.
- **Thinking it's a decision between no children and two children.** Many of us assume that we must have two children, to provide the first child with a companion and as a hedge against having a spoiled only child. However, only children are no more or less spoiled, lonely, or maladjusted than children with siblings. For many people, a one-child family is just right.
- **Making the decision without knowing what children are really like.** How do you feel when you're with babies and children? Get to know your friends' kids or your nieces, nephews, and cousins. Take them to the park. Have a sleepover. Spend an afternoon playing games. Do you have a good time? Do you feel drawn to them?
- **Worrying that you won't be a good parent.** It is common to doubt your ability to parent. Be assured that you can learn, grow, and change by talking with supportive people in your life, reading parenting books or taking parenting classes, or discussing your fears and concerns with a counselor.

ISSUES FROM CHILDHOOD

Most of us bring issues from our childhood into adulthood. It is often difficult to think seriously of having a child until you work through the issues of most concern. Counseling can help make your past less burdensome and give you the space to consider parenthood. Some feminist counseling centers, family service agencies, community health centers, and other community organizations offer free or low-cost professional help.

Women who had particularly difficult childhoods often find it especially hard to make decisions about whether to have children.

For a long time I didn't want children. My desire to not have children was motivated by how messed up my parents were. I didn't want to bring a child into the world with that kind of baggage.

If you feel distressed or damaged by events when you were younger, you may wonder if you will be able to nurture a child. Many women who have lived through incest or physical abuse fear the physical changes of pregnancy, and medical examinations and inseminations can feel invasive. Some women with abuse histories find that pregnancy and childbirth sometimes trigger flashbacks or feelings of helplessness.

Taking time to reflect on and to address these issues can provide an opportunity for healing and growth, whether or not we become parents, and, if we do, help make the transition to parenting easier.

MAKING THE DECISION

Three women reflect on how they made the decision to have children and how they felt in the aftermath of their decisions:

I spent a lot of time being the oldest child and helping my mother out with my siblings. I don't remember being a happy child or ever wanting or thinking I would have children. Then I became a social worker and youth worker. One day I realized I spend all my time caring for children, exactly what I thought I didn't want! After getting over my fears, I finally had a child, and it is the best thing that ever happened in my very wonderful life. She is a complete joy, and I feel so lucky. My biggest regret is getting started too late and only having one child.

I love kids, but I've never had a strong urge to have them myself. I always wondered: How do you fit together the pieces of taking care of yourself and being a parent? I was single for most of my thirties, then got involved with someone who was sure he didn't want children. But I still felt it was important for me to make an active choice for myself—I didn't want to say no just because he said no. I talked with a lot of women, looked at both sides, then decided against having a child. The hardest part was

Read more stories about deciding whether to have children (p. 127) and how children affect dating and relationships (p. 129).

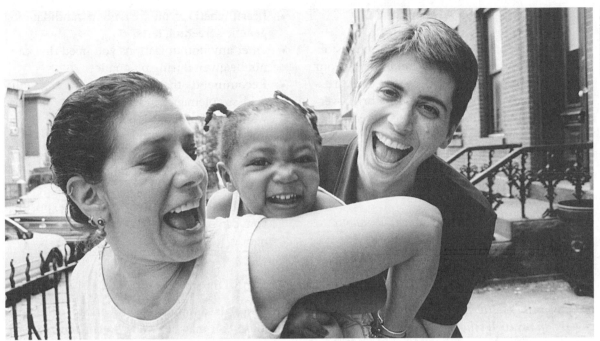

telling my parents, because I felt like they'd be so disappointed in me. But when I did, I felt a tremendous relief, and really, I haven't thought about it much since.

I had a child at forty-six. Before that, although I loved being with other people's children, anytime something went wrong and the child irritated me, I would think to myself, How could I ever stand the full-time responsibility of being a mother? Somehow, becoming a mother changed that. There is an intangible, indescribable bond intrinsic to the relationship that in the long run transcends the petty everyday irritating occurrences.

DECIDING NOT TO HAVE A CHILD

Once my husband and I had been married a few years, there were constant questions about when *we would start a family—particularly from our parents, whose friends were all grandparents. Then there was additional pressure when our friends were all having children—this changed the dynamics of our friendships and was an unexpected result of deciding not to have children.*

The societal and familial pressures on women to have children can be intense. Our culture sees having children as an intrinsic part of being a woman, and many people assume that a woman cannot be truly fulfilled if she doesn't have a child. Those of us who choose not to have children are often judged as selfish by those around us. Many of us find it helpful to join a support group or find others ways to connect with people who support and validate our choice. For more information and support, see the Childless by Choice Project at childlessby choiceproject.com.

PATHS TO PARENTHOOD

In becoming parents, we embark on a transformative journey. Welcoming children into our lives brings moments of elation, fear, grief, frustration, and joy. This section offers a brief overview of several different paths to parenthood: conceiving and bearing a child; adopting; or caring for a foster child.

TRYING TO CONCEIVE

It's amazing how little we are taught about our own bodies in health class. We get a few basic lessons on birth control, but that's it. Where is the detailed information on predicting the timing of ovulation and learning to monitor your own unique fertility patterns? It certainly wasn't covered in my high school health curriculum.

Once you decide to try to get pregnant, you may be surprised to find that you know much more about preventing pregnancy than about achieving it. Charting your menstrual cycle is one way to learn about fertility "signals" and optimize your chance of getting pregnant. (To find out more, see "Charting Your Menstrual Cycles," p. 26.)

If possible, it's good to meet with your health care provider or a maternity care provider before you begin trying to get pregnant. A preconception visit can help you learn about how to best prepare for pregnancy. During this visit, a good health care provider will do the following:

- Learn about your past pregnancies and births, take a family history, and examine you to assess for potential problems during pregnancy.
- Identify ways to help you manage current medical conditions and avoid pregnancy complications.
- Review all medications you are taking and recommend changes, if necessary.

- Learn whether you are a good candidate for genetic screening tests.
- Offer any immunizations you need that cannot be given during pregnancy.
- Recommend that you start taking folic acid supplements (400 mcg a day for most women) a few months before you start trying to conceive.
- Offer support and help for substance abuse, such as smoking cessation and/or alcohol or drug abuse.
- Identify any unsafe environmental exposures you can reduce or eliminate during pregnancy.

ADOPTION

Adoption is another way to create or extend families. You may be unable to conceive, or you may have a medical condition that would make pregnancy and childbirth unsafe. Some women prefer not to become pregnant or choose adoption over giving birth out of concern for children who need loving families.

Adopting Katy has been the greatest joy of my life. She is 11 months old now and was born in Kazakhstan. Several people have said how lucky Katy is or how brave I am to be doing this alone. In all honesty, though, I am the lucky one to have such a fabulous daughter, and courage has nothing to do with it. A mother's love and desire are what made (and continues to make) this family happen. I have never been more sure of anything and am thrilled that she is my daughter.

Another woman says of her experience adopting after infertility:

The time between finding out you cannot or should not have a pregnancy and deciding to follow a new dream is the saddest time. In life there are no guarantees, but if you go with an adoption agency with a good reputation, you can be almost certain you will become a parent. And once you make the decision, it is as if a rainbow appears. We call this our paper pregnancy, a child born in our hearts. Instead of running out of stores at the sight of a pregnant woman and avoiding the baby-product aisle at the market. I smile, hold my head up. I am on cloud nine.

Adoption entails logistical, emotional, and financial challenges. Though our options are often limited by finances, the requirements of adoption agencies and foreign countries, or the availability of children to adopt, learning about the various choices and being honest about whatever limits exist will help create a situation that will work for everyone.

My partner and I were present at the birth of our son, which we considered an incredible gift after years of infertility and a long adoption process. After a difficult birth, I was allowed to carry the baby to the neonatal unit, where he was measured and tested. It was in this intense moment that we learned that our birth mom had tested positive for drugs, so they were going to test our baby, too. I experienced an amazing tug of mixed emotions—I was furious at the birth mother for lying to us about her drug use and worried that the baby would have some problem that we weren't prepared to take on . . . [The baby] also looked terrible—so huge and puffy from the birth mom's untreated diabetes—and I worried whether I could love this ugly baby. Over the next few days, as it became clearer that the birth mom was going to follow through with the adoption, I still freaked out about my mixed feelings about the baby. Ironically, my partner, who had always been more ambivalent about being a mother, was the one who immediately and fiercely bonded with the baby. My feelings gradually resolved themselves as I spent time holding and talking to this little person in the

LESBIAN FAMILIES AND ADOPTION

Though increasing numbers of lesbian and bisexual women are choosing to adopt children, many of us still encounter discrimination as we expand our families. Although some adoption agencies will work with openly lesbian singles and couples, most of us are forced to adopt simply as "single, straight" mothers. However, once the adoption has taken place, several states allow a same-sex partner to be legally recognized as a parent through a second-parent adoption.

The Human Rights Campaign (HRC) website has extensive materials on the specific decisions and legal issues facing lesbians and bisexual women considering adoption (hrc.org/issues/parenting /adoption.asp). HRC also maintains a database to help you search for LGBT-friendly adoption agencies.

NICU [neonatal intensive care unit], where he spent six days. He began to lose his puffiness and turned into my beautiful baby.

There are a number of things to think about in planning to adopt. How would you feel about having and maintaining contact with your child's birth parents? Would you want to have a child who resembles you as much as possible, or would you embrace a child of another race or ethnicity? Do you want to adopt a newborn baby or an older infant or child? Are you willing to welcome a child with medical or emotional challenges? Are you open to parenting any child you are able to adopt?

The process of adoption can force us to confront complex ethical questions rarely considered by those who produce biologically related children: Why are home studies and other measures of parental fitness reserved only for adoption? How much control should we be allowed to exercise over the selection of a child? How can we be aware of, avoid, and work to prevent situations that might exploit or coerce birth mothers? How do we balance the potentially different needs of the child, birth parents, and adoptive parents regarding the degree of openness in adoption? Are those of us who live in wealthier nations "entitled" to raise children left homeless in other parts of the world by poverty or social stigma? How can we help our children deal with the racial, cultural, and identity issues they may face?

Many of us find it helpful to connect with a community of other adoptive and prospective adoptive parents or an adoption organization. They can answer questions, direct you to resources, and support you in the joys and frustrations of the adoption process. These groups are available in many cities, and many adoption websites offer online support.

Finances

Adoption is often an expensive process. To help offset the cost, the federal government provides a tax credit of up to $13,170 per child (as of 2011) to adoptive families; many states also provide tax credits or deductions. The military provides some reimbursement for adoptive families. Low- or no-interest loans are also available for adoptive families, and many employers offer adoption benefits.

Emotions and Relationships

The process of adoption can be an emotional journey. It is exciting to welcome our children, but there are also many times when we experience frustration, sadness, powerlessness, anxiety, and impatience. If you have been infertile, you may discover that adoption doesn't "fix" that experience. You may be elated at finally becoming a mother, yet still grieve for the pregnancies you will never have.

If you come to adoption purely through choice or preference rather than infertility, your primary struggles are likely to be logistical. The time it takes to find your child can feel as though it will never end, and it is difficult to plan ahead.

Women entering parenthood through adoption need as much support as women who are pregnant. The logistics of your life, your sense of identity, and your relationships will all change. In addition, you face challenges unique to adoption. You won't *look* pregnant, so you can choose not to discuss the ins and outs, ups and downs of your adoption process. On the other hand, others may discount your experience because they can't see that you are in the process of becoming a parent. In addition, some people still have misunderstandings and negative judgments about adoption.

FAMILIES AND PARENTS NEED A LOT OF SUPPORT

Parenting is hard work, both emotionally and physically. Our technological, fast-paced society does not serve the complex needs of parents and children, nor does it truly support and value caregiving within families. In order for women to balance the demands of family and work, we need a public commitment to family policies that make women's and children's needs a priority.

Child rearing is important and valuable work that deserves social and economic support. Whether or not we individually choose to have children, we all have a shared stake in the next generation and must work together to advance better family policies. For more information on the social policies that affect families, see "Being a Mother Today," p. 459.

We bring to childbirth our histories, our relationships, our rituals, our needs and values that relate to intimacy, our sexuality, the quality and style of family life and community, and our deepest beliefs about life, birth, and death.[1]

Pregnancy and birth are as ordinary and extraordinary as breathing, thinking, or loving. Whether you are having your first baby or are already a parent, each pregnancy calls on all your capacities for creativity, flexibility, determination, intuition, endurance, and humor. Similarly, each pregnancy should be accompanied by high-quality prenatal care, accurate information about pregnancy and birth, access to the full range of safe and healthy care options, and enough time for maternity leave. You deserve encouragement, love, and support from those close to you; a safe work and home environment; nourishing food; and time for rest and exercise.

Ideally, you will experience your pregnancy and birth within what childbirth advocates call "a climate of confidence" that reinforces your strength and innate abilities and minimizes fear. Some of the factors that contribute to such a climate can be achieved only through collective efforts to fix major problems in our maternity care system; others are more likely to be within your personal control. This chapter focuses on how to prepare for a safe and healthy birth and how to understand and navigate the U.S. maternity care system. It provides guidance for choosing caregivers who listen to you and respect you as an active participant in your pregnancy and birth and selecting a birthing environment in which you feel comfortable and safe.

Because of space restraints, this chapter doesn't address the physical changes of pregnancy, normal fetal development, ways to cope with pregnancy discomforts, or the symptoms and treatments of pregnancy complications. Many excellent books cover these topics in depth, including *Our Bodies, Ourselves: Pregnancy and Birth; Pregnancy, Childbirth, and the Newborn;* and *The Working Woman's Pregnancy Book* (see Recommended Resources). There are also many organizations whose websites feature trustworthy information, including Childbirth Connection (child birthconnection.org).

NINE MONTHS OF CHANGE AND GROWTH: PHYSICAL AND EMOTIONAL CHANGES

Pregnancy is a natural process. A new life develops inside you without any conscious work on your part. Cells divide, brain synapses develop, a new heart starts to beat.

The nine months of pregnancy are a full-body experience that can bring major emotional changes as well. Every organ system adapts. Your heart literally grows as it pumps extra blood throughout your body. Digestion patterns change as your body delivers nutrients from the food you eat to your growing fetus. Hormonal changes that support the pregnancy cause changes to your skin and hair. Your ligaments soften to allow your pelvis to enlarge to accommodate your baby as he or she is born. Your breasts grow, and you begin to produce colostrum, the earliest milk that will deliver nutrition and immune factors to your baby soon after birth when you breastfeed.

When it is time for your baby to be born, a remarkable cascade of hormonal signals between you and your baby trigger labor and allow it to progress. After birth, your body continues to offer your baby safety and comfort. Skin to skin, your baby will stay warm and quickly adapt to the many demands of life outside the womb. You and your baby will together experience hormonal shifts and physical sensations that set the stage for healthy attachment and breastfeeding. These same stimuli assist your body to recover from birth and minimize bleeding.

These remarkable changes assist with an even greater transformation: becoming a mother. Being pregnant transforms your identity and calls on your emotional strengths and resources. You may gain confidence in your own abilities as your body accommodates to the new life growing within you. Learning to trust ourselves and our bodies during the changes of pregnancy, birth, and parenthood may help us as we face other challenges throughout life.

As a woman who struggled with so many body image issues and an eating disorder as a younger woman, my first pregnancy was an exercise in body acceptance. Watching my stomach and hips grow and change in ways I could not control, I felt an alternating sense of disgust and amazement. When I began to look obviously pregnant, something changed. I was able to inhabit my body proudly, touching my hands to my belly knowing that my child needed this body to grow, develop, and give him life—never did I feel such love and pride about my physical body, and it was pure magic!

Many women report heightened perceptions, increased energy, and feelings of being in love, special, fertile, potent, and creative while pregnant. You may also have surprisingly strong negative emotions or feel ambivalent about this baby growing in you. These thoughts and feelings are common, even in planned and desired pregnancies.*

Sometimes it seemed like I had gotten pregnant on a whim—and it was a hell of a responsibility to take on a whim. Sometimes I was overwhelmed by what I had done. A lot of that came from realizing that I had chosen to have the baby without the support of a man. I was scared up until the third trimester that I wasn't going to make it.

You may have questions: How will my pregnancy change me and my life? How do I feel about my body changing shape? What supports do I have? How long can I keep working? Will I get laid off? Can I physically handle labor and birth? Do we have enough money? Will my baby be healthy? Will I be a good parent?

It is common to have fears and anxieties while standing on the threshold of the enormous and permanent change of becoming a

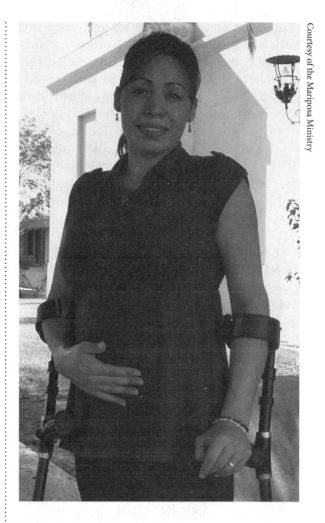

Courtesy of the Mariposa Ministry

mother. Many of us find it helpful to talk with other women who are navigating the changes that pregnancy and new parenthood bring. You may be able to find support in childbirth classes, exercise classes, and peer support groups designed for pregnant women, as well as on online social networking sites used by expectant and new parents.

Pregnancy and childbirth raise perfectly natural fears of pain and the unknown, and we can never be completely sure of the outcome, no matter how we care for ourselves in pregnancy, where or how we give birth, or how much we've

---

* If your pregnancy was not planned, or if you are deeply ambivalent about whether you want to raise a child, see Chapter 12, "Unexpected Pregnancy."

planned or prepared for it. Yet pregnancy and birth are intrinsically healthy processes, successful in the great majority of instances when understood, respected, and supported. Our own confidence can be enhanced when our providers offer intelligent guidance and support, so that, when possible, labor unfolds on its own. Used in conjunction with appropriate medical interventions for managing complications, these practices help ensure that we experience pregnancy and birth safely in a true climate of confidence.

CHOOSING A PRACTITIONER AND A PLACE FOR YOUR BIRTH

Although our maternity care system as a whole has major limitations, there are many providers who consistently offer high quality, woman-centered care as well as birth settings where staff share a commitment to supporting safe, healthy, and satisfying birth experiences. Take time before becoming pregnant or early in your pregnancy to learn about your options.

An optimal provider and birth setting will offer you:

- Care that is consistent with the best available research on safety and effectiveness
- An environment and treatments that support or enhance, rather than interfere with, the natural process of pregnancy and birth
- Individualized care that takes into account your health needs and those of your baby, as well as your personal preferences and values
- Abundant support, comfort, and information
- Access, either directly or through an efficient referral mechanism, to treatments for complications, should the need arise

Identifying your priorities, learning about the differences among various approaches

to childbirth, and finding out which options are available to you can help you make decisions that fit your circumstances and preferences.

CHOOSING A PROVIDER

Most providers are part of group practices, which means that you will be attended at birth by whichever provider is on call at that time. In addition, the provider on call will respond if you have any concerns during pregnancy that come up outside regular office hours. This can be frustrating if you have a good relationship with a particular provider but are offered care by another whom you do not know as well. On the positive side, working in such teams can give midwives and doctors more predictable, limited work hours; this entails less fatigue and can reduce medical errors. Some groups have you see one doctor or midwife for the whole pregnancy, while others rotate you through the group so you get to meet everyone. If you will be working with a group practice and have a choice, look for one in which all members have comparable philosophies of care that are well matched to your needs and preferences. Some practices host public events to introduce all the providers.

TYPES OF PROVIDERS

Midwives
Midwives have been attending and supporting women during pregnancy and childbirth, and teaching other women to do so, for centuries. All midwives are trained to provide women with prenatal care, care during labor and birth, and follow-up care after the baby is born. In the United States today, midwives attend approximately one in ten vaginal births, primarily in hospitals.

MODELS OF MATERNITY CARE

Before choosing a care provider and place of birth (the two usually go hand in hand), it is helpful to understand the two main paradigms in maternity care education and practice, described as the midwifery model and the medical model.*

The classic midwifery model is based on the assumption that most pregnancies, labors, and births are normal biological processes that result in healthy outcomes for both mothers and babies. It focuses on maximizing the health and wellness of a woman and her baby, identifying and managing medical problems early on, and attending to the emotional, social, and spiritual aspects of pregnancy and birth. Midwifery care seeks to protect, support, and avoid interfering with the unique rhythm, character, and timing of each woman's labor. Midwives are trained to be vigilant in identifying women with serious complications. Medical expertise and interventions are sought when necessary but are not used routinely.

A strict medical model of care focuses on preventing, diagnosing, and treating the complications that can occur during pregnancy, labor, and birth. Prevention

strategies tend to emphasize the use of testing, coupled with the use of medical or surgical interventions to avert a poor outcome. Medical expertise and interventions are vital for women and babies with complications. However, routine interventions on women at low risk of problems can actually lead to problems. Training in the medical model does not typically focus on developing skills to support the natural progression of an uncomplicated birth.

Although it is crucial to understand the differing philosophies and training among practitioners, it is also important to note that the letters after someone's name do not tell you much about her or him as an individual. Some doctors have attitudes, styles, and approaches that fit the midwifery model, and some midwives incorporate the medical model that is more common for doctors.

The midwifery model and medical model also give rise to two different ways of organizing maternity care systems. In most industrialized countries, midwives coordinate the care for the majority of childbearing women and collaborate with obstetricians or other specialists when a woman has medical complications or risk factors. Healthy women often give birth in midwife-led hospital units or birth centers or at home. In contrast, in the medical model prevalent in the United States, doctors manage the care of most women, almost all of whom give birth in hospitals. When midwives do provide the care, they are usually supervised by doctors and working under medical rather than midwifery protocols.

* These terms derive from the kinds of care physicians and midwives have historically provided. However, their use is not meant to imply that all midwives follow a midwifery model or that all physicians follow a medical model. Some people believe it is more accurate to refer to the different models of care as a physiologic model (that is, care in accord with the normal functioning of a woman's body) versus an interventionist or pathology-driven model.

Most communities in the United States fail to promote a midwifery model of care despite powerful evidence in numerous studies that underscore the benefits of midwifery care and the heightened satisfaction of women who use midwives. A 2008 Cochrane systematic review comparing midwife-led to physician-led models of care concluded, "Midwife-led care confers benefits and shows no adverse outcomes. It should be the norm for women classified at low and high risk of complications."[2]

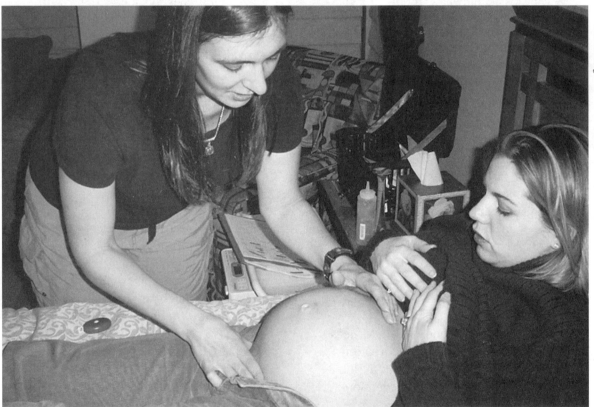

© Traci Palagi

Certified Nurse-Midwives and Certified Midwives

Certified nurse-midwives (CNMs) are educated in nursing and midwifery. Certified midwives (CMs) are educated only in midwifery. Both CNMs and CMs are specialists in the care of healthy women in pregnancy and childbirth.

They also provide well-woman care, which includes gynecological checkups, pelvic and breast exams, Pap tests, and family planning services. CNMs and CMs are certified by the American Midwifery Certification Board.

CNMs and CMs are able to attend births in hospitals, birth centers, or homes, and they typically have established relationships with doctors with whom they can consult as needed and who will assume care during pregnancy or labor if certain complications develop. Their services are usually covered by health care insurance policies. Depending on their style of practice, a CNM or CM might be with you for your whole labor or might function more as physicians do, coming in periodically to check on you and then being present when you give birth.

Because I had conceived through in vitro fertilization and had previously had a miscarriage, I was worried about my pregnancy. The reproductive endocrinologist I worked with frowned on any birth setting but a hospital. In addition, I had a serious gastroesophageal complication and wanted my providers to be on equal footing with each other. All this led me to choose an obstetrician. But when she announced she was leaving the practice (in my sixth month), I took the opportunity to reexamine my situation.

Not only had my OB and my gastroenterologist never communicated with each other, they gave me contradictory advice. I met with the other members of the obstetric practice and was uncomfortable with how they discussed epidurals and C-sections. I realized that no matter how I had conceived, I now had a normal pregnancy. Well into my third trimester, I switched to a midwifery practice and was able to have a natural childbirth like I wanted.

Certified Professional Midwives

Certified professional midwives (CPMs) specialize in healthy pregnancy and natural childbirth. They attend births at home and, in some states, birth centers. They learn their profession by attending freestanding midwifery schools or through apprenticeship to other midwives, combined with reading and study. CPMs have nationally recognized credentials through the

Recommended Reading: To learn more about your state's rules concerning CPMs, check out Citizens for Midwifery (cfmidwifery.org/states). To find out about efforts to change legislation in states that do not yet regulate CPMs, visit The Big Push for Midwives (thebigpushformidwives.org).

North American Registry of Midwives. The licensing of CPMs varies from state to state, and in some states this type of midwifery is illegal or unregulated.

CPMs may or may not have formal relationships with individual physicians and/or hospitals. It is important to carefully explore the issues of medical backup and emergency care with your provider, because you may need to arrange for physician or hospital backup yourself. (For information on who is a good candidate for home birth, see "Birth Places," page 367.)

Insurance coverage of CPMs differs from state to state and insurer to insurer. It is more common where home birth midwives are licensed.

Other Midwives

Some midwives are not certified and consider themselves "traditional," "independent," or "direct entry" midwives. Although many such midwives are experienced and practice safely, the lack of a national credential and, in most cases, a license to practice makes it difficult to evaluate their skill and safety record. If you are considering a midwife who is not certified, ask careful questions about the midwife's training and experience and her arrangements for referral and transport if complications develop.

Physicians

In the United States, physicians attend 90 percent of all births. Here's a look at the different type of physicians who commonly provide care to pregnant women.

Family Physicians

A family physician is a medical doctor who is trained to provide basic, comprehensive care to people of all ages. Some family physicians provide maternity care and have hospital delivery room privileges. A few are trained to perform cesarean sections. These doctors often know the whole family, which can enhance planning for a woman's care as well as the care of the baby after birth. Studies have shown that family physicians' use of common interventions such as episiotomy, cesarean, and labor induction tends to fall between that of midwives and that of obstetrician-gynecologists.[3]

Obstetrician-Gynecologists

Increasingly over the last several decades, obstetrician-gynecologists (ob-gyns) have replaced family practice doctors in providing maternity care. Ob-gyns have completed a four-year medical and surgical residency program in obstetrics and gynecology after completing medical school. Because ob-gyns are trained to diagnose and manage complications of pregnancy and birth, they are appropriate providers for women or babies who have serious medical conditions. (For examples of these conditions, see "Hospital," p. 369.) Women with such health problems may benefit from shared care with a midwife. Ob-gyns also provide care for childbearing women without specific medical concerns who either prefer to work with an obstetrician-gynecologist or must do so because of limited options.

Ob-gyns commonly provide prenatal checkups and oversee labor but rarely stay with you throughout labor and may be present only at the time of birth. (During labor, your hands-on care is generally provided by labor and delivery nurses.) Because obstetrics is a surgical specialty, OB care typically involves much higher rates of intervention than midwifery or family practice–based care.

Maternal-Fetal Medicine Physicians

Maternal-fetal medicine physicians (MFMs) are subspecialists in the obstetrics field who have additional training in complicated obstetrics. They often assume care of women with serious conditions such as diabetes or heart disease. These doctors usually practice in large academic medical centers or urban areas and see women only on referral from a physician or midwife. Many perform prenatal and genetic testing procedures and have expertise in the field of genetics. Frequently, they devise a plan of care in collaboration with a pregnant woman's midwife or physician in her home community. If you are referred to a maternal-fetal medicine specialist, find out whether she or he actually attends births; many no longer do.

FINDING A PROVIDER

The vast majority of us enter pregnancy as healthy women, with no major medical problems. If this is true for you, you can choose from the full range of providers and birth settings available in your area. If you have a serious medical condition or are at risk of developing such a condition, an obstetrician or maternal-fetal medicine specialist should be on your team and you should plan to give birth in a hospital, but you still may have midwives involved in your care. Choosing a clinician and birth setting that fit with your beliefs and preferences will be more effective than writing a birth plan and hoping to influence routine practices in medical settings.

To get names of practitioners, ask your family and friends for recommendations and, if you have insurance, find out which providers and services your health care insurance covers. Doulas and childbirth educators can provide excellent guidance about caregivers in the community. Interview the people who you think are most likely to be a good fit for you. (Some insurers will cover an interview visit, and some practices will not charge for the interview; this varies.) For a list of questions to ask, see p. 368.

Setting up a counseling visit before you become pregnant is one way to get to know a doctor or midwife you might consider for your pregnancy care. You can also choose your birth setting first and select a provider from those who attend births in that location. If you are not happy with the care you receive, you have the right to change providers at any time, but be aware that some care providers have a cutoff point for accepting new clients.

BIRTH PLACES

The environment, culture, and routine practices used in different birth settings can affect the process of labor and birth. If you are healthy and have not experienced complications in your pregnancy, you can choose from any of the options in your community, which may include giving birth at home, in a birth center, or in a hospital. Some communities have several hospitals that provide maternity services, so if you are planning a hospital birth you may want to evaluate each one.

Home

Home birth is a good option for healthy women who have healthy pregnancies, a safe and supportive home environment, and easy access to backup medical care. Two critical characteristics of home birth are that you rely on your body's natural abilities (not technology or drugs) to get you through labor and that you can receive continuous sup-

ONLINE HOSPITAL AND CARE PROVIDER RATING SITES

Many websites allow health care consumers to rate and provide feedback on care providers and facilities. Other sites provide safety and performance data for hospitals. These sites, in turn, help consumers looking for health care evaluate the choices in their communities.

The Birth Survey is a grassroots project that aims to increase transparency in maternity care. The site invites women who have given birth to provide feedback about care providers and birth settings. Survey questions are designed to assess whether care is evidence-based and mother-friendly, as defined by the nonprofit Coalition for Improving Maternity Services. In addition, project volunteers have been working with state health departments to obtain and publish facility data such as rates of cesarean section, induction, and episiotomy. You can view consumer feedback and intervention rates for the providers and facilities in your area at thebirthsurvey.com.

port from attendants of your own choosing. Home birth is associated with a very low likelihood of having a cesarean, episiotomy, medications to speed up labor, and pharmacologic pain relief and with high rates of satisfaction.

Midwives are specifically trained to monitor mother and baby's well-being during labor and to handle complications that may arise. Sometimes complications or a desire to use pain medication may require transport to a hospital.

QUESTIONS TO CONSIDER ASKING MIDWIVES AND DOCTORS

- What is your philosophy of childbirth?
- How long have you been practicing? How many births have you attended as the primary attendant?
- Do you practice alone or with others? If with others, what is their experience? Do they share your beliefs and manner of practice?
- Who attends births for you when you are away?
- Where do you attend births, and can I take a tour?
- How can I reach you?
- How often will I see you during these next months?
- What kind of childbirth preparation do you recommend?
- What tests do you recommend for pregnant women? Why?
- How do you define and handle complications?
- Do you provide labor support and stay with women throughout labor? If not, do the nurses provide one-on-one care for women during labor?
- How do you feel about doulas, labor assistants, or family and friends being present?
- Do you support moving around during labor, changing positions, and eating and drinking?
- Will I see you after the birth takes place?
- If I want to hold my baby right after birth, breastfeed, and not be separated, will that be supported?
- If I plan to breastfeed and experience problems, what support will you offer?
- Under what circumstances do you recommend IVs, continuous electronic fetal monitoring, Pitocin, episiotomy, forceps or vacuum, cesarean section, or immediate clamping of the baby's umbilical cord? What is your cesarean rate? Episiotomy rate? Induction rate?
- What is your protocol for the birth of twins and breech births?
- Do you attend vaginal births after cesareans (VBACs)?
- How much do you charge? Are your services covered by my insurance?

Additional Questions for Care Providers Who Attend Home and Birth Center Births

- Are you licensed and certified?
- What are your requirements for accepting patients to give birth in this setting?
- What drugs and equipment do you have available?
- What are the qualifications of your birth assistant?
- Do you have a formal agreement with an obstetrician-gynecologist to provide care if complications occur?
- Do you recommend that I meet the physician who will assist me in case of a complication?
- What hospital will I be transported to if a complication occurs during labor? What about in an emergency?
- Under what conditions would we go to the hospital?
- Would you stay with me if we transfer?
- What percentage of your clients transfer to a hospital during labor?
- Are you trained in newborn resuscitation?
- What kind of postpartum care can I expect? Do you provide follow-up care for the baby as well?

Many home birth midwives carry equipment to help address these needs before and during a transfer. In most studies of planned home birth, 10 to 20 percent of women who begin labor at home will transfer to a hospital before birth, but most of these transfers are for nonurgent situations, such as exhaustion, slow labor progress, or need for pain relief.[4]

Birth Center

Freestanding Birth Centers

Birth centers provide comprehensive family-centered care for women during pregnancy, childbirth, and the time following birth. In the birth center philosophy, pregnancy and birth are normal and healthy processes that should be interfered with as little as possible.

Usually birth centers are homelike places, in contrast to the more institutional setting of hospitals, with added comforts such as birth tubs and birthing balls for relaxation and to relieve pain. Midwives provide personalized, continuous care to laboring women. Birth centers have systems in place to deal with complications during labor and birth and to transfer you to a hospital if necessary.

As with home birth, at a birth center you can expect greater reliance on your own physiology rather than on technology, a focus on individualized care, and staff available to give you continuous support.

Birth centers vary in their rates of using tests and procedures, in their policies and restrictions, and in their medical backup arrangements. There are certain situations in which you may be required to switch to hospital care before or during labor—or even after giving birth—either as a precaution due to complications or in the rare event of an emergency.

Not all women are eligible to give birth at a birth center, and each has its own screening guidelines. Most commonly, this affects women seeking vaginal births after cesarean sections (VBACs). (For more information on VBACs, see p. 388.) You can find out if there is a birth center in your area through the American Association of Birth Centers (birthcenters.org).

Birth Centers in Hospitals

A birth center located within a hospital may have a philosophy and practice anywhere on a continuum between that of a typical freestanding center and that of a hospital. Though many hospitals call their traditional labor and birth units "birth centers" in marketing materials, an in-hospital birth center is separate from the general labor and birth unit and is designed for healthy women who desire midwifery-model, low-intervention care. In most cases, women who need medical interventions—such as intravenous Pitocin or electronic fetal monitoring—or women who desire epidural analgesia will move to the general labor and birth unit for these procedures.

One advantage of in-hospital birth centers is the close proximity to surgical and anesthesia facilities, should they be needed. However, in-hospital birth centers are more likely than freestanding birth centers to place restrictions on laboring women, such as requirements for a period of continuous fetal monitoring before admission or certain routines for newborns.

Hospital

A hospital is the standard setting for many women who prefer to be close to medical care while giving birth or who intend to use an epidural for pain relief. It is also the setting of choice for women and babies who have medical conditions that increase the chances of needing special care. Hospital care is considered safest for women with high blood pressure, diabetes, or seizure disorders; women carrying multiple babies; women who are delivering prematurely or who are more than two weeks beyond their due date; and women whose babies are not in a

IS IT SAFE TO GIVE BIRTH AT HOME?

The media tend to portray childbirth as a high-risk event where anything could go wrong at any time. It is therefore not surprising that most of us feel that the safest labor and birth setting is the hospital, where we can be constantly monitored for problems and an operating room and surgical staff are available in case anything goes wrong.

But the reality is that most complications that occur in labor and birth are predictable. They tend to occur in women with high-risk pregnancies, develop slowly, or are known side effects of labor interventions such as medications to strengthen contractions or reduce pain. Although urgent complications can occur without advance warning, these are the exception rather than the rule.

Still, many women wonder if home birth can be as safe as hospital birth. Researchers have been studying this question for decades. Until recently, virtually every study suffered from major flaws that resulted in promising data but no clear answer to the safety question. More recently, three studies have been published that meet the highest standard for home birth research.[5] One of these, a study from the Netherlands, where home birth is common, looked at the outcomes of more than a half-million planned home births. These studies show no difference in death or serious injury to babies and much better outcomes for mothers in planned home births.

Importantly, the three recent studies came from countries where only healthy women at term, with no risk factors for complications, may plan home births. In addition, midwives in these settings are highly skilled and regulated and have established relationships with consultant physicians and hospitals, so women or babies who need hospitalization can access it easily.

For these reasons, the outcomes of the studies cannot necessarily be applied to the United States, where there are no standard eligibility requirements for planned home birth. Laws regulating midwifery vary across the United States, and some midwives work without any formal arrangements for consultation and referral. Still, the largest study of planned home births in the United States showed excellent outcomes for both mothers and babies with low rates of obstetric complications, although the study did not meet the rigorous standards of other studies because hospital data on low-risk women in the United States are inadequate.[6]

In practice, the safety of home birth depends on the health of the woman and fetus, the skill of the home birth care provider, the distance to a hospital, and the ability to get safe, timely care at that hospital should a complication develop. Consider each of these carefully when exploring the option of planned home birth.

head-down position or have problems that have been identified during the pregnancy. If you have one of these conditions, you will want to be with practitioners and facilities with experience handling your situation.

For some women, there are disadvantages to giving birth in a hospital. Hospital routines, which are set up to promote efficiency and to facilitate emergency medical treatment, are sometimes not flexible enough to accommodate an individual woman's needs. Providers who work in hospitals, even if they believe in informed choice and supportive, low-intervention care, are often constrained by hospital protocols—such as policies forbidding vaginal birth after cesarean section or restricting what women can eat or drink in labor. Interventions such as cesarean surgery, vacuum- or forceps-assisted vaginal birth, and episiotomy are significantly more common in hospitals than in birth centers or the home birth setting.[7]

If you don't have a doula or other knowledgeable support person, assistance with nonmedical pain management will depend largely on the skill and availability of the labor and delivery nurses. You may be able to request a nurse with such experience when you arrive at the hospital, if that is important to you.

There is wide variation among hospitals. Some adhere to best practices, attending to the emotional and physical comfort of women and honoring informed choice, while others impose rigid routines and impersonal care. Likewise, rates of procedures such as cesarean surgery and outcomes such as infection vary across hospitals. If you live in an area with more than one hospital, it is best to ask knowledgeable people, such as childbirth educators or doulas, for their opinions of area hospitals and to check published quality reports if these are available. (Search online for "maternity care quality" and your state or region, or contact your state department of health.) The Birth Survey (thebirthsurvey.com), a nationwide grassroots project, offers intervention rates (where available) and consumer feedback on hospitals as well as birth centers.

I almost never hear of the totally natural, completely positive hospital birth experience, and that's why I'd like to share our story. . . . We chose the hospital we did because of the fact that there were many nurse-midwives on staff that I hoped would be supportive of my desire to have a natural birth. I . . . felt very supported by my husband's medical knowledge and he knew how strongly I wanted to do it drug free—he would be my advocate. He also shared a very empowering piece of advice with our birth class: that should you be in a hospital and not comfortable with the plan, you are entitled to say that you understand the risks and benefits of a procedure and [you] can refuse it. That is your right.

When my contractions had not kicked in . . . twelve hours after my water broke and the usual time they give before they start to induce, we said we wanted to wait a bit. We walked, delaying the Pitocin, but [later] . . . negotiated half the normal dosage. . . . By that time, my husband looked at the monitor and noticed the contractions were getting stronger and more frequent without being induced. Despite the suggestion to continue as planned, we decided to go natural, asserting our right. The doula arrived, and after four hours of intense labor. . . . I reached a point where I said that I couldn't go on. She said to me, "No, you are there. Let's get ready to start pushing!"

Like a set change in a play, there was a whole new team, the bed changed position, and we started to push. Our incredible nurse-midwife was on her knees for the entire two hours while I pushed, holding a warm compress to my perineum so I wouldn't tear—which I didn't. At 5:40 P.M., Sadie was born. It was the single most incredible moment of my life. We feel very blessed to have had the seemingly elusive wonderful, natural hospital birth.

MATERNITY CARE IN TODAY'S HEALTH CARE SYSTEM

For many of us, pregnancy is our first serious contact with the medical system. Whether you have a healthy pregnancy or experience complications, with excellent information, care, and support, you can emerge from your maternity care experiences as an empowered, savvy health care consumer, better prepared to take control of your own health and that of your children.

I started my pregnancy with so much fear and mistrust of doctors and hospitals and decided on a home birth to avoid even having to deal with them. Well, best laid plans . . . at thirty-three weeks, I developed severe preeclampsia and HELLP syndrome. I had to accept that we needed doctors and hospitals to do this safely, but I wanted to be involved in making decisions about my care and not just accept every medical intervention just because I had a complicated pregnancy.

I was induced at thirty-four weeks, and even though I was on magnesium sulfate, which made me feel woozy and sick, and Pitocin, which strengthens contractions, had electronic fetal monitors, couldn't eat, and had to stay in bed, I was able to labor on my terms—with my husband and doula by my side. Against what seemed like all odds, I delivered my healthy daughter vaginally with no pain medication and was able to hold her skin to skin after birth. She did end up going to the NICU for a couple of days, but I think the fact that I held her right away made breastfeeding easier and helped me cope with the separation. I thought I'd feel traumatized by a "medicalized" birth, but I felt ecstatic and like I could take on whatever life throws my way. I think the experience prepared me for the intensity of motherhood, and I would even say it strengthened my marriage.

Unfortunately, too often the opposite is true. The maternity care system frequently offers fragmented, impersonal care that does not reflect what research has shown for decades produces the best health outcomes for mothers and babies. Maternity care in the United States is characterized by several problems:

Too few women get adequate prenatal care. In the past decade or so, care options—such as testing for pregnancy complications or pain relief options in labor—have become much more complex. Fewer women are taking prenatal education classes and more women are experiencing high-risk or complicated pregnancies. Yet the time a woman spends in prenatal visits has been reduced. The typical woman may have as little as two hours of total interaction with her doctor or midwife during her entire pregnancy.[8] Many women also enter prenatal care late, especially low-income women who have Medicaid insurance.

Too many women are exposed to the risks of high-tech procedures, even when they are healthy and unlikely to benefit from them. The most visible example of this is the U.S. cesarean section rate: one in every three women gives birth by C-section. Cesarean sections can be lifesaving and health-enhancing in emergency situations, but unnecessary cesareans expose more mothers and babies to the risks of major surgery, without any clear gains for maternal and infant health overall.

Too many women are subjected to these potentially harmful procedures without giving informed consent. In Childbirth Connection's national survey of women who had given birth in U.S. hospitals, Listening to Mothers II, participants overwhelmingly agreed that women should know the potential harmful effects of procedures. Yet far fewer than half of women were able to correctly answer basic questions about the risks of labor induction or cesarean surgery, even if they had experienced these interventions themselves.[9]

U.S. MATERNITY CARE: ROADBLOCKS TO CHANGE

Why are some medical interventions still being overused in the United States today, despite the evidence against them? And why aren't approaches that are known to be helpful offered to all women? Advocates for improving maternity care point to the following roadblocks to change.

Obstetrical training and the medical system. Obstetricians provide care for the vast majority of pregnant women in the United States. Obstetricians' training emphasizes identifying and managing the complications of pregnancy and childbirth. They generally receive much less instruction in the natural progression of childbirth or in low-technology techniques that minimize problems. While doctors trained years ago learned to safely deliver breech and twin babies vaginally, newer doctors have not learned these skills, as the standard of care has shifted to require cesarean for such births.

Economic incentives. Surgical interventions can save doctors time and money. Many payment systems offer a single or fixed fee to doctors, regardless of whether a baby is born vaginally or by cesarean, and others offer a larger fee for a cesarean. Therefore, doctors who patiently support natural labor, which starts at unpredictable hours and generally requires more time, are penalized financially. Scheduled inductions and cesarean sections help hospitals make nursing staff schedules more predictable and shift more of health care providers' work to convenient weekday hours. Nondrug methods of pain relief and the one-on-one nursing care that enables natural labor are not billable to insurance, while epidurals and other anesthesia services are major sources of revenue for hospitals.

Fear of lawsuits. If something goes wrong, doctors may be blamed for not doing something, but rarely are they blamed for doing something that is not necessary. For example, malpractice lawsuits for not performing a cesarean section are much more common than lawsuits for doing one when it wasn't necessary. To avoid litigation, many doctors and some midwives report that they feel compelled to do "too much" rather than be accused of doing "too little."

A rushed, risk-averse society. The desire to eliminate pain and control outcomes may cause both health care providers and expectant parents to embrace unneeded and potentially harmful procedures. Healthy women with low-risk pregnancies receive treatments that were designed for use by women with high-risk pregnancies. The widespread use of epidurals also has transformed childbirth in the United States. Though epidurals are in most cases a very effective form of pain relief during labor, they sometimes have adverse effects and require the proactive use of other interventions to keep mothers and babies safe and labor progressing.

In addition, nearly three-quarters of women who had episiotomies (a surgical cut to make the vaginal opening bigger during birth—a painful procedure associated with known harms when used routinely) did not give consent.

Too few women have the benefit of low-tech supportive care practices that help them safely cope with the demands of pregnancy, labor, and birth. In the Listening to Mothers II survey, most women said they were not allowed to drink or eat food, were confined to bed once admitted to the hospital and in "active" labor, and gave birth lying on their backs (a position that is more painful than upright positions and poses challenges for giving birth). Only 2 percent of women experienced a set of five supportive care practices that research shows benefit mothers and babies.*

Too many women end up with physical and emotional health problems after giving birth. In a follow-up survey of Listening to Mothers participants, many women experienced pain, physical exhaustion, and sexual problems lasting months after birth, as well as shorter-term problems such as infection and rehospitalization. Most had some symptoms of postpartum depression in the two weeks prior to the survey, and 9 percent of mothers appeared to be suffering from childbirth-related post-traumatic stress disorder.[10]

PRENATAL CARE

Prenatal care consists of three interrelated elements: regular visits with your midwife or doctor; the care you give yourself; and the care you receive from friends, family, and other support people. This section focuses on prenatal visits with a care provider.

WHAT TO EXPECT FROM PRENATAL VISITS

Prenatal care by your midwife or doctor will encompass regular health assessments, coordination of care with other providers or services, and establishing a plan of care for labor, birth, and your postpartum recovery and adjustment to motherhood.

---

* These practices are: labor begins on its own; the woman has the freedom to move and change positions; the woman has continuous labor support from a partner, family member, or doula; the woman does not give birth on her back; and the mother and baby are not separated after birth.

RIGHTS OF WOMEN DURING PREGNANCY AND BIRTH

No matter what situations you face when you are pregnant and in labor, understanding your rights is key to making good decisions and being better able to act on them. The statement below is excerpted and adapted from Childbirth Connection (childbirthconnection.org), a nonprofit group that works to improve maternity care for all U.S. women and families.*

The statement outlines a set of basic rights for childbearing women, applying widely accepted human rights to the specific situation of maternity care. Most of these rights are granted to women in the United States by law, yet they are not always honored. In addition, the wider social, political, and economic organization of health care, parenting, and the workplace makes it difficult or impossible to consistently exercise these individual rights.

Every Woman Has the Right to:

Choose her birth setting from the full range of safe options available in her community, on the basis of complete, objective information about the benefits, harms, and costs of these options.

Receive information about the professional identity and qualifications of those involved in her care and know when any are trainees.

* For the full text of this statement, see Childbirth Connection's "The Rights of Childbearing Women" at childbirthconnection.org/rights.

Communicate with caregivers and receive all care in privacy (which may involve excluding nonessential personnel) and have all personal information treated according to standards of confidentiality.

Receive maternity care that is appropriate to her cultural and religious background and receive information in a language she clearly understands.

Leave her maternity caregiver and select another if she becomes dissatisfied with the care.

Receive full advance information about harms and benefits of all reasonably available methods for relieving pain during labor and birth, including methods that do not require the use of drugs.

Accept or refuse procedures, drugs, tests, and treatments. She has the right to have her choices honored and to change her mind at any time.

Enjoy freedom of movement during labor, unencumbered by tubes, wires, or other apparatus. She also has the right to give birth in the position of her choice.

Be informed if her caregivers wish to enroll her or her infant in a research study. She should receive full information about all known and possible benefits and harms of participation, and she has the right to decide whether to participate, free from coercion and without negative consequences.

Have unrestricted access to all available records about her pregnancy, her labor, and her infant; obtain full copies of all records; and receive help in understanding them, if necessary.

A woman who had planned a home birth but discovered late in pregnancy that her baby was breech describes how she exercised her rights in a hospital setting:

Through all our research, we found out that there were several doctors at this hospital who were experienced in delivering breech and that while hospital staff would try to pressure me into having a C-section, it was my right to decline a cesarean. We showed up at the hospital the next day to try a version [where doctors try to manually turn the baby] with a letter that specified that we were not giving consent to a C-section unless mine and/or the baby's lives were at risk. The version didn't work, and the doctors tried to convince us to have a C-section. The biggest reason they could give us was that it would be challenging to schedule staff who were experienced at delivering breech to be available when I went into labor. That did not seem like a good enough reason to cut me open.

Once the doctors realized that we were not going to consent to a C-section, a very nice female doctor offered to be on call for me. She spent over an hour talking with me, trying to get me comfortable with delivering in a hospital. As I became more comfortable, my labor kicked into high gear. My third daughter was born less than four hours later. It was the easiest and quickest labor I have had. We were back home less than three hours after giving birth.

All prenatal care is not alike. Some prenatal care providers, especially midwives who practice in home and birth center settings, offer long visits with plenty of time to answer questions, address concerns, celebrate joys, and explore fears. We may be encouraged to participate in aspects of our visits, such as taking our own blood pressure or writing our weight in our own medical records.

My 6-year-old daughter, Lucia, often came to my appointments with me, and I think it was an important part of making her the great big sister that she is. Our midwife, Elizabeth, was really patient with all of Lucia's questions, let her try all of her tools, and always had a doll for her to hold that was the same size as our growing baby. After Savina was born, Lucia was really sad that we couldn't go visit Elizabeth anymore.

Some provider visits are brief and emphasize tests and procedures. While most of us have one-on-one appointments with a care provider, more women are participating in supportive group prenatal care with other women due around the same time. Be prepared to take a proactive role to get the most out of your visits. For more information, see Chapter 23, "Navigating the Health Care System."

PRENATAL VISITS

In the first trimester, prenatal visits to your health care provider are recommended every four to six weeks. The timing of your visits may vary depending on your individual needs. Visits will typically include measuring your weight and blood pressure, listening to the baby's heartbeat (after ten to twelve weeks), and measuring his or her growth by feeling the uterus or plac-

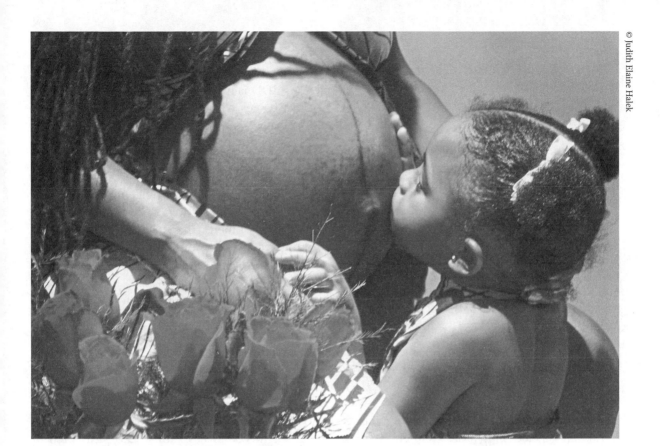
© Judith Elaine Halek

ing a measuring tape on your abdomen. Ideally, you will have enough time to talk about any concerns, review test results if tests were done, and discuss future plans.

If you participate in group prenatal care with other women, your visits will also include time to learn together the information you will need to make informed choices about your care. If you have traditional one-on-one prenatal visits, you will likely benefit from childbirth education classes, including early pregnancy and breastfeeding or parenting classes, especially if your care provider offers relatively brief prenatal visits (less than thirty to sixty minutes with the midwife or doctor). For more information see "Childbirth Classes," p. 383.

YOUR FIRST VISIT

If your first prenatal visit is the first time you will meet your care provider, come with questions that will help you decide if she or he is a good fit for you. (See suggested questions on p. 368.) If possible, bring your partner, other family member, or a friend for support.

At the first visit, you will be asked about your health history and your family's history, your background, your occupation, and what support you have at home. You will talk about your diet, exercise, and drug and alcohol use. The purpose of this visit is to help you identify any problem areas, such as physical and psychological concerns. If you are experiencing physical or sexual abuse, consider telling your midwife or doctor.

He or she may be able to help by giving you referrals and scheduling more frequent visits if needed.

Another important goal of the first prenatal visit is to establish a reliable estimated due date (EDD). Your EDD is thirty-eight weeks from the day you conceived the pregnancy. If you don't know when you conceived, you can determine your EDD by reviewing your menstrual cycle. If you have regular, twenty-eight-day menstrual cycles, your EDD is forty weeks from the beginning of your last menstrual period. Many women, however, don't have regular menstrual cycles, or their cycles are longer or shorter than twenty-eight days. If this is true for you, tell your provider how long your menstrual cycles usually are, whether they are regular, and whether you have recently been on a hormonal birth control method or breastfeeding (these can both alter your menstrual cycle.)

Pregnancies usually last about thirty-seven to forty-two weeks, with most women giving birth between thirty-nine and forty-one weeks. Your EDD is merely the middle of that window. Most babies will not actually be born on their due date.

Some doctors' offices and clinics have ultrasound machines and use them at this first visit to see the fetal heartbeat and estimate how far along you are. However, office ultrasounds are not routine in all settings or necessary for most pregnant women. The quality of the pictures produced by ultrasound machines is unlikely to provide useful information about your baby's well-being.

At the first prenatal visit, your doctor or midwife may ask you to get undressed. The examination typically includes a pelvic exam to collect specimens for tests—which may include a Pap test and gonorrhea and chlamydia cultures—and to feel the size of your uterus. If you want to see your vagina and cervix, ask for a mirror. (For more information on pelvic exams, see "The Gynecological Exam" p. 35.) If it is ten to twelve weeks after your last period, you may be able to hear the baby's heartbeat with an electronic Doppler (ultrasound wave device). Later in pregnancy, the baby's heartbeat can be heard with a simple device called a fetoscope.

Before leaving, ask when to return, what to expect from future visits, and where and whom to call with problems and concerns. The practitioner should provide you with any other information you may need, such as written materials and referrals to classes and nearby resource centers. You should leave feeling listened to and well cared for—off to a good start. If you don't think this person is a good fit for you, seek a different provider, if possible.

Your subsequent visits will generally be shorter than the first one. Your care provider will check your weight, blood pressure, and

CARE FOR PREGNANT WOMEN WITHOUT HEALTH INSURANCE

Finding appropriate medical care and services can be difficult if you do not have health care insurance. Some women who lack health care insurance become eligible for Medicaid coverage after becoming pregnant. Eligibility requirements in all states are expanded for pregnant women, and there is a special program called "presumptive eligibility" that pays for medical care for pregnant women whose Medicaid applications have not yet been approved. To find out if you are eligible for Medicaid, visit benefits.gov. To see if your state has a presumptive eligibility program, go to statehealthfacts.org and search for "presumptive eligibility."

In 2014, as a result of new health care legislation, many more of us will become eligible for federal subsidies to purchase health care insurance, and all plans will be required to cover maternity and childbirth services as part of an "essential health benefits" package defined by the federal government. Medicaid will also cover many younger adults who currently lack coverage, enabling women to have insurance before becoming pregnant. These insurers will not be allowed to charge women who are pregnant higher rates.

Your local medical assistance, welfare, social services, or public health office can help you find a clinic that will offer you care or refer you to an insurance program that is available to you.

One program available everywhere in the United States is the Special Supplemental Nutrition Program for Women, Infants, and Children (WIC). WIC provides milk, fruit, vegetables, whole grains, juice, cheese, and eggs and offers some prenatal and breastfeeding education. The program may be housed in the local health department, schools, or free clinics. It is available to everyone and is often the best place to start when you're looking for affordable prenatal care. People in the WIC office can refer you to health care providers and other programs and services that are available to you during pregnancy. The WIC website (fns.usda .gov/wic) lists toll-free phone numbers for WIC agencies in each state.

If you aren't able to find insurance coverage, you might consider working with a midwife at home or at a birthing center. These midwives often provide the most affordable care; your out-of-pocket costs will likely be lower than those at a hospital or ob-gyn office. For more information about finding low-cost care or accessing Medicaid, see Chapter 23, "Navigating the Health Care System."

urine; measure your belly to evaluate the baby's growth and position; and listen to the fetal heartbeat. You will occasionally have other tests or procedures, which your care provider should discuss with you ahead of time. All prenatal visits should include plenty of time to talk about your pregnancy, discuss plans for labor and birth, and get your questions answered.

TESTS DURING PREGNANCY

Some prenatal tests give information about the mother's health, while other tests provide information about the characteristics of the developing fetus. While some tests are routine and generally helpful, every test does not make sense for every woman. Ideally, tests will be selected based on your individual circumstances and personal preferences.

TESTS THAT GIVE INFORMATION ABOUT YOUR HEALTH

Prenatal tests that provide information about your health, such as blood testing to find out if you are anemic or are HIV-positive, are important because they detect conditions that often can be treated.

Your state health department may require certain tests, such as blood tests for syphilis or HIV. If you do not want certain tests, you may have options for refusing them in most states, although states differ in procedures for refusing such tests.

After your first prenatal visit, blood tests are not needed at each visit. In your sixth month, a blood test that measures the level of sugar in your blood is routine in many practices. The blood is drawn one hour after you drink a measured amount of sugar (glucose). If your blood sugar level is higher than normal after you've drunk the sugar solution, you will be asked to do a second, three-hour test to determine if you have gestational diabetes. Some women find that the testing makes them feel nauseous, lightheaded, or weak. Blood tests before and after a high-carbohydrate meal may be an appropriate alternative way to screen. Gestational diabetes occurs in about 4 to 7 percent of women and is associated with higher rates of cesarean section and larger babies. It also puts you at increased risk for developing diabetes later in life.

About a month before your estimated due date, your care provider will offer you a vaginal culture for group B streptococcus (GBS). GBS is not an infection; it is one of the bacteria that can be found normally in the vagina. Ten to 30 percent of pregnant women carry this bacterium. Because in rare cases a baby will become ill from GBS infection contracted during birth, your practitioner may test you for GBS and recommend treatment during labor to prevent your baby from becoming sick. Women with GBS are usually given intravenous penicillin during labor.

There is controversy in the obstetrical community about the value of recommending screening for GBS to all women. The test is not offered routinely in many other countries. That's because the downstream effects of the tests—such as the use of antibiotics and separation of mothers and babies after birth—can be harmful, and many women need to be screened and exposed to these interventions to prevent a single newborn illness or injury.

TESTS FOR FETAL IMPAIRMENTS

Ever since the 1970s, it has been possible to get some information during pregnancy about the characteristics of the developing baby. In recent years, the number of tests available to pregnant women has multiplied, allowing increased scrutiny of the fetus for specific disorders. Women may choose prenatal testing to learn about health problems, diseases, or disabilities that might occur. If you learn through prenatal testing that your baby will likely be born with a correctable, treatable, or lifelong impairment, you may want to make special plans before the child's birth. Or you may decide to end the pregnancy if you know that your future child would have a disabling condition or be unlikely to survive after birth.

Though prenatal tests may offer useful in-

CAN YOU REFUSE A TEST?

You have the right to refuse tests and procedures in pregnancy and on behalf of your baby after birth. However, many women feel intense pressure to agree to whatever interventions the provider recommends. Sometimes women are told that if they refuse certain tests (the gestational diabetes screening test or a GBS culture, for example) the baby will be subjected to painful tests and possibly separated from the mother after birth.

If you are facing scare tactics and have other care providers available to you, consider transferring your care. Seek out unbiased sources of information such as knowledgeable childbirth educators or reputable books and websites. You may decide that you do want to go ahead with the test and that you simply needed to feel fully informed before agreeing to it. Or you may discover alternative approaches to testing that feel more comfortable to you. If you decide to refuse a test given around the time of birth, make sure you have excellent labor support from companions or a doula with whom you have shared your choice. They may be able to help you stand up for yourself and avoid extra tests and procedures the hospital wants to impose.

I decided against getting the test to see if I carried group B strep. If you have GBS, they give you antibiotics, which need to be started four hours before birth. My entire first labor was less than four hours, so it seemed really unlikely that I would even be able to have the treatment. (I was right—I barely got to the birth center in time.) I figured—why do the test if you can't do anything about the results? Knowing I was colonized with GBS and that I wouldn't be able to do anything about it was not the kind of stress I wanted at the end of pregnancy.

formation, they also raise concerns if the report is false-positive. Most of the noninvasive tests (blood tests and ultrasounds) are screening exams that are not perfect, and they can indicate a problem that with further testing will turn out not to be there. Invasive tests such as amniocentesis or chorionic villus sampling (CVS) can give you a 100 percent true answer about some genetic conditions, but these tests involve drawing fluid out of the amniotic sac by inserting a needle through the abdomen or vagina. These tests carry a small risk of miscarriage. Even when they do not cause medical problems, tests can create anxiety and expense and add to the medicalization of pregnancy and birth.

I had a CVS [chorionic villus sampling] done, which was both physically and emotionally painful. We found out there were some irregularities, so I ended up needing an amnio as well. It turned out the irregularity was some fluke in the test, and we finally got a clean bill of health [for the fetus]—six months into the pregnancy. The waiting was excruciating. To be pregnant but not be able to let yourself feel the joy and hope of it was truly horrible.

Tests for fetal impairments give us both the opportunity and the responsibility to decide whether we want to become parents of a child with a particular set of characteristics. Some

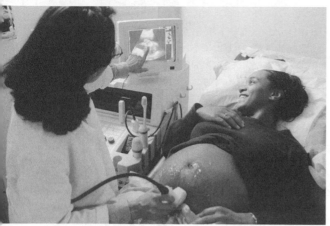

© Keith Brofsky / Getty Images

of us may decide that we don't want this information. Others of us will be extremely eager to know all we can about our developing baby. Your doctor or midwife may strongly recommend testing, but it should not be automatic; decisions about testing are up to you.

Types of Tests

Three types of tests screen for or diagnose disorders in the fetus:

- **Genetic carrier testing** is blood tests that can be performed before you get pregnant or in early pregnancy. The tests determine if you or your partner is a carrier of diseases that can be inherited by your children. Examples of genetic carrier tests are blood tests for sickle-cell anemia or cystic fibrosis.
- **Screening tests** measure the likelihood that your fetus has a particular condition but cannot tell for certain whether the fetus has the condition. Examples of screening tests are ultrasounds and "maternal marker" blood tests. Screening tests are typically used to determine if a diagnostic test is necessary.
- **Diagnostic tests** give a yes-or-no answer, identifying whether the fetus does or does

not have a particular condition. Examples of diagnostic tests are amniocentesis and chorionic villus sampling.

It is important to note that none of the tests guarantees that the baby will be healthy; instead, they are designed to ask, and answer, one specific question, such as: "Does my baby have cystic fibrosis?"

For more information about specific tests for fetal anatomy and well-being, visit the March of Dimes (marchofdimes.com) and see the chapter on prenatal testing in *Our Bodies, Ourselves: Pregnancy and Birth.*

QUESTIONS TO CONSIDER ABOUT TESTING

Before choosing whether or not to have any test, find out what information the test is capable of providing and its advantages and disadvantages. Ask your health care provider, and do your own research, to find out the following:

- Does the test pose any risk to you and/or your developing baby?
- Why is this test recommended for you? Are you in a group that makes you or your baby more likely to have this condition?
- When can you expect the results to come back?
- How reliable is this test? What is the incidence of false-positive results? If you get a result described as abnormal or unusual, what kind of follow-up testing or counseling will be offered?
- What are your options after receiving the result? Are there any treatments available for you or for the fetus if the result is abnormal?
- How much will this test cost? Will your health care insurance cover part or all of the cost of this test? If not, can you get any financial assistance?

Additional questions for tests that give you information about the baby's characteristics:

- Would knowing that my baby will have a particular condition make a difference in my decision to continue my pregnancy? If so, how?
- What do I know about life with these conditions?
- Would knowing any other characteristics detectable by prenatal testing, such as the sex of my baby or the identity of the father, affect my decision about continuing my pregnancy? If so, how?

CHILDBIRTH CLASSES

Prenatal visits rarely provide enough time to discuss preparation for labor, birth, breastfeeding, and early parenting in detail. Childbirth classes can help fill this gap. In the past thirty years, childbirth education has evolved. Today, women can choose from Lamaze, Bradley Method, ICEA, Birth Works, HypnoBirthing, Birthing from Within, and mindfulness-based childbirth preparation methods, among others. Childbirth classes teach you about the process of labor and birth and offer techniques to help you relax and cope with it.

Techniques that improve confidence can help you prepare to cope with labor sensations. Meditation, visualization, movement, and rhythmic techniques are tools you might use to help ride the waves of labor.

Hospital-sponsored classes tend to focus upon medical interventions and are less likely to give you details about all of their risks and benefits or your rights. Seek out an independent childbirth educator to get unbiased information and help with making decisions and having a childbirth experience that meets your needs. A doula may also provide you with one-on-one education and preparation classes. If these options aren't available or are unaffordable, arrange a get-together with pregnant friends to explore childbirth information and stories together. Many large cities have independent childbirth educator or doula organizations that can provide a list of alternative class options. Childbirth education organizations can often direct you to educators in your community, and some of their websites include directories.

SPECIAL CONSIDERATIONS

WHAT IS A HIGH-RISK PREGNANCY?

Some women have preexisting medical conditions such as diabetes, high blood pressure, epilepsy, autoimmune disorders, HIV, or heart or kidney disease that increase the risk of problems during pregnancy. Others begin pregnancy healthy but develop a complication that needs closer monitoring, such as placenta previa, preterm labor, gestational diabetes, or preeclampsia.

When I first became pregnant, I envisioned having a healthy pregnancy and a natural birth with midwives—I'd already done that once before. But after experiencing serious bleeding in my seventh month of pregnancy, I was diagnosed with placenta previa. I spent the rest of my pregnancy on bed rest, hospitalized for most of that time, and eventually gave birth by emergency C-section when the bleeding started again. I never wanted to have hospitals, high-risk specialists, and surgeons so involved in my pregnancy, but I am eternally grateful that they were there when I needed them.

If you have a high-risk pregnancy, you may need to be seen by or consult with an obstetrician, maternal-fetal medicine physician, or relevant specialists and have more frequent prenatal visits or adjust your daily activities. But even though your risk of complications during pregnancy is higher, you may not actually develop any worrisome complications.

Some of us are labeled "high risk" but are actually healthy, and with good supportive care we can expect to remain healthy and give birth safely to healthy babies. Being considered high risk can affect our confidence and expose us to extra testing and procedures that we may not need. If you don't think you are high risk, talk to your care provider about what that means for your care. If you believe a high-risk label will limit your choices unnecessarily or lead to overuse of interventions, consider switching care providers.

If your pregnancy requires attention from a specialist, a midwife or family practice doctor may still be able to provide the general care you need.

PREGNANT AND PARENTING TEENS

Becoming pregnant as a teenager can present many challenges. Younger teens (thirteen to fifteen years old) have a higher rate of complicated births, but you can help prevent problems by taking good care of yourself and getting support.

It will be especially important that you gain enough weight, so don't diet while you are pregnant. If getting enough food is difficult for you, contact the Special Supplemental Nutrition Program for Women, Infants, and Children (WIC) in your community or call your local food bank. (For more information, see p. 379.)

You may have many plans to make as you prepare to give birth. You will need to know where you and the baby will live, and you may need to figure out how to stay in school or at your job, arrange for health insurance, and ensure that you will have enough money. It can seem overwhelming. The more helpful people (family, friends, the baby's father, school counselor, public health nurse, social worker, midwife, or nurse-practitioner) you can surround yourself with, the better. They can encourage you to be and to stay healthy, to feel positive about pregnancy and birth, and to plan for and make decisions about your and your baby's future.

I'm 15, and when I got pregnant, it was really hard for me in school to do gym. You know, the running and all. The gym teacher was kind of mean, so I talked to my counselor, and she got me into this school that is just for girls who are pregnant. It is better for me, 'cause we just walk for exercise and everybody helps you.

Just because you are having a baby does not mean you have to leave school. Ask your school guidance counselor or health care provider if there are schools in your community especially for pregnant or parenting students. Many communities have such schools. They may offer classes in parenting as well as day care for your baby so that you can attend classes.

I'm 16, and this is my first baby. My mom had me when she was 16, too. When I went into labor, I told my mom I wanted my little sister to be with me. She's 12. After my baby was born, I told my sister, "You are smart and pretty. Don't do this. Don't do what me and mom did. You can be anything you want." I love my baby, but I want my sister to have a better life. Later, my midwife told me I was smart and pretty, too, and that I could do anything I want. She said I could still go to college. I hope I can. I know it will be a lot of work, but I would like to be a lawyer.

PREGNANCY IN YOUR LATE THIRTIES OR FORTIES

Many of us become pregnant for the first time in our late thirties and early forties, and, rarely, even in our middle or late forties. If you are over age thirty-five, medical providers may label you as an "elderly primigravida"—a woman of "advanced maternal age"—and consider you high risk. Most of this increased risk is not related to your age itself but to the fact that older women are more likely to have health problems such as high blood pressure or diabetes, which can affect pregnancy outcomes. In addition, the risk of some fetal impairments, such as Down syndrome, increases as a woman ages. However, the vast majority of women thirty-five and older have healthy pregnancies and births.

Because you are over age thirty-five, your health care provider will offer you blood testing, ultrasounds, and/or an amniocentesis to help determine if there are any chromosome problems in your baby. For more information about these tests, see "Tests for Fetal Impairments," p. 380.

Some of us find our age and experience a benefit as we progress through our pregnancies and motherhood:

For much of my life, I had been convinced that I didn't want kids. Then I settled into my career and found myself in a really great relationship. We talked about kids and realized that we really wanted them. We got married when I was 38, and I got pregnant three days later. . . .

As an older mom I think—no, I know—I'm a better mom than I would have been at a younger age. I'm healthy, so I'm still able to do all the active things with the kids—biking, snowboarding. And I am much more patient than I used to be. We do struggle a bit with balancing preparing for retirement with trying to save for the kids' college, but in the grand scheme of things, that's a pretty good challenge to have.

WEIGHT AND PREGNANCY

Women considered overweight or obese are at increased risk for certain complications, including gestational diabetes, high blood pressure, a larger-than-average baby, and cesarean sections. Of most concern is the sky-high rates of cesarean sections. Many providers work under the assumption that being fat interferes with a woman's ability to give birth vaginally and that cesareans are necessary when women are obese. But other providers and activists question whether the high rate is medically necessary and believe that it is caused in part by misguided assumptions about obesity and by unneeded interventions and protocols commonly used with big women.

Cesareans involve major abdominal surgery and thus pose risks for women of any size. They are even more risky for big women. Obese women who have surgical births have higher rates of anesthesia problems, severe bleeding, and infections than non-obese women who have surgical births.[12] If you are considered overweight or obese, there are things you can do to lower your chances of having a cesarean section. These include being proactive about your health habits, choosing a provider who is size-friendly, avoiding routine medical interventions during labor unless clearly needed, and not intervening when a big baby is suspected. (The fear of big babies is one of the strongest factors driving the high rate of cesareans in heavy women; however, having a big baby is not in and of itself a valid medical reason for having a cesarean.) For more detailed information, see "Women of Size and Cesarean Sections: Tips for Avoiding Unnecessary Surgery" at the Our Bodies Ourselves website, ourbodiesourselves.org.

IF YOU ARE EXPERIENCING ABUSE OR VIOLENCE

Some studies find that one in six women is battered during pregnancy. Unfortunately, this figure may be misleadingly low, because many women do not report abuse—or even recognize that they are being abused.

Many women experience abuse for the first time during pregnancy. The stress of a pregnancy and jealousy over the baby may trigger violent or controlling behavior in a partner who hasn't behaved violently in the past. Abuse can involve any type of physical violence (slapping, hitting, shoving, squeezing, choking), sexual violence (forcing you to have sex when you don't want to or making you have sex in ways that are painful or make you feel bad about yourself), or emotional abuse (keeping you away from friends or relatives or saying things that make you feel bad about yourself).

Many health care providers do not notice or recognize the signs of abuse (bruises, depression, drinking to cope) and therefore fail to address it. But if you tell your care provider about the abuse, she or he can direct you to community resources that can help. You can always get help by calling the National Domestic Violence Hotline (thehotline.org) at 1-800-799-7233. This free, confidential service is available twenty-four hours a day, and translators are available for those who don't speak English. Hotline advocates can provide crisis intervention, safety planning, and information on and referrals to local domestic violence agencies in all fifty states.

For more information about partner abuse and getting help, see "Intimate Partner Violence," p. 709.

IF YOU HAVE EXPERIENCED SEXUAL ABUSE

The effects of previous sexual abuse may resurface during pregnancy and labor and after the baby is born. For example, you may feel invaded or violated during prenatal checkups, feel extraordinarily vulnerable in the midst of labor, or have unsettling flashbacks while nursing or bathing your baby. Try to find a health care practitioner who listens carefully to you—and with whom you feel comfortable enough to tell at least part of your story. Find a family member or friend to talk with, or a therapist if possible. Though having a history of sexual abuse may be emotionally difficult, with good support, pregnancy, birth, and motherhood can be empowering and healing, both physically and emotionally.[13]

IF YOU HAVE A DISABILITY

Women with physical, intellectual, or psychiatric disabilities have the right to the same choices as women without disabilities.

However, you may encounter inaccessible facilities, insensitive practitioners, ignorance, or discrimination when attempting to get care. There have been limited research, data, and training about disability and pregnancy. Be prepared to advocate for yourself and to educate your health practitioner, or to find someone who can help.

People may try to talk you out of having a baby, unable to imagine how you could cope. Don't let their ignorance affect your decision. Asking yourself questions beforehand can help clarify your thoughts and wishes: Will pregnancy and birth put my health at risk? If so, how? Are there ways to lessen the risk? If my disability is genetic, how do I feel about the possibility of passing my disability on to the baby? Contact organizations that deal with your specific concerns.

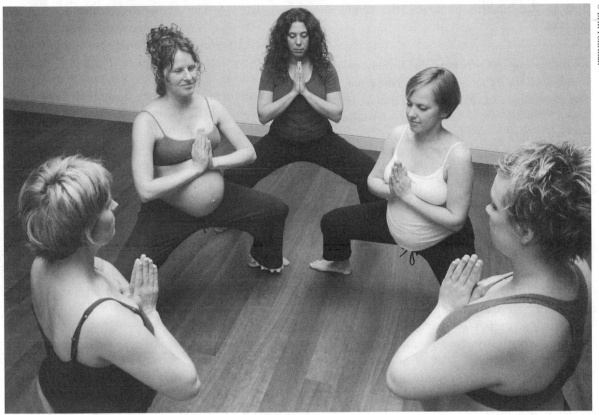

Being in the hospital and experiencing the intense physical changes of labor may trigger feelings of vulnerability or helplessness. Remember that you are the expert about your own needs. Trust yourself to handle difficult situations and people, and ask for help. Make sure someone accompanies you to act as your advocate. You may want to tour the hospital or birth center in advance. You also may want to write a brief statement about yourself and include a paragraph describing how you want to be treated (for example, "Don't talk to me through my attendant/interpreter; talk to me directly"). Hand out copies to everyone so that you won't have to answer the same questions over and over.

IF YOU HAVE A CHRONIC ILLNESS

If you have a chronic illness, you may wonder both how the pregnancy will affect the illness and how the illness will affect the pregnancy. Some chronic illnesses are unaffected by pregnancy, some may be made worse, and others may actually improve. If possible, arrange for a preconception consultation with a maternal-fetal medicine specialist or a physician with expertise in your particular condition.

Carefully choose the people who know you and your needs best to help you decide where you want to have your baby and who you want to be with you during childbirth. If your health care insurance plan doesn't allow you to make these decisions, try to meet all of the members of the health care team who might care for you.

I found a diabetes educator who listened to me and helped me assemble a health care team. She encouraged me to learn more and be more involved in my care. I was started on insulin and a diet and given blood sugar goals and supplies.

It was not easy, but I did it all—testing eight times a day, insulin shots five times a day, and the diet. I didn't have a baby yet, but I lugged a large insulated diaper bag everywhere I went. It was filled with my needles, insulin, log, meter, snacks, ice, and other supplies.

I became an active member of the team who had a good idea of what was going on and even offered suggestions. I am thankful my body responded favorably to my efforts and I was able to keep hitting my goals without complications. After my son was born, it was scary to no longer have such intense support, but the knowledge I gained will allow me to continue to care for myself in order to care for him.

IF YOU ARE DEALING WITH ADDICTION

If you are struggling with addiction to tobacco, drugs, or alcohol, it's important to get help. Some of us find added motivation to quit in knowing that our babies will be affected by our use. Finding treatment may also be easier, as federal laws require that Medicaid and most private insurance plans cover smoking cessation counseling and drug therapy for pregnant women.

The following resources can help you find the care you need:

- To find a smoking cessation program, call 1-800-QUITNOW, or go to smokefree.gov or quitnet.com.

- The U.S. Department of Health and Human Services' Substance Abuse Treatment Facility Locator (findtreatment.samhsa.gov) provides detailed listings of treatment programs near you, including their particular focus and forms of payment accepted.
- To find help if you are abusing alcohol, visit Alcoholics Anonymous (aa.org), Narcotics Anonymous (na.org), or Women for Sobriety (womenforsobriety.org) to find local groups and meetings as well as online support. All are free and guarantee anonymity. Volunteers can answer questions and help you get connected with support people, meetings, treatment centers, and other help. Even if alcohol is not the drug you are using, AA can connect you with a counselor or support person in your area who is familiar with the drug you are using.

Many pregnant women are afraid to seek treatment for alcohol or drug addiction. You may not know whom to trust or if by telling someone about your use you could get into legal trouble. Women with addictions deserve support and access to safe, affordable treatments—not punishment.

IF YOU HAVE HAD A PREVIOUS CESAREAN SECTION

Most women who have given birth by cesarean section in the past can safely give birth vaginally in a following pregnancy, thus avoiding the complications associated with cesarean surgery. These complications include infection, excess bleeding, and problems associated with blood clots. Vaginal birth is also associated with an easier and shorter recovery than cesarean surgery. The risks of pregnancy and likelihood of problems during cesarean section increase the more C-sections a woman has had, so women who intend to have future pregnancies can reduce the chance of problems by planning vaginal birth.

However, about one out of every four women who plans a vaginal birth after cesarean (VBAC) will have a cesarean because of problems that arise during labor. Cesareans that take place during labor are somewhat riskier than cesareans occurring before labor. In addition, a small number of women who plan VBAC—about 1 in 200—will experience uterine rupture during labor. Uterine rupture—a tear through the complete thickness of the uterus, usually at the site of a previous C-section incision—requires immediate delivery of the baby and surgical repair of the uterus to control bleeding. Although most women and babies who experience uterine rupture recover fully, studies show that for every 100 uterine ruptures, about 6 babies will die and 25 women will have hysterectomies (removal of the uterus). Overall, death of the baby during labor or soon after birth is very rare but slightly more common with planned VBAC versus planned cesarean.

Not every woman faces the same chances of experiencing harms and benefits. For instance, if you have given birth vaginally in the past, you are more likely to give birth vaginally and less likely to have a uterine rupture than women who have not. If your cesarean section was for slow progress in labor, your chance of giving birth vaginally is lower than if your C-section was for a problem such as fetal distress. You need accurate, unbiased information about *your* likelihood of various outcomes to make an informed choice. In addition, you must consider the risks and benefits of different choices within the context of your own life and priorities.

I hated the idea of recovering from surgery with a toddler in the apartment and a new baby to take care of, especially since my partner could only take a few days off of work. I also wasn't sure we were done having kids, and I was afraid of some of the complications you hear about with third and fourth C-sections. I'm so glad I was able to have a VBAC.

Unfortunately, in the United States today, most women are discouraged from planning VBAC. As of 2009, half of hospitals in the United States *required* women with prior cesareans to consent to cesarean surgery in order to give birth there, and a large proportion of maternity caregivers are unwilling to attend VBACs, a clear violation of the right of informed refusal.[14] In 2010, the National Institutes of Health convened a Consensus Conference to review all of the scientific evidence on planned VBAC and planned repeat cesarean and affirmed that both options have important risks and benefits and that VBAC is a reasonable and safe choice for most women.[15] Several months later, the American Congress of Obstetricians and Gynecologists (ACOG) released a practice guideline encouraging greater access to VBAC and reaffirming women's right to autonomy and choice.[16] Based on strong evidence, the guidelines recommend that most women with one or two previous cesareans receive counseling and be offered the choice of VBAC. These developments have paved the way for consumer advocacy to improve access to the full range of safe birth options for women with prior cesareans.

For more information about the advantages and risks of both VBAC and repeat cesarean section and how to advocate for the best care for either choice, visit Childbirth Connection (childbirthconnection.org) or the International Cesarean Awareness Network (ican-online.org).

DEPRESSION AND OTHER MENTAL HEALTH CHALLENGES DURING PREGNANCY

Despite the stereotype that all pregnant women are glowing, for some women pregnancy is a difficult time. Symptoms of depression include loss of pleasure in activities that you used to enjoy; persistent feelings of worthlessness, sadness, or hopelessness; prolonged periods of appetite change or fatigue; uncharacteristic tearfulness; or suicidal thoughts. It is possible to be depressed without actually having feelings of sadness. Though depression can affect any pregnant woman, it is more common in women who have experienced depression in the past.

It can sometimes be hard to differentiate between feelings of sadness that are part of the normal range of response to challenging life experiences and serious depression that calls for more than basic support and help with problem solving. The medical definition of depression typically ignores the cause(s) of a woman's distress, and thus often fails to address specific issues such as poverty, discrimination, sexual assault, abusive relationships, or the end of a relationship that contribute to feelings of sadness, poor self-image, and despair.

Too often women experiencing reasonable responses to difficult life situations are treated by health care professionals with mood-altering medications that can have unwanted side effects. These medications—whose popularity is fueled by simplistic and unrealistically optimistic advertising—are often prescribed before women are offered more holistic approaches that have been demonstrated to be equally or more effective. However, when social support systems are not readily available or talk therapy is not helpful, some women do find that medications can provide relief, especially by helping them return to normal function in the short term.

Currently, in North America, pregnancy is treated as though it is an at-risk situation for depression, and routine prenatal care includes screening for depression. Nonetheless, evidence shows that pregnant women experience no more depression than women who are not pregnant. According to one large systematic review,

about one in every thirteen pregnant women experiences some depression.[17] In a survey of U.S. women of reproductive age, there was not a significant difference in rates of depression between pregnant and nonpregnant women, and the trend was actually toward pregnant women experiencing less depression.[18]

Why is there potential harm with screening? Screening large, generally healthy groups of people inevitably produces false positives that may result in healthy people being labeled as having a mental health disorder and exposing them to the unnecessary risks of treatment. Furthermore, although many believe that detection and treatment of depression in pregnancy have been shown to prevent depression after birth, there is little scientific evidence to support this view.

Symptoms of serious depression may develop in the context of challenging life circumstances, or they may arise with no apparent cause.

Ever since my eighteenth week of this pregnancy, I have been feeling depressed. I feel flat/unhappy all the time, I cry a lot, I can't sleep, I can't concentrate, I'm impatient with everyone, and not even playing with my toddler makes me happy anymore. This is a much-wanted pregnancy, and there is nothing going on in my life that should be making me so unhappy.[19]

If you are pregnant and experiencing feelings of mild to moderate sadness, the first things to do are to try to get enough sleep and exercise, eat well, and reach out to friends, family, religious counselors, and/or specialized support groups for practical and emotional support. If these strategies do not ease the depression, seek help from a health professional, such as your primary care provider or ob-gyn, or a psychotherapist, social worker, or psychologist with experience treating depression during pregnancy. Depression is treatable, and a good therapist can provide support and guidance as well as help assess whether additional treatment may be helpful. If you have concerns about hurting yourself or others, or an acute sense of hopelessness or inability to function, seek medical attention immediately.

Antidepressants are commonly prescribed during pregnancy. Although these medications are widely believed to be very effective, a recent review of *all* the clinical trials submitted to the FDA—including negative studies pharmaceutical companies chose not to publish—found that antidepressant medications are only slightly more effective than placebos.[20]* For people experiencing mild to moderate depression, they were no more effective than a placebo. Among people who were suffering from major depression, only one of ten people treated with antidepressant medication significantly improved as a result of taking the medication. Among people whose depression was categorized as "very severe," one out of four responded to antidepressant medication.

Furthermore, antidepressants have not been shown to be more effective for mild to moderate depression than nondrug options such as psychotherapy, cognitive behavioral therapy, and exercise. The clinical trial evidence strongly supports a model of symptomatic treatment focusing on life situation, rather than a model of an imbalance in brain chemistry that is "fixed" by antidepressant medication. Most depression is episodic, generally resolving (even without treatment) in about four to six months.

Although some clinicians believe that antidepressants are more effective than shown in clinical trials, the only scientifically valid way to determine whether and by what margin medication is superior to treatment with a placebo is from the results of randomized, double-blind, controlled trials.

In addition to the question of effectiveness, there is some concern about the possible risks of taking antidepressants during pregnancy. For example, can they cause birth impairments? Do they increase the risk of miscarriage? Several studies suggest that there is an increased risk of heart defects in infants whose mothers take antidepressant medications, especially paroxetine (Paxil and generic equivalents),[21]† and some evidence that women taking certain antidepressant medications have an increased risk of miscarriage.

There have also been reports of some harmful effects on infants of women who took antidepressants in the last trimester of pregnancy, including effects such as jitteriness, crying, and feeding problems that may be withdrawal effects, and very rarely, a serious disorder called persistent pulmonary hypertension.[22] There has been controversy surrounding all of these risks and the medical evidence is being hotly contested in legal cases. More research is needed to answer questions about potential risks, including risks that may be due to underlying differences (unrelated to drug use) between women who do and don't take antidepressants.

For women who become pregnant while taking antidepressant medication, these concerns must be weighed against the risk that stopping antidepressant medication during pregnancy will lead to worsening of depression or the symp-

* Estimates of higher efficacy are possible when one selects a subset of clinical trials that omits studies showing less efficacy or when an analysis puts a positive spin on negative results. It is also true that many studies show a considerable response rate to a placebo. Moreover, most depression episodes are temporary and resolve on their own, and in many cases it is hard to distinguish between the effects of drugs and those of other forms of social support and care.

† The FDA has classified paroxetine as class "D" in pregnancy. This means that the FDA has determined good evidence of human fetal risk and thus recommends "do not use" during pregnancy. The other SSRIs are classified as "C," indicating that there is only animal evidence and/or lack of human studies. Therefore, the FDA recommends their use with caution. Drugs classified as "A" or "B" are generally considered appropriate for use in pregnancy; "D" and especially "X" drugs should be avoided if possible.

toms of drug withdrawal. One study showed a high rate of depression relapse when pregnant women were taken off their antidepressant medication, but the study did not gradually taper the dose of medication and failed to distinguish between symptoms of drug withdrawal and recurrence of depression.[23]

Depression in pregnant women is associated with low weight gain, alcohol and substance abuse, and sexually transmitted infections, all of which can harm mothers and babies. Although there is no evidence that taking medications will prevent any of these problems, women with severe depression clearly need professional help.

In the United Kingdom, the National Institute for Health and Clinical Excellence (NICE) recommends the use of older and less expensive tricyclic antidepressants rather than newer drugs such as Prozac, Paxil, and Zoloft because of the longer experience with their use and because of concerns that the newer antidepressants may be less safe overall during pregnancy.

Pregnant women who are struggling with other mental health problems, such as bipolar disorder, anxiety, or post-traumatic stress disorder may be offered medications other than antidepressants. If medication is recommended, make sure that you are fully informed about its benefits and adverse effects, as well as the full range of alternatives—both drug and non-drug. Also, check the FDA's assessment of the safety of each medication for use in pregnancy. (This information is included in the package insert of each prescription medication, which is available from your pharmacy.) You and your health care providers can also get free information on the possible risks of medication on your pregnancy from the Organization of Teratology Information Specialists* (otispregnancy.org).

---

* Teratology is the study of the causes and biological processes leading to abnormal fetal development and birth impairments.

PREPARING FOR LABOR AND BIRTH

As the weeks pass and you get closer to the day your baby will make his or her long-awaited arrival, it's a good time to ask yourself, "What do I want out of my birth experience?"

Every woman hopes for a safe birth and a healthy baby. Beyond that, you may prefer strongly to have a natural childbirth, or you might know you prefer an epidural. You may have cultural or religious customs you would like to integrate into your birth. If you have other children, you may be particularly motivated to have an easy recovery. If you have had a prior traumatic birth or other past trauma, you may wish to avoid certain triggers during this birth. These are just a few examples of the many hopes and expectations we bring with us to the birth-planning process. It is important to ask yourself questions to clarify your values and preferences and, if you have a partner, to discuss these and find out about his or her hopes as well.

As you learn more about pregnancy, childbirth, and early motherhood, you may find that your values and assumptions have changed since early pregnancy. As you begin to think about your upcoming birth and transition to motherhood, ask yourself if your midwife or doctor still seems like a good fit. It is common for women to switch care providers or birth settings in mid- or late pregnancy, and most women who do switch are happy they did.

The major labor and birth choices you will need to consider ahead of time are who you want to have with you for support, strategies for coping, and which labor interventions you will agree to under which circumstances.

IF YOUR CARE PROVIDER RECOMMENDS INDUCTION OF LABOR OR CESAREAN SECTION

In a survey of women who gave birth in U.S. hospitals in 2005, fully half of respondents had labor induced (34 percent) or underwent a planned cesarean before labor began (16 percent). Though some of those were necessary procedures, experts agree that both interventions are overused.

Every week of pregnancy matters for proper development of the fetal heart, lungs, and other organs, and women who have inductions who are first-time mothers and/or have an unready cervix are vulnerable to ending up with unneeded cesarean.

With exceptions such as placenta previa, severe high blood pressure, or a baby whose growth is significantly restricted, letting labor begin on its own is generally safer than induction or planned cesarean. If your care provider suggests inducing labor or scheduling a C-section, take time to carefully consider the recommendation and ask plenty of questions, such as:

- Why are you recommending an induction or cesarean?
- What are the risks to my baby and me if I wait for labor to begin naturally?
- Can you provide me with a high-quality research study that shows that induction/cesarean in this situation is safe and will reduce my risk of an unhealthy outcome?
- Is induction likely to be successful for me? If not, how much time will you wait for labor to start, or will you expect me to have a cesarean?
- What other aspects of my care are affected by the choice to have an induction/cesarean (e.g., restrictions on food and drink or movement in induced labor, separation from the baby after birth)? How can my birth team support me in making sure my baby and I get the supportive care we need?

DOULAS

Having continuous, high-quality supportive care from others during labor and birth is one of the best ways you can ensure a safe and satisfying experience. Studies demonstrate that women who receive continuous labor support while giving birth need less medication, have lower cesarean section and assisted vaginal birth (vacuum extraction, forceps) rates, and are more satisfied with their birth experiences.[24]

Many of us count on and receive excellent support from our partners or our health care providers. Yet our partners are probably inexperienced at attending births and need their own support, especially in long labors. Midwives, doctors, and nurses in hospitals may not be able to provide continuous care because of the many different demands on their time. (Midwives who attend women at home or in a birth center typically do provide continuous support.) For these reasons, some women choose to be accompanied by a doula (a trained labor support person) or a relative or friend who is knowledgeable about and comfortable around birth and who can stay through the whole process.

Birth doulas provide continuous emotional support, comfort techniques, and encouragement throughout labor and birth. Doulas complement midwifery and medical care, offering a wide range of services, sometimes including home visits after the baby is born. To find a doula in your area, try doulamatch.net or the websites of any of the doula-certifying organizations.

Doulas usually make an initial visit during pregnancy and then arrange to be with you during labor. Some doulas specialize in certain situations, such as teen mothers, women whose native language is not English, women who have experienced a prior loss, VBAC mothers, women whose partners are deployed overseas, or women who cannot afford traditional doula services.

PLANNING FOR PAIN MANAGEMENT

During pregnancy, most of us wonder how we will cope with the intensity and pain of labor and birth. You and those who will support you during labor can learn relaxation routines and other strategies from classes, books, or audio or video resources and practice them before you go into labor. These strategies range from comfort measures such as changing positions, using touch, or relaxing in water to mental strategies such as focused breathing or hypnosis to medication such as opioids (narcotics) or epidurals.

The pain relief methods you choose to use can affect your experience and memories of labor. Learning about the potential advantages and disadvantages of different methods, thinking about your preferences with regard to pain control, and talking with your provider and support people about what you want before you go into labor will help you make sound decisions.

While preparing is important, labor itself is unpredictable. You can't know in advance what you will experience or what you will want or need. Your labor may be easier or more complicated than you imagine. You might plan to give birth without medication and then find yourself needing greater relief, or you might plan on having an epidural but then find you don't need one.

I was determined to have a total "medical buffet" during my delivery. I'd start with Nubain and then move to an epidural and be blissfully pain free. However, when I arrived at the hospital, my OB told me that it was too late for any medical intervention and it was time to push. In fact, I had been lucky not to have had him in the car on the way. I had to throw my "imagined delivery" out of the window and have this baby. I labored for sixty-four minutes in the hospital, and he was born. I was swearing like a sailor and yelled at everyone within a two-foot radius, including my husband. (I swore at my OB so atrociously that when I returned to the same hospital three years later for baby number two, the nurses remembered me.) At one point my OB nonchalantly said, "If you focused that energy on pushing instead of yelling at us, you'd have a baby by now." I got all huffed up at her and my husband, and then my son crowned. She smiled and said, "I told you." It was the most powerful moment of my life; I delivered him, cut the cord, and held him in my arms . . . all before breakfast.

Because it is often challenging to make specific decisions about pain relief before labor, and because all pain-relieving medications can have adverse effects, it is generally best to approach normal labor with the idea of using no-risk or very-low-risk strategies first and then proceeding to the next higher level of intervention if needed. It's also helpful to rest as much as possible during early labor and conserve your energy, as exhaustion can diminish your capacity to tolerate pain and thus increase the need for pain medication. The "Pain Medications Preference Scale" on pp. 396–397 can help you clarify your feelings about pain and pain management during labor.

Your choice of birth setting and provider can affect your options for pain management; for more information, see "Choosing a Provider," p. 362, and "Birth Places," p. 367. For more information on specific coping strategies and pain relief methods, see "Coping with Pain," p. 410.

PLANNING WITH CONFIDENCE, KNOWLEDGE, AND FLEXIBILITY

Learning about our options for coping with labor and working with a knowledgeable support team can help us feel less anxious as we anticipate labor and birth. We can arrive at informed decisions about the approaches we prefer, recognizing that we may need to make changes based on how our labor unfolds.

I was scared of the pain. I wanted to avoid interventions if possible, but I also wanted my limits to be respected. I wanted to see a midwife because I believed that her philosophy of birth, practical techniques, and continuous support would help me have the kind of birth I wanted. But I needed to know that if my labor was really hard or lasting forever, or if I was totally exhausted, she would support me in getting an epidural.

The first midwife I interviewed when I was pregnant didn't seem to hear my fears; she just said that women's bodies were designed to give birth and that my body would do so also. The second midwife, the one I chose, was more reassuring: she said she knew lots of nondrug techniques to help me cope and manage with the pain but that she was committed to helping me have a good birth, whatever that meant to me. She said that there were times when epidurals

were extremely helpful. In the end, I didn't have an epidural, but knowing that it was an option—and knowing that my midwife wouldn't see me as a failure if I had one—may have been part of what helped me avoid one!

PREPARING FOR BREASTFEEDING

Breast milk is the best food for babies; it provides all the nutrients your baby needs to grow, as well as antibodies that protect against infection. Nursing also provides numerous health benefits to you. Whether you are undecided about breastfeeding or committed to it, take time to talk with midwives, childbirth educators, and other mothers and to read available books during your pregnancy. Having good support and plans in place before you give birth can help smooth the way. (To read more about breastfeeding, including how to get off to a good start, see "Breastfeeding Your Baby," p. 436.)

YOU ARE READY FOR BIRTH!

The transition to motherhood can be challenging, both physically and emotionally. Learning as much as you can and listening to other women's stories will give you information and inspiration to face the challenges of pregnancy and childbirth with greater confidence.

A woman planning a home birth said:

My mother gave birth to me at home. Her mother had given birth to five children and had considered her labors her finest, strongest moments. I know I can give birth and it is hard work, but I trust my body. At night I sit still, close my eyes, breathe deeply, and picture myself opening up. . . . My birth will be unique.

PAIN MEDICATIONS PREFERENCE SCALE

This table, created by the childbirth educator Penny Simkin, can help you clarify your feelings about pain and pain management during labor.*

NUMBER	WHAT IT MEANS	YOUR PARTNER, DOULA, NURSE, OR CAREGIVER CAN HELP YOU BY
+10	I want to be numb, to get anesthesia before labor begins. (An impossible extreme.)	• Explaining that you will have some pain even with anesthesia. • Discussing your wishes and fears with you. • Promising to help you get medication as soon as possible in labor
+9	I have a great fear of labor pain and I believe I cannot cope. I have to depend on the staff to take away my pain.	• Doing the same as for +10 above. • Teaching you some simple comfort techniques for early labor. • Reassuring you that someone will always be there to help you.
+7	I want anesthesia as soon in labor as the doctor will allow or before labor becomes painful.	• Doing the same as for +9 above. • Making sure the staff knows that you want early anesthesia. • Making sure you know the procedures and the potential risks.
+5	I want epidural anesthesia in active labor (4-5 cm). I am willing to try to cope until then, perhaps with narcotic medications.	• Encouraging you in your breathing and relaxation. • Knowing and using other comfort measures. • Suggesting medication when you are in active labor.
+3	I want to use some medication but as little as possible. I plan to use self-help comfort measures for part of labor.	• Doing the same as for +5 above. • Committing herself or himself to helping you reduce medication use. • Helping you get medications when you decide you want them. • Suggesting half doses of narcotics or a "light and late" epidural.
0	I have no opinion or preference. I will wait and see. (A rare attitude among pregnant women.)	• Helping you become informed about labor pain, comfort measures, and medications. • Following your wishes during labor.

−3	I would like to avoid pain medications if I can, but if coping becomes difficult, I'd feel like a "martyr" if I did not get them.	• Emphasizing coping techniques. • Not suggesting that you take pain medication. • Not trying to talk you out of pain medications if you request them.
−5	I have a strong desire to avoid pain medications, mainly to avoid the side effects on me, my labor, or my baby. I will accept medications for a difficult or long labor.	• Preparing for a very active support role. • Practicing comfort measures with you in class and at home. • Not suggesting medications. If you ask, suggesting different comfort measures and more intense emotional support first. • Helping you accept pain medications if you become exhausted or cannot benefit from support techniques and comfort measures.
−7	I have a very strong desire for a natural birth, for personal gratification along with the benefits to my baby and my labor. I will be disappointed if I use medication.	• Doing the same as for −5 above. • Encouraging you to enlist the support of your caregiver. • Requesting a supportive nurse who can help with natural birth. • Planning and rehearsing ways to get through painful or discouraging periods in labor. • Prearranging a plan (e.g., a "last resort" code word) for letting her or him know if you have had enough and want medication.
−9	I want medication to be denied by my support team and the staff, even if I beg for it.	• Exploring the reasons for your feelings. • Helping you see that they cannot deny you medication. • Promising to help all they can but leaving the final decision to you.
−10	I want no medication, even for a cesarean delivery. (An impossible extreme.)	• Doing the same as for −9 above. • Helping you gain a realistic understanding of risks and benefits of pain medications.

* Used with permission from Penny Simkin and Childbirth Graphics.

CHAPTER 16 ▪ ▪ ▪ ▪ ▪ ▪ ▪ ▪ ▪ ▪ ▪ ▪ ▪ ▪ ▪ ▪

W omen's experiences with labor and birth vary widely from woman to woman, from one phase of labor to another, and from one labor to the next. Your labor will be unique, influenced by many factors: the size, position, and health of your baby; your health and medical history; your expectations and feelings; the people who support and attend to you; and the place in which you labor and give birth.

But despite the variations, there is a common theme: the natural flow of labor. This process involves interplay between you and your baby. During your pregnancy, your body has held and protected your baby. Now, under the influence of hormones that you and your baby release, your body will soften, open, and yield to allow the baby to pass through. Labor contrac-

This chapter emphasizes normal physiological labor and the care choices and birth setting practices that help women have safe and satisfying birth experiences. Unfortunately, far too few women in the United States experience optimal births. A survey of women who gave birth in U.S. hospitals in 2005 found, for example, that most women had unnecessary medical and surgical interventions, did not walk or move around in active labor, and gave birth on their backs; and nearly half of babies spent the first hour after birth with hospital staff, usually for routine care.[1]

For women with chronic medical conditions, pregnancy complications, or a particularly complicated labor, medical interventions can be lifesaving. However, many medical interventions routinely used during labor and birth are unnecessary and may cause harm. For more information, see "Maternity Care in Today's Health Care System," p. 372, and "U.S. Maternity Care: Roadblocks to Change" p. 373.

We need to work to reduce unnecessary, routine interference with physiological birth while recognizing that some women and babies need such interventions to experience birth safely. Women with high-risk or complicated pregnancies must be able to access effective treatments without forfeiting the emotional support, physical comfort, and respect for informed choices all women deserve.

tions, your body movements, and your pushing efforts will guide the baby down while the baby flexes, stretches, and rotates to navigate the birth canal. The birth process progresses from the softening (ripening) and opening (dilation) of your cervix to your baby's descent and birth to the delivery of the placenta.

Giving birth was life-changing for me and for many of the women I have attended as a midwife. In a world in which we may often feel ineffective and pessimistic, working through labor under our own power can transform our sense of self. We experience ourselves as strong, sturdy, resilient, and able. We tap on inner strengths we may never have tapped before and are amazed by what we are able to accomplish. Once we become aware of how powerful we can be in giving birth, we can call on this throughout our lives, in all sorts of situations.

A woman who gave birth in a hospital birthing center says:

The day before she was born, I'd done everything: cooked, mopped, even put up a new mailbox in the bitter cold weather outside. At three A.M. my waters broke. We didn't sleep much after that. We had an already scheduled appointment with Lucy at ten. Since I was only 1 centimeter dilated, she said, "Go on home." . . . Off we went, and all of a sudden, there I was in hard labor, doubled over. Back we drove to the hospital birth center. No one was expecting us; the place was empty.

We got a room. I took a shower and curled into the yoga "child's position," letting hot water run down my back, relatively comfortable. Lucy finally arrived, saw I was completely dilated, and said, "Impressive! Good show!"

LOWERING YOUR CHANCE OF A CESAREAN BIRTH

In the United States today, about one in three women gives birth by cesarean section. While most mothers and babies who have cesarean births do fine, cesarean sections involve more risks than spontaneous vaginal births (births that do not involve the use of forceps, vacuum extraction, or a cesarean). The following tips can help lower your chances of having a cesarean section:

- Choose a care provider who follows the midwifery model of care. (See "Choosing a Provider," p. 362.)
- If you're healthy and haven't had complications in your pregnancy, consider giving birth at home or in a birth center (see "Birth Places," p. 367).
- Ask what the C-section rate is for your provider and birth setting. If the C-section rate is above 15 percent, the provider or setting probably uses C-sections in women who could safely birth vaginally.
- Be proactive in your health habits. Eating well and exercising regularly may reduce the risk for complications such as gestational diabetes that often lead to cesareans.
- Don't induce labor unless there is a clear medical need. Concern that the baby is big is not a medical reason to induce, nor is being up to a week beyond your estimated due date.
- Don't go to the hospital until you are in active labor. If you go to the hospital and have not yet dilated to 4 centimeters, return home or go for a walk nearby.
- Have continuous labor support from a companion who trusts your ability to give birth. This can be a friend, a volunteer doula, or a doula you hire. (For more information, see "Doulas," p. 393.)
- Avoid routine medical interventions during labor, especially continuous electronic fetal monitoring, unless clearly needed.
- Resist any pressure to have a cesarean if there is no good rationale. (For more, see "If Your Care Provider Recommends Induction of Labor or Cesarean Section," page 393.)

I pushed for two hours. I never doubted that I could do it, but it took so long, I was exhausted. Finally, Rosa crowned. Margaret caught her; I remember she put her on my belly. Since she didn't cry, they worried, took her to another room, but Marg said, "That's ridiculous: Bring her back!" And so they did. We stayed two nights. It was an amazing moment finally to bring her home.

SIGNS OF APPROACHING LABOR (PRELABOR)

Labor continues the process begun at conception. The finely tuned biological system that nurtures developing babies guides labor as well. Just before labor begins, your body and your baby get ready for birth. The joints in your hips and pelvis further relax and open, ligaments increasingly

WHEN WILL LABOR BEGIN, AND WHAT MAKES IT START?

No one can predict or determine exactly when labor will start. The baby's size and maturity, as well as multiple hormonal and placental changes, affect the onset of labor, but the biological mechanisms that cause labor to begin are not well understood.

soften, and the baby may drop deeper in your pelvis. Toward the end of pregnancy—for some women, even earlier—you may occasionally feel a painless tightening of your uterus, the Braxton Hicks contractions. You may also feel increased pressure in your pelvis and on your bladder as the baby settles deeper into your pelvis.

You may notice that your emotions are nearer the surface and that your interest in anything unrelated to the birth of your baby wanes. Your baby is getting ready, too, removing fluid from the lungs, wriggling into position, and responding to the shifting hormones that increase resilience for the work ahead. Other signs of approaching labor may include loose stools, more mucus discharge, or cramping. Most of these signs are not specific enough to be obvious, and some women don't experience them at all, but in retrospect, you may recognize signals that your body and mind were gearing up for labor.

One woman describes how her focus shifted as labor approached:

During my pregnancies, I always tried to take a walk during lunch. The bigger I got, the shorter my walks became, and in retrospect, they also became more focused. In the days leading up to my daughter's birth, I went like a homing

WHEN TO CALL YOUR HEALTH CARE PROVIDER

You and your care provider should discuss when you should call. Specific recommendations will be based on your health, how far along you are in your pregnancy, and whether or not this is your first baby. In general, you should call your provider if:

- Your bag of waters breaks (membranes rupture).
- You experience strong, painful contractions that are difficult to talk through and are steadily getting more painful and closer together.
- You are experiencing severe pain.
- You think that your labor has started and you are less than thirty-seven weeks pregnant.
- You experience bleeding that is as heavy as a period or bright red.
- You have any questions or concerns.

If you are planning to give birth in a hospital, talk with your provider about when you should go in. In general it is best to wait until you are in active labor (see "The Stages of Labor," p. 403). This can help you avoid a cascade of unnecessary interventions that can lead to avoidable cesarean surgery and other undesirable outcomes.

IF YOUR WATER BREAKS BEFORE LABOR

The sac containing the amniotic fluid that surrounds your baby (the membranes, or "bag of waters") usually breaks shortly before contractions start or during labor or birth. In a small percentage of women, though, the waters can break many hours or days before labor starts. This causes the fluid to leak out before contractions begin. You may experience a large gush of fluid, followed by continuous leaking.

If the sac breaks on its upper side, the fluid may trickle out slowly. A slow leak may be confused with urine leaking or with discharge of mucus.

Call your midwife or doctor to make a plan when your bag of waters breaks or if you think you are leaking amniotic fluid. Your provider will probably want to see you to confirm that the bag has broken and to check the baby's position and heartbeat. At this time, there will likely be a discussion of the pros and cons of waiting for labor versus inducing labor.

Health care providers have differ-ent opinions about how long to wait for labor to start after the bag of waters has broken. The American College of Nurse-Midwives (ACNM) says that waiting for labor to begin on its own is a safe option unless there are signs of or risk factors for infection, and as long as the woman and baby are otherwise healthy.[2] With this approach, eight out of ten women will begin labor naturally within twenty-four hours. In contrast, the American Congress of Obstetricians and Gynecologists (ACOG) advises immediate induction of labor after water breaks, which is a reversal of its previous recommendation. ACOG made this change without citing any new evidence that induction is safer than waiting for labor to begin on its own.[3]

If you wait for labor contractions to start spontaneously, you should avoid having intercourse or putting anything into your vagina and decline vaginal exams unless there is a clear medical need, to reduce the risk of infection. It may be best to avoid taking a bath until active labor has begun.[4]

---

pigeon to a local bookstore that always seemed to have some must-have cookbook on sale. The Food and Cooking of Thailand; The Complete Spanish Cookbook; One-pot, Slow-pot, and Clay-pot Cooking; Slow Cooker; and Russian, German & Polish Food & Cooking—I simply had to have them all. These books are now fondly known as my "nesting collection."

Another woman was surprised by how little warning she had before labor began in earnest:

It was July 4, and while eating breakfast I said to my husband, "I guess we're not going to have a Fourth of July baby." I just felt so normal. I'd had Braxton Hicks contractions for a few weeks and some mild indigestion the night before, but everything seemed to be status quo, and I figured that even if I began having the early signs of labor, I'd still have a long road ahead. Little did I know that my "independence baby" would be in my arms by four o'clock that afternoon!

One woman describes the beginning of her labor:

I went into spontaneous labor in the wee morning hours during a rainstorm. My contractions started waking me up at two A.M., so I got out of bed and started cleaning. . . . I did some organization around the apartment for a bit and then took a wonderful bath in our Jacuzzi tub. I deep conditioned my hair and carefully shaved my legs, knowing that I might not have the luxury to do these things in the busy weeks to come.

THE STAGES OF LABOR

STAGE/PHASE	HOW LONG WILL IT TYPICALLY LAST?	HOW DILATED WILL MY CERVIX BE?	WHAT WILL MY CONTRACTIONS BE LIKE?	WHAT ELSE MIGHT BE HAPPENING?
Warm-up labor (prelabor, prodromal labor)	On and off for days or weeks	0 to 3 cm	Vary greatly in length and intensity.	Mucus discharge, backache. It's hard to tell when you move from this into latent-phase labor.
Stage 1: Latent phase	A few hours to a day or more	0 to 4-5 cm	Vary widely. Usually short (about 30 to 60 seconds), spaced relatively far apart (anywhere from 5 minutes to over 20 minutes apart). You may be able to ignore or distract yourself from them.	Mucus discharge (with "bloody show"), backache, upset stomach.
Active phase	Between 2 and 10 hours	4-5 to 7-8 cm	Last about a minute or more, spaced regularly. You probably will not be able to walk or distract yourself.	You may feel tired or discouraged, wondering if you can do it. Pressure in your lower back, need to change positions often.
Transition phase	A few contractions to 1-2 hours	7-8 cm to full dilation (about 10 cm)	Occur about every 2 minutes and last at least 60 seconds so you have short rests in between contractions.	Intense emotions and physical sensations. You may feel restless, irritable, and exhausted. Trembling, nausea, and vomiting are common just before the cervix becomes completely dilated. Water is likely to break if it hasn't already.

(continued on next page)

STAGE/PHASE	HOW LONG WILL IT TYPICALLY LAST?	HOW DILATED WILL MY CERVIX BE?	WHAT WILL MY CONTRACTIONS BE LIKE?	WHAT ELSE MIGHT BE HAPPENING?
Stage 2: Pushing, giving birth	A few contractions to over 3 hours	Fully dilated, 10 cm ("complete")	Powerful contractions about every 3 minutes. (Some women experience a break in contractions for 10-25 minutes once the cervix is fully dilated, before feeling the urge to push.)	Pain lessens, and you may be able to rest for a brief time before the urge to push becomes uncontrollable. You may also become more clearheaded and energetic. As baby descends, you will feel strong pressure in the vaginal and rectal areas, resulting in a strong urge to push. Stinging, burning sensation as baby's head crowns.
Stage 3: Delivery of placenta	May last up to 30 minutes or longer, usually completed in 10 minutes or less		No contractions, then one to several strong cramps.	Provider may massage uterus to cause it to contract and reduce bleeding; this can be painful.
Stage 4: Recovery	May last 1-2 hours if birth was unmedicated and not prolonged or difficult; longer if otherwise		Mild or moderate cramps as uterus contracts.	Thick, bloody vaginal discharge (lochia) that may last 2-4 weeks. Uterus will tighten to prevent bleeding. Swelling and discomfort in your perineum. Trembling legs.

I told my partner, Brian, at around four A.M. that I was starting labor. We snuggled in bed, and he put on one of my favorite movies. I held on to him tightly through my contractions, which were not that close together yet. I called Melissa, my nearest and dearest friend, who lives three hours away. She was one of my labor support team. She would head down right away to help me through this.

LABOR BEGINS AND EARLY (LATENT) LABOR

The latent phase of labor may feel much the same to you as prelabor, but during this time your cervix will open up (dilate) to 4 to 5 centimeters and will usually completely thin out (efface). Labor contractions will be short and spaced relatively far apart (from five to twenty minutes apart). During the latent phase, your contractions will become longer, more painful, and more regular. This is not yet the time to go to a hospital or birthing center. However, most women at this stage want some kind of care, such as the reassuring presence of a partner or close friend or a care provider or other guide familiar with birth. Some women say that this phase of labor is the hardest psychologically. One midwife explains:

It's like starting a hike and no one is telling you how long it is. The trail has lots of meandering switchbacks and hills, and you don't know where you're headed or how long it will take to get there, but you just keep going. Later, it may get physically more difficult, but at least then you can see the end in sight, the peak of the mountain, and you can push on.

Sometimes contractions build up gradually, starting with any of the signs mentioned above, with menstrual-like cramps evolving into stronger contractions that grow closer together over a long period of time, sometimes even over a period of days. At the other extreme, labor can begin abruptly, with strong regular contractions no more than five minutes apart, causing you to stop everything you are doing and concentrate.

Everyone responds differently to early labor. Walking, showering, taking long baths, or cuddling with loved ones can relax you and help labor progress. These early hours may be sweet as you lie with your partner or sit alone, the baby still within you in the quiet of your home. It is important that you continue to eat nourishing foods to prepare you for the work ahead. And sleep is critical for much the same reason, particularly with a first baby, for which labor may be longer. Some women feel too excited or apprehensive to sleep. Try to save your energy for active labor. Don't worry if contractions slow down when you lie down to rest; it's still early. If you truly don't feel up for rest, spending time with friends and family can be a nice distraction, but check in with yourself frequently and consider whether you would rather be resting.

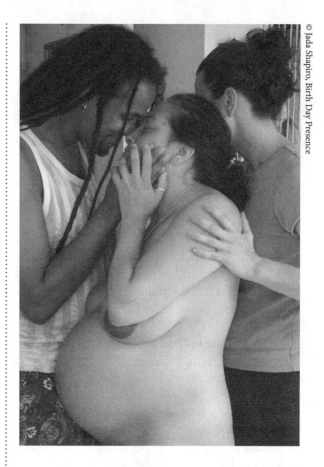

If you begin to feel like a "watched pot," ask for some time alone.

When we went for a walk, we ran into friends. "What are you doing up? I thought you were in labor." It was fun changing people's image of a woman in labor.

LABOR PROGRESSES (ACTIVE FIRST STAGE)

For many first-time mothers, it can take a day or more to get to about 4 centimeters dilation, which signals entry into the active phase of labor. When you feel painful, wavelike, regular,

Your water may break at any time before or during labor. Some women will notice their water break before labor or during early labor. If you start active labor and your water hasn't broken yet, it most likely will during transition or while pushing.

rhythmic contractions that last forty-five to sixty seconds and that are so intense you can't talk or walk while you are having one, you are likely in active labor. The contractions may begin in your back, you may feel them only in the front, or you may feel them in both the back and front. Your uterus feels hard to the touch.

Though you may have heard that labor will get more and more painful as it progresses, this is not necessarily true. Some women say the active phase of labor was the most painful, some say the transition phase, and others say pushing was the most painful. In general, women feel the most pain during periods when the cervix is dilating fast or when the baby is descending quickly. These events can happen at different phases of labor for different women.

I spent most of the night laboring alone in the dark, like a cat. It was marvelous. Not easy—it's hard work; that's why it's called LABOR. It was intense. Not painful—I can't call it painful. But it's . . . inevitable. Inescapable. Uncontrollable. You can't get away. I kept thinking of that kids' game "Going on a bear hunt": "Can't go over it, can't go around it, have to go through it!"

This is the time to gather your support people, to call your provider if you are having a home birth, or to prepare to go to the birth center or hospital. If you are not sure if you are

in active labor yet, your care provider can help you know for sure. A careful phone consultation, a home visit, or a visit at the office can help determine your progression. Staying home or in another familiar, comfortable setting until active labor is well established is an important strategy for reducing your chance of interventions. Studies show that being admitted to a hospital in early labor increases the chances of having medications to speed up your labor or a cesarean section.[5] Travel can be an uncomfortable challenge during active labor, but you can regain your rhythm once you are settled in your chosen birth setting.

Progress in the active phase of labor, both for first-time mothers and for women who have given birth before, is widely variable. In many hospital birth settings, expectations for labor progress are based on outdated studies that showed average dilation rates in women with medically managed labors (known as the "Friedman curve") or driven by financial incentives to get labor done more quickly and make room for the next patient to be admitted. The traditions of natural or expectant management and current evidence show that normal labor can be significantly longer than previous studies suggested, and "plateaus"—when the woman's cervix doesn't actively dilate for several hours—are common.[6] As long as the mother and baby are doing well, labor should be allowed to progress on its own.

One woman describes her experience of getting "stuck" temporarily at a certain point in active labor:

I got stuck at about 8 to 9 centimeters for a really long time. I wasn't aware how long, except that it was hours. [The doctor] who was on call suggested Pitocin to speed things up, but I refused. Part of my concern was that the contractions were already so intense that I felt if they were

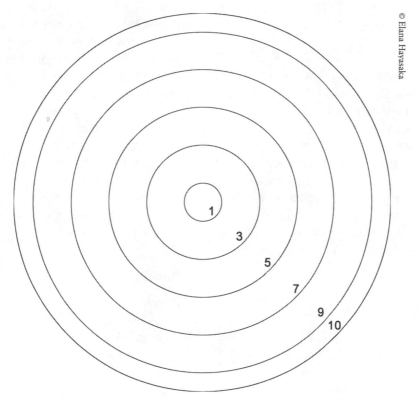

Cervical dilation shown in actual size (in centimeters). When you reach about 10 centimeters, you will be ready to push.

stronger and closer together I wouldn't be able to cope, and I did not want to do anything that put me at risk for a C-section . . .

. . . In the end, I realized that though it was hard, it was never more than I could take, and I had been prepared to keep pushing for even longer if necessary. I had not reached the end of my strength. We never would have been able to do it without our doula's help—she was worth her weight in gold.

The last few centimeters from 8 cm to complete dilation (about 10 cm) can be the hardest, most intense phase of labor, but it is also usually the shortest. In first pregnancies, this period generally lasts no more than a couple of hours.

The transition is when many women get discouraged and feel that they have hit a wall and can't go on. Excellent labor support from a loved one or doula can help you discover deep wells of strength to finish birthing. If you experience challenges at this time, keep in mind that this is the home stretch. Your body has already accomplished most of the difficult work. Do whatever makes you feel more comfortable and helps you handle the intensity of labor. When transition is over, you will be pushing your baby out. One woman recalls how she shed her usual inhibitions during transition:

The hospital's birthing pavilion was like a good hotel. But I didn't get to kick back with a book

MEDICAL APPROACHES TO SPEEDING UP LABOR

Active labor may be over in several hours, or it may take a day or longer. As long as the mother and baby are doing well, there is no reason for concern. Efforts to stimulate labor should be used only if they reduce the likelihood of a poor outcome such as infection or a cesarean section or prevent exhaustion and suffering. The two most common methods used in hospitals for stimulating labor arguably achieve neither of these outcomes reliably.

Artificial Rupture of Membranes

If you are in active labor with a bulging sac of water in front of your baby's head and the baby is deep in your pelvis, your doctor or midwife may recommend rupturing the membranes to strengthen contractions or to speed up a prolonged labor. This procedure, known as amniotomy, is performed during a vaginal exam using a small tool that looks like a crochet hook. Breaking the membranes is thought to release chemicals and hormones that stimulate contractions, and the direct pressure of the head rather than a cushion of fluid on the cervix is thought to assist dilation. However, a systematic review of the better-quality published research on routine amniotomy found that it is ineffective at speeding labor and may increase the likelihood of cesarean surgery.[7] None of the studies assessed pain, but women commonly report increased pain after membranes are broken. Amni-

otomy may also predispose a woman to infection and increases the chance that the umbilical cord will be compressed enough to temporarily reduce oxygen flow to the baby.

Amniotomy is required if internal fetal monitoring is planned. Some women very late in labor find that amniotomy provides relief if a large pocket of fluid is bulging in front of the baby's head. Most women's membranes release spontaneously during pushing, if they haven't broken earlier in labor.

Pitocin

Pitocin (synthetic oxytocin) is sometimes used to make labor progress more quickly. It is given through an IV and makes contractions more frequent and forceful. Pitocin is on a small list of high-alert medications (drugs that have a high risk of causing injury when they are misused) identified by the Institute for Safe Medication Practices, and the use of Pitocin requires continuous fetal heart rate monitoring. Pitocin is begun at a low dose, which is gradually increased to achieve contractions that are close enough together to continue opening the cervix and moving the baby forward into the birth canal.

Negative consequences of having labor augmented with Pitocin include being attached to an IV and the electronic fetal monitor, which may limit your freedom to move into different positions. With Pitocin, contractions may reach their peaks more rapidly. If this occurs, the contractions may be more painful. In addition, you may get too much medication for a short time, and this can cause contractions that come too close together. As a result, the baby may get less oxygen between contractions than she or he would with typical contractions. Turning the Pitocin off, lying on your side, and/or receiving extra IV fluids can quickly remedy this situation.

Since using Pitocin requires continuous fetal heart rate monitoring, fetal heart rate changes that appear alarming but are nonetheless tolerated by the baby may result in other interventions. Research is mixed on whether and under what circumstances Pitocin augmentation affects the likelihood of cesarean section.

Pitocin also interferes with the production of a woman's own natural oxytocin. Oxytocin is the hormone that regulates the emotional responses of connection and bonding. It is crucial for giving birth, breastfeeding, and attachment. More research is needed to understand whether the use of Pitocin in labor affects the emotional health and behavior of women and babies.

Pitocin may be used if labor progress slows and other efforts are not effective. Because epidurals disrupt a woman's own oxytocin levels, Pitocin is often needed to keep labor progressing after an epidural is placed.[8] Some hospitals have a low-dose Pitocin protocol based on the peak action time of the drug. In this case, Pitocin is increased very slowly and over a longer period of time. This mimics natural labor more closely and makes the contractions easier to deal with.[9]

In Childbirth Connection's 2006 Listening to Mothers II survey, 59 percent of women had their bag of water artificially ruptured and 55 percent received intravenous Pitocin to speed up or strengthen contractions after labor started.[10] When more than half of women receive interventions to treat "abnormal" labor, there may be something wrong with the definition of abnormal. Choosing a care provider and setting in which these interventions are used infrequently and arranging to have excellent labor support are good strategies for ensuring you will not be exposed to them unnecessarily. (For more information, see Chapter 15, "Pregnancy and Planning for Birth.")

and some room service. All through the night, I heaved around on the floor in a variety of positions—on my side Jane Fonda aerobics style, on all fours with ass and yoni to the wind, on the floor, and then up on the bed. I was desperate for comfort, relief and a baby in my arms.

Shift changes were going on, and people were coming and going. It was like Grand Central Station. . . . They asked me if I minded having a nursing student watch the birth. By this time, I didn't care if the security guard from the parking lot brought in popcorn and Raisinettes to watch the event.

Another woman says:

The peak of each contraction was such that I needed to close my eyes and really concentrate

DIFFERENCES BETWEEN PERIODIC AND CONTINUOUS FETAL MONITORING

The baby's heart rate and rhythm provide information that care providers can interpret to make a judgment about the baby's health. The baby's heartbeat can be assessed periodically (intermittent monitoring or intermittent auscultation) or continuously throughout labor. Intermittent auscultation involves using a handheld fetoscope (an instrument like a stethoscope) or, more commonly, a handheld ultrasound (Doppler) to record the baby's heart rate.

Hospitals generally use continuous external fetal monitoring, which produces a continuous electronic record of the baby's heart rate. This provides more data about the baby, but more data do not necessarily lead to better ability to make judgments about the baby's well-being. In fact, in healthy women without labor complications, and even in some higher-risk labors, continuous electronic fetal monitoring dramatically increases the likelihood of a cesarean section.

If you have an epidural, are receiving Pitocin for induction or augmentation, or have health problems such as high blood pressure, you will be required to use continuous electronic fetal monitoring. Many hospitals now have wireless units that allow you to stay reasonably mobile even while your baby's heartbeat is continuously monitored.

In healthy women without labor complications, intermittent monitoring is associated with equally good infant outcomes and reduced likelihood of cesarean surgery, compared with continuous monitoring.[11] Intermittent auscultation allows the woman to remain mobile and keeps the attention of staff and labor support companions on the woman herself rather than machines.

Unfortunately, intermittent monitoring is very infrequent in hospitals, due to staffing issues, liability concerns, and the frequent use of other interventions that necessitate continuous monitoring. In a nationally representative survey of women who gave birth in U.S. hospitals in 2005, just 6 percent were monitored intermittently throughout labor.[12]

on the number of deep breaths I was taking, knowing that at the count of five or eight, depending on the length of the sensation, it would start to ease up. There's a sureness in numbers— the logic overwhelmed the raw wildness of the sensation. I knew time was my only ally in dealing with the pain. With time each contraction would be over, with time the baby would be born.

COPING WITH PAIN

Labor and birth are intense and unpredictable, and can push us to places within ourselves that we've never been. Many of us fear the pain and wonder how we will manage.

Fortunately, many techniques are available to ease and help manage pain. These techniques range from comfort measures such as walking, touch, and submersion in water to mental strategies such as focused breathing and hypnosis to medications such as opioids and epidurals.

THINKING ABOUT LABOR PAIN

In everyday life, physical pain, especially intense pain, is usually a warning that something is wrong in our bodies. But the pain of labor is not a sign of danger, nor is it a symptom of injury or illness. It is a sign that your body is working hard to birth your baby.

Labor pain is different in many ways from other kinds of pain. For one, the pain is self-limiting—it will end when the baby is born. It is also intermittent, not continuous, which means you will usually have periods of no pain between contractions. In addition, labor sensations intensify gradually over time, and this allows your body time to adapt. These differences often make labor pain easier to cope with than other kinds of pain.

Because pain and suffering often go hand in hand, we tend to think they're the same thing. But they're not. Pain is a physical sensation, while suffering is an emotional experience. We may suffer (feel helplessness, anguish, remorse, fear, panic, or loss of control) even when there is no physical sensation of pain. And we may experience physical pain without suffering. As Penny Simkin and April Bolding, longtime advocates for birthing women, write, "One can have pain coexisting with satisfaction, enjoyment, and empowerment."[13] By the same token, they say, suffering can be caused or increased by factors other than physical pain: "Loneliness, ignorance, unkind or insensitive treatment during labor, along with unresolved past psychological or physical distress, increase the chance that the woman will suffer."

While it is commonly believed that a woman's satisfaction with her birth experience is linked to how much or how little pain she feels, this isn't typically so. Our satisfaction seems to be highest when we trust that we are getting good information, we are given opportunities to participate in decisions regarding our care, and our caregivers treat us with kindness and respect.[14] Pain and pain relief seem to have less effect on our overall satisfaction than the quality of support we receive from our caregivers.

My labor felt like a marathon that lasted over two days. There were easy periods, where I sailed along (I was even able to sleep), but there were stretches when it felt like a steep, uphill climb that would never end. But just like in a marathon, you just keep putting one foot in front of the other. You don't think about reaching the end, you just think about taking the next step. Having the support of a great midwife, my husband, and a few close loved ones made all the difference. I had such a HUGE sense of accomplishment when my daughter emerged and made her first tiny sounds. I was exhilarated by meeting such a great physical (and mental) challenge and felt I had earned a marathon "crown."

STRATEGIES TO HELP YOU COPE WITH LABOR

Certain strategies lay the foundation to help you cope with the pain of labor. These include working with a provider you trust; knowing ahead of time what pain relief strategies are available in your chosen birth setting and maximizing your range of safe options; and giving birth in a safe, comfortable space, surrounded by people who will provide you with good support.

Most women labor best in a calm, nurturing environment. For instance, having privacy, dim lights, quiet voices, and/or music of your choosing can contribute to your sense of ease and safety.

Some of the strategies listed below can help reduce pain, while others can help you cope better with it. Women's responses to these techniques vary; you may find that some techniques are helpful while others are not. Your support team can help you try different strategies and see what works. An experienced nurse, midwife, or doula will have suggestions for specific techniques to assist you. In some cases, there is little scientific evidence that a particular strategy is helpful, but it is included as some women find it comforting and it poses no risks.

Movement, Positions, and Rhythm

Having the freedom to move and change positions makes labor more manageable for many women. Upright movements, such as walking, swaying, lunging, moving on a birthing ball, and dancing, can help reduce discomfort and help move the baby down into a good position for birth.[15] As labor progresses, you may find yourself staying in one place or gravitating to a bed, but you are unlikely to want to lie on your back. Upright positions may be more comfortable and may open your pelvis to help the baby descend. Being on your hands and knees can help relieve back pain. Lying on your side helps you rest your legs and may help the baby to rotate into a good position for birth.

In active labor, you turn inward, and you develop a rhythm that takes you through each contraction and rest period. You may rock back and forth, moan, curl around a partner's hand during each contraction, and then want massage or total silence in between. The pattern that works for you will be uniquely yours. While the woman is in this zone, she can benefit when her support team reinforces her rhythm/ritual and keeps interruptions to a minimum.

The two things that helped me through the labor were mooing and yelling at the top of my lungs. Mooing was the only sort of deep moaning noise

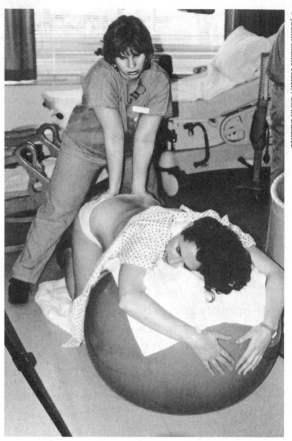

that made my whole body feel good, but it did not fit into my mental picture of myself as a chic, polite woman, so I kept making myself laugh. I would do these big low bellows and then burst out laughing because I was so embarrassed, but then that felt really good, so I would just keep laughing.

Many hospitals may restrict your movement, especially if you are alone, so try to have a support person with you and try to maintain your freedom to move during your labor. If you are encumbered with multiple attachments such as blood pressure cuffs, IVs, a bladder catheter, and electronic fetal monitoring equipment, it may be impossible to move freely. You have a right to

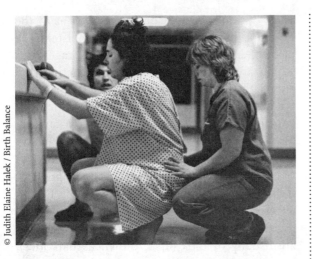

© Judith Elaine Halek / Birth Balance

refuse all these monitors. If you do accept them, you can adapt by standing by your bed, sitting in a chair, swaying in your partner's arms, and so forth. If you have an epidural or have taken medicines that can make you feel dizzy, you will likely be restricted to bed.

The Comfort of Water

Being in water during labor can be wonderfully soothing and can help you relax. Many studies have shown water immersion during labor to be safe for both mother and baby while also reducing the mother's pain and her need for pain medication. Women who bathe or shower during labor have high satisfaction with this method.

When using a tub, work with your midwife or physician to determine when and for how long you can be in the bath, so that you can avoid any negative effects. If a woman enters the bath before she is in active labor or stays in for more than one or two hours, labor progress can be slowed.[16] Drink plenty of fluids, and keep the tub water at body temperature to avoid getting dehydrated or overheated.

If a tub is not available, showers are also a good option during labor. Standing and swaying under the water or holding an extended show-

erhead and letting the water run over your belly can be very helpful.

Breathing

Focusing on your breath, a calming and centering technique used in meditation and yoga, may help in labor as well. Classic strategies include a deep, sighing breath at the beginning and end of each contraction to release tension. During contractions, you can pay attention to your breath, letting it anchor you to the moment as your contraction begins. Or breathe along with the contraction, matching your breathing to the rise and fall of the contraction as it becomes stronger, peaks, and subsides. Repeating affirmations may also be helpful. Focusing on exhaling slowly between contractions as you relax muscles and get rid of tension can help as well.

Hypnosis

The use of hypnosis in labor has undergone a recent renaissance. Self-hypnosis involves practicing techniques before labor begins that you can use to help trigger deep relaxation when the contractions start. You can practice these on your own or with a partner. Several kinds of prenatal classes are available to learn hypnosis for birthing.

Touch

The human touch is a powerful way to relieve pain and reduce anxiety in labor.[17] Touch may range from a supportive hand placed for reassurance in one spot, such as on your arm, to light stroking on your back and arms as you have a contraction to a firm massage on your neck and shoulders between contractions. Counterpressure is using a special kind of touch to help relieve back pain in labor. Someone places the palms of her or his hands over your lower back where the sacrum (the triangular area at the base of the spine) is and then firmly presses in and supports your back during a contraction, holding it until the contraction is over. Another technique is squeezing in on both hips, which places pressure on the outside of your pelvic bones.

In the midst of the wildness of transition, as I was on hands and knees throwing up into a bowl, my midwife placed her hand right at the small of my back. After giving birth, I couldn't conjure up in my mind what a contraction felt like, but I will always remember just how that touch felt.

Heat and Cold

At times during labor, an ice pack on your lower back or a warm compress on your abdomen or back may be just the right thing. (Wrap an ice pack so that the ice is never directly in contact with your skin, and a warm compress should never be too hot to hold comfortably in the hand.) At other times, a cold washcloth on your forehead or on the back of your neck may feel perfect. The changing sensations can sometimes distract you from labor pain.

When I was home-birthing my baby daughter, my four-year-old son, Alex, held an ice-cold wet washcloth to my forehead during the most intense part of my labor. It was extremely soothing and also allowed me to direct my focus to a single place without distraction. It was definitely one of the best tools for birthing comfortably and calmly. Not to mention, it was a wonderful way for my son to participate in the birth of his sister!

MEDICATIONS FOR PAIN RELIEF

Pain medications can be extremely helpful at certain times and in certain situations in labor. They can dramatically ease the pain of labor and can be vital in managing complicated or difficult labors. Yet, like most medical interventions, they have some risks for mothers and babies and should be used only with full knowledge of all options and alternatives as well as of the risks and benefits. Medications do not take the place of emotional support and encouragement, which are essential regardless of whether you are using medication or not. These medications are not available at outside-of-hospital births; if you are giving birth at home or in a freestanding birth clinic, you will have to transfer to a hospital if at some point you need or want them.

There are two basic ways that pain medications are used during labor: systemically, that is, affecting the entire body, and regionally, affecting a targeted area. The systemic medications are usually opioids (also known as narcotics), but they also include nitrous oxide. (See box.) Epidurals use a mixture of local anesthetic (numbing medicine) and usually add an opioid.

Injectable or Intravenous Opioids

Opioids (also called narcotics) are the most commonly used systemic medicines given to relieve pain during labor. They include morphine (usually used only in early labor to help women get some sleep when this stage of labor is long), meperidine (Demerol or Pethidine), nalbuphine (Nubain), butorphanol (Stadol), and fentanyl (Sublimaze). Specific medicines used vary by provider and location.

When used systemically, opioids are given through an intravenous line (IV) or by an injection into your arm, leg, or buttock. They work by being absorbed into the bloodstream and going to the receptors in your body that diminish pain perception. In general, they make you feel relaxed, sleepy, and possibly a little dizzy, and you tend to feel your contractions less. They may make it easier for you to rest for longer periods of time between the contractions.

Each opioid works for only a limited length of time and can be safely given only at certain times during labor. After a peak of effectiveness, the medicine begins to wear off. The length of time varies from one medicine to an-

NITROUS OXIDE

Nitrous oxide (N_2O) is an odorless, tasteless gas that you inhale through a mask. You may know nitrous oxide as "laughing gas" or a tool for pain relief during dental care. Exactly how nitrous oxide works is not well understood, but many women who use it during labor find it beneficial. In the United Kingdom, where midwives use it in hospitals and carry it with them to home births, N_2O is the most commonly used form of analgesia, with three of every five women using it at some time during labor.[18]

Used with current equipment and procedures, nitrous oxide is safe, is effective for many women, and has important advantages compared to other much more commonly used methods of labor analgesia. It provides better pain relief than opioid medicines and doesn't have any of the adverse side effects for mothers or babies that can occur after using opioids or epidurals.[19] N_2O takes effect very quickly (about a minute after breathing in the gas), wears off quickly, and is controlled by the laboring woman.

Unfortunately, nitrous oxide is rarely available for use in labor in the United States. In 2010, the American College of Nurse-Midwives issued a position statement calling for an increase in the availability of nitrous oxide for laboring women. A growing number of advocates and care providers are working to make nitrous oxide widely available to birthing women in the United States. For more information, see "Nitrous Oxide for Pain Relief in Labor" at the Our Bodies Ourselves website, ourbodiesourselves.org.

other. One to two hours is common, with the peak often being less than half an hour after the medicine is given.

Advantages and Disadvantages of Opioids

One advantage of systemic medicines is that they are short-acting. They therefore can be used at a time in the labor when you just need some help to make it through a challenge. The use of morphine for women who are exhausted in early labor is one example. Another common example is a onetime dose of systemic medicine if you are in the middle of labor and feel exhausted or like giving up; it may be what you need to get through this short but tough time. Mothers who try this may get a second wind and do fine without further medication. Others may have an even harder time coping with labor because of the way the medication makes them feel ("high" or disoriented). Another advantage of using systemic medicine over regional medicine such as an epidural is that you can either avoid the possible adverse effects of the epidural altogether or delay getting the epidural until later in the labor, which may diminish the impact of some of the epidural's negative effects.

The main disadvantage of systemic opioids (narcotics) is that their use in labor has generally been found to have limited effect on controlling women's pain. When women rate the effectiveness of all the techniques used to minimize pain during labor, systemic opioids are less effective than immersion in water.[20] They are also much less effective for pain relief than epidurals. They will not take the pain away completely. The medicine may "knock you out" between contractions, or it may "take the edge off" by decreasing the intensity of the contraction at its strongest. Some women experience a welcome feeling of relaxation; others feel a bit out of control.

Other disadvantages of opioids are:

- The use of these medicines may decrease the production of your own endorphins (hormones that reduce your perception of pain).
- They are short-acting, and there is a time limit for when you can get another dose. So after you have been given one dose, there is usually a waiting period before you can have more if the first dose doesn't work as well as you want. Some women find this waiting period very difficult.
- Just as they circulate throughout your body, systemic medicines get into the baby's circulation. There, they have the same effect on the baby that they do on you. If a baby is born too soon after this type of drug is given to the mother, she or he may need help to breathe or may have to be given medication to wake up. For this reason, many care providers will not give systemic pain medication if birth is likely to occur soon.
- Babies of mothers who receive these medicines can also have trouble initiating breastfeeding successfully and may not be able to suck correctly during the first few hours or days of life.[21]

Epidurals and Spinals

Epidurals and spinals cause numbness below the level of the back at which they are placed. In an epidural, medicine is infused just outside the outermost of the two membranes covering the spinal cord (the epidural space); in a spinal, the medicine is injected between the two membranes. Either epidurals or combined spinal-epidurals are offered for labor pain. These methods may involve the use of local anesthesia, which works by taking away sensation through a numbing effect on nerves. Or it may involve opioid medications only or a combination of local anesthesia and opioid medications.

To place an epidural or spinal, an anesthesiologist or nurse-anesthetist first numbs a small area of skin on your back. For an epidural, she or he uses a needle to place a catheter (a tiny, flexible plastic tube) into the epidural space. With the catheter in place, an anesthetic, or more usually a combination of anesthetic and opioid, can be infused through a pump that controls the dose and the rate throughout your labor. In patient-controlled epidural anesthesia, you have access to a button that activates the pump. (It has controls that won't allow you to overdose yourself.)

A spinal is a single injection usually used for short-term pain relief in situations when pain control is needed faster. A spinal uses local anesthetic and sometimes an opioid that is injected into the spinal fluid that surrounds the spinal cord. Loss of feeling below the site of injection occurs quite quickly. Spinals are often used for cesarean surgery and sometimes for forceps or vacuum extraction deliveries.

Some hospitals offer a combined spinal-epidural: a onetime dose of opioid or anesthetic is injected into the woman's spinal fluid, and then a catheter is left in place in the epidural space for use when the spinal medicine wears off. The advantage of the combined spinal-epidural is that the spinal component offers relief without numbing, and if relief wears off before the birth, the anesthesia staff can add anesthetics to the epidural catheter and avoid a second procedure.

An epidural or a spinal will be accompanied by continuous electronic fetal monitoring of the baby. In addition, women who have an epidural or spinal will have an IV and equipment to monitor blood pressure. Most women will need a temporary urinary catheter to empty the bladder and will be confined to bed, because this type of medication also affects the nerves that control the hip and leg muscles.

Advantages and Disadvantages of Epidurals and Spinals

The greatest advantage of epidurals (and spinals) is that they can take away the greater part of the pain in labor and while giving birth for most women who use them. An epidural can provide much-needed rest for an exhausted mother, especially when other approaches have failed. An epidural can be helpful in the case of a very long labor. Psychological issues or individual circumstances may make experiencing the physical sensations of labor too difficult for some mothers at some point. Finally, some women choose epidurals simply to eliminate all labor pain.

However, regional analgesia can change the course of labor in many adverse ways. The disadvantages of regional medications used for labor pain include:[22]

- Sometimes the insertion of the epidural is ineffective, and the process has to be repeated. Epidurals sometimes fail to work or fail to relieve pain in a small area of your abdomen or back (also known as an epidural window). Such areas sometimes can be anesthetized with higher doses of medication but some women never do get complete pain relief.
- You are more likely to have a short episode of low blood pressure right after the epidural or spinal is injected, which may be associated with a drop in the baby's heart rate. If this happens, your providers will increase fluids through the IV, help you change position, or administer medicine to raise your blood pressure. If the drop in the baby's heart rate lasts for more than a few minutes, your

provider will likely give you oxygen and may place an internal monitor (which involves breaking your membranes, if they are not already broken) to better track the baby's response. These episodes of low blood pressure usually resolve quickly and do not cause any lasting effect on you or the baby.

- Spinal and epidural opioids can cause itching. This is generally mild but can be quite bothersome for some women.
- This type of medication can increase the amount of time that you are in labor, including a longer pushing phase.
- You may be more likely to receive Pitocin, a synthetic form of the hormone oxytocin, to make your contractions stronger. (See "Medical Approaches to Speeding Up Labor," on p. 408.)
- The longer you have an epidural, the more likely you are to develop a fever during labor. Because your providers cannot know if a fever is from an infection or from the epidural, if you get a significant fever in labor, your providers will start antibiotics and your baby may be separated from you and subjected to more tests in the first hours after birth.
- You are more likely to have forceps or vacuum delivery. Instrumental vaginal deliveries are more likely to lead to tears into or through the anal sphincter muscle.
- Between one and two of every one hundred women who get an epidural, and fewer than one of every one hundred women who receive a labor spinal, get a severe headache called a spinal headache. The headache usually doesn't start until the next day; if it occurs, effective treatment is available.

Evidence is mixed on whether there is an association between epidurals and problems in establishing breastfeeding; such problems seem more likely to be linked to epidurals that include high-dose opioids in the mixture.[23]

GIVING BIRTH

The active phase of labor is complete when your cervix is open wide enough to accommodate the baby's head (about 10 cm, or 4 inches) or there is full or complete dilation. Around this time, you will likely feel a strong urge to begin pushing your baby out the final few inches. Often, after transition and just before you feel like pushing or bearing down, your contractions may space out or even stop for a while, allowing you to rest.

The contractions were coming hard, [but] I could actually sleep between them. It was all very surreal and otherworldly. Immense pain and then total relaxation. I felt like I was in a scene from The Red Tent *[a novel set in biblical times; the title refers to a tent in which women gave birth]. I pushed from somewhere buried inside me. Deep, guttural, almost animal-like noises came from within me. Loud noises. Noises I soon had no control over. My body was pushing out my baby, and I was merely providing the sound track.*

More rapid, intense contractions, a powerful opening-up feeling, and rectal pressure (a sense that you need to have a bowel movement) are signs that you are completely dilated and ready to push your baby down through your vagina and give birth. Pushing can be a great relief because it requires you to become an active participant, in contrast to the yielding and letting go necessary for active labor.

After a few pushes, I somehow realized that I had to change gears. Pushing was up to me. *I wasn't supposed to lie there and cope with it, counting and breathing and moaning until it was over. It*

was time to be active, to decide when to push, when to breathe, when to rest.

Pushing your baby out works best when you do just what your body wants, without external direction. Bear down when you feel the urge—an innate reflex stimulated when your body produces high levels of oxytocin in response to pressure from your baby's head low in your pelvis. In the past, women were taught to hold their breath and push during each contraction. Many providers may still tell you to hold your breath and push down as hard as you can for a count of ten. But breath holding and sustained, directed bearing down can be exhausting and frequently do more harm than good. Studies of women in labor have shown that holding your breath can increase the chance of worrisome fetal heart rate patterns because your baby does not get as much oxygen when you push this way.[24] With gentle support and positive feedback, you can follow your own urges and find a rhythm that feels right and moves your baby down. You or your labor support companions may need to tell your care providers not to direct you how and when to push.

When I was pushing, really pushing, I felt powerful. When I realized that I was in charge of pushing, and when I felt my contractions as guides to how often and for how long I should push, I started to reel in my mounting panic and to harness my energy.

Depending on the baby's position, pushing can sometimes be very painful and very hard work. Change positions to relieve pressure points and to find positions that are more comfortable for you. Sometimes pushing while sitting on the toilet can be effective, as we are psychologically conditioned to relax our pelvic muscles there. Being upright (leaning, squatting, hanging from something or someone) may

PUSHING WITH AN EPIDURAL

An epidural changes the second stage of labor considerably. The urge to push is often delayed and sometimes absent entirely. Pushing takes longer and can be more tiring, it's harder to change positions, and instrumental (vacuum or forceps) delivery is more common. Some of these challenges can be overcome with a more relaxed and patient approach that allows plenty of time for the baby to descend and be born.

You can decrease your chance of having a vacuum or forceps delivery or a cesarean and avoid overexhaustion by not pushing immediately when your cervix is completely dilated. If you wait until you feel the urge to push or until your baby's head has descended further, you will have more energy and will be able to push more effectively. Research suggests that the length of time before the baby is born is the same whether you allow an hour or two of passive descent of the baby (when you relax and don't consciously try to push) or start pushing immediately after you are fully dilated.[25]

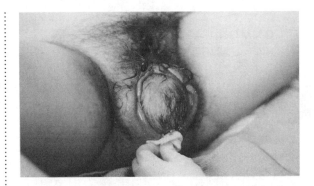

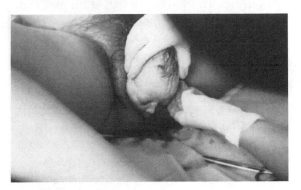

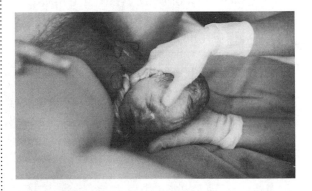

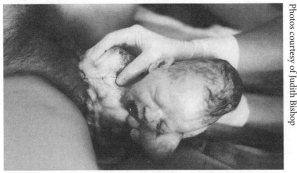

lessen pain and backache. Upright positions may also help align the baby in your pelvis better and open the pelvic bones a bit to give the baby more room, allowing her or him to navigate through the birth canal more easily.

It may take only a few pushes, or it may take a few hours of pushing, to birth your baby. As long as both you and your baby are doing fine and the baby is moving down, there's no reason to limit this phase of labor.

Between pushes, breathe slowly and rest.

COMMON LABOR INTERVENTIONS THAT CAUSE HARM WITH LITTLE OR NO BENEFIT

Although almost all interventions can be helpful in certain circumstances, harm is associated with their overuse. The interventions listed below are used in large numbers of U.S. births, despite evidence that their routine use makes labor and birth riskier for women and babies.

- **Laboring or pushing on your back:** The flat-on-the-back position tends to be more painful, slows down labor, results in more trauma to the perineum and vagina during birth, and reduces oxygen flow to the baby.[26] It may also make you feel like a passive recipient of medical care rather than an active participant in the birth of your baby. Even if you have a medical condition that makes walking unsafe or choose an epidural, you can still use a variety of positions in bed, such as lying on your side.

- **Episiotomy,** a surgical cut straight back into the perineum to enlarge the vaginal opening, has been shown to increase postpartum pain and the risk of a tear extending into the anal sphincter muscle, which can lead to incontinence (involuntary loss of urine, gas, or feces). The best evidence suggests that episiotomy should be used only when the baby is showing severe signs of distress late in the pushing phase of labor.[27]

- **Immediate clamping of the umbilical cord** after birth deprives babies of up to one-third of their blood volume. Although most babies can withstand this amount of blood loss, it is associated with an increased likelihood of anemia for several months after birth. Delayed cord clamping has additional benefits for preterm and low-birth-weight infants and may also reduce the mother's blood loss after birth.[28]

You might even fall asleep for a few minutes. Remember that—just as in earlier phases of labor—your uterus works involuntarily to move the baby down and out. Work with it, and give it time. Your labor may not progress as quickly as you had imagined or as others around you expect.

When the pushing stage of labor is nearing its end, the baby moves under your pubic arch, and your perineum, the area between the vaginal opening and the rectum, stretches slowly to accommodate the head. Gentle guidance to push slowly and with short pushes at this stage, encouragement of favorable positions, and techniques such as touch, hot compresses, and warm oils applied to the perineum for comfort all work with this process and may prevent or minimize tearing. When you feel a burning sensation, breathe lightly so as not to push too rapidly and risk tearing. Reaching down to touch your baby's head for the first time often produces an "Ahhhh" that opens you up even more.

A midwife who gave birth at home says:

I often tell women in labor that they will feel a second wind—a surge of energy—when it is time to push. I found that this didn't really happen when I started pushing. But I definitely felt this when I started feeling the stretching and knew [my baby] would be born soon. It was like the only thing I needed to do in the world was push with all of my might. And that was true! It was the only thing I had to do. All the wonderful people supporting me were taking care of every single other thing.

I pushed and the burning peaked, and then, all of a sudden, nothing. My baby's head was out. It is truly amazing how quickly you can go from the most intense pain to no pain at all.

YOUR BABY IS BORN!

Within seconds of birth, babies make a remarkable transition from life in the womb, where all of their needs were met by the placenta, to life outside the womb, where they must regulate their own breathing, temperature, and digestion. These transitions happen most easily when the baby is placed on your chest for skin-to-skin contact with you, with the umbilical cord intact (not clamped immediately) and in an environment of peace and calmness. Sometimes hospital routines or medical complications make it difficult or impossible for the mother and baby to remain in such close contact right after birth. Babies can overcome these disruptions when they are medically necessary, but it is best to keep the mother and baby together barring extreme circumstances.

Some babies breathe as they are being born and look pink immediately. Others take a few moments to begin breathing, a process that unfolds as blood continues to flow through the umbilical cord.[29] Gentle stimulation such as rubbing the baby's back can also help a baby begin breathing in a regular, sustained way. Healthy babies are usually able to clear their own airways of fluid and mucus without suctioning. If there was meconium (the baby's first bowel movement) in the amniotic fluid and the baby isn't breathing immediately, she or he may need suctioning right after birth to prevent the meconium from getting into her or his lungs.

Not all newborns cry. Some do for a moment and then stop. Often they breathe, blink, and look around or cough, sneeze, and snuffle. Your baby's head may appear oddly shaped, having been temporarily molded by coming through the birth canal. Her or his body may be covered with patches of vernix, a white, waxy substance that coats and protects the baby's skin inside the uterus. All babies arrive wet with amniotic fluid.

Mothers and babies belong together during this precious time. When you feel ready, hold your baby naked against your belly and breasts, near the familiar sound of your heart, so that she or he can touch your skin and smell, hear, and see you. You and your new child need as much peace and quiet time together as you can create. In any setting, well-meaning providers and others can interrupt this important personal time because they want to know how you and your baby are doing. In a hospital, medical personnel

© Britt Fohrman

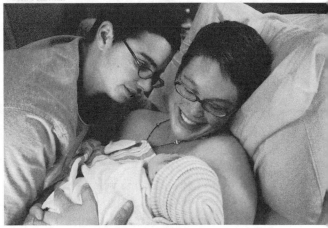

MECHANICAL INTERVENTIONS IN BIRTH: VACUUM EXTRACTOR AND FORCEPS

The vacuum extractor and forceps can help when babies need to be born quickly or when a woman would benefit from assistance to allow vaginal birth to continue. They are important tools in skilled hands. They can be used only when the cervix is fully dilated and the baby has descended well into the vagina. With both vacuum extractors and forceps, the mother must continue to push with contractions. In most instances, anesthesia is given prior to the use of these instruments so the pelvic area is numb.

The vacuum extractor is a small, flexible suction cup that fits on the baby's head. Use of the vacuum extractor will result in an exaggeration of the natural elongation of the baby's head caused by labor for a short period. Even when done properly, it can cause a blood-filled swelling (cephalohematoma) on the baby's head.

Forceps are two metal branches that are slipped onto each side of the baby's head and then locked together so as to fit snugly. Forceps are much more likely to cause injury to the woman's vagina and perineum (the tissue between the vagina and rectum) than a vacuum delivery and can also cause injuries in babies. They are particularly risky when used inappropriately or by unskilled providers.

The use of vacuum extraction has increased. A number of factors account for this, including the increase in the use of epidural anesthesia, which lengthens the pushing stage; a maximum time limit for pushing allotted to women in some hospitals; hospital efforts to lower the cesarean section rate; and reduction in the use of forceps as fewer providers have forceps skills. Vacuum extraction is often used with epidurals because epidurals can interfere with pushing.

Before using an extraction delivery method, if there is no immediate emergency, move into different positions that open your pelvis. Try squatting to make your pushing more efficient or nipple stimulation to increase the strength of contractions.

---

may have their own schedules for evaluations. Providers can often unobtrusively examine your baby in your arms. It is usually not necessary to have tests done right away. If there is a medical reason to take your baby away from you for a short time, your partner or support person may accompany the baby.

Writing to her child, one woman recalls:

You were perfect, of course. Sue caught you and placed your warm, wet body on my chest. You immediately gave out a healthy, albeit short, cry and then just looked around and took it all in. The three of us just sat there getting to know each other. We were so in awe and in love with you that we forgot to check to see whether you were a boy or girl!

You may approach labor and birth with a vision of how you will react when you first meet your baby. It is common to have a reaction that does not match up with a vision of instantaneous bonding. Often disbelief, shock, wonder, or an overwhelming sense of pride are the first emotions. As you spend quiet moments with your baby over the next hours and days, the bonding process will intensify.

DELIVERY OF THE PLACENTA

Delivering the placenta completes the birthing process. After five to thirty minutes or so, the umbilical cord lengthens, a contraction occurs, and the placenta is expelled, often with a gush of blood. Breastfeeding or simple skin-to-skin contact in a quiet and undisturbed environment stimulates this process. It's important that your providers not pull on the placenta before it has separated from the uterine wall. It is very important that no fragments of the placenta remain in your uterus, as these fragments may allow blood vessels to remain open, causing hemorrhage. Retained fragments can also put you at risk for

infection in the uterus. Your care provider will inspect your placenta carefully to make sure it is complete and intact.

Once the placenta comes out, blood vessels close off. Your uterus contracts and begins to shrink. After the placenta is out, your baby's suckling helps keep your uterus firm and contracted.

Some view the placenta as a beautiful organ, with its pattern of blood vessels resembling a tree of life. Many cultures have rituals surrounding the afterbirth, including planting trees or flowering bushes above it. Let the staff know if you want to see and/or keep the placenta.

THE BEGINNING OF A BREASTFEEDING RELATIONSHIP

The first few hours of a baby's life are a time of heightened alertness. Breastfeeding will be easier to establish if your baby nurses at least briefly

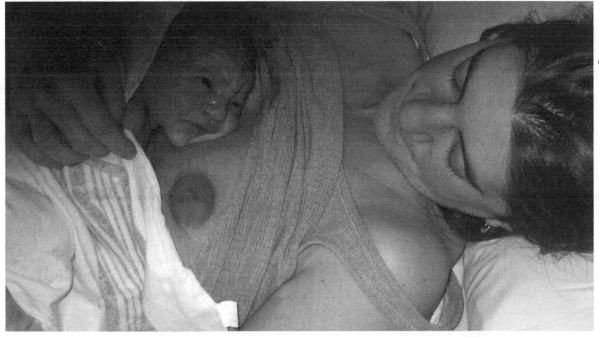

© Eric Silverberg

within the first hour or two after birth. Babies have an instinctive sucking reflex but show varying degrees of interest and take different amounts of time to nurse. Some latch on to the breast immediately; others learn to do so more gradually. Smelling, licking, and exploring your breasts are part of the process. Allowing your baby to suckle, even if you don't plan to breast-feed, will give her or him the benefit of antibodies and nutrients from colostrum, the first milk. After a few hours, your baby will fall asleep, and when he or she wakes up the next time, breast-feeding may not be as easy as it was the first time. Over the first twenty-four to seventy-two hours, your baby will learn all the coordinated moves used to latch on to your breast and nurse effectively. If she or he was able to nurse initially right after birth, the learning process will be a little faster and can set you on the path of a long, fulfilling breastfeeding relationship.

You might want to ask your midwife or doctor in advance to help you start breastfeeding by placing your baby onto your belly or chest, skin to skin, right after birth. Also, if you are planning to breastfeed, it is important to insist that the baby not be given any water or formula without a clear medical need.

THE FIRST HOURS AND DAYS AFTER THE BABY IS BORN

At home and in birthing centers, it is usually easy for you both to be together, sleeping and waking together, getting to know each other, the baby nursing whenever she or he desires. In the hospital, specifically request that your baby remain with you. If a practitioner thinks that separation is needed, ask for an explanation and remind hospital staff that you want your baby to remain with you. Even if medical observation or treatment becomes necessary, it is usually pos-sible for you or your partner to stay with your baby.

BIRTH BY CESAREAN SECTION

My first baby was a face presentation, mentum posterior, and there was no way he would have made it out alive vaginally; that position wedges the baby's face between the sacrum and the pubic bone, with no room to descend. I had a C-section in a small local hospital. The OR [operating room] was actually warm. . . . My midwife and my partner were with me, right in the OR! It was a good way for this skeptic to learn that yes, a surgical birth can be a positive event. I had minimal anesthesia and had the baby back with me within an hour or so of his birth.

In certain circumstances, cesarean sections are clearly needed for the safety of the mother and/or the baby. In other circumstances, it can be difficult to determine whether or not the surgery is medically necessary and a different care path might have resulted in healthy vaginal birth. The risks and benefits of a cesarean vary according to your specific situation. Ideally, you will discuss during prenatal visits the possibility of having a cesarean section, although many of the circumstances that require birth by cesarean section emerge only during labor.

I'd always dreamed of having a home birth and, if that wasn't possible, to give birth in a birth center with a midwife. At thirty-two weeks, I had some bright red spotting. My midwife came to the hospital with me for an ultrasound, which showed that my placenta was partially covering my cervical opening. The obstetrician held out the possibility that the placenta might still move away from the cervix, although he was doubtful. I returned home with directions to call immediately if there was any more bleeding. At thirty-five weeks, I woke to find blood pouring. With a towel between my legs, I called my midwife, jumped in the car, and headed to the hospital, where my lovely five-pound daughter, Chiara, was delivered by cesarean section.

If you are giving birth by cesarean section, whether planned or not, the process will start in an operating room, where you will usually receive spinal or epidural anesthesia to make you completely numb below the level of your ribs. Your partner or support person may be asked to wait outside the operating room while the spinal or epidural is being set up, but in most instances he or she can return to the room to support you during the surgery. If an epidural catheter (tube) is already in place when the decision for surgery is made, the level of anesthesia will be increased so that you are completely numb.

In the rare instance when a cesarean section needs to be performed very quickly, you may be given general anesthesia (which makes you unconscious), because it is faster than making you numb with a spinal or epidural. General anesthesia is also used in the rare instances when an adequate level of anesthesia is not obtained with a spinal or epidural.

For most cesarean sections, your belly will be scrubbed and you will be given a dose of antibiotics before or during the procedure to reduce the risk of infection. In addition, a small tube (catheter) will be placed in your bladder to keep it empty during the procedure. A drape will be placed between your chest and the lower part of your body to create a sterile area for the operation. The drape also prevents you from seeing the surgery as it happens, although you can ask to have it lowered enough to see the baby emerge, if you prefer. Sometimes the drape is close to your neck, but you can turn your head to the side if it makes you feel claustrophobic.

Orgasmic Birth authors Elizabeth Davis and Debra Pascali-Bonaro also suggest:

You may be able to have music in the room, aromatherapy on a tissue at your nose, touch support from your partner or doula, the opportunity to see the baby emerge by watching in a mirror, and photos (taken by your partner or doula) of your first few moments with your baby.[30]

Your arms may be strapped down at either side to keep you from inadvertently touching the sterile field, although some hospitals are doing away with this requirement because it makes some women feel vulnerable and helpless. If you prefer to have one or both arms free, say so. Operating room staff will attach a sticky patch to your skin and place a small clip over one of your fingers that monitors your vital signs. In most hospitals, if you do not have general anesthesia, a support person or partner as well as a doula or midwife can be present during the surgery. He or she will likely stay at the head of the bed, next to your head, behind the drape.

After the anesthesia has taken effect, the surgeon will usually make a horizontal incision in your skin, low down near the pubic bone—the so-called bikini cut. The surgeon will then open up the layers inside your abdomen and cut through the uterine muscle to lift your baby out.

I looked up at my husband. There he was, looking quite ridiculous in his blue scrubs and hairnet. He was standing slightly, just enough to see over the draped curtain. His eyes [were] intently staring. I can't even be certain he blinked. When the doctor announced the birth of our daughter, there was no need for him to say it. I saw it on my husband's face, the birth of his daughter. His eyes widened at first, almost as if someone had stomped on his toe, then he began to cry. The look

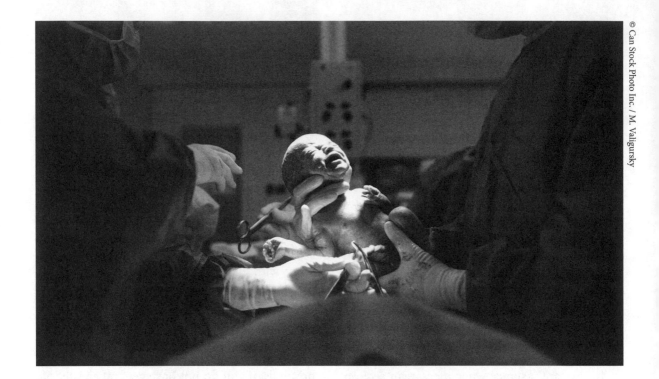

on his face was amazement, pride, love. I saw the birth of our daughter that day, too . . . through the eyes of my husband. It was beautiful.

The surgeon will clamp and cut the umbilical cord and hand your baby to a nurse or other attendant, who will suction your baby's nose and mouth if needed and assess the baby's breathing. Once the baby is breathing normally and has been bundled into a warm blanket, your partner and you can hold your baby next to you cheek to cheek and you can welcome your child even as the doctor removes the placenta, sews up the incision, and closes the skin with sutures or staples. The entire procedure usually takes about an hour.

Following your surgery, you will be cleaned up in the operating room and taken to a recovery room, where you can focus on getting to know your baby. This is an important time to start breastfeeding. The baby is usually alert

for the first hour or two after birth. Ask for help if you feel that you cannot start breastfeeding on your own. The surgery and recovery pose extra challenges for getting breastfeeding off the ground, and good support and your determination can make all the difference. During this time, if you have had a spinal or epidural, the anesthesia will gradually wear off. If you received a long-acting medication in the spinal/epidural catheter, you shouldn't have much pain the first twenty-four hours. If you did not have the long-acting medicine, you will be given IV pain medication as needed. Usually, after a few hours you are ready to go to your postpartum room.

Women who have complicated labor and obstetric emergencies understand the necessity of a cesarean section. Some experience a cesarean section as a relief, even while wondering whether or not it was truly necessary. Some fault themselves, feeling guilty or defensive that they

Although everyone hopes for a healthy baby, in rare cases babies are born with serious medical problems. You may face challenges that you never anticipated. Very rarely, the unthinkable happens: A baby dies at birth. At such a time, your grief may feel unbearable. For more about childbearing loss, see Chapter 18, "Miscarriage, Stillbirth, and Other Losses."

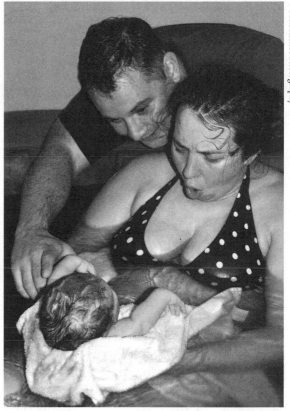

didn't do "everything possible" to have a vaginal birth even though they did the best they could, given their physical circumstances and the information and support available. It's normal for women to have a wide variety of emotional responses to a cesarean. Honor your feelings, whatever they are. If you feel you need additional support after a cesarean, visit the website of the International Cesarean Awareness Network (ican-online.org).

A midwife says:

I tell women who begin labor at home and end up in a hospital, "Who you are never changes. Your planning, ideals, beliefs, and principles never change just because you end up with a cesarean. You are stronger than you would have been, because you've gone through all these decisions and made the choices you did."

AFTERWORD

We relive the births of our children many times during the days, weeks, months, and years afterward. Looking back upon your birth experience may call up a wide range of emotions. You may feel fulfilled, ecstatic, and immensely close to your loved ones and your baby, especially if you felt supported and respected throughout the process. You may feel joy, wonder, and a great sense of accomplishment.

On the other hand, if unexpected complications, medical interventions, or insensitive comments and behaviors of medical personnel dominated your birth experience, you may feel a bewildering mix of joy and disappointment. You may feel distant from your baby. It is not uncommon to apologize for having wanted more ("It doesn't matter—after all, my baby is healthy, and that's all that counts") or to feel sad or guilty about not having had the birth you wanted. Worst of all, you may blame yourself—"My body just didn't work right"—instead of recognizing that you did not get the support that might have resulted in a different outcome or that birth is, in the end, unpredictable.

Even though I was relieved that everything was okay and thrilled with my baby, I had the nagging sense that I had failed somehow. Later I got over feeling that it was my fault, but I still felt cheated out of the birth experience we had hoped and planned for. Sometimes I still can't help feeling a little jealous when I hear women talk about their wonderful birth experiences.

It is normal to have doubts, regret, grief, or anger rising to the surface over time. Talk with your partner, good friends, or a counselor for comfort, understanding, and support. Women's groups and online discussion groups or chat rooms may also be helpful.

If you are dissatisfied and want to learn more about what happened, get a copy of your baby's birth records. Check them against your memories. Talk to the practitioner and others who attended your labor. Write letters to those you feel did not meet your needs; it may help them to become more responsive and respectful in the future. Going through some of these processes may make it possible for you to feel more at peace.

The transformation to becoming a mother is profound; the demands are huge. With a new baby you experience a new identity and responsibilities, a connection with someone who, having been part of yourself for nine months, now becomes an individual outside of yourself who needs your help and support twenty-four hours a day. Our society provides mothers with few if any rituals, resources, or social supports for this transition. Most other Western industrialized societies offer generous paid maternity and paternity leave, flexible working conditions, quality state-run day care programs, and well-organized midwifery services. Though there is little government support for new parents in the United States, many communities have active doula groups, birth networks, breastfeeding support, or new parents' organizations. These groups offer much-needed help with the joyful, difficult, passionate, challenging work of being a mother.

Even now, twenty-four years after my daughter's birth, I am still learning how powerful that event was. It is amazing how the experience of pregnancy, labor, and birth keeps reaching across the years of my life to open doors in my heart.

CHAPTER 17

Becoming a mother changes everything in your life—turns it upside down—and makes you wonder who you are and whether you are the same person you used to be. Our feelings range from exhilaration to exhaustion, from confidence to uncertainty. Many factors affect how we experience this time in our lives: our physical and mental health and the health of the baby; our feelings about the birth or adoption experience; our ability to feed and nourish our baby; our readiness to be mothers; and the amount and kind of resources we have and support we receive from partners, families, friends, and health care providers.

Many of us find that being a mother brings deep pleasure, intimacy, and insight. Birth and breastfeeding give us a new

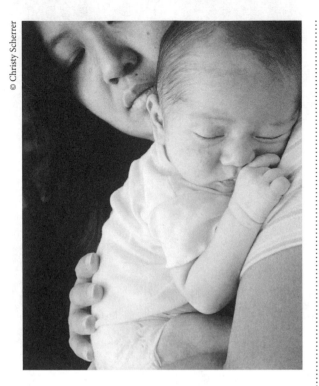

respect for our bodies. Caring for and cuddling our babies, we discover new dimensions to loving.

All three of my postpartum experiences have been among the sweetest times of my life. I felt centered and essentially satisfied in a way I have never felt before or since. Being with my babies gave me such incredible joy.

At the same time, almost all women experience some difficulties navigating the changes new motherhood brings.

During those early weeks, sometimes I wasn't sure where the baby ended and I began. I felt that I had lost my old self and was too tired, physically and emotionally, to find her again. But I was also discovering a new part of myself that I hadn't known about before: unexpectedly intense

feelings for my new baby, a resurgence of love for my mother, connection with other women. I went from despair to overwhelming feelings of tenderness, all within the space of an hour.

This chapter focuses on the first few months of parenting, including the physical recovery from pregnancy and birth; breastfeeding, health, and well-being; changes in our relationships; emotional concerns; and some of the more common mental and physical health conditions we may face during these months.

YOUR PHYSICAL RECOVERY

The moments and hours after giving birth are an important time for resting and recovering from the hard work of bringing your child into the world. Though the initial exhilaration that often follows birth can leave you feeling energized, resting in these early days can help you have a faster, easier, and more complete recovery.

I had my baby in a birth center and was home in my own bed four hours after my daughter was born. Friends brought meals over for the first week so my partner and I could revel in the experience of our new family. My mother came later, when my partner had returned to work, and having those extra hands and caring presence around really helped me in those early days.

If you have given birth somewhere other than in your home, you and your health care provider will discuss when you should go home. The standard hospital practice is for women to go home one to two days after a vaginal birth and three to four days after a cesarean birth. These numbers are guidelines; the length of your stay may depend upon how you and your baby are doing as well as upon your insurance coverage. If you give birth in a birth center, you may be discharged just a few hours after giving birth, but postpartum care typically includes home visits and frequent phone contact from a midwife or nurse in the first week. Postpartum home visits are also typical after a home birth.

BODY CHANGES

Whether you had a straightforward birth or required numerous medical interventions, your body will go through many physical changes in the hours and days after giving birth.

For at least the first couple of weeks, your uterus will still be enlarged and you will still appear pregnant and probably be most comfortable wearing maternity clothing or other loose-fitting clothes. Whether or not you breastfeed, your breasts will swell and may leak milk, especially at night, when your body produces higher levels of the hormone prolactin. A supportive nursing bra and absorbent cotton breast pads can keep you comfortable during these changes, which for most women last just a few weeks. Be sure to change breast pads frequently to keep your breasts dry. Swelling in the legs, feet, and hands is common for several days after giving birth. If swelling is severe, you experience pain in one or both of your legs, or you are swollen more on one side than the other, tell your midwife or doctor, as these could be signs of a blood clot.

Soreness

Nearly all women experience some kind of body soreness after labor and birth. Back pain or other body aches can result from the physical exertion of labor or from particular labor positions. These aches and pains during the first few days are completely normal. Soaking in a tub, getting a massage, and moving around can help alleviate general soreness. Pay attention to your posture as your body readjusts your center of gravity, and use pillows to support your body's alignment while resting and nursing.

Vaginal Discharge (Lochia)

Both women who have vaginal births and women who have cesarean sections experience vaginal discharge after childbirth. This discharge, called lochia, is blood mixed with material from the uterine lining that supported the baby in the womb. It is initially red, then will lighten to pink, then brown, before becoming clear or yellowish and finally stopping four to eight weeks after the birth. Women who have cesarean deliveries may have lochia for a shorter period of time, because much of this material is removed during surgery.

Your bleeding may become slightly heavier for a day or two when you become more active. If this happens, you may be doing too much; try resting for a day.

No one ever talks about it, but a postpartum woman's best friend is a box of high-quality overnight maxi pads—with wings! A friend told me to bring my own before I went into the hospital—and double up on them, front and back—so that I wouldn't have to rely on the hospital's awful ones that move and don't absorb anything anyway. It was great advice.

Cramping

Like lochia, uterine cramping (pains and feelings of tightness in your belly) is a normal part of recovery from childbirth. This cramping is a sign that your uterus is contracting and returning to its usual size. Uterine cramping is often more intense for women with the second baby and babies after that. These "afterpains" generally stop being painful by the third day after giving birth.

While few women have serious problems after giving birth, the first several days are an important time to be on the alert for signs of complications such as excess bleeding, infection, or surgical complications related to cesarean section. Call your provider immediately if you have any of these symptoms:

- You have soaked through more than one large maxi pad in less than an hour or pass clots larger than an egg.
- You have a fever higher than 100.4°F.
- Your abdomen hurts when you press on it.
- You have severe pain in the area of your cesarean incision or in your perineum or vagina.
- You have pain or severe swelling in one of your legs.
- You have bad-smelling vaginal discharge (the normal odor is similar to that of a menstrual period).

To relieve the cramping, hold a pillow or a heating pad over your abdomen, lie on your stomach if this is comfortable, or lie on your side with a pillow between your legs and over your stomach. Over-the-counter pain medicines such as ibuprofen (sold under brand names such as Motrin or Advil) can be taken. If the cramping is worse during breastfeeding, try taking ibuprofen about fifteen minutes beforehand. Aspirin should be avoided because it can increase bleeding.

Perineal Pain

Perineal pain due to episiotomy, tears, stitches, or just the stretching of vaginal birth is also very common. It may be uncomfortable to walk or sit.

During the initial period of recovery (the first twenty-four hours), most women find it helpful to apply ice, which not only assists with pain relief but can help reduce the swelling in the area. Keep a squirt bottle next to the toilet to spray on your perineum as you urinate. This will dilute the urine and reduce the stinging. After twenty-four hours, you can soak the vulvar/perineal area in tepid water in the bathtub or in a sitz bath, a special insert that can be placed on the toilet. Some women find that adding herbal infusions of comfrey or witch hazel to the sitz bath promotes healing and decreases swelling. You may also use pain medication for perineal pain.

Pain After Cesarean Section

If you have had a cesarean section, you will likely need stronger pain relief medication than women who have had vaginal births. Talk with your health care providers about postsurgical pain relief, both for the first few days and then for the first two to three weeks after going home. During the first day in the hospital, you may require intravenous medication, followed by a gradual change to pain medication you can take by mouth. You may be given a liquid or light diet initially; solid, heavier foods should be added slowly. Eat what you feel you can tolerate. When you go home, usually four to five days after surgery, you likely will need to continue to take prescription medicines for pain relief. It is best to take opioid pain medication only when it is really needed, because such medicines can cause constipation and other side effects. Be sure that you get enough pain relief to be able to comfortably care for yourself and your baby.

Bowel and Urinary Changes

You may not move your bowels for a day or two after birth. This is normal. To make the first bowel movement easier and prevent future constipation, drink plenty of water, move around as soon as possible after birth (it will probably take a day to begin walking again after a C-section), and eat plenty of fruits, vegetables, and fiber. Prunes, prune or cherry juice, or a stool softener can also help with constipation.

Bowel movements will likely be uncomfortable if you had an episiotomy or tear, or if you developed hemorrhoids during pregnancy or birth. Holding some folded toilet paper gently against your perineum when you have a bowel movement can help reduce discomfort. Witch hazel pads—especially ones that have been chilled in the refrigerator—and sitz baths can ease the discomfort of hemorrhoids, as can over-the-counter medicines. If your hemorrhoids are very uncomfortable, talk with your provider about prescription creams and suppositories that can help.

After giving birth, your body gets rid of the excess fluid volume you built up during the pregnancy. You will likely need to urinate frequently and in large amounts. A few women have difficulty emptying their bladders after birth because of swelling; this can occasionally require getting a temporary urinary catheter.

You may experience pelvic muscle weakness, which can lead to urinary incontinence (leaking urine). You may also have bowel or gas incontinence due to weakened pelvic floor muscles. Kegel exercises can help you recover pelvic muscle tone. (For more information on Kegels, see page 643.) If incontinence persists, ask your provider about a referral to a pelvic floor physical therapist who can help you restore strength with various exercises.

FATIGUE

Fatigue is a major factor in the days and weeks after you give birth. You are recovering from the physical demands of labor and birth and, at the same time, your sleep is being interrupted by your baby. If possible, have your partner or a support person sleep in the room with you—even if you are in a hospital or birthing center—to help support you in your recovery and facilitate your bonding with the baby.

In the first days either at home or in the hospital, be choosy about the visitors you see. Their job is to help you, not the other way around. A visit that interferes with a much-needed chance to rest should be avoided. Ask friends and relatives to stay for a few minutes only or to delay their visits. Many will be happy to share their concern and generosity in other ways, such as volunteering to care for your other children, doing simple errands, or dropping off meals for your family. For some new mothers, however, visits from family and friends are welcome. The important thing is that you be aware of your needs and ask others to be considerate—or ask someone to be a buffer for you.

My midwife told me to stay in pajamas or even in bed when visitors came. This was such great advice. People don't want to stay long when you look and act like you need rest (which you do when you've just had a baby!). Some friends stayed longer but visited with my older daughter or my husband in another part of the house while I slept or nursed. After a week or so, I was ready to put on real clothes and visit with friends and family downstairs. But I was glad I was protective of those early days.

POSTPARTUM CARE

You may have a postpartum visit at your care provider's office one to two weeks after giving birth, especially if you had a cesarean. Your care provider will check your blood pressure, ask about your bleeding, assess your breastfeeding, and, if necessary, discuss birth control options with you. If you had a laceration, episiotomy, or cesarean section, she or he will also check to see that you are healing properly. If your cesarean incision was closed with skin staples, they will be removed at this visit. This is rarely painful.

A visit to the midwife or doctor is usually scheduled at six to eight weeks. This visit usually includes an internal pelvic exam to make sure that lochia has stopped or nearly stopped and that the cervix is closed and the uterus is back to its nonpregnant size. If you are sexually active with a male partner and don't want to immediately become pregnant again, discuss options for birth control with your care provider, if this was not done immediately after the birth (see "Birth Control," p. 450).

For many of us, postpartum care on this schedule is adequate, and after six weeks we feel well enough to manage any persistent health concerns ourselves. But for other women, the U.S. model of postpartum care falls short. A survey of women who gave birth in 2005 found that many women had significant health problems related to pregnancy or birth that lasted six months or longer.[1] This was especially true of women who had cesarean surgery: Nearly one in five had pain at the incision site for longer than six months. Some women also reported new onset of chronic illnesses, such as high blood pressure, diabetes, or mood disorders during or soon after pregnancy. Just because your postpartum period has ended according to medical milestones, don't hesitate to follow up with your regular health care provider when you are experiencing ongoing discomfort or other health problems. Unfortunately, many women become ineligible for Medicaid after pregnancy and have no insurance to pay for health care for

FOR WOMEN WHO HAVE ADOPTED

The women in the new mothers' circle eyed me warily. I'd sat silently and politely listening as they discussed their C-section scars, cracked nipples, and nighttime feedings, and now, apparently, it was my turn. I had suffered insomnia, jet lag, and a radical life change, but I didn't feel I had a right to complain; after all, I'd been reminded more times than I could count, "You're lucky, you did it the easy way."

Though many of the issues of adoptive mothers—exhaustion, isolation, adapting to a new baby—are the same as those of women who gave birth, women who adopt also face different logistical, emotional, and financial challenges. For more on these issues, see "Adoption," p. 356.

ongoing problems, even if the problems are related to pregnancy.

MEETING YOUR BABY

EARLY ATTACHMENT: CREATING A HEALTHY BOND WITH YOUR BABY

Attachment is a natural, biological process that occurs between human beings to create an emotional bond. Just like other mammals, human newborns are born with behaviors that help ensure that they are protected and nourished. Parents learn how to respond to cues such as the baby's hunger signs or distress cries. Over days, weeks, and months, the attachment strengthens.

Although attachment occurs as part of the continuum of pregnancy, labor, and birth, we need not have given birth to our children in order to experience attachment. Fathers, partners, and adoptive parents form deep emotional bonds with babies, although these may evolve on a different rhythm from attachments made between a biological mother and her newborn.

Research indicates that there is a sensitive period around the time of birth when it is easier for secure attachments to be made. Procedures in labor and after the birth may disrupt this sensitive period. These include medications given to women in labor,[2] cesarean surgery,[3] and separating mothers and babies after birth.[4] These disruptions can be overcome, especially if the woman has excellent emotional support in labor and after birth.[5] But all efforts should be made to keep these disruptions to a minimum so that mothers and babies get off to a good start.

Most babies are quite alert during the first hour or two after birth. This is an ideal time to share skin-to-skin contact with your baby and to begin breastfeeding. After the initial alert period, most babies experience a sleepy period that usually lasts for three to five hours. This is a great time for you to recover—to rest, bathe, and relax.

You may encounter unexpected circumstances that delay contact with your baby. Be patient and creative in your efforts to connect with your baby. If your baby requires special medical care and cannot be held for a while, talk to your baby, sing to your baby, and just be there, to the extent possible given your situation and your baby's health. If you have medical complications that delay the contact, ask another close family member to hold your baby. If you have conflicting emotions that complicate your ability to connect with your baby right away, give yourself permission to connect with your baby at your own pace. You will grow into the relationship with your baby over time.

SLEEPING

Increasingly, hospitals have a policy of rooming in, where mothers and babies stay in the same room after birth and both are cared for together. Still, many hospitals take babies to a central nursery right after birth for a short observation period, especially if the mother has had a C-section, and take babies to the nursery for procedures such as weight checks or medications throughout the hospital stay. However, if you and/or your support people are able to take care of the baby, you can request that your baby stay in the room with you.

After the surgery, I know that Andrew and my midwife, Maria, met up and she gave him advice on how to get the baby to me as soon as possible. She gave him the confidence that it was possible despite their usual policies. The hospital staff said, "Well, we don't really allow the baby to go right away." But Andrew said repeatedly, "I understand, but how about we just take him." And it worked. Andrew remembers pushing Luke down the hall in the little rolling crib feeling as if he'd just committed a felony—crazed and exhilarated. When he delivered him to my breast, with Maria's encouragement all the way, he felt he was returning a lost jewel to a crown! And that's how it felt, as if a piece of me had returned. He latched on right away, and I felt a new joy on my baby's birthday.

Rooming in will help you and the baby get to know each other. Often, for instance, a mother rooming in with her baby will quickly become familiar with the signs that her baby is hungry, wet, or otherwise in need of attention well before the infant begins to cry. Rooming in can also facilitate more frequent breastfeeding and touch. Whether you are at home or in a hospital or birthing center, you can cuddle with your baby and keep her or him skin to skin after feedings. You may also wish to bring a sling with you to the hospital so that you can comfort your baby with your warmth, smell, and movement while still having your hands free.

Once you are home, the baby can sleep in a crib, bassinet, or co-sleeper (a three-walled, criblike baby bed that attaches to your bed) or in bed with you (this practice is known as bed sharing). To reduce the risk of sudden infant death syndrome (SIDS), always have the baby sleep on her or his back. Create a safe space where the baby is secure from falling and from things that could accidentally smother the baby, including quilts, comforters, crib bumpers, sheepskin pads, stuffed toys, and pillows.

Some research indicates that bed sharing may increase the incidence of SIDS, particularly if the baby is sleeping on soft bedding or on her or his stomach. This is a controversial issue. One review of the research suggests that the increase in SIDS that has been associated with bed sharing is likely related to other factors, such as an adult in the bed drinking alcohol, smoking, or being extremely tired; overcrowded housing conditions; and/or when sleeping takes place on a water bed or soft sofa or the infant is placed under a heavy comforter.[6] Many health care providers and researchers suggest that when bed sharing is practiced safely, it has benefits for infants and parents, including better sleep and easier nighttime feedings.[7]

Though bed sharing may be controversial, room sharing is not. Having your baby in close proximity to you allows you and your baby to respond to each other more easily than if you are in separate rooms. It also may reduce the risk of SIDS.[8]

BREASTFEEDING YOUR BABY

I had read all the books about how good breast milk is for babies, and I wanted to nurse my child,

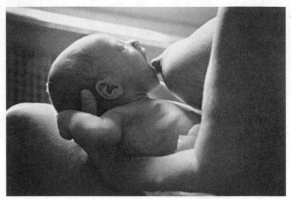

but before he was born I still felt a little strange about it. I never had any experience like that before, so I didn't know what it would be like to have this little person sucking on my breast almost twenty-four hours a day. I was almost wishing deep down that formula was better for babies. Then, after the birth and when we were in the hospital and started trying to breastfeed. I had this total change in attitude. I was like "This isn't as weird as I thought it would be. This is a bonding thing."

Many of us find great pleasure and pride in our body's ability to nourish new life. In addition, breastfeeding offers many benefits to both mothers and babies. Breast milk provides exactly the right balance of nutrients, adapting to your baby's changing requirements as she or he grows in the first months of life. It has unique nutritional properties that benefit infant health and that are not available in formula. Babies who are formula-fed are more likely than babies who are breastfed to develop ear infections, diarrhea, asthma, diabetes, lower respiratory tract infections, and eczema. Both sudden infant death syndrome (SIDS) and childhood leukemia, though rare, are more common in babies who are formula-fed.[9]

Mother's health is also affected by breastfeeding. Women who do not breastfeed are more

addition, some of us prefer not to or are unable to breastfeed. In these circumstances, formula is a vital alternative (see p. 446).

DECIDING TO BREASTFEED

I remember at age 5 watching my mother breastfeed my youngest brother. He was born by forceps, and he had a scrape on his cheek by his ear from the forceps blade. My mom told me that she would take extra vitamin C that would go through her breast milk to help Scott heal and grow. I remember her saying, "Even though a lot of women don't breastfeed, in this family, we breastfeed all our babies!" Every time she nursed him, I would climb on the sofa next to her and watch his cheek heal. And years later, when I was handed my own newborn, I felt my mother and my grandmother's love through that memory of "in this family, we breastfeed all our babies!"

The attitudes and assistance of the people who surround you play a significant role in supporting breastfeeding. Many of us make the decision to breastfeed before our babies are born, although many women don't plan in advance and are still able to breastfeed just fine. Planning ahead can be helpful, though. We may sign up for a breastfeeding class, purchase nursing bras and nursing pillows, and choose birth settings and pain relief options that will maximize our chances of successfully breastfeeding. Having the phone numbers of local lactation consultants and your local La Leche League (LLL) can also be useful.

likely to develop breast cancer, ovarian cancer, and type 2 diabetes.[11] Women who do not breastfeed or breastfeed for only a short period of time are also more likely to experience postpartum depression.[12]

In addition to being good for our babies' and our own health, breastfeeding has practical advantages: When you breastfeed, you don't have to spend money on formula or deal with bottles (except when you're separated from your baby). Breastfeeding means that your baby's food is always available—at the right temperature and with the right nutrients for growth and development.

In several specific circumstances, breastfeeding is not recommended (see sidebar, above). In

Some of us hesitate to breastfeed, for a variety of reasons. We may feel concerned about exposing our breasts in public, we may not know other women who nurse, or we may never have witnessed anyone breastfeeding before. If you are trying to decide whether to breastfeed your baby, learn more about breastfeeding. Ask nurs-

FINDING HELP WITH BREASTFEEDING

Whether you just have a simple question, need some mild troubleshooting, or are facing more serious challenges with breastfeeding, reliable sources of help and resources are available. Friends, neighbors, sisters, cousins, and others who have breastfed can sometimes provide immediate, practical, and wise advice. In addition, your midwife, pediatrician, or ob-gyn may be able to answer your questions. (However, some providers have very little experience and may recommend weaning or supplementing your baby unnecessarily.)

Other good sources of breastfeeding help include:

- La Leche League International has more than three thousand groups in at least sixty countries. It holds local meetings that are free, providing information and peer support from other mothers who have taken training in basic breastfeeding support and group facilitation. For more information, visit llli.org, or call 1-877-452-5324.
- The Office of Women's Health free Breastfeeding Helpline is staffed by trained peer counselors. You can reach them Monday through Friday, 9 A.M. to 6 P.M. EST, at 1-800-994-9662.
- Lactation consultants are trained and certified breastfeeding professionals whose services may be covered by private and public insurance companies. You can search for certified consultants at the International Lactation Consultant Association, ilca.org.

ing mothers, female friends, or relatives to share their stories with you and answer questions and concerns you might have. You may also want to consider attending a La Leche League meeting to meet other nursing mothers and ask any questions you might have.

If your hospital doesn't provide sufficient breastfeeding support, or if you must return to work in a matter of weeks, you may feel as if the decision not to breastfeed—or not to continue an extended period of time—has been made for you. But breastfeeding for any length of time is better than none, because of the health benefits to both you and your baby. You may also find that you are able to overcome some of the physical or emotional inhibitions and obstacles that initially discouraged you from trying.

GETTING BREASTFEEDING OFF TO A GOOD START

Breastfeeding is about building a relationship with your infant, and, like any long-term relationship, establishing it requires patience, give-and-take, and sometimes hard work. Most healthy newborns will be ready to nurse within the first hour after birth. Right after your baby is born, hold her or his belly skin to skin with yours. Most babies held in this position can locate the nipple and begin feeding on their own. Babies who have the opportunity to initiate the feeding process themselves are more likely to feed well as they grow.[13] Your colostrum (sometimes called the "first milk") is the best fuel for your baby during this learning phase. Frequent skin-to-skin contact in the early days and keeping your baby in your room at night can make breastfeeding easier and help you get more rest.

LATCHING ON

I was lucky. My kids latched on right away after they were born. It's like they were showing me how to do it.

Establishing a good "latch" or seal for breastfeeding is the single most important thing you can do to prevent sore nipples and other breastfeeding problems. A healthy latch is not painful and allows the baby to draw an adequate amount of milk from the breast. For most mother-baby teams, patience and practice are the keys to establishing a pain-free latch. To begin, it is important for you to know what a good latch looks like. Ask someone knowledgeable about breastfeeding, such as a nurse, midwife, or lactation specialist, to look at your baby's latch and give you feedback. You can also consult books and online resources that show images of correct latch.

Watch your baby and follow her or his signals. Learn to respond to the more subtle signs of hunger before your baby becomes agitated and starts to cry. Among the newborn's first signs of interest in food are little movements of the body, especially the hands moving near the head, smacking the lips, mouthing movements, seeking with the lips, rooting (turning the head in response to anything that touches the cheek), and bobbing the head. Babies who are awake and somewhat hungry will respond to the smell of their mother's milk and the closeness of her nipple by opening their mouths widely and sealing onto the breast and nipple. During the early days, breastfeeding frequently helps increase your chance of breastfeeding success. Put your baby to the breast at any sign of hunger. Rooming in with your baby at the hospital will help you learn to recognize and respond to these hunger signs.

Babies draw both nipple and breast tissue into their mouths when breastfeeding. To help your baby do this, line the baby up so that you are belly to belly and her or his neck is not turned to the side. When your baby's mouth is open wide, gently bring your baby to your breast, and insert your entire nipple and as much of the areola (the darker skin around the nipple) as possible into her or his mouth (flattening your breast with your thumb and index finger makes this easier). It is important to bring the baby to the nipple rather than leaning forward and pushing your breast toward the baby. The baby's lower jaw should be on the breast as far as possible from the nipple, so that the lower jaw and the tongue can draw milk from the breast (see p. 440).

Once the baby has established a seal, pause to look and listen. Your baby's cheeks should touch your breast, hiding her or his mouth. Your baby's lips, if you can see them, should be rolled slightly outward, away from your breast. If your baby's lips are curled in or under, gently break the suction by putting your pinkie between the nipple and the baby's mouth, and then try again (if just the bottom lip is turned in, you can pull down slightly on the jaw rather than relatching). Your baby's chin should be firmly planted on the breast. A good latch position will allow you to have good eye-to-eye contact with your baby. Listen for the sounds of swallowing and a shift in breathing between sucks. Watch to see if the baby's ears move, a sign that she or he is swallowing. If your baby is correctly positioned, you should not feel any pain. If feeding is painful, ask a nurse or lactation specialist for help.

She took right to the breast. Ahhhh, such a glorious feeling! Nothing in the world can match it. Such relief physically and mentally.

HOW TO BRING A BABY TO BREAST

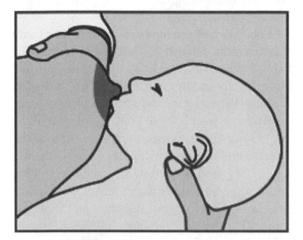

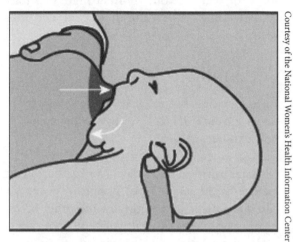

Courtesy of the National Women's Health Information Center

1. Tickle the baby's lips to encourage her or him to open wide. 2. Point your nipple to the roof of the baby's mouth and when she or he opens wide, pull her or him onto the breast, chin and lower jaw first. 3. Watch the lower lip and aim it as far from base of nipple as possible, so the baby's tongue draws lots of breast into the mouth.

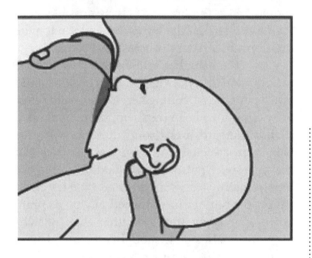

Another important part of establishing a healthy latch is getting comfortable with a few basic ways to cradle your baby while breastfeeding. Nurses and lactation consultants often encourage mothers to start newborns out with the "crossover" and "football" holds; both of these nursing positions are relatively easy to master and provide a mother with good control of her baby's delicate head and neck. Large-breasted women may be presented with specific chal-

lenges or need to experiment with different holds. In any position, it is important to keep the baby's head in alignment with her or his body and keep the baby horizontal, with her or his head, chest, navel, and knees all facing you.

If detailed instructions about latch and positioning make your head spin, it's important to remember that breastfeeding is, at heart, a human instinct. While it may take time and effort to get a healthy nursing relationship started, within a matter of days or weeks, you and your baby will learn about each other and establish a relationship. Rather than worrying about picture-perfect holds, listen to and look to your baby for cues. Trust yourself and your baby. Filter out unhelpful, unsolicited opinions. Respond to your baby's—and your body's—needs. And don't hesitate to seek help if you need it, as many women do.

Some babies, especially those born prematurely, may not have a strong enough sucking action to draw the nipple fully into the back of the mouth. This is necessary in order to draw milk from the breast and initiate the suck-breathe-swallow cycle. They may also tire more easily than full-term infants. Sleepy or jaundiced babies may prefer napping to nursing during the first few days of life and may need to be woken frequently to nurse. In rare cases, babies have anatomical conditions that can interfere with the establishment of a healthy latch. An experienced lactation specialist should be available for all women and babies experiencing such problems, as they can usually be overcome with individualized care and support.

He had trouble nursing right off the bat and was grunting for air a bit. He would latch on, but he had a weak suck. I had him latched on wrong for the first day or two and wound up with sore nipples and spoon-feeding him the colostrum because it hurt so badly. The nurse/lactation consultant came out on the second day to check up on us . . . It took me a couple weeks to fully adjust to nursing him; it was still uncomfortable but not painful. After that, I was able to nurse him for nearly two years without problems. I am so glad I did.

EARLY BREASTFEEDING PATTERNS

Breastfed newborns need to nurse at least eight to twelve times within a twenty-four-hour period. All that suckling, while providing nourishment for your baby, is also stimulating your breasts to ramp up their milk production, so as your baby grows, your supply will grow, too.

Frequent nursing is important for your baby's health and development as well as for building your milk supply, but this does not mean that you need to stick to a strict schedule. Breast-feed whenever your infant shows hunger cues. Sometimes babies cluster-feed (nursing every thirty to forty-five minutes right after or before sleeping) and then take long naps in between.

You may wonder if your baby is getting enough milk. Usually, you do not have to worry about this. Your baby will drink what she or he needs, and your body will make whatever your baby needs. Breastfeeding works on the principle that the more your baby sucks, the more milk you will make. If your baby is nursing and growing, she or he is doing fine. Still, in the first few days it makes sense to watch for other signs that the baby is getting enough.

The common guide for many years was "at least six wet diapers a day" once mature milk comes in. However, some babies urinate and pass stool at the same time, and it can be difficult to tell how many times your baby has urinated. Diapers holding only urine should be well saturated every couple of hours.

Breastfed babies generally have fairly watery bowel movements. The color will progress from greenish black in the first day or two to mustard yellow when they are getting milk. During the first two weeks after birth, your baby should have four or more stools every day; if not, contact your pediatric care provider.

CHALLENGES OF BREASTFEEDING

Sore Nipples
It started well for me—the baby latched on right away and sucked well—but then I got a cracked nipple and it was incredibly painful every time he nursed. And then the milk got stuck in some of the ducts in that same breast. So I needed him to nurse more on that side to get the milk moving, but every time he latched on it felt as if someone had set fire to my nipple. It took six weeks to get through all that. I didn't think I'd make it, but luckily I had a lot of support from my husband,

RESOURCES ON MEDICATIONS AND BREASTFEEDING

If a doctor suggests that you take medication while you are breastfeeding, learn as much as you can about the effects of the medication on breastfeeding mothers and babies. Some doctors, because they lack knowledge about the safety of taking medicines while breastfeeding, will err on the side of caution and tell women they must disrupt breastfeeding or stop entirely. In reality, few drugs are truly incompatible with breastfeeding, although sometimes caution or close monitoring is necessary. Talk with your maternity care provider, your baby's pediatrician, a lactation specialist, or your local La Leche League leader.

The best source of information is the book *Medications and Mothers' Milk* by Dr. Thomas Hale (Pharmasoft Publishing, 2010). Ask your provider if she or he has a copy, or look for it in your local library. The book is also available online for a fee at ibreastfeeding.com. Another excellent resource is LactMed (toxnet.nlm.nih.gov/lactmed), a free online database of research on the effects of different drugs on breastfeeding.

my family, the midwives, and the lactation nurse at the clinic.

Some mothers complain of sore nipples for the first days or weeks—and some limited discomfort or tenderness is normal. But if it is getting worse rather than better, or if you experience severe pain or cracked or bleeding nipples, consult with a health care professional or lactation specialist immediately. These can be signs of an incorrect latch or of something more serious, such as an infection, that should be treated promptly.

The most common cause of nipple soreness is a poor latch. Your baby may be getting milk by "chewing" on the tip of the nipple, rather than opening wide and compressing as much of the areola as possible. Pain often stems from incorrect positioning, the baby not opening his or her mouth wide enough, or tongue tie (ankyloglossia). If you have pain in your nipple every time the baby sucks, take the baby off your breast and reposition yourselves so that your nipple moves farther back in your baby's mouth. If that does not resolve the issue and you continue to have pain, contact a lactation consultant for advice about improving the latch and ask to be checked for possible tongue-tie (which can be corrected with a simple procedure).

Another cause of nipple soreness is a yeast infection commonly known as thrush. Thrush is caused when an infection in the baby's mouth spreads to the mother's nipples. A newborn can get thrush if the mother had a vaginal yeast infection when giving birth or if the mother was treated with antibiotics after the birth. A thrush infection can make a woman's nipples itchy, red, swollen, tender, and sometimes cracked. Many mothers with thrush complain of a severe burning or cut-glass sensation while nursing. If your baby has thrush, you may see white, cheesy patches on the inside of the baby's mouth that do not come off if you wipe them with a soft cloth or your finger. Check with your pediatric and obstetric care providers for diagnosis and treatment of this problem. It is important that both you and your baby receive treatment; otherwise you can pass the yeast infection back and forth between you.

Engorgement
(When Your Breasts Are Too Full)

Engorgement is a state of overfullness in the breast that is accompanied by swelling, redness or shininess of the skin, increased temperature of the breast, and marked discomfort when the breast is moved or touched. Engorgement may occur in the first few days while your milk comes in or after breastfeeding is well established, particularly if you go for longer periods of time without nursing or pumping, such as when the baby sleeps for longer stretches or you return to work.

If your breast is very hard and the nipple has become flat, you may want to express a small amount of milk manually until your areola softens so that it is easier for your baby to latch on. Soaking your breasts in a basin of warm water may help your milk to flow. Cool compresses or cool packs (wrapped in a clean dishcloth) may provide comfort before and after nursing. Having the baby nurse as often as she or he wants to is the best way to prevent and treat engorgement. Pumping your engorged breasts may overstimulate them and cause your body to make more milk than is needed. If you are engorged, keep your breasts comfortably supported, use cool packs for comfort, and let the baby breastfeed, allowing him or her to determine how much milk your breasts need to make.

Plugged Ducts and Mastitis
(Breast Inflammation)

A red, sore, or possibly even swollen spot on your breast may signify a plugged milk duct. To clear the blockage, try to gently massage the area while nursing, taking care to massage toward the nipple, nurse frequently from that breast, and start each feeding session from that breast. Apply moist heat or direct the shower spray to the area when bathing. Changing the infant's positions for feedings may also help drain the area more effectively.

If the blockage does not clear, you may develop a breast infection called mastitis. A full-blown case of mastitis feels like a bad case of the flu. In addition to pain and redness on the breast, you will be achy, feverish, and shivery. You may be tired and sore and not feel the least bit like breastfeeding, but whatever you do, don't stop. You've got to keep your breasts draining, or the mastitis could advance to a breast abscess, a rare but serious condition that can require surgical drainage.

If you think you have mastitis or have a temperature over 100.4°F, contact your health care provider immediately. You will likely need antibiotics, which can be taken safely by nursing mothers. Your health care provider may also recommend a nonsteroidal anti-inflammatory medication, such as ibuprofen (Advil or Motrin), which is also considered safe when you are breastfeeding. While mastitis symptoms are present, try massaging your affected breast in the direction of the nipple and changing nursing positions to drain your breasts more effectively. Also get plenty of rest and plenty to drink. You should start to feel better within twenty-four hours. If you are not starting to feel better, still have a temperature, or are feeling worse after three to four doses of an antibiotic, call your health care provider.

At a well-baby checkup for my baby, I showed my doctor my cracked and swollen breasts. There were a few warm red spots on them. Other than my breasts and nipples being sore, I felt fine. My doctor gave me a prescription for antibiotics just in case I developed mastitis. I picked up the prescription immediately since we live a fair distance from the closest pharmacy and headed home. Within an hour of arriving home, I had a high fever and felt like I had been run over. I started the antibiotics immediately and lay down for a nap. By the time I woke, I was already feeling much better.

Low Milk Supply

Though the vast majority of mothers produce enough breast milk to provide all the nourishment the baby needs, a small percentage of mothers do not. This can be incredibly difficult.

I so wanted to breastfeed my baby. All through my first pregnancy, I dreamt about it. So, when my son came five weeks early, after a difficult birth followed by formula in the hospital and then jaundice, my romantic ideas about nursing quickly faded. We tried everything—nurse-ins, support, a lactation aid, constant pumping, domperidone . . . it was just crushing and completely exhausting. He was supplemental from the beginning. I really gave it all I could for five months, but my supply and his suck never got to where they needed to be. I am so glad I stuck it out with him as long as I did; I know what he got from me serves him well. But I carried a sense of sadness and loss about it. Our breastfeeding relationship was so wrapped in the experience of the struggle. I was really consumed with fear and feelings of inadequacy when I was pregnant with my second child—would it be the same? I was bracing myself against the pain and grieving for the loss of this potential beauty again. Thankfully, I had no need to worry. I am positively thrilled that his little sister, born big and term at home, has been a vigorous and committed nurser from her first latch!

Concerns about possible low milk supply usually arise several days after birth, often if a baby has lost a significant percentage of her or his birth weight and has soiled or wet only a few diapers. In many cases, the cause of this may actually be poor latch or some other common breastfeeding difficulty. Mothers are often con-cerned that they have low milk supply because their baby is fussy at the breast or nursing frequently, but these are generally not indicators of a low milk supply.

In rare cases, low milk production is caused by a medical condition or by the effects of previous breast surgery. In addition, certain kinds of medications, including combined hormonal birth control pills, can affect how much milk your breasts produce.

Women experiencing low milk supply can sometimes generate enough milk by pumping between feedings or using herbal supplements, teas, or prescription medications to increase the supply. Sometimes it is necessary to supplement with formula or with donated breast milk to meet the baby's nutritional needs. Consult a breastfeeding-friendly pediatric care provider or a lactation specialist if you are experiencing low milk supply.

BREASTFEEDING UNDER SPECIAL CIRCUMSTANCES

Breast Surgery

If you have had breast surgery, successful breastfeeding may still be possible. Breast reduction surgery or a lumpectomy (breast cancer treatment) can sometimes cause problems with milk supply. Breast augmentation surgery is usually less problematic. If you have had a mastectomy (breast removed), you can probably still nurse with the milk produced by the remaining breast. Inform your health care providers about your surgery, and be sure to monitor your baby's weight carefully. Even if you do not have sufficient glandular tissue to produce a full milk supply, you can usually breastfeed if you choose to and supplement with formula or donor milk.

Adoption

Adoptive mothers may also wish to breastfeed, and in some cases it may be possible to create a milk supply even without giving birth. Putting the baby to the breast frequently can sometimes help stimulate the nipple and affect hormone levels that control milk supply. Using a quality double electric pump might also help to build your milk supply. A supplemental nursing system (SNS) can be used to allow adopted babies to drink their infant formula at the mother's breast while simultaneously stimulating the mother's milk supply. Some women who are expecting an adopted child prepare for possible breastfeeding by beginning a pumping regimen in advance of the baby's arrival or taking prescribed medications that stimulate milk production. It's a good idea to make enjoyment of the nursing relationship the main goal and to regard milk supply as a bonus rather than a necessity, as the amount of milk produced is generally small.

BREASTFEEDING IN PUBLIC

Many mothers breastfeed their babies wherever they are. In most parts of the world, it is common to see women breastfeeding on the bus or in a park. But in the United States and some other Western countries, cultural taboos and the sexualization of the female breast sometimes make us feel uncomfortable about nursing in public.

Nursing wherever we are makes it easier to go out with the baby without advanced planning. If you nurse only at home or in private places, you may feel constrained and wean earlier than mothers who feel comfortable nursing in public. Part of becoming more relaxed about public nursing is trying it out and experimenting. Specially designed nursing clothes now make it easier to breastfeed discreetly (if discretion is your goal). You can also try nursing in front of a mirror, just to see what others see. In addition, certain baby carriers (e.g., slings) and nursing covers can provide privacy for you and your nursing child.

I went to a La Leche League meeting when my daughter was just a few weeks old. It was one of the first times I left the house after giving birth, and it was the first time I nursed in front of people I didn't know. I was so comfortable because I was around other nursing mothers and it gave me so much confidence. I have now breastfed two kids for a total of five years and can't even begin to count the number of public places we've nursed.

Women in the United States have a constitutional right to breastfeed in public, and almost all states now have laws that specifically address public breastfeeding as a legal right. A growing number of mothers identify as lactivists— lactation activists—and advocate for the legal right to breastfeed in public. Many mothers' groups have formed to make our culture more

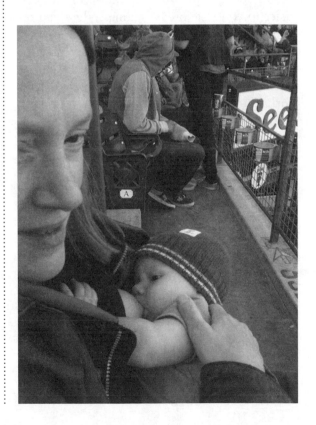

accepting for breastfeeding mothers and babies. Some have filed lawsuits against public facilities where women have been asked to stop nursing and have participated in public nurse-in protests against coffee shops and restaurant chains that have asked nursing mothers to leave or cover up.

BREASTFEEDING AND WORK

Returning to work after your baby is born doesn't mean you have to stop breastfeeding. Unless you work at home, work for only short periods of time, or have on-site day care in your workplace and can take breaks to breastfeed your baby, you will likely need to express (pump) your breast milk, refrigerate it, and then have your partner or a caregiver feed your milk to your baby. Many mothers have continued breastfeeding for months—even years—after returning to work.

A good-quality breast pump will make it easier to continue breastfeeding. When you return to work, breastfeed your child before leaving home each day and try to take two or three pumping breaks during an eight-hour workday. When you are reunited with your child after work, nurse frequently to maintain your milk supply.

As a working mother, I always nursed my baby after waking in the morning and then pumped the remaining milk for her first bottle of the day. I also woke her before I went to sleep at night or pumped before going to bed in an effort to build my supply and decrease the amount of milk I had to pump at work. I also found that co-sleeping and night nursing was a beneficial way for us to bond, despite my extended daily absences, and it also helped build my milk supply.

The 2010 health care reform legislation requires companies with more than fifty employees to provide a lactation room and unpaid break time for breastfeeding mothers. Individual states and employers may have additional protections. If you are planning to pump after returning to work, explain your plans to your supervisor or human resources department prior to your maternity leave, so that your employer has the opportunity to make the necessary arrangements for you. Many employers are eager to retain their employees and may be able to help you work out a plan to take pumping breaks.

Unfortunately, many workplaces and jobs have not yet made the appropriate changes to support breastfeeding women. Mothers who are paid hourly to work in fast-food restaurants, in stores, or on assembly lines—disproportionately African American and Hispanic—are often not provided with lactation rooms or paid pumping breaks. Women who work in salaried positions are more likely to have such benefits. This division establishes a group of women who can afford to breastfeed beyond the first weeks and another group who often cannot.

FORMULA AS AN ALTERNATIVE TO BREAST MILK

I felt like I was cut loose from the system way before I was ready. I was discharged before my milk had even come in. Some of the people who trained me at the hospital had not even nursed themselves. I felt like each individual tried her best, but it never came together for me. He never latched correctly. I never produced much milk. After a few days, it felt like time was ticking away and my baby wasn't getting enough to eat. When I finally made the decision to say, "I'm done with this. We're going to give you some formula," it was a huge relief. I felt like I could finally start trying to enjoy this new life.

In the not-so-distant past, many nursing mothers felt as though they were singled out for choosing to breastfeed. Now that health care providers and government officials are touting the benefits of breast milk, many formula-feeding mothers now feel that we are judged each time we feed our babies from a bottle.

Many of us who want to breastfeed but can't for medical reasons, or who lack the support we needed to get off to the right start, feel deeply disappointed that our bodies are not doing what we think they are "supposed" to do. These feelings may be similar to the grief and sense of loss some of us feel when labor and delivery did not go as we hoped.

There was always an assumption that I was going to breastfeed, and every time I pulled out the bottle, I always felt like I had to explain myself. People assume that everyone can nurse their babies. But not everyone can. I don't want to be judged for that.

CHOOSING A FORMULA

Infant formula is sold under different brand names and can be purchased in most large grocery stores and drugstores. Typically, there are only minor differences between standard formulas made by different companies, despite some of their advertising claims. Unless your infant has a health problem, you may feed her or him any of the commercially available formulas.

All formula is made from either modified cow's milk or soy products, with additional nutrients added. (Because soy milk and cow's milk are not appropriate foods for human newborns, they are altered when used in formula to make them safer for babies.) Some formulas are modified to feed babies with special needs, such as premature babies or infants sensitive or allergic to cow's-milk protein. Allergy symptoms may include eczema or skin rash, abdominal pain or cramps, and vomiting or diarrhea. Soy formula gained popularity in the 1990s because of concerns about allergies to cow's milk protein. But babies can be intolerant of soy protein as well, and there are no known advantages of soy formula over other formula, except for kosher and/or vegan families that want a formula without cow's milk or babies who cannot tolerate cow's milk–based formula.[14] If your family has a sensitivity to cow's milk or soy products, consult with your baby's care provider to choose the formula that is best tolerated.

Recently, formula companies have begun adding omega-3 fatty acids to formula. The companies claim that these fats (which are present in human milk) will increase visual development and intelligence in children who consume them, compared to babies who consume formula without these fats. However, the most recent research does not appear to support this. The same companies that market formula are now marketing the fats for use by pregnant and nursing women, with little evidence that using them has positive effects on the baby. Pregnant and nursing women and their babies can benefit from a diet rich in omega-3 fatty acids.

MOTHERS' HEALTH AND WELL-BEING

As new mothers, we face changes in our relationships, sexual health, and emotional well-being. Meeting the challenges of new motherhood is easiest when we are able to attend to our own health and well-being, communicate openly and honestly with our partners and other loved ones, and get support from the people around us.

Unfortunately, these things aren't always under our control. Our partners, other family members, and employers may expect us to bounce back from birth after just a few weeks. Whereas in other countries, new mothers can easily and freely access community-based or even home-based health care and support, in the United States, postpartum care is fragmented and often inadequate. For more information, see "Being a Mother Today," p. 459.

BODY IMAGE

Our bodies change dramatically during pregnancy and childbirth and continue to change postpartum. Our culture emphasizes the need to lose the baby weight and get our bodies back—as if it were possible or desirable for pregnancy and childbirth to leave our bodies entirely as they were before. These attitudes devalue the fact that our bodies have done the incredible feat of growing a whole other human being. Even when we are in awe of our bodies, our shape and appearance after giving birth can be difficult to get used to.

My body now is a lot different than before I had my son. But it is also a body that has served a purpose. I look at my belly, a little looser than before, and remind myself that it carried him while he grew. I look at my breasts, lower and less full than before, and remind myself that they nourished my tiny premature baby into a rough-and-tumble toddler. *

The postpartum months are not a time to diet. A healthy, well-balanced diet with plenty of protein, calcium, and fiber is important for postpartum recovery. Extra calories are needed to support breastfeeding. Opt for easy meals, frequent snacks, and fresh, healthy foods. Ease back into exercise slowly, beginning with light walks and abdominal exercises.

Pregnancy and new motherhood can sometimes trigger eating and exercise disorders, especially in women who have struggled with those disorders previously. If you find yourself turning to unhealthy behaviors as a way of coping with the emotions and challenges of new motherhood, seek help from a qualified counselor or health care professional.

SEXUALITY

After recovering from childbirth, some of us experience increased sexual desire. Many new moms, however, feel less interested in sex, at least for a while. Some women forgo sexual activity entirely during the postpartum period and focus instead on bonding as a family. Others of us miss being as sexual as we were before.

Often a woman and her partner experience mismatched levels of desire:

All that first year, our old forms of go-to-it sexuality were just too much. I was too tired and I'd fall asleep in the first five minutes, leaving Jack frustrated, even angry. Other times I've have the nursing and holding of the baby on my mind and intercourse seemed rough and crude. Also, I think that by the end of the day I had had a lot of skin-to-skin rubbing and touching and didn't feel sexually hungry at all. But Jack hadn't had much at all. The unevenness was driving us nuts.

How we feel sexually is affected by many factors, from our physical recovery to the strength of our relationship. Many of us need time to adjust to our new role of mother. Sleep deprivation and shifts in hormone levels can decrease our sexual desire. Our emotions are also key ingredients in how we respond sexually. Depression (and some of the drugs used to treat it) can negatively affect libido (see "Postpartum Mood Disorders," p. 455). In addition, feeling insecure about our bodies can affect our sexuality; those of us with poor body image are often less interested in being sexual.

* Excerpted from Claire Mysko and Magali Amadeï, *Does This Pregnancy Make Me Look Fat? The Essential Guide to Loving Your Body Before and After Baby* (Deerfield Beach, Fla.: Health Communications, Inc., 2009).

Understanding the physical and emotional changes you are experiencing can help ease the transition, as can talking with other mothers and recognizing society's mixed messages about sex and motherhood. Sharing your concerns openly and honestly with your partner, asking for help, and maintaining a sense of humor can also help you feel comfortable with your sexuality.

When Can I Have Sex Again?

Most health care providers suggest waiting four to six weeks, or until your perineum has healed and discharge has stopped, before engaging in vaginal or anal penetration. (This is true whether you gave birth vaginally or by cesarean section.) Before that, your cervix is still dilated (more open than usual), leaving you vulnerable to infection. Making love without penetration, snuggling, and solo sex (masturbation) are all okay.

Just because it's okay to have sex doesn't mean you're ready. Many of us don't want to have sex for quite a while after birth. Give yourself permission to take however much time you need.

Relationship Issues

Frustration about everyday issues can be a roadblock to good sex when there's a new baby in the house. Anger or resentment about housework, role confusion, differing parenting styles, frequency of sex, not having enough time alone, and many other factors can lead to a lack of closeness and a limited sex life. Talking with your partner about these may help. If contact with your baby fulfills your desire for physical intimacy, your partner may feel jealous or left out.

When I nursed at night, the sight of me holding my full breast to this sleepy little baby used to drive Les nuts. When I'd get back into bed, he'd be wild to make love, fast and hard. It got to be quite a thing because I'd come back to bed feeling mild

and sleepy. Les wanted to [have sex] and I wanted to snuggle. We fought over it a lot.

Talking about your differences and setting aside special time to reconnect emotionally with your partner can lead to rediscovering physical intimacy together. Using "I statements" ("I feel——when you——") to share your concerns and listening without judgment or blame can open the door to a healthy discussion, as well as to the bedroom.

After months and months of snarling, we just had to invent "middle ways" of being physical with one another. I think I picked it up from watching each of us with the baby—the nuzzling and snuggling that goes on with no expectation of orgasm, just affection.

Back rubs, snuggling, massages, hugging, and invigorating conversation are all ways to feel close to your partner without the pressures of sexual performance or enjoyment.

Physical Considerations

Vaginal Discomfort

Many new mothers experience vaginal pain or a pulling sensation at the perineum, particularly if stitches were needed, when first resuming penetrative sex. Decreased estrogen levels may cause vaginal tissues to become thin and sensitive and lead to decreased lubrication, even when you are sexually aroused.

Taking things slowly and using lots of lubricant can help lead you back to pleasurable sex. If you want to have intercourse, experiment with different positions. Sometimes the pulling is less if you're on top. Starting with finger penetration first may help you adjust to the changes and reduce anxiety.

Scar tissue from sutures will soften and perineal discomfort will likely ease within two to six months. Vaginal dryness is linked to changing hormone levels, especially when breastfeeding, and will likely ease with weaning. If either problem persists after you have stopped breastfeeding, and over-the-counter lubricants don't work, talk with your health care provider.

If you had a vaginal birth, your vagina may feel stretched and less sensitive than before.

Abdominal Pain

If you had a cesarean birth, certain sexual positions may cause or increase abdominal pain. You may want to experiment with different positions or delay sex until you have healed more.

Breast Changes

Your breasts may become either more or less sensitive while you are nursing. If you experience heightened sensation, you may find that you enjoy it or that you prefer that your breasts be left alone for anything but breastfeeding, due to tenderness, feeling "touched out" from nursing all day, or difficulty separating the breast function of nursing from sexuality.

If you are breastfeeding, your breasts may leak or spray during orgasm. Some women enjoy this experience, while others find it unsettling. If it's a problem, you can wear a bra with nursing pads while having sex.

Some women experience sexual arousal while nursing. This is a normal sensation and is related to the release of oxytocin, which is associated with both orgasm and the letdown that happens as breast milk comes in.

Nursing mothers have higher levels of prolactin and lower levels of estrogen, which may result in less frequent or less intense desire. While many women find that breastfeeding reduces overall sexual drive, most women note that sexual drive returns when weaning or while continuing to nurse a toddler who does not nurse frequently. However, some women who nurse have a strong sex drive, and mothers who

don't breastfeed may still have a lowered sex drive after becoming mothers.

There were times when I got into bed, gave my husband a peck on the cheek, and leaned back onto my pillow relishing the prospect of some sleep. Sex was the last thing on my mind, and usually I conked out in minutes. But he would sometimes gently stroke my body in a few choice spots, and before I knew it, I actually felt aroused and suddenly interested in making love. Where that energy came from, I still can't fathom.

Birth Control

If you are having vaginal intercourse with a man, it's important to think about family planning before you are fertile again. Regular breastfeeding inhibits ovulation and will delay the return of your period. Most women who are breastfeeding will resume menstruation between three months and two years after giving birth. If you are not breastfeeding, your menstrual cycle usually resumes one to three months after giving birth. This means that you may ovulate (release an egg from the ovary) as soon as twenty-five days after delivery and could become pregnant again even before your period resumes.

When deciding on a birth control method, you face special considerations as a new mother. Some methods of birth control, such as hormonal methods that include estrogen, should not be used by nursing mothers; some methods, such as diaphrams and cervical shields, need to be refitted due to changes in the uterus, cervix, and vagina after childbirth; and some are less effective once a woman has given birth. For a full discussion of the efficacy, benefits, and potential harms of all birth control methods, see Chapter 9, "Birth Control," especially "Breastfeeding as Birth Control," p. 249, and "Suitable Contraceptive Methods to Use While Breastfeeding," p. 251.

THOUGHTS AND EMOTIONS

In the first hours and days after giving birth, you will likely experience a range of feelings. It is not unusual to feel multiple, contradictory emotions, all at the same time.

She was placed on my chest, and I began to cry from the overwhelming sense of emotions I felt. I was feeling so many things simultaneously: relief, love, excitement, awe, astonishment, pride, and achievement. It was truly a momentous occasion, very surreal and very beautiful. When I looked deeply into my newborn daughter's eyes for the very first time, I kissed her softly and whispered: "Hi, Baby. Welcome to the world, we've been waiting for you."

EARLY ADJUSTMENT

During the first few months after giving birth, we learn what it means to have a baby in our lives. Our babies eat and sleep at unpredictable times, and we find ourselves on call around the clock.

Thoughts and emotions in the early weeks and months of motherhood can be influenced by many factors, including our physical recovery from being pregnant and giving birth, our feelings about the birth, the health of our babies and how "easy" they are, how ready we feel to become a mother, our financial resources, the other demands we face, and the amount and kind of support we get from people around us.

GETTING SUPPORT

Flight attendants on airplanes explain that in the event of an emergency, when oxygen is needed, passengers with children should first secure their own oxygen masks before fitting masks on their children. This is a lesson we can apply to the turbulence of our experience with moth-erhood: We cannot properly care for our children unless we properly care for ourselves.

As new mothers, we may focus on our babies to the exclusion of ourselves. We may feel ashamed to ask for help, not realize that help is needed, or not even realize that asking for help is acceptable or possible. Some mothers may believe that the involvement of a partner or support from family members means we aren't good enough. Our culture idealizes mothers who are eternally self-sacrificing. But help and support are crucial, and being attentive to your own needs can boost your ability to meet your child's needs. It is important not to think of the mother's needs and the baby's needs as mutually exclusive and instead to find creative ways to meet both people's needs without sacrificing the other.

Because I am single and have a disability, I could not and cannot get away with trying to be a supermom. I knew then and know even more clearly now that it does indeed take a village. I have relied heavily on my community of friends, some family, and a key group of child care providers. I am reminded how people enjoy being part of an emerging family, that isolation is the bane of parenthood, and that letting others help is a gift to everyone, especially the child. Asking for help has brought friends closer to me and my son in a more intimate way. I am grateful for that.

Mothering is hard work, and new mothers need many different kinds of care: practical help, emotional support, financial support, nurturing, and guidance. Unfortunately, it can be hard to find the care and community we need. Our society provides little concrete help, whether in terms of paid maternity or paternity leave, subsidized child care, or other forms of support. In addition, aspects of our culture, such as families living far apart rather than in intergenerational households and neighbors often not knowing

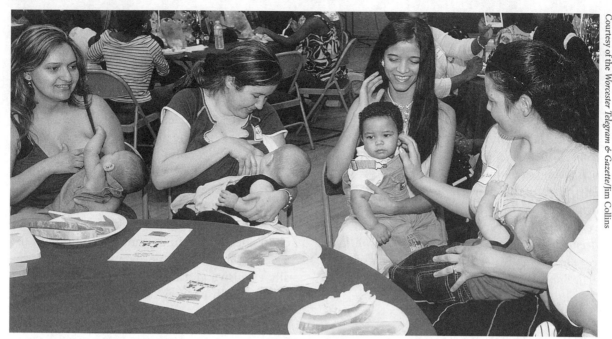

Several mothers and babies celebrate the sixth birthday of the Worcester (Massachusetts) Healthy Start Initiative. The initiative receives federal funding to promote community-based programs for uninsured and low-income women and their babies.

one another, make it likely that we will be alone with our babies for long stretches of time. Independence and self-reliance are prized in the United States, even though it is unrealistic for new mothers.

When we feel helpless or lost or confused, talking about what we're feeling may seem like the wrong idea. But often telling someone—your partner, a family member, a close friend, or your midwife, physician, or therapist—how you feel can help ease the stress and isolation that so often characterize new motherhood.

[My partner] was working hard all the time and feeling stressed out about his new responsibilities as sole financial provider for the family. We argued a lot. There were times when I couldn't even believe I had a baby with him! . . . I remember saying "No one told me about all this!"

to a friend, and she told me that she thought the same thing after she had her first baby. Then I realized that the more I talked to other mothers, the better I felt. I was not alone! One of my friends gave me Sheila Kitzinger's book The Year After Childbirth. *I read it cover to cover. . . .*

I made a point to go over to the house of a friend who also had children a couple times a week. Getting out of the house and with other moms really helped. My partner and I started going to a really great therapist. Just taking the time to focus on our relationship felt so good. In a short time, we were communicating well again and our therapist told us that many new parents go through this. . . . If I could give one piece (or two!) of advice to a new mama, it would be to get together with other like-minded mamas often, and be patient with yourself. You are doing a great job!

TIPS FOR THE FIRST WEEKS

- **Ask for help.** As much as possible, get family and friends to clean, cook, and take over your other responsibilities, so that you are free to focus on your baby and your recovery.
- **Sleep or rest when the baby sleeps.** Respecting your need to sleep and rest is one of the most important ways to recover, heal, and ease the stress of life with a newborn.
- **Nurture yourself with good food.** Eating well and staying well hydrated are important ways to recover from giving birth and have the energy to meet the demands of being a new parent. Eat whole foods and go easy on sugar and caffeine, which may sap your energy over time.
- **Take time to relax and make time for some physical activity.** Rest and relaxation, balanced with gentle activities such as talking a walk, can add to your sense of physical and emotional well-being.
- **Talk to other new mothers about your experience—and listen to what they have to say about theirs.** Hearing other people's stories can help normalize what's happening and ease isolation. You can do this by attending a new-mom group, by using online discussion boards and social media networks, or by spending time with friends who are mothers.
- **Remember that you have added a whole new 24/7 job to your life.** Be patient and gentle with yourself as you adjust. As you get to know your baby better and become more confident, it will get easier.

Ways to Get Support

You can find support for yourself and your family in different ways. Many of us turn to family and friends or parenting, breastfeeding, or new-mother support groups both in our communities and online. Others draw on the help of paid caregivers.

Family and Friends

Talking to your partner, your family, and close friends ahead of time about what you think you might need once the baby arrives helps set the stage for support. It is hard to know exactly what your needs will be, but having a support group of willing family members and friends is a good place to begin. Even if you didn't make plans in advance, turn to those people for help once the baby is born. It might also be helpful to talk with other women about what they thought was most helpful when they first became mothers.

As much as possible, ask for *concrete* help. Sometimes you are not even sure what you need when friends ask what they can do for you. Saying yes to small things—your partner offering to be with the baby and/or watch your other children while you sleep; friends who ask if they can bring you food, watch your kids, or clean your house—helps you to recuperate and to learn what kind of help is actually useful to you. Practicing can also help you know when to say no—for instance, to people who offer things you don't really want or need or whose company drains you.

Parenting Support Groups

Your local hospital may offer support groups for new mothers through its social services or childbirth education department. Often these groups are free. Libraries, children's bookstores, coffee houses, places of worship, and YWCAs and YMCAs sometimes host weekly meetings for new mothers and babies. You can find these groups by checking your local library or community center, looking online, or asking friends, neighbors, or other new mothers. If you take a childbirth class, the instructors may have a list of community resources.

There are many websites devoted exclusively to the experience of new mothers; some feature online support groups or schedule local, in-person meet-ups. And there's no limit to the number of blogs and online communities offering real women's stories about their day-to-day experience of motherhood. For more links and resources, visit ourbodiesourselves.org/childbirth.

Social Service Organizations

Your local family services agency, public health department, community health center, mental health agency, or hospital providing maternity services may offer counseling in a group or individual setting, often for a sliding fee.

Paid Caregivers

A postpartum doula, a caregiver whose role is to mother the mother, can help with everything from providing breastfeeding support to caring for your baby day or night to making sure you are fed and well rested. Some doulas charge an hourly or flat rate, while others offer a sliding scale, and occasionally doula support will be covered by health insurance. To find a certified doula in your area, visit DONA International (dona.org) or call 1-888-788-3662. You can also contact the Childbirth and Postpartum Professional Association (cappa.net) or

1-888-692-2772. (For more information about doulas, see page 393.)

Night nannies, home health aides, and part-time or full-time child care providers can provide relief, even if it's just a few hours a couple of times a week so you can rest or get out of the house for a while. Small breaks can make a big difference.

EMOTIONAL CHALLENGES

Emotional highs *and* lows are normal during the first few weeks after giving birth. Many women have times of feeling irritable, moody, weepy, and overwhelmed. These "baby blues" are very common. They usually occur in the first two weeks after birth and can last for days or a few weeks. Typically new mothers feel better after these down times and don't remain stuck in one continuous emotional rut.

Some new mothers, however, struggle with more painful feelings for a longer period of time, experiencing what are classified as postpartum mood disorders.

POSTPARTUM MOOD DISORDERS

I know that I don't exude excitement and joy, but I don't know how to process what I am feeling. I just want to have one really good cry and let it all out, but I'm ashamed to. I'm afraid that if I start crying I won't be able to stop. There's so much love going on around me, and all I feel like doing is screaming until my head explodes. I don't know how to share any of this with anyone, so I cry alone when I get a chance; just a few minutes here and there.

Many women who experience postpartum emotional difficulties are afraid to discuss their negative feelings for fear of being seen as a bad mother or crazy. But postpartum mood disorders are both common and treatable, and it is important, both for our own sake and for the sake of our families, to seek help.

Postpartum mood disorders can include severe depression (sometimes mixed with anxiety), as well as other seriously disabling problems labeled with terms such as anxiety/panic disorder, obsessive-compulsive disorder, post-traumatic stress disorder, and, very rarely, psychosis. Postpartum depression is by far the most common of postpartum mood disorders, affecting about one in seven new mothers. It can start anytime in the first year after giving birth. Symptoms of postpartum depression can include hopelessness, suicidal thoughts, sleep

POSTADOPTION DEPRESSION

As an adoptive mother, I sometimes seemed to have little in common with other new moms. My baby was ten months old, not a few weeks. She didn't look like me. I hadn't given birth to her. And I had other different issues—insensitive comments, for example, or fears about a shortened parental leave (which at that time was seventeen weeks instead of the six months' maternity leave for biological mothers), not bonding with her, or she with me. There was only one thing that I was certain I shared with some biological mothers: I was extremely depressed.

Is it possible to get postpartum depression without having given birth? Though few studies have been done, postadoption depression clearly exists. Physical exhaustion, isolation, financial worries, and stress from the adoption process have all been cited as causes of postadoption depression. Sometimes unresolved feelings about infertility arise. Some adoptive parents see the adoption as bittersweet and focus on the loss experienced by the child's birth mother or the child. There is also a huge disconnect between outsiders' assumptions about adoptive parents and the real stresses that any new parent experiences. Adoptive mothers often hesitate to ask for help because of comments such as "Don't be silly, you had it easy, you didn't have to give birth or breastfeed" or "Isn't this what you wanted for so long?"

Strategies for coping with postadoption depression are similar to those for coping with postpartum depression: Acknowledge that this sort of depression exists; seek support, especially from other mothers; ask for help; and take care of yourself.

SIGNS TO WATCH FOR

Although many of us may experience one or two of the warning signs below at various times, experiencing a combination of them for an extended period may indicate depression or another postpartum mood disorder.

If you are experiencing any of the following problems for longer than two weeks, consider seeking help from a therapist:

- Feelings of inadequacy, worthlessness, or guilt, especially failure at motherhood
- Loss of interest or pleasure in activities that used to bring pleasure
- Excessive anxiety over the baby's health or, conversely, lack of interest in the baby
- Inability to care for yourself or your baby
- Restlessness, irritability, or excessive crying
- Changes in appetite, such as forgetting to eat or overeating
- Changes in sleep, such as waking in the night, having racing thoughts, and not being able to go back to sleep
- Difficulty concentrating, remembering, or making decisions
- Hopelessness and profound sadness
- Uncontrollable mood swings, including feelings of rage or anger
- Feeling overwhelmed or unable to cope
- Fear of being alone

If you are experiencing even one of these more serious symptoms, contact your health care provider immediately:

- Unusual headaches, chest pains, heart palpitations, numbness, hyperventilation, panic
- Fear or recurrent thoughts of harming the baby or yourself
- Scary thoughts about the baby getting hurt (different from thoughts of you being the one to hurt the baby)
- Compulsive behaviors such as washing your hands excessively or constantly checking to see if your baby is breathing
- Recurrent thoughts of death or suicide; feeling that the baby would be better off without you
- Hallucinations

and eating problems, inability to feel good or be comforted, and withdrawing into oneself. A woman experiencing postpartum depression may have a hard time caring for her baby or meeting the other demands of daily life.

Besides postpartum depression, women sometimes experience other postpartum mood disorders. Feelings of intense anxiety, fear, or panic, along with rapid breathing, an ac-celerated heart rate, hot or cold flashes, chest pain, and shaking or dizziness are symptoms of an anxiety/panic disorder. Recurrent frightening thoughts, including obsessing over the baby's health or acting out repetitive behaviors such as compulsive hand washing, are symptoms of an obsessive-compulsive disorder. A combination of depression with anxiety/panic disorder or obsessive-compulsive disorder is also possible.

Women who experienced fear, powerlessness, or a sense of being mistreated during labor and delivery are at greater risk of developing post-traumatic stress responses. These women may develop unpleasant repetitive thoughts, nightmares, agitation, fear of interactions with others, or an ongoing sense of panic.

A very small percentage of women (about one or two per thousand new mothers) experience a serious illness called postpartum psychosis. Women with postpartum psychosis may experience hallucinations and delusions and other symptoms including insomnia, agitation, and bizarre feelings and behavior. Postpartum psychosis generally develops within one to four weeks after giving birth and is considered a medical emergency.

WHO IS AT RISK?

Any women can develop a postpartum mood disorder. The hormonal changes that occur during pregnancy and birth appear to play a strong role in the development of these problems.

However, certain factors are linked with a greater likelihood of experiencing a postpartum mood disorder. These include severe or ongoing postpartum pain; health problems in the mother or baby; a high-needs baby; relationship, financial, or other major stresses; isolation; and a lack of social support. Ongoing sleep deprivation is also a risk factor.

Women who have a past history of physical or emotional trauma, depression, sexual abuse, severe premenstrual syndrome, substance abuse, or other mental health issues are at increased risk of postpartum mood disorders. Adolescent mothers are also at increased risk of postpartum depression.

GETTING HELP

If you are experiencing postpartum emotional problems, ask for support and practical help taking care of your baby and yourself. If you have a partner—or other support people—available, ask him or her to share household chores and nighttime feeding duties. Do only as much as you can, and don't blame yourself for leaving nonessential things undone. (For other ideas on practical help and self-care, see "Tips for the First Weeks," p. 453.)

Isolation can contribute to depression and anxiety, so try to find at least one family member or friend with whom you can honestly share your feelings and your experience of motherhood. Meeting with a new-mother group can be a great way to connect with other women facing the same challenges. Many support groups and online chat rooms focus specifically on helping women with postpartum depression. (See "Ways to Get Support," p. 453.)

Sometimes, however, the support and help of friends and family is not enough. If this is true for you, consult with your primary care physician or ob-gyn or seek out a social worker, psychologist, or psychiatrist who is knowledgeable about postpartum mood disorders.

TREATMENT

Besides getting more support from the people around you, the two basic types of treatment offered by mental health professionals for postpartum depression and anxiety disorders are talk therapy and medication. Talk therapy involves regular sessions with a counselor or therapist, discussing your feelings and developing constructive ways to meet the challenges of being a new mother. Medications—including antidepressants, antianxiety drugs, sleep medications, or a combination of the three—can sometimes be helpful.

In the rare event that you experience postpartum psychosis, you will likely need to go to a hospital for a short time for appropriate therapy.

Counseling or Therapy

Therapy sessions can help you express and understand your feelings more fully. They can also help you explore possible solutions for postpartum challenges and learn better ways to communicate your needs and get them met. Therapists and counselors can direct you to other community resources for new mothers and families.

Medications

Although antidepressant medications are commonly prescribed for postpartum mood disorders, surprisingly there has been only one small study (involving eighty-seven women) that actually tested the effectiveness of drug therapy for postpartum depression. This study showed that fluoxetine (Prozac) and six sessions of counseling (cognitive behavioral therapy) were equally effective in relieving depression. Cochrane Reviews summarizes this limited evidence about drug therapy for postpartum depression as follows:

It is not possible to make any recommendations for antidepressant treatment in postnatal depression from this single small trial. More trials are needed, with larger sample sizes and longer follow-up periods, to compare different antidepressants in the treatment of postnatal depression, to compare antidepressant treatment with psychosocial interventions and to assess adverse effects of antidepressants. Treatment of postnatal depression is an area that has been neglected despite the large public health impact.[15]

Despite the lack of good scientific evidence about such an important issue in women's health, many health care providers and the general public *believe* antidepressant therapy to be a proven treatment for postpartum depression. And drug companies have little incentive to do clinical trials that risk having a negative effect on sales of their drugs.

Especially in light of the paucity of scientific evidence supporting antidepressant therapy for postpartum depression, it is important to remember that antidepressants (like other medicines) can produce negative effects, such as sleep, digestive, and sexual problems, and, rarely, more serious effects. Unfortunately, finding unbiased information about the effectiveness and safety of antidepressants is challenging, as much of the widely available material on the Internet and elsewhere is produced or sponsored by drug companies.

Women in severe crisis sometimes find that only talk therapy combined with medication is helpful. (For more information on the potential benefits and harms of antidepressant medications, see "Depression and Other Mental Health Challenges During Pregnancy," page 389.) If you are breastfeeding, be sure to tell your provider. Though commonly used antidepressants do pass into breast milk, their short-term negative effects on babies, if any, appear to be transient. Additional research, particularly on the long-term safety of antidepressants for breastfed babies, is needed. To learn more about the effects of medication on breast milk, work with a provider who is knowledgeable about medications and breastfeeding and consult Thomas Hale's book *Medications and Mothers' Milk*. (For more information, see "Resources on Medications and Breastfeeding," p. 442.)

Depression can make bonding with your baby difficult, which can adversely affect your baby's overall development. So finding a solution that works for you is important. Therapeutic decisions should be guided by your preferences, the severity of your illness, the risks of the medicines in question, and the known risks of depression for you and your baby.

BEING A MOTHER TODAY

Through digital media, books, blogs, and parenting magazines, mothers today have more access to one another's stories and ideas about mothering than our foremothers did. Thanks to the voices of those brave enough to share their experiences, we have a fuller picture of the physical changes and emotional landscape of motherhood. And thanks to changing laws and cultural attitudes, women can more easily pursue single motherhood or coparent with a female partner, and can continue a career after having kids.

But the myth of the supermom who is perpetually cheerful, all-knowing, and self-sacrificing lives on, and it's hard to resist. We—both as individuals and as a society—still have certain expectations about what it means to be a mother.

Everyone's like "This is the best time of your life, aren't you so happy?" There's no room to say no. . . . You're not allowed to have the negative emotions. You love and hate your child so much, all together, all at once.

It's important to be able to talk about how it feels trying to live up to others' expectations. Traditionally, though, mothers have been expected to talk only about the positive; voicing frustrations with some of the more difficult moments can be tough. We expose not only our ambivalence but our vulnerability.

I was afraid I wouldn't be a good mother or would forget to feed him or change him. I was afraid he wouldn't like me. I was afraid of everything in the world and yet was so happy at the same time. It was the strangest feeling in the world. I still sometimes feel that way and think that every mother does at some point. We doubt ourselves all the time and really need to just relax and go with it, because chances are we're doing a really good job.

MOMMY WARS AND OPTING OUT

I'm a single mom. My son's father has just disappeared. My main support is my family, but it comes with a cost. My mom and aunt seem to feel they can tell me how to parent, especially since they are providing me with free babysitting while I work. . . . I really wish I didn't have to work, but I have no choice. I would much rather be home with my son, because I just love being his mother.

In addition to feeling the pressure to be a supermom, many mothers are conflicted about balancing work and family. Those of us who work outside the home often contend with the stress of arranging for full-time child care and may feel guilt and judgment about the choices we make. Those of us who stop working to care for children may be frustrated by the loss of identity and advancement opportunities that often come with leaving the workforce.

My brain is melting and coming out my ears. I feel like everything I was trained to do, all my hopes and aspirations, are frozen in time. My husband goes about his life and his job and then gets to come home and be a great daddy. [Sometimes] he says things like "You seem really touchy today," and all of a sudden I'm like "Did you pee by yourself today? Did you go to the bathroom alone? That's how I'm rating the quality of my days right now."

For many women, working is not optional; it is a financial necessity. For other women, the cost of child care may make staying home a financially sensible choice. Some women make great financial sacrifices to stay home. These are complex decisions based on our values, priorities, and needs.

The media-driven talk of the mommy wars polarizes mothers into two camps: those who work outside the home and those who stay at home. In reality, many of us cycle into and out of these roles. Too often, public discourse either praises working mothers for their multitasking abilities or condemns them for neglecting their children; similarly, it often either praises stay-at-home moms for being devoted to their children or condemns them for giving up so much of their identity and career potential. No wonder all of us feel judged.

While our society idealizes motherhood, our government provides little concrete support for children and families. Unlike most other industrialized countries, the United States has no guaranteed paid family leave, no guaranteed health care, and little affordable high-quality child care. We need public policies that value and support families and caregivers, who are mostly women. We also need to push for a society that recognizes that fathers, like mothers, need to strike a balance between their career and their family life.

It's often said that it takes a village to raise a child. Finding *your* village, gathering support around, and allowing other nurturing adults into your circle will ultimately enrich both you and your child's world. As your child's first role model, leading the way with a sense of balance, a commitment to your priorities, and a strong network of support will provide a road map for your child as he or she navigates the road to healthy adulthood.

Whenever I feel guilty or start worrying that I'm doing it wrong, I remind myself that in the end, it usually turns out okay. Because a huge part of our kids' emotional and physical health as adults is due to what kind of parents we are. But an even huger part is because of the kids themselves: their temperaments, abilities, intelligence, etc. And their teachers and peers also play a big role. There's no One True Path to successful motherhood.

Miscarriage, Stillbirth, and Other Losses

Despite their frequency, pregnancy and childbirth losses are not widely recognized or understood in our culture. Many pregnancy books barely cover the topics, and when they do, they tend to sequester the information at the back. Most health care providers are understandably reluctant to inform women of the possibility of loss or discuss medical options until a problem occurs. Yet this lack of knowledge means we learn about our options and make choices only in the midst of the crisis.

The loss of a pregnancy or the death of a baby during pregnancy or after childbirth is often an immense and shocking blow. The grief that follows can be intense.

We went home from the hospital dazed and tired. I was weak and enormously sad. I don't know that I've ever experienced such deep emotional pain. The loss was so great and so complete. . . . For the first few days I couldn't talk to anyone, but at the same time, it was painful to be alone. I would just cry and cry without stopping.

Another woman says of her miscarriage:

I was hysterical with grief and jealous of all those pregnant moms and moms pushing strollers. I didn't know anyone who had had a miscarriage. That was a terrible thing. Even though intellectually you know miscarriage is quite common, there is still a great deal of secrecy and shame surrounding the experience.

Women who experience the loss of a pregnancy or a baby need emotional support and sensitive care and attention from health care providers, families, and friends, both during the loss and afterward. Some hospitals now have bereavement teams and organize pregnancy-and-infant-loss support groups. Sensitive providers and in-person or online groups can help us and our partners with the isolation that often follows a loss and support us in grieving, healing, and making decisions about future childbearing.

The vast majority of women who experience loss go on to have successful pregnancies and give birth to healthy babies. Having a subsequent successful pregnancy, however, does not necessarily erase the pain of earlier losses.

TYPES OF PREGNANCY AND BIRTH LOSSES

Pregnancy and infant loss occurs in many different ways, including miscarriage, ectopic or molar pregnancy, loss in a multiple-gestation pregnancy, the decision not to carry to term a fetus with genetic anomalies, stillbirth, and early infant death.

MISCARRIAGE

Miscarriage, the loss of a pregnancy before the twentieth week, is by far the most common type of pregnancy loss.* An estimated 15 to 20 percent of known pregnancies end in miscarriage.† The risk of miscarriage increases as we age: Women under age 30 have about a 12 percent chance of miscarrying; women between ages 30 and 34 about 15 percent; women between 35 and 39 about 25 percent; women ages 40 to 44 an estimated 40 percent; and women ages 45 and older about 80 percent.[1]

Most miscarriages take place within the first twelve weeks of pregnancy. The chance of miscarriage decreases significantly once a heartbeat has been detected.

The vast majority of miscarriages cannot be prevented. Early losses often occur without a detectable embryo. Between 50 and 70 percent of first-trimester miscarriages and about 30 percent of second-trimester miscarriages are caused by chromosomal anomalies in either the sperm or the egg. Other conditions that can result in miscarriage include infection; abnormalities of the uterus or cervix; smoking; substance abuse; exposure to environmental or industrial toxins; and chronic diseases, including diabetes, kidney disease, and autoimmune processes. In rare cases, women miscarry after certain tests during pregnancy, such as chorionic villus sampling (CVS) or amniocentesis.

Many women learn about an impend-

---

* The medical term for miscarriage is spontaneous abortion. If your provider uses this term, he or she does not mean that you chose to terminate the pregnancy.
† The actual number is likely significantly higher because many miscarriages occur very early on, before a woman knows she is pregnant, and may simply seem to be a heavy period on or near schedule.

ing miscarriage at a routine prenatal visit, before experiencing any physical symptoms of loss. Some women first notice that early signs of pregnancy—nausea, fatigue, breast tenderness—have diminished or gone away. The first symptoms that a miscarriage has begun are usually spotting or bleeding, followed by cramps in the lower back or abdomen.

Roughly two to three out of ten pregnant women experience some vaginal bleeding or spotting during the first trimester of pregnancy, and only half of those women will miscarry.[2] Bleeding in the second trimester is more likely to be a sign of miscarriage. If you have any vaginal bleeding during pregnancy, your health care provider can help determine if the bleeding is likely to result in miscarriage or if it has another cause that does not threaten the pregnancy.

If a blood test or sonogram indicates that you are going to lose the pregnancy, you and your care provider will need to decide whether to allow the miscarriage to occur and complete itself naturally or to schedule a procedure to discontinue the pregnancy.

There are several different ways to end the pregnancy. Medical treatment, which can be used only early in the pregnancy (generally before ten weeks), involves taking a drug, such as misoprostol, that causes uterine contractions and expulsion. In early pregnancy loss, this works more than 80 percent of the time, but failure rates are higher after about ten weeks.[3] Surgical procedures include what is commonly referred to as a D&C (dilation and curettage), D&E (dilation and evacuation—used when the pregnancy is further along), or MVA (manual vacuum aspiration). These are all suction (aspiration) techniques that remove the pregnancy tissue, and they can be performed on an outpatient basis in a clinic, obstetrical office, hospital, or emergency room.

If you miscarry naturally or take medication, you will probably not be in a health care facility when the miscarriage begins. The process may be over in a day, or it may take several days. It is best to work with your doctor or midwife, since there is a risk that the bleeding will be heavy enough to necessitate an emergency procedure to complete the miscarriage. The fetus, amniotic sac, and placenta, along with a large amount of blood, will be expelled.

If you are less than eight weeks pregnant when the miscarriage occurs, the expelled tissue may look no different from heavy menstrual bleeding. If you have reached eight to ten weeks, more tissue will be expelled and miscarrying can be more painful. In this instance, if you have chosen to allow the miscarriage to occur spontaneously, try to arrange for a trusted, knowledgeable person to be with you through the process—and throughout the night, if needed. If you were planning on having a doula for your birth, consider arranging to have one help you through this. Think about where you will be most comfortable, and have supplies such as bed liners, sanitary pads, and hot water bottles or a heating pad on hand. You may want to ask your provider to prescribe pain medication in case you need it.

I was much better prepared for my second home miscarriage. My doctor had provided me with good pain medicine, and I was better prepared for dealing with all the blood. I had also been

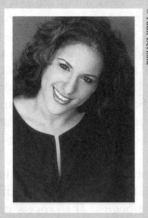

© Fadil Berisha

"I EXPECTED TO HEAR THE BABY'S HEARTBEAT."

CATHERINE MCKINLEY

It took me eight months to conceive. Then suddenly I was having my encounter with the magical: a routine eight-week sonogram where I expected to hear the baby's heartbeat for the first time. My ob-gyn tried to mask his concern as he moved the wand across my quiet belly. He was strangely nonchalant as he told me that the office equipment was not always able to get sensitive readings early in pregnancy. He wrote out a referral for a hospital sonogram, and I tried to brush off my anxiety.

The radiologist performing the sonogram was very pregnant. I laughed at her crankiness because she was so stunning, with a stomach so large her belly button was pointing toward the floor. But then her body almost seemed to be mocking me as she told me that she was unable to find a heartbeat. "You've miscarried," she said emotionlessly. It was difficult to process what she was saying. There had been no sign of blood; my body had not pushed out anything.

For weeks I'd felt this blooming feeling. But the night before, I had noticed that my skin had a funny new smell and I was suddenly feeling achy all over. Now I felt my body turning in on itself, betraying itself. I was admitted to the hospital for a D&C the next afternoon. That wait and the days after were some of the hardest moments of my journey to motherhood.

The loss roused old griefs: the eight months of wild fear that conception was impossible; the legacy of an illegal abortion, registered as a D&C while I was a college exchange student in Jamaica; birth family lost through adoption; and later the family I recovered whose inabilities rendered them as good as lost to me. An older friend who had had five children and twice as many pregnancies told me to embrace the heartache; I was being seasoned for motherhood. "You won't always get it easy," she said, "But the difficulty is what gives you the desire and the heart to mother better."

I got pregnant two months later and held my breath until the end of my first trimester. I was healthy and enjoying my pregnancy, but there was that lingering grief. I have come to like the idea of being seasoned. All of the trials have inscribed a kind of passion and will in my mothering.

There will be some blood clots, and you may notice tissue that is firmer or lumpy-looking, which is placental, or afterbirth, tissue. You may or may not see tissue that looks like an embryo or fetus.

Once everything in your uterus has been expelled, bleeding will continue, lessening over several days. If bleeding increases or stays bright red, or if you have foul-smelling discharge or a fever, contact your health care provider. If fetal tissue remains in your uterus, your provider can perform a D&C or a D&E to remove it, so as to prevent infection. These procedures involve dilating the cervix and using suction and/or a medical instrument to remove remaining fetal and placental tissue.

Once bleeding has ceased and the cervix is closed, you can have sexual penetration without risk of infection. Since it is difficult to know when the cervix has completely closed, most providers recommend waiting two weeks. A repeat blood pregnancy test after a few weeks is important to make sure your hormone levels are normal. If you feel dizzy or tired, ask to be checked for ane-

informed about how to tell if the amount of bleeding was dangerous. But I was alone, and it was a horrible thing to go through on my own. I really wish I'd had sense enough to make sure I had a friend with me to hold my hand or rub my back or bring me tea during those horrible hours.

mia. If you do not know your blood type, get a blood test within a few days of miscarrying. If your blood type is Rh-negative, you may need a shot of Rh immune globulin within seventy-two hours of the miscarriage, as if you were carrying an Rh-positive fetus, there is a small chance that you were exposed to Rh-positive blood cells from the fetal tissue during the miscarriage. The shot prevents your body from producing antibodies to Rh-positive blood that could harm a fetus during a future pregnancy.

Physical recovery from a miscarriage ranges from a few days to a couple of weeks. Your period will likely return within four to six weeks. Emotional recovery often takes longer. Give yourself time to grieve, search for medical explanations if there are any, and seek out other women who have miscarried. Remember that most miscarriages are single episodes and do not mean that you will have another.

ECTOPIC PREGNANCY

In an ectopic pregnancy, the fertilized egg implants outside the uterus, usually in the fallopian tube, where it cannot develop normally. This can be a life-threatening condition requiring immediate treatment. Ectopic pregnancies occur in about one in fifty to one in one hundred pregnancies.[4] The rate of ectopic pregnancy has increased over the past several decades, most likely because women are conceiving at older ages and more women are using advanced reproductive technologies—both risk factors for ectopic pregnancy. Most ectopic pregnancies are caused by an infection or inflammation of the fallopian tube, scar tissue or adhesions from previous tubal or pelvic-area surgeries, or a tubal abnormality. If you have had a previous ectopic pregnancy, pelvic surgery, or pelvic inflammatory disease, or if you conceived using assisted reproductive techniques, your risk of having an ectopic pregnancy is higher.

RECURRENT PREGNANCY LOSS

A minority of women experience multiple miscarriages or later losses and are unable to carry a pregnancy to term. Pregnancy loss is considered recurrent when a woman has had more than two losses. Between 50 and 75 percent of recurrent loss remains unexplained. However, for known causes, some treatments may be available. For more information, see "Patients' Fact Sheet: Recurrent Pregnancy Loss," at the American Society for Reproductive Medicine's website, asrm.org, and "Recurrent Early Pregnancy Loss" at emedicine.medscape.com/article/260495-overview.

If you have had multiple losses, support is crucial.

Friends encouraged me to call their friends who had been through similar situations. This helped me tremendously. I loved talking to the woman in Oregon who had had four miscarriages before they discovered she had a blood-clotting disorder, or the woman in Boston who had three miscarriages and now had two small boys. These women became my friends.

If you have an ectopic pregnancy, you will have a positive pregnancy test and may feel all the usual signs of early pregnancy. Vaginal bleeding, dizziness, weakness, and gastrointestinal discomfort are common early symptoms. As the pregnancy progresses, the pressure in the tube or abdomen may cause stabbing pains, cramps, pain in your shoulder, or a dull ache that may vary in intensity and come and go. It is critical to contact your provider if you have vaginal bleeding and/or sharp pain in the pelvic area, abdomen and/or neck and shoulders. If an ectopic pregnancy is not diagnosed early, the fallopian tube can rupture, causing severe blood loss and shock.

If you have any of the symptoms of ectopic pregnancy, your health care provider should check your hormone levels every two to three days and do a vaginal ultrasound as early as possible (at about six weeks). Ectopic pregnancy is occasionally misdiagnosed as an early miscarriage. This is why your provider may ask you to get a blood pregnancy test after a suspected miscarriage. The test can help confirm the presence or absence of residual fetal tissue.

If an ectopic pregnancy is found early, physicians can give you the drug methotrexate, which dissolves the embryonic tissue. If your pregnancy is more advanced, you may need a laparoscopy, which requires small incisions in your abdomen to insert a fiber-optic light (laparoscope) and other instruments to view the pelvic area and to remove the embryonic tissue. Doctors will try to save the fallopian tube if it is possible to do so. In some cases, laparoscopy is unsuccessful or unsafe (if, for example, the fallopian tube has ruptured), and then the surgical procedure is a laparotomy, which involves a larger incision and does not involve fiber-optic light. With either a laparoscopy or a laparotomy, the whole tube can be removed if necessary. Blood tests will be performed to check changes in your levels of hCG (human chorionic gonadotropin, the hormone produced by placental tissue) after any of these treatments in order to confirm that no ectopic tissue remains.

The loss of an ectopic pregnancy may bring on feelings like those that follow miscarriage, as well as fear that such a pregnancy could happen again. If you have had internal bleeding or a traumatic emergency surgery, seek additional support and talk with your provider about how this may affect future conception and pregnancies and how to minimize future risks.

MOLAR PREGNANCY

Molar pregnancies (also called gestational trophoblastic disease and hydatidiform mole) happen when the cells that are supposed to develop into the placenta instead develop into a tumor made of trophoblastic (placental) cells. The growth must be removed so that it does not spread. The chances of a molar pregnancy are very small—about 1 in every 1,000 to 1,200 pregnancies.[5] A partial molar pregnancy means there is some fetal development along with an abnormal placenta. In a complete molar pregnancy, there is no fetal development, just an abnormal placenta.

Signs and symptoms, usually identified through routine pregnancy visits, include first-trimester vaginal bleeding, high blood pressure, and a uterus that is too large for the gestational age. Molar pregnancies are treated by a D&C to remove the abnormal tissue and, in rare cases, by chemotherapy to treat any remaining abnormal cells. Close follow-up after a D&C is very important to ensure that no more abnormal tissue remains. A molar pregnancy does not affect your chances of having a subsequent normal pregnancy. But, like any other pregnancy loss, it is likely to bring grief, fears, and questions. In addition, after a molar pregnancy, you should avoid getting pregnant again for a period of time (up to a year), because the best way to know whether all the abnormal tissue is gone is to measure hCG, and a new pregnancy will make that test useless.

The news of the trophoblastic tissue put me into high gear. Keep busy. Or sleep. Can't stop to think, can't stop to cry. I feel driven. I need to stop and mourn, but how can I feel it necessary to mourn when there wasn't even anybody in there!?

MULTIPLE-GESTATION PREGNANCY LOSS

Pregnancy loss is more likely in multiple-gestation pregnancies—those with two or more embryos or fetuses. There has been a dramatic increase in the number of multiple-gestation pregnancies because more women are conceiving after age thirty and because more women are using infertility treatments, both of which increase the chance of having a multiple-gestation pregnancy.

Because of the level of early testing in standard prenatal care, women sometimes learn about a multiple-gestation pregnancy only to later discover that one fetus, or more than one, has died. If this occurs in early pregnancy, it is sometimes called vanishing twin syndrome and may be associated with some vaginal spotting during the first months.[6] It can be hard to know how to acknowledge and mourn such a loss.

Early on in my first pregnancy, I found out I was pregnant with twins. The news was overwhelming and scary but also exciting. Then one twin stopped developing. I had no signs or symptoms of miscarriage, and eventually the fetus was reabsorbed by my body. Most people don't know what to say when you tell them you've lost a baby. Several people said, "Well, you were only trying for one." That was not at all helpful to hear. I was worried about the health and viability of the "healthy" twin and about what had gone wrong in my body. I was thrilled and relieved when I gave birth to my son six months later, but I think sometimes about my son's twin and about the anxiety of that pregnancy. It's taken me a long time to acknowledge how that loss affected me.

Multiple-gestation pregnancies, particularly those with more than two fetuses, are far riskier than single pregnancies for both mothers and babies. In some situations, women must decide whether to selectively terminate one or more of the fetuses to increase the chances of the remaining fetus or fetuses surviving.

LOSS AFTER PRENATAL DIAGNOSIS OF ABNORMALITIES OR IMPAIRMENTS

Some of us choose to end a pregnancy after discovering that we are carrying a fetus with severe impairments or a fatal abnormality. Loss from terminating a pregnancy is different from other pregnancy losses because it arises out of our own decision, but it can be just as painful and difficult.

Religions, cultures, communities, and individuals vary widely in their beliefs about the ethics of ending a pregnancy in these circumstances. Those of us who experience this kind of loss may not speak openly about it for fear of being judged. Support from other women with similar experiences can help many of us come to terms with our decision. Honoring the loss, even when it stems from our own choice, and acknowledging the validity of grief can also help the healing process.

There wasn't one moment when it became clear that we were going to terminate the pregnancy. It was just something that slowly, and very painfully, came to feel like the right thing to both of us. . . . I was deeply upset by the loss of the baby and felt like the only way to get back on my feet was to get pregnant again. I got pregnant again about four months later and gave birth to my second daughter. Sometimes when I see my children, I have this vision of the boy we didn't have being with them. He is really present in our lives in these unexpected ways, and I imagine he will stay there for a long time.

STILLBIRTH

Stillbirth, a loss after twenty weeks' gestation, is much less common than miscarriage; in the United States, it occurs in about 1 out of 160 pregnancies.[7] This figure varies with a woman's age, with women under 15 and over 40 having the highest rates. Race is also a factor. African-American women face a significantly higher chance of stillbirth than Hispanic or non-Hispanic white women, with stillbirth occurring in about 1 out of 89 pregnancies.[8] (For more information, see "Disparities in Loss," p. 471.)

Stillbirths are generally divided into early loss (between twenty and twenty-eight weeks) and late stillbirth (twenty-eight weeks or greater). The most common causes of early loss are congenital anomalies, placental problems leading to bleeding and fetal growth restriction, and preterm infection in a fetus too young to survive. Stillbirths after twenty-eight weeks often involve apparently healthy fetuses but may also be due, as with earlier stillbirths, to placental problems such as poor fetal growth or premature separation of the placenta.

Some factors that put women at increased risk of stillbirth include being over age forty or under age fifteen, having a multiple-gestation pregnancy, obesity, smoking, and using drugs. In addition, babies with chromosomal anomalies and nonchromosomal structural impairments are also at higher risk of stillbirth.

Most fetal deaths are detected before labor begins, usually at a routine prenatal check or when a woman notices an absence of the usual kicks and movement. An ultrasound will confirm that the baby has died. If a stillbirth is detected, you will need to make some decisions about how to proceed. If there is no medical need for immediate delivery, you can either wait for labor to come naturally or have labor induced. If possible, take time to prepare yourself for the experience and to gather your support network.

Emilio III was stillborn at almost twenty-four weeks. I was going to go through labor knowing that I wouldn't have a new life in my life. It was the worst eight hours of my life. The labor was painful both physically and emotionally. In the end we delivered a beautiful baby boy. At the nurses' urging, we agreed to see and hold him. We got to hold him for a long time. We have pictures of him and share them with our daughter, who was born a little over a year later. She talks about her big little brother all the time, which reminds us that he is a part of our family.

After the birth, you will need to decide whether you want to see and hold your baby. You may want to name the baby if you haven't already done so, take photos or have a professional photographer do so, and take some time to say your good-byes. It may seem at first that seeing or holding the baby will be too much to handle, but many women later feel grateful to have done so. Such acts help to acknowledge the infant's existence and to preserve her or his memory. Some hospitals now offer a memory box to bereaved parents; it can include footprints and handprints, along with any items that were in contact with the baby, such as a blanket. If you will be staying in a hospital for more than a few hours after childbirth, you should consider whether you would prefer to be in a hospital ward that is not filled with pregnant women or new mothers.

You will be faced with a number of difficult and pressing decisions, including how you wish the baby's remains to be handled and whether you want to have an autopsy performed. In some cases, autopsy can provide important information about the cause of the stillbirth, provide information for future pregnancies, and help researchers figure out how to prevent stillbirths in the future. Unfortunately, even after a thor-

FINDING INFORMATION AND SUPPORT

- **Share Pregnancy & Infant Loss Support** (nationalshare.org) aims to provide support for those whose lives are affected by the death of a baby. This encompasses emotional, physical, spiritual, and social healing, as well as sustaining the family unit. Includes helpful suggestions for friends and family members on how to support a parent whose baby has died.
- **Wisconsin Stillbirth Service Program** (www2.marshfieldclinic.org/wissp) works to increase general awareness and knowledge about stillbirth, including its causes, frequency, and the parental needs following such an experience, and provides access to links, resources, and medically sound information.
- **International Stillbirth Alliance** (stillbirthalliance.org) is a nonprofit coalition of organizations dedicated to understanding the causes and prevention of stillbirth and to enhancing bereavement care of families who experience stillbirth.

ough evaluation, in more than half of stillbirths a cause cannot be determined.[10]

If you choose to have an autopsy done, the person performing it should be a pediatric or neonatal pathologist or be working with one. If the person is not, you may want to ask for a referral to a pathologist with the necessary expertise to review the findings. It can take up to six weeks to schedule and get the results from an autopsy. If you do not want an autopsy done, ask whether X-ray or CT scanning of the baby can be performed as an alternate way of getting information.

For women who experience stillbirth, an additional pain can come when our breasts fill with milk for a baby who will not be drinking it. Talk to your health care provider about ways to cope with your milk. Some women choose to pump and donate the milk to other women who need it, through breast milk banks and organizations. For more information, see the website of the Human Milk Banking Association of North America (hmbana.org).

EARLY INFANT DEATH

When a baby dies during the first twenty-eight days of life, it is called neonatal death. Some babies die during or shortly after childbirth, due to impairments that may or may not have been previously detected, to something that goes wrong during labor, or to unknown causes.

The shock of a death that comes so quickly after birth is hard to bear. It is devastating to meet a baby only to lose him or her so soon.

Depending on cultural norms, newborn babies who die can be given the same rites and ceremonies as other people who die, though arranging funeral services for a tiny baby can feel very cruel. Ask for others to step in to help with arrangements, meals, care for older siblings, and whatever else you need to get you through this time.

COPING WITH LOSS

Losing a pregnancy or a baby evokes many emotions. You may feel buffeted and torn by confusion, relief, shame, anger, sorrow, fear, powerlessness, or despair. You may need to withdraw at first, or feel numb about a reality that seems too much to bear. Some of your friends and family may not be able to handle the loss. Others may offer platitudes such as "You'll

DISPARITIES IN LOSS

Those of us who are African American are far more likely to experience loss during pregnancy, birth, and early infancy than women in other racial/ethnic groups. Ectopic pregnancies are more common, and non-Hispanic black women are nearly twice as likely to have a stillbirth.[11]

Black women are also nearly two and a half times as likely to experience an infant death.[12] One of the chief contributing factors to infant mortality is low birth weight associated with preterm birth (less than thirty-seven weeks); babies who weigh less than three pounds, four ounces are about 100 times more likely to die in the first year of life than babies of normal birth weight. Black women are two to three times as likely to give birth to infants that are low birth weight.[13]

The reasons for these disparities are not fully understood. Many factors—including poverty, education, and access to quality care, as well as stress, infection, biological differences, and environmental exposures—likely play a role. More research is needed to fully understand and address these significant racial disparities. For more information, see "Disparities in Women's Health," p. 761.

have another baby" that can fail to comfort you or to acknowledge the importance of your baby's existence.

Most people didn't know how to give me support, and perhaps I didn't really know how to ask for it. People were more comfortable talking about the physical, and not the emotional, side of miscarriage. I needed to talk about both. It was also difficult for my husband, because people could at least ask how my body was doing. Unfortunately, he would sometimes be completely bypassed when someone called to talk with us, despite the fact that he, too, was in deep emotional pain.

A tremendous void and a sense of loneliness often follow a loss. If you have a partner, your feelings may differ from his or hers in strength or content. Grief may be mixed with guilt; both can cause tension between you. You may blame yourselves and wonder if either of you did something "wrong" (too much activity, too much sex, not enough good food, etc.), but this is rarely the case.

I had so many people to celebrate with when the test was positive, but now that I was unpregnant I was more alone than ever. I felt like a little baby's soul had rejected me. That maybe I was just too lame for the soul to cling to or maybe I wasn't enough of a parent for it to thrive. Maybe my anxiety had killed it. Maybe it was the lack of red meat in my diet. Maybe . . . well, it could have been anything.

In addition to these emotional responses, your body will be going through changes. It is important to have a follow-up visit with your provider not only for physical reasons but as an opportunity to ask questions. Request the first appointment of the day or one before the day officially starts, so that you don't have to face a room full of pregnant women. Ask a support person to go with you if you think that might be helpful. Bring your questions with you in writing, and take notes—or ask your support person to do the note taking so you can focus on the conversation.

The depth of grief is not simply related to the duration of the pregnancy or the age of the infant; unexplained loss can be especially hard to accept, and healing from the loss can be a long process. You may feel a strong resurgence of grief on the date when your baby would have been born or when you see children the same age as your child would have been.

Our society has few formal ways of dealing with loss. Some of us find solace in creative expression—sewing a memorial quilt, creating artwork, or writing. Creating a ceremony or ritual helps us recognize the significance of the loss and honor the memory of the one who died. Some women mark the anniversary of important days in the lost baby's life—such as the date of conception or of her or his birthday—to acknowledge the baby's existence and place in the family.

This summer we will be planting a tree in front of our house in memory of Kyle. Summers will forever bring mixed emotions for us, July especially. Growing up in Brazil, summers were such a highlight of our lives. I like to think that there is a reason why we lost Kyle in the summer. Perhaps slowly we will be able to hold his memory as one of those forever-treasured childhood memories of joyful and innocent summers. With time, we are better able to embrace the full cycles of life even when it feels unnaturally "wrong" that some life cycles are not as long as we expect.

Some of us heal by working to improve the way that women who experience loss are treated by hospitals and providers, or by creating resources on pregnancy or infant loss. As a result of such efforts, many hospitals now have bereavement teams and pregnancy-and-infant-loss support groups. There are also a number of support organizations and books on loss—most formed or written by women with personal experience of it—that offer guidance on grieving as well as on coping during future pregnancies (see "Recommended Resources"). You may be the beneficiary of such work; or, if you experience loss, you may also feel moved to use your sorrow, anger, and determination to help others.

Trying to get pregnant again as soon as possible helps many of us to cope. Others may decide not to try again. There is no right decision; there is only a decision that feels right for you.

SUBSEQUENT PREGNANCY

Many women who have experienced a pregnancy or infant loss find that future pregnancies are emotionally challenging. Despite achieving a long-desired pregnancy, you may find that grief for your previous losses and anxiety about whether this pregnancy will be healthy dominate your experience. You may embrace the use of technologies such as home pregnancy tests, home Dopplers, and ultrasounds that may help you feel more connected to the pregnancy, or you may choose to forgo technologies that did nothing to protect your last pregnancy. Being pregnant again can raise all sorts of feelings: detachment, worry, guilt, hope. Be gentle with yourself, and give yourself permission to cope in ways that work for you. If the pregnancy results in a baby to bring home, there will be plenty of time for love.

Depending on your experience, you may want to remain with your health care provider or find a new one. Either way, talk with your provider about her or his policy for dealing with pregnancy loss and monitoring a woman who has had a prior loss. If the provider brushes off your questions or does not respond compassionately to your concerns, consider finding a new provider.

You are likely to feel most anxious around the time in the pregnancy when the previous loss occurred. It may help to remind people around you as you approach that point, so that they are prepared to support you or give you the space you need—and to celebrate with you when you pass that point, while recognizing that fears remain. And you may experience a resurgence of grief around the time of childbirth. If possible, talk with women who have had the same experience to learn how they managed their feelings and found the courage and optimism to try again. Pregnancy-after-loss support groups and therapists knowledgeable about pregnancy loss can be especially helpful. For more information, see "Pregnancy After Infertility or Previous Pregnancy Loss," at the Our Bodies Ourselves website, ourbodiesourselves.org.

It was six months after the second miscarriage before we felt ready to try again. We became pregnant easily. Understandably, we were terrified. We tried to face every test with guarded optimism. Pregnancy test, hormone levels, first sonogram, heartbeat, nuchal translucency, amniocentesis. By the time we made it through the twenty-week sonogram, I believed we were actually going to have a baby. I never complained about any of the discomforts of pregnancy. I didn't want to jinx it. I loved being pregnant, loved giving birth. . . . I felt and still feel such gratitude for our two sons. Because the path to motherhood was more bumpy than I imagined, it feels especially miraculous, especially precious.

CHAPTER 19 ■ ■ ■ ■ ■ ■ ■ ■ ■ ■ ■ ■ ■ ■ ■ ■ ■

When we started trying to become pregnant four months before our wedding, we expected that I would be pregnant on our wedding day. I was in my prime childbearing years. After nine months, I saw my family doctor, sure there must be something wrong with me. Sometimes it can take twelve months, she said. . . . [But] the twelve month mark came and went.

Many of us grow up dreaming about the day when we will have children. The forces that contribute to these desires are complex, powerful, spiritual, and sometimes unexplainable. Our longing for children is a deep primal need, and being unable to conceive or carry a pregnancy to term can be devastating.

Infertility can rock our very foundation—our sense of control over our futures, our faith in our bodies, and our feelings about ourselves as women.

I've been infertile since I was twenty-two and had a hysterectomy. . . . It feels like a pretty cruel fate. I've always been enthralled with what women's bodies can do. I know there are other options for having families and that at some point I will choose one of them, but it doesn't make my situation of being infertile much easier.

It can be a source of frustration, as we find ourselves on the wrong side of the statistics.

I always believed that I would have children without any problems—as many as I wished and when I decided it was the right time. Unfortunately, after four years of trial and error, tests, and operations, my husband and I are realizing that life does not always happen the way we plan it.

Societal pressures intensify the pain of infertility. In many religions and cultures, our worth and power as women are measured by our ability to procreate. Some of us are viewed as irresponsible for having "too many" children, while others are pitied or perceived as not being truly fulfilled if we choose not to or are unable to bear a child.

Infertility treatments have allowed millions of people around the world to build the families they so deeply desire. Yet, as with other medical treatments, they have limitations. Glossy media images of fifty-year-old celebrities who just gave birth to twins can lead us to believe that infertility treatments are universally successful and accessible; unfortunately, this isn't true. The success rates of infertility treatments vary greatly, depending on the kind of procedure used, the skill and expertise of the treatment clinic, and the health and age of the woman treated. Infer-

tility treatments also include risks, are physically and emotionally demanding and are expensive.

This chapter offers information on the causes of and treatments for infertility, as well as guidance and support for women navigating the world of infertility.

WHAT IS INFERTILITY?

Infertility is medically defined as the inability to become pregnant after twelve months of regular sexual intercourse without birth control or, for women over age 35, six months. Infertility also refers to women who are unable to carry a pregnancy to term. The Centers for Disease Control and Prevention (CDC) estimates that at least

SOCIAL INFERTILITY

While there is no standard definition for "social infertility," the term is used to describe postmenopausal women, singles, and same-sex couples who turn to fertility treatments and/or adoption for family building.

Before you begin any kind of fertility testing or treatment, it's important to be sure you are timing intercourse or inseminations properly. Charting your menstrual cycle and observing your body's fertility signals can tell you if and when you are ovulating and help you maximize your chances of conceiving. (To learn more, see "Charting Your Menstrual Cycles," p. 26.)

THE PREVALENCE OF INFERTILITY

Though it may seem that infertility is on the rise, infertility rates have remained fairly consistent over time. Societal and behavioral shifts in the last quarter of the twentieth century have certainly allowed us to become increasingly aware of and concerned about infertility. This is largely due to women steadily postponing the age at which they give birth to their first child and because new technologies make it possible for many to overcome infertility

It's unclear whether infertility disproportionately affects certain populations. Even though research does not show large disparities in infertility across different groups, social and racial disparities in health status and in the prevalence of certain risk factors (e.g., sexually transmitted infections) suggest that many preventable causes of infertility disproportionately affect the less privileged. Financial barriers also limit access to appropriate diagnosis, evaluation, and treatment and may lead to underestimating the frequency of infertility in the same population groups. On the other hand, delaying childbearing may be more common among professionals and other higher-income groups, making those groups more vulnerable to the effect of aging on fertility.

one in ten U.S. women age fifteen to forty-four has difficulty getting pregnant or staying pregnant.[1]

WHAT CAUSES INFERTILITY?

For pregnancy to occur, many complex processes and factors need to line up. A woman must produce a healthy egg; a man must produce healthy sperm. Favorable cervical fluid needs to be present so that sperm travel from the vagina to meet the egg while it's still in the fallopian tube. Timing of intercourse or insemination is critical, since an egg generally lives only twenty-four hours. Once the sperm and egg join, this single cell divides to become an embryo, which must implant properly in the uterine lining before it can grow.

Couples can experience infertility when there is a problem with any one or more of these delicate phases of conception. The CDC estimates that about one-third of infertility cases are associated only with female factors and another one third of problems are associated only with male factors. The remaining cases are caused either by a mixture of male and female problems or by unknown causes.[2]

WHY A WOMAN MAY EXPERIENCE INFERTILITY

I am 39 years old; finally, my life is settled enough to start having a family . . . the doctor did a blood test and told me even though I had regular menstrual periods, my ovarian function was poor, I was premenopausal, and my chances of getting pregnant and not miscarrying were low.

Age is the most important factor affecting a women's fertility. Long before menopause, our bodies' reproductive capabilities slow down. This natural decline of fertility happens in all women, though it happens at different ages for individual women. Though women can experience other causes of infertility at any age, infertility among older women is often the result of normal age-related changes occurring in the reproductive hormones that make a woman's ovaries less able to release eggs, decrease the number of healthy eggs she has left, and increase her risk of miscarriage. (For more information, see "Aging and Fertility," p. 351.)

Overall, one of the most common causes of female infertility is linked to problems with ovulation, the physiological process by which eggs mature. An important sign that a woman is not ovulating normally is irregular or absent menstrual periods. However, a woman can be having regular periods and still have problems with ovulation. One cause of ovulation problems is polycystic ovarian syndrome (PCOS), a metabolic disorder affecting nearly 10 percent of all women, that can interfere with hormone production and ovulation. (For more information, see p. 647.) Premature ovarian insufficiency (POI) is also linked to ovulation problems and occurs when a woman's ovaries stop functioning fully before the age of forty. POI, which affects about 1 percent of all women, is not the same as early menopause. (For more information, see p. 524.) Ovulation problems may also be due to thyroid disorders, adrenal gland disorders, benign pituitary tumors, excessive exercise, diabetes, weight loss, obesity, or medications such as for cancer treatments.

Another common cause of infertility is blocked fallopian tubes or other structural problems. This can be due to endometriosis, pelvic inflammatory disease (PID), or scarring due to surgery or repeated injury. Some women are born with structural abnormalities affecting their reproductive organs that may also prevent the egg from traveling down the fallopian tube, inhibit the growing embryo from implanting in the uterus, or increase the risk of an ectopic pregnancy. Uterine fibroids, which are noncancerous growths in the uterus, are also associated with obstructions in the uterus and/or fallopian tubes as well as repeated miscarriages.

Other possible causes of infertility include immune system problems, issues with the cervical fluid, and luteal phase defects.

WHY A MAN MAY EXPERIENCE INFERTILITY

Sometimes a man is born with a condition that causes male infertility and other times problems emerge later in life due to illness or injury. More than 90 percent of male infertility is due to sperm abnormalities affecting sperm count, sperm motility (movement), or sperm morphology (shape). Some causes of male infertility include:

- Varicocele, which occurs when the enlarged veins on a man's testicle(s) cause temperature increases that can affect the number or shape of the sperm.
- Retrograde ejaculation, which occurs when the muscles of the bladder wall do not function properly and sperm are forced backward into the bladder instead of forward out the urethra. This can be caused by surgery, spinal cord injury, certain medications, or aging.
- Structural abnormalities that damage or block testes, the ducts that carry the mature sperm, or other reproductive structures.
- Underdeveloped, undescended, or injured testes.

UNEXPLAINED INFERTILITY

Sometimes, even after extensive testing, physicians are unable to find any medical reason for the infertility. You seem to be ovulating normally, your fallopian tubes are open and healthy, your partner has a high sperm count with good motility, and neither of you has any other underlying health issues. This type of diagnosis provides hope to some—maybe, if there is no known problem, pregnancy will happen after all—while it leaves others extremely frustrated—if we don't even know what's causing the problem, how can we address it?

THE EMOTIONAL SIDE OF INFERTILITY

Infertility affects us not only physically but also emotionally. When faced with infertility, many of us react with shock, anger, and denial.

I am incredibly pissed, after being fantastically shocked, that the second blood test shows there is no longer a pregnancy. There is anger at my body, at God, at my own intuition. . . . I hang up on my sisters and mom when they call me to console. I am inconsolable. It feels [like] the grief and anger will consume me.

It's normal to have a wide range of emotions about infertility. You may feel something you or your partner did in the past caused your present inability to conceive or to stay pregnant. One or both of you may feel guilty and responsible for your childless state. Could drug or alcohol use, masturbation, past abortions (even though properly performed), or unusual sex practices be "responsible"? Though these do *not* cause infertility, it's easy to place the blame on anything we can think of, because we want explanations for the unexpected and inexplicable. Try to have compassion for yourself. Infertility is not your fault.

Many of us find it difficult to spend time with our friends' or relatives' children. Child-centered holidays may become stressful, lonely, and depressing times as we wonder, "Why them

SECONDARY INFERTILITY

Secondary infertility occurs when a woman who has previously been pregnant is unable to conceive again. Many of the same causes mentioned above may be a factor with secondary infertility; however, the most common issues are usually related to age, tubal damage, male factors, or a combination of factors.

MEN AND INFERTILITY

Because of the very nature of infertility, women experience the bulk of the responsibility for treatments, regardless of whether the infertility is caused by male or female factors. Women usually begin the process of seeking out a diagnosis or treatment, while our male partners follow along, sometimes in denial of their need to seek care or be involved. It is easy for men to feel that infertility is a threat to their virility or manhood, and there's very little social support or information geared toward men struggling with infertility.

Yet male infertility can occasionally indicate a underlying medical condition in need of treatment, such as heart disease or cancer. A thorough examination of your partner by a urologist trained in male infertility is an important step in the evaluation of any infertility problem and a good investment in his health.

MAXIMIZING YOUR FERTILITY

Certain factors can affect fertility in both women and men. Some of these factors can be modified, while others are not under our individual control.

- **Alcohol, tobacco, and other drugs.** Drinking, smoking, or using drugs while trying to conceive can delay conception and increase miscarriage. The good news is that these risks begin to reverse immediately upon quitting.
- **Weight.** Women at a healthy weight are more likely to be fertile. Being excessively over- or underweight can disrupt ovulation and lead to hormonal imbalances for both women and men. If you are overweight, losing even 5 percent of your body weight is sometimes enough to improve fertility.
- **Sleep and relaxation.** Try to get plenty of sleep and do what you can to reduce stress. While there is no scientific evidence that stress *causes* infertility, reducing stress may help you feel better able to cope.
- **Your environment.** Exposure to radiation, metals such as lead, chemicals such as pesticides, and other toxins can lead to reduced fertility or infertility. When possible, avoid exposures to known or suspected toxins. (For detailed information, see Chapter 25, "Environmental and Occupational Health.")
- **Your overall health.** Illnesses such as diabetes, kidney disease, autoimmune diseases, high blood pressure, and genetic disorders can contribute to infertility. Previous sexually transmitted infections and other infections can impair fertility for both men and women. Before you begin infertility treatment, review any medications you are on with your provider. Over-the-counter and prescription drugs, including antibiotics, painkillers, antidepressants, steroids, and hormonal treatments can all impact fertility.
- **Healthy sperm.** Activities and practices that cause the testicles to overheat can damage sperm. Because of this, men—particularly those with a marginal sperm count—may want to avoid hot tubs and hot baths, minimize long bike rides or horseback riding, and keep electronics (cell phones, computers, etc.) away from their laps.

Although taking good care of yourself is important, self-care usually cannot address the root cause of infertility. Infertility is often beyond our personal control.

and not me?" It's common to feel envious and jealous of others' fertile state.

[During that time] two more friends announced their pregnancies, and one friend who had become pregnant five months after we started trying gave birth. I was shocked at how much they affected me. I stayed in bed and cried all day after the second one. I felt like a terrible friend, full of envy.

In addition to the stress of going for tests and treatments, you may be subject to other pressures at home and at work. Friends and family

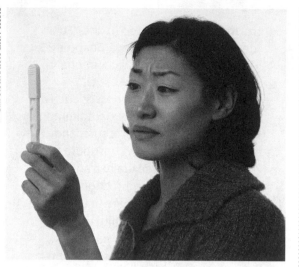

© Can Stock Photo Inc. / Iofoto

may ask you, "Well, has it happened yet?" Perhaps worse is when they don't say anything but look at you and sigh a lot. People you hardly know may provide unwelcome comment.

I have found it quite hard dealing not only with our infertility problem but also with the reactions of people around me. I'm sick of people telling me to "relax," "stop thinking it out," "adopt and you'll get pregnant," and all the other wonderful clichés, although said to be comforting, ring of insensitivity.

With the myriad of feelings surrounding infertility, good coping skills are essential. Here are some tips to help manage and lower the stress of infertility.

- Acknowledge your feelings.
- Don't blame yourself.
- Work as a team with your partner.
- Communicate openly with your clinic and health care providers.
- Seek support through friends, family, and professionals if needed.

- Educate yourself about your infertility diagnosis and treatment.
- Don't let infertility take over your life.

INFORMING YOURSELF AND FINDING SUPPORT

No one should face infertility alone. Other women and couples who have already been diagnosed or treated can supplement the information you receive from your physician with firsthand knowledge and provide you with additional resources that may help buoy your spirits during treatments.

Our clinic, and other friends going through fertility treatments, advised us to keep the process to ourselves. Seven years later, my wife and I looked at each other and realized that the pain we endured could have been greatly reduced if we had shared our experience with others rather than keeping it bottled up inside of us. Once people learned what we were going through, they threw their arms around, and they all said, 'Oh, I wish I had known. I would have gone out of my way to support you.' "

Joining a weekly or monthly infertility support group made up of others going through similar experiences may also be helpful to you and, if you have one, your partner. For a list of support groups in your area, visit resolve.org. You might also want to talk to women who decided not to pursue infertility treatments or chose to stop after a certain number of tries, or women or couples who made the decision to adopt or remain childless. Be on the lookout for knowledgeable and compassionate support that will help you make decisions that will serve *you* best in the long run.

You may also want to work with a professional counselor who can provide ongoing support. There are many well-trained clinical social workers or psychologists with expertise in the unique psychological, emotional, and ethical issues related to infertility. They can also offer strategies for coping and provide guidance as you decide whether and how to continue treatment. Some fertility clinics provide counseling at the clinic; you can also find knowledgeable independent counselors.

ONLINE ADVICE AND SUPPORT

Infertility websites offer all kinds of information about the causes, diagnoses, and various treatments for infertility. Online support groups and infertility blogs are tremendously popular and can help you stay connected with others going through similar experiences.

Because anyone can post just about anything on the Internet, it's important to be a critical consumer. Be wary of sites that are strictly commercial, such those sponsored by specific infertility clinics or drug companies, as they may downplay the risks of treatments, exaggerate success rates, or exploit in other ways your deep desire to bear a child. For more information, see "Health Information Online," p. 661.

SEEKING APPROPRIATE FERTILITY CARE

Finding a physician who specializes in infertility can be challenging. Though there are more than four hundred fertility clinics in the United States, your options will largely depend upon where you live; whether you have health care insurance and, if so, what it covers; and your financial resources.

For most women, seeing a family practitioner or gynecologist is the first step. These primary care physicians can perform the initial testing and perhaps even start you off with some basic treatments.

If these first measures are not successful, ask for a referral to an infertility specialist or a reproductive endocrinologist (RE). REs are ob-gyns who have several years of additional training in treating infertility and are board-certified in reproductive medicine and infertility. The Society for Reproductive Endocrinology and Infertility (SREI) (socrei.org), the Society for Assisted Reproductive Technology (SART) (sart.org), and the American Society for Reproductive Medicine (ASRM) (asrm.org) websites all list members who are infertility specialists.

WORKING WITH YOUR HEALTH CARE TEAM

It's crucial to have a good relationship with your fertility care team from the start. Your providers should describe any tests and procedures, and their risks and costs, clearly and patiently so that you understand what to expect. Choose a doctor with whom you feel comfortable as well as one who will take the time to listen to your hopes and fears, answer your questions, be sensitive to your specific feelings and needs, and respect your decisions. Most important, make sure whoever you decide to work with on your infertility journey has good quality control and strong ethics. For a list of questions to ask your fertility clinic or specialist, go to the American Fertility Association website (theafa.org) and search "Important Questions for Your Doctor."

DECIDING WHAT'S RIGHT FOR YOU

Most of us never expect to be faced with infertility. Decisions about infertility treatments are complex; there are no easy answers. Do you want to try only hormone therapies and minor surgeries, or are you willing and economically able to try more invasive procedures, such as IVF, donor eggs, or surrogacy? How long do you want and can you afford to undergo treatments? If they aren't succeeding as you had hoped, how will you and your partner, if you have one, decide whether to continue or stop? These are questions to keep in mind as you go through the infertility process.

THE INFERTILITY WORKUP

An infertility workup tests all the links in the chain of events from ovulation to an established pregnancy. Because many tests are conducted separately and scheduled at specific times in your cycle, the workup can take several months to complete. These tests can be invasive, painful, and emotionally exhausting as well as expensive, since medical insurance coverage is limited, even for initial diagnosis. Many insurance companies do not cover infertility treatments or offer only limited benefits. As of 2010, only fifteen states mandated some degree of health care insurance coverage for infertility.[3]

Although the sequence of diagnostic tests may vary with different doctors or clinics, the infertility workup will include some or all of the following.

A general and medical history of you and your male partner, if you have one. This should include a review of your menstrual history as well as details about any previous pregnancies, episodes of sexually transmitted infections, and abortions; your family history related to infertility, DES exposure, menstrual irregularities, or early menopause; your use of birth control; whether you have been exposed to any toxins that may have affected your repro-

ductive system; and behavioral factors, such as stress, nutrition, smoking, drinking, and use of drugs, both prescribed and recreational.

Semen analysis. Because the semen analysis is probably the simplest and least invasive of the tests and male factors account for about a third of all infertility, this is usually the first test recommended. The man will be asked to ejaculate into a clean container, and the specimen will be examined under a microscope to assess sperm count, shape, and motility.

A thorough gynecologic examination. Your uterus, ovaries, breasts, and general pelvic area will be checked. This will include a transvaginal ultrasound in which a slender probe is inserted into your vagina to look at your reproductive organs.

Monitoring ovulation. A thorough clinician will make sure you understand your menstrual cycle and will help you track your ovulation, usually by taking your temperature every morning, monitoring your cervical fluid, or using a urine test kit that can detect the hormone surge occurring right before ovulation. (For more information, see "Fertility Awareness Method," p. 26.)

Hormonal profile. This involves blood tests to check the levels of all hormones related to your menstrual cycle, ovulation, and fertility, including follicle-stimulating hormone (FSH) and luteinizing hormone (LH), as well as testosterone, dihydroepiandrostone sulfate (DHEAS), prolactin, estrogen, and progesterone levels.

Ovarian reserve testing. The term ovarian reserve refers to the number and quality of eggs in the ovaries. It can be measured in two ways: by checking blood levels of the hormones anti-Mullerian hormone (AMH), inhibin B, follicle-stimulating hormone (FSH), and estradiol; and by conducting an antral follicle count using ultrasound scans to observe the number and size of the growing follicles that contain the eggs. How best to interpret ovarian reserve tests is controversial, since clinical experience with these tests is still evolving. Even so, most infertility patients should be periodically evaluated for the possibility of impaired ovarian reserve before pursuing any advanced fertility treatment.

Hysterosalpingogram (HSG). An HSG is almost always needed during the initial fertility-testing phase. This test can show any impairments in the uterus, cervix, and fallopian tubes by injecting a radio-opaque dye into the vagina and uterus while a series of X-rays is taken. Such problems may dictate the type of fertility treatment needed. If a woman delays this test, it could result in wasted time, energy, and money if she learns she had a structural problem that was missed. Though an HSG is not an infertility treatment, women have a slightly increased chance of conceiving in the cycles immediately following this test, perhaps because the dye "cleans out" any minor blockages in the fallopian tube.

Hysteroscopy. During a hysteroscopy, a lighted viewing instrument is inserted through the vagina and cervix and into the uterus, typically under general anesthesia. This is done to examine the lining of the uterus, help collect a biopsy sample if needed, and guide surgery to remove growths in the uterus.

Laparoscopy. Laparoscopy allows a practitioner to view the tubes, the ovaries, the exterior of the uterus, and the surrounding tissue of the pelvic cavity. It is the only test that can confirm endometriosis. Performed under spinal or general anesthesia, usually on an outpatient basis, laparoscopy involves making a tiny incision near your navel (belly button). Carbon dioxide gas is used to inflate the abdomen and allow the practitioner to view the pelvic organs. Sometimes a dye is flushed through the fallopian tubes to see whether they are open. If endometriosis, polyps, or scar tissue is found, it can be removed during the procedure as well.

TREATING INFERTILITY

Once you have pinpointed the most likely cause of your infertility, you can work with your practitioner to decide the right treatment path for you. Infertility treatments don't always involve expensive high-tech methods such as IVF. In fact, the vast majority of infertility cases are treated though less expensive, lower-tech treatments. Since not all treatments work for everyone and it's impossible to predict exactly what will work for you, treating infertility is as much an art as a science. Carefully consider the pros and cons of all your options.

DRUGS

A variety of drugs is used to correct hormonal imbalances, induce ovulation, suppress ovulation, and prepare the uterus. They can consist of natural hormones or synthetic drugs designed to mimic or block the action of natural hormones. Some are taken orally, while others require injections. Depending on your diagnosis and clinic experience, there are many fertility drug protocols involving several different types of medications, dosages, and schedules. Some of the most commonly prescribed infertility drugs are:

Clomid. Clomiphene citrate (brand names Clomid or Serophene) is usually the first choice for treating infertility because it's relatively cheap and effective and has been around for more than forty years. Clomid is a pill given to women who are not ovulating normally. Approximately 60 to 80 percent of women taking Clomid will ovulate, and about half will become pregnant, with most pregnancies occurring in the first three months. Like all fertility drugs, Clomid can increase your chances of multiple births, although it's less likely than with some injectable fertility drugs.

Femara. Femara, also known by its generic name letrozole, was not originally meant to be a fertility drug. Instead, it is commonly used to treat postmenopausal women with breast cancer. Many clinicians have concluded that Femara is as effective as Clomid when inducing ovulation. However, this medication is used less frequently because studies have shown a risk of birth impairments if taken while a woman is actually pregnant. To eliminate any potential problems, clinicians who prescribe Femara for ovulation induction need to ensure that it's used only before conception and not during an actual pregnancy.

Follicle-stimulating hormone (FSH) (Follistim, Fertinex, Bravelle, Gonal-F, Metrodin). These injectable hormones mimic FSH and promote ovulation. They can be created in a lab using recombinant DNA technology or extracted and purified from the urine of postmenopausal women.

Human menopausal gonadotropin (hMG) (Pergonal, Repronex, Humegon, Menopur). These injectable drugs combine both ovulation hormones FSH and LH to increase egg production.

Gonadotropin-releasing hormone (GnRH) agonist (Lupron, Zoladex, Synarel). These injectable drugs work to prevent ovulation from occurring naturally, allowing doctors to control ovulation via other drugs. Sometimes GnRH agonists are also used to affect the growth of the uterine lining.

One of the drugs, Lupron, is commonly used but has never been approved by the FDA for this particular purpose. Many women have reported serious problems with the drug. More information about its potential harms is available at Lupron Victim's Hub (lupronvictimshub.com).

Gonadotropin-releasing hormone (GnRH) antagonist (Antagon, Cetrotide). These injectable drugs work quickly against the hormones LH and FSH, suppressing ovulation to prevent the eggs from being prematurely released before they can be retrieved.

Human chorionic gonadotropin (hCG) (Pregnyl, Novarel, Ovidrel, Profasi). These injectable drugs are generally used along with other fertility drugs to mimic LH and trigger the ovaries to release the mature egg or eggs.

Progesterone. If a pregnancy occurs after infertility, some clinicians recommend progesterone supplementation. Progesterone can be taken orally, by injection, or as a vaginal suppository or gel for as long as ten to twelve weeks to help maintain the pregnancy until the placenta is fully functional.

Most of these medications, especially the injectables, can be very expensive, costing thousands of dollars. The cost is often not covered by insurance. Because all fertility medications contain hormones, a variety of side effects can occur, such as hot flashes, cramping, bloating, discomfort, nausea, breast discomfort, headache, uterine bleeding, and mood changes.

As with all medications, fertility drugs come

with risks. The most common risk is the risk of multiple pregnancies. Carrying twins, triplets, or high-order multiples presents risks to both mothers and babies. To minimize the chance of multiples, careful monitoring of ovulation is critical. Your doctor should always keep track of how you are responding to the medications and take the necessary precautions to limit having too many eggs fertilize.

Another potential complication of fertility drugs is ovarian hyperstimulation syndrome (OHSS). OHSS happens when the ovaries, after being stimulated, become large and produce too much fluid. Women with mild OHSS may experience abdominal distension, nausea, diarrhea, and some weight gain. With moderate OHSS, women can have substantial weight gain and abdominal distension because of the enlargement of the ovaries and liquid accumulating in the abdominal cavity. In addition, vomiting and diarrhea can cause symptoms of dehydration, including decreased urine volume, thirst, and skin dryness. Severe OHSS may also lead to accumulation of liquid in and around the lungs, shortness of breath, and in extreme cases lead to acute respiratory distress syndrome. Moderate to severe OHSS occurs in about 1 percent of all ovarian stimulations. In most cases, the administration of hormones is stopped and the cycle canceled to help your body recover. Infertility treatment can often be resumed later on, changing the stimulation protocol.

Before taking any medication, discuss costs, possible side effects and health risks with your clinician and do your own research. If you take the medication, let your provider know if you have an adverse reaction.

The long-term safety of many of these drugs has not been adequately studied, although some good large studies are now under way. Some epidemiologic studies have suggested an increased risk of ovarian and uterine cancer among women treated for many cycles with some infertility drugs. It is not known whether the excess cancer risk is due to the drugs or to the underlying infertility. The International Agency for Research on Cancer has stated that there is inadequate evidence from animal or human studies to tell whether Clomid is carcinogenic, but it has not reevaluated the evidence in more than ten years. More research is needed to fully understand the possible long-term risks of these medications.

SURGERY

Surgical techniques can sometimes correct structural problems of the cervix, uterus, and tubes. Microsurgery may repair tubes and remove adhesions. Balloon-catheter techniques have also been successful in outpatient settings to open blocked fallopian tubes. Laser surgery using the carbon dioxide or argon laser, often in combination with microsurgery, may remove scar tissue or endometrial adhesions. However, if there is significant tubal damage, in vitro fertilization (IVF) may provide a higher chance of a successful pregnancy than surgical repair of the fallopian tubes.

INTRAUTERINE INSEMINATION (IUI)

IUI, or intrauterine insemination, is a relatively simple infertility treatment in which a very thin flexible catheter is used to place specially washed and prepared sperm directly into the uterus. IUI may be used in some cases of male-factor infertility, such as low sperm count, or if a sperm donor is being used. IUI may also be used if the woman's cervical mucus is not ideal. In cases of unexplained infertility, IUI may also be tried, especially before moving on to more advanced treatments. Sometimes doctors recommend that prior to IUI, women take drugs that are known to stimulate egg production. (These drugs require monitoring to prevent multiple births.) Success rates with IUI vary greatly but are typically between 4 percent and 20 percent. IUI generally costs about $1,000 per attempt. It is increasingly common (and some health care insurance plans require it) for women to try several cycles of ovarian hyperstimulation (via medication) combined with IUI before attempting IVF. These treatments are expensive, given the cost of the drugs, but less expensive than a cycle of IVF.

ASSISTED REPRODUCTIVE TECHNOLOGIES

Assisted reproductive technologies (ARTs) are procedures used to treat infertility in which both eggs and sperm are manipulated outside the body. ART procedures involve surgically removing eggs from a woman's ovaries, combining them with sperm in the laboratory, then returning the fertilized eggs or embryos to the woman's body or donating them to another woman.

The best-known ART is in vitro fertilization, also called IVF. In 1978, Britain's Louise Brown was the first baby born as the result of IVF. (The British physiologist Robert Edwards, who invented and carried out the procedure, was awarded the Nobel Prize in Physiology or Medicine in 2010.) Today approximately 1 percent of all children in the United States are born each year via ARTs such as IVF, egg donation, and surrogacy.[4]

FERTILITY PRESERVATION AND EGG FREEZING

Unfortunately, many treatments for cancer can cause infertility. In an effort to preserve their ability to have children in the future, an increasing number of people are using techniques such as egg or sperm freezing before beginning cancer treatments. Research regarding how cancer affects reproductive health (also called oncofertility) and fertility preservation options are growing, sparked largely by the increase in the survival rates of cancer patients. For more detailed information about cancer and fertility preservation, see fertilehope.org.

One method for fertility preservation that has expanded beyond cancer patients is egg freezing. Some fertility clinics are promoting this option to all women interested in extending their fertility. The goal is to freeze your unfertilized eggs when you are in your twenties or thirties to use later in life when you are ready to build your family. However, this is still considered experimental as well as controversial. The American Society for Reproductive Medicine feels that there are not yet sufficient data to recommend the freezing of eggs for the sole purpose of circumventing reproductive aging in healthy women. The medications used to stimulate egg production carry health risks, and the high cost of egg freezing—about $13,000 per cycle—puts it out of reach for many women. In addition, the high water content of eggs means that egg freezing is far more difficult and unpredictable than freezing sperm or embryos, and success rates are not yet clear. Some people fear that fertility clinics that promote expensive egg-freezing services are selling women false hope.

IN VITRO FERTILIZATION (IVF)

IVF is a multistep treatment process. Several weeks prior to the actual procedure, you will take hormonal contraception to suppress your own ovarian function. Following that you will receive one or a combination of fertility drugs, often by injection, to stimulate the production of eggs. During this time, you will have to make several visits to the clinic, where providers will carefully monitor the number and size of the eggs in each ovary.

Once the eggs are ready, the actual IVF procedure consists of two major steps: egg retrieval and embryo transfer. During the egg retrieval, you will be sedated while the mature eggs are surgically removed from your ovaries. This typically takes place at your local fertility clinic. Follicles from both your left and right ovaries are retrieved through a process called follicular aspiration. Follicular aspiration involves inserting a hollow needle through the cervix and into the ovaries. The needle is then used to suction out any follicles that may be present in the ovaries. In order to guide the needle into the appropriate area of the ovary, a transvaginal ultrasound will be used. Once the needle is in the proper position, any follicles inside the ovary will be aspirated out. The follicle aspirates will be immediately examined under a microscope to ensure the presence of viable eggs. This is different from the typical menstrual cycle, in which the ovaries process many eggs but only one mature egg is released into the tubes and can be fertilized.

After the egg retrieval process you may feel a little tender in your abdomen. You will also feel fatigued as a result of the anesthetic. After several hours of monitoring, you will be allowed to go home. You may notice some light vaginal spotting. You will also receive antibiotics to prevent infection.

After the retrieval process, your eggs will be joined with sperm from your partner or a donor in the lab. If the eggs are fertilized, they will be allowed to divide for three to five days, then placed back into your—or a gestational carrier's—uterus. This is called the embryo transfer. The embryo transfer catheter is loaded with the embryos and passed through the cervical opening up the middle of the uterus. An abdominal ultrasound is used simultaneously to view the catheter tip and ensure its proper placement. When the catheter tip reaches the ideal location, the embryos are released out of the catheter to the lining of the uterus. Again, this is different from the natural conception process, when typically the sperm meets only one egg in the tubes and after fertilization the one embryo falls into the uterus and implants in the uterine lining to establish a singleton pregnancy. Exceptions occur, and in about 2 percent of all natural pregnancies more than than one embryo grows in the uterus. However, because the norm is to transfer more than one embryo, in IVF more than 30 percent of the pregnancies are multiple.

For most women, the embryo transfer procedure feels similar to a Pap test and does not require any sedation or other drugs. You will likely feel no or minimal pain or discomfort.

About nine to eleven days after the transfer, a blood pregnancy test can be done. If one or more embryos have successfully implanted into the uterus, hCG hormone will be detectable.

If there are more viable embryos than are transferred, families may choose to freeze (cryopreserve) the extra embryos for future use. In addition to saving thousands of dollars in costs, this decision protects women from having to repeat stressful and potentially risky drug therapies to stimulate ovulation again. With recent technological advances, IVF cycles using frozen embryos have the same chance of success as those using fresh embryos.

The success rates of IVF vary greatly, based

on many factors, including the quality of the implanted embryos, the skill of the clinic, and, most important, a woman's age. On average, a woman younger than 35 who is using her own eggs and fresh embryos has about a 40 percent chance per cycle of getting pregnant and giving birth to a live baby. Women between the ages of 35 and 37 have about a 30 percent chance, women 38 to 40 about a 22 percent chance, and women 41 to 42 about a 12 percent chance.[5]

In general, IVF costs about $10,000 to $15,000 per cycle. Insurance coverage for ART is patchy. Many employers, in an effort to contain costs, don't purchase such benefits for their employees. Some states have laws mandating that employers offer infertility treatment benefits. Medicaid does not cover ART, not even in states where by law employers must offer the benefits. To learn more about benefits you might be eligible for, check with your health care insurance plan. The infertility association Resolve keeps track of the states that mandate coverage of infertility treatment and describes the various laws. To find out more, see resolve.org/family -building-options/.

INTRACYTOPLASMIC SPERM INJECTION (ICSI)

Intracytoplasmic sperm injection is a technique that involves injecting sperm directly into the middle of the egg. ICSI was originally developed for couples in which the male partner either has sperm that are unable to fertilize an egg or has very few sperm in his semen (as may happen after cancer treatment). In the most severe cases—when no sperm can be found in the man's semen—the sperm can be surgically removed from the epididymis (the duct that houses immature sperm); the mature sperm are then injected into a woman's removed egg.

In most cases, about 50 to 80 percent of eggs injected using ICSI become fertilized, but the procedure itself might damage some eggs or the egg might not grow into an embryo even after it is injected with sperm. ICSI usually costs about $2,000 on top of the price for IVF. There are some concerns about the risks to babies conceived via ICSI, with some research suggesting that they have a higher-than-expected rate of birth impairments, including, in boys, infertility. Since ICSI is frequently used with men who have the poorest sperm quality, it is possible that genetic factors may play a role. Further research is needed to fully understand the risks.

ICSI increases the success rates of ART when male-factor infertility is present. However, national ART data do *not* show that using ICSI increases success rates when male-factor infertility is not present. Because there is no clear standard of care, clinics vary widely in their use of ICSI. Despite there being no clear evidence that it leads to better outcomes in the absence of male-factor infertility, more than 50 percent of IVF procedures in the United States are performed with ICSI.

PREIMPLANTATION GENETIC DIAGNOSIS

Preimplantation genetic diagnosis (PGD) begins with the creation of an embryo using IVF. At its earliest state of development, one or two cells are removed from each embryo—similar to a biopsy—and are examined for genetic differences before the embryo is placed in the uterus to develop. PGD was originally developed for families with a history of genetic impairments, including Tay-Sachs disease, Down syndrome, cystic fibrosis, sickle-cell disease, spinal muscular dystrophy, Huntington's disease, Marfan syndrome, hemophilia, and fragile X syndrome. PGD is most often recommended when either parent is a known carrier or may be at risk of a genetic disability.

Some people are concerned that PGD is

SINGLE-EMBRYO TRANSFERS

When reproductive medicine was in its infancy, many fertility clinics transferred multiple embryos during each cycle, attempting to increase the rate of pregnancy. This technique resulted in many twin, triple, and even higher-order multiple births. Unfortunately, multiple births—including twin births—greatly increase the chances that a woman and her children will have poor health outcomes.

The most common problems in the short term are that multiples are often preterm and the babies often have a low birth weight. Preemies are more likely to need intensive care and longer stays at the hospital and are at higher risk of dying shortly after birth. Birth impairments are also more common among multiples, although they affect a minority of the infants. The longer-term consequences of preterm delivery and low birth weight include developmental disabilities such as cerebral palsy (CP). Whereas the rate of CP is about 2 percent among singletons, some studies have found that the rate is about five times as high among twins and about twenty times as high among high-order multiples. These risks are not limited to multiple births: babies that are born singletons but were part of a multiple pregnancy have some of them as well. Multiple pregnancies also carry a higher risk of health complications for the mother during pregnancy and birth.

And there are effects on the health of the family as well: studies show that divorce is much more common among couples that have had multiples than among couples who have had singletons.

Finally, there are consequences for society at large, because the costs of the medical care for multiple pregnancies and infants born in multiple births are huge compared to the costs associated with caring for singletons.

Because of these risks, many experts in the field now encourage the strategy of transferring only one embryo at a time. A 2010 meta-analysis of clinical trials comparing the outcomes of double embryo transfers with the outcomes of a sequence of one single-embryo transfer followed by a thawed embryo transfer if the first cycle has not succeeded found single-embryo transfer more likely to lead to the birth of a single, healthy baby.[6] Though the first strategy—double-embryo transfer—leads to pregnancy faster, it is associated with multiple births and the related adverse health outcomes. The second strategy—single-embryo transfer—may require more attempts but almost invariably yields singleton births and better health outcomes for both mother and baby. The chance of a woman giving birth to a single full-term baby (over thirty-seven weeks) following single-embryo transfer is almost five times greater than her chance of doing so following double-embryo transfer.

The main barrier to elective single-embryo transfers is cost. Many families are unable to pay for multiple IVF cycles, so they opt to have multiple embryos transferred in a single cycle. The first insurance company to address this problem, Aetna, recently marketed a benefit that offers a free "rescue" IVF cycle to women who choose elective single-embryo transfer if the first cycle fails.

CLINIC STATISTICS AND SUCCESS RATES

Success rates for ART vary greatly, as many factors affect them, including the kind of procedure performed, the health and age of the individuals involved, and the skill and experience of the clinic. The Centers for Disease Control and Prevention (cdc.gov/art) and the Society for Assisted Reproductive Technology (sart .com) gather and publish yearly statistics on the success rates of various procedures. Though all IVF clinics are required by law to report their data to the CDC each year and about 85 to 90 percent do so, the only penalty for clinics that don't is that the CDC publishes their names as "nonreporters."

The CDC warns against using just the report to rank clinics, because despite the standard format, differences in success rates are tricky to interpret. Still, the numbers give you a place to start and contain some important information that can help you evaluate fertility clinics. It is important to ask several questions as you view infertility statistics:

• How is "success" defined? Success can be defined many different ways—by the number of embryo transfers, the number of pregnancies, or of births. What you are interested in is the live birth rate (preferably single births) among women of your age and diagnosis using the same treatment you are undergoing.

• Are there parameters excluding certain women from the clinic? Some clinics may refuse to take on particular women, such as women above a certain age or women who are unlikely to conceive, in the hope of bumping up their statistics. Pay careful attention to the ages, diagnoses, and other characteristics of the patients the clinic routinely treats. Select one that has had good success with patients like you.

• What is the average number of embryos transferred per IVF cycle? What is the singleton live-birth rate? Responsible ART programs try to maximize their pregnancy rates while minimizing the multiple-pregnancy rate. Needing to transfer too many embryos may indicate suboptimal laboratory conditions or a less refined embryo transfer technique.

• Does the clinic offer elective single-embryo transfer (e-SET)? What is its live-birth rates after e-SET?

• What are the frozen embryo pregnancy and birth rates? In order to maximize the number of pregnancies that can be achieved from a single egg retrieval (and lessen your need to take additional fertility medications), it's important to assess your clinic's experience with frozen embryos. Increased pregnancy rates from frozen embryo transfers are also an indirect indication of a high-quality laboratory and transfer procedures.

• Numbers count! If a clinic performs only a few ART cycles every year, all of its measures of success will be statistically imprecise, and a high (or low) success rate may be that way because of chance rather than skill. Choose a clinic that has a high success rate based on large numbers of cycles.

For more information about IVF clinic statistics, see the CDC's video "Infertility: A Tutorial on the ART Report" (cdc.gov/art/PreparingForART/) or read its fact sheet at cdc.gov/art/PreparingForART/Tutorial.htm.

being or will be used not only to detect serious medical problems but also to detect a whole array of undesirable attributes or to select for gender or certain physical characteristics or the ability to perform well in sports or music. The American Society for Reproductive Medicine (ASRM) uses different terms for the procedure depending on how the procedure is used. The term PGD is used only when the procedure is performed on embryos from men and women who are known to carry a serious hereditary condition. ASRM uses the term "preimplantation genetic screening" (PGS) to describe the same process when it is done to search for mutations or other traits. ASRM recommends the use of PGD but says that the evidence is insufficient to know if PGS is useful and does not recommend it.

Many people worry that PGD and PGS may fuel eugenic tendencies and make it harder to preserve a society in which people with disabilities will be fully valued for who they are.

The procedure does not appear to have any effect on overall pregnancy rates for IVF. It generally costs an additional $5,000.

COLLABORATIVE (THIRD-PARTY) REPRODUCTION

One thing I find runs through my head (completely unbidden) is that I am a bad feminist for lamenting the fact that I can't have biological kids; that I know well enough that there are many nontraditional ways to have families that are not lesser than biological families (I have a three-year-old brother adopted from the foster care

system, so I have firsthand knowledge of this) and that I need to get over this. But having that option removed feels like a violation of my body by my body, if that makes any sense. Feeling this, feeling like a bad feminist—these are uncomfortable places to dwell in.

The phrase collaborative or third-party reproduction refers to the process when another person provides sperm, eggs, or embryos or when another woman provides her uterus so that a family can have a child. The donor's or surrogate's involvement is limited to the reproductive process and does not extend to raising the child. Collaborative reproduction is complicated and involves a number of important considerations to ensure a safe and successful experience.

Donor Sperm

Insemination with donor sperm involves using the sperm of a man who is not your partner to conceive. Families interested in donor sperm can use a known donor (a friend or relative) or find an anonymous donor through a sperm bank.

Sperm from sperm banks have been tested for numerous infections and genetic diseases. Usually you can find out basic information on potential anonymous donors, including their physical characteristics, ethnic and/or racial background, educational level, and career. You may also be able to read a personal profile on the donor and see a photo.

Success rates vary based on your age, past pregnancy history, and infertility diagnosis (if

Group: Women's Health Initiative in Bulgaria

Country: Bulgaria

Resource: Нашемо мяло Ние самиме (Our Body, Ourselves), a Bulgarian edition of *Our Bodies, Ourselves*

Website: ourbodiesourselves.org/programs/network/foreign/

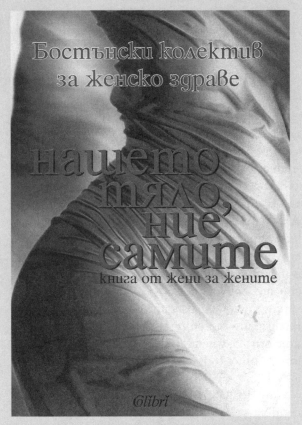

The cover of the Bulgarian adaptation of *Our Bodies, Ourselves.*

In Bulgaria, it's considered a woman's duty to bear children, and assisted reproductive technologies are widely used by infertile couples. With eighteen clinics in the country and more on the way, women spend years saving money for the treatment and navigating the health care system to learn more about different treatments, risks, and outcomes.

As the demand for these services increases, Women's Health Initiative in Bulgaria (WHIBG), an OBOS partner that published an adaptation of *Our Bodies, Ourselves* in 2001, reports that women's health care activists have successfully advocated for better regulation of treatment procedures and government subsidies for women unable to afford care. In 2009, almost one-quarter of the 6,000 couples who underwent in vitro procedures received monetary assistance from the Bulgarian government.

In addition to being concerned about safety and access, WHIBG is researching the context in which women decide to seek assisted treatment. The organiza-

tion notes that the majority of Bulgarian women feel that assisted reproductive technologies embody hope and empowerment, despite the emotional and physical risks they might face. As a result of these attitudes, WHIBG makes policy recommendations to decrease the stigmatization of childlessness and to ensure that women can access the resources they need to exercise their full range of reproductive options.

WHIBG is also drawing attention to how a deregulated health care system, combined with a socially biased view of motherhood, leads to problems with care and has underscored the importance of providing emotional support to women

undergoing treatments. Due to WHIBG's work, several clinics have been encouraged to include psychologists on their infertility treatment teams.

you have one). Costs associated with sperm donation vary greatly from a few hundred to several thousand dollars, depending on the process you plan to utilize, which fertility clinic you are being treated at, and whether you use a known or anonymous donor. Because no one keeps track of sperm donation, it is not known how many children have been born through donor sperm over the years.

Donor Eggs

Conceiving a baby via egg donation is becoming increasingly common, with more than ten thousand women and families using donor eggs each year. Egg donation allows the possibility of becoming pregnant through the use of another woman's eggs. It is most often used by women who experience primary ovarian insufficiency, age-related infertility, poor egg quality, unexplained infertility, or disorders that may be transmitted genetically. Once a donor's eggs have been retrieved and fertilized by your partner's or donor's sperm, any resulting embryos will be placed either in your uterus or in the uterus of a gestational carrier.

Because the eggs of healthy young women are used, success rates are usually over 60 percent for most clinics. Babies born through this expensive procedure—often totaling between $30,000 and $40,000—are not genetically related to the woman who bears them. Coming to terms with this modern phenomenon can be difficult, as it means accepting that you will likely never conceive your own biological child.

You and your partner, if you have one, the fertility clinic, and/or an independent egg donor agency may work together to locate a potential donor. Sometimes a relative or friend will offer to donate her eggs. In some lesbian relationships, one partner may donate the egg and the other serve as the birth mother, enabling both women to have a biological connection to the child. In most cases, however, egg donors are unknown to the recipient family.

Regardless of how you find your egg donor, it's important she be properly screened, both physically and emotionally. An egg donor should be between the ages of 21 and 30, healthy, and fertile. She will also need to have a thorough psychological screening to identify any emotional problems, evaluate her motivations for donating, and verify that she understands the physical, psychological, and legal risks. It's imperative that you consult an attorney who specializes in egg donation to ensure that all involved are protected.

I felt like an eggless sociopath for even considering asking one of these young women if I might purchase their eggs. How and why do they decide to sell their eggs to someone like me? How do the donor agencies and these young women determine that their eggs are worth $8,000 while someone else's eggs are worth only $5,000?

Egg donors are paid a fee typically ranging anywhere between $5,000 and $10,000. There are also many ads advertising compensation

WORKING WITH A DONOR OR SURROGACY AGENCY

The donor and surrogacy industry in the United States is a more than $38 million a year industry that is growing by 6 to 8 percent each year.[7] Currently, there are few guidelines or monitoring for sperm donors, egg donors, or surrogacy agencies. Anyone, regardless of background or credentials, can recruit potential donors or surrogates and charge a fee to match them with intended parents.

As a result, there is great variability in these types of agencies, what they offer, and how much they charge. Agencies range from Internet-only sites to brick-and-mortar offices run by lawyers, health care professionals, well-intentioned former infertility patients, or previous donors or surrogates.

If you are choosing to pursue egg donation, it's important that you carefully evaluate any agency you are considering working with. Ask about its experience and credentials. Request references and talk with former donors, surrogates, and intended parents. Understand the agency's donor or surrogate recruitment, selection, and payment policies, as well as all costs that you will be responsible for. The agency should have strong relationships with local fertility clinics, mental health professionals, and attorneys specializing in reproductive law and be well respected within the field.

Compare several agencies so you can recognize any differences or red flags. Above all else, agencies offering third-party reproduction services should be open, honest, and ethical, committed to protecting the interests of donors, surrogates, and intended families.

above $20,000 and even a few approaching $100,000 for young women with very specific desirable characteristics, such as proven fertility, certain physical characteristics or ethnic backgrounds, attendance at prestigious colleges, or high SAT scores. The egg donor fee is intended to compensate the donor for all costs associated with the time and energy needed for donating her eggs, including undergoing medical and psychological screenings, taking drugs to hyperstimulate her egg production, and undergoing a sedated surgical procedure to retrieve the eggs. Almost all egg donor programs encourage anonymous egg donation, although it's possible for you to meet the egg donor in some cases.

Because these procedures carry some health risks, and because the long-term risks of egg donation have not been adequately studied, egg donation raises ethical concerns. Some people believe that while it is acceptable for a woman who desperately wants to become pregnant to accept the health risks involved, it is exploitive to encourage women who receive only money and not a potential baby to donate eggs, especially when there is not sufficient information available to make an informed choice.

Surrogates and Gestational Carriers

A surrogate is a woman who is willing to be impregnated using IVF and carry a baby for the intended parents to help them build their family. Surrogacy is most often considered a family-building option among women who have lost their uterus, were born with a uterine anomaly

EMBRYO DONATION

Some couples that become pregnant through ART treatments may end up with additional frozen embryos. Many couples opt to freeze the remaining embryos, particularly if they hope to have additional children, but some decide to donate the embryos to other families who have not been successful conceiving. The donated embryos are then transferred into a woman's uterus using frozen embryo transfer.

Embryo donation is also chosen by many families who are unable to afford IVF or egg donation. Embryo donation is available at some fertility clinics and is typically less expensive than other types of ARTs. The embryo donor receives no payment for the embryo; however, you must pay the clinic or agency for stor-ing the embryo, testing the embryo, and transferring the embryo into your uterus. These procedures cost about $3,000 to $5,000 per transfer. Only a few hundred children have been born via embryo donation so far, and the success rates are not yet known.

If you choose to use donor embryos or to donate your embryos to another family, you will need to investigate the legal implications involved. You should consult an attorney specializing in fertility as well as a mental health professional knowledgeable about the complex facets of birthing a child with no genetic tie to either parent. For an up-to-date and helpful legal reference book, see *Legal Conceptions: The Evolving Law and Policy of Assisted Reproductive Technologies* by Susan Crockin and Howard Jones.

that would make carrying a child exceedingly difficult, or are unable to carry a pregnancy to term for other health reasons.

There are two types of surrogacy: traditional and gestational. Traditional surrogacy is when a woman offers to use her own eggs *and* carry the child as well for the intended parents, thus maintaining a genetic connection. A gestational surrogacy is when an egg (from a donor or the intended mother) is fertilized outside the body and then implanted into the gestational surrogate, who has no genetic connection to the child. In both cases, a woman goes through a pregnancy and bears a baby destined for another person or couple.

A surrogacy pregnancy can easily cost over $100,000, including agency fees, escrow fees, attorney fees, insurance, medical bills, medical and psychological testing, clinic fees, cycle medications, travel, missed work, surrogacy compensation, and any miscellaneous expenses. Depending on the state, once the baby is born the contracting parent(s) must legally adopt the child, making appropriate legal counsel imperative. A surrogate is typically compensated between $25,000 and $35,000 for her time, inconvenience to her own life, and all expenses associated with pregnancy and childbirth. Some surrogates develop lifelong relationships with the families they are helping, even exchanging periodic updates and pictures of the family they helped build.

Surrogacy is a highly complex ART procedure, both legally and ethically. Since 1976, there have been about 25,000 surrogate births in the United States. This includes several high-profile

TELLING THE CHILDREN

A growing number of women and couples struggling with infertility are choosing to use donor sperm or donor eggs to conceive a child. These technologies have allowed millions of people the opportunity to have a family. They also raise complex questions about the role and importance of genetic ties and the rights of children conceived with donor gametes.

In the past, parents were advised to keep using a donor a secret, perhaps thinking this would protect the couple from embarrassment. Today, the results of surveys of thousands of offspring conceived via sperm donation show that such secrecy can cause great distress.

An increasing number of people are recognizing that children conceived using donor sperm or donor eggs—like children who are adopted—deserve to know their origins and genetic histories. Organizations such as the Donor Sibling Registry (donorsiblingregistry.com) and the Infertility Network (infertilitynetwork.org) offer excellent books, newsletters, video documentaries, support groups, and seminars (live and on DVD) to help families deal with the issue of disclosure.

cases where surrogates changed their minds about surrendering the baby once the child was born. Heart-wrenching public discourse took place in dramatic courtroom settings where the most controversial aspects of ART were debated, sometimes for months or years. In response, Washington, D.C., and Arizona have banned surrogacy altogether, and Michigan, New York, Indiana, Kentucky, and Nebraska have declared surrogacy contracts void and unenforceable.[8]

THINKING ABOUT INFERTILITY

INTIMACY AND INFERTILITY

We were supposed to make love at seven o'clock in the morning, and then I had to run to my doctor's for the postcoital test. Who feels like making love at seven in the morning during a busy week anyway?

During the months or years of testing and treatments, you will have to plan your sex life around your menstrual cycle and fertile days. Documenting when you have sex and having sex at prescribed times may make you feel as if nothing is private or sacred in your life anymore.

Many couples find that spontaneity in lovemaking decreases. Men may experience performance anxiety and be unable to get an erection. Women may feel physically violated, due in part to the increased amount of prodding and probing experienced in the exam room.

Though many couples find their relationship grows stronger during infertility treatment, even the strongest of couples may experience pain and confusion. No matter how difficult it is, try to find a way to stay intimate. Concentrate on pleasure for pleasure's sake. Focus on all the good and positive aspects of each other. Remember that there is a life beyond infertility.

HEALTH RISKS OF INFERTILITY TREATMENTS

There are risks associated with taking any medication or undergoing a medical treatment, especially when anesthesia or surgery is involved.

COMPLEMENTARY AND ALTERNATIVE TREATMENTS FOR INFERTILITY

Complementary and alternative treatments such as massage therapy, acupuncture, traditional Chinese medicine, herbs, vitamins, mind-body approaches, yoga, visual imagery, and relaxation techniques may improve your ability to manage treatments and cope better with the emotional challenges they present. Some research suggests that some of these treatments might also improve your chances of becoming pregnant, but unfortunately there is little high-quality research.

Still, more and more fertility clinics are including complementary and alternative treatments alongside conventional medical options. Other clinics have developed relationships with practitioners or programs to which they regularly refer patients. If you chose to utilize complementary and alternative therapies, try to find a provider who is well trained (and licensed when appropriate) and experienced and has a solid reputation within the fertility field. For more information, see "Complementary and Alternative Therapies," p. 674.

Many people feel that the potential risks associated with fertility treatments are worth the opportunity to possibly become a parent.

The most common and underappreciated risk of infertility treatments is multiple gestation pregnancies. Women who undergo infertility treatments are much more likely to become pregnant with more than one fetus than women who conceive naturally. ART-conceived infants account for about 1 percent of all infants born in the United States, but they account for about 18 percent of twins and triplets. Multiple gestation pregnancies, including twin pregnancies, pose increased risks for pregnancy complications, premature delivery, low birth weight, long-term disability among infants, and even infant death.[9]

In ART, multiple births are largely due to the practice of transferring multiple embryos back into the uterus during IVF. They are preventable by limiting the number of embryos transferred. In the past few years, the American Society for Reproductive Medicine and the Society for Assisted Reproductive Technology have issued increasingly stricter guidelines for the numbers of embryos that should be transferred back into the uterus. The fertility clinics have been responsive: in 1996, more than 60 percent of ART procedures entailed the transfer of four or more embryos, whereas in 2008 that proportion was reduced to 14 percent. Currently, the largest number of procedures entails the transfer of two embryos. This trend has had an important impact on the number of high-order pregnancies. In 1996, 7 percent of ART births were triplets or higher-order multiples, and this proportion came to slightly less than 2 percent in 2008. That is the main reason why the number of high-order multiples has declined nationally since 2003. What has not happened, however, is a decrease in the number of twin births in ART: this can be accomplished only by promoting single-embryo transfer (see p. 489), and the United States has been slow at adopting this standard of care. The percentage of single-embryo transfers increased from 6 percent in 1996 to 12 percent in 2008. In contrast, in Sweden about 75 percent of embryo transfers are now single-embryo transfers. In Japan, all women under 37 years of age who have experienced no previous failure with ART must transfer only one embryo.

THE EVOLVING FIELD
OF INFERTILITY

The field of infertility diagnosis and treatment is evolving rapidly. As drug companies, hospitals, and physicians introduce new technologies and drugs into medical practice and the marketplace, diagnoses and treatments of infertility continue to change. New causes of infertility will likely be revealed as we learn more about environmental toxins and about how our genes interact with the changing environment.

Unfortunately, new techniques and treatments are rarely studied in controlled, randomized trials that could establish their safety and effectiveness. Some procedures used today are tried and true; many others are still considered experimental. Practitioners will agree about the efficacy of some drugs and procedures and differ about others.

You have a right to know whether your treatment is new or experimental and whether and how it has been studied scientifically. You also have the right to know about the possible risks and side effects of each treatment and about the amount of time and money that will be required. Try to determine the safest and least invasive treatments. Whenever possible, develop with your doctor a written course of treatment, including when to stop, that is tailored to your needs. And work to understand all you need to know to give truly informed consent to diagnostic and treatment approaches.

As a growing number of clinics in the United States limit the number of embryos implanted, an increasing proportion of multiple births will be the result of using injectable fertility medications that hyperstimulate ovulation. When too many eggs develop and are fertilized through either regular intercourse or an IUI, a multiple pregnancy results. Many families pursue injectable medications over IVF because of cost. Infertility treatments are usually not covered by insurance. Though still expensive, fertility medications alone are a fraction of the cost of an IVF cycle. The high out-of-pocket expenses associated with fertility treatments cause many to try to cut corners to build their families as quickly as possible, including taking fertility medications without proper monitoring or fully understanding the risks involved.

Unfortunately, there is still much that is unknown about the other risks various fertility treatments pose to women and the children born from these procedures. Good-quality research that follows large numbers of women and babies for long periods of time is needed. The Infertility Family Research Registry (IFRR) is a nonprofit organization that monitors and advocates for research on the health of people and families that have faced a diagnosis of infertility or dealt with infertility treatments. For more information about the IFRR, visit ifrr-registry.org.

THE ETHICS OF
FERTILITY TREATMENTS

Assisted reproduction can raise complicated ethical challenges for the individuals involved, health care professionals, and the greater society. Infertility treatments today create new definitions of parents and children and require a rethinking of the conventional notions of family. For families facing infertility, decisions about family building become complex.

One ethical dilemma associated with ARTs involves the politics of embryos and what to do with unused embryos. Many couples fertilize as many eggs as they can during their treatments and freeze any remaining embryos for later use. It's estimated that about a half a million cryopreserved embryos are being stored in fertility clinics across the United States. Many are eventually used for family building, but many remain unused, and often couples are ill equipped to make a decision about what to do with their embryos once their families are complete. Some just stop paying the storage fees or lose contact with the clinics. For both ethical and legal reasons, clinics are reluctant to dispose of embryos without a couple's consent. Couples who want to donate them to research are confused by varying laws and restrictions stymieing their ability to donate. Very few couples opt to donate their embryos to other couples due to lack of education about the option and ethical and moral concerns about giving one's genetically related embryos to an unknown couple. Moreover, many couples have a hard time coming to terms with permanently disposing of them, even through a compassionate transfer in which the remaining embryos are thawed and placed into the vagina at a time when conception is not possible.

It's important for couples to think about what they will do with their remaining embryos before they undergo fertility treatments and begin to create embryos. If not, they may struggle with the uncertainty about what to do with them for years or even decades. Further conflict occurs in situations of divorce or death. Laws are not consistent from state to state about who is ultimately responsible for embryos and what can be done with them. Given the length of time some embryos have been cryopreserved, some people have even included them in their wills, further delaying any conclusion.

Third-party reproduction, in which another person enters into the baby-making mix, also involves risks and raises many important ethical concerns. Though the FDA ensures the overall safety of the gametes, there is much more involved with such treatments than the passing of genetic material from one person to another. There is no consensus about how to appropriately and ethically recruit donors and surrogates or how to eliminate the risk of coercion or exploitation. Since money (often large amounts) is exchanged, commodification of reproduction is suggested. Furthermore, there is no guarantee that donors and surrogates fully understand the risks involved or are able to provide informed consent, especially given the lack of standards for education and screening. Further complicating matters, the intended parents pay for all costs involved, creating a great deal of pressure for donor programs and surrogacy agencies to quickly find matches for their clients—the intended families—and creating a conflict of interest in terms of whose interests are being protected. Even though recommendations exist as to how many times one can donate or be a surrogate and under what conditions, they aren't enforced.

Some women's health activists have concerns about the health risks to egg donors from using the drugs that stimulate ovulation. There is a lack of long-term safety data and too little research on the serious, occasionally irreversible problems experienced by some women using the drugs. Some people fear that the risks of egg donation have been underplayed and feel that regulations are needed to better ensure that the long-term consequences of donation are better understood. Several advocacy groups are calling for a national egg donor registry to better track the effects of these drugs.

In addition, there has been little research on what happens to donors, surrogates, intended families, and children after donation or birth—

physically or emotionally. People who have built their families through collaborative reproduction are not followed. There is also no method for donors to contact families they helped to build or vice versa later on. This is especially concerning if a medical need arises or information about their own personal or family health history changes. In fact, most sperm and egg donors never know if their donation even resulted in a pregnancy. We need to know more about what happens down the road for donors, surrogates, recipient parents, and their children so we can minimize any negative consequences, including unintentional ones.

Treating infertility in the United States has become an extremely technical, competitive $4-billion-a-year business.[10] Physicians providing treatment are often also business owners aware of profit margins. Many fertility clinics feel pressure to produce statistics that show potential patients the highest possible pregnancy and birth rates. This sometimes affects their choices regarding treatments. Likewise, fertility doctors struggle with trying to appease patients (rather than lose them to another clinic) who want to proceed with certain treatments when the chances of a good outcome are remote and other more appropriate options such as using donor eggs, surrogacy, adoption, or stopping treatment do not appear to be acceptable.

The business side of infertility treatments also restricts access to care for many families who don't have the necessary financial resources, since infertility treatment is not typically covered by insurance. Many people seek out other options, such as traveling to other countries for cheaper treatment. Several countries have severely restricted infertility treatments or require long waiting times, causing many families to travel elsewhere for treatments. Some are able to get good state-of-the-art care by well-trained physicians at an affordable price. Others find themselves in situations that may be unethical or unsafe, particularly with regard to egg donation or surrogacy, where very poor and uneducated women may be exploited for their reproductive potential. Unfortunately, guidelines, standards, and sources of unbiased information protecting donors, surrogates, and families struggling to have a baby are inadequate.

As technologies continue to proliferate, ethical and social challenges multiply, with complex questions of justice, rights, and conflicting principles continually raised. As a society, we are long overdue to discuss these issues and to guard against leaving them solely in the province of researchers and biotechnology entrepreneurs. We also need to devote resources and energies to identify and remove the environmental and physical causes of infertility. Prevention, education, and increased access to appropriate and cost-effective fertility care, including insurance coverage, are also imperative so that more families throughout the world are able to safely have children when they are ready. For more on the social and ethical issues raised by assisted reproductive technologies, see "Emerging Issues: Biopolitics, Women's Health, and Social Justice," p. 801.

RESOLUTION

IF YOU GET PREGNANT . . .

Getting pregnant will undoubtedly bring great joy and relief. Unfortunately, infertility doesn't end with getting pregnant. The experience of infertility often brings its own baggage to a pregnancy: grief for previous losses, anxiety, and fear that your body, unable to conceive on its own, may not be able to carry a pregnancy.

Other than brief spurts, I couldn't get excited until the very end, and even that was guarded. I've had friends who've seemed to go through pregnancies with an air of expectation that everything will work out, and I'm envious of the joy they seem to have had. I felt like all the commercials and cards out there about the joys of pregnancy were written for someone other than me. It made me feel defective a bit, that I couldn't get into fully loving being pregnant, even though my pregnancy was easy.

For many of us, pregnancy and parenting after infertility are a balancing act—caution and breath holding on one hand while trying to appreciate every moment on the other. For more information on the common experiences of women who conceive after infertility, see "Pregnancy After Infertility or Previous Pregnancy Loss" on the Our Bodies Ourselves website, ourbodiesourselves.org.

THINKING ABOUT WHEN TO STOP

I've been working through my feelings over my failed procedure, over the probability that I will never be pregnant. . . . I am feeling really sad, very discouraged . . . angry, [and] frustrated at the fact that we did the best we could but hit another brick wall. I am really uncertain how to proceed. Does it make sense to put more money into a procedure with no guaranteed outcome? How will we feel if we do this one more time and [fail again]? Maybe I should cut my losses and proceed with adoption. On the other hand, I have been pursuing the dream of raising a birth child for a decade. I still deeply want to raise a child I give birth to. I may always wonder if I could have been successful on my second try.

If fertility treatments don't succeed as you had hoped, you may feel extremely disappointed, angry, vulnerable, and desperate to try any intervention that offers a glimmer of hope. Some of us find ourselves, after every failed intervention, undergoing treatments that become increasingly physically invasive and emotionally debilitating.

If there's always something more that you can do, it becomes a situation where you don't even have control over when is enough.

On top of our own pain, many of us feel pressure from partners, family, friends, and colleagues to pursue more technically and socially complex treatments. This seemingly never-ending journey may lead some of us into a spiritual and ethical labyrinth that forces us to make quick rather than well-thought-out decisions concerning hormone therapy, IVF, donor egg, sperm and embryos, surrogacy, adoption, and living child-free.

MOVING FORWARD

If treatments are unsuccessful, we face difficult decisions: Should we continue trying, pursue adoption or foster parenting, or make the decision to not raise children?

For many of us, adoption provides another path to having children.

For more information, see "Adoption" on page 356.

Some of us decide—generally with a lot of grief and conflicted feelings—not to pursue parenthood.

The challenges of living child-free aren't always easy, and there are definitely still ups and downs. But the downs are helped tremendously by realizing there is much more to life. I also feel blessed to have the support of my wonderful and loving husband and close and caring friends. Overall, I feel that I have grown as a person and can now face the future, whatever it holds.

For more information, see "Understanding What It Means to Live Childfree After Infer-

tility" at blogher.com/understanding-what-it
-means-live-childfree-after-infertility.

As you decide on the next step, give yourself permission to be uncertain and cautious, change your mind, and grieve. Figuring out how to move forward is hard. But many of us find a way to live with the pain and disappointment of infertility and move on.

Our daughter is now 4 months old. We continue to heal from our six years of infertility and the loss of our son. I have come to believe that there will always be some pain associated with the battles we fought—and so often lost. At the same time, we love our daughter with all our hearts and we are happier than we have been in a very long time.

Postreproductive
Years

CHAPTER 20

Just as our bodies changed during puberty and we began to menstruate, so again—usually at midlife—we transition from our reproductive years to the natural end of monthly menstrual cycles. The transition usually begins in our forties and ends by the early fifties, although any age from the late thirties to sixty can be normal.

In keeping with the focus of this edition of *Our Bodies, Ourselves*, this chapter focuses on the reproductive health aspects of perimenopause and the social and cultural context of this significant transition.

WHAT DO WE MEAN WHEN WE SAY "MENOPAUSE"?

People commonly use the word "menopause" to mean different things, which can lead to confusion. For some women, "I'm in menopause" means they're somewhere in the months or years from the first night sweat until periods have stopped for good. This phase is more usefully called perimenopause, as is done in this book. Others use menopause to mean the literal moment of the final menstrual period (FMP), which we can't know was truly final until a further year has passed. Strictly speaking, this moment is menopause. To add to the confusion, some say "I'm menopausal" to mean that periods are over and they're somewhere in the last third of life, while others call this last phase postmenopause, as is done here.

You'll see in the table on p. 507 that the term "menopausal transition" is also used for much of the phase we are calling perimenopause.

I'd finally gotten my PMS and horrible cramps under control after trying everything—vitamins, yoga, massage, eliminating most caffeine, antidepressants, acupuncture—when my gynecologist told me I was perimenopausal. I started getting two periods a month, and they weren't light, either. I was fatigued, cranky, irritable, and I cried easily. Sometimes my short-term memory faltered.

For some reason I expected a very emotional perimenopause with mood swings and general despondency. Lo and behold, in my midforties I had a few hot flashes, some skipped periods, and that was it as far as I could tell. My two last periods came on April Fools' Day and the Fourth of July.

Perimenopause* is the one-to-ten-year stretch during which the ovaries function erratically and hormonal fluctuations may bring a range of changes, such as hot flashes, night sweats, sleep disturbances, and heavy menstrual bleeding. Perimenopause is a natural transition that affects each woman differently; for about 20 percent of us, the discomforts are so disruptive that we need major support and/or medical interventions.

Menopause is marked by the final menstrual period, known to be final after twelve months with no periods. After no flow for one year, the ovaries settle down and the reproductive hormones—estrogen and progesterone, which the body no longer needs for possible reproduction—have declined to low, steady levels. Most of us will live a third of our lives in what many call postmenopause. (Chapter 21, "Our Later Years," explores the possibilities and issues of that time, including sexuality and relationships.)

Some of us reach the end of menstrual periods early owing to chemotherapy or radiation therapy, surgical removal of the ovaries, or special health conditions. More discussion of early or premature menopause starts on p. 524.

---

* The definition of perimenopause has been through many versions. The World Health Organization has defined it as three years before menopause, but this can be determined only in retrospect. In 2001, a committee of experts met to try to define the process more clearly. The committee noted that in a woman's late reproductive years, her menstrual cycle was often reduced by up to two days. Early menopause transition was defined as variation in cycle length of seven days, and late menopause transition was defined as having skipped two periods, or going sixty days without a period. This does not adequately describe all the ongoing changes, but it is one way of defining the process.

Climateric: The Journal of the International Menopause Society 10, no. 115 (2007): 115.

	Menarche				Final menstrual period (FMP)			
Stages	-5	-4	-3	-2	-1	+1	+2
Terminology:	Reproductive			Menopausal transition		Postmenopause	
	Early	Peak	Late	Early	Late*	Early*	Late
				Perimenopause			
Duration of stage:	Variable			Variable		1 yr	4 years	Until demise
Menstrual cycles	Variable to regular	Regular		Variable cycle length (*persistent 7 or more day difference in length of consecutive cycles*)	*An interval of amenorrhea ≥ 60 days*	Amenorrhea ≥12 mos	None	
Endocrine	Normal FSH		↑ FSH	↑ FSH	↑ FSH (≥ 40 IU/l)			

* *Stages most likely to be characterized by vasomotor symptoms*

↑ = *Elevated*

Adapted from Soules et al., *Fertility and Sterility* 76 (2001): 874–78.

CHANGE OF LIFE: CULTURAL AND PERSONAL CONTEXTS OF MIDLIFE PERIMENOPAUSE

Midlife involves emotional, social, and physical changes, with the biological transition of perimenopause being just one of its aspects. It brings the end of the childbearing years, perhaps a time of relief, or of sadness at the loss of children we never had or never raised. Many of us reach menopause caught among the responsibilities of raising teenagers, launching grown children, caring for aging parents or other relatives, and working at demanding jobs—a stressful balancing act. Changes in living circumstances may couple with the hormonal fluctuations that often emerge during perimenopause to pose new challenges and problems. Everything from a new sort of loneliness to a profound sense of new freedom may emerge.

Women who are now making the menopause transition are pioneers in that more of us are living longer with better health, so the postmenopausal life stage may be nearly as long as our reproductive years. The menopause transition may offer opportunities to take stock of our lives, to be more self-directed, and to make the most of our time and relationships: What do I want to do? What am I not able to do? What can I control? Now that I know myself pretty well, how do I want to live? What do I want to learn? How can I improve my self-care for the next portion of my life?

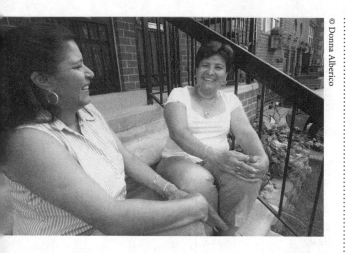

I just want more! More time free of kids to focus on my work; more time to myself; more passion in my marriage or from somewhere else.

Our experience can be profoundly influenced by our social/cultural context, in which we often encounter negative stereotypes of aging and discrimination against women. In a society that seems to value us primarily for our reproductive role, the end of our biological capacity to reproduce (unless we resort to the more extreme assisted reproductive technologies) can diminish our worth in others' eyes. Economic realities impair the ability of many of us to get the exercise, sleep, food, and medical care that are part of taking good care of ourselves. And Western society overvalues youth and beauty, setting them as a sexist standard for measuring women's worth. Once we are perceived as aging, we become prime targets for expensive or risky antiaging treatments, from wrinkle creams and Botox to face-lifts and liposuction.

The most important signs of midlife for me were the physical changes that made me realize that I was not young: vision loss, lack of sexual appetite, hair texture thinning, skin changes, and some wrinkles. I couldn't count on my looks anymore. My body was changing; what was the rest of my life going to be like?

The social realities of sexism and ageism can make it more difficult to deal with the sexual and reproductive changes that occur naturally in the middle years. These cultural messages have little to do with hormones and can't be treated with medication. We need to educate ourselves about the menopause transition and develop a critical perspective in order to resist the cultural messages that surround us. We can proceed with increased confidence as we become informed consumers and know that we are not alone. In fact, the support we receive from friends, family, and colleagues is critical in navigating this life transition well.

AM I THERE YET? HOW TO TELL IF YOU'VE REACHED PERIMENOPAUSE

The transition of perimenopause begins anywhere from your late thirties to age sixty and can last from one to ten years. Women who smoke tend to reach menopause earlier than nonsmoking women. Other than that, the only consistent factor that roughly predicts when you might start perimenopause is the age at which your mother went through what used to be called "the change."

It can be difficult to know whether you've entered perimenopause, because the hormonal fluctuations of that transition begin while menstrual periods are still regular. And it is difficult to use estrogen and progesterone or other hormone tests to indicate whether you are in perimenopause. These tests are not reliable indicators, because the ovaries often work unpredictably during perimenopause and reproductive hormone levels normally vary from hour to hour and day to day.

Endocrinologist Jerilynn Prior, founder of the Centre for Menstrual Cycle and Ovulation Research (cemcor.ubc.ca), a nonprofit research center in Vancouver, British Columbia, developed the following list of nine changes common to early perimenopause. If, despite regular pe-

EXPLORING CULTURAL DIFFERENCES IN WOMEN'S EXPERIENCES

Do women's experiences of perimenopause and menopause vary with ethnicity or cultural background? Most research done about menopause has been with white women, says Dr. Eun-Ok Im, a professor of nursing at the University of Texas at Austin. Dr. Im's four-year national study looked at ethnic differences in menopausal symptoms reported by white, Hispanic, African-American, and Asian-American women. Among the study's 2010 findings: African-American women were more likely to report hot flashes; white women were more likely to report more mood and memory changes; and women of Japanese and Chinese origin were more likely to report fewer menopausal symptoms in general.

Dr. Im notes that while past studies have shown white women to be concerned about menopause as a "harbinger of physical aging taking them away from society's youthful ideal," the study found they are becoming more optimistic about menopause, with many seeing it as an opportunity to rethink their lives and redefine themselves. Some even mentioned relief and benefits when going through menopause.

"A possible reason for the positive changes in the way white women look at menopause might be that the recent women's health movement has educated women to accept menopause as a normal developmental process, allowing them to refocus on themselves," said Dr. Im.

African-American, Hispanic, and Asian-American women already reported being more optimistic and positive about menopause than white women. In Dr. Im's study, many black women said that they were raised to be strong and accepting of a natural aging process. They viewed menopause—compared with other difficulties in their lives—as just another part of life to endure. Hispanic women spoke about getting support from family and friends during the menopausal transition. Findings also strongly suggest that there are subethnic—Chinese, Korean, Indian, Filipino—differences in the menopausal symptom experience of Asian-American women, and more studies are needed in this area.

How much the reported variations are due to genetic makeup, diet, expectations, or something else is still unknown, but Dr. Im believes findings like the ones in her study will work to eliminate ethnic biases and inequity in menopausal symptom management and promote culturally competent care for menopausal women.

An ongoing multiethnic study, the Study of Women's Health Across the Nation (www.swanstudy.org), also found that "African American women are more positive towards the idea of menopause than women of other ethnicities."[1] White women in this study noted more muscle aches, difficulty sleeping, and irritability than women of other backgrounds.

riods, you have any three, she suggests you can assume you have begun perimenopause.[2]

1. New-onset heavy and/or longer flow
2. Shorter menstrual cycles (less than twenty-five days)
3. Newly sore, swollen, or lumpy breasts
4. New midsleep wakening
5. Increased cramps
6. Onset of night sweats, especially around menstrual flow
7. New or markedly increased migraine headaches
8. New or increased premenstrual mood swings
9. Weight gain without changes in exercise or eating

PERIMENOPAUSE

Many women breeze through perimenopausal changes, while for some the hormone fluctuations create a range of mild discomforts discussed in detail below. For about 20 percent of us, the hormones fluctuate wildly and unpredictably, with spiking and falling estrogen and declining progesterone causing one or more years of nausea, migraines, weight gain, sore breasts, severe night sweats, and/or sleep trouble in what one researcher who experienced these discomforts calls "ovarian chaos."[3] For this group, perimenopause can be enormously disruptive both physically and emotionally.

Most women successfully alleviate any discomforts of perimenopause and beyond through nonmedical self-help approaches such as meditation, yoga, relaxation, regular exercise, healthful food, enough sleep, and support from family and friends. It helps, too, when colleagues at work are understanding of sudden hot flashes or the days when lack of sleep makes it harder to concentrate.

Other women—especially those for whom perimenopause is particularly difficult—may choose a balance of nonmedical and medical solutions. Health care providers who are well informed about perimenopause can be important partners in thinking through the options. This chapter presents what is known about the risks and benefits of different approaches so that you can choose the approaches that work best for you. It's important to remember that perimenopause and postmenopause are not diseases; they are life phases for every woman. And even the most difficult perimenopause does end.

The following figure, based on work by the gynecologist Nanette Santoro, helps to explain the hormonal fluctuations of perimenopause. The first row shows what happens to the four major female reproductive hormones—estrogen, progesterone, FSH, and LH—in a typical menstrual cycle. The second row is based on samples collected by a perimenopausal participant every day for six months. Notice that the estrogen levels for this woman go up higher relative to progesterone levels than is ever seen during regular cycles. This is probably why some perimenopausal women experience "estrogenic" effects such as fibroid growth, heavy menstrual bleeding, breast tenderness, and an increased response to psychological stressors.[4] The perimenopausal years have often been seen as a time of estrogen deficiency, but this information gives us a more complex and accurate picture.

PERIMENOPAUSAL SIGNS

Premenstrual Syndrome (PMS)

Some women report more severe premenstrual discomforts (PMS) during early perimenopause, when cycles are still reguar, such as swollen or tender breasts, water retention (bloating), anxiety, sleep disruption, or irritation. Whether you have had such discomforts for years or are just beginning to have them now, you can typically

HORMONE LEVELS

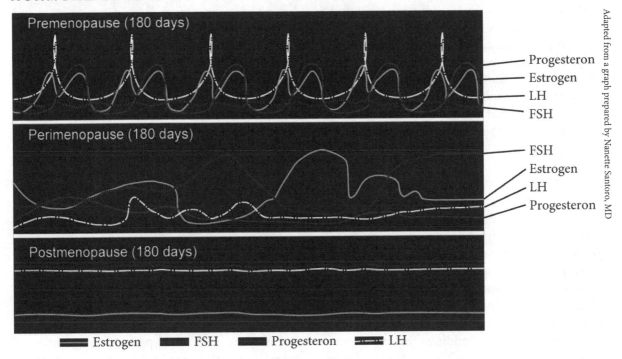

Adapted from a graph prepared by Nanette Santoro, MD

Premenopause (180 days)

- Progesteron
- Estrogen
- LH
- FSH

Perimenopause (180 days)

- FSH
- Estrogen
- LH
- Progesteron

Postmenopause (180 days)

Estrogen   FSH   Progesteron   LH

look forward to relief later in perimenopause, when your periods become irregular, and certainly by postmenopause, when the hormones level out. For more information on menstrual discomforts such as mood changes and severe cramps, see "Physical and Emotional Changes Through the Menstrual Cycle," p. 23.

Menstrual Cycle Changes

One common menstrual change in early perimenopause is shorter cycles, usually averaging two or three days less than usual but sometimes lasting only two or three weeks. It can feel as though you're starting a period when the last one has barely ended. In later perimenopause, you may skip a period entirely, only to have it followed by an especially heavy one (this is known as flooding). Occasionally, menstrual periods will be skipped for several months, then return as regular as clockwork.

The hormonal ups and downs of perimenopause can be the cause of almost any imaginable bleeding pattern. When estrogen is lower, the uterine lining gets thinner, causing the flow to be lighter or to last fewer days. And when estrogen is high in relation to progesterone (sometimes connected with irregular ovulation), bleeding can actually be heavier and periods may last longer.

Menstrual irregularities are a normal part of this stage in a woman's life and rarely require medical intervention. (For abnormally heavy bleeding, see below.) If you and your caregiver decide that efforts should be made to regulate your cycles at this time, be aware that while oral contraceptives are sometimes prescribed for menstrual irregularities, the use of progesterone alone can be a milder intervention. Progesterone can be used to manage the imbalance of estrogen and progesterone. A clinician can prescribe progesterone or its synthetic cousins, progestins, to be taken the last fourteen days of the cycle. This replaces the progesterone that would normally be secreted in an ovulatory cycle and helps to create a more regular bleeding pattern. (See p. 535 for a discussion of peri- and postmenopausal hormone therapy in the United States, the potential harms and benefits, and differences among the hormonal treatments currently available.)

Abnormally Heavy Bleeding

About 25 percent of women have heavy bleeding (sometimes called hypermenorrhea, menorrhagia, or flooding) during perimenopause. Some women's menstrual flow during perimenopause is so heavy that even supersized tampons or pads cannot contain it. If you are repeatedly bleeding heavily, you may become anemic from blood loss. During a heavy flow you may feel faint when sitting or standing. This means your blood volume is decreased; try drinking salty liquids such as tomato or V8 juice or soup. Taking an over-the-counter NSAID such as ibuprofen every four to six hours during heavy flow will decrease the period blood loss by 25 to 45 percent.

Don't ignore heavy or prolonged bleeding—see your health care provider if it persists. Your provider can monitor your blood count and iron levels. Iron pills can replace losses and help avoid or treat anemia.

Other medical treatment may include progesterone therapy or the progestin-releasing Mirena IUD, which is known to reduce menstrual bleeding. If your health care provider suggests hysterectomy as a solution to very heavy bleeding during perimenopause, you may want to try these and other less invasive approaches first. Removal of the uterus is an expensive and irreversible step with many effects (see p. 628).

Heavy bleeding during perimenopause may be due to the estrogen-progesterone imbalance. Also, polyps (small, noncancerous tissue growths that can occur in the lining of the uterus) can increase during perimenopause and can cause bleeding. Fibroid growth during perimenopause can sometimes cause heavy bleeding, especially when the fibroid grows into the uterine cavity. If very heavy bleeding persists despite treatment, your provider should test for possible causes of abnormal bleeding. (See p. 611 for more about the causes of abnormal uterine bleeding as well as the pros and cons of various treatment options.)

BIRTH CONTROL DURING PERIMENOPAUSE

A popular myth is that once your periods become irregular in perimenopause, you can't get pregnant anymore. Because of this myth, women in perimenopause have a much higher rate of unplanned pregnancies than you would expect. Even if your periods are lighter or shorter than they used to be or you are skipping them for months at a time, you may still be fertile and can potentially get pregnant. If you have sex with men and don't want to become pregnant, you will need to use birth control until you have gone without a period for at least a full year—and some experts recommend up to two years for women who reach postmenopause in their forties. For more information, see Chapter 9, "Birth Control."

Some experts question the use of estrogen-containing birth control methods during perimenopause. According to Jerilynn Prior, "Estrogen levels average higher in perimenopause because the feedback loops that normally control it are not consistently 'working.'" That could mean that using hormonal forms with four-times-higher estrogen doses may not reliably suppress the body's estrogen levels. Thus these methods could produce an estrogen "overdose."[5] She suggests barrier methods (condom, diaphragm, cervical cap) plus vaginal spermi-

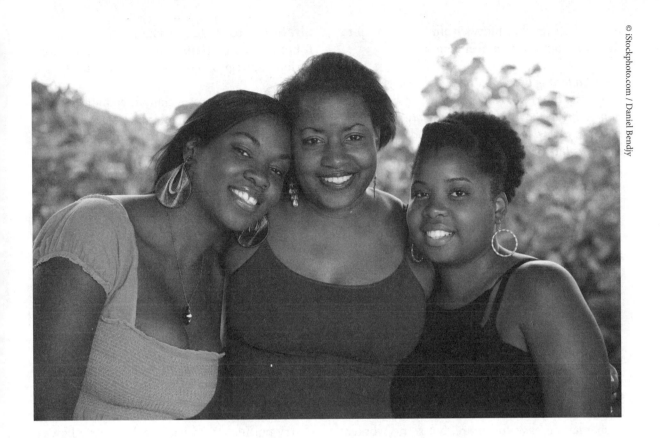

cide, or the Mirena progestin-carrying IUD, as other possible contraceptive options.

HOT FLASHES AND NIGHT SWEATS

Hot flashes are legendary signs of perimenopause and for some women can continue well into postmenopause, though 20 to 30 percent of women never have them at all. A woman experiencing a hot flash will suddenly feel warm, then very hot and sweaty, and sometimes experience a cold chill afterward. Hot flashes are thought to be due to a change in the brain's control mechanism for body temperature.* Some women ex-

perience a more rapid pulse rate, a feeling that the heart is jumping (palpitations), or increased or decreased blood pressure. There is increased blood flow to surface blood vessels, so the hands get hot, and sometimes there is a visible redden-

* Factors that may be involved in hot flashes include the body's core temperature regulation and brain chemicals. The body's thermostat has an upper set point, at which the blood vessels open up and

perspiration occurs in an effort to release heat. There is also a lower threshold, at which shivering begins to generate heat. Between these two extremes is a temperature zone known as the thermoneutral zone, at which the body normally functions. Researchers now theorize that the zone between the high and low set points in perimenopausal and postmenopausal women who experience hot flashes is narrower than in women who don't experience them. A slight increase in core body temperature (from having a cup of tea or getting upset, for example) could cause a sensitized woman to experience a hot flash as her body tries to reduce its temperature. Another factor that could be affecting the body's core temperature regulation is the brain neurotransmitter norepinephrine, which has been shown to reduce the thermoneutral zone in animals. Levels seem to be higher in some perimenopausal and postmenopausal women who experience hot flashes.

ing of the skin that moves from the chest up to the face. Some women feel panicky.

If I get a feeling of mild nausea and a surge of anxiety that isn't related to anything that's happening at the moment, this usually means I'm about to have a hot flash. Oh yes, and it starts to feel as though the shirt on my back is made of weighty material, even if I'm wearing a summer blouse.

Hot flashes may begin long before cycles become irregular; you may start to feel warmer at night before other changes begin. They may even occur around your period or after childbirth. Hot flashes can continue for some years after periods end. Forty-five percent of women still have them five to ten years after periods stop, and a few of us have them into our seventies. Each woman has her own hot-flash script: the frequency; the triggers; how the hot flash starts and finishes; how often flashes come; and how long they last. An occasional mild hot flash may be easy to ignore, but some women find flashes acutely uncomfortable, distracting, and even embarrassing. One fifty-two-year-old woman describes her hot flashes:

It's not like I'm feeling "a little warm"—it's like I'm on fire, and I don't care if anybody else is around, I still want to strip off all my clothes to get cooler.

Hot flashes sometimes cause enough perspiration to soak nightclothes and sheets (night sweats), and they can disturb sleep.

Heavier women's hot flashes tend to be more frequent and severe than thinner women's, because the increased subcutaneous tissue acts as insulation and prevents heat loss. Hot flashes are the body's attempt to get rid of heat, and those of us who are better insulated often have more difficulty doing so. Recent studies indicate that weight loss can reduce hot flashes.[6]

Strategies to Reduce Discomfort

If hot flashes are bothering you, you can adopt various strategies to reduce the discomfort.

- Dress in layers (especially breathable or natural fibers), so you can shed or add clothes according to how you are feeling.
- Identify your personal triggers, and attempt to avoid them. Spicy foods, hot drinks, alcohol, caffeine, and anxiety are common triggers.
- Carry cool water with you and drink it regularly. Keep your environment cool with fans or air-conditioning.
- Avoid stress as much as possible. Learn to decrease your response to stress—through meditation, or practicing slow, deep abdominal breathing several times a day, for example. When a flash starts, use the slow, deep abdominal breathing method or other forms of the relaxation response.
- Do something active that increases your heart rate for thirty minutes a day.
- Try putting a cold pack under your pillow at night so when you wake up with a hot flash you can turn your pillow over and it is nice and cool.
- Wash your hands in cool water at the start of or after a hot flash; it will cool you off and make you feel cleaner.
- If you are a smoker, get help in quitting. Smokers tend to have more frequent and more intense hot flashes.

Alternative Remedies

Some women try nutritional supplements (such as soy products), botanicals (such as red clover), antioxidant vitamins (such as vitamin E), and herbal preparations (such as black cohosh, Saint-John's-wort, and Chinese herbal medicine). Most are safe for short-term use (up to six months), although if you are trying phytoestrogens they are probably more safely used when taken as food rather than as pills or supplements. Some of these remedies seem to help, but well-designed studies have often been unconvincing. All studies of hot flashes using a placebo show a placebo effect (as many as 30 percent or more of women feel better even on inert tablets). Women taking alternative remedies should tell their health care providers so they can stay alert to possible interactions with other medications.

Hormones

Taking estrogen has been shown in multiple randomized trials to relieve hot flashes in post-menopausal women, and progestins such as medroxyprogesterone are effective as well. (No study has proved anything more effective for perimenopausal hot flashes than a placebo.) However, data from the Women's Health Initiative show that the most widely used estrogen-progestin preparation increases the risk of stroke and other serious illness. Recently presented but not yet published randomized control trial data show that oral micronized progesterone (Prometrium) effectively treats night sweats and hot flushes in postmenopause.[7] If you are considering hormones, it is important to be aware of the most recent research on which forms are safest. For a detailed discussion, see "Hormone Therapy—Yes or No?," p. 535.

Nonhormonal Medications

There are various nonhormonal medications that women have tried for problematic hot flashes. Keep in mind that there is no evidence at this point that using any of the nonhormonal medications for months or years is safer than hormone therapy.

Antidepressants. Studies have indicated that relatively low doses of some antidepressants can be more effective at preventing hot flashes than a placebo (and about 70 percent as effective as estrogen). The drug tested most extensively has been low-dose venlafaxine (Effexor), although others such as paroxetine (Paxil) and fluoxetine (Prozac) also seem to work. However, long-term safety data on such use are absent. In addition, the studies producing the most positive results were conducted with women who had breast cancer, and negative results were reported more often by women without breast cancer. Further study on women without breast cancer is needed.[8] Antidepressants are perhaps most appropriate for hot flashes if you also need treatment for depression. They come with their own unknowns and potential side effects, including sleep difficulties, lowered sexual interest, and difficulty reaching orgasm, and some women have difficulty when they try to stop taking them.

Gabapentin. A seizure medication used for pain control, gabapentin has been used with some success to treat hot flashes, but it, too, has side effects to consider, including nausea and fatigue. It is often most appropriate for hot flashes in women who also need the medication for pain.

Clonidine. The antihypertensive clonidine has also been used to treat hot flashes. Antihypertensives are perhaps most appropriate for hot flashes if you also need treatment for high blood pressure. If this treatment is taken in doses that are effective, women without high blood pressure may experience dizziness or dry mouth.

New methods. There have been reports of success in treating recalcitrant (stubborn) hot flashes using a nerve block in the neck (stellate ganglion block), although this more invasive approach demands caution and further study.[9]

SLEEP DISTURBANCES

Sleep disturbances are common in both perimenopause and postmenopause. Most commonly, a woman will fall asleep without a problem, then wake up in the early-morning hours and have difficulty getting back to sleep.

Women who experience hot flashes or night sweats tend to have insomnia more often than those who don't. Sleeplessness can cause fatigue, irritability, and a feeling of being unable to cope. Getting enough sleep is critical to overall good health.

For more dependable sleep, you may want to try these lifestyle changes:

- Cut out caffeinated beverages (coffee, tea, colas, and chocolate), especially after about three P.M., as caffeine stays in the bloodstream at least six hours. Caffeine is a stimulant that interferes with sleep and leads to more frequent urination.
- Avoid smoking. Tobacco is a stimulant.
- Avoid or limit alcohol consumption. Although alcohol is initially a sedative and makes one sleepy, it becomes a stimulant as it is metabolized, resulting in fragmented sleep and the need to urinate during the night.
- Go to sleep at about the same time every night.
- Exercise regularly. Exercising during the day or early evening can relieve tension and help promote sleep. Avoid doing anything strenuous just before bed.
- Take a hot bath, listen to music, or read before bed.
- Filter out noise and light. Close doors and windows, use earplugs, or use a soothing sound machine. Use room-darkening shades or an eye mask to block light.

Valerian has long been used as an herbal sleep remedy and has shown benefit in some, but not all, clinical trials. Evidence is strong that melatonin works for jet lag and sleep problems due to changing work schedules such as shift work, but the data are not clear on regular insomnia.[10] (Using melatonin that is synthesized rather than made from animal products avoids the theoretical risk of exposure to viruses.) Some women find antihistamines such as dimenhydrinate (for example, Dramamine), diphenhydramine (Benadryl), and chlorpheniramine maleate (Chlor-Trimeton) helpful. Some women try sleeping pills, but as these can be habit-forming and stop working after prolonged use, they are best used occasionally, not regularly.

If your sleep disturbances persist, you may want to discuss medical relief with your health care provider. In some women, oral micronized progesterone helps to decrease the time it takes to fall asleep, increase early night rapid eye movement sleep, and increase total sleep time without causing morning changes in alertness or brain function.[11] Both estrogen and low-dose antidepressants in the tricyclic family can relieve insomnia for some women. Be sure to learn about the effects and long-term impact of these medications.

Sometimes it is worth consulting a sleep specialist. Sleep conditions such as apnea and restless leg syndrome can contribute to sleep difficulties, and a sleep study may be necessary to diagnose them.

VAGINAL CHANGES

Vaginal dryness is sometimes a problem in early perimenopause. This could be related to the fact that some women do have low-estrogen episodes during this stage.

As estrogen and progesterone levels decline in late perimenopause and postmenopause, vaginal walls frequently become thinner, drier, and less flexible and more prone to tears and cracks. (This can be particularly true for women who have never given birth or have had only C-sections during childbirth, as vaginal birth gives the walls a lasting stretch.) Less lubrication is produced, so it can also take longer to become moist during sexual activity. Penetration may be uncomfortable or even painful and can lead to irritation. If tissues become very delicate, vaginal wall bleeding may result from friction associated with sexual activity. Women who have what many clinicians refer to by the term vaginal atrophy (thinning and inflammation of the vaginal walls, also known as atrophic vaginitis) may end up completely avoiding intercourse or other insertive sex because of the discomfort. One fifty-six-year-old woman says:

Forget intercourse! After menopause, I couldn't even ride my bicycle anymore—my vagina always felt sore.

Some prescription and over-the-counter drugs may cause or contribute to vaginal dryness. Antihistamines, for example, dry vaginal tissue as well as nose and eye tissues. Douches, sprays, and colored or perfumed toilet paper and soaps can irritate vaginal and vulvar tissues. There are also a variety of skin conditions that can cause pain and/or irritation with insertive sex. Consult a clinician if this is a persistent problem for you. (See "Painful Intercourse/Penetration," p. 185.)

The following tips can relieve vaginal dryness and resulting discomfort with sex:

Lubricants and vaginal moisturizers, such as Silk-E, Albolene, Astroglide, or Slippery Stuff may be helpful during sex. Vegetable oil is another option. For more information, see "Lubrication," p. 177. If dryness persists, try an over-the-counter moisturizer, such as Replens, which may be used one or more times a week but *not* at the time of penetration. Avoid scratching, which can irritate delicate tissues and lead to infections and further problems. Itching can be a sign of a yeast or fungal infection that needs treatment (see p. 637). Applying prescription steroid ointment to the pubic and vaginal area can relieve itching.

Regular sexual activity also helps maintain vaginal flexibility and pliability, presumably because it increases blood supply to the vagina and can have a stretching effect.

Wait until you are fully aroused before penetration. Vaginal dryness during sexual activity at any age may simply mean that you need more stimulation and maybe even an orgasm before penetration. You may want to tell your sex partner(s) that you will need lots of varied stimulation and experimentation to find out what is arousing.

Drink more liquids—some recommend eight or more cups each day.

Graduated dilators may be used to gently expand your vaginal walls and increase elasticity. Start with a small size, and work your way up. As a sixty-year-old woman puts it, "Ah, the dilators. I call them my white plastic boyfriends. And do not forget the lube!"

Other options to consider if lubricants and other strategies are not sufficient include:

Low-dose local (vaginal) estrogens, in very small amounts, are highly effective at relieving vaginal dryness. They can also restore thickness and flexibility to the tissues in the vulva and vagina. Preparations include: Estring (a Silastic ring that you insert like a diaphragm and leave in for up to three months), Vagifem tablets, and Estrace and Premarin creams. There is also Estriol, a bioidentical vaginal cream made by compounding pharmacies. These products have a local effect, and far less estrogen gets into the bloodstream than it does with oral or transdermal (patch) estrogen medications.

The ring delivers a minuscule amount of estrogen to the bloodstream and the tablets send a little more, though the dose delivered in the tablet has recently been reduced. Regrettably, there are no long-term studies that demonstrate if even these small amounts of estrogens have risks, but they definitely improve the quality of life for many women.

If you use a vaginal estrogen cream, keep in mind that it can send a larger and somewhat unpredictable amount of estrogen into the bloodstream, depending how much is used and how often it is used. Most women initially require nightly treatment, but many women find that a smaller dose than prescribed works fine, especially if they are sexually active. Try using just enough to cover a fingertip and apply it to the opening of the vagina; the applicators tend to deliver a systemic dose of estrogen and deposit it higher than necessary. Estrogen cream should not be used as a lubricant for intercourse because it can be absorbed through a partner's skin.

If you're among the small number of women who have persistently sore breasts while using vaginal estrogen, try decreasing the dose to see if that will eliminate the soreness. If soreness persists, consult your health care provider.

Hormone therapy that includes systemic estrogen is also effective at relieving vaginal dryness. However, since low-dose local estrogens work well, it is typically not necessary to resort to systemic HT.

If vaginal dryness is an issue, getting help can make a big difference. A sixty-three-year-old woman recalls a time when she had not had sex for a number of months and sex was very uncomfortable:

I was so dry and tender that it felt like my partner had gravel on his fingers. I was really alarmed but started to use vaginal estrogen. I love sex, and it was such a relief to feel like I had my clit and my vagina back as a place of pleasure!

URINARY CHANGES

Some women at midlife report having to pee more often and needing to get up a few times during the night. Some also experience urinary incontinence (UI), of which there are two types.

Urge incontinence is a sudden strong urge to urinate followed by an involuntary flow; it begins for some women in perimenopause and improves after menopause. Stress incontinence is the involuntary leaking of urine when coughing, sneezing, laughing, or exerting oneself during strenuous activity.

Urinary incontinence is more common at older ages. Lower estrogen levels seem to be involved in some types of UI but not all. In the Women's Health Initiative (WHI) trials (see p. 535), higher estrogen levels caused incontinence and worsened already existing incontinence. It doesn't seem to be just synthetic estrogens that are the culprit—even studies of estrogen patches or gels show mixed results. Some medications and caffeinated beverages can make you pee more often, and even as little as 500 mg of vitamin C may cause urinary urgency and sometimes incontinence. Mobility problems can be a factor, too, when you can't get to a toilet fast or on your own at all.

Urinary incontinence and having to pee frequently can sometimes indicate that you have a urinary tract infection. The low estrogen and progesterone levels in late perimenopause and postmenopause can result in thinning of the urinary tract tissues and a weakening of the bladder and urethra (the tube from the bladder to the outside), increasing susceptibility to urinary infections. So if you are having urinary problems, make sure to check for an underlying infection (see "Urinary Tract Infections," p. 639).

Incontinence can be successfully managed, treated, and sometimes even cured. Besides wearing panty liners, you can try these self-help and medical approaches:

Kegel exercises. At all ages, strengthening the muscles of the pelvic floor will help control urine leaks. If you have never done Kegel (perineal) exercises, this is a good time to start and keep doing them (for details, see p. 643).

Bladder training. Teaching yourself to go longer and longer without urinating can also be very helpful. Sit on the toilet every two hours, whether you have to go or not. Then, every two days, extend the interval by thirty minutes until you're doing it every four hours. Try to maintain the schedule whether or not you have an accident. If you have an urge to urinate, stay still and use the muscle-strengthening exercises until the urge passes, then move slowly to the bathroom. Sometimes it helps to relax the body rather than tense up all over in an attempt to hold the urine back. Avoid drinking a lot of fluid before you go out or while you're away from home, and catch up with liquids when you return home.

Medications. Some medications help decrease bladder contractions (hyperactive bladder) that produce leaking. Some are relatively new, and they may not help your particular urinary problem, so it's a good idea to get more information before deciding to take them. Certain medications (Detrol and Ditropan) may have a negative impact on memory and the central nervous system.

Vaginal estrogen in the form of tablets, cream, or rings. Vaginal estrogen can sometimes help with urgency, frequency, and urge incontinence and in the prevention of urogenital atrophy and recurrent urinary tract infections. But studies don't agree on whether taking whole-body (systemic) estrogen/progestin therapy reduces incontinence in postmenopausal women or makes it worse.[12] The most common type of estrogen pills used in the past, conjugated equine estrogens (Premarin), appear to make it worse—with or without a progestin.

Other Treatments for Urinary Incontinence

Some leaking of urine is caused by anatomical problems (see "Pelvic Relaxation and Uterine Prolapse," p. 646). Weakening of the tissues with age is sometimes related to damage from childbirth. To treat this, a pessary (which resembles a diaphragm) can be inserted into the vagina to help keep the bladder and urethra in their correct positions and prevent leakage.

One of several types of surgery might correct anatomical issues causing urinary incontinence, but if you are thinking about this, be sure to have a thorough discussion of the risks and benefits with an experienced gynecologic surgeon or a specialist in female urology. As with any major surgery, understand what is proposed and get another opinion before agreeing to any procedures. Ask about alternatives, the success rate, complications, and whether you might need to repeat the procedure if it doesn't work. Ask, too, how many of this kind of procedure the surgeon has done.

Finding help can be challenging, because female reproduction and urology are separate medical specialties. Most urologists know little more than the basics about female reproductive organs, while not all clinicians in either specialty know much about treating middle-aged and older women with urinary problems. Urogynecology is a relatively new subspeciality of ob-gyn in which gynecologists have additional special training in urogynecologic surgery.

SEXUAL DESIRE AND SATISFACTION

Sexual problems are by no means universal in perimenopause and postmenopause. For example, one woman reported happily that "my libido was stronger than ever, and I was fortunate to have a husband who enjoyed pleasing me." But many women in perimenopause report decreased sexual interest, lack of arousability, lack of sufficient vaginal lubrication (see above for ways of handling this), and sometimes even aversion to sex. These can be affected by perimenopause-related problems such as heavy, unpredictable menstrual periods or mood swings and may improve with the arrival of postmenopause if you continue to be sexually active with yourself or a partner.

Sexual desire and function can be affected by other health problems, such as high blood pressure or diabetes, or life changes, such as the death of a partner or having a partner who is no longer interested or able to engage in sex.

If you have problems with changing sexual desire or experiences that are troubling to you, try to address specific problems before linking them to perimenopause or postmenopause. If you or your partner takes a medication that seems to be reducing sexual desire, discuss your concerns with your health care provider. Often substituting a different drug will help. If sex is uncomfortable, discuss it with your health care provider. The section on "Painful Intercourse/Penetration," p. 185, may also be helpful.

Be aware of the range of nonmedical factors that might be affecting your sexual satisfaction, including relationship issues, inadequate sex education, or difficulty talking about what you like or need for full satisfaction. The brain is an important sex organ, and if you are feeling stressed, tired, or annoyed (or angry) at a partner, you might not feel at all sexual. If there are issues in your relationship, seek a way to spend time with your partner to see whether you can sort things out. Finally, if you have also lost interest in other activities, consider whether or not you might be depressed, as not taking pleasure in activities you have enjoyed in the past is a com-

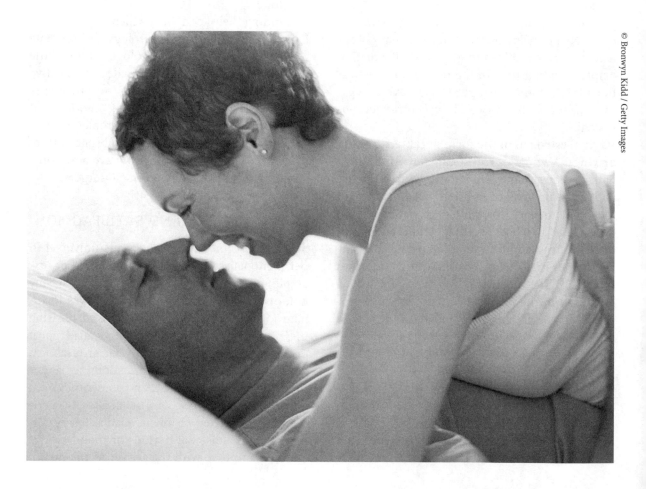

HOW DRUGS AND DISEASE AFFECT SEX

Some drugs—such as Prozac and related antidepressants and some antiepileptic medications—depress sexual function or interest. Medication for high blood pressure can prevent erections and women's arousal, as can too much alcohol. (The depressive effect of alcohol becomes more pronounced as people get older.) Fear often interferes with sex after a heart attack or a diagnosis of heart disease, but most women find that after an initial recovery period, sex is as enjoyable as ever. Ask your health care practitioner and pharmacist about the effects on sexual interest, arousal, or functioning of any medications that are prescribed for you or your partner; look them up in the *Physicians' Desk Reference* or on MedlinePlus (medlineplus.gov) (See "Sex with a Disability or Chronic Illness," p. 194, for the effects of some conditions and medications.) If your clinician cannot answer your questions about sexuality, ask to be referred to someone who can.

SAFER SEX DURING PERIMENOPAUSE AND POSTMENOPAUSE

If you are sexually active, you are at risk of getting a sexually transmitted infection, including HIV. Dryness of the vaginal lining (and, in postmenopause, the thinning of the lining) may result in irritation from insertive sex, resulting in increased access for bacteria or viruses. Practicing safer sex—that is, using condoms or latex dams for protection—can reduce the risk of STIs. For information on how to protect yourself, see Chapter 10, "Safer Sex."

mon sign of depression. For more on desire, including a discussion of testosterone treatment as well as the effects of hormones and medications, see "Sexual Challenges," Chapter 8. For more on sexuality in postmenopause, see "Sexuality," p. 560 in Chapter 21, "Our Later Years."

MEMORY AND THE MIND

Many women report memory gaps or lowered ability to concentrate during perimenopause and postmenopause. The relation among cognitive function, memory, and hormones is not fully understood. Occasional forgetfulness—those "senior moments" so many of us talk about—may also reflect general stress, specific worries, depression, lack of sleep, not having paid attention to details, or being distracted by things such as a phone ringing, a child yelling, or a dog barking. A fifty-two-year-old woman says:

With all the changes that are going on in my body, no wonder I can't remember other things! And no wonder I sometimes get a bit weepy—a whole part of my life is behind me now. Luckily, these feelings don't last long. I've heard that postmenopause is a breeze after perimenopause.

In fact, the brain's capacity to reorganize its cells and grow connections continues throughout life. Brain exercises such as reading, doing crossword or other puzzles, and engaging in social activity or stimulating conversations can sometimes improve memory.

Sleep deprivation—from whatever cause—should not be underestimated as a cause of memory and concentration issues. If you're having trouble sleeping, resolving that issue may also improve your memory and ability to think.

Some women report that hormone therapy helps with their perceived loss of cognitive function,[13] but it is not yet clear whether estrogen or progesterone (alone or together) is helpful for memory.

MOOD

Clearly, hormonal shifts can affect our moods. Current research suggests that during perimenopause, when reproductive hormones are unpredictable and erratic, women may become moody and even depressed. Those with a history of postpartum depression, a family history of depression, or severe PMS may be particularly at risk, especially those who are not physically active and do not take time for themselves or pay attention to their bodies' signs and signals. Of course, sleep deprivation and midlife stresses can contribute as well. The relationship between perimenopause/postmenopause and mood, or the more serious and sometimes debilitating condition called depression, is complicated and not fully understood.

Most women find that emotional ups and downs smooth out well with the low and steady hormone levels of postmenopause, although being postmenopausal, especially in a youth-oriented culture, brings its own challenges. Even if you've never needed counseling or medication, you may want to consider getting help if mood swings or depression before or after menopause are seriously disrupting your life. However, though the ad campaigns of drug companies have touted—and individuals have reported—the positive effects of HT on mood,

the Women's Health Initiative data showed that the most prescribed combined oral estrogen and progestin had no clinically meaningful effect on participants' overall vitality, mental health, or depressive symptoms—at least on average.

REACHING POSTMENOPAUSE

After the ups and downs of perimenopause, some women scarcely notice postmenopause. The periods end, period. If you have had uterine problems, such as heavy bleeding or fibroids, they may clear up without treatment when your estrogen levels drop. Endometriosis will usually get better. A fifty-six-year-old woman says that reaching menopause is "wonderful":

No more bloating, sore breasts, menstrual migraines, back pain, greasy hair, and zits. I now realize I felt like I had been pregnant for thirty-five years!

Despite the continuation for some of us of a variety of effects such as hot flashes and vaginal dryness, many women find the evenness of the postmenopausal decades energizing as they begin a new phase that will last the rest of their lives. See Chapter 21, "Our Later Years" for a discussion of some of the dynamics, issues, and health questions of this time.

TAKING CARE OF OURSELVES DURING PERIMENOPAUSE AND BEYOND

Many of the changes associated with aging and the postmenopausal years that were once thought biologically inevitable are actually preventable and sometimes even reversible. Heart disease and osteoporosis are two examples. During perimenopause and earlier, you can take active steps to maintain good health and lessen the impact of these and other chronic conditions associated with aging. Acquiring healthy habits—exercising, eating healthfully, quitting smoking, and reducing dependence on caffeine, sugar, and alcohol—is always a good place to start.

ACTIVITY AND MOVEMENT

Physical activity becomes increasingly important in midlife. The ratio of body fat to muscle mass increases as we grow older, and without exercise we lose more muscle mass. We typically begin to lose bone mass in our thirties, often because of physical inactivity and sedentary jobs. Happily, an increasing number of women of every age have rejected this norm and are on the move. A woman in her fifties says:

I took up tae kwon do, Eastern self-defense, which appealed to me as a Japanese American. To my amazement, after a few months of kicking and hitting an imaginary opponent, my chronic insomnia and stiff neck disappeared. Gone also were the painful attacks of gastritis. I began feeling more energetic. . . . That was more than five years ago. Today, all the ailments that I thought I would have to live with the rest of my life are gone.

Aerobic exercise, such as walking, swimming, biking, and dancing, makes your heart work harder and strengthens the muscles and ligaments that support the skeleton. Weight-bearing exercise builds bone. Strength training with weights helps maintain muscle strength and improves balance. Yoga promotes flexibility and balance. There's exercise to fit almost any kind of physical limitation, including isometric muscle toning and chair yoga if you are not mobile. It's important to exercise the whole body, so as to keep up strength and flexibility everywhere.

Exercise can lower blood pressure and reduce the risks of heart attack and stroke, arthritis, emphysema, and osteoporosis. It is essential to maintaining a healthy weight (although exercise alone will not generally lead to weight loss). It can help improve posture, sleep, and bowel function and relieve depression and hot flashes, and it makes most people feel better overall. After exercise, blood rushes to the skin, bringing with it extra nutrients, raising skin temperature, and increasing the collagen content. Skin actually thickens, becoming more elastic and less wrinkled. Some women find that regular exercise improves their sexual response and feelings of sensuality.

WEIGHT GAIN AT MIDLIFE

Women in midlife often complain of difficulty controlling weight gain. This is probably due to a combination of slower metabolism, decreased activity, and increased caloric intake. The ten-

PREMATURE MENOPAUSE

If a woman's periods cease before the age of forty, it is known as early or premature menopause. Premature menopause can be caused by certain surgeries and medical treatments, and by early changes in ovarian function that are not yet well understood.

Surgical menopause

In women who have not yet reached menopause, surgical removal of the ovaries (oophorectomy) will lead to an abrupt drop in hormone levels. This results in the same changes as those in natural menopause except that testosterone levels are lower after oophorectomy, but the abruptness can make the transition more difficult. Removal of the uterus (hysterectomy) with the ovaries left in place does not bring premature menopause, although menstrual bleeding stops and fertility ends and the hormonal changes of perimenopause may occur at a younger-than-average age. (For discussions of hysterectomy and oophorectomy, see p. 628.)

Treatment-induced menopause

Premature menopause can occur as the result of chemotherapy, pelvic or whole-body radiation therapy, or other drug therapies used for cancer treatment. Some women who have undergone cancer treatments experience a temporary alteration of ovarian function; for others, the impact is permanent.

Premature ovarian insufficiency (POI)

Approximately 1 percent of women under the age of forty will experience the unexpected onset of night sweats, hot flashes, sleep disturbances, and other perimenopausal symptoms. Periods may dwindle or stop. Once known as premature ovarian failure, this condition is now referred to by many as premature ovarian insufficiency (POI), because the ovaries rarely "fail" entirely. Instead, ovary function becomes insufficient to maintain a regular menstrual cycle.

Causes of POI include genetic factors (chromosomal irregularities, particularly fragile X syndrome and Turner syndrome) or an autoimmune process. Viral infection may also play a role. Some women with POI also suffer from other autoimmune disorders, such as Addison's disease (adrenal problems), or experience other endocrine disruptions, such as thyroid disease. Diabetes, lupus, rheumatoid arthritis, and inflammatory bowel syndrome are also thought to be connected to POI, as are environmental toxins. Still, more often than not, researchers are unable to determine an exact cause for premature menopause. Family history can be important, in that some women come from families where it is common.

If you are under the age of forty and begin to experience irregular menstrual cycles and/or other symptoms of perimenopause (such as hot flashes, insomnia, headaches, or vaginal dryness), a health care provider should assist you to track your experiences, cycles, and ovulation. (See the Centre for Menstrual

Cycle and Ovulation Research website, specifically the "Help Yourself" section [cemcor.ubc.ca/help_yourself], for a daily perimenopause diary.) Other possibilities may need to be ruled out, such as pregnancy, an eating disorder, thyroid disease, endocrine tumors, or other hormone disturbances. Since most primary care providers do not see a large number of women with POI, they may not have enough experience to diagnose, answer questions about, or provide the best evaluation of your condition. In fact, most women report having visited several health care providers before receiving the diagnosis of POI. This means that it's very important for you to understand your body, note any changes or concerns, and seek a specialist if needed.

It is a mistake to assume that POI is the same as normal menopause except that it occurs earlier. There is a distinctive set of physical and emotional concerns when a woman's ovaries become insufficient at a young age. This includes a higher risk of cardiovascular disease and osteoporosis. Fertility is affected, and this is a major concern for many women with POI. Because young women with diminished ovarian function may see a return of ovulation periodically, approximately 5 to 10 percent of women with POI who have unprotected intercourse do become pregnant spontaneously. For others who want to become mothers or add to their families, many turn to assisted reproductive technologies, such as egg donation, embryo donation, surrogacy, or adoption.

Treatment

Though there is no cure for diminished ovarian function, many good treatment options are available that can alleviate symptoms and minimize complications. Most clinicians recommend that women with premature menopause, if they have no contraindications such as cancer, go on hormone therapy until they reach the age of fifty-one to fifty-two or the natural age at menopause.[15] (Therapy with transdermal estradiol and oral progesterone is one example.) More research is needed on the benefits and risks of hormone therapy for premature menopause, but some recent evidence supports the use of transdermal rather than oral estrogen for POI.[16]

Coping with early or premature menopause

Most women who experience early or premature menopause describe it as a shock. They suddenly feel "out of step" with other women their age and never expected to have to face these types of challenges and decisions at this point in their lives. It is very important to allow yourself to grieve and to have your emotions acknowledged and validated. A good support network can help you successfully manage the long-term impacts throughout your life. Increased support for women with premature menopause is becoming available. One example is Early Menopause (earlymenopause.com), a well-done noncommercial support website for women. Also visit the National Women's Health Center (womenshealth.gov/menopause/early-menopause).

IN TRANSLATION: MENOPAUSE IN OTHER CULTURES

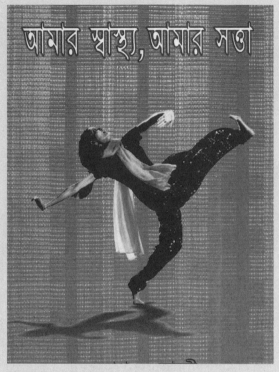

Bengali booklet.

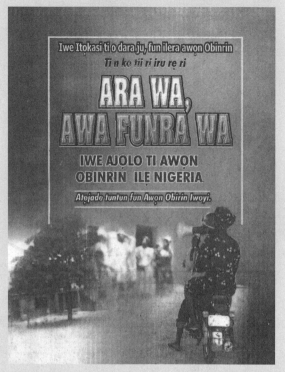

Nigerian booklet.

Group: Sanlaap (India) and Manavi (USA)

Country: India

Resource: "Aamaar Shaastha, Aamaar Sattaa" (My Health, My Self), a Bengali booklet based on *Our Bodies, Ourselves*

Websites: sanlaapindia.org; manavi.org

Group: Women for Empowerment, Development, and Gender Reform (WEDGR)

Country: Nigeria

Resources: Print and nonprint materials based on *Our Bodies, Ourselves* in pidgin English and Yoruba

Website: ourbodiesourselves.org/programs/network

"The effects of menopause on the sexual, reproductive health and lives of women [have] been our major work," says OBOS's partner in Nigeria, Women for Empowerment, Development, and Gender Reform (WEDGR).

In Nigeria, a primary goal of marriage is to have children. Women who do not have children are often blamed for infertility and ostracized by family and community. This attitude, which stems largely from a lack of information, also applies to postmenopausal women, who are no longer able to become pregnant.

In a survey conducted by WEDGR, 85 percent of men who did not have children and whose wives were approaching or in postmenopause freely admitted to having sex with other women with the intent to reproduce. The men were unaware that infertility can be ascribed to both men and women or that menopause is part of every woman's life cycle. After adapting and translating content from *Our Bodies, Ourselves* into pidgin English and Yoruba, WEDGR used the materials to educate the community about the social and biological impact of menopause and the health implications of unprotected sex. As a result of this outreach, there is a growing awareness of menopause as a natural stage, rather than a problem or taboo.

In comparison, OBOS's partner in India, Sanlaap, a feminist nongovernmental organization, reports that though gender segregation and restricted mobility are the norm for women throughout their childbearing years, women past menopause actually gain power and status within the family and society. This power is increased if they have given birth to sons. Older women are allowed more freedom to interact with men. They are often seen as matriarchs and wise advisers in their families. In the rural contexts of West Bengal, a state on the eastern coast, older women often play the roles of arbiters and negotiators to resolve conflicts within and between families.

dency to gain weight during midlife is important for women's health because of the relationship between high body mass index (BMI) or high waist-to-hip ratio and high blood pressure and diabetes.[17] Women with a 35-inch or more waist are more likely to have metabolic changes that increase their risk of diabetes. The factor most consistently related to this midlife weight gain is a decrease in physical activity; exercising regularly can make a difference.

If weight gain has you feeling bad about your body and your looks, even questioning your sexual attractiveness, you are not alone. Many of us are working out a balance between staying fit and accepting our body as it changes.

EATING WELL

Although the same basic principles of healthful eating apply throughout life, nutritional requirements change somewhat with age. Good nutrition is essential to health, independence, and quality of life for women at midlife and older, and it is one of the major elements in suc-

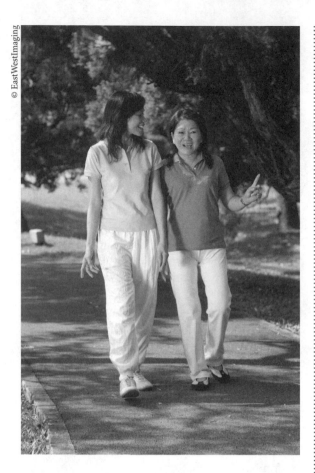
© EastWestImaging

cessful aging. Eating well can also help prevent or manage chronic diseases and even enhance sexuality.

Because women living in low-income communities face obstacles to locating and purchasing fresh fruits and vegetables and other healthful foods, some innovative projects are now taking on the critical issue of food equity. Having been ignored by food retailers for decades, inner-city neighborhoods suffer the most from our unequal food distribution system. Some communities have started urban farms and gardens as a way to improve health and to change the social landscape in both literal and figurative ways. See the documentary *Food Fight* (foodfightthedoc.com) for more details.

PREVENTING BONE LOSS AND OSTEOPOROSIS

Bone, like all the other living tissues in our bodies, is constantly replacing itself throughout life. If you are physically active and eat a healthful diet with adequate calcium during youth, you build bone when it matters most and give yourself a lifelong advantage. Some bone loss is normal in women and men as the years go by. By the mid-thirties, we start to lose bone more quickly than we replace it. Most women lose bone even faster from the start of irregular periods in perimenopause until four years after the final flow. Another period of increased bone loss occurs in our seventies. This is important because bone loss is associated with an increased risk for fracture—a potentially devastating injury as we age.

Osteoporosis—a condition of significantly low bone density—is a somewhat arbitrary designation of the World Health Organization (WHO) of a level of bone loss that is 2.5 standard deviations below the average bone density of a healthy young woman at her maximum bone density. Not all bone loss is osteoporosis. Many of us who develop osteoporosis will never know about it unless we break a bone. Publicity campaigns by drug companies that make medications to treat bone loss give the impression that *all* women will get osteoporosis unless we take medication (although the ads target mostly middle-class women, who are assumed to have money for these products). It is important to focus on preventing fractures, not just on taking drugs that might prevent osteoporosis.

Prevention

It is never too late to begin strengthening your bones. Weight-bearing exercise builds and maintains adequate bone density, muscle mass, and balance; yoga, jogging, strength training with weights, special back exercise regimens,

COMPARING CALCIUM SUPPLEMENTS

You can use calcium supplements to help fulfill the daily recommendation of 1,200 to 1,500 mg. Calcium supplements come in various forms.

COMPOUND	HOW MUCH CALCIUM	FORM	EFFECT ON DIGESTION
Calcium carbonate	40 percent calcium	Tablets	May upset stomach
Calcium citrate	21 percent calcium	Tablets	May be easier to digest
Calcium phosphate	39 percent calcium	Added to orange juice or soy milk	Easily absorbed without upsetting digestion

and physical therapy also help. Exercising in water provides beneficial resistance to movement while placing less stress on joints, but swimming itself is not weight-bearing, so it does not build bone strength.

What you eat and drink can help build bones (see below). Avoid harmful habits such as smoking, and drink no more than one alcoholic drink a day on a daily basis. Keep foods with low nutrient density ("empty calories") to a minimum.

You can also prevent early osteoporosis by avoiding, when possible, medical interventions that contribute to bone thinning, such as oophorectomy (removal of the ovaries). Women on steroids for more than three months, or on high doses of thyroid medication or some anti-seizure medications, are at increased risk for osteoporosis. The following commonly used drugs are also associated with an increased risk of osteoporosis: corticosteroid medications (long-term use), aromatase inhibitors to treat breast cancer (long-term use), a class of antidepressant medications called selective serotonin reuptake inhibitors (SSRIs), the cancer treatment drug methotrexate, the acid-blocking drugs called proton pump inhibitors, and aluminum-containing antacids.[18]

Many fractures are preventable with commonsense safety measures. These include wearing low-heeled shoes, using handrails, and getting rid of scatter rugs. For a complete list of indoor and outdoor safety tips, see "Preventing Falls and Broken Bones" at the National Osteoporosis Foundation (nof.org/aboutosteoporosis).

Eating to Limit Bone Loss and Reduce Fractures

Calcium

Calcium helps prevent bone loss, which can lead to osteoporosis, and is critical for skeletal health. Since women over age thirty-five absorb calcium less easily, it is important to exercise more (necessary to absorb calcium) and get enough calcium in your diet, along with other nutrients that help your body absorb calcium. If you can't tolerate milk products, owing to lactose intolerance or other sensitivities, don't worry; many other sources of calcium are available, such as dark leafy greens, beans, and calcium-fortified orange juice. Interestingly, long-term studies consistently show *no* reduction in fractures for people with high consumption of dairy products. (The addition of retinol/vitamin A to milk is currently being considered as a possible explanation for this. See ncbi.nlm.nih.gov/pubmed/20599880.)

Vitamin D

Many experts suggest 800 and up to 1,200 IU of vitamin D a day for optimal calcium and phosphorus absorption.[19]* The main sources of vitamin D are sunshine, oily fish such as salmon and mackerel, fortified milk, and cereal. Yogurt and cheese, though good sources of calcium, contain no vitamin D. As we age, we absorb less of the vitamin D we eat, and those of us who live in the north or spend much of the day indoors don't get much sun exposure. Vitamin D deficiency, which is common in adults in the United States, can both cause and increase osteoporosis. Blood tests for vitamin D levels are available. Especially if you live in a northern climate, you may want to take a vitamin D supplement or combination calcium/vitamin D pills.[20]

Magnesium

Many researchers recommend that calcium be balanced with magnesium in a two-to-one ratio, although healthy adults without serious bowel disease are not magnesium-deficient. If your magnesium level drops lower, calcium will not be absorbed as well. Fruits and vegetables contain magnesium, as do some calcium supplements.

Other Nutrients

Although most prevention messages have focused on calcium and vitamin D, recent research has shown that several additional nutrients and food constituents are important. And supplementing with calcium and vitamin D has not always produced as good results as hoped for, suggesting that other factors need to be kept in mind. Eating fruits and vegetables has emerged as an important way to protect bone health. Several other nutrients, including magnesium (discussed above), potassium, vitamin C, vitamin K, some of the B vitamins, and carotenoids, have emerged as more important than researchers initially thought. In June 2010, *Osteoporosis International* published a study showing that the antioxidant lycopene (from tomato juice or supplements) can help to reduce bone loss.[21]

The thinking has changed on protein: Rather than having a negative effect on bone, protein intake appears to benefit bones in older adults. Drinking carbonated soft drinks such as cola is associated with negative effects, and modest alcohol intake (one glass of wine per day) shows positive effects on bone density, particularly in older women. The current data on diet and bone health support balanced diets with plenty of fruits and vegetables, adequate dairy products and other protein foods, and minimal consumption of unhealthful foods with low nutrient density.

MEDICAL APPROACHES TO OSTEOPOROSIS PREVENTION AND TREATMENT

Do You Need a Bone Density Test?

The recommended age for beginning periodic bone density tests is sixty-five, although if you and your health care provider identify risk factors for osteoporosis you may choose to be tested sooner. The dual-energy X-ray absorptiometry (DEXA) test compares your bone density with that of a healthy young adult. Following this test, some of us are told we have osteopenia, which refers to bone loss that is usual with aging and could potentially lead to osteoporosis but presents no immediate danger. This diagnosis is controversial among women's health activists, as it has led to early and unnecessary medications. (See p. 531.)

Bone testing is useful primarily for those at high risk, and even then it might not improve

---

* Officially recommended levels remain lower than this. Despite calls by some experts for people to take in much more vitamin D, a November 2010 report from the Institute of Medicine (IOM) declared that most people are getting enough of the nutrient each day. The IOM did bump up the recommended dietary allowance of vitamin D from the amount cited in its last report, released thirteen years ago: 600 international units (IU) of vitamin D for people age 51 to 70 (up from 400 IU recommended in 1997), and 800 IU daily for those over 70 (up from 600 IU).

outcomes. Early detection is meaningless unless women learn how to reduce bone loss and make necessary changes in eating habits, exercise, and lifestyle patterns. Since these changes can benefit all women, we should be doing them anyway.

Medical Treatments for Osteoporosis

Hormone treatments—both estrogen alone and estrogen-progestin combinations—have been shown to reduce the risk of osteoporosis and bone fracture while women are taking them. The protective effect of estrogen disappears within two years after the cessation of hormone therapy (HT), and for those who stop HT, the short-term risk of hip fractures increases compared with that of women who stay on HT.[23] Since the results of the Women's Health Initiative (WHI) study were announced in 2002 with a finding that one popular hormone therapy can cause breast cancer, blood clots, and stroke (see below), a search has been on for alternatives.

Many women with thinning bones have been prescribed bisphosphonates—a new class of nonhormonal drug that slows bone breakdown—in the hope that they would be safer than hormone treatments. There was a hope not only that women with osteoporosis could use this medication to prevent further bone loss but also that it would prevent osteoporosis. All bisphosphonates have been shown to decrease spine fractures, compared with a placebo, and some of them decrease hip fractures, compared with a placebo. However, they can make bones denser but more brittle and have been associated with very rare but severe jaw ulcers and deterioration and unusual fractures in the middle of the thighbone.

In October 2010, the FDA announced that bisphosphonates used to treat osteoporosis must include a warning about risk of atypical thigh fractures. (Drugs mentioned in the FDA report are Fosamax, Fosamax Plus D, Actonel, Actonel with Calcium, Boniva, Atelvia, and Reclast.) The FDA also acknowledged that problems with bisphosphonates may increase with length of use, and it encouraged health care providers to "consider periodic reevaluation of the need for continued bisphosphonate therapy, particularly in patients who have been treated for over five years."

If you are taking bisphosphonates, be sure to inform your dentist before any dental surgery (but don't delay if you have a toothache or abscess or another urgent need); also, report new jaw, hip, or thigh pain to your health care provider. If you are considering starting on bisphosphonates, compare the latest data on their risks with the risks of other forms of osteoporosis prevention and treatment, including a bone-healthy lifestyle and monitoring of bone density. Understanding the risks and benefits of these drugs is definitely a work in progress. No one who is now eighty took bisphosphonates in her fifties, for example, since they were not approved until the 1990s.

Selective estrogen receptor modulators (SERMs), such as the drug raloxifene (sold as Evista), can prevent bone loss and reduce the risk of spine (but not hip) fracture without the increased risk of breast or uterine cancer that HT has. However, raloxifene may increase hot flashes and creates a risk of blood clots similar to the risk with pill estrogens. It is not a good choice for women with high risk of blood clot or stroke.

A mixed estrogen-progestin-testosterone-derived steroid called tibolone is widely used in European countries to treat hot flashes and night sweats and to increase bone density. Tibolone has a side effect similar to estrogen in pill form: it increases the risk of stroke in older women. The "Million Women" British study has shown that it increases the risks of endometrial cancer,[24] and it has been shown to increase recurrence in women with breast cancer.[25] Whether tibolone increases or decreases new cancers is still being debated. Unless there is conclusive reassuring evidence on this point, tibolone is unlikely to be approved for use in the United States.

Since the risk of debilitating fractures becomes significant after age seventy, women who start taking any of these drugs during perimenopause or in early postmenopause will probably have to take them for decades for the benefit of reduced fractures to become apparent. Further research into the long-term effects of these medications is needed.

SEEKING CARE AND TREATMENT FOR PERIMENOPAUSAL DISCOMFORTS

COMPLEMENTARY/ALTERNATIVE THERAPIES

Some women turn to alternative therapies for help during and after perimenopause, including herbs or botanicals, such as black cohosh, and food supplements, such as soy products.

The same questions we ask about drugs need to be posed for any complementary and alternative therapy: What is the specific reason to take it? Are there well-designed, sufficiently large randomized trials showing that it is effective for the recommended purpose? What are the side effects and harms associated with it? Has it been recommended to you by someone who may earn money from its sales?

Often these products are touted as a natural way to cope with discomforts without studies that adequately demonstrate their value. These remedies may not be produced in consistent strengths or doses because they are not regulated the way FDA-approved drugs are. They may not be safe for everyone. Be sure to tell your health care providers if you are taking alternative remedies; seemingly harmless remedies such as Saint-John's-wort or valerian can interact with other medications.

A plant extract called black cohosh is one of the most widely sold menopause treatments (it is found in over-the-counter products such as Remifemin). It appears to be reasonably safe for those who don't have liver problems,[26] and some studies show benefits, but a large study by the National Center for Complementary and Alternative Medicine (NCCAM) found it no more effective than a placebo.[27] Ginseng, evening primrose oil, dong quai, and vitamin E do not appear to reduce hot flashes.[28] A full review of the evidence can be found on the NCCAM menopause page (nccam.nih.gov/health/menopause). NCCAM summarizes a 2005 National Institutes of Health (NIH) State-of-the-Science conference on the management of menopause-related symptoms by saying, "There is very little high-quality scientific evidence about the effectiveness and long-term safety of CAM (complementary and alternative medicine) therapies for menopausal symptoms. More research is needed."[29]

One thing researchers agree on is that soy in food has weak estrogenic effects; these phytoestrogens have shown mixed results in studies of hot flashes and vaginal dryness—probably because of the diversity of products as well as individual variations in how women respond to soy. Some oncologists have concerns about soy for breast cancer survivors. Although the data are not clear, food-based soy (rather than supplements) is most likely safe. For more information on how to evaluate CAM therapies, see "Complementary and Alternative Therapies," p. 674.

PERIMENOPAUSE/MENOPAUSE AND WESTERN MEDICINE

In much of U.S. culture, natural biological transitions such as childbirth or menopause are considered by many in the medical field to be medical conditions likely to need treatment through drugs or surgery. Ironically, this medicalization can lead to both overtreatment and undertreatment in perimenopause. Overtreatment comes when providers prescribe (and we ask for) medications for every kind of perimenopausal or postmenopausal problem, when in many cases a healthful lifestyle and self-care are safer and may well be more effective. When joints stiffen and ache, for example, this may be a result of aging or lack of adequate stretching and exercise, not just hormone imbalances. On the other hand, undertreatment is likely when we and our providers attribute almost every symptom we experience to perimenopause, rather than thoroughly investigating symptoms that may point to serious conditions.

FINDING THE RIGHT HEALTH CARE PROVIDER

One of the most important things you can do to improve your health care is to establish a relationship with a health care practitioner or clinician whose philosophy resembles yours, who has pertinent up-to-date expertise, and who is open-minded. If possible, do so *before* perimenopause begins. Women's physical needs are as varied and individual as their personalities. You need a provider who will listen to what you know and feel and who will take the time to answer questions completely and without prejudice. If your current practitioner won't do that, ask friends, coworkers, and other health care providers to recommend someone else. If you can't change practitioner, at least speak up, ask questions, and insist on participating fully in all decisions concerning your care.

For those of us who have a particularly difficult menopause transition, finding a clinician who specializes in perimenopause and postmenopause can be helpful. The North American Menopause Society (NAMS) has a certification process for such clinicians, and its website (menopause.org) can give you more information. NAMS clinicians tend to be practitioners of mainstream medicine. Some CAM providers have experience helping women navigate the menopause transition with other approaches. If alternative practitioners suggest non-FDA-approved and otherwise less conventional treatments, be sure to request evidence of dependable research to back up the recommendation before making your decisions.

INSURANCE AND ACCESS TO HEALTH CARE

National health care legislation enacted in 2010—the Patient Protection and Affordable Care Act—has led to better coverage of certain services used by peri- and postmenopausal women. Many midlife women in the United States have experienced a gap in health care insurance coverage, being too young for Medicare (under age sixty-five) and not quite poor enough for Medicaid. The United States is the only industrialized country in the world that does not provide access to basic health care for all. Because most health care insurance is tied to benefits offered on a voluntary basis by employers, unemployed people and even many workers are uninsured. Many women lose health care insurance coverage after divorce. It is increasingly difficult to keep jobs as we grow older. Then we are faulted for needing so-called entitlements such as Social Security, Medicare, and disability benefits, though we may have been contributing to these funds for many years. Medicare is criticized as being too expensive, when it should be considered a model for a universal, single-payer health care insurance system. See Chapter 21, "Our Later Years," and Chapter 26, "The Politics of Women's Health," for more.

NONHORMONAL MEDICAL TREATMENT OPTIONS

For those of us who have tried the nonmedical approaches, choose not to use hormone therapy (HT), and still have problems that seriously disrupt our work, sleep, or relationships, there are nonhormonal treatments that address many of the discomforts of perimenopause and beyond. Some of these are FDA-approved and others are considered off-label, which means clinicians may prescribe them for unapproved uses.

Drug companies now heavily market several nonhormonal medications to treat many conditions that were previously treated with estrogen. These include bisphosphonates for bone loss (see above for serious risks of bisphosphonates); anti-inflammatory drugs for joint pain, heavy flow, and cramps; antidepressants for hot flashes and mood problems; sleeping pills for insomnia; statins for high cholesterol; and so on. Many of these medications are even less well understood than HT for long-term use. If you have distressing symptoms but decide to forgo hormone therapy, ask a knowledgeable clinician for other options—but be aware of what else is in your medicine cabinet and the potential interaction risks.

HORMONE THERAPY— YES OR NO?

For many women, nonmedical self-help approaches can alleviate the discomforts of perimenopause and beyond. For others, a balance of nonmedical and medical solutions is needed, and well-informed health care providers can be important partners in thinking through the options. We need to be well informed as consumers, because there are many unanswered questions about the safety of hormone therapy, which is one of the primary medical treatments offered.

What follow are sections on the history and politics of hormone therapy, what we know so far about research on safety issues, and a discussion of the options that may be presented to you.*

HORMONE THERAPIES: A BRIEF HISTORY AND POLITICS

You may have heard about the Women's Health Initiative (WHI), a large study of HT use by women during and after the menopausal transition. The WHI study ended three years early (in 2002), because it had already documented serious health risks to women from certain commonly used forms of HT. Since that time, there have been ongoing discussion and contro-

Each woman considering whether to use hormone therapy should educate herself, find an informed health care provider who is hopefully not overly influenced by drug company marketing, and carefully weigh the risks and benefits for her own situation. According to most current expert advice in the United States,[30] if you decide to use HT, use the smallest dose for the shortest amount of time possible, taper off gradually when you stop, and review the regimen regularly with your health care provider.

If you already have a history of heart disease, blood clots, or breast cancer, you will probably be advised against taking HT. Having a family history of clotting problems or breast cancer (especially premenopausal breast cancer) may also put you at more at risk of complications of hormone therapy. Review your personal and family history with your clinician.

versy about what the WHI study actually proved about the dangers of hormone therapy and what it didn't. To understand what the WHI study can mean for health care decisions before and after menopause, the following history may be helpful. The hormone therapy story illustrates many lessons about medical care, science, business, and profit making in medicine and women's health. For study findings, visit the National Institutes of Health (www.nhlbi.nih.gov/whi).

In 1942, the FDA approved Premarin, an estrogen product made from pregnant mare's urine, for treatment of hot flashes. Drug companies soon began marketing estrogen as a magic pill not only for short-term relief from

---

* Until recently, taking hormones for perimenopausal and menopausal discomforts was called hormone replacement therapy (HRT). This term made it sound as though menopausal women are missing something—that we are somehow deficient without the hormones we had in youth. Yet most hormone therapy prescribed today does *not* provide the same levels of hormones that our ovaries were making during our menstruating years. The term "hormone therapy" (HT) avoids the implication that all women should be replacing something essential that is now missing.

hot flashes, night sweats, and vaginal dryness but also for maintaining youthfulness, preventing diseases associated with aging, and keeping women "feminine forever"—without adequate evidence about longer-term effects.* Then, in 1975, it became clear that estrogen administered without progesterone caused a dramatic increase in cancer of the uterine lining (endometrial cancer)—the first big shock about hormone therapy. After that time, progestins (synthetic forms of progesterone) were added to standard hormone therapy for women with a uterus, to prevent overgrowth of the uterine lining that can lead to cancer.

Barbara Seaman's 1977 book *Women and the Crisis in Sex Hormones* suggested that the hormone treatment currently in use for menopause could cause breast cancer, stroke, and blood clots. Although Seaman and the growing women's health movement warned against the overpromotion of hormones, flawed research and drug company marketing efforts through the 1990s pushed HT for the prevention of a variety of ills, from cardiovascular disease and osteoporosis to Alzheimer's disease, colon cancer, tooth loss, and macular degeneration. Estrogen-based HT for perimenopause and menopause became the most prescribed drug treatment in the country.

In the 1990s, some observational studies (in which women who chose to take or not take HT were followed over time) suggested that HT prevented heart disease, while other studies suggested that HT increased the risk of breast cancer and blood clots. Most medical professionals, including many who received funding from the pharmaceutical industry, advocated hormones for all women, reasoning that many

more women died from heart disease than from breast cancer. (In the observational studies, healthier women were more likely to take hormones, and that could skew the results; this also biased physicians' prescribing practices.)

The first randomized control trial to challenge the theory that HT was beneficial for heart disease was the Heart and Estrogen/Progestin Replacement Study (HERS), a study of women with cardiovascular disease in which older women with heart disease took HT or a placebo. In 1998, HERS found no benefit of the top-selling HT formulation for preventing cardiovascular events.[31] There remained a critical absence of dependable research to tell us whether or not HT prevented heart disease and should be recommended to all women.

In 1993, the Women's Health Initiative set out to answer that question. WHI enrolled women age fifty to seventy-nine in a thirteen-year, large randomized trial of Prempro, the most widely used combination of estrogen and progestin. In 2002, the trial was stopped early because it had demonstrated more breast cancer, stroke, cardiovascular disease, and blood clots in the women on hormones. Continuation of the study was considered unethical because of these effects, even through the same women had less colon cancer and fewer fractures. The estrogen-alone arm of the study (which didn't prescribe a progestin because those women had had hysterectomies and didn't need progestin protection in their uterus) also showed an increase in blood clots and stroke, while fractures were prevented. No significant increase in breast cancer was shown for estrogen alone. Women on estrogen alone had no difference in colorectal cancer risk. Women sixty-five and older taking HT had no protection against mild cognitive impairment, and there was a small increased risk of dementia.

When the results of the WHI came out, many women felt outraged and baffled—especially

---

* Search "Robert Wilson" at ourbodiesourselves.org for more on Wilson's 1966 book, *Feminine Forever,* and the decades-long fascination with using synthetic estrogen for a wide spectrum of age-related conditions.

those who had been taking HT, sometimes for years—as the results seemed to indicate that they had been misled about both the benefits and the risks of the drugs. Many women stopped taking HT abruptly, preferring to return to hot flashes and other discomforts rather than continue with the medication.

There is significant debate about how to interpret many of the results of the WHI, and ongoing analyses of the large amount of data collected continue. One important limitation of the WHI was that it tested only Premarin, a synthetic estrogen made from the urine of pregnant mares, and PremPro, a combination of Premarin and the progestin Provera (medroxyprogesterone acetate). Those products were used at the time by the vast majority of U.S. women taking HT. (The choice of Premarin and PremPro for the WHI was in part the result of their product being donated by the company, Wyeth-Ayerst, now a part of Pfizer.) As a result, the WHI findings did not answer questions about the safety and effectiveness of other hormone formulations, regimens, and delivery methods (such as patches).

A third of the women in the WHI were in their fifties, making this the largest randomized controlled trial ever done of women in this age group. However, the majority of the participants were more than a decade past their final menstrual period, raising a question as to whether the trial's results apply only to older women. In fact, later analysis of the results for the more newly menopausal women showed a somewhat better safety profile.

The results of the WHI contributed to an evolution away from the concept that menopause begins a time of estrogen deficiency and that hormone "replacement" is a necessary thing. Rather, low levels of reproductive hormones after menopause are normal and may not be problematic.

Understanding of HT continues to change—and tomorrow's headline may contradict today's. In the meantime, decades of drug company ads and promotions have influenced both women and health care providers. You will see many claims being made in the coming years—both pro and con—about different products, including ones sold without a prescription that are unregulated by the FDA. Watch, too, for advertising that tries to redeem the image of PremPro in the minds of the public. Although it's true that the WHI study had many flaws, it's also true that horse estrogens and chemically altered progestins no longer appear to be the best option. Until research identifies the harms and benefits of the variety of available hormone regimens, women should be cautious about unproved claims.

The hormone controversy raises an important bioethical issue. Many of us believe that the standards for using unproved treatments on healthy populations should be more stringent than those for treating people who are ill and are willing to take risks in hopes of a cure. The marketing of bisphosphonates to women with osteopenia is an example of encouraging women to use drugs for a nondisease condition, as was the pre-WHI marketing of HT to women for prevention of possible future problems.

Perimenopause and menopause are not disease states; if we feel well, treatments should not be pushed on us. On the other hand, a certain number of women don't feel healthy during this time, and it's important to have options for treatment. Any type of medication—whether hormones or newer drugs such as bisphosphonates, antidepressants, and statins—may result in unanticipated negative effects, so every woman's decision to use hormones and other medications needs to be a personal, well-researched assessment of potential harms and benefits. And the decision needs to be revisited regularly as more is learned about the drugs and their effects.

HORMONES: NOT ALL THE SAME

Many people use the terms estrogen, hormones, and hormone therapy (or the outmoded "hormone replacement therapy") interchangeably, as though they are all the same thing. But in fact, research beginning with the WHI has revealed that there are types that pose more risk and some that may pose less. If you decide to use hormones, it's important to learn about the differences.

Many benefits and safety issues may turn out to depend on important details about the type of hormone, who's using it, in what form, and when. As you read through the following information, keep in mind that a great deal more research is needed before much can be said with 100 percent certainty about the risks and benefits of the many kinds of hormone therapy. And each of us is different, and may react differently, to HT.

Estrogens

The three major naturally occurring estrogens in women (made primarily by the ovaries) are: estradiol (es-tra-DYE-all), estriol, and estrone. Estradiol is the predominant estrogen during the pre- and perimenopausal years, whereas estrone predominates after menopause. Estriol is a weak human estrogen usually found in substantial amounts only during pregnancy. Some clinicians believe that estriol is safer for the breast than its more powerful cousin estradiol, but there aren't strong data that argue for or against using estriol. Estrone is produced when fat acts on adrenal estrogens after menopause—perhaps explaining why women with a high body mass index suffer from more estrogen-related cancers such as breast and endometrial.

The role of estrogen therapy in perimenopause is one of the many crucial issues on which there are many opinions and insufficient research. There are those who believe that because perimenopausal estrogen levels average higher than premenopausal levels and occasionally surge to double or triple those levels, estrogen-based therapy (including oral contraceptives) in perimenopause may not be safe and may cause harm.[32] On the other hand, there are clinicians who have extensive experience treating symptomatic perimenopausal women with oral contraceptives and other estrogens with apparently good effect.

Use with More Caution: Estrogen in Pill Form (Oral Estrogens)

Pills in which some estrogen comes from pregnant mares' urine (conjugated equine estrogens, brand name Premarin) are commonly used in the United States. Other oral estrogens contain the primary estrogen found in reproductive-age women (estradiol) synthesized in the lab from plants. When estrogen first came on the market decades ago, pills were the only option. But now we know that when the body processes oral estrogen through the liver, it stimulates the liver to make clotting proteins, which increase the chances of blood clots. Even with pills made of estradiol and not the urine of pregnant mares, the process of going through the liver converts the estradiol to other substances (such as estrone) and incites the liver to produce some detrimental proteins.

May Be a Better Choice: Estrogen Through the Skin

Some data now exist to support the view that estrogen given through the skin (transdermal estradiol) bypasses the liver and is less likely to cause blood clots and possibly strokes than oral preparations (pills), even if the pills are made of estradiol.[33] However, transdermal estrogen appears to carry the same breast cancer risk as oral estrogen.[34] Watch in 2011 or 2012 for the results of a large randomized study of newly menopausal women called Kronos Early Estrogen

Prevention Study (KEEPS) (see p. 545), which is comparing transdermal with oral estrogen.

Look for transdermal products that contain estradiol. This comes in estrogen gels (such as EstroGel and Divigel), a spray (Evamist), and many patches. These all appear to have similar risk profiles, so the choice is based on convenience and cost (this can vary depending on insurance coverege). Two benefits of the patch: Most can be cut to adjust or slowly taper your dose, and the patch delivers even levels of hormones twenty-four hours a day. If the patch you are prescribed causes skin irritation, ask to try another one.

Note: Over-the-counter creams in supermarkets and health food stores claiming to be estrogen are not permitted to contain real estradiol, but they may contain the weaker estrogen called estriol. Strengths and standardization vary.

Another Option: Estrogen Vaginal Ring
A soft, plastic-like ring releases estradiol into the vagina slowly over the course of three months. This is an option for women who are comfortable enough with their bodies to insert it (it's not much different from inserting a tampon). One type, called Estring, is meant to affect primarily the vagina, for women with only vaginal symptoms such as dryness; the other, Femring, is a higher dose meant to reach the whole body and work systemically.

Progestogens (Progesterone-Type Products): Natural and Synthetic
Women with a uterus who go on estrogen therapy should use a progestogen (progesterone-like product) along with estrogen. Progesterone mimics the work of the body's progesterone in preventing overgrowth of the uterine lining that may lead to endometrial cancer. Progesterone is also used on its own by some practitioners to treat discomforts and irregularities caused by the reduced progesterone levels in perimenopause. (See "What About Progesterone Used Alone?" p. 540.)

Some progestogens are bioidentical—meaning they're the same as in the human body—while others, called progestins, are chemically altered synthetic versions that may resemble progesterone only in how they change the uterine lining and preserve a pregnancy. (See "Bioidentical Hormones and Compounding Pharmacies," p. 541, for more discussion.)

Use with More Caution: Medroxyprogesterone Acetate (Provera)
In the Women's Health Initiative controlled trial and in large observational studies from England and France, this synthetic progestin given with estrogen increased the risk of breast cancer or appeared linked to increased breast cancer risk. Provera is also in the combination product PremPro and is heavily marketed for HT in the United States.

A Progestin in What Is Probably a Safer Form: Progestin-releasing IUD
The progestin-releasing IUD (Mirena) releases a low dose of progestin that works primarily within the uterus. This is an effective treatment for heavy bleeding in many women, and because it releases a low dose that works locally, it avoids some of the risks and side effects of progestin taken in pill form. Some women do report systemic effects from Mirena such as headaches and acne. Some clinicians prescribe Mirena to deliver progestins in women on hormone therapy, but it is not FDA-approved for this. For more information on Mirena, see "Intrauterine Devices," p. 238.

May Be a Better Choice: Bioidentical Micronized Progesterone, Orally or Vaginally
For many years no one knew how to make natural, non-chemically-altered progesterone

survive the digestive tract, so pharmaceutical companies invented chemically altered versions that not only survived the digestive tract but had the profitability advantage of being patentable. It wasn't until the 1980s that researchers discovered that they could grind lab-created progesterone extremely fine (micronize it) and put it in oil in a gelcap to keep it from being broken down by the digestive tract.

Prometrium, the first (and so far only) micronized progesterone product to be approved in the United States, was approved in 1998. By that time, Provera and other chemically altered progestins were well established as standard, so the use of micronized progesterone is, to date, less widespread in the United States than in Europe. Bioidentical micronized progesterone is molecularly the same as your body makes and may have a better breast safety profile than its synthetic progestin cousins such as Provera.

Prometrium comes dissolved in peanut oil in a 100-mg or 200-mg gelcap. (For women with peanut allergy, a compounding pharmacist—see below—can dissolve it in olive oil instead, with similar doses and absorption.) A third option, a vaginal progesterone gel called Crinone, is extremely expensive in the United States.

The WHI showed an increase in breast cancer for estrogen and progesterone used together, though not for estrogen used alone; therefore, many suspect progesterone of causing breast cancer even though only the progestin Provera was used in the study. However, in a very large observational study of European women, Prometrium given with estrogen was not associated with an increased risk of breast cancer, while estrogen alone and estrogen with progestin were. This fits with what we know from animal, human, and cell studies, which show that chemically altered progestins have different effects than progesterone does on how cells grow, insulin sensitivity, and other risks of breast cancer.[35]

Reactions to progesterone vary—a dose that's calming to one woman may make another feel mildly depressed or as though she has PMS—so experimenting with different routes (oral or vaginal) and doses may be necessary. Prometrium capsules can be used vaginally; this results in a slower, steadier release of hormones and has less sedative effect.

What About Progesterone Used Alone?

Some clinicians think the waning levels of progesterone relative to levels of estrogen during perimenopause are a major factor in the symptoms of perimenopause, and that progesterone therapy is often the best approach. Both the lab-made "natural" progesterone and lab-made progestins can help manage the erratic bleeding in perimenopause.

In addition, there is recent randomized controlled trial evidence that Prometrium in a dose of 300 mg just before bed decreases hot flashes in healthy normal-weight postmenopausal women more than a placebo.[36] The Centre for Menstrual Cycle and Ovulation Research is just starting a similar trial for hot-flash treatment in perimenopausal women.

When taken by mouth, Prometrium acts as a sedative and is helpful for increasing sleep time and reducing night waking. (For this purpose, one practitioner recommends a 300-mg dose, which keeps the blood level in the normal range for the progesterone-rich second half of the cycle; another recommends trying the 100-mg dose first.) Take it right before bed to avoid dizziness—the sedative effects usually wear off by morning. If you are sleep-deprived when you start it, you may feel sluggish or tired in the morning because your body is trying to catch up on lost sleep.

Use with More Caution: Progesterone Cream

Progesterone creams made in compounding pharmacies (see sidebar) are made with natural progesterone, which may have a better safety/

BIOIDENTICAL HORMONES AND COMPOUNDING PHARMACIES

The term "bioidentical" has been used to refer to hormones that are the chemical equivalent of those made by women's bodies—notably estradiol, estrone, and estriol (instead of horse estrogens) and progesterone (instead of the chemically altered progestins). Although chemically synthesized in a lab from plant-based building blocks, these hormones can be considered more natural to women than horse estrogens or progestins that have been chemically altered to make them digestible and patentable. The oral micronized progesterone called Prometrium is an example of a bioidentical hormone.

Many bioidenticals are made by compounding pharmacists, who mix hormones into gelcaps, gels, or creams. The hormones in many compounded products (estradiol and progesterone) are also found in FDA-approved products, whereas additional hormones such as estriol and testosterone are found only in compounded products.

Theoretically, both compounded and pharmaceutical industry products are acceptable options; however, the quality control of compounded products varies widely. In the United States, an industry has arisen to promote and commercialize bioidentical hormones and a particular approach to HT that includes compounded products that are not FDA-approved. Promoters of compounded products often recommend frequent monitoring of hormone levels with saliva or blood tests. However, hormone level tests are not a particularly useful way of judging how a therapy is working. A better gauge is how a person feels in response to the therapy.

If you choose to use compounded hormones because your provider suggests a hormone such as estriol or testosterone that is not available in a commercial product or because you need a different dose than is commercially available, choose a licensed pharmacist who has taken the Professional Compounding Centers of America course in compounding of medications and who is registered with the Pharmacy Compounding Accreditation Board.

risk profile than progestin. However, it's difficult to know the right dose because blood levels do not reflect the actual exposure of tissues. When used as part of estrogen-progesterone hormone therapy, progesterone creams used instead of oral progesterone may not be in a high enough dose to balance the estrogen and protect the vaginal lining from cancer, so they are not a particularly safe option. It's possible, however, that progesterone cream used alone can be effective for hot-flash treatment in menopause.[37]

When progesterone creams are sold over the counter and not prescribed, there is no quality control, and the cream may contain anywhere from too much progesterone to none at all.

Combination Products

There are several combination HT products with both estrogen and progestin (none contains progesterone). Although they seem convenient, they provide clinicians with less opportunity for careful individual dosing of each hormone.

Use with More Caution: PremPro

PremPro, the most widely used HT in the United States for many years, is a combination of Premarin (conjugated horse estrogens) and Provera (a progestin). The WHI trials showed that women taking estrogens with progestins by mouth significantly increased their risk of strokes and blood clots in the lungs or legs, with a trend toward increased breast cancer. A memory substudy of the WHI found that women sixty-five and older taking PremPro had a heightened risk of developing dementia.[38]

Convenient Though Not Proved Safer: Patches

Combination estrogen/progestin patches, such as CombiPatch and Climara Pro, contain a synthetic male hormone–derived progestin (norethindrone acetate or levonorgestrel) with transdermal estrogen. Though they have not been proved to be safer than oral combinations of estrogen with progestin, some women use patches because of convenience and because continuous absorption may provide more effective control of the discomforts for which the therapy is being used.

IT'S YOUR DECISION IN THE END

It's your decision whether to take hormones. Consider your own history, values, health status, and preferences, as well as what's known and not known about harms and benefits. Keep up with new research findings. Women can have quite different reactions to the same hormonal regimen and what is good for some women may not be good for others. Furthermore, what is best for a population of women may not be best for an individual—thus the importance of each woman weighing both the knowns and the unknowns in making her own decision.

Keep the risks in perspective. For most women, smoking, poor diet, and lack of exercise are the most important risk factors for heart disease and osteoporosis. You can change those. Ask for help from your friends, family, and health care provider to support better habits.

If you decide to stop taking hormones, tapering off slowly may minimize the return of discomfort.

RESEARCH ON MIDLIFE WOMEN'S HEALTH

Until recently, medical research paid little attention to the health concerns of aging women. Even today, it focuses on the medical aspects of peri- and postmenopause, as though reproductive organs were the center of a woman's life. It continues to overlook the basic biology of aging, occupational and environmental damage, racial and ethnic differences, and the influence of socioeconomic factors on our health. Studies are often designed and funded by corporate interests rather than objective researchers, and tend to focus on drugs rather than nonmedical interventions. They often neglect the needs of women of color, undermining the ability of health care practitioners to provide appropriate care. Three important studies are under way to remedy this long-standing neglect.

The Study of Women's Health Across the Nation (SWAN) (www.swanstudy.org) is the first major longitudinal study of women of different racial and ethnic backgrounds as they transition through menopause. Since 1994, about 3,300 U.S. women from diverse backgrounds—white, African American, Hispanic, Chinese, and Japanese—have participated in SWAN at seven centers around the United States. The study examines psychological, social, and economic factors, in addition to health and medical com-

KEEPING UP WITH NEW RESEARCH

To keep up with new information and research findings on perimenopause and menopause, visit the websites of the following organizations. For more on how to understand study findings, see Chapter 23, "Navigating the Health Care System."

The Centre for Menstrual Cycle and Ovulation Research: cemcor.ubc.ca

National Institutes of Health (NIH): nih.gov

National Women's Health Information Center: womenshealth.gov/menopause

American Menopause Foundation: americanmenopause.org

National Women's Health Network: nwhn.org

The North American Menopause Society* (NAMS): menopause.org

Society for Menstrual Cycle Research: menstruationresearch.org

* The North American Menopause Society has strong ties to the pharmaceutical industry, but many of its members have tried to minimize the direct influence of drug companies over the content of NAMS educational programs.

ponents, including ovarian aging, its effects on bone and body composition, and risk factors for cardiovascular disease.

SWAN has generated a wealth of information about how women age. In 2010, the women in SWAN were fifty-six to sixty-six years old, and most had transitioned into postmenopause. By following various health issues, including diabetes, osteoporosis and fractures, osteoarthritis, heart disease, and depression, SWAN will continue to deepen our understanding of how menopause and other factors may play a role in later disease, disability, and quality of life, with the goal of finding better ways to prevent disease and maintain the health of older women.[39]

The Black Women's Health Study (BWHS) (bu.edu/bwhs), funded by the National Cancer Institute and administered by the Slone Epidemiology Center at Boston University School of Medicine, enrolled 59,000 African-American women in 1995. The focus of the study is to identify and evaluate causes and preventives of cancers and other serious illness for African-American women. Although it focuses primarily on younger women, it is also looking at conditions more typical of midlife and older women, such as cardiovascular disease, diabetes, and breast cancer, which affect black women earlier.

The BWHS has identified modifiable risk factors for both breast cancer[40] and type 2 diabetes.[41] Mortality rates of breast cancer are greater in black women than white women. The BWHS found that the use of menopausal hormones was associated with an increased risk of breast cancer, as has also been found in white women. A high intake of vegetables, especially cruciferous vegetables such as broccoli and collard greens, was associated with a reduced risk of breast cancer. Future research in the BWHS will address the causes of urinary incontinence, another condition that affects older women. BWHS has been funded through 2013.[42]

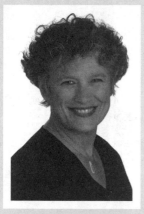

JERILYNN PRIOR

The endocrinologist and clinician-scientist Jerilynn Prior, M.D., is founder and director of the Centre for Menstrual Cycle and Ovulation Research at the University of British Columbia. She is a key contributor to recent research exploring the significance of higher estrogen and declining progesterone levels in perimeno-pause. She studies the use of progesterone in its bioidentical, oral micronized form to treat severe hot flashes and other disruptive discomforts experienced by women in perimenopause and beyond. She works to counter the commonly held belief that perimenopause is a time of estrogen deficiency and questions the appropriateness and safety of estrogen therapy during this time. Her work, much of which you can find at cemcor.ubc.ca, runs counter to many of the conventional views of peri- and postmenopause.

In speaking out for "a newer, clearer meaning" for the word "menopause" and arguing against use of the term "postmenopause" for the last third of a woman's life, Jerilynn offers insight into what might motivate a scientist and clinician to swim so hard against the tides of established thinking.

What we currently have is outdated language about women that reenforces our "deficiencies" as women. Why not, as women, start making language that fits our experiences and isn't disease-oriented? Why subject ourselves to those physicians who want to give us routine estrogen treatment in perimenopause and beyond, treatment we may not need at all?

It is long past time for a revision of outmoded language about midlife. I could cite instances from at least a dozen scientific articles that use the terms—menopause, menopausal transition, perimenopause and FMP—in mutually contradictory ways. That is not science—it is confusion. Who does confusion serve? Certainly not women.

The actual final menstrual flow can't be determined to be final for a further year, so why give it a name or initials? I remember my final, final flow very well because it came 14 months after my last "final" flow. I had cramps and sore breasts for weeks on end and began to wonder what on earth was happening to me. But, nevertheless, that flow was a non-event. I celebrated being menopausal when one further full year had passed. I don't want to be POST a non-event for the rest of my life.

Though this edition of *Our Bodies, Ourselves* sticks with the words and usages currently in practice—perimenopause, menopause, and postmenopause—Jerilynn Prior's scientific work on behalf of women has a passion and intelligence that suggests that these changes may yet come.

The Kronos Early Estrogen Prevention Study (KEEPS) (keepstudy.org) includes 729 newly menopausal women of ethnic makeup intentionally similar to the women in the WHI study, with 70 percent non-Hispanic Caucasian, 8 percent African American, and 7 percent Hispanic. This large randomized study is comparing a low dose of the estrogen pills used in the WHI study (Premarin), a transdermal estrogen (a patch), and a placebo. (Those receiving active estrogen will also be given oral micronized progesterone to avoid increasing the risk of uterine cancer.) In effect, KEEPS is trying HT using what many now believe to be the safest approach.

A limit of KEEPS is that it is studying only disease markers such as lipid levels and calcium in the heart and arteries, not heart attacks and strokes. But as many researchers now believe that transdermal estrogen may not increase the risk of thromboembolic events, a risk with oral estrogen, KEEPS findings could be quite significant. (For more on what's known about the risks and benefits of transdermal estrogen, see "Hormones: Not All the Same" on page 538.) Results should be available in 2011 or 2012.

HORMONE TOPICS FOR FURTHER STUDY

Are pills that use estrogen synthesized in the lab from plant substances safer than pills synthesized from the urine of pregnant mares? Are nonoral modes of administration safer because they avoid metabolism by the liver? We have too few conclusive answers because no blinded randomized trials have yet directly compared these products head-to-head. Given the high cost and large numbers needed for such trials, none is likely to be performed soon.

Two practicing gynecologists and an endocrinologist who contributed to this chapter wrote the following wish list of further studies they'd like to see. These items for further study give a sense of how much still needs to understood.

- Head-to-head comparison of safety and effectiveness of transdermal versus oral estrogen.
- Birth control pill use during perimenopause: Does it suppress the estrogen produced by the body or not?
- Vaginally applied estrogen: Does it improve or worsen perimenopausal urologic symptoms such as incontinence? How about systemic estrogen? What systemic estrogen levels result from vaginally applied estrogen?
- Head-to-head comparison of the safety and effectiveness of estriol and estradiol when used vaginally.
- The mechanism of hot flashes and nonhormonal treatments for them.
- The role of progesterone in perimenopause, in bone formation and loss, and in treatments for perimenopausal discomforts.

CONCLUSION

Perimenopause, during which our fertility is ending, ushers in what many call postmenopause, a new stage of life that often spans several decades in which our identity and value go well beyond our biologically based reproductive capacity. In postmenopause, we may rethink our roles and find new kinds of creativity and productivity, a new relationship to our bodies and sexuality, and new configurations of family and friends and of work and meaningful activities.

The menopausal transition, in spite of its physical trials for some, offers us an opportunity to think about what we want in the next phase of our lives. By finding and giving support among friends and women our age at work or in support groups, we can share experiences and information, especially about the more difficult aspects of perimenopause. Perimenopause and menopause need to be discussed. There is no need to feel isolated as we go through this life episode. A woman who joined a support group says:

There's a lot of mutual help; people really listen to each other and laugh a lot. Now I don't worry about menopause or growing older the way I used to.

Many women are also turning to websites and blogs for information, advice, and support. Organizations are cropping up that recognize the importance of midlife and the older years as a time of engagement, contribution, and advocacy. (See Chapter 21, "Our Later Years," for more on this movement.)

By being informed and proactive as we go through these transitions and by taking good care of our bodies and our health, we can enter postmenopause without buying into ageist and sexist notions. A fifty-five-year-old woman says:

Intellectually, I know some of my physical and mental capacities will diminish as I age, but I want to deal with this with a sense of self-acceptance [and] not lower expectations. I hope my generation of feminist boomers will not deny the limits of aging and not give in to internalized ageist attitudes towards others and ourselves as we age.

Recommended Reading: Here are some suggested blogs and websites that provide information, resources, and community.

Menopause Chit Chat: menopausechitchat.com

Menopause the Blog: menopausetheblog.com

Project AWARE: project-aware.org

Red Hot Mamas: redhotmamas.org

The Perimenopause Blog: theperimenopauseblog.com

Women's Voices for Change: womensvoicesforchange.org

By actively advocating for policies and programs that improve the health, well-being, and financial and social status of women through the menopause transition and beyond, we can ensure that more and more women will go through these experiences of aging with plenty of community support and the best years ahead.

■ CHAPTER 21

A s we age, we may question whether society fully grasps the complexity and diversity of our lives. We're either trim and tan adventurer-grandmothers, with lives as busy and meaningful as ever and an active sex life to match, or we're cast in the more prevalent role of decline, our later lives a pitiful epilogue that depicts us as inevitably frail, vulnerable, and alone.

We know that this stage—like every stage—is more complicated than either story line and traverses decades with highs and lows. As more of us live longer, we are challenging negative myths about aging and redefining what it means to be old— and doing so on our own terms with our own stories. But we're up against a youth-oriented mind-set that devalues and marginalizes women after our reproductive years. As Ashton Applewhite writes:[1]

We call people out for racist and sexist attitudes, but few blink at the suggestion that older people are befuddled or disabled or dependent or creepy, even repulsive. After all, that's how people over 65 tend to be depicted in entertainment and advertising (if they make an appearance at all).

Our culture has so far failed to recognize the massive transition that is under way related to aging and the opportunities it presents for both young and old. A number of recent studies[2] signal a shift from an exclusive focus on the problems and deficits of aging to new models that focus on health, growth, development, and meaningful engagement. It is imperative for us to raise awareness, reframe issues, and present practical, women-centered information that challenges the status quo.

This chapter discusses some aspects of aging that affect our health and social/emotional well-being, with an emphasis on reproductive health and sexuality, the focus of this edition of *Our Bodies, Ourselves*. Questions to be addressed include: How can we make the adaptations needed to maximize good health and maintain independence and quality of life? How much medical intervention are we comfortable with in the later years of our lives? What preventive health care exams, including breast and vaginal exams, do we need when we are in our sixties—or in our eighties? How do sex and sexual pleasure fit in?

While the chapters on relationships, sexuality, and sexual identity include stories from women over sixty, this chapter takes a closer look at how aging affects sexual health, relationships, and well-being. It also identifies numerous resources that provide trustworthy information on caregiving, housing, and economic concerns, among other issues.

THE NEW OLD AGE

Historically, most people did not have an extended old age; for many of us, our life spans will extend decades beyond those of previous generations. Consider that between 1900 and 2007, life expectancy at birth[3] increased from forty-eight to eighty years for women (closer to eighty-one for white women and seventy-seven for black women; life expectancy varies by race, but the difference decreases with age). Life expectancy at older ages has also increased: Between 1950 and 2007, life expectancy at age sixty-five rose from fifteen to twenty years for women.

By the year 2030, when all baby boomers (those born between 1946 and 1964) are at least age sixty-five, nearly 20 percent of the U.S. population will be sixty-five or older, up from 13 percent in 2010[4] and just 4 percent in 1900.

It is up to us to change the aging paradigm—to create purposeful roles for ourselves and positive role models of aging and elderhood for younger people—and to question how our communities can best address the complexities that accompany growing older.

Many of us are asking: How can we balance affirming the positive aspects of aging with recognizing the problematic realities without giving in to age bias? How can we tap into the vast knowledge and insights of women about the aging process and end the potentially oppressive effects of imposed cultural constructs? How can we address health care gaps, which include inequities in care and health disparities, and advocate for changes in policies, institutions, and programs so that everyone can experience better health and improved quality of life?

The road map for navigating these issues isn't always clear. What is certain, however, is that we are a growing force, and our influence can't be ignored. Our numbers will give us extra clout as voters and activists in our communities—clout we can use to press for social policies that improve the lives of all women, so that what some call the bonus years are experienced more universally.

AGING HAS BECOME FEMINIZED

Although we are living longer than ever before, the quality of our lives as we age depends on many factors: our health, the losses we have suffered, our finances and living arrangements, our family situation and networks of support, and how well we adapt to new changes and, perhaps, new limitations.

Statistically speaking, the problems of aging are predominantly women's problems. In 2008, women accounted for 58 percent of the population age sixty-five and older and for 67 percent of the population eighty-five and older.[5] We have the benefits—and the potential disadvantages— of living longer. Though we'd like to think we'll all have longer life/health spans, most of us will experience some loss, illness, and increased dependency on others, perhaps as we're still considered caregivers ourselves. We need to incorporate this reality into our view of aging and find ways to plan for and cope with these challenges.

Financial concerns especially add to the stresses of daily living. Among women age sixty-five and older, 12 percent are living in poverty.[6] For married women, the number is much less, around 4 percent. Unmarried older women have considerably less income and a lower standard of living than do married women. For women living alone, the poverty rate jumps to 20 percent overall and varies greatly by race: 16 percent of white women, compared with 39 percent of black women, 33 percent of Asian women, and almost 40 percent of Hispanic women.

OUR BODIES IN CONTEXT

Some cultures value and honor older people. Generally speaking, U.S. society is ageist; that is,

it idealizes the young and marginalizes and segregates older adults. Ironically, ageism is a form of bigotry unlike any other; most of us will fall victim to it sooner or later.

Many of us have felt discriminated against on the basis of age, sometimes from midlife on at work, in relationships, in media representations, and even in medical care. Women are still valued mostly for their reproductive and sexual capacity and are often held to impossible standards of youth and physical attractiveness. This makes us vulnerable to age discrimination at an earlier age than men. Ageism is bad for everyone—but especially for women.

A sixty-three-year-old woman describes her frustration with the limitations of the commonly used phrase "postmenopausal women":

I think the term is far too narrow. It defines us by the lack of blood dripping out of our vaginas every month, by our lack of reproductive ability. My 20-something feminist self in the mid-1960s would be appalled at the label; my 60-something self looks at the term quizzically and becomes equally appalled. The time from our early fifties until death, "the postmenopausal years," may span thirty to fifty years. For many women, they may be some of our most productive and fulfilled years. For me, my life has not stopped getting better. But this time in my life needs a different label from "postmenopausal" that describes its richness and breadth. Years of maturity, years of more harmony, years of moving beyond? While my body may not able to do all that it once could, my life is a tremendous adventure—not waning.

Though the term "postmenopausal" may be useful in a biological or life context, some women advocate doing away entirely with biologically based terms to describe older women. After all, "postandropausal" is not a term used for men.

Advertisements play on and exaggerate our

fears and anxieties about the natural changes in our bodies as we age. Businesses—especially the pharmaceutical, plastic surgery, and cosmetic industries—exploit and profit from these attitudes. Meanwhile, we are more likely to be put down for things that are admired or ignored in older men, such as pride in our achievements or having wrinkles on our faces or extra weight on our bones. The bottom line is that all of us are growing older and all our lives are touched by aging, but society in many ways doesn't accommodate or value the needs and perspective of older women.

Aging itself is often seen as a condition that we have to do something about—giving rise to the phrase "medicalization of aging." The natural changes in our bodies associated with growing older become defined as diseases or conditions that always (rather than sometimes) need medical supervision or intervention, including drugs or surgery. Self-acceptance as we age can be hard-won but invaluable.

A popular newspaper column by Shirley Haynes has made many rounds via email. In response to a young person asking how she feels about being old, Haynes wrote, "I was taken aback, for I do not think of myself as old." Then she thought about it some more:

I would never trade my amazing friends, my wonderful life, and my loving family for less gray hair or a flatter belly. As I've aged, I've become kinder to myself, and less critical of myself. I've become my own friend. . . .

Old Lesbians Organizing for Change (oloc.org) works to challenge ageism and other oppressions. Visit OLOC's website for information on regional and national gatherings.

I will walk the beach in a swim suit that is stretched over a bulging body, and will dive into the waves with abandon if I choose to, despite the pitying glances from the bikini set. They, too, will get old (if they're lucky). . . .

So, to answer the question, I like being older. It has set me free. I like the person I have become.[7]

RELATIONSHIPS

MAINTAINING CONNECTIONS

As we grow older, we create new patterns and adjust to changes, sometimes with a heightened awareness of the passage of time and the preciousness of present moments. Some of us in long-standing marriages or partnerships may experience renewed pleasure at having shared so many life experiences and be enthusiastic about growing even closer.

It may be time to redefine roles and to set new goals as our relationships change. What new interests do we develop as individuals or as a couple? What kind of lifestyle do we want to have in our retirement years? Where do we want to live? What are our long-term support and service needs in case of illness?

Reaching this stage of our lives may also be cause for assessing our relationships. Some women leave relationships that they previously tolerated. Older women who initiate divorce after having a put a lot of thought into it can feel exhilarated by a new beginning. If a partner initiated the dissolution of a long-term marriage or partnership, it may be difficult, at least at first, to take these next steps alone or to consider dating again.

Family relationships—and our place in the generational hierarchy—also shift and change. Our families may be genetically and biologically related, blended, or extended. Many of us are getting used to becoming grandmothers, great-aunts, or godmothers to the children in our lives; 80 percent of those age sixty-five and older have grandchildren, as do 51 percent of those age fifty to sixty-four.[8] We may have developed ties to families into which our grown children have married or to the grown children of new partners, as well as to the second families of former spouses.

These experiences can be trying as well as fulfilling. One sixty-five-year-old woman says:

My life feels full, and with an open heart I develop evolving relationships with my sons and daughters-in-law and their families, but I do find it hard that my husband and I are the oldest generation with no buffers.

A lesbian woman in her seventies describes this decade as the most fulfilling she's experienced:

I live close to my family, including five grandchildren, and I am in a live-in relationship, so I am very fortunate to have a strong social support system. Retirement has opened up many choices, and I am very active.

Once our children leave home, we may think we have more space and freedom, only to find they are returning home, at least temporarily. More of us are caring for younger generations, too. According to a 2010 Pew Research Center survey,[9] one child in ten in the United States lives with a grandparent; about four in ten of those children are being raised primarily by that grandparent.

For some of us, our friends are our family, and we will care for them (and they for us) as we age. These important bonds are often overlooked or minimized by others who see our lives as lacking if we aren't close to our families or don't have relatives living nearby.

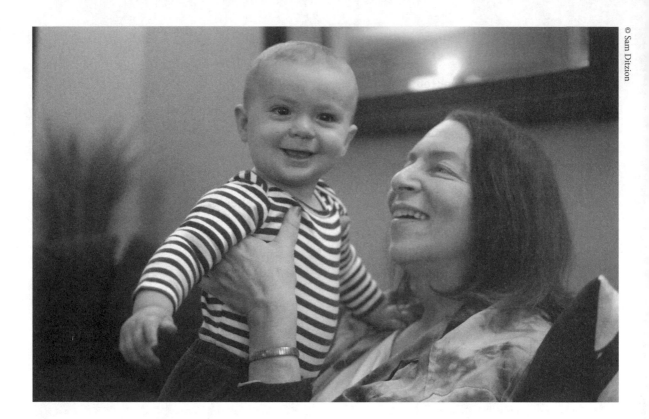

No matter how we define our relationships, social connections can have a positive effect on our health. As many of us know, isolation can be very hard to endure. Bonding and renewing bonds with spouses, lovers, family members, friends, and neighbors can improve our well-being and even longevity. Even pets can have a positive effect on our outlook.

A ninety-eight-year-old woman says that in addition to taking care of her health through sleep and diet, she continues to spend time with friends: "I socialize with other people, not just in my building. And I laugh—a lot!"

A seventy-three-year-old describes the importance of keeping connected with her spiritual community:

Last week I sat in a group of older women discussing religion and spirituality and was reminded of our midweek prayer meetings sixty years ago. . . . I nourish my spirit through music, nature, and meditation, but mostly through relatedness to people I love.

FAST FACT:
OLDER SAME-SEX COUPLES

There are an estimated 2.4 million gay, lesbian, or bisexual Americans over the age of fifty-five[10] and 1.5 million over sixty-five.[11] The number of gay men and women over fifty-five in same-sex couples almost doubled between 2000 to 2006, from 222,000 to 416,000.[12] In almost one quarter of same-sex couples, both partners are at least fifty-five or older.[13]

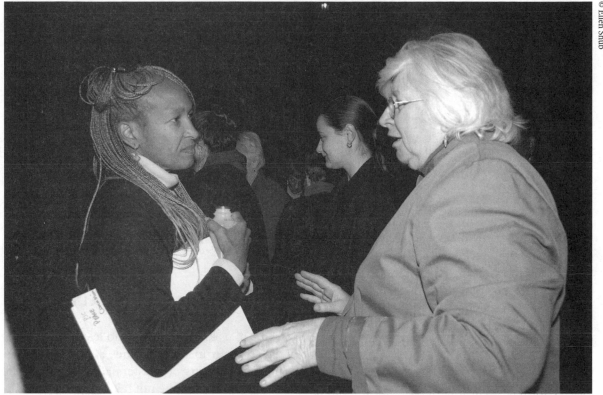

DEALING WITH LOSS

These are the years when we are likely to experience and mourn the deaths of friends and loved ones in increasing numbers. Many women live longer than their male spouses or partners, often by a decade or two. Nearly 42 percent of women age sixty-five and older are widowed,[14] compared with 14 percent of men. Looking closer at the age demographics, 25 percent of women and 7 percent of men between sixty-five and seventy-four are widowed; 52.5 percent of women and not quite 19 percent of men age seventy-five to eighty-four; and 76 percent of women and not quite 38 percent of men age eighty-five and older.

In addition to the official widows, millions of us have lost unofficial partners—female and male. Grieving may be complicated when un-conventional situations make it hard to be open about loss and to receive essential social support from friends and community. One woman reflects on her partner's suicide:

Years ago, when Trudy discovered that she had cancer . . . she drove to the hills above our home early one Sunday morning and put a bullet through her heart. It pierced my heart, too, for it ended our eighteen years of life together. Trudy's death caused me to close the door in denial of my lesbian feelings. It took eleven years for me to begin to creep cautiously from the closet.

Support that does come through makes it easier for us to grieve and helps us to find solace in our day-to-day lives. A core group of friends can make all the difference:

*We have a women-over-70 group. We let down
our hair and talk about our problems and help
each other by providing a sustaining set of
relationships.*

GOING IT ALONE

At this point in our lives, some of us would
rather not have one special partner. Maybe we've
been single all along. Maybe we have been divorced or widowed and have grown accustomed
to being on our own. We may have achieved a
satisfying and deeply erotic relationship with
ourselves spiritually or through self-pleasuring,
or we may enjoy celibacy and create intimacy
through friendships or social outreach.

Forty percent of women age sixty-five and
older live alone, compared with 19 percent of
men in this age bracket.[15] Some women would
prefer to have a partner but don't. If you are over
sixty, it may be hard to find a suitable partner of
either sex. Straight women are subject to a double whammy, because with each decade of age
there are fewer men in our age range, and those
men may prefer to date younger women.

One woman in her early seventies says:

*An older woman tends to know what works and
doesn't, is independent and more self-sufficient.
Older men don't like being by themselves.*

Being older does not have to mean remaining unattached for the rest of our lives, nor does
it have to mean forgoing sex. Some of us have
met compatible partners with whom companionship and pleasure are possible. In addition to
reaching out to family and friends for help making connections, matchmaking services and online dating sites for older adults have multiplied
in recent years. Social networking sites can be
a way to develop relationships based on shared
interests.

Sometimes connections happen when we
aren't even looking. Women meet old flames or
potential partners in volunteer activities or in
new jobs. A widow of twenty years met someone in her building when she was almost ninety:

*Some of it is dumb luck, of course. He thought
he was a one-woman man. I thought I was too
old! We first got to like each other over time.
Then it took us by surprise and developed into
love. At first we hesitated to admit we had
feelings for each other. Now, even though our
backgrounds are very different, we seem to be
on the same wavelength without trying very
hard.*

AGING AND HEALTH

Some of us know women who learn to walk and
dance again in their eighties after hip replacement operations or masters athletes who excel
in their fields, despite not taking up a sport until
they were past midlife. People begin healthier
lifestyles at every age, but many of us also encounter health challenges with increasing frequency and severity as we age. These issues
affect many aspects of living. A sixty-nine-year-
old woman living in New York City says:

*As I age, I am more aware of the potential of a
life-altering health event or a life-threatening
illness. One friend has a terminal illness, and
another recently fell, developed back problems,
and is temporarily somewhat physically limited.
I try to keep this in perspective, but it's certainly
more on my consciousness than it was when I was
younger.*

A woman who is sixty-three adds:

*I have been with age-mate friends and family as
they have been diagnosed with type 2 diabetes,*

hypertension, skin cancer, breast cancer, uterine cancer, arthritis, and other chronic diseases, as well as loss of strength and stamina. I have seen how it takes longer for all of us to heal after a minor illness or injury.

An eighty-one-year-old woman describes how she and her friends have learned how to incorporate health issues into a discussion without making it the only discussion:

I find that, like most women my age, I have frequent doctors' appointments for eyes, teeth, chronic conditions, etc. Going to the doctor always raises mortality issues: What does this ache or pain mean? I started bunching my appointments together because health issues can take over your life, and I want to focus on the many activities I enjoy. I have a group of friends I get together with regularly, and we have ten minutes of "health reports"—and then on to other things.

She also outlines her efforts to be prepared:

I am aware that an unexpected emergency room visit could happen at any time, and so I carry my cell phone with me at all times and have picked up on the ICE (In Case of Emergency) campaign. I have programmed ER contact information into my cell phone under the acronym ICE which, when activated, speed dials my ER contact. Also, I have at all times with me a list of medications that I take, my doctors' names, my blood type, any allergies to medications or foods, and a health care proxy.

We all age differently; some women have disabilities from an early age, while more of us develop disabilities in midlife and our older years as a result of chronic conditions and diseases. Often our fears of aging are fears of disability

and dependency and the isolation that results. We may feel stigmatized if we require an assistive device for mobility, hearing, or vision. Just as the disability movements have done, we need to work for change so society is more supportive as we adapt to physical changes.

PREVENTIVE MEASURES: TAKING CARE OF OURSELVES

Some of the effects of aging, once thought biologically inevitable, are preventable and sometimes even reversible. Prevention is the key word—doing what we can to take care of ourselves so as to avoid or ease the chronic conditions associated with later life. Acquiring healthy habits—reducing dependence on nicotine and alcohol; exercising; and eating nutritious, balanced meals—can help many of us achieve a more fulfilling quality of life.

There are, however, numerous obstacles to making lifestyle changes, including financial insecurity, home and community safety, and our own current health. Many factors are beyond our control. Years of exposure to occupational health hazards may result in chronic and/or debilitating disease. Women of color, 40 percent of whom work in physically demanding or hazardous occupations, are at higher risk for chronic diseases in later life. Between 60 and 80 percent of women over age sixty have high blood pressure, with rates for black women higher that those for white or Latina women. Among women ages sixty to seventy-four, one in three black and Mexican-American women has type 2 diabetes, compared with about one in six white women. We must strive to make the changes that are within our power and advocate for labor, environmental, and health care policies that will improve conditions everywhere so that more people can age in better health.

Some basic preventive measures that can make a difference in our later years include:

Start or continue exercising. Exercise can help maintain or improve some chronic conditions associated with old age, including diabetes, high blood pressure, and cardiovascular disease. It can lower blood pressure and reduce the risks of heart attack, stroke, arthritis, and osteoporosis, and even helps to improve sleep and bowel function. Exercise has also been shown to improve mental ability, and studies indicate that it can help relieve mild to moderate depression. Walk, swim, or move in any way possible. Gentle exercises such as yoga, tai chi, or the Alexander Technique can help with posture, balance, and stress.

Many exercises can be adapted as we age or modified to match our capabilities. A sixty-seven-year-old woman says:

I go to the gym five times a week (doing aerobics, spinning, and weight lifting). I started going in my fifties, and since then I have developed arthritis and chronic back problems and have a little less energy. I have adapted my routines to these changes. I love exercising—it's central to my sense of vitality, well-being, and taking care of my aging body.

Engage your mind. Activities that stimulate brain activity—such as doing crossword puzzles, reading, and playing trivia games—may offer some protection against the cognitive decline that comes with aging. Brain exercises don't help people who have already been diagnosed with Alzheimer's disease, a study found.[16] Minor memory lapses and slowing of cognitive processes are a result of normal aging and need to be distinguished from serious neurological disorders such as Alzheimer's.[17]

Get to bed. Older adults require the same amount of sleep as younger adults. Sometimes sleep patterns might change—you may find yourself going to bed earlier and rising earlier—but sleep disturbances and decreased sleep are

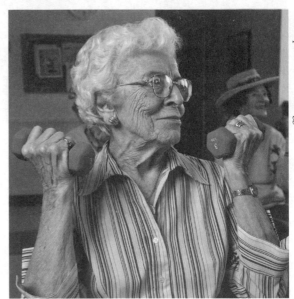

© iStockphoto.com / Rich Legg

not a natural part of aging and should be discussed with your health care provider.

Schedule a checkup. Under the 2010 health care reform act, Medicare will pay for annual wellness visits and preventive screening tests, including Pap tests; mammograms; bone density, blood pressure, and cholesterol tests; and colorectal screenings. Older women are also encouraged to get an annual blood test to check triglycerides and homocysteine levels, as well as blood sugar level (for diabetes), thyroid function, general electrolytes level, liver and kidney output, vitamin B levels (especially vitamin B_{12}), and vitamin D levels. Dental checkups are also recommended but are not covered by Medicare.

COMMON CHRONIC DISEASES

As we live longer, we become more at risk of acquiring one or more chronic conditions such as heart disease, osteoporosis, diabetes, arthritis, some cancers, and urinary incontinence. These conditions can affect our ability to live inde-

Good places to learn about chronic diseases and to find help managing these conditions include:

- **CDC Chronic Disease Prevention and Health Promotion:** cdc.gov/chronicdisease
- **National Council on Aging:** ncoa.org
- **The National Women's Health Information Centers:** womenshealth.gov

pendently and participate in daily activities. In addition, older women are often caregivers and may be taking care of a loved one also suffering from one or more chronic health conditions.

Successful management of chronic conditions is one of the hallmarks of healthy aging. Our health care system, which devotes more resources to acute problems and late-stage chronic illness, is not designed for an aging population. Resources need to be focused more on the following areas: prevention; support for self-care and ongoing maintenance of chronic conditions; slowing the progression and reducing the symptoms, complications, and functional limitations of conditions; coordination of preventive, medical, and management interventions; and optimum communication between ourselves and our families and health care providers.

GUIDELINES FOR SEXUAL AND REPRODUCTIVE HEALTH CARE

If you have had access to routine health care, by the time you're in your sixties you have probably had decades of regular screening tests for common sexual and reproductive health problems, including cervical cancer and breast can-

cer. As we age, screening guidelines change. What follows are some recommendations concerning tests and treatments in our sixties and beyond.

Since greater longevity is a recent phenomenon, there is not yet an abundance of good data on screening guidelines for women over the age of eighty-five. We need to advocate for more research for this age group.

Vaginal Health

It's important to maintain vulvovaginal health in postreproductive years. Medicare pays for gynecological visits every other year. If you are experiencing any problems such as vaginal dryness or dyspareunia (pain before, during, or after intercourse), consult a gynecologist who is trained to identify and address specific problems. For a fuller discussion, see "Vaginal Changes," p. 516; and "Painful Intercourse/Penetration," p. 185.

Mammograms

Guidelines issued by the U.S. Preventive Services Task Force in November 2009 recommend regular screenings to detect possible cancer once every two years for women age fifty to seventy-four.[18] This guideline refers only to screening mammograms, not diagnostic. Studies have found no benefit from more frequent screenings for women who don't have a history of breast cancer, though women are urged to talk with their health care providers if they experience any changes in their breasts. The task force concludes that the current evidence is insufficient to assess the additional benefits and harms of screening mammography in women age seventy-five or older. For more discussion of mammograms, see p. 590.

SOCIAL SERVICES FOR LGBT ELDERS

The health care needs of LGBT elders are often more magnified. For instance, lesbians are at greater risk for cancer, obesity, and drug and alcohol addiction, and male-to-female transgender people are at higher risk for HIV/AIDS. Health care and social service providers may lack experience working with diverse older communities. The good news is that this is rapidly changing.

In 2010, the U.S. Department of Health and Human Services and the Administration on Aging awarded a three-year grant to Services and Advocacy for Gay, Lesbian, Bisexual & Transgender Elders (SAGE) to establish the National Resource Center on LGBT Aging (lgbtagingcenter .org). SAGE also provides caregiving services and started the nation's first home visitation program for LGBT elders. Visit sageusa.org for more information.

Two recent reports—"Outing Age 2010: Public Policy Issues Affecting Lesbian, Gay, Bisexual and Transgender Elders," from the National Gay and Lesbian Task Force Policy Institute;[20] and "Improving the Lives of LGBT Older Adults,"[21] from SAGE, the LGBT Movement Advancement Project, American Society on Aging, Center for American Progress, and National Senior Citizens' Law Center—present in-depth looks at public policy issues and the challenges facing millions of aging LGBT people in the United States.

"LGBT elders remain a highly vulnerable and largely invisible aging population," said NGLTF Executive Director Rea Carey. "We know that invisibility leads to greater social isolation, which can lead to increased vulnerability in many areas. We also know that discrimination across the lifespan leaves LGBT people economically and socially vulnerable as they age. 'Outing Age 2010' shines a laser beam on these needs and offers concrete recommendations on how aging advocates, policy makers and social service agencies can meet them."

Pap Tests

The Pap test (also known as a Pap smear or cervical cytology screening) is a simple test that can detect abnormal cervical cells that could lead to cervical cancer. According to the American Congress of Obstetricians and Gynecologists,[19] if you are age sixty-five or older, you should discuss with your health care provider whether cervical cancer screening is still necessary. It is reasonable to stop screening at sixty-five or seventy if you have had three or more negative cytology results in a row and no abnormal test results in the past ten years.

If you have had a hysterectomy, talk to your provider about whether you still need routine Pap tests. The answer may depend on the reason for your hysterectomy, whether your cervix was removed, and whether you have a history of moderate or severe dysplasia.

Bone Densitometry

Older women are more at risk for osteoporosis because bone loss is accelerated by the decline of estrogen at menopause. As bones weaken, fractures and breakage are more common. It is

For a comprehensive discussion of osteoporosis and osteopenia, see "Preventing Bone Loss and Osteoporosis," p. 528. For more on medical problems affecting only women, including ovarian cancer, endometrial cancer, pelvic organ prolapse, and hysterectomy, see Chapter 22, "Selected Medical Problems."

recommended that all women over age sixty-five be screened. Studies have not evaluated the optimal intervals, but women should allow a minimum of two years or more between tests to review changes. There are no data regarding at what age to stop testing.

If you are told you have osteopenia, consider your options before taking prescription medicine. This relatively new term means only that your bone mineral density (BMD) is less than the average for young adult white women. In other words, your bone mineral density may be perfectly normal for you. Osteopenia is not a disease state, and not all women who have osteopenia will develop osteoporosis. For women with a "–1" or a "–2" BMD screening result, a bisphosphonate such as Fosamax shows no clear benefits, and longer-term use has been associated with decay of the jaw and unusual fractures of the thighbone. For more information, see

HEALTH INFORMATION SOURCES

Accurate and trustworthy health information is a necessity at any age. For information on how to find reliable information and obtain the health care you need, see Chapter 23, "Navigating the Health Care System." Here are some websites and newsletters that offer information specific to women and aging:

Websites

- **CDC Aging** (cdc.gov/women/az/aging .htm): Provides numerous health publications as well as current statistics.
- **The AGS Foundation for Health in Aging** (www.healthinaging.org): A service of the nonprofit AGS Foundation for Health in Aging, this site features well-organized sections with links to additional resources.

- **The National Women's Health Information Center** (womenshealth .gov/aging): Includes physical health resources as well as a mental health section with information on loss and grieving.

Newsletters

- **Focus on Healthy Aging** (focuson healthyaging.com), a publication of Mount Sinai School of Medicine, reports on the newest and best tools of healthy aging. The cost is $29 per year for an eight-page monthly publication.
- **Harvard Women's Health Watch** (health.harvard.edu/newsletters), also an eight-page monthly publication, covers prevention strategies, new diagnostic techniques, and new medications and treatments. The cost is $24 per year for online access, $28 for print and online.

"Medical Approaches to Osteoporis Prevention and Treatment," p. 530.

SEXUALITY

When we've got wisdom, connection, logistics, time, intimacy, a sense of humor, ease of communication, resilience of body and spirit, and no kids barging in, who needs youth?
      —*Joan Price, author of* Better Than I Ever Expected: Straight Talk About Sex After Sixty [22]

THE SEX CONTINUUM

It is a myth that sexual desire and activity fade as a natural, irreversible part of aging. Our society's view of aging women as "dried up" and sexless is perpetuated by a hypersexualized, youth-oriented culture that doesn't know enough about the sex lives of older women and doesn't view older women as sexual. Sexuality, unlike fertility, can continue throughout our lives. Henry Wadsworth Longfellow understood and expressed the opportunities of aging very well when he wrote:

For age is opportunity no less
Than youth itself, though in another dress,
And as the evening twilight fades away,
The sky is filled with stars, invisible by day.

While we may have to accommodate changes that can make sexual enjoyment more challenging (such as arthritis or loss of energy), with good communication and a deeper understanding of our needs—as well as more creativity—we can continue to give and receive pleasure.

Appreciating our bodies and sexuality more fully can happen at any age. Many women enjoy sex more in middle and later life:

I'm no longer worried about pregnancy; the children are gone; my energy is released. I have a

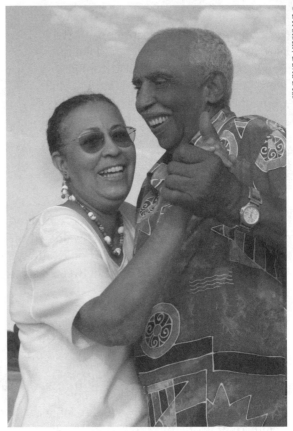

© DK Stock / David Deas

new surge of interest in sex. But at the same time, the culture is saying, "You are not attractive as a woman; act your age; be dignified," which means, to me, be dead sexually.

A seventy-three-year-old woman says:

My sexual drive doesn't burst out, unasked for, anymore. But it's there. It just needs a particular environment in order to emerge: candles and wine at dinner, a long postdinner kiss, a rub against my husband's thigh, and then music. Not just any music, but certain songs and groups that over the decades have always turned me on. For me, it's UB40, Santana, and Manu Chao. A few minutes of dancing and slowly stripping, a bit of licking, and I am fully aroused.

Sexual feelings often depend more on how we feel about our bodies and our relationships than our age. Some women discover their sexuality when they discover a new sexual identity or when they leave abusive or indifferent partners. Some make peace with parts of their bodies they didn't like. Sometimes health improves, either naturally or from making changes.

During partnered sex, we may have to overcome years of conditioning to initiate sex or consider alternatives to routine patterns. It is possible to change old habits and assumptions by talking and exploring together. Some of us have been with the same partner for years and are used to working things out:

My libido was down, as was Tom's. We were having less frequent sex, and I was waiting for him to take the initiative. Finally, I said to myself, "I can do something about this, I am a sexual being"—and I began to initiate sex and we had a great time.

Inhibitions often lessen with age.[24] We may give ourselves more freedom to experiment in relationships or to be more open about them. Some older women have relationships with younger men. Some have sexual relationships with women for the first time. Others who quietly have been lesbian or bisexual for many years may feel more comfortable coming out.

I am eighteen years into what I hope will be a lifelong relationship with a woman. Sex for us is a steady friend. During our busy workweek, we cuddle, and that's good. On weekends and

PLEASURE IN OLD AGE

As Meika Loe's research shows in her new book, *Aging Our Way: Lessons for Living from 85 and Beyon,*[23] women age eighty-five and older desire and experience a range of pleasure. With broader definitions of pleasure, opportunities for sexual intimacy and sensory pleasure do not disappear in late life.

Lillian, ninety, is hearing impaired and uses an oxygen tank. She describes intimacy with her second husband:

We enjoy spending time together and [we enjoy] a little bit of sex. It is very satisfactory, by the way. It always has been for me. Bernie said I can't offer you much in the way of physical things but a lot of hugs and kisses, and I thought okay. . . . Well the first night I felt like I was back to being a virgin again in his bedroom wondering what's coming on your wedding night and he comes in and it was just lovely and I said to him, Bernie, you sold yourself short! . . . I wish I felt better now, but Bernie and I love each other very much. We watch romance movies every night on cable.

Alice, a ninety-two-year-old widow, thrives on physical touch with friends and loved ones and cherishes hugs.

Hugs are good for people, especially old people . . . I remember as a 30-something visiting old people who would hold onto my hand, and I just wanted to get away. But now I understand it. It is a need—almost involuntary.

on vacations, we make time for lovemaking and cherish how it reconnects and refreshes us.

Others continue a lifelong enjoyment that has brought them much happiness and satisfaction:

The biggest reason my sexual life remains so vital is that I have multiple partners. My relationship with my husband has been nonmonogamous for all of our thirty-two years together. This is a very complex lifestyle and not for everyone; it has been a great challenge and brought much richness to my life. Sexual freedom has been incredibly liberating for me and has contributed to my staying younger in mind, body, and spirit. It has enriched my relationships with all my various partners, whether short or long term. I got the impression from my mother that at this age she was tolerating sex, but it was not a life-giving activity in her life. How sad for her!

Of course, not everyone wants to be sexual. A seventy-three-year-old woman writes:

I frankly don't need it, and I don't miss it at all. I had a very, very full sex life, and I was mad about my husband, which is a nice way to be. When he died, it was a real shock. I haven't discovered another person that I had that desire for in twenty-five years now. I'm used to my life the way it is now, and I don't think that my life is incomplete.

For some, sex is laden with abuse and pain that can never be overcome. Others are less interested in sex, even in a good relationship. And our partners may lose interest, too. Adjustments, disruptions, or feeling less sexual can also result from chronic or acute illness or surgery. It can take a while to adjust to new circumstances and resume a pleasurable sex life. But there are many ways to have sex and experience sexual pleasure,

regardless of our relationship status or physical capacity.

PHYSICAL CHANGES THAT AFFECT SEXUALITY

A 2010 Harvard Medical School Special Health Report, *Sexuality in Midlife and Beyond*,[25] identifies the following possible age-related sexual changes for women:

- Physical changes: decreased blood flow to genitals, lower levels of estrogen and testosterone, thinning of the vaginal lining, loss of vaginal elasticity and muscle tone
- Desire: decreased libido, fewer sexual thoughts and fantasies
- Arousal: slower arousal, reduced vaginal lubrication and less expansion of the vagina, less blood congestion in the clitoris and lower vagina, diminished clitoral sensitivity
- Orgasm: delayed or absent orgasm, less intense orgasms, fewer and sometimes painful uterine contractions
- Resolution: body returns more rapidly to a nonaroused state

For those of us with male partners, age-related effects on men's sexuality matter as well. Men over age fifty may have difficulty getting an erection sufficient for intercourse, and erections may require more direct stimulation. In addition, the need to ejaculate is less urgent, and the rest period between erections grows longer.

Such changes may affect our sexual relationships. It can be common, for example, to worry that vaginal dryness, less intense orgasms, or erection difficulties mean a partner is feeling less attracted to us or losing interest in sex. These perceptions can trigger feelings of rejection and resentment. ("Am I no longer sexually attractive?" "Is she or he having an affair?") If you are starting a new sexual relationship after divorce or the death of a spouse, it is also quite common to fear that you will not become aroused or will not be able to have an orgasm with a different partner. Or you may be self-conscious about baring your changing body in front of someone new. Sometimes we simply tire more easily, as this sixty-five-year-old woman writes:

I still need about the same amount of clitoral stimulation as in my earlier years, but I get tired so much more quickly. I joke with my partner that we will need to get a vibrator soon if he finds that his hands start getting too tired. Sometimes I start to fall asleep even as I am getting quite aroused. That would never have happened a few decades ago!

A 2007 study on sexuality and health among older adults found that the most prevalent sexual problems cited by older women were low desire, difficulty with vaginal lubrication, and inability to climax. Only 22 percent of women (and 38 percent of men) reported having discussed sex with a physician since turning fifty.[26] Many women are reluctant to talk about sexual difficulties with their gynecologists or other health care providers; it's also probable that physicians are uncomfortable discussing sexuality with older patients—particularly women, since we are often perceived as sexless—and need more training about older women and sexuality. One woman notes that her doctor never brought up sex after a recent surgery:

I had a stent put in last summer, and I was concerned about resuming sexual activity with my husband. The doctor didn't mention sex in his long list of dos and don'ts. I had to bring it up.

In a separate 2007 study on older women's sexual desire and agency, many of the women interviewed had internalized societal assumptions that led them to value their male partners' sexual needs over their own.[27] We all deserve positive relationships with partners who love us for who we are and who care about our fulfillment.

PRACTICAL APPROACHES TO AGE-RELATED SEXUAL CHANGES

Declining health or bodily changes can affect sexuality. Chronic illnesses such as diabetes can decrease blood flow to the genitals; arthritis, back pain, and limited mobility can restrict the range of comfortable sexual positions; and medications for chronic diseases such as hypertension and heart disease can affect energy levels and sexual functioning (see "Sex with a Disability or Chronic Illness," p. 194). It is also common to feel initial embarrassment over the loss of a breast, or over a colostomy bag or some other apparatus, especially with a new partner. In a 2004 AARP survey, respondents ranked better health for themselves or their partners at the top of a list of features that might improve their sexual satisfaction.[28]

At the same time, sexual activity has health benefits. If one moves and expends energy during sex, the heart and joints get a workout. Active sex can also burn calories and cause the brain to release endorphins, which help to reduce stress.[29] Sexual activity may help people sleep better, owing to the release and sedative effects of oxytocin and endorphins. The clenching and unclenching of vaginal muscles during sex and orgasm condition the vaginal walls and work the muscles of the pelvic floor (known as the pubococcygeus, or PC, muscles). The movement also strengthens these muscles and may help delay or minimize incontinence. And research has shown that orgasms can decrease pain for hours.[30] Having orgasms regularly can help to maintain vaginal lubrication, and regular vaginal penetration can help to maintain vaginal elasticity.

While I was married there was never an issue about "using it or losing it," as we had sex at least two to three times a week, and that kept my vaginal tissues well lubricated. After my husband died, I didn't have a regular sexual partner for more than a decade, but I did enjoy having orgasms while by myself and also discovered along the way that taking cod liver oil daily had a major impact on keeping my vaginal tissues lubricated.

If the sensitivity of your nipples, clitoris, or vagina changes, you may want to adjust the intensity of stimulation and possibly experiment with the use of a vibrator. Shifting positions—and bed cushions—can protect joints and tissues and lead to more comfortable sex, especially if you have problems with mobility, flexibility, or painful joints. More time and stimulation may be needed for arousal and reaching orgasm, but that's okay. Set aside a time that works best for you. Some people use late afternoons for sexual activity, for example, because medications have kicked in and fatigue hasn't.

LOSS OF DESIRE

Most women experience fluctuations in levels of desire throughout their lives. There are many reasons for experiencing less sexual desire: overwork and anxiety; the loss of newness in a long-term relationship; a past history of abuse; gradual changes and accommodations reached in a long-term marriage; or the fact that somebody we're dating for companionship just doesn't attract us in that way. Sometimes, though, lack of sexual desire or responsiveness can be caused by medications, lower hormone levels, or other medical problems, such as low thyroid function or cardiovascular disease.

If you want to be sexual but are experiencing difficulty, or if you're experiencing pain or anxiety about sexual activity, talk to a health

Recommended Reading: For more on women and sex, check out "Sexuality and Spirituality in Women's Relationships" by Gina Ogden (ginaogden.com.media/2AWP .pdf), an analysis of the first large-scale survey that investigated the connections between sexuality and spirituality; and *Sex Is Not a Natural Act and Other Essays* by Leonore Tiefer (leonoretiefer.com).

care provider or counselor and let that person know that sexual activity is important to you. Depending on the cause, there may be steps you can take to improve your sexual experiences, including modifying your medications.

If you think your relationship is causing the problem and communication with your partner is difficult, consider getting help together—or alone, if your partner is unwilling to go for counseling. A licensed sex therapist or counselor specializing in relationships and sexuality may provide useful advice or recommend workshops or support groups on older women's sexuality. If no workshop or support group is available, consider organizing one.

Couples can learn to handle changes in desire. A woman writes of having "no libido" at sixty-three:

I did the creams (which worked wonderfully) but now want to be as drug-free as possible. On the fingers of my wonderfully patient and determined husband, or on my very occasional own, any oil-based cream works wonders on the clitoris. Combined with plenty of skin-to-skin coziness as we sleep, this is plenty of satisfaction for me.

The author Joan Price writes about the importance of planning for sex:

We've discovered that sex works best when we schedule it, make time for it, clear away our busy calendars for it. We turn off our computers and phone ringers. We make dates, anticipate our times together, plan for them, fantasize about them, and tantalize each other by phone by murmuring about what we'd like to do. What we give up in spontaneity, we make up for with constant mental foreplay.[31]

PLEASURING OTHERS– AND YOURSELF

Sex is whatever gives you erotic, sensual pleasure, either with an intimate partner or by yourself.
—Carol Rinkleib Ellison, the author of Women's Sexualities: Generations of Women Share Intimate Secrets of Sexual Self-Acceptance[32]

As in our younger years, we can explore sexuality without a partner, satisfying ourselves and discovering what turns us on by enjoying fantasies and/or self-stimulation. Sex toys and erotica are available online. See Chapter 7, "Sexual Pleasure and Enthusiastic Consent," for good sources.

With a partner, do whatever pleases you both. If your partner is a man of middle age or older, it may be difficult for him to get or keep an erection. Impotence in men is often an unspoken secret.

Studies have shown that that only 30 percent of women regularly climax from vaginal intercourse alone. In a 2009 study[33] of women age sixty to seventy-five, many women reported that there are a wide range of sexual activities that could be equally pleasurable. Touching, kissing and caressing all over, mutual masturbation, and oral sex can give both women and men pleasure and satisfaction.

I still miss being with my late husband, even close to twenty years after he died. But now that I am again in a steady, loving relationship with someone who understands my body so well, I experience deep and satisfying sexual pleasure once again. Sometimes I think he knows more about my clitoris than I do!

HIV INFECTION IN WOMEN

Jane Fowler founded HIV Wisdom for Older Women (hivwisdom.org), an organization dedicated to awareness, prevention, and care, in 2002. She was diagnosed with the virus in 1991, at age fifty-five, and remains committed to discussing STI risks. Because older women no longer need pregnancy protection, condom use among this population is low. Also, older women are often overlooked in prevention messages for safer sex.

"The prevailing, naive attitude that senior women are not at risk for the viral infection and don't need prevention information, must be reversed—in everyone's mind," Fowler told Women's eNews.[34]

Her strategy includes encouraging teenagers to talk to their grandparents. "Once people get past their own embarrassment and understand grandparents today are still sexually active, they realize I'm right," she said in an interview.[35] "Their grandparents face the same risks of sexually transmitted diseases as they do."

For more on protecting yourself at any age, read Chapter 10, "Safer Sex."

If you love intercourse and your partner's age-related sexual changes are affecting the experience, you and/or your partner might talk with a health care provider about Viagra and other erectile-function medications. If he's doing fine but intercourse is uncomfortable for you, see Chapter 8, "Sexual Challenges."

NAVIGATING HEALTH CARE

TWENTY-FIRST-CENTURY MEDICAL CARE

At any age, we may have to consider the medical tests we are willing to have, which of several possible treatment options is best for us (and which ones we can live without), and how much intervention we want—or don't want—if our condition is not likely to improve. These issues are even more important now with high-tech medical advances. Overtreatment is sometimes considered as big a problem as undertreatment in the U.S. health care system.

Many of us will enjoy better health and longevity than previous generations, but the rates of gain are inconsistent across income levels and racial and ethnic groups, and there are disparities compared with other industrialized countries.

According to the U.S. government report *Older Americans 2010: Key Indicators of Well-Being*,[36] in the 1980s, a sixty-five-year-old woman living in the United States had one of the highest average life expectancies in the world, but twenty years later the life expectancies of older women in many countries surpassed that of women in the United States.

Older people face physical, emotional, and social changes and challenges that require special attention. We may need a multidisciplinary team to help us manage medical conditions so we can be as vital, active, and independent as possible. Unfortunately, there is a great shortage of doctors, nurses, psychologists, psychiatrists, dentists, and other health care professionals trained in caring for older adults.

In 2010, there were about 7,100 geriatricians in the United States, a 22 percent decline from 2000. According to a 2008 study by the Institute of Medicine (IOM), a larger shortage is looming. By 2030, when more than 71 million people in the United States will be age sixty-five or older, there will be only an estimated 8,000 geriatricians.[37] The Association of Directors of Geriatric Academic Programs predicts that the nation will need 28,000 more geriatricians—for a total of 36,000—to meet the demand.

If the IOM predictions hold true, there will be only one geriatrician for every 4,254 older adults, compared with one for every 2,546 older adults in 2007, and one geriatric psychiatrist for every 20,195 older adults, compared with one for every 11,372 older adults in 2007.

WRONG DIAGNOSIS, WRONG TREATMENT

Providers without adequate training may interpret emotional or mental confusion as normal aging when it may actually indicate poor nutrition, chronic dehydration, lack of stimulation (interesting daily activities), treatable physical problems, grief, or a reaction to medicine.

Health care providers may judge older women's concerns about pain and health problems to be neurotic, imaginary, or the inevitable result of aging, far more than they judge men's this way. Sometimes providers do not fully treat chronic conditions, misdiagnose and/or fail to manage reversible conditions, and overprescribe drugs. Time after time, older women receive antidepressants and pain relievers instead of a full exam to determine what's really wrong.

Conversely, simpler things such as diet, exercise, and therapy (including physical, occupational, and psychological therapies) get less attention, even when we need them most. Complicating things further, health care insurance plans may limit access to certain tests, treatments, and health care practitioners.

People over age sixty-five take 34 percent of the medicines prescribed annually in the United States, though they currently make up only 13 percent of the U.S. population.[38] Health care providers sometimes neglect to find out what drugs we are taking, including over-the-counter products, before prescribing others. Older adults are more likely to be taking multiple prescriptions, have fewer physical reserves to combat adverse drug responses due to incorrect dosage or drug interaction, and are more likely to be hospitalized owing to an adverse response.

Aging may cause increased sensitivity to drugs, since the kidneys and liver break down and excrete drugs more slowly. You may need lower doses adjusted to your size, age, activity level, and nutrition needs. Women at any age may require lower doses than men because of physical differences. Some drugs can cause depression (for which you may be offered more drugs) or mental confusion, though the symptoms often stop when you stop taking the medicine.

A friend of mine who lives in a nursing home was recently diagnosed as having various ailments that require anywhere from three to ten pills a day. She was never told what the pills were or what they were for. When the nurse came to her room to give her the pills, my friend looked her squarely in the eye and said, "The doctor only knows my body and how it works for a short time. I have known it for ninety-four years, and nothing is going in it until I know what it is!"

When you visit a health care provider, it's good to bring a list of physical changes and the medications you are taking, as well as a list of questions and concerns. Or send the information to the provider's office in advance of the appointment. Some doctors now have interactive websites that enable patients to ask questions ahead of time. A sixty-nine-year-old woman says:

I told my new doctor about what I eat, all the vitamins I take, why I dislike going to a gym, and what I do for physical activity. I also explained why I don't want to have all the invasive tests everyone my age seems to be having. Even though she's under 40, she seemed to get it and didn't push me. Most important, she took the time to listen to me.

We sometimes feel intimidated by health care providers and are afraid to ask questions, inquire about alternative approaches, or request a second opinion. Remember, you have the right to do all those things. If your practitioner is not well informed about managing the diseases and chronic conditions of aging, or is not caring toward you and not responsive to your concerns, try to find someone else who can be more helpful.

I had lower back problems. My neurologist sent me to an orthopedic surgeon, who told me to have an operation which, he informed me, had some risks. I didn't feel comfortable with his assessment and sought a second opinion. It was hard to find a doctor to do this. The opinion of the second doctor was that I didn't need an operation. I agreed, as did my husband and children. I started physical therapy and feel much better.

If you're not comfortable raising questions, ask an advocate to accompany you. Having a significant other, family member, or friend with you can be helpful, particularly if you are going to have a surgical procedure. This person needs to know what to ask and watch for and should

If you want more information about the drugs you're taking, visit the National Library of Medicine online (nlm.nih.gov/medlineplus/druginformation.html) for drug side effects and interactions.

be persistent with each provider, especially if multiple health care providers are involved. Paid advocates are becoming increasingly necessary to navigate health care settings.

For more information on the topics discussed above, see Chapter 23, "Navigating the Health Care System."

PLANNING AHEAD

Planning ahead involves integrating all aspects of our lives: work/retirement, health/health care, long-term care, finances, housing, meaningful relationships, activities, and community. It's best to be proactive and to talk about living arrangements and health care before a crisis arises so you can age in line with your values.

Sharing your desires with family and friends can help you clarify plans and goals and learn what roles you might need others to play. Sometimes talking about your future with a social worker, life planning coach, mental health professional, or clergyperson can be helpful. If you have financial resources to pay for counseling, an organization such as the Life Planning Network (lifeplanningnetwork.org) can help you identify a coach or consultant.

You can't predict the future, but the more prepared you are, the more likely it is that your wishes will be respected. Following are some useful resources to help with the planning process.

RETIREMENT AND SOCIAL SECURITY

Since 2003, the official retirement age at which we can collect full Social Security has been phased upward gradually from sixty-five to sixty-seven, depending on your date of birth. You can collect reduced benefits as early as age sixty-two or delay collecting until age seventy. Planning ahead is critical to deal with gaps in earning power during employment years. If you have taken time off for raising children or elder-parent care, you may have less in savings put aside or retirement income. If you collect early, the law limits how much you can earn from working in retirement. If you decide to keep working after full retirement age, your earnings will not result in a reduction in Social Security benefits. For more information, visit Women's Institute for a Secure Retirement (WISER) (wiserwomen.org).

Social Security benefits may be based on your own earnings or those of a husband. Wives, widows, or divorced women may be entitled to a higher benefit from a husband's or ex-husband's Social Security than from their own. Unmarried women, even in long relationships, and women in same-sex marriages are not yet entitled to benefits from a partner's Social Security or, in most states, from job-related pensions or insurance.

HOUSING

As you get older, you may consider moving to smaller quarters or share living space with friends or other relatives. Cohousing movements are becoming more popular with retirees. Naturally Occurring Retirement Communities (NORC), where older adults age in place with community services, are cropping up. And Volunteers of America (voa.org) launched an Aging with Options initiative in 2009, helping people to stay in their own homes while receiving care.

MEDICARE BASICS

Medicare is the federal insurance program administered by the Centers for Medicare and Medicaid Services (CMS) for all people age sixty-five and over and for people with disabilities under age sixty-five.

Part A, which applies to everyone, covers acute medical care in hospitals (sixty days at full cost, after which a patient copay is required) and short-term nursing home or home care. Part B, which is optional, covers 80 percent of follow-up and outpatient medical treatments, as well as tests and some equipment. It doesn't cover vision or dental care. Part D, also optional, covers prescription drugs and is made necessary by the high cost of medicines.

You have to pay for Parts B and D yourself. Monthly payments for Part B can be deducted from your Social Security benefits. Medigap, the supplemental insurance sold by private insurers, or Medicare Advantage (which contracts with Medicare), covers the deductibles for parts A and B and 20 percent of costs of procedures and supplies *not* covered by Medicare Part B. Some retirees obtain these supplemental policies from employers as part of a benefits package, but most of us have to buy this insurance ourselves. People under age sixty-five with disabilities who are unable to work are eligible for Supplemental Security Income (SSI).

Part D is purchased through a private insurance stand-alone drug plan or Medicare Advantage, or it may be covered by Medicaid (the government insurance plan for people with low incomes). Prior to implementation of the Patient Protection and Affordable Care Act (the health care reform bill enacted in 2010), after you and your plan together spent a certain amount on co-payments, deductible, and insurance combined, you reached a coverage gap (the so-called donut hole), and you would have to pay 100 percent of total drug costs up to the catastrophic coverage limit. Once that limit was reached, you'd pay a small co-payment for each drug.

The new health care law addresses this by providing Medicare beneficiaries who reached the donut hole in 2010 with a $250 rebate, after which they receive a pharmaceutical manufacturers' 50 percent discount on brand-name drugs. The discount will increase to 75 percent off brand-name and generic drugs to close the donut hole by 2020.

The same law requires everyone in the United States to have health care insurance. Depending on your income level, you may be eligible for Medicaid or a subsidy to help you pay for insurance. The new law also forbids private insurers to deny coverage to people with preexisting conditions and to make women pay higher premiums just because they tend to live longer than men. Age rating (charging higher rates for older adults) is still permitted, and premiums can vary by as much as a three-to-one ratio (they previously varied by as much as six to one).

Some providers do not accept Medicare patients because the reimbursement rate is too low. Medicare's major limitations are that it focuses on acute care

In addition, more thought is being given to supporting elder-friendly communities that provide opportunities for people to age in place by ensuring the accessibility of community resources, such as shopping, medical care, transportation, and places of worship. Partners for Livable Communities (livable.org), a national nonprofit organization, has long focused on older adult populations in its work on urban development and community planning and has formed partnerships with municipal organizations for an Aging in Place Initiative (agingin placeinitiative.org). Such communities, which are deemed livable for older citizens, are livable for *all* ages.

Some neighborhood residents are banding together to form intentional communities, in which residents stay in their homes as they age, supported by local programs and services. One such community is Beacon Hill Village (beacon hillvillage.org), a membership organization located in the heart of Boston that was founded in 2001.

You may be eligible for subsidized housing when you reach a certain age or if your income drops below a certain level. Contact Administration on Aging (aoa.gov) and National Council on Aging (ncoa.org) to find local affiliates. Your state department on aging also can provide information about subsidized housing options and combined housing and services options.

HOUSEHOLD HELP AND LONG-TERM CARE

Long-term care services are currently fragmented and expensive. Out-of-pocket expenses for long-term care represent the greatest financial risk for older adults, especially those who have cognitive, physical, or mental problems. Medicare covers only short-term home or nursing home care for acute illness after a hospital stay. All other expenses must be paid out of pocket, including long-term care at home, in the community, or in a nursing home.

Medicaid is a primary source of funding for home care and nursing home care, but only those of us with very low incomes or who spend down most of our assets are eligible. Private long-term care insurance usually has strict limits on the kind of care covered and where it must occur for it to be reimbursed. Most people age sixty-five or older lack such coverage.

The Community Living Assistance Services and Supports Act (CLASS Act), instituted under the 2010 health care reform law, establishes a national, voluntary long-term care insurance program to help seniors and those with disabilities pay for nonmedical services and support. It is the first step toward publicly financed long-term care supporting aging in place, with both home and community-based options. After contributing for five years, participants will be eligible for benefits on the average of $50 a day to apply toward the daily cost of care. The program, effective in 2011, is financed through voluntary payroll deductions. All working adults will be enrolled unless they choose to opt out. Proponents argue that this program will reduce medical costs in the long run. It remains to be seen whether the amounts provided will really be enough to help most of us pay for the care we need. Various organizations can help you find services and people to assist you or other family members. Use the Eldercare Locator (www.eldercare.gov) or call 1-800-677-1116 to find resources in your area.

HEALTH AND LEGAL DECISIONS

Designating someone you trust to make legal and health care decisions for you if you are unable to communicate your wishes can help ensure that your preferences will be respected. Check with your state attorney general's office for the specifics of state laws and for copies of forms to use for health care proxies, advance directives forms and/or living wills. For more information concerning state laws and hospital policies, visit estate.findlaw.com/estate-planning.

A durable power of attorney gives someone you trust the authority to act on your behalf in financial and other legal matters if you are unable to take action yourself.

A health care proxy document gives someone you trust the authority to make medical testing and treatment decisions for you if you are unable to make them for yourself. The proxy is sometimes referred to as a health care agent or durable power of attorney for health care. Choose a health care proxy in advance and talk about your values and wishes with that person.

A medical advance directive or living will describes the medical treatment you wish to receive (or refuse), and under what conditions. This makes your wishes clear to your proxy person, family members, and medical care provid-

ers. It can be written as a letter to the person who has your health care proxy and to your lawyer. Share the information with at least one trustworthy person who does not live in the same home as you. Federal law requires hospitals to give patients information about their right to make health care decisions and to appoint proxies and complete advance directives and do not resuscitate (DNR) documents. Living wills are not legal documents in some states; even so, it's better to put your wishes into writing and communicate those wishes to your loved ones than to stay silent.

END-OF-LIFE CARE

We need to do more to normalize discussing end-of-life issues. Sometimes medical science, rather than concern for quality of life, shapes the advice we receive about death and dying. It's up to you to say what you want or don't want, and it's essential to talk with your doctor or health care provider about your wishes. Even then, however, it's a good idea to also talk with someone who can advocate on your behalf, if needed. Researchers have found that black patients tend to receive life-prolonging measures even when they have DNR orders or state a preference for symptom-directed care.[39]

You may choose palliative care to relieve, reduce, or soothe the symptoms of disease or disorders while keeping your dignity. You may refuse inappropriate, aggressive treatment. Some people who say they want to die are really saying they can't bear living with severe pain or depression, for which treatment may make life satisfactory. Medical professionals are trained to save lives, but they are also bound by oath to do no harm.

It may be possible to choose where you die—at home or in a hospital or a hospice facility. Hospice workers are specially trained to provide support and comfort to the dying, rather than trying to prolong life by whatever means possible. They can help manage pain and improve the quality of life for patients with serious, advancing illness. They can assist with dying comfortably at home if primary caregivers are available, or in hospice facilities, which may be self-contained or attached to a hospital or nursing home. If your priority is to have your wishes and values respected and your symptoms controlled, allowing you to spend meaningful time with the ones you love, this is your right.

Compassionate end-of-life care that addresses your emotional, spiritual, and practical needs is essential, regardless of the type of treatment or care you choose. Though legal, medical, and theological controversies abound, the right to make decisions about our quality of life is part of our basic right to control our bodies and our lives.

CAREGIVING

Women have been the primary caregivers for generations. With increased longevity, a growing number of us will see our parents live to old age as we head there ourselves. Though caregiving can be immensely fulfilling, the resulting responsibilities, which may involve years of care, have to be balanced with workplace and other family commitments.

Sixty-six percent of all caregivers are women; 41 percent of these women work full-time, and 13 percent work part-time.[40] The average age of the adult care recipient is sixty-nine years old. Sixty-seven percent of working women who are caregivers have had to make workplace adjustments, such as going in late, leaving early, or taking time off, while 22 percent have had to take a leave of absence. Often the caregiving is taken for granted, with little support or appreciation. The economic value of caregivers' unpaid contributions is estimated at $375 billion.[41]

Research shows that caregivers have higher rates of depression, chronic disease, infection, and exhaustion than peers of the same age who don't look after others.

SALLY AND BETH

When Sally Gabb and her partner of twenty years, Beth Grossi, wed in 2005 in Massachusetts, they expected to be together, finally married, for many more years.

In September 2009, Sally, sixty-six, felt her body undergoing changes. "Bladder control," she said to herself. "I'm just getting to be an old lady." She was later referred to a urologist, who took a urine sample and called her in for a ureteroscopy.

"The first one to mention the C-word," Sally recalls, "was my urologist, who said, 'You definitely have a growth that is pressing against your bladder, and it's probably cancer.'"

Sally was scheduled for a biopsy that December. The same month, two large lumps appeared on her neck, requiring a second biopsy. Both came back malignant. Sally, who had no other health conditions, learned she had Stage IV uterine cancer.

"It's very scary. I think in some ways the person who you're with has to deal with the possibility of being left behind," she says, thinking back to her initial conversation with Beth about the diagnosis. "And whereas the person with the diagnosis—you're kind of going off into the unknown. So it's different unknowns."

Beth, too, feels the weight of the unknown. Sally's illness serves as a reminder that cancer, which took Beth's brother's life, can happen to anyone.

"It has made me aware that we weren't as Teflon as youth leads you to believe," says Beth. "It has put a lot of

fear and reality inside me, and makes me realize that we have to live every moment and not take things for granted."

Even though their home state of Rhode Island does not recognize their marriage, Sally's health care providers have treated them as spouses. Beth stays with Sally in doctors' offices and emergency rooms. If there's a meeting with Sally's oncologist, he always asks Beth to attend.

"There's never a question," Sally says, emphasizing the support she feels that she and Beth have had through her treatment.

But because the state treats them as separate individuals, Sally has taken care of property and financial matters. She and Beth own their house together, so to keep Beth from having to go through probate court, Sally placed the property in a joint trust. She also signed a living will.

"Starting to deal with that stuff is really odd," she says, "but after a while it normalizes, and you start thinking practically. It isn't something that upsets me anymore. I just want to make sure things are taken care of for her."

The couple has avoided talking about assisted living facilities because Sally has remained healthy through treatments. Sally wants to remain at home, but if she experiences a widespread recurrence and Beth is unable to care for her, they would try to find a facility where both women could live.

"If we decide to try to look for something in Massachusetts, could we even afford it?" Sally asks, referring to the state that would recognize their marriage. "Beth would do anything she could to keep me in a place where she could be with me all the time."

Sally and Beth have been talking more about some of Sally's other wishes.

"I tell her I want her to have a wild party, something to celebrate my life," says Sally.

"As for aging," Beth says, "I realize how lucky you are to get old."

We rushed my husband to the hospital with a stroke, and it was a medical miracle. Now I am not so sure it was a blessing. He is not always rational and cannot be left alone. . . . I had to give up my job. Financially, we are in terrible shape, but disaster will strike when he dies. I am 57 and won't be eligible for anything. I can't see my way out.

THE NEEDS OF PAID CAREGIVERS

Women make up the vast majority of workers in long-term care occupations such as nurses, nurses' aides, personal care attendants, and home care workers—and are grossly underpaid for their services. Many of these jobs are held by women of color and recent immigrants. These jobs require a great deal of standing and lifting, and workers are more likely to develop chronic conditions such as leg and back pain. Yet these same workers are also more likely to lack adequate health care insurance to pay for their own care.

All women concerned with caregiving—whether as family caregivers, as paid workers, or as care recipients—must join together to affirm the value of this work and advocate for decent wages and benefits.

One of a caregiver's greatest challenges is to balance self-care with her multiple responsibilities. The need for support for family caregivers cannot be underestimated.

People often think of caregivers as looking after spouses, forgetting that many of us are single. The essayist Margaret Nelson writes with great compassion and insight about taking on the care and end-of-life decisions of a friend, called "Anna," who was diagnosed with what turned out to be terminal cancer. Anna was single, lived alone, and had no close family. She asked Nelson and another friend to share the role of exercising a durable power of attorney.

A few weeks after Anna's death, Nelson ran into a colleague, who wanted to acknowledge Anna's death with a card of sympathy:

Did I know to whom it should be sent? When I responded that he could send it to me, he missed my meaning, assuming that I meant that I would forward it to her family. When I tried to explain that I would keep the card myself, he again misunderstood.[42]

RESPITE AND RESOURCES

With increased numbers of women in the workforce, fewer siblings to share extended years of caregiving, and increased geographic distance between family members, it is often difficult for primary caretakers to get help. Yet we cannot do it alone.

Resources exist to help caregivers, but waiting lists can delay services for low-income families. The National Family Caregiver Support Program, the first universal federal program created in 2001, provides information, counseling, respite care, and other services to all family caregivers. For information in your area, visit www.eldercare.gov or call the Eldercare Locator at 1-800-677-1116. Other resources include:

Family Caregiver Alliance (caregiver.org) offers information, services, and advocacy for caregivers.

National Alliance for Caregiving (caregiving.org) is a nonprofit coalition of national organizations focused on family caregiving. Alliance members include grassroots organizations, professional associations, service organizations, disease-specific organizations, a government agency, and corporations.

Rosalynn Carter Institute for Caregiving (rosalynncarter.org) establishes local, state, and national partnerships committed to building quality long-term home and community-based services. The website offers a good list of caregiver resources.

Share the Care (sharethecare.org) offers information about a creative model in which neighbors help family members with caregiving.

ACCEPTING CARE WHEN WE NEED IT

Many of us accept and even expect that others will depend on us, yet many of us fear becoming dependent ourselves. We need to learn how to accept help without feeling diminished, and others need to learn to provide help as our relationships change and become more dependent. Chronic illness or a new disability may be a blow to our pride and habits of self-sufficiency.

ELDER ABUSE AND NEGLECT

Older women and individuals who are dependent on others for care and protection are at increased risk of abuse, neglect, or abandonment. The overwhelming majority of abuse and neglect cases occur in home settings, and in more than half of all reported cases, a family member is identified as the abuser. Many elder abuse cases involve spouse/partner violence.[43]

Financial exploitation—the illegal or improper use of a person's funds, property, or resources—is considered abuse and is a growing concern. According to the U.S. Administration on Aging,[44] an estimated $2.6 billion or more is lost annually because of elder financial abuse and exploitation.

More specific data on elder abuse and neglect are woefully inadequate; state statistics vary widely, as there is no uniform reporting system and comprehensive national data are not collected. The National Institute on Aging funded a series of grants starting in 2003 to develop survey methodologies for abuse and neglect surveillance. A new indicator is being included in the Healthy People 2020 initiative (healthypeople.gov), increasing the number of states that collect and publicly report incidents of elder maltreatment. A national study of elder abuse and neglect would increase public awareness of the problem.

Though one sign does not necessarily indicate abuse, the Administration on

Aging lists these possible warning signs[45] that there could be a problem:

- Bruises, pressure marks, broken bones, abrasions, and burns may be an indication of physical abuse, neglect, or mistreatment.
- Unexplained withdrawal from normal activities, a sudden change in alertness, or unusual depression may be indicators of emotional abuse.
- Bruises around the breasts or genital area can occur from sexual abuse.
- Sudden changes in financial situations may be the result of exploitation.
- Bedsores, unattended medical needs, poor hygiene, and unusual weight loss are indicators of possible neglect.
- Behavior such as belittling, threats, and other uses of power and control by spouses or partners are indicators of verbal or emotional abuse.
- Strained or tense relationships or frequent arguments between a caregiver and the care recipient are also potential signs.

Sexual assault and nonconsensual sexual contact–including unwanted touching, suggestive talk, forced nudity, and forced exposure to sexually explicit content–are possible at any age. Service providers may overlook signs of assault, and we may feel embarrassed to discuss it. This fear can contribute to the underreporting of sexual assault among older women.

We may encounter particular obstacles to leaving or getting help including wanting to keep the family together. It may be difficult to leave because the abuser depends on you financially or on your care. Many of us face poverty or diminished income as we age; we may lack the financial resources or affordable and appropriate housing we need in order to leave.

Complex health care needs, mobility issues, or disabilities may combine with a lack of accessible community services to make living on our own difficult or impossible. Abusers have been known to damage assistive devices or prevent medical visits, further limiting mobility and access to help.

If we try to tell family or friends what is happening, the abuser may try to discredit us and persuade others that he or she is looking out for our well-being. Some caregivers (family or others), claiming to be unraveled by the stress of caregiving, use stress as an excuse to continue abusive behavior without intervention by social services or law enforcement.[46]

If you experience or suspect elder abuse, neglect, or exploitation, call 911 or contact the national Eldercare Locator at 1-800-677-1116. The National Center on Elder Abuse (ncea.aoa.gov) offers a list of state reporting numbers along with information on all forms of elder abuse, including domestic violence. Other resources include the National Committee for the Prevention of Elder Abuse (preventelderabuse.org) and National Clearinghouse on Abuse in Later Life (ncall.us).

This may be our first time accepting assistance, and doing so without resentment or loss of pride may be challenging. If helpers provide choices when possible, it may be easier to accept that help graciously.

As a widow at age 80, I had been living alone, and it was becoming harder for me to get around. A lot of my friends had died. . . . The solution for me was to relocate to a long-term care community close to my daughter. This gave me independence with family support nearby. My move has enabled my daughter and me to renew our relationship. We have built up a friendship based on a deep understanding of each other. I truly treasure this in my old age.

Another woman remarks:

Whether we have our own grandchildren or not, being in connection with babies, children of relatives, friends, neighbors, or clients puts life in perspective. I think about my grandson's vulnerability and how his overwhelming needs will be met. Wouldn't it be nice if we lived in a world where dependency in older adults would be met with such care and love?

LIVING FULLY: BUILDING COMMUNITY, CONTINUING ADVOCACY

From the bottom of my heart: Life gets greater and more surprising after 40, 50, 60, and, yes, 70.
—Gloria Steinem (at age seventy-six)[47]

The recipe for good health reaches beyond the basics of physical and emotional health. It includes having a sense of purpose and an enthusiasm for life. The strengths we develop by navigating the challenges of adulthood provide the foundation for successful living with meaning and fulfillment during our later years.

Getting old can be wonderful if you're not imposed on by other people's rules about how you should be when you're old. I consciously break as many as I can, because then I'm breaking through oppression.

We deal with less time left, we clarify our priorities, and we figure out what really matters to us. As we develop a sense of purpose, we may find we have the freedom to open up to more

Recommended Reading and Resources:
As you make your transitions, a book you might find useful is *Project Renewment: The First Retirement Model for Career Women* by Bernice Bratter and Helen Dennis. The first part of the book addresses the challenges women may face when looking to retire. The second part teaches readers how to start and maintain their own Project Renewment group for support and connections. See projectrenewment.com for more information. Other resources include:

The Transition Network (thetransition network.org) is a community of women over fifty who join forces as they navigate the transition from one career to another or whatever is next.
WomanSage (womansage.org) provides support for women in midlife through educational programs and social philanthropy.

creative expression than we had time for earlier in our lives.

I have returned to art after many years. I am in conversation with the paint, paper, and the visual world, sometimes responding realistically and sometimes abstractly. At age 67, this inner urge to paint feels like a more authentic, core response than it did in the early days, and I know that it will sustain me for the rest of my life.

Dr. Gene Cohen, a geriatric psychiatrist who was the first chief of the Center on Aging at the National Institute of Mental Health and the first director of George Washington University's Center on Aging, Health & Humanities, was convinced that older people have untapped wells of creativity and skills. He called creative activities "chocolate for the aging brain."[48] Cohen conducted the first national longitudinal study on the impact of creativity, aging, and well-being. Sponsored in part by the National Endowment for the Arts, the study demonstrated a positive link between creativity and healthy aging. Visit the National Center for Creative Aging (creative aging.org) to learn more.

A sixty-eight-year-old woman describes the steps she took after deciding she wanted to sing folk songs to her granddaughter. First, she had to learn how to play the guitar:

I went to the nearest music school, got a 28-year-old guitar teacher who plays jazz and blues, and told him I wanted to learn to play three chords. After many weeks he kept saying, "Aren't you bored?" He began to improvise with me as I played. From then on, he started teaching me twelve-bar blues and progressions and I moved to another level. I started playing in jazz clubs and joined a jazz group. I'm a beginner, but I love the process.

Those of us who grew up in the women's movement know we have more opportunities and possibilities before us than previous generations had at the same age. Are we as old as we look or as old as we feel? When does getting old even start? According to a 2009 Pew Research Center study,[49] survey respondents age eighteen to twenty-nine believe that the average person becomes old at age sixty. Middle-aged respondents put the threshold closer to seventy, and respondents age sixty-five and above say that the average person does not become old until turning seventy-four.

As for the age one feels, nearly half of all respondents age fifty and older say they feel at least ten years younger than their actual age. Among those age sixty-five to seventy-four, a full 16 percent say they feel at least twenty years younger than their age, and 34 percent say they feel ten to nineteen years younger.

One woman describes attitudes at her assisted living community:

We are so stuck on numbers! I don't think of aging in terms of numbers. People here up to 100 years old come to exercise classes. We don't use the word "old." We think the eighties are young. If you're active and vital and life is interesting, this is what counts. It gives others courage.

Many of us are asking how we can live with passion, purpose, hope, and meaning until our last breath. We are charting new territory in our later years and creating new norms for aging. Through support groups and other collectives, we are finding ways to affirm our gifts and define our legacies. The more we can give voice to the full experience of our aging process without feeling "less than," the more we can support one another to resist ageist attitudes. Our sense of ourselves changes in our older years, especially when we don't have familiar roles and we are balancing losses and gains and reinventing meaning and self-worth.

At 80, I'm more focused on being rather than doing. My outer world shrinks as my inner world expands. I embrace this stage of life, trying to accept new limitations and reflect on what enriches me, nourishes me, and what is the meaning of living now given I can't do and be the way I used to be.

WORK AND RETIREMENT

Many women are working into their seventies and beyond. According to the U.S. Bureau of Labor Statistics, the number of workers age fifty-five and older is projected to grow by more than 46 percent by 2016, more than five times as fast as the overall workforce. Some of us may not have planned to work that long, but financial security is rarely a given, especially in a volatile economy. It may be necessary to work to procure health care insurance for a spouse, even after reaching sixty-five and becoming eligible for Medicare. Or other family members may be out of work. We need to advocate for institutional policies that make flexible work options more available to older workers.

Retirement, even if welcomed, may lead to loss of status and structure, as well as loss of income. Yet patterns of retirement are changing as more of us seek meaningful activity throughout our lives. These later years can be a time for rewiring, renewal, and continued growth; we may be exploring entirely new fields or activities or pursuing volunteer opportunities that strengthen self-esteem, community connections, and a sense of purpose.

INTERGENERATIONAL LIVING

As we look for positive models for elderhood and think about what we can leave to future generations, consider building intentional connections with young people in your family or your community. A woman in her sixties describes being a grandmother to a new baby boy:

When I saw him, I immediately felt a visceral feeling of attachment and unconditional love for this baby. This is one of the gifts of aging. Loving him puts me in touch with aging in a new way. He pulls me into my future and a new chapter in my life. I feel rejuvenated.

Our wisdom and skills may be much needed by younger generations. Intergenerational programs that pair elders with younger women or with children who don't live close to their own grandmothers can give our spirits a lift and remind us that we have earned every wrinkle. Intergenerational connection may involve sharing family recipes, healing relationships with those we love, writing memoirs, researching and drafting family histories, and creating ethical wills that express our values and wisdom.

Programs such as the Intergenerational Center at Temple University (templeigc.org) provide national training and services for nonprofit organizations, foundations, and government agencies interested in applying intergenerational strategies. Generations United (gu.org) also focuses on improving the lives of children, young people, and older people through intergenerational strategies, programs, and public policies.

One eighty-five-year-old woman who lives in a cohousing development says that the experience has enabled her and her now-deceased husband to age in an intergenerational community:

We have potlucks, community events, and engage in socially conscious activities. We recently housed a family from Uruguay for six months while their son got medical treatment. In this environment, I fully experience deaths, births, children growing up—all aspects of the life cycle which is not typical in our age-segregated society.

As we work toward building a society that celebrates and supports elderhood, fostering intergenerational relationships and participating in advocacy organizations are essential to building supportive networks. We can share, celebrate, and continue our work on behalf of social, political, and economic justice.

Going to the March for Women's Lives was one of the most thrilling and exciting things I have ever done in my eighty-five years. The local League of Women Voters had organized buses that would drive from our retirement community to

Washington, D.C., and then drive along slowly at the rear so that those of us who couldn't walk that far could participate. Being part of such an important event with all those young women was electrifying.

WORKING TOGETHER TO CREATE CHANGE

The growing numbers of aging women (including nearly 40 million baby-boomer women)[50] could give us more clout as a political constituency if we organize or work for organizations that promote our issues. Government agencies such as the Office on Women's Health, the White House Council on Women and Girls, and the Department of Health and Human Services are paying more attention to us and to organizations that advocate on our behalf, such as the National Council of Women's Organizations (womens organizations.org).

Grassroots groups that welcome and encourage our voices include OWL, the Voice of Midlife and Older Women (owl-national.org), Raging Grannies International (raginggrannies. org), and the Gray Panthers (graypanthers.org) (see p. 583 for more organizations and website addresses).

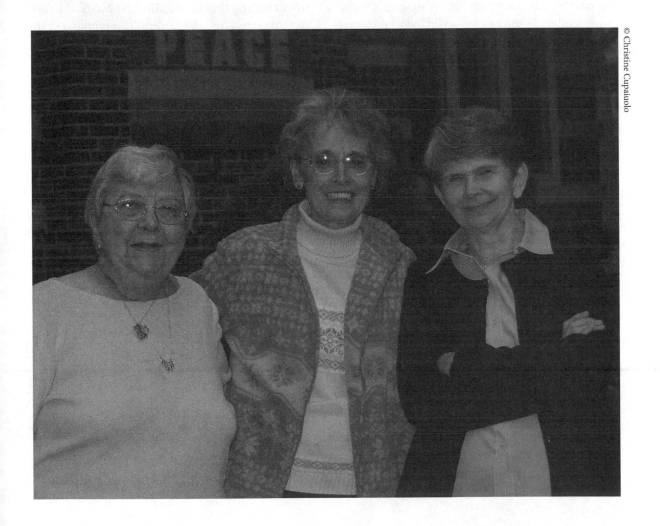

© Christine Cupaiuolo

In the years to come, we need to build on our strength in numbers by creating and supporting programs that meet older women's needs, including:

Long-Term Care: We need a continuous care system in which everyone receives care appropriate to her condition, provided promptly and efficiently in a setting of her choice and adjusted as needs change. We must keep pressuring policy makers and health institutions to support long-term care and the social services needed by an aging population.

Better care for older people requires better pay for all the providers who care for the chronically ill—including social workers, case managers, and sitters. It requires more social recognition of the role of family caregivers, some of whom have given up paid jobs to care for family members, and finding ways of paying them for providing long-term care.

Health Care: Protecting and maintaining Medicare, as well as expanding access to medical care not covered under Medicare, is crucial to women's health. Health care reform moved us in the right direction, but we won't have full, comprehensive coverage unless the government plays a larger role and we move toward a single-payer health care system.

For now we need to expand Medicare coverage to women ages sixty-two to sixty-five, and we must press for more affordable health care insurance policies that cover what we really need and don't reduce us to poverty. We must also support states' efforts to expand eligibility for Medicaid and push for adequate funding.

Work-Family Balance: The United States lacks policies that adequately support a reasonable work-family balance. We aren't paid for housework, child care, and eldercare, which keep some of us out of the paid workforce when our children are young and again when we are needed to help with aging parents and other family members. These gaps in paid work reduce our retirement benefits and pensions later on. We need to advocate for institutional policies that make flexible work options more available to older workers.

Expanding the Family and Medical Leave Act and passing a paid sick leave act is necessary so women can take time off for caregiving without risk of job loss. Those who quit jobs or take unpaid leave to care for a family member need some kind of insurance coverage to make up for lost income, now or in retirement. It is worth noting that the Family and Medical Leave Act, enacted in 1993, requires employers to grant twelve weeks of unpaid leave each year to care for a newborn or adopted child or a seriously ill family member, or to recover from one's own serious health condition. The law does not cover temporary or part-time workers and applies only to companies with more than fifty employees.

Retirement Security: After all this time, and in spite of laws and cultural shifts that have opened many occupations to women and enabled many of us to reach higher positions, we still confront ceilings in status and pay. Women still earn on average only 78 cents for every dollar paid to men; the disparity grows with age. That translates to a lifetime of wage discrimination and affects how much we receive in Social Security benefits and pensions. Retirement security can be even more difficult for never-married women with limited incomes, divorced women who were married less than ten years and who therefore can't get Social Security based on their ex-husbands' earnings, and women widowed before age sixty.

Women are more dependent on Social Security because they reach retirement age with fewer resources. It should provide enough to live on for women who have spent their lives making homes for their families, independent of marital history. Any proposals to address the future solvency of the Social Security Trust Funds must be assessed for their impact on women. Moves to cut benefits, raise the retirement age, or privatize Social Security will undermine women's economic security.

Most women do not receive employer-provided pensions. We need to expand access to employer-based part-time and temporary workers' retirement programs, institute portability of pension plans, and extend spousal rights to everyone. We must call on Congress to close the gender wage gap by passing the Paycheck Fairness Act, which will close the loopholes in and strengthen the Equal Pay Act of 1963.

Though some states recognize the marriage of same-sex couples, the Defense of Marriage Act (1996) still blocks Social Security benefits for same-sex spouses. Many older women would benefit from extending spousal pension rights to all. We need to increase benefits for widows and give Social Security credits for caregivers.

Aging touches everyone's life. Together we need to tell our stories and push our local, state, and national governments to provide a continuum of services for our older years—and to ensure that public and private programs acknowledge the diversity of our lives and economic resources. The steps we take as we age will influence attitudes and policy now and for future generations.

ADVOCACY ORGANIZATIONS

In addition to the organizations identified in this chapter, contact the following groups to become more involved with health care reform and gender equity policies that address work-family balance, retirement security, and caregiving:

Institute for Women's Policy Research: iwpr.org

League of Women Voters: lwv.org

National Committee on Pay Equity: pay-equity.org

National Committee to Preserve Social Security and Medicare: ncpssm.org

National Organization for Women (NOW): now.org

National Partnership for Women & Families: nationalpartnership.org

National Women's Law Center: nwlc.org

Pioneer Network: pioneernetwork.net

Raising Women's Voices: raisingwomens voices.net

Medical Problems and Navigating the Health Care System

CHAPTER 22

This chapter looks at procedures and problems that are particular to women's organs and the female body. It covers some of the conditions that affect large numbers of women—conditions for which it is sometimes difficult to get reliable women-centered information. Much is still unknown about many of these conditions, though new research findings emerge regularly.

These conditions are organized by anatomy. Some problems, of course, will involve more than one area of the body. The chapter focuses on benign (noncancerous) diseases or problems and on cancer prevention and diagnosis. It deals less with cancer treatments, since they tend to change quickly.

Other chapters in this book cover many topics related to

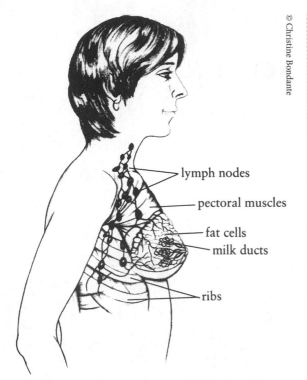

lymph nodes

pectoral muscles

fat cells
milk ducts

ribs

A breast, showing the structure of milk ducts, lymph nodes, and fat cells.

medical concerns. In particular, see Chapter 2, "Intro to Sexual Health" for information on preventive care for sexual and reproductive health and what to expect in a gynecological exam, and Chapter 23, "Navigating the Health Care System" for information on how to find good care, how to work collaboratively with a health care provider, and where to find trustworthy and up-to-date health information.

BREASTS

Our breasts are dynamic organs. They change considerably during our lifetime in response to aging and to variations in our body's hormone production. Understanding these changes can help reassure us when we think something is going wrong.

The breasts respond to estrogen and progesterone during each menstrual cycle, with growth and fluid retention that may be barely noticeable for some women but painful for others. The individual differences in breasts, along with the changes caused by age and menstrual cycles, can produce needless anxiety. We may worry that every change or pain is a symptom of cancer, when in fact most conditions causing change, lumps, or pain are benign.

Small cysts (a lobule or duct with fluid inside) may form, but they are usually smaller than a pea. Benign (noncancerous) tumors, such as fibroadenomas, may form during the teens and twenties and grow large enough to feel like smooth, mostly round, rubbery marbles that can be moved back and forth in place.

As we mature, small cysts may fill up further with fluid, sometimes causing tenderness and growing to sizes that can be felt with the fingers. By our fifties, dense glandular tissue and stroma begin to decrease (a process called involution), and fatty tissue increases. During perimenopause (see p. 510), hormone levels begin to fluctuate, and our usual cycles may become irregular. Effects of hormone changes on the breasts may include increased pain and lumpiness, which might be worrisome if we are looking for signs of breast cancer. Cancer rarely forms within cysts, but we may feel anxious while awaiting proof that a cyst is not cancer.

Some women's breasts remain lumpy after menopause. Most benign lumps are caused by hormone stimulation, so if you are taking hormones after menopause, the breasts will continue to feel as they used to. Cysts rarely form after menopause, so if a new lump does form, it's a good idea to have your health care provider examine it. Breast pain in the postmenopausal years may be coming from the chest wall, arthritis of the spine, or, only rarely, cancer.

BENIGN BREAST CONDITIONS

Breast Lumps

There are several kinds of breast lumps. Cysts are fluid-filled sacs that develop from dilated lobules or ducts, most commonly during our forties or fifties. They can be identified by ultrasound or by removing the fluid and making sure no lump remains. Simple cysts—those that are just fluid, for example—don't have to be removed unless they are causing pain or are so big that you can't feel the surrounding breast tissue. A breast ultrasound is the best way to be sure a cyst is simple.

Treatment involves numbing the skin with a local anesthetic, inserting a thin needle into the cyst, and drawing the fluid into a syringe— a process called aspiration. The fluid may look gray and cloudy, dark and oily, or clear yellow or green. If a lump remains after aspiration, or if the fluid looks dark and bloody, you'll need to have the area biopsied (tissue will be removed and examined under a microscope for further diagnosis). Cysts may refill with fluid after aspiration. If the same cyst continues to refill, removal may be recommended.

Fibroadenomas are benign growths that form mostly during our teens and twenties; some that form early may last throughout life. They may develop in one or both breasts. A fibroadenoma that's getting larger is usually removed surgically. These growths sometimes shrink at menopause, as hormone levels decrease. Fibroadenomas are rarely associated with cancer, although some breast cancers can feel like fibroadenomas. The younger you are, the more likely it is that you have a fibroadenoma and not a cancer. Often a mammogram can confirm that the lump is a fibroadenoma, but the only way to be certain is by doing a biopsy and looking at the tissue under a microscope.

Pseudolumps are areas of dense normal breast tissue. They develop in many women during the premenopausal years. To make sure there is no cancer, these areas should be evaluated with good breast imaging and follow-up breast exams.

Cancer in the breast usually feels firm and hard. It often does not have clear edges but blends into the surrounding breast tissue. Breast cancers are usually about 1 centimeter (half an inch) in size before you can feel them; in women with firmer, lumpier breasts, they must be even larger to be felt.

What If I Have a Lump?

First of all, don't panic! More than 80 percent of all breast lumps are *not* cancer, especially in women under forty. Lumps in our breasts big enough to feel may be cysts, benign tumors such as fibroadenomas, pseudolumps, *or* cancers. It is impossible to tell the difference with physical examination alone. A lump that gets smaller over time is unlikely to be cancer. A lump that remains the same size or gets bigger could be cancer, so it should be medically evaluated.

Many women feel anxiety and fear upon finding a lump and immediately think it's cancer. Our reactions may vary from wanting to go to the doctor immediately to being immobilized by fear. Finding a lump requires taking some decisive actions for yourself and your health. Tell someone you love about your concerns, so you can get some support and not have to go through the next steps alone. Then, contact your health care provider. Tell the appointment person or nurse that you have found a new breast lump and ask to be seen promptly.

Your clinician will do a physical examination of your breasts and determine whether further evaluation is necessary. She or he may suggest following the lump for one or two months, schedule you for diagnostic breast imaging (mammogram or ultrasound), and/or refer you to a breast specialist (usually a surgeon). If more information is needed, a biopsy may be recommended, since only a tissue sample determines for sure whether a lump is cancerous or benign.

This can be a very stressful time. Even though it's likely that a breast lump is benign, statistics don't always calm our fears. It helps to speak frankly with your health care provider about your concerns and to have the support of friends and/or family. It is also important to have confidence in your health care provider. If you are not comfortable with his or her recommendations, particularly a "wait and see" approach, be sure to say so. Getting a second opinion may be a good idea in this situation.

Breast discharge, itching on the areola, breast pain, and a breast infection are some of the other benign conditions of the breast that women experience. Nipple discharge, especially if it is bloody or coming from just one breast, should always be evaluated because it can be associated with cancer. Consult your health care provider for any persistent and troubling symptoms.

SCREENING FOR BREAST CANCER

Mammography

Mammography is the primary means of screening women at average risk for breast cancer. It utilizes a low dose of radiation to identify malignant tumors, especially those not easily felt by hand. A mammogram can also further investigate breast lumps that have already been identified, as well as other symptoms. Mammography involves X-ray radiation passing through the breast, producing an image on film or on a digital recording plate.

From 1975 to about 1990, the age-adjusted mortality rates from invasive breast cancer increased. In about 1990, they began to fall. By 2007, mortality had fallen by about one-third compared with its peak in 1989 and by 28 percent compared with 1975.[1] It is not clear how much of the decline in mortality is due to screening mammography. (See p. 591 for a discussion of routine mammogram screening for all women over age forty).

Digital Mammography

Digital images can be enlarged and the contrast adjusted, enabling radiologists to concentrate on suspicious areas. This improves their ability to detect tumors in dense breast tissue. Digital images can also be stored and transmitted electronically, making it easier to consult with experts at a distance. For women under age fifty, women who are pre- or perimenopausal, and women who have dense breasts, digital mammography may work better, but for most women over age fifty, the use of digital mammography does not seem to catch cancers earlier or improve outcomes.

Ultrasound

Ultrasound imaging—also called sonography—may be used to evaluate abnormalities that appear on regular mammograms. This technique excels in distinguishing solids from liquids, so it's useful for differentiating solid tumors from fluid-filled cysts, which are benign. Ultrasound can also be used to guide needle biopsies. Ultrasound works by creating an image from reflected high-frequency sound waves emitted by a device called a transducer, a microphone that helps magnify the sound. Ultrasound is not useful as a screening tool by itself.

Recently, two medical devices have been developed to address the problem of missed tumors following mammography in women with dense breasts, a condition present in about one-third of women having mammograms today. One of these automated whole-breast ultrasound devices has been shown in a large, well-designed study to significantly improve cancer detection compared with mammography alone.[2] This technique is not yet widely available.

Magnetic Resonance Imaging (MRI)

MRI is quite effective in detecting invasive breast cancer, but it also can falsely identify benign lesions as malignant. It is not a substitute for regular mammography, nor is it for screening of the general population. Some recommend it for screening women at very high risk for breast cancer. MRI uses a powerful magnetic field and radio frequency pulses that are processed by a computer to create images of organs and tissues. It does not use ionizing radiation (X-rays) but does require an intravenous contrast injection.

Positron Emission Mammography (PEM)

PEM is used in addition to mammography to identify small invasive cancers and ductal carcinoma in situ (DCIS)—cancer that is confined to the milk ducts. PEM is not yet widely available and may not be covered by insurance. It uses gamma rays to detect "hot spots" of rapidly growing cells, and a computer analyzes the image to determine the size, shape, and location of the mass. The efficacy of PEM is still under study.

Breast-Specific Gamma Imaging (BSGI)

Like PEM, BSGI is used along with mammography. It is not widely available and needs more research to determine how well it works. It may not be covered by insurance. BSGI employs a radioactive tracer to identify cancer cells.

Thermography

Thermography is used to assist in the diagnosis of breast cancer, but it produces too many false-positive and false-negative results to be used alone as a screening tool. It records the temperature of different areas of the body by measuring infrared radiation. Malignant tissue generally has a higher temperature than normal tissue because of its richer blood supply and higher metabolic rate.

In the future, as less invasive and more effective approaches are sought for early diagnosis and treatment of breast cancer, newer imaging technologies that look at breast cancer at the cellular level may become more widely used if there is clear evidence of their effectiveness as screening tools. Currently, BSGI and PEM involve fairly high doses of radiation and are therefore not appropriate for routine breast cancer screening.

DEBATE AROUND BREAST CANCER SCREENING GUIDELINES

All experts agree that mammograms can find breast cancers when they are small, are more curable, and need less treatment. But there is disagreement among experts over how many are found or missed, how many are successfully treated when found, how many don't need treatment at all, when to begin a regular mammogram schedule, and when to end it.

Screening for Women Age Forty to Forty-nine

For women between age forty and forty-nine, there is wide disagreement about screening mammograms.

The United States Preventive Services Task Force (USPSTF), a highly respected expert group, issued new guidelines in November 2009 recommending that women in this age group discuss with their clinicians when to start screening and whether to begin screening at age forty after considering the benefits and risks and discussing personal preferences.

In doing so, the USPSTF retracted its previous guideline for this age group, which recommended *routine* (that is, automatic) screening every one to two years starting at age forty.

The American Cancer Society (ACS) and

the American College of Radiology (ACR), however, both continue to recommend routine screening every year starting at age forty for all women.

There is agreement that mammography reduces death from breast cancer, even in women between the ages of forty and forty-nine. The USPSTF agreed that screening in this age group was responsible for at least a 15 percent decrease in mortality. So why the different recommendations?

The USPSTF used a rigorous method of evaluating mammography studies. It relied almost exclusively on prospective randomized trials comparing death rates from breast cancer in those randomized for screening against those randomized for observation only. Since the benefits of screening mammography have been widely acknowledged, only one randomized trial started during the last twenty years (because randomizing would have to assign some women to "no mammography," which most researchers would consider unethical). Critics of the USPSTF position assert that the weight of the USPSTF review is based on radiology studies that are out of date, but other experts dismiss this criticism.

In addition, different expert groups give different weight to the factors against and for routinely screening forty- to forty-nine-year-old women.

Factors against routine screening starting at age forty: Breast cancer is much less common in this group than in older women; the number of false-positive tests (in which the mammogram suggests a woman has cancer, but a biopsy shows no cancer) is higher for younger women; and starting mammograms at forty would mean having exams every two years for an average of thirty-four years. Over a lifetime, a woman's chances of needing a biopsy to prove she didn't have breast cancer might be as high as 50 percent.

Factors for routine screening in women starting at age forty: Cancers that are found in this age group tend to be more aggressive than those found in older women, and screening done every year, instead of every two years, may catch more of these aggressive cancers. While women may have to endure more biopsies, or anxiety with false-positive diagnoses, not getting screened can also produce anxiety.

It may be helpful to consider the comment of Dr. Ned Calogne, who chaired the USPSTF: "If I take 1,000 women age 40, over their lifetimes, 30 of them will die from breast cancer if we do no screening. If I screen every one of those women beginning at age 50 until she's 74, we reduce the deaths from 30 to 23. And if I reach down and screen them in their forties, I can increase that by one additional life saved—at best."[3]

Most experts agree that if a woman between the ages of forty and forty-nine is identified as being at high risk, she should be regularly screened (see "What Are the Risk Factors Associated with Getting Breast Cancer?" p. 593).

Screening for Women Age Fifty to Seventy-four

All experts agree that women age fifty to seventy-four should be screened regularly.

Some experts say women in this group should be screened every year; others say every one or two years.

The USPSTF proposes screening every two years. It argues that the additional lives saved by screening yearly are not enough to justify an annual procedure. Screening at two-year intervals would preserve 81 percent of breast cancer mortality reduction seen with screening at one-year intervals.

The American Cancer Society and the American College of Radiology recommend screening every year. They argue that the 19 percent increase in breast cancer deaths that comes with screening only every two years is not acceptable.

WHAT ARE THE RISK FACTORS ASSOCIATED WITH GETTING BREAST CANCER?

- **Age:** A woman's risk of developing breast cancer increases with age. Women from age fifty through age fifty-nine have a one in forty-two chance of being diagnosed, while at age eighty-five, one in eight or nine women will be diagnosed. The incidence of breast cancer in women younger than fifty is about 2 percent of all breast cancers diagnosed, but the chance of dying from this disease at a younger age is greater than that for women after menopause (who tend more to die from other diseases). Breast cancer is the leading cause of cancer death in women thirty-five to fifty-four years old, because women in that age bracket do not have a high death rate in general.

- **Personal history of breast cancer:** Such history increases one's risk of developing a new breast cancer in the other breast by about 0.8 to 1 percent a year up to ten years and then levels off.

- **Genetics:** A woman with an inherited BRCA1 or BRCA2 mutation or two or more first-degree relatives (a sibling, parent, or child) with premenopausal breast cancer has a significantly increased risk of developing both ovarian and breast cancer.

- **Reproductive factors:** The following factors are associated with increased risk of breast cancer: age at first menstrual period younger than twelve years; birth of a first child after age thirty; no full-term pregnancies; older age at menopause (greater than fifty-five years); not having breast-fed for at least six months.

- **Hormonal factors:** Postmenopausal obesity (thought to increase one's estrogen levels); recent oral contraceptive use, with some evidence suggesting that oral contraceptives slightly increase the risk of breast cancer among women under thirty-five years old;[4] long-term use of combined hormone therapy (see p. 541); long-term use (more than five to seven years) of estrogen alone (see p. 538); and high bone density after reaching menopause (suggesting high estrogen levels).

- **Other factors include:** Alcohol consumption (more than one drink per day or five per week); lack of exercise in adolescence as well as adulthood; a breast biopsy showing certain pathologies such as atypical ductal or lobular hyperplasias (where the cells lining the milk ducts of the breast or the cells that produce breast milk grow abnormally); and a history of high-dose radiation exposure to the chest area (often used in the treatment of Hodgkin's disease or lymphomas). Research in both the United States and Europe has shown a relationship between nocturnal light exposure (such as working night shifts) and breast cancer.

While white women are more likely to have breast cancer than African-American women, young African-American women are at greater risk for an aggressive form of breast cancer. Incidence data among various ethnic groups have been collected only since 1992, and research continues to question whether breast cancer development varies among these groups, even after disparities in access to care are taken into account.

Unfortunately, although risk factors for breast cancer have been identified, none is a "big red flag" that shows a direct relationship or cause in the way cigarette smoking is for lung cancer. Many women have no known risk factors.

Screening for Women Over Age Seventy-four

For women over seventy-four, there is disagreement.

The USPSTF makes no recommendations, because there are no randomized studies for this age group. The ACS and the ACR recommend annual screening as long as a woman has a life expectancy of five to seven years (most experts believe that the benefits of mammography compared with no mammography show up only after five years). They also note that it is easier to find breast cancer in older breasts and breast cancer risk increases with age. They also believe that the risks of screening are small.

The decision to screen or not screen in this age group, all agree, should rest on a discussion with one's clinician/primary care provider. Whether it's better to be screened every year or every two years is disputed. The incidence of breast cancer continues to increase into one's eighties, although most of these breast cancers are not as aggressive as those found in younger women.

Clearly, mammography can find curable breast cancers, even though there are disagreements about when to start routine screening. Weighing your personal preferences and concerns along with the recommendations of experts can be confusing and very stressful, especially if you have personal risk factors or friends or relatives who have faced breast cancer. Nevertheless, informed deliberation will help you make the best decision for you.

BREAST CANCER

Incidence Rates

A woman living in the United States has a one in nine lifetime risk of developing breast cancer. While any woman can develop breast cancer, the chances increase with age. Breast cancer in men is extremely rare but does occur (about 1 in 100 individuals diagnosed with the disease will be male). Most breast cancer occurs in women with no family history or known genetic risk. In fact, 70 to 80 percent of women with breast cancer have none of the known risk factors besides age. Only 5 to 10 percent of cases are in women with high-risk mutations of the BRCA1 and BRCA2 genes (see p. 597). About 255,000 women per year are diagnosed with breast cancer, both noninvasive ductal carcinoma in situ (approximately 62,000) and invasive breast cancers (approximately 192,000). The National Cancer Institute estimates that there are more than 2.5 million women living with breast cancer in the United States.

Breast cancer incidence is highest in the United States and in western and northern Europe. The lowest rates are in Asia and Africa, although incidence rates have been rising in areas such as Japan, Singapore, and urban China. These regions are moving toward more Western economies and patterns of reproductive behavior. Although the influence of dietary patterns is complicated, higher caloric intake at younger ages can lead to earlier onset of menstruation, which *is* a risk for breast cancer.

PROBABILITY OF DEVELOPING
INVASIVE BREAST CANCER AMONG WOMEN[5]*

CURRENT AGE IN YEARS**		RISK PER 1,000 WOMEN***			
		in 10 years	in 20 years	in 30 years	Lifetime
30		4	17	41	123
40		14	37	68	120
50		24	56	86	109
60		34	67	86	91
70		37	58	–	65

*Based on an analysis of data from the Surveillance, Epidemiology and End Results registry for 2005-2007.

**Women who are free from invasive breast cancer at their current age.

***Number of women in 1,000 who would develop invasive breast cancer in the next period of time.

The established risk factors for breast cancer do not account for all of the breast cancer cases. Despite the billions of dollars spent on breast cancer research, we have much to learn about why some women develop breast cancer and others don't.

Starting in the 1970s, the incidence of breast cancer rose at alarming rates. Much of this long-term increase is believed to be due to delayed childbearing and having few children. Obesity is also a factor. And as more women have screening mammograms, more cases are found; that accounts for some of the increase.

Between 2002 and 2003 there was a decrease in the incidence of breast cancer, particularly among women ages fifty to sixty-nine. This drop in the number of breast cancer cases coincides with the release of research findings from the Women's Health Initiative study (nhlbi.nih.gov/whi), which prompted many women to discontinue their use of hormone therapy.

Many people believe that the industrial processes and environmental damage that began during or after World War II play a major role in rising rates of breast cancer in Western countries. Research into environmental connections to breast cancer is the focus of organizations and foundations such as Silent Spring Institute (silentspring.org). Such research is difficult and frustrating because it entails identifying geographic breast cancer patterns in a population that is very mobile and hard to track.

Hormones and Breast Tissue

Reproductive hormones play a role in the development of breast cancer because they can affect cell growth as well as promote the growth of an existing cancer. As women age, the effect of estrogen on breast tissue decreases. As we go through perimenopause and become postmenopausal, breast tissue changes to fat.

On mammograms, young normal breast tissue appears thick and white, but as the breast ages and turns to fat, it shows up dark on breast imaging. In part, this accounts for why breast cancers, which appear white on a mammogram, are more easily detectible in women after fifty, who are usually approaching completion of perimenopause. As Dr. Susan Love has commented, "Looking for cancer on a young woman's mammogram [is] like looking for a polar bear in the snow."[6] Having denser breasts—with more glandular tissue in relation to fatty tissue—is a risk factor for the development of breast cancer. More research is being done to try to figure out why dense breast tissue is a risk factor and what, if anything, can be done for women with dense breasts.

The Women's Health Initiative (WHI) was the first randomized controlled study looking at women and hormone therapy (HT, formerly called hormone replacement therapy or HRT). It began in 1991 with the first results released in 2002 (see nhlbi.nih.gov/whi for more information). The major objectives of the WHI were to study cancer, osteoporosis, and heart disease among older women. The trial was stopped early in 2002 when researchers found that women who had taken a particular estrogen and progestin had a greater incidence of several diseases compared with women receiving a placebo.

For healthy women who took estrogen plus progestin, the research demonstrated an increased risk of heart attack, stroke, blood clots, and breast cancer. This same group also had a decreased risk of colorectal cancer and fewer fractures. After 2002, hormone therapy use declined in the United States and around the world. Many believe that this decline explains in large part the decline in incidence of breast cancer shortly afterward.

In 2006, the National Cancer Institute reported on the Women's Intervention Nutrition Study (WINS), which included women who had undergone hysterectomy and were given estrogen without progestin. (Women with a uterus who take hormones usually include a form of progesterone along with the estrogen, to reduce the chances that estrogen "unopposed" will lead to endometrial cancer.) Results from this study comparing women receiving estrogen with women receiving a placebo found that there was no difference in the risk of heart attack, but there was an increased risk of stroke and blood clots among the estrogen group. The effect on the risk of developing breast cancer was uncertain. (Estrogen made no difference in risk for colorectal cancer, but there was a reduced risk of bone fractures in women who took it.) The Million Women Study conducted in the United Kingdom[7] did show a clear increase in breast cancer among women on estrogen alone.

Follow-up studies have shown that the increased risk for breast cancer with hormone therapy—including both estrogen and progestin—diminishes within five years of discontinuing hormones. Recent studies report that the breast cancers developing in women taking both estrogen and progestin are more aggressive and more lethal than doctors previously thought.

What all of this means for women is that long-term use of hormones (greater than five years) increases breast cancer risk.[8] Each woman needs to discuss hormone use with her health care provider to determine what makes the most sense for her own situation. Some women consider using bioidentical hormones as an alternative to conventional hormones. Bioidentical hormones are chemically identical to the hormones produced by your body; there are many FDA-approved hormones that fit the definition of bioidentical, and their long-term safety has yet to be established. (See Chapter 20, "Perimenopause and Menopause," for more discussion.)

Genetic Testing and Inherited Risk

Breast cancer develops when changes occur in genes in breast cells. In that sense, all breast cancer has a genetic element. But genetic does not mean inherited. Only an estimated 5 to 10 percent of breast cancer cases result from an inherited genetic predisposition. In other words, more than 90 percent of all breast cancer cases result from factors that are not inherited and, in many cases, are unknown.

We all inherit half our genes from our mother

CAN BREAST CANCER RISK BE REDUCED?

Even though the causes of most breast cancer are unknown and nothing is guaranteed to prevent cancer, some studies have shown that certain health behaviors are associated with lower risk:

- Using hormone therapy during perimenopause only if needed and for a limited time (excellent evidence)
- Breastfeeding: the longer we nurse, the more protective the effect against premenopausal breast cancer (strong evidence).
- Delaying menstruation in girls by avoiding excessive caloric intake and increasing exercise in prepuberty (good to strong evidence). Girls used to start menstruating on average around age sixteen, a century ago; now the average age is around twelve, with some girls starting younger.
- Getting more than three hours of exercise every week (good evidence)
- Limiting alcohol to no more than one drink a day (good evidence)

- Limiting postmenopausal weight gain (good evidence)
- Eating more fruits and vegetables (evidence for direct connection is mixed)
- Consuming less saturated and trans fats, which are associated with health problems (evidence for direct connection is mixed)

Silent Spring (silentspring.org) and other environmental and health organizations have pointed to a growing body of evidence linking breast cancer to exposures to environmental pollutants and toxins. They recommend precautionary measures such as these:

- Microwave in glass or ceramics, not plastic. Don't let plastic food wraps touch high-fat foods such as cheese or meats during heating.
- Avoid plastic containers and bottles that contain endocrine disruptors—chemicals that disrupt the endocrine system in animals, such as bisphenol A (BPA).

and half from our father. There are some genes that dramatically increase the risk of breast cancer. Two of them are called BRCA1 and BRCA2 gene mutations. Blood tests have been developed—and are now aggressively marketed commercially—that can identify these mutations. A positive test result (having one of these mutations) does *not* mean that an individual will definitely develop breast cancer. Nor does a negative test mean that a woman *won't* develop breast cancer; it means only that her lifetime risk is the same as that of most other women in the industrialized world. But for those individuals who have an inherited BRCA1 or BRCA2 mutation, there is a significantly increased lifetime risk of developing breast, pancreatic, and ovarian cancers. BRCA1 carriers have an average cumulative breast cancer risk (up to age seventy) of 65 percent, compared with 45 percent for BRCA2 carriers.

It's important to consider the family history of breast and ovarian cancer from both your

ENVIRONMENTAL POLLUTION AND BREAST CANCER

Despite our decades-old war on cancer, women today are much more likely to develop breast cancer than any previous generation.
—*Silent Spring Institute*[9]

The consistent link between estrogen and breast cancer is one reason that scientists and activists continue to call for more research into environmental connections to cancer. The decline in breast cancer incidence that followed women's reduced use of hormone therapy strengthens the hypothesis that exposure to other external hormones and hormone-mimicking chemicals increases the risk of breast cancer. The Silent Spring Institute is a well-recognized research foundation that specifically focuses on the impact of environmental exposures, especially the effects of pollutants that mimic or disrupt estrogen and other reproductive hormones.

Even with strong evidence that chemical pollutants may affect breast cancer risk, it's difficult to apply what is learned in the laboratory setting to studies of girls and women. For one thing, it would be unethical to design a study where half of the participants were exposed to a chemical and the others were not, just to find out whether it caused cancer. Also, researchers need to be able to estimate a woman's exposures to multiple chemicals dating back to the years when a tumor started. We can't really know what's in our processed food and drinking water, what's off-gassing from the new carpet, or what's being tracked into homes from the outdoors. Finally, corporations hesitate to fund research unless patentable chemotherapies or medical procedures are likely to emerge from it. Public and philanthropic support is needed to fund environmental studies investigating underlying problems and their relation to cancer.

To find out how you can get involved with a breast cancer or environmental advocacy organization and make a difference for future generations, see Chapter 25, "Environmental and Occupational Health," and Chapter 27, "Activism in the Twenty-first Century."

mother's and your father's sides of the family. Genetic testing should be considered only in limited circumstances.[10] It is usually recommended that individuals with breast and/or ovarian cancer undergo testing for BRCA mutations because if the results are negative, their children would not need to be tested. Individuals without breast and/or ovarian cancer who are most likely to benefit from genetic testing are those of us who believe—because of a family history of two or more first-degree relatives (such as a mother or sister) with breast and/or ovarian cancer—that we may be mutation carriers and, if so, who want to take some action to try to reduce our cancer risk.

All genetic testing should be accompanied by written, informed consent; complete information about benefits and risks; and professional counseling about options. This is best done through one of the many cancer risk assessment programs located throughout the country. A comprehensive list of programs can be found on the websites of the National Society of Genetic Counselors (nsgc.org) and American Board of Genetic Counseling (abgc.net).

Cancer Risk Reduction for Women with Gene Mutations

If you have BRCA gene mutations, several possible strategies can reduce your risk of breast and ovarian cancer. These include taking drugs such as tamoxifen or raloxifene; prophylactic—that is, preventive—mastectomy; and having the fallopian tubes and ovaries removed. Because the science behind these strategies is changing so rapidly, and because these are major decisions with important risks to consider, it's best to consult experts, pursue the latest information about these options, and consider their possible effects on your life.

Breast Cancer Diagnosis

When you find out you have cancer, it's normal to feel shock, disbelief, fear, and anger. This psychological trauma comes exactly when you need to focus all your energy on learning about your treatment options. The most important thing to remember is that a diagnosis of breast cancer is usually not a medical emergency. This means that you have time to seek out opinions about the best way to proceed and to choose physicians with whom you feel comfortable. You have the right to have all of your questions answered and to understand your treatment options fully before deciding what to do.

Doing whatever your doctor suggests may be appealing at a time when you need to be taken care of, but it does not always result in the best care. Although most doctors have good intentions, they tend to offer only the treatment they know best. It's wise to get a second opinion before committing yourself to a plan, even if you feel confident with your first doctor. This is especially true if your physician has not fully explained your surgical treatment options.

> *If we genuinely hope to defeat the breast cancer epidemic, we must find ways to prevent the disease from even developing. And we must view environmental toxics as possible targets for our prevention efforts.*
>
> —*Silent Spring Institute*[11]

Lumpectomy and radiation therapy (also called breast-conserving therapy) when compared with mastectomy (removal of the entire breast) has the same survival rates; that is, the same percentage of women who don't die of breast cancer. If your surgeon is not explaining this to you, then you should definitely seek a second opinion. While in some circumstances a mastectomy may be recommended and be better for keeping the cancer from spreading, you should fully understand why your doctor is recommending it. Some physicians may be slow to accept new therapies until there's more experience with them; some may be unwilling or unable to discuss all available treatments. Some states, including Massachusetts, California, and Minnesota, have laws that require patients to be informed of all medical options.

Even though you may have a good relationship with your health care provider, if you live in a small town you should strongly consider going to the nearest large city with a research-oriented or university hospital. These institutions generally keep up with ongoing studies, use a team approach, and may be more flexible about treatment. A local women's health center, the National Cancer Institute (cancer.gov), or the American College of Surgeons (facs.org) can help you find appropriate cancer centers and specialists. Cancer centers usually have special breast cancer centers. The advantage of getting a second opinion or of being treated at a breast cancer center is that a team of specialists—medical, surgical, and radiation oncologists—will be involved with your care from the beginning. Private oncologists may not practice in teams, making coordination of your care more difficult. Certain breast cancer centers offer more treatment choices, including clinical trials testing new therapies.

If you meet income guidelines and were diagnosed under a federally funded screening program for uninsured or underinsured women, Medicaid will cover treatment for breast cancer. Some communities have local support groups for women with cancer, where you may be able to get help with transportation to medical appointments and with child care, as well as encouragement from other women who have had or are having similar experiences.

Surgery is usually recommended within six to eight weeks of the biopsy, so it's okay to take time to adjust, ask questions, and find out about your options. In some cases, chemotherapy is used over several weeks or months to reduce the size of the tumor prior to surgery (this is called neoadjuvant chemotherapy).

When you are trying to decide about treatment, the most pressing question is likely to be "How can I maximize my chances of disease-free survival?" But you will also want to understand the long-term effects of cancer therapy. To decide on the best treatment, you also need to know the size of the tumor, whether or not there is cancer in the lymph nodes, the hormone status of your tumor (called ER/PR), and what the HER-2/neu* status of your tumor is. These are specific for each woman's cancer, and these tumor markers can help individualize and optimize your

---

* HER-2/neu stands for "human epidermal growth factor receptor 2." It is overexpressed in 20 to 30 percent of breast cancer tumors and is associated with more aggressive disease.

therapy. Most of this information is available after the biopsy, and it is used to recommend systemic therapies (endocrine/hormone therapy or chemotherapy) and/or radiation. Usually the medical oncologist is the one who discusses appropriate treatment options based on the biopsy or surgery results.

It is important to learn about all the available options. The entire field of breast cancer medicine is changing rapidly. Old, established theories and treatments are being questioned, while newer techniques have not been used long enough to be completely evaluated. The 2010 edition of *Dr. Susan Love's Breast Book* and her website (dslrf.org) contain up-to-date and credible information on breast cancer treatment as well as important current research. The National Breast Cancer Coalition website (breastcancer deadline2020.org) takes an activist approach. Getting balanced information on the pros and cons of various treatment options will help with knowing what questions to ask and how best to proceed with your care.

Stages of Breast Cancer

Cancers are classified in stages. These stages provide some information about prognosis for an individual, as well as a mechanism for comparison of treatments and outcomes in different populations. Staging for breast cancer is based on three elements: tumor size or extent (T); which lymph nodes, if any, contain cancerous cells (N); and metastases—cancer detected by X-rays or scans in other parts of the body (M).

When cancer is first diagnosed, the clinical stage is identified by physical exam and some testing for metastatic spread. After surgery, lab analysis of the breast tissue and lymph nodes removed will determine the pathologic stage. The stage is important because doctors usually base their recommendations for treatment on how well other women with cancer at the same stage

BREAST CANCER STAGES*

STAGE	SIZE	AXILLARY LYMPH NODES	COMMENT
O	DCIS	Negative	Noninvasive
I	Less than 2 cm	Negative	
IIA	2-5 cm Less than 5 cm	Negative Positive	
IIB	More than 5 cm	Negative	
IIIA	Less than 5 cm More than 5 cm	Positive and matted Positive	
IIIB	Any size and spread to chest wall, skin	Negative or positive	
IIIC	Any size	Spread to other nodes	
IV	Any size		Spread beyond breast and nodes to other organs of the body

*For more information on breast cancer stages, see cancer.gov/cancertopics/wyntk/breast/page 7.

and similar history have responded to various treatments. The TNM stage is then grouped into five categories or overall stages.

CLASSIFICATION OF TYPES OF BREAST CANCER

Breast cancers are classified by whether they are noninvasive (or in situ) or invasive breast cancer. In situ tumors are made up of cells that when seen under a microscope look like but do not behave like cancer. They remain encapsulated within their usual environment—inside the duct or the lobule. There are no blood vessels or lymphatic vessels there, so these cells have no access to other parts of the body. In contrast, invasive (also known as infiltrating) breast cancer goes through the walls of the ducts and lobules, invading the surrounding fatty/fibrous portion of the breast tissue where blood vessels and lymphatic vessels lie.

Lobular Carcinoma in situ (LCIS)

LCIS is not cancer now—it's considered a risk factor for the development of breast cancer someday. Because LCIS is not preinvasive, there's no need to remove it unless it is found on a core biopsy. Because a core biopsy is a limited sample, the recommendation in this case is to have more tissue removed and examined to be sure there is no neighboring in situ or invasive cancer.

In studies of women with LCIS, 20 to 40 percent developed cancer (mostly invasive ductal carcinomas) over twenty years or more. Such cancers may occur anywhere within either breast, not only in the area where the biopsy was done.

Ductal Carcinoma in situ (DCIS)

DCIS is a noninvasive cancer. Many scientists believe DCIS will become invasive cancer if enough time passes. But it may never become an invasive cancer in your lifetime. More women get this diagnosis now because improvements in technology have made it possible to find more and more DCIS with screening mammograms. Because DCIS can become an invasive cancer, treatment is usually recommended. There is unfortunately no way yet to tell which women really need treatment.

If you receive this diagnosis, get a second pathology opinion—preferably with a breast pathologist—before agreeing to any treatment. If possible get an opinion from a breast cancer center where you could meet with a multidisciplinary team of breast specialists.

Women diagnosed with DCIS have approximately a 1 percent risk of developing metastatic disease and 96 to 98 percent are alive ten years after diagnosis.[12] Treatment aims to remove the area of DCIS and reduce the chance of a local recurrence within the breast. For years the customary treatment for DCIS was mastectomy. Early studies comparing a more breast-conserving approach with lumpectomy combined with radiation therapy showed similar rates for local recurrence of disease and no difference in survival. Now women have a choice regarding treatment options. For breast-conserving therapy, a procedure similar to lumpectomy, called wide excision or partial mastectomy, is performed with the goal of clearing the margins of DCIS (meaning no DCIS is found at the edges of the tissue removed). For some women, even after several excisions, DCIS remains at the margins and mastectomy is recommended.

There is a lack of consensus in the medical community regarding whether radiation therapy is needed for all women diagnosed with DCIS. Studies have not yet provided strong evidence suggesting that adding radiation therapy is more or less effective than wide excision alone.

Invasive Breast Cancer

In invasive or infiltrating breast cancer, the breast cancer cells have moved outside the ducts or lobules into the surrounding tissue. Because the tumor cells can spread to other parts of the body, through either the blood or the lymph system, treatment usually requires both local surgical and possibly radiation therapy, along with systemic treatments, such as hormone-locking medicines and/or chemotherapy.

An unusual but very aggressive form of breast cancer is known as inflammatory breast cancer (IBC). The first symptom is usually redness of the skin, along with an orange peel appearance of the skin called *peau d'orange* (which is why it is called inflammatory). Usually an antibiotic is prescribed to see if the redness is caused by an infection. If it doesn't get better, a biopsy of the breast and the skin will diagnose the cancer. The usual treatment is chemotherapy first, followed by mastectomy and radiation.

Overview of Breast Cancer Treatments

As researchers discover more about the biology of breast cancer, treatment theories change. Breast cancer, in general, grows slowly. Most breast cancers have been growing for six to ten years before they are large enough to be seen on a mammogram or felt during an exam. During this time, cancer cells could be spreading (metastasizing), through blood vessels and the lymphatic system, to other places within the body. This doesn't always happen—not all breast cancer cells survive outside the breast. Also, the size of the cancer doesn't always correspond to how aggressive it is; the type of cells in it will affect what happens, too. However, there is no sure cure. A classic saying among breast cancer survivors is that you don't know you're cured until you die from something else. Women who have been successfully treated "so far" refer to being NED, or having No Evidence of Disease.

Current treatments for breast cancer are either local (therapy to the breast) or systemic (therapy to the whole body). Surgery and radiation are local therapies; chemotherapy, endocrine/hormone therapy, and biologic/targeted therapy are systemic therapies because they reach other parts of the body beyond the breast.

Almost all women with breast cancer get some kind of local therapy, typically a combination of surgery with or without radiation therapy. The two usual surgical treatment options are (1) lumpectomy (breast-conserving therapy) followed by localized radiation to the affected area or (2) mastectomy. Some sort of lymph node testing is done for invasive cancers or noninvasive cancers that are more than 5 centimeters in size. A sentinel node procedure can be done when there are no palpable nodes (nodes that can be felt) under the arm. This involves removing only the nodes closest to the cancer, called the sentinel nodes. If those nodes do not show a spread of the cancer from the breast, then the more extensive operation removing more axillary nodes, which used to be standard, is not needed.

Overall survival depends on whether cancer cells have already spread beyond the breast to other parts of the body, and if so, on the effectiveness of systemic therapy. Local therapy may make a difference in the risk of local recurrence within the breast or how likely the cancer is to come back within the breast/chest area. In general, deciding whether it's a good idea to have systemic therapy (such as hormone/endocrine therapy) depends on what testing suggests about whether the cancer might spread and on how you feel about the risks and side effects.

Questions to ask your health care team so that you can be as well informed as possible include the following.

At initial diagnosis:

- Please explain to me the type of breast cancer that I have. Is it noninvasive DCIS or invasive cancer?

- How can I get an appointment with a breast surgeon? Are there hospitals near where I live that have multidisciplinary breast cancer programs with a team of breast specialists I can meet in one visit?
- What information do I need to bring with me to my visit?
- Do you have a breast pathologist who can review my slides? How would we get a second opinion on the pathology?
- Can we review my pathology report? What is meant by "grade"?
- What is staging and what is my stage of disease?
- Do I need any additional testing and if so, why?
- What support services are available for me and whom can I talk with?
- Is there someone who can follow me through treatment and be available to answer questions?

When discussing local surgical treatment options:

- Can I have a breast-sparing lumpectomy and radiation therapy?
- If not, why not?
- Can you walk me through the surgical procedure?
- Will there be a lymph node procedure, and if so, what kind?
- Explain your technique for a sentinel node biopsy (used to determine if cancer has spread into the lymphatic system). What does it mean when a sentinel "lights up"? How many of these procedures have you done? How many false-negative cases are there?
- What is the risk of a local recurrence in my breast or chest wall if I have a mastectomy?
- What is my risk of developing breast cancer in my other breast?

- If mastectomy is recommended or if I choose to have a mastectomy, can breast reconstruction be done? What types of reconstruction would be available?
- If I have a lumpectomy (also called partial mastectomy and wide excision), what are the chances you will not get clear margins?
- How many breast surgeries do you do in one month?
- How will the pathology results of my surgery influence my overall treatment?
- Walk me through the recovery process. What will I be able to do and not be able to do?
- What restrictions will there be on my activity? Can I exercise?
- How long do I need to miss work?
- If I have a mastectomy, how long will I be in the hospital? Will I need help at home afterward?
- What are possible short-term and long-term complications of the surgery?

Questions for the radiation oncologist:

- What happens during the radiation treatments?
- What will the side effects be?
- Will I be tired from my treatments? Can I work during my radiation therapy?
- How many treatments will I need?
- I hear there is a shorter course of radiation therapy that takes less than six weeks. Can I have the shorter treatment? If not, why not?

Questions for the medical oncologist:

- Please explain to me what ER and PR and HER-2/neu mean.
- How are these markers used in planning my treatment?
- When would chemotherapy begin?

- What are the immediate (short-term) and long-term side effects of the drugs I'm supposed to take?
- What happens to my veins? What is a port, and will I need a port during treatment?
- Is there a clinical trial appropriate for me?
- If I need chemotherapy, can someone give me a tour of the treatment area?
- Are there integrative therapies such as Reiki, acupuncture, and massage that I might use to help manage the side effects?

Lifestyle questions:

- What exercise can I do during my treatment?
- Can I dye my hair during treatment? Will I lose my hair during treatment?
- Can I travel during treatment?
- Will I gain weight or lose weight during treatment?
- Are there special foods that I should eat or avoid during my treatment?

Prosthesis, Reconstruction, or Scar?

Some women who have had a mastectomy feel comfortable doing nothing to "fill in" the place where a breast is missing, choosing not to get an external prosthesis or have breast reconstruction surgery:

I refuse to have my scars hidden or trivialized behind lambswool or silicone gel. . . . I refuse to hide my body simply because it might make a woman-phobic world more comfortable. . . . I am personally affronted by the message that I am only acceptable if I look "right" or "normal."

Others of us don't want a visible scar, and some worry that other people may be repelled by it. Some decide to use a prosthesis inside a bra, to fill in the area and "match" the other side under clothing. Some prefer to have breast reconstruction done by a plastic surgeon; this is done by using your own tissue and/or an implant.

Prosthesis

With an external prosthesis, you may look as if nothing has changed, as long as you wear your bra, which holds the prosthesis in place. It may shift under your clothes or feel heavy; it may be hot in the summer and cold in the winter. However, the feel, fit, and comfort of prostheses are continually improving. Stores and online companies that specialize in prosthesis fitting can custom-make one to fit your anatomy. You can get a temporary prosthesis after surgery; once your scar has healed, you can be fitted for a permanent one. Many health plans cover all or part of the cost of a prosthesis. Medicare will pay for one every year or two if you get a prescription from your doctor. If you have health care insurance, ask your insurance company what costs it will cover.

Reconstruction

Breast reconstruction is a surgical option either at the time of the mastectomy or later. Some physicians pressure women to start reconstruction at the same time that they undergo a mastectomy. Although this may provide a psychological boost and slightly reduce the number of surgeries, it's also okay to wait and see how you feel. If it seems that you have too many decisions to make all at once—sorting out your cancer therapy as well as whether to have reconstruction and what kind—then don't rush into it. You will also want to learn about important safety considerations, especially regarding silicone breast implants.

Surgical reconstruction involves using either an implant under the chest muscle or your own tissues, with blood vessels, moved from your back, abdomen, or buttocks to your chest area (called a flap reconstruction). Sometimes an implant is used to supplement the tissue transfer operation. Reconstruction is not without risks, both during surgery (risk of blood loss or infection) and later on, but it also may have physical and emotional benefits.

An implant is a flexible synthetic envelope made of silicone and filled with salt water (saline) or silicone gel. The implant is placed behind the pectoral muscle or a flap of your own tissue and then the skin is sewn together. If there's not enough space for the implant, a flexible expander is put in first to stretch the overlying tissues with saline injections over three to six months. Once the space is the right size, the expander is removed and replaced with a permanent implant.

Implant Risks

Many women have developed debilitating conditions after breast implant surgery. The two major breast implant manufacturers have both reported a very high rate of complications after reconstruction with their implants. Here are the statistics from one company, for women two or three years after surgery: 46 percent needed additional surgery; 25 percent had their implants removed; 6 percent had substantial breast pain; 6 percent had necrosis (death of tissue); and 6 percent had ruptured implants, often with "silent" and prolonged leakage of silicone into their bodies.[13] These complications were expected to increase over the following years.

Both manufacturers also reported a significant increase of symptoms associated with autoimmune diseases, including joint pain, fatigue, hair loss, and muscle pain. This increase happened within two years of getting implants.[14] Unfortunately, the companies never published those findings in medical journals.

We need more research on women who have had breast implants for at least ten to twelve years, since most leakage or rupture occurs after that period of time. Some research has found an increase in fibromyalgia and some autoimmune diseases among women with leaking silicone gel breast implants. We need better research to determine how often women with leaking silicone implants suffer from autoimmune symptoms, not just autoimmune diseases.

Reconstruction: Questions to Ask

Make sure you consult a board-certified plastic surgeon to find out what type of reconstruction is best for you. If the reconstruction uses muscle from somewhere else on your body (such as a TRAM flap), you will lose strength at the spot it came from. This is less likely if you have a tissue transfer that does not use muscle, such as the DIEP flap, which instead uses fat and skin tissue from the abdomen. If you want to consider a TRAM flap or DIEP flap, it's especially important to find a plastic surgeon who is very experienced at that type of procedure, because experience increases the chances of success in these more complicated surgeries.

For any reconstruction, ask how long the recovery period is for the operation being recommended. If you smoke or have diabetes, complications may be more likely, as your blood vessels may be narrower or damaged, and healing can be more difficult. If you are active, especially in a particular sport, ask your surgeon to try to make it possible for you to return to this activity eventually. Once you get a recommendation, ask to speak with other women who have had the same procedure, both with this surgeon and with others. You can find other women to talk to through oncology social workers as well as through breast cancer support groups and other organizations. Breast Cancer Action (bcaction.org) is a great place to start.

If you have one breast removed, the plastic surgeon will probably try to make your two breasts look as similar as possible. This is difficult with implants, which tend to make the new breast much higher and rounder than the remaining breast. Some plastic surgeons recommend a breast lift and/or an implant in the remaining breast, so that the two breasts will be more symmetrical.

Consider the possible problems that can result from additional surgery and its risks. Further recovery time and side effects, such as loss of nipple sensation, should be taken into account. It is also important to know that an implant in the remaining (healthy) breast is likely to interfere with the accuracy of mammography, since the implant shows up as a solid white shape on the mammogram, hiding any cancer above or below it. To try to improve the accuracy, whenever you go for a mammogram, the technician should take additional mammography views (called displacement views). These views are important to detect cancer, but they expose you to more radiation and could thus increase your risk of breast cancer in the future. In addition, the pressure from a mammogram can cause an implant to break or leak. For those reasons, women who undergo reconstruction should seriously consider whether they want the additional risk of an implant in the remaining breast.

If you are considering reconstruction, make sure the surgeon understands what you want;

she or he may have something different in mind. It's important to mention what size you would like to be and make sure the surgeon agrees. If you are planning a TRAM flap or DIEP flap, talk to your surgeon about how you feel about having a second scar where your own tissue will be taken for the operation. Your body size and how much flesh you can spare may be a factor in whether these procedures work for you. Some plastic surgeons suggest a tissue flap with an implant, but that means you have the longer recovery time of the flap surgery and all the long-term complications of the breast implant. Ask about newer procedures that may be less damaging. Take time to become as well informed about reconstruction as you are about treatment.

Whatever type of reconstruction you choose, the surgeon can create a nipple and areola using darker, grafted skin or a tattoo. This is usually done several months after the reconstruction surgery.

Future Promise: The Prognosis for Breast Cancer

More than 200,000 new cases of breast cancer are diagnosed every year in the United States; more than 44,000 women in the United States die of breast cancer each year. Currently, about three-quarters of women who get breast cancer are still alive ten years later, and almost two-thirds are still alive fifteen years later. Many women live long, healthy lives after a breast cancer diagnosis. But even with all the indicators available, it is difficult to make predictions for any specific woman. An individual's immune system and general health are part of the picture, but there are still many unknown factors.

Current research is focusing on identifying biomarkers—proteins in the blood that indicate the presence of cancers and how they will behave. Research is also looking at ways to keep cancer cells from reproducing, such as cutting off the blood supply to tumors and changing the genetic instructions that make them grow out of control; and developing drugs that can target cancer cells without killing healthy ones. In the foreseeable future, further work in these areas should result in more individualized and effective treatments—and perhaps even a cure. Participating in research such as comparative studies or clinical trials of new treatments is an opportunity to contribute to progress in breast cancer research and can be meaningful for some women.

THE UTERUS AND CERVIX

The uterus (womb) is a pear-sized organ made up of muscle that sits in the lower abdomen. It is lined with endometrium, hormonally sensitive tissue designed to nourish a developing embryo. Each month that a woman doesn't conceive, this lining is shed through a menstrual period. The uterus can stretch to accommodate a growing fetus, then push the baby out and return almost to its former state. The cervix is the opening to the uterus. It protects the inside of the uterus from the outside world and then opens during labor to let a baby out.

This section covers some of the major conditions and problems we may experience with these parts of our body. For more information on the anatomy and function of the uterus and cervix, see Chapter 1, "Our Female Bodies."

FIBROIDS (LEIOMYOMAS, MYOMAS)

Fibroids are solid benign smooth-muscle tumors* that appear, often in groups, on the outside, inside, or within the wall of the uterus, possibly changing the size and shape of it. Many

---

* The word "tumor" used to be a euphemism for cancer, but in fact, tumors are just growths of cells that serve no purpose. Over 90 percent of all tumors are benign (not cancerous) and harmless.

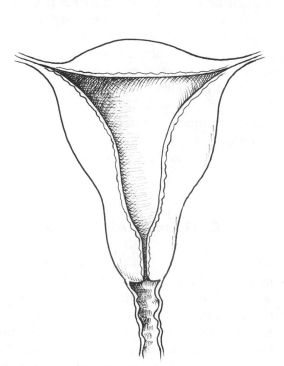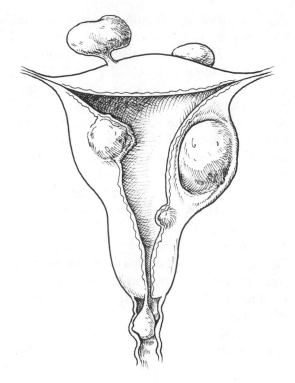

A uterus without fibroids, left, and a uterus with fibroids (benign growths), right

fibroids cause no problems at all, and many woman do not even know that they are present. Most women with fibroids can conceive and carry a pregnancy to term without any special treatment.

Some fibroids, depending on size and location, can cause heavy vaginal bleeding, abdominal or back pain, urinary problems, and constipation. Sometimes they may make a woman's belly look bigger. Fibroids that bulge into the uterine cavity (submucous fibroids) may make it difficult to conceive or to sustain a full-term pregnancy. There are several way to remove fibroids—which one is best depends on the size and location of the fibroids, as well as the skills of your surgeon. In at least 10 to 50 percent of cases in which fibroids are removed, new fibroids grow. However, only about 20 percent of women will require more treatment.

About 30 percent of all women get fibroids by age thirty-five and almost 80 percent of women will have fibroids by age fifty. Black women are more likely to have them, and to get them at a younger age. The cause of fibroids is unknown. About 40 percent of fibroids will grow during pregnancy, usually within the first three months. Some researchers used to think that using oral contraceptives made fibroids grow, but this is not as clear with low-dose pills. Very rarely, taking estrogen after menopause might affect fibroids.

Fibroids may be discovered during a routine pelvic exam. Because fibroids can grow, they should be monitored. If they haven't grown any more by the time you have your next monitoring exam several months later, a yearly checkup will be enough. Ultrasound can give more definite information about the number and size of fibroids, but this is not always necessary.

If you have fibroids and abnormal bleeding, be sure to get carefully checked for other possible causes of the bleeding (see "Abnormal Uterine Bleeding," p. 611).

Medical Treatments for Fibroids

In many cases, no treatment is necessary for fibroids; this is called watchful waiting. If you are nearing menopause, the natural decline in estrogen levels at that time usually shrinks fibroids. Although many physicians recommend hysterectomy—removal of the uterus—(see p. 631) as a treatment for fibroids, this is usually not necessary.

Myomectomy. If you have excessive bleeding, pain, urinary difficulties, or problems with pregnancy, you may want to have an operation called a myomectomy to remove the fibroids. Done by a skilled practitioner, myomectomy avoids some of the problems associated with hysterectomy and poses no greater risks. Even large, multiple fibroids can be removed with a myomectomy. There are several approaches, depending on the size and location of the fibroids.

Embolization of the uterine arteries. This procedure, performed by an interventional radiologist, cuts off blood supply to the fibroids, making them shrink. It reduces bleeding and tumor or uterus size in most women who have it done. The recovery time is typically shorter than for surgical removal of fibroids, if the procedure goes smoothly. Complications may include severe pain and fever that might require an emergency hysterectomy, damage to the uterus or other organs, and loss of ovarian function due to a constricted blood supply (this leads to premature menopause). For these reasons, this may be a risky approach for a woman who still wants to get pregnant.

Focused ultrasound surgery. Also called focused ultrasound ablation, this is another less-invasive option, but it can be used only for smaller fibroids and is not widely available.

Other treatments. Sometimes the drug leuprolide acetate (Lupron) is recommended to help shrink fibroids in women approaching menopause or planning to have surgery. However, Lupron has many negative effects, some of which may last many months beyond use of the drug. These include hot flashes, vaginal dryness, trouble with memory and concentration, and bone thinning. Also, after the Lupron is stopped, the fibroids can grow back.

The newest treatment, a medicated intrauterine device (IUD) called Mirena put into the uterus, can reduce bleeding and possibly enable you to avoid surgery.

Self-Help

Some women try to prevent or reduce fibroids by avoiding processed foods and the hormones usually found in commercial meat, dairy, and egg products, but there is no evidence that this will work. If your fibroids cause heavy bleeding, see the self-help treatments on p. 613. Yoga exercises may ease the feelings of heaviness and pressure; some women find visualization techniques helpful, too.

POLYPS

Polyps are a focal buildup of the uterine lining. Sometime benign polyps can grow in the uterine lining and cause a woman to have heavy periods or bleeding between periods. Once they are diagnosed—usually by ultrasound, and sometimes by a procedure with a thin fiberoptic instrument called a hysteroscope—they are typically easy to remove. Removal is usually recommended because of the small risk (fewer than 3 out of 100 polyps) that they may be precancerous, and to treat abnormal bleeding.

HYPERPLASIA

The endometrium can also become hyperplastic owing to abnormal growth of the endometrial cells. This condition can cause abnormal uterine bleeding, especially in women who are not ovulating regularly or who are taking estrogen without progesterone (or a progesterone-like substance like a progestin). While endometrial hyperplasia is benign, another condition called atypical endometrial hyperplasia can be a precursor of cancer of the lining of the uterus (endometrial cancer). In this circumstance, a hysterectomy is sometimes recommended to prevent the development of uterine cancer. Benign endometrial hyperplasia may be treated with high-dose progesterone, depending on the woman's age or intention to become pregnant, or with the Mirena IUD, which contains a progestin.

UTERINE CANCER (ENDOMETRIAL CANCER)

Endometrial cancer is the most common pelvic cancer, affecting fourteen out of every ten thousand women yearly. Most women with this cancer are over fifty and past menopause; 10 percent are still menstruating. If you are heavy for your size, take synthetic estrogen without a progestogen, or have diabetes, high blood pressure, or a hormone imbalance that combines high estrogen levels with infrequent ovulation, your risk of uterine cancer is increased.

During the early 1970s, there was a sharp rise in the incidence of uterine cancer because of estrogens prescribed for menopausal women without any additional progestogen (progestin or progesterone) to reduce the chances of endometrial hyperplasia. Taking progestogens usually prevents the development of this condition in women taking estrogen.

Symptoms

Bleeding (including light staining) after menopause is the most common symptom of uterine cancer. However, most women who bleed do not have cancer. For women who are still menstruating, increased menstrual flow and bleeding between periods may be the only symptoms. Unfortunately, the Pap test, while effective at detecting cervical cancer, is not reliable for detecting uterine cancer. If you have the above symptoms, your medical practitioner will probably recommend an aspiration or endometrial biopsy to sample the uterine lining—this is a simple office procedure. In some cases, a dilation and curettage (D&C) is preferred (performed with intravenous sedation or general anesthesia). Make sure that you have discussed the risks and benefits of these alternatives before making a decision.

Prevention and Self-Help

Because endometrial cancer appears to be influenced by factors such as obesity, hypertension, and diabetes, controlling these conditions with self-help methods may prevent this type of cancer from developing. Exercise and a healthy diet with plenty of fruits and vegetables is the best strategy.

Medical Treatments for Uterine Cancer

When uterine cancer is found early, the success rate of conventional treatments is very high. Medical treatment for uterine cancer includes surgery, radiation, and chemotherapy. There is wide disagreement about which is best. Outside the United States, radiation is used frequently with good results. Hysterectomy is the most common treatment in the United States. Follow-up radiation after surgery is possible if the tumor was large, if it is found or suspected to have spread to the lymph nodes, or if cellular changes suggest a fast-growing tumor. Hysterectomy can often be done laparoscopically. If the cancer comes back after one of these treatments, progestogen treatment may help slow it down.

ABNORMAL UTERINE BLEEDING (AUB)[15]

Heavy menstrual bleeding (which may include clots of blood) or bleeding happening outside the normal cyclic menstruation is referred to as abnormal uterine bleeding (AUB). AUB is a common gynecological problem, but its causes can be tricky to diagnose. The most likely cause of AUB for any woman depends on whether she is premenopausal, perimenopausal (near menopause), or postmenopausal.

Some causes of AUB include hormonal imbalances, pregnancy, the use of hormonal contraceptives (birth control pills or Depo-Provera, for instance), fibroids, endometrial polyps, infection, and, more rarely, precancerous or cancerous growths. Infrequently, bleeding that seems to be coming from the vagina may actually come from the urinary tract or gastrointestinal tract. For severe bleeding without an obvious explanation, ask to be screened for von Willebrand disease, especially if you have a history of other bleeding problems (see p. 613).

Fibroids can cause heavy, longer periods, sometimes with cramping and clots. More commonly, this occurs when the fibroids are submucosal and impinge on the uterine lining. Such periods are usually not irregular.

In addition to being a sign of a possible physical problem, heavy and/or irregular bleeding is a nuisance. It can also result in anemia from low iron and thus cause fatigue. Sometimes, heavy and prolonged bleeding may be part of the normal transition to menopause.

ABNORMAL UTERINE BLEEDING IN MENSTRUATING WOMEN

If you are menstruating and notice any of the following patterns, contact your health care provider:

- An episode of menstrual bleeding that lasts three or four days longer than usual
- More than one menstrual cycle that is shorter than twenty or twenty-one days
- Bleeding after intercourse
- Heavy monthly bleeding, especially with clots (if you are soaking through ten sanitary products a day you are bleeding heavily)
- Spotting or bleeding between menstrual periods

Abnormal Uterine Bleeding at Perimenopause

During perimenopause (the transition to menopause), new and different bleeding patterns are common. That makes it hard to decide when the menstrual cycle is normal and when there is a problem. The amount of blood flow may vary from month to month. Women sometimes skip their period for a few months, and then have regular periods again. However, if you are experiencing many episodes of irregular bleeding as described in the box above, it could be a sign of a medical problem that should be addressed.

Abnormal Uterine Bleeding in Menopausal Women

Women who take hormone therapy may experience normal or abnormal uterine bleeding.

You should understand what pattern is expected with your hormone prescription and contact your health care provider if your bleeding is different from what you've been told to expect.

Vaginal bleeding is abnormal in any woman who is postmenopausal (has gone a full year without any menstrual periods), unless she is taking hormones.

Diagnosis

Clinicians will review a woman's medical history. For premenopausal women who are missing periods, the bleeding pattern may suggest pregnancy or ovulation (producing an egg). A pregnancy test can find out whether an abnormal pregnancy is causing AUB. Blood tests can check for anemia, thyroid function, and female hormone levels. Other symptoms, such as pelvic pain or hair growth, can suggest other particular causes of AUB.

A clinician may be able to detect uterine abnormalities such as fibroids through a pelvic exam. Women with AUB should get a Pap test if one has not been performed recently.

Adenomyosis (endometriosis in the wall of the uterus, a condition affecting about 10 percent of women) is another cause of heavy and painful periods. It can be diagnosed only with an expensive MRI or a surgical specimen during a hysterectomy.

Four special tests are often used to evaluate AUB, as follows.

Endometrial biopsy: This is a quick office procedure involving the removal of tissue from the uterine lining (endometrium) to check for precancerous and cancerous cells. A thin tube, which is a suction device, is inserted into the uterus through the vagina and the cervical opening. It withdraws samples of uterine tissue for analysis. This may cause cramping, and some women will need pain medication, including anesthesia.

Transvaginal ultrasound: In this test, a wand placed in the vagina produces sound waves that create an image of the pelvic organs. The test can identify uterine fibroids. It measures the endometrial lining and may indicate abnormalities in the endometrium.

Sonohysterogram, or saline infusion sonography: This special kind of transvaginal ultrasound involves putting saline (salt water) into the uterus through a thin tube, to improve the image and detection of abnormalities.

Hysteroscopy: Diagnostic hysteroscopy involves threading a thin flexible scope into the uterus to view the contents of the uterine cavity. It can be done in the office or at a surgical procedure unit. Operative hysteroscopy is done at the hospital with anesthesia. A slightly larger scope is used to look at the uterine cavity and remove abnormal tissue such as fibroids or polyps.

Medical Treatments of Abnormal Uterine Bleeding

The treatment for abnormal bleeding depends on what is thought to be its cause. A woman's age and plans for childbearing, as well as her preference, are important in planning the treatment. Treatments range from observation (and taking iron, if a woman is anemic) to hysterectomy, or removing the uterus.

Various medications can reduce or regulate abnormal bleeding and relieve pain. Nonsteroidal anti-inflammatory drugs (such as ibuprofen) taken for pain may also reduce bleeding. Tranexamic acid is a medication that significantly decreases menstrual bleeding. Only recently introduced in the United States, it has been available in other countries for many years. Birth control pills make the cycle more regular and reduce bleeding, but there is some controversy about using them during perimenopause (see the Centre for Menstrual Cycle and Ovulation Research for more information: cemcor .org).

An IUD (intrauterine device) treated with a progestin, such as the levonorgestrel-releasing Mirena, can be a nonestrogen hormonal option for controlling bleeding. Some other drugs, such as danazol and Lupron, reduce bleeding even more but also have serious negative side effects (see above); they are typically used for only a short time, to postpone or prepare you for surgery.

Noninvasive outpatient surgery (endometrial ablation) may be done with several techniques that cauterize, freeze, or remove the lining of the uterus to reduce bleeding. These include operative hysteroscopy (where the uterine lining is surgically removed) or the use of specially designed instruments such as the thermal balloon (ThermaChoice) or NovaSure to cauterize or even freeze the uterine lining. Endometrial ablation is an option after more serious causes of abnormal bleeding are ruled out. It may be less effective in the presence of fibroids. Hysterectomy is the only known effective treatment for adenomyosis.

Always discuss the particulars of your situation and your choices with your clinician. If you are uncomfortable with the options offered, try to get a second opinion.

Self-Help

If you are premenopausal, you may be able to stabilize your menstrual flow by reducing stress and changing your diet. Cutting down on animal fat and adding fiber helps to restore normal hormonal balance by lowering cholesterol, which is converted to estrogen in your body.

There is controversy about whether soy products—and which types—are beneficial for AUB or may help to regulate periods. Supplements of vitamins A, E, and C with bioflavonoids may help if your diet does not include enough of these vitamins. (Take no more than 10,000 IU of a vitamin A supplement twice a day, since larger doses can be toxic. One carrot contains 8,000 IU, and dark green leafy vegetables contain a lot, too, so you can get enough vitamin A from food.) If you are bleeding heavily, increase your iron intake to prevent anemia.

Some women find that Chinese medicine, including acupuncture and Chinese herbs, helps to restore hormonal balance. If you are approaching menopause, the bleeding may stop by itself as your hormone levels get lower.

VON WILLEBRAND DISEASE, A BLEEDING DISORDER

The underlying cause of very heavy periods may be von Willebrand disease (VWD), the world's most common inherited bleeding disorder. It's a deficiency in the amount or quality of a protein that is required for blood to clot. VWD affects about 1 percent of people of all racial and ethnic backgrounds. Both men and women can inherit it from either parent. Because of our monthly periods, VWD affects females more frequently than males, but health care providers don't always realize that is what's wrong. The bleeding can range from being simply annoying to interfering with school, work, sleep, and mood.

VWD bleeding can be described as "oozing and bruising." Bleeding typically occurs in the mucous membranes (for example, in the mouth after dental work, or in the rest of the gastrointestinal system). The most common symptoms are heavy or prolonged periods, easy bruising, prolonged nosebleeds, and prolonged bleeding following surgery, injury, dentistry, and childbirth. Other signs can be bleeding into the joints and urine. VWD may result in miscarriage and unnecessary surgery, including D&C, uterine ablations, and hysterectomy at a young age. Affected family members can have different bleeding patterns, as can people with the same type of VWD. Absence of bleeding does not rule out the disease. People with severe VWD have the same level of joint damage as do those with moderate hemophilia.

The American Congress of Obstetricians and Gynecologists (ACOG) recommends screening all women with severe uterine bleeding for VWD. A federally supported U.S. hemophilia treatment center, if near you, may be a good place to seek help.

There is no cure for VWD, but there are effective treatments. Treatment varies according to how severe your condition is, and may include hormones, a synthetic nasal spray, or medication that is injected under the skin or infused into a vein. You may need to see a hematologist (blood specialist) familiar with VWD for accurate diagnosis and appropriate treatment.

BENIGN CERVICAL CONDITIONS

Cervicitis is a general term for inflammation of the cervix. A Pap test report or cervical biopsy may mention it, but it's not always a real disease or disorder. Cervicitis may accompany vaginal infections, pelvic inflammatory disease, and sexually transmitted infections.

Cervical eversion (also called ectropion) occurs when the kind of tissue that lines the cervical canal grows on the outer vaginal part of the cervix, making it red, with a bumpy-looking texture that is smooth to the touch. If the inside (columnar epithelium) puckers out, that is referred to as eversion. This is a common physical variation. Most women do not have any symptoms, although eversion can cause bleeding during a Pap test. Eversion requires no treatment unless it is accompanied by infection. Those of us whose mothers took diethylstilbestrol (DES) during pregnancy are more likely to have this condition.

Cervical erosion is a pinkish-red sore on the cervix, next to the cervical opening. This rare condition causes little discomfort. Most cases referred to as erosion in the past were really eversion.

Cervical Polyps

Cervical polyps consist of excess cervical cells that "pile up" within the cervical canal. They appear as bright red tubelike protrusions from the cervical opening, either alone or in clusters. Polyps are very common and usually benign. Most polyps contain many blood vessels with a fragile outer wall, so bleeding may occur after intercourse or other vaginal penetration, douching, or self-exam. Polyps may also bleed during pregnancy, when hormonal changes stimulate growth of blood vessels in all cervical, vaginal, and uterine tissue.

Cells from the polyps will be collected as part of a Pap test. Cervical polyps are almost never cancerous.

Polyps do not necessarily require treatment. When they are small and there is little or no contact bleeding, you or your clinician can usually just keep track of them with regular exams. Removing cervical polyps is often recommended as a preventive measure but is not required. You may want to have them removed if the polyps begin to grow. This is a simple office procedure where your practitioner twists the polyp off and scrapes or cauterizes the base. If your polyp is very large (this is rare), or if you have several of them, you may have to go to the hospital for removal. Sometimes polyps grow back after removal.

CERVICAL DYSPLASIA AND CERVICAL CANCER

Cancer of the cervix is responsible for the deaths of half a million women around the world every year. In some countries, it is the leading cause of cancer death in women. Cervical cancer deaths are on the decline in the United States, probably

RISK OF DYSPLASIA (PRECANCER) AND CERVICAL CANCER

The following factors may increase a woman's risk of cervical cancer:

- Never having a Pap test or not having had one for five or more years. Over half of new cervical cancer diagnoses every year are in women who have been exposed to HPV and who don't get this screening test. Therefore, they do not get early intervention to prevent cancer from developing.
- History of sexually transmitted infections, since HPV is often transmitted along with other STIs
- Smoking, which has been linked to cervical cancer in large population studies
- Synthetic hormones such as those in birth control pills or exposure to DES in your mother's uterus
- Unprotected sex at an early age. Young cells in the vagina are more vulnerable to whatever may cause cervical abnormalities; these cells are gradually replaced during the teen years with more resilient cells.
- Exposure to infection. It takes only one sex partner with HPV to get an infection, but having more sex partners increases the chances of infection. If you or your partner have (or have had) multiple sex partners, your risks of developing abnormal cervical cells are greater. Barrier contraceptives (especially condoms) reduce such risks.
- Contact with cancer-causing substances (in mining, textiles, metalwork, or chemical industries) or sexual contact with a partner who has worked with these substances
- A compromised or weakened immune system, which can result from being HIV-positive or using immune-suppressing medications such as chemotherapy. Yearly Pap tests are recommended for these women.
- Unhealthy living and working conditions and environmental hazards, often the result of having limited income. Women without access to a safe, clean environment are more likely to develop dysplasia and cancers—and at earlier ages—than other women.

as a result of Pap tests (which can catch cervical cancer early) and the treatment of precancerous cervical problems called dysplasia. Most cervical cancer results from human papillomavirus (HPV) infections that are transmitted through sexual contact (see p. 298 in Chapter 11, "Sexually Transmitted Infections). The Pap test, often done as part of a routine gynecologic exam (see "Pap Tests," p. 40), is a screening test for precancerous or cancerous changes in cervical cells.

Most of the cellular abnormalities we call dysplasia are now thought to be caused by HPV, but only some types of HPV are associated with cervical cancer. Tests that can identify the presence of these "high-risk" HPV types are now available (see p. 299).

The results of the Pap test are classified according to what kinds and degrees of cell changes you have, if any. Many systems have been used over the years. At one end of all the

HPV VACCINES

In 2006, the FDA approved the use of Gardasil, the first vaccine designed to prevent cervical cancer. FDA approval of Cervarix followed four years later. Both vaccines are highly effective against two types of HPV known to be associated with cervical cancer. Gardasil also protects against two other HPV types associated with genital warts (see p. 298). Newer HPV vaccines are being designed to protect against more HPV types.

Gardasil's introduction was highly controversial, because its manufacturer (Merck) initially lobbied some states for school mandates, which would require vaccine distribution in certain grades. Because the vaccine is so much less effective if administered after exposure to HPV, and because so many girls have their first sexual experience in their early teen years (when exposure to HPV is highly likely), these mandates were proposed for girls eleven to twelve years old.

Some parents objected strongly to these proposed mandates. Media coverage portrayed the objections as coming mostly from socially conservative groups and individuals, yet many parents who actively support school-based comprehensive sex education also objected primarily because the vaccine was tested mostly in older girls and women (age fifteen to twenty-five) instead of the group to which the vaccine is marketed. Only a few hundred girls in the eleven- to twelve-year-old range were included in the clinical trials that led to approval of the vaccine. Parents understandably wanted more evidence of safety before seeking the vaccine for their daughters. As of 2011 millions of young girls have been vaccinated with Gardasil and Cervarix, so five-year safety profiles for the vaccine will soon be available.

Even the chair of the CDC Advisory Committee on Immunization Practices pointed out that a school mandate for this vaccine was not appropriate when it was initially introduced. First, although genital HPV infections cause nearly all cervical cancer, they are not transmitted by person-to-person contact normally encountered in typical school or classroom settings. Simply sitting next to a student with an HPV infection will *not* transmit the HPV virus. Intimate contact is required. Second, new vaccines are generally introduced more slowly—not with universal school mandates—to determine what kinds of problems may emerge that need to be considered before rolling out a new vaccine campaign for a very large population.

Disparities in Access

Most women who die of cervical cancer never had regular Pap tests, had false-negative results, or did not receive proper follow-up.

In the United States, socioeconomic and racial disparities are evident in statistics for cervical cancer. Vietnamese immigrants are five times more likely to be diagnosed with cervical cancer than white women. African-American and Native American women are twice as likely to die of the disease as are white women.

In one study, Hispanic women had about twice the cervical cancer incidence of non-Hispanic women in border counties near Mexico.[16] Disparities are due, at least in part, to women of color having less access to Pap screening. It is quite possible that those women with the highest rates of cervical cancer will also have less access not only to Pap screening but also to the HPV vaccine. Until our health care system addresses such disparities in access, girls and women likely to benefit the most from this vaccine may well not be able to choose it.

To ensure more equal access to any adolescent vaccine, adequate infrastructure and resources must be made available. Some recommend implementation of school-based adolescent immunization programs similar to those formerly in place for delivery of hepatitis B vaccines. The United Kingdom and Australia have volunteer, nationally supported school-based campaigns that have resulted in high HPV vaccine coverage for about 70 percent of teenage girls.

Currently, school-based health programs and routine preventive care visits for adolescents are limited in the United States, making it highly difficult to provide good access to HPV vaccines, especially the type of access needed to ensure all three required vaccine doses are administered. Available data suggest HPV vaccine coverage in the United States is low (less than 50 percent) and the proportion of girls receiving all three doses of HPV vaccine is even lower (less than 25 percent).

Pap Tests Essential for Prevention and Treatment

HPV vaccines do not protect against all types of HPV associated with cervical cancer. Thus, regular Pap tests among sexually active women remain essential for cervical cancer prevention. Resources should not be diverted away from Pap screening programs to pay for the unusually expensive cervical cancer vaccine. Because Merck marketed Gardasil with a campaign that unnecessarily frightened girls, young women, and parents, many people now have a distorted view of this disease, the vaccine, and the continued importance of Pap screening.

There is no question that HPV vaccines represent an important scientific advance in the field of vaccine research, but exaggerating their potential benefit in places such as North America will not serve us well. In countries where there is little or no access to Pap screening, current HPV vaccines might have much more potential for saving lives if their costs were reduced considerably and if adequate infrastructure to provide them responsibly were securely in place.

Important questions will be answered over time as use of the HPV vaccine expands and improved vaccines are developed. For example, will successful prevention of infections and disease caused by the types of HPV targeted by this vaccine be replaced by disease caused by other HPV types, which now account for a smaller percentage of cervical precancer and cancer? Are three

scales is normal, and at the other end is cancer. In between are grades of dysplasia. Sometimes it can be difficult to distinguish one stage or grade of dysplasia from the next, and different laboratories or practitioners may interpret a given cell sample differently. Since the addition of the HPV DNA test in 2003, many clinicians interpret results of the Pap test in conjunction with this newer test.

As many as 40 percent of all tested women will have an abnormal Pap test at some time during their life. We often feel anxious when we hear our results are "abnormal," because we fear cancer, but there is no need to panic. Most cervical cell changes are very slow. Dysplasia is not cancer, and in about 80 percent of cases, dysplasia does not develop into cancer. The cells of most women diagnosed with mild dysplasia will return to normal. But all cases of diagnosed dysplasia should be watched closely—with repeated Pap tests and other recommended procedures. If abnormal cells are found, many women get tested again after six months to see if the abnormalities are still present. Dysplasia should be treated if it is severe or if it progresses.

Clinicians sometimes recommend a colposcopy after an abnormal Pap test. This is an office procedure during which the cervix is swabbed with an acetic acid (dilute vinegar) solution to make the abnormal areas stand out. Selected biopsies of the most abnormal areas are then examined under a microscope by a pathologist to better define the extent and severity of the abnormalities.

Treatments for cervical dysplasia are based on age, severity of the dysplasia, and each woman's personal history.

Medical Treatments for Cervical Dysplasia

Treatments for dysplasia (precancer) of the cervix vary widely. Different practitioners may have varying preferred treatments for each diagnosis, making it difficult sometimes to get appropriate treatment for your condition and avoid unnecessary or pointless diagnostic tests, treatments, and surgery. That's why second and even third opinions may be important. Procedures such as colposcopy, punch biopsy, and cone biopsy should be done only by medical practitioners who have special training, skills, and sufficient experience.

Minimal abnormalities often require no treatment. Mild (low-grade) abnormalities are usually managed with watchful waiting. Moderate or severe (high-grade) abnormalities require treatment or further evaluation. Treatments include:

Cryotherapy, which destroys abnormal tissue by freezing, can be done in the clinician's office. **Laser,** which uses a high-intensity light beam to evaporate abnormal tissue, is most often performed in an outpatient procedure center or occasionally in a hospital on an outpatient basis. Often, local anesthesia is given to numb the cervix.
Loop electrical excision procedure (LEEP),

which uses a wire loop charged with a small electrical current, is usually performed in an office or outpatient procedure center with local anesthesia. Clinicians use LEEP to remove abnormal tissue. The sample can also be sent to a pathology lab for evaluation. Sometimes this procedure is also called a LLETZ (large loop excision of the transformation zone).

Cone biopsy, which removes a cone-shaped portion of the cervix, can be done in an outpatient procedure center, or in the hospital on an outpatient basis, with local or general anesthesia. Clinicians may use a scalpel, laser, or electrical loop as used in LEEP to remove the tissue. Because cone biopsy does not destroy tissue, the sample will be sent to the pathologist for evaluation.

Hysterectomy is not appropriate for cervical dysplasia, but it is recommended as the appropriate treatment for invasive cancer (see "Uterine Cancer," p. 610). This is major surgery, with serious risks and other health consequences.

Long-term negative effects of laser and LEEP on the cervix are uncommon. Tissue damage may, on rare occasions, weaken the cervix, so it can be harder to carry a pregnancy to term. (This is more common with a cone biopsy, which also can produce scarring that might later interfere with dilation of the cervix during labor and birth, sometimes leading to a cesarean section.)

CERVICAL CANCER

Since the 1940s, the U.S. cervical cancer mortality has decreased by 75 percent. Currently, between 10,000 and 11,000 cervical cancer cases occur yearly, resulting in 3,000 to 4,000 deaths. (In comparison, about 40,000 women die yearly from breast cancer.)

In its early stages, cervical cancer is almost always curable, depending on the severity of the lesions and the treatment used.

If severely abnormal cells have spread beyond the upper tissue layer (surface epithelium) of your cervix into the underlying connective tissues, you have invasive cervical cancer. A Pap test followed by a biopsy can determine whether that has happened. At first the spread is very shallow and may not involve the lymph or blood circulation systems.

Medical Treatments for Cervical Cancer

For invasive cervical cancer, most physicians recommend a hysterectomy with removal of lymph nodes in the pelvis. If the cancer has spread into the lymph or blood vessels, doctors usually suggest radiation or hysterectomy plus removal of the ovaries. Sometimes a combination of the two is used (chemotherapy is not as effective as local radiation). Recently, there have been efforts to find fertility-sparing surgeries for cervical cancer.

You should be involved in your treatment and have the final say in all decisions. If you have any doubts about treatments recommended by your health care provider, try to get second and third opinions.

OVARIES

OVARIAN CYSTS

Ovarian cysts are relatively common and may result from normal ovulation. They develop when a follicle (the fluid-filled sac that nurtures a developing egg) has grown large but has failed to rupture and release an egg. Often, cysts don't cause any symptoms or discomfort, but you may experience a disturbance in the normal menstrual cycle, an unfamiliar pain, or discomfort on one side in the lower abdomen. Pain during intercourse is another symptom. Cysts are sometimes found by a routine bimanual pelvic exam, then diagnosed with ultrasound. Often they disappear by themselves, though some types may have to be removed.

To determine whether a cyst requires treatment, wait a cycle or two for it to disappear. If it persists, a medical practitioner may use ultrasound to monitor it. Practitioners disagree about whether removing benign cysts is necessary, but small ones do not usually cause problems and may be left alone.

A large cyst is more of a health risk because it can rupture, causing severe abdominal pain and sometimes bleeding. A large cyst may also twist and damage the blood supply to the ovary. These two uncommon situations require prompt surgery. Pathological cysts, such as a dermoid cyst or a cyst of endometriosis, should usually be removed.

If your physician advises removal of the ovary along with a benign cyst, get a second opinion. Removing the ovary, though a conventional practice in the past, is unnecessary in many cases. Ovaries perform many functions, even after menopause.

Recurrent cysts may indicate a hormonal imbalance and/or life stresses. Changing your diet, learning how to reduce stress, and using acupuncture may also help to get your system back in balance.

OVARIAN CANCER

Cancer of the ovaries accounts for only 3 percent of all cancers in women in the United States. About 22,000 cases were estimated for the year 2010 (with about 14,000 deaths expected). It is the ninth most common cancer among women in this country, but it is the deadliest among gynecologic cancers. Most ovarian cancer occurs among midlife and older women; more than half of all women diagnosed with ovarian cancer are over age sixty.

The exact causes of ovarian cancer are still unknown. Possible risk factors include a family history of ovarian cancer; few or no pregnancies; the use of fertility-stimulating drugs; a history of breast, colorectal, or endometrial cancer; exposure to industrial products, including asbestos, or to high levels of radiation; a diet high in fat; and the use of estrogens other than the birth control pill. (In one large study, the risk of developing ovarian cancer was higher in women who used menopausal hormone therapy than in women who never used such therapy, but the increased risks varied by type of hormone and regimen, as well as by whether a woman had had a hysterectomy).[17]

Using talcum powder in the genital area has long been suspected as a risk factor, but so far evidence points to an elevated risk for only one type of relatively rare ovarian cancer. Oral contraceptive use is protective against ovarian cancer, as is having multiple pregnancies. Having a tubal ligation also appears to reduce risk.

One reason the death rate is so high is that most ovarian cancer is found in the later stages, when it is harder to treat effectively. When it is found early, about 90 percent of the women treated survive at least five years.

Diagnosis

Ovarian cancer does not always have clear symptoms. Its warning signs—which may be vague and are frequently dismissed as stress or nerves—include indigestion, gas, bowel disturbances, loss of appetite or weight, a feeling of fullness, enlargement or bloating of the abdomen, lower abdominal discomfort or pain, unexplained weight gain, frequent urination, fatigue, backache, nausea, vomiting, nonmenstrual vaginal bleeding, or pain during intercourse. Most of these are relatively common complaints in midlife women.

If you have persistent symptoms or a family history of ovarian cancer, your gynecologist should do a thorough evaluation. In some cases, you may need to be referred to a gynecological oncologist, who specializes in cancer diagnosis and treatment. The screening tests now available for ovarian cancer are not very accurate, so there is still no good routine testing method for women with no symptoms and no risk factors. A blood test for a protein called CA-125 is not enough to diagnose ovarian cancer, because many other conditions can also raise the level of CA-125 in the blood; therefore, it needs to be used in combination with other tests.

Diagnostic tests for cancer of the ovaries include pelvic ultrasound, computerized tomography (CT or CAT scan), magnetic resonance imaging (MRI), and surgery, the only conclusive diagnostic tool. Exploratory surgery (laparotomy) is used for diagnosis, staging, and, frequently, tumor reduction. (For more information on stages and different types of ovarian cancer, including borderline tumors not likely to become malignant, see Recommended Resources.)

About 5 to 7 percent of ovarian cancer cases are associated with an inherited risk factor, and removal of an ovary or ovaries (oophorectomy, see p. 630) has been shown to be an effective way to avoid breast cancer in women who carry a BRCA1 or BRCA2 gene mutation. Discuss all the benefits and harms of a prophylactic oophorectomy with your health care provider.

Medical Treatments for Ovarian Cancer

Early detection, prompt diagnosis, and accurate staging are necessary for the successful treatment of ovarian cancer. Treatment depends on the stage of the disease at the time of diagnosis, the type of cells that make up the tumor, and how fast the cancer is growing. The current standard medical options for treating ovarian cancer include surgery, chemotherapy, and/or radiation. Immunotherapies, including interferon, interleukin, bone marrow or stem cell transplants, and monoclonal antibodies, are also available in clinical and/or research settings.

New cancer therapies often become available to patients through clinical trials. Information about some of these investigational treatments is registered with the National Cancer Institute (cancer.gov). Many women also explore supplemental or alternative treatments, alone or in conjunction with mainstream treatments. More research is still needed to better understand the causes of ovarian cancer and to find more effective diagnostic tests and treatments.

SELECTED REPRODUCTIVE TRACT PROBLEMS

PELVIC INFLAMMATORY DISEASE

I had been complaining of the same problem— pain in my lower right abdomen—for a couple of years. I had severe menstrual irregularities, fevers, bleeding between periods, bleeding after intercourse, pains, and general malaise. Several times I was treated with antibiotics, which brought only some temporary relief. Never was the issue resolved as to what was causing this. Never were my sexual partners or practices mentioned.

Pelvic inflammatory disease (PID) is a general term for an infection that affects the lining of the uterus (endometritus), the fallopian tubes (salpingitis), and/or the ovaries (oophoritis). It is caused primarily by sexually transmitted infections that spread up from the opening of the uterus to these organs (see Chapter 11, "Sexually Transmitted Infections"). Nearly 1 million women in the United States develop PID every year, and 300,000 women are hospitalized for it.

This may be a low estimate, because PID is underdiagnosed.

Symptoms

The primary symptom is pain in the lower abdomen. It may be so mild that you hardly notice it, or so strong that you may not even be able to stand. You may feel tightness or pressure in the reproductive organs, or an occasional dull ache. Part of the reason PID is so underdiagnosed is that women may also have some, most, or none of these other symptoms: abnormal or foul discharge from the vagina or urethra, pain or bleeding during or after intercourse, irregular bleeding or spotting, increased menstrual cramps, increased pain during ovulation, frequent or burning urination, inability to empty the bladder, swollen abdomen, sudden high fever or low-grade fever that comes and goes, chills, swollen lymph nodes, lack of appetite, nausea or vomiting, pain around the kidneys or liver, lower back or leg pain, feelings of weakness, tiredness, depression, and diminished desire to have sex.

The intensity and extent of the symptoms depend on which microorganisms are causing the problem, where they are located (uterus, tubes, lining of the abdomen, etc.), how long you have had PID, what if any antibiotics you have taken, and your general health. Doctors characterize PID as acute, chronic, or silent (when symptoms are not noticeable).

Causes

Most cases of PID are caused by microorganisms responsible for sexually transmitted infections. They can get into the body during sexual contact with an infected man or woman.[18] If you are carrying these microorganisms, certain procedures or reproductive events can push them farther into your body, including miscarriage, childbirth, abortion, or other procedures in-

volving the uterus, such as endometrial biopsy, hysterosalpingogram (X-ray of the reproductive tract), IUD insertion, or donor insemination. If you have chronic PID and antibiotic treatment doesn't help, your sexual partner(s) may be reinfecting you. Men can be carrying the organisms that can cause PID without having symptoms, so they must be tested and treated, too, and they should use a condom during intercourse.

The risk for developing PID is higher if you are exposed to infected secretions—especially infected semen—during menstruation and ovulation, when your cervix is more open and your mucus is more penetrable. Women using some IUDs are also at higher risk during the first four months after insertion. In some parts of the United States, gonorrhea still causes most PID. In other areas, chlamydia is more often the cause of PID. Current guidelines recommend annual chlamydia screening for women age twenty-five and under who are having sex, to find and treat this infection before it causes PID.

The complications of PID can be very serious. If untreated, PID can turn into peritonitis—a life-threatening condition—or into a tubo-ovarian abscess. It can affect the bowels and the liver (causing perihepatitis syndrome). Months or years after an acute infection, infertility or ectopic pregnancy can result if your fallopian tubes were damaged or clogged by scar tissue. PID can also cause chronic pain from adhesions or lingering infection. In the most extreme cases, untreated PID can result in death.

Preventing PID

Because so much PID is caused by sexually transmitted organisms, preventing PID involves preventing sexually transmitted infections. You can reduce your risk by using condoms and engaging in safer sex practices. For more information, see Chapter 11, "Sexually Transmitted Infections."

Diagnosis

If you could know right away exactly which organisms were causing your PID, you could get the right antibiotics. But pinpointing the organisms often takes some tests that may be expensive and not readily available. Sometimes organisms infecting the uterus and fallopian tubes don't show up in a cervical culture. You may be told that your chronic cystitis is caused by trauma to the urethra during intercourse when it's really a sign of PID, or that you got infected by wiping yourself from back to front, when you really have a sexually transmitted infection. You may be told that you have a spastic colon or an emotional, not a physical, problem, when that is not true. Try to have your situation thoroughly assessed, particularly if symptoms persist despite treatment, or seek a second opinion.

Blood tests can help indicate whether you have an infection but won't always tell you which one. Sometimes an endometrial biopsy can find hard-to-culture organisms, but if it is not done carefully, this procedure can spread germs from the cervix and vagina to the uterus. In some cases, ultrasound, including vaginal ultrasound, may be useful. A definitive diagnosis often requires laparoscopic surgery.

Medical Treatments for PID

Most experts seem to agree that since your health and fertility are at stake, you should start treatment while waiting for test results. Both you and your partner must be treated. If your partner continues to carry the microorganism(s), you will be reinfected. Taking the wrong drugs can make organisms more difficult to get rid of; however, the practical strategy is to begin treatment, then adjust it according to what cause is found. Once you start taking antibiotics, you cannot get an accurate culture again until at least a couple of weeks after you stop taking them.

Therapy lasts at least ten to fourteen days. You should receive two different kinds of antibiotics, since more than one organism may be involved. Remember to take all your antibiotics, even if your symptoms are gone, so that antibiotic-resistant strains of microbes will be less likely to develop. (See the Centers for Disease Control and Prevention website for more information about antibiotic resistance: cdc.gov/drugresistance.) Antibiotics can cause yeast overgrowth in the vagina, so you may need something to keep the yeast in check while trying to cure the much more serious PID (see "Yeast Infections," p. 637).

Many experts recommend that all women with PID be hospitalized for treatment, but not all physicians follow these recommendations. Most women are hospitalized in the event of an acute attack, to get intravenous (IV) antibiotics. If you're still not cured, it may be because you got the wrong antibiotic, have a pelvic abscess, or were reinfected by a partner.

You may be urged to have a hysterectomy if the doctor thinks that PID has damaged your pelvic organs beyond repair. Also, emergency hysterectomies are done in some cases of acute PID (for example, when an abscess ruptures). If the infection is in your urinary tract, as it often is, then hysterectomy does not eliminate it. Hysterectomy is rarely necessary for PID, except in cases of persistent, debilitating PID.

Avoid intercourse until you have felt completely well through an entire monthly cycle and your partner(s) have had negative test results for all STIs. You can have a recurrence of PID months after the initial infection is cleared up, particularly if you don't keep up daily health routines or are under too much stress.

Self-Help

There are some things you can do to help alleviate discomfort while you wait for test results to come back and for antibiotics to start working. Very hot baths and a heating pad applied directly to the lower abdomen help relieve pain and bring disease-fighting blood to your pelvis. You can soak a cotton cloth in castor oil, place it on the abdomen, cover it with plastic wrap, and then put a heating pad or hot water bottle on top to bring a maximum amount of heat to the pelvic area. Ginger root compresses and taro root poultices may relieve pain, keep the area loose and freer from adhesions, and dissolve already formed adhesions. Do not douche or use tampons; doing so may force microorganisms up into your uterus. Do not reuse a douche bag that may be harboring infectious organisms.

Certain herbs and teas may be useful against infection of the reproductive and urinary tracts. Raspberry leaf tea can strengthen the reproductive system; cranberry juice may help with UTIs. Try to eat wholesome, fresh foods and reduce stress as best as you can.

ENDOMETRIOSIS

Endometriosis is a puzzling hormonal and immune system disease in which tissue like that which lines the inside of the uterus (endometrium) grows outside the uterus. It affects girls and women from before a first menstrual period to postmenopause and can cause pain, infertility, and other problems. There are an estimated more than 6 million girls and women in the United States alone who have endometriosis.

The most common symptoms of endometriosis are pain before and during menstrual periods, pain during or after sexual activity, infertility, fatigue, and heavy bleeding. Other symptoms such as lower-back pain with periods and intestinal upset with periods (including di-

arrhea, painful bowel movements, and/or constipation) are also common.

Many with endometriosis also experience a range of immune disorders, including allergies, asthma, eczema, and certain autoimmune diseases. Other symptoms may include irregular bleeding, pain related to urination, yeast infections (gastrointestinal or vaginal), and abdominal bloating. Infertility affects 30 to 40 percent of women with endometriosis, and about a third of women with infertility have endometriosis. (If you know you want to conceive, be aware that delay in diagnosis and treatment may make pregnancy less likely if the disease advances.)

Women and girls with endometriosis appear to be at higher risk for developing autoimmune diseases such as chronic fatigue syndrome, fibromyalgia, hypothyroidism, lupus, multiple sclerosis, rheumatoid arthritis, and Sjögren's syndrome. Currently, researchers are studying whether there is a greater risk for certain types of cancers. Because of these risks, and because symptoms seem to worsen with time, early diagnosis is important.

Like the lining of the uterus, endometrial growths usually respond to the hormones of the menstrual cycle, building up tissue and then breaking it down. The result is internal bleeding, inflammation of the surrounding areas, and formation of scar tissue and adhesions. Complications of endometriosis can include formation and even rupture of cysts (which can spread endometriosis to new areas), intestinal bleeding or obstruction, or interference with bladder function. Symptoms often worsen with time, though cycles of remission and recurrence are sometimes the pattern.

The extent or size of endometrial growths may not have any correlation with the intensity of pain. Even tiny growths can produce substances called prostaglandins that are involved in pain (as well as in menstrual cramps).

Endometrial growths (also referred to as

nodules, tumors, lesions, or implants) are usually inside the abdomen—on the ovaries, in the fallopian tubes, in the ligaments supporting the uterus, in the area between the vagina and the rectum, on the outer surface of the uterus, and on the lining of the pelvic cavity. The implants can also be found in internal abdominal surgery scars, or on the bladder, intestines, vagina, cervix, and vulva. Rarely, they develop in the lung, arm, thigh, and elsewhere in the body.

"Don't be a baby, honey; all girls get cramps. Take two aspirin and go back to class," the nurse at my high school told me when I was bent over double in tears. . . . I'm not a baby. I'm not a hypochondriac. . . . It took six years to find out. Looking back, I wish I had been a more aggressive patient. I should never have allowed myself to believe these occurrences were all in my head. . . . Don't listen to the people who tell you to go away. Be persistent. Listen to your body.

Endometriosis is a major factor in decreasing the quality of life for many girls and women. It can be chronic and its seriousness is often underestimated. The Endometriosis Association (endometriosisassn.org), an international self-help organization founded in 1980 that conducts research collaboratively with the National Institutes of Health and Vanderbilt University School of Medicine, has collected data from four thousand women diagnosed with endometriosis and found that 79 percent said that they were unable to carry on normal work and activities at times, yet 69 percent had been told by a gynecologist that nothing was wrong.

I was diagnosed too late, though I complained bitterly about very painful, heavy periods since my midteens. I think it's disgraceful that doctors aren't more interested in treating this disease before things get so out of hand. . . . I am 36 and too destroyed (physically and emotionally) to carry on the fight to preserve my fertility.

Many doctors still don't take menstrual pain seriously. The average time between onset of symptoms and diagnosis is more than nine years because doctors are slow to diagnose and, in part, because girls and women delay reporting their symptoms. A compelling reason to push for earlier diagnosis is that those who had taken a long time to be diagnosed were more likely to end up having a hysterectomy, according to Endometriosis Association data.

Diagnosis

A definitive diagnosis of endometriosis currently requires a laparoscopy—an outpatient surgical procedure done under anesthesia, in which the patient's abdomen is distended with carbon dioxide and the abdominal organs are checked by using a laparoscope (a fiber-optic tube with a light in it). Though growths can sometimes be detected during a manual pelvic exam or on ultrasound, endometriosis is sometimes confused with other disorders that have similar symptoms (PID, ectopic pregnancy, cysts, appendicitis, diverticulitis, irritable bowel

THE ENDOMETRIOSIS ENVIRONMENTAL CONNECTION

Research has strongly suggested a causal relationship between dioxin, often called the most toxic chemical ever made by humans, and endometriosis. Dioxin and similar chemicals disrupt hormones and stimulate immune system reactions. Dioxin accumulates in our food from environmental sources, including pesticides and herbicides, industrial waste, and incineration. For information on how to reduce your exposure, see Chapter 25, "Environmental and Occupational Health."

syndrome, or even cancer). The Endometriosis Association has a diagnostic kit that helps.

Medical Treatments for Endometriosis

There are a number of treatments for endometriosis, but not one that works for everyone. The most important thing to know is that you must educate yourself and make your own decisions about your treatments, and find the right health care practitioner(s) for you. In the process, you may want to consider your age, your symptoms, where and how severe the growths are, whether or not you want to get pregnant, your past experiences with hormones, and family history.

Hormonal treatments aim to stop or stabilize the production of various hormones for as long as possible. Recently, aromatase inhibitors have also been used to stop estrogen production in lesions and in fat cells. Hormonal treatments include gonadotropin-releasing hormone (GnRH), agonists (such as Lupron), testosterone derivatives (danazol), progesterone-like drugs (Provera), the Mirena IUD (which releases a progestogen, a progesterone-like substance), and oral contraceptives. New drugs are currently in development. Medications can be very expensive, and all cause side effects that are problematic for some women. All tend to work while you are taking them, but the disease usually returns when you stop.

Surgery ranges from conservative (removing growths) to radical (hysterectomy and removal of the ovaries). Radical surgery has been called the definitive cure for endometriosis, but the disease can continue or recur even when the ovaries are removed with the uterus. Minimally invasive gynecologic surgery through the laparoscope has largely replaced major abdominal surgery. As with any surgery, the skill and experience of the surgeon are of paramount importance.

Self-Help

Complementary medicine—especially nutritional approaches, traditional Chinese medicine, environmental medicine, and other treatments—has proved helpful for some women. Contact the Endometriosis Association for more information and refer to comprehensive books on the subject.

Getting Support

Connecting with other women who also have endometriosis can be very helpful. One way is through the Endometriosis Association Facebook page (facebook.com/EndoAssn) or local meet-ups. Getting support can decrease feelings of isolation and provide opportunities to counteract misinformation or a lack of information, as well as to share experiences with others who understand what you're going through.

DES

The DES story is a cautionary tale of medical care gone awry.

DES (diethylstilbestrol) is a powerful synthetic estrogen that crosses the placenta of pregnant women and can damage the reproductive system of the developing fetus. DES may also affect other body systems: endocrine, immune, skeletal, and neurological. This drug was prescribed to an estimated 4.8 million U.S. women between 1938 and 1971 (and sometimes beyond) in the mistaken belief that it would prevent miscarriage. In fact, DES was untested for pregnancy use or safety, and studies showing that it did not prevent miscarriage were ignored for almost two decades. It was aggressively marketed and used worldwide, under more than two hundred brand names, in pills, injections, and suppositories, and sometimes in pregnancy vitamins, until it was found to be linked to a rare form of vaginal/cervical cancer (clear cell adenocarcinoma of the vagina or cervix) in women who were exposed when their mother took the drug during pregnancy.

DES exposure during an embryo's development has lifelong effects that can't be reversed. For example, the cells of the endometrium (uterine lining) of an adult woman who was exposed to DES in the womb will act differently from those of a woman who wasn't exposed.

Outside the United States, DES was also prescribed during pregnancy in Canada, Ireland, France, the United Kingdom, the Netherlands, Australia, New Zealand, Israel, Russia, and Poland. Other countries may include Belgium, Czechoslovakia, Finland, Germany, Italy, Norway, Portugal, Spain, and Switzerland. DES use in some of these countries extended beyond the 1970s. Large generational studies of DES mothers, daughters, sons, and granddaughters by the National Cancer Institute DES Follow-up Study continue in the United States as a result of efforts by DES advocacy groups.

Who Is Exposed and How to Find Out

Several million people have been exposed to DES, most without knowing it. If you were born between 1938 and 1971, if your mother had problems with any of her pregnancies or remembers taking anything when she was pregnant with you, you could have been exposed. (DES was most widely used between 1947 and 1965, when "wonder drugs" were popular.) However, with the passage of time it has become increasingly difficult to be sure by finding medical records. Some health care providers or facilities no longer have old records or refuse to give out the information. Any women in the appropriate age group should try to find out if she is at risk. See DES Action (desaction.org) for the latest information about DES exposure.

Medical Problems and Care for DES Daughters

One out of every thousand DES daughters is likely to develop clear-cell adenocarcinoma, a rare type of vaginal or cervical cancer. It has occurred in girls as young as seven and women up to age forty, with the peak at ages fifteen to twenty-two. Although the number of cases of clear-cell cancer has declined in the last three decades (mirroring decreased use of DES beginning in the 1970s), it continues to be found in DES daughters, some in their fifties. There is a suggestion of a possible increase in the number of cases as DES daughters reach menopause. If you are a DES daughter, you need a special yearly DES exam (see p. 628) for the rest of your life.

Annual DES exams can find clear-cell cancer early, so it can be treated. This cancer grows quickly and sometimes has no symptoms in the early stages. Typical treatment for clear-cell cancer may include a radical hysterectomy, surgical removal of all or part of the vagina, and reconstruction of the vagina. Radiation treatment may be added. Eighty percent of women survive this cancer.

Studies show that DES daughters have a greater risk for a more common vaginal cancer, squamous cell carcinoma. You may also have adenosis—columnar cells where the usual squamous cells should be—around the cervix. If you do, you may be more vulnerable to precancerous or cancerous changes. Annual monitoring is recommended until any adenosis disappears; discuss this with your gynecologist and be sure she or he knows about your exposure. Dysplasia (abnormal cell change) is more common among DES daughters, but normal cell changes may be mistakenly seen as abnormal when your cervix is checked, leading to unnecessary treatment with possibly harmful effects. That's why it's important to find a health care provider with experience in DES screening.

Structural changes in the uterus and cervix are common in DES daughters. Cervical "collars" or "hoods" (adenosis) do not have to be treated and may disappear after age thirty. A smaller or T-shaped uterus may contribute to pregnancy problems (see below).

If you are a DES daughter over age forty, your risk for breast cancer may be almost two times greater than that of unexposed women.[19] DES mothers, too, have developed more breast cancers than unexposed women—sometimes as long as twenty years after exposure—so both mothers and daughters should get a clinical breast exam every year, in addition to doing self-exams to become familiar with the normal look and feel of their breasts. Women exposed to DES should report any changes to their health care provider. Annual mammography or other additional screening exams are also appropriate for DES daughters.

Contraception for DES daughters poses some special considerations. Birth control pills may be risky, since they increase estrogen exposure in someone already at higher risk of hormone-related cancer. IUDs may not be safe because of cervical and uterine abnormalities. Barrier methods (condom, diaphragm) are probably the safest choice overall.

Pregnancy problems have resulted from structural abnormalities in the uterus and cervix of DES daughters. You might have trouble conceiving, or be more likely to miscarry, deliver prematurely, or have an ectopic (tubal) pregnancy (in the fallopian tube instead of the uterus). A pregnant DES daughter needs high-risk obstetrical care. Checking early in pregnancy for signs of problems may help prevent serious complications.

The doctor [who] was doing my DES exams didn't know anything about pregnancy problems for DES daughters. So I brought him seven articles that DES Action gave me. We both read them, and as a result, he checked my cervix at every prenatal visit. It took fifteen seconds and took away tons of anxiety.

Other problems, including endometriosis, menstrual irregularities, and pelvic inflammatory disease, have been reported by many DES daughters. DES sons have increased risk of urogenital problems. Recent studies have shown that DES granddaughters may have delayed menstruation regularity and DES grandsons may have an increased risk of hypospadias (in which the urethral opening on the penis is in the wrong place). Tell your doctor if you are a DES grandchild and be vigilant for any new information about DES.

The DES Exam

The annual DES exam for DES daughters is similar to a regular Pap test and pelvic exam, but it is more comprehensive, because changes caused by DES do not usually show up in routine exams. A copy of directions for doing the exam is available from DES Action for you to show your doctor. The exam should include careful visual inspection of the vagina and cervix, gentle palpation of the vaginal walls, Pap tests from the cervix and from the surfaces of the upper vagina, and a bimanual pelvic exam (see p. 39). Sometimes iodine staining (Schiller's test) of the vagina and cervix is used to distinguish normal tissue (which stains brown) from adenosis (which does not stain). These tests will indicate anything that might need further testing by colposcopy or biopsy. Even after a hysterectomy, DES daughters still need an annual gynecological exam. Daughters can contact DES Action at 1-800-337-9288 or info@desaction.org.

HYSTERECTOMY AND OOPHORECTOMY

The United States has the highest hysterectomy rate in the industrialized world. Statistics from

WHEN IS HYSTERECTOMY NEEDED?

Hysterectomy may be recommended for several life-threatening conditions:

- Invasive cancer of the uterus, cervix, vagina, fallopian tubes, and/or ovaries. Only 8 to 12 percent of hysterectomies are performed to treat cancer.
- Severe, uncontrollable pelvic infection (PID)
- Severe, uncontrollable uterine bleeding (rare, usually associated with childbirth)
- Rare but serious complications during childbirth, including rupture of the uterus

If you have any of these conditions, hysterectomy may save your life and also free you from significant pain and discomfort.

Hysterectomy may be justified as treatment for some conditions that are not life-threatening, but these usually can be treated without resorting to major surgery:

- Precancerous changes of the endometrium, called hyperplasia. (Remember, however, that hyperplasia can often be reversed with medication.)
- Extensive endometriosis causing debilitating pain and/or involving other organs. (More conservative surgery and/or medication is usually an effective treatment in these circumstances.)
- Fibroid tumors that are extensive, are large, involve other organs, or cause debilitating bleeding. (However, fibroids usually can be removed by myomectomy, thereby preserving the uterus.)
- Pelvic relaxation (uterine prolapse) that is causing severe symptoms. (Another treatment option in this case is uterine suspension surgery or a pessary—see p. 646.)
- Severe bleeding leading to anemia and not correctable with iron supplementation. (Birth control pills, the Mirena IUD, and endometrial ablation are alternative treatments that can be used before resorting to hysterectomy.)

Hysterectomies should not be performed for mild abnormal uterine bleeding, fibroids without symptoms, and pelvic congestion (menstrual irregularities and low back pain). These problems typically respond to cheaper and safer alternatives.

2004 indicate that about one-third of all U.S. women have had a hysterectomy by the age of sixty. Today, about 90 percent of hysterectomies are done by choice and not as an emergency or lifesaving procedure. Various studies have concluded that anywhere from 10 percent to 90 percent of those operations were not really needed, but many physicians continue to recommend them. This surgery has certainly saved lives and restored health for many women, but unnecessary operations have needlessly exposed women to risks. There is increasing understanding that a woman's uterus and ovaries have value during midlife and beyond, so the view of a woman's uterus and ovaries as "expendable" during later periods in our lives is now obsolete.

Both hysterectomy (removal of the uterus) and oophorectomy (removal of the ovaries) are major surgery and may have long-term effects on our health, sexuality, and life expectancy. Because of the controversy over high hysterectomy and oophorectomy rates, many insurance plans now require a second opinion from another physician before agreeing to pay for the procedures. Because some surgeons recommend hysterectomy routinely, women need to understand when the surgery is truly necessary (see sidebar, p. 629).

Fortunately, diagnostic and therapeutic techniques such as sonography, Pap tests, hysteroscopy, endometrial ablation, and laparoscopy make it possible to avoid or delay many hysterectomies that might have been done in the past. It is important to consider and utilize these techniques before resorting to major surgeries.

The most recent data suggest that black women have a somewhat higher hysterectomy rate than white women, possibly because black women are more likely to have fibroids. In the past, hysterectomy was performed solely for the purpose of sterilization among many poorer women and women of color in the United States, and this history affects the overall rate of hysterectomy among women of color. The problem of sterilization abuse led to federal sterilization guidelines in 1979, but the practice of performing medically unindicated hysterectomies continued for many years. It is likely that the rates of unnecessary hysterectomies have dropped only relatively recently.

Whenever you have any doubts about the need for a hysterectomy and/or oophorectomy, seek one or more other opinions about possible alternative approaches (such as a myomectomy, which removes fibroids without removing the uterus).

Oophorectomy

Oophorectomy is removal of either one (unilateral) or both (bilateral) ovaries. The fallopian tube(s) may be removed as well. Common reasons for oophorectomy include benign tumors of the ovary such as an endometrioma or dermoid; ovarian cancer; pelvic infection; and ectopic pregnancy (a pregnancy that occurs outside the uterus). In many cases, benign tumors, dermoid cysts, and endometriomas (cysts of endometriosis) can be removed without taking out the ovaries. Large functional cysts (fluid-filled sacs that often form during a menstrual cycle) can also be removed in this way, if they are not reabsorbed on their own. Women who have mutations of the BRCA1 or BRCA2 genes are at higher risk for ovarian cancer and sometimes have their ovaries removed as prevention.

If only one ovary is removed and not your uterus, you will continue to be fertile and have menstrual periods. However, you may experience an earlier menopause. If both ovaries are removed, you will experience surgical menopause (see p. 524). Even if one ovary is retained, you may have menopause-like symptoms due to loss of blood supply to the remaining ovary. (Such symptoms are also possible when both ovaries are retained after a hysterectomy.)

The ovaries usually continue to produce some hormones after menopause. Routine removal of healthy ovaries of women over forty-five during a scheduled hysterectomy should no longer be done,[20] even though some doctors still try to justify an oophorectomy to prevent the possibility of future ovarian cancer. Evidence now shows that removing ovaries in this way does far more harm than good, because so many more women will die from heart disease and osteoporotic fractures resulting from the surgery than from the relatively small number of ovarian cancers that would be prevented. For more information, see "Hysterectomy and Ovarian Conservation" at ourbodiesourselves.org.

Risks and Complications

Although the death rate from hysterectomy is low (under 1 percent), surgical complications include the following:

- **Infection.** Most infections can be treated successfully with antibiotics, but some can be severe or even uncontrollable.
- **Hemorrhage** at the time of surgery or afterward (a transfusion or second operation may be necessary).
- **Damage** to your internal organs, most frequently the urinary tract and sometimes the bowel. Sometimes there is damage to the ureter (tube connecting the kidney to the bladder) or the bladder.

Less common surgical complications include blood clots, complications from the anesthesia, and intestinal obstruction from postsurgical scarring.

Long-term Risks

For those of us who are in our early forties or younger, removal of the uterus and ovaries may increase the risk of heart attack. Even if our ovaries are not removed, there is an increased chance of an earlier menopause. This is usually due to the decreased supply of blood to the ovaries, so that they lose their ability to produce hormones, either immediately or over time. Many physicians assure us that we can avoid these risks by taking estrogen, but estrogen therapy does not substitute for functioning ovaries (see Chapter 20, "Perimenopause and Menopause").

Hormonal effects of hysterectomy with oophorectomy vary from one woman to the next. Some women suffer severe hot flashes and lack of lubrication. Some women use hormone therapy for a while, then gradually taper off. Long-term symptoms sometimes associated with hysterectomy and/or oophorectomy include constipation, urinary incontinence, bone and joint pain, pelvic pain, and depression.

Hysterectomy, Oophorectomy, and Sexuality

Many women are concerned about the effect that hysterectomy, with or without oophorectomy, will have on sexual response. Some physicians and popular literature suggest that any sexual difficulties we may experience are "all in our head." In fact, there is some physiological basis for these problems. For women who experience orgasm primarily when a partner's penis or fingers push against the cervix and uterus (causing uterine contractions and increased stimulation of the abdominal lining), that kind of sensation may be lost if the uterus and cervix are removed. This is probably an individual response and has not been proved in studies. In addition, if the ovaries are removed, hormone levels drop sharply, and that can affect sexual feelings:

I had a hysterectomy two years ago at the age of 45. I went from being fully aroused and fully orgasmic to having a complete loss of libido, sexual enjoyment, and orgasms immediately after the surgery. I went to doctors, all of whom denied ever having seen a woman with this problem before and told me it was psychological. Before surgery, my husband and I were having intercourse approximately three to five times a week, simply because we have an open and loving relationship. Now I find that I have to work at becoming at all interested in intercourse. And I no longer have the orgasm that comes from pressure on the cervix, although I still have a feeble orgasm from clitoral stimulation.

Testosterone, a hormone that contributes to muscle strength, appetite, and sex drive, can increase sexual desire in women whose ovaries have been removed, but it may have masculinizing side effects, such as a lowered voice, acne, and facial hair. Side effects can be limited by using low-dose testosterone cream or gel. However, even in low doses, these products have not been adequately tested for long-term safety.

Local effects of surgery may occasionally cause problems. Vaginal lubrication tends to lessen after hysterectomy and oophorectomy, and intercourse may be uncomfortable if your vagina has been shortened by the operation, or if there is scar tissue in the pelvis or at the top of the vagina. In order to minimize scarring, preserve nerve function and ligament support, and avoid shortening the vagina, some physicians recommend leaving the cervix in if no cancer was involved.

However, for many women, sex is unchanged or even more enjoyable after hysterectomy, since painful symptoms are gone. In the words of a woman who had a hysterectomy because of huge fibroids:

I had terrible cramps all my life and genuine feelings of utter depression during my periods. My ovaries were not removed, and my libido was not affected. My sexual response, if anything, improved. I also had for the first time no fear of unwanted pregnancy and more general good health.

Consider the benefits of surgery against the possibility of changes in sexual desire or response that can't be predicted in advance. Treatments less drastic than a hysterectomy can usually reduce pain and bleeding from benign uterine conditions and improve overall well-being.

Hysterectomy Procedures

Total hysterectomy, sometimes called complete hysterectomy: The surgeon removes the uterus and cervix, leaving the fallopian tubes and ovaries. You may continue to ovulate but will no longer have menstrual periods; instead, the egg will be absorbed by the body into the pelvic cavity.

Total hysterectomy with bilateral salpingo-oophorectomy: The surgeon removes the uterus, cervix, fallopian tubes, and ovaries. One ovary may be left in, if it is not diseased. In rare cases (usually to treat widespread cancer), the surgeon will remove the upper part of the vagina and perhaps the lymph nodes in the pelvic area. The latter is called radical hysterectomy.

Supracervical (or subtotal) hysterectomy: This procedure leaves in the cervix, to limit the effect of surgery on the function and anatomy of the vagina. It's also less likely to interfere with nerves and arteries as well as ligaments that support the vagina. If the cervix is left in, you still need Pap tests.

Abdominal or Vaginal?

The uterus can be removed either through an abdominal incision or through the vagina. Surgeons sometimes prefer an abdominal approach because it enables them to see the pelvic cavity more completely. The incision is made either horizontally, across the top pubic hairline, where the scar hardly shows afterward, or vertically, between the navel and the pubic hairline. Vertical incisions tend to heal more slowly.

Vaginal hysterectomy has the advantage of a shorter recovery period and faster healing. Because the incision is inside the vagina, you won't have a visible scar. Laparoscopically assisted vaginal hysterectomy (LAVH) enables the surgeon to see an image of the pelvic cavity without the downside of a large incision. Vaginal hysterectomies are performed increasingly frequently and require greater skill, so it's important to find a surgeon who does them regularly. Mistakes during surgery can result in permanent urinary tract difficulties. Other disadvantages include a possible shortening of the vagina, which can result in painful intercourse afterward and temporary (but severe) back pain.

Minimally invasive loparoscopic techniques (where the pelvic organs are visualized through a small scope placed through the belly button) are used more frequently now to avoid the long recovery and large scar associated with the abdominal approach. Because only small incisions are required, the recovery is dramatically better. Just be sure to find a surgeon experienced in these relatively new techniques.

Self-Help: Recovering from Hysterectomy/Oophorectomy

After a hysterectomy, you may be in the hospital for as few as one or as long as several days, depending on the kind of procedure, the amount of anesthesia, and your general health. For the first day, you will probably have an IV and a catheter inserted in your bladder. You will usually be given medication for pain and nausea. Within a day, you can expect to be on your feet and encouraged to do exercises to get your circulation and breathing back to normal. You may also be told to cough frequently to clear your lungs. (Holding a pillow over an abdominal incision, or crossing your legs if you had a vaginal incision, will help reduce pain from coughing.) You may also have gas pains to contend with. A self-help technique to dispel abdominal gas uses heat applied to an acupressure point beneath the navel. Walking, holding on to a pillow and rolling from side to side in bed, and slow deep-breathing exercises may help, too. You can begin to have light solid foods, as well as fluids, when you feel able to keep them down. Hospital stays are growing shorter and shorter. This can be scary, but once your IV is out and you can keep down oral pain medications, being at home with good help may provide many comforts and avoids the risk of catching an infection in the hospital. Plan ahead to make sure you have the support you need (family, friends, or community support services).

Recovery at Home

After you go home, you may have light vaginal bleeding or oozing that gradually tapers off. You may also have hot flashes caused by estrogen loss, even if your ovaries were not removed. You will probably continue to have some pain, despite taking pain medication. Consult your medical practitioner if you have fever, nausea and vomiting, or foul vaginal discharge, as this may signal an infection.

Try to arrange for someone to take care of you for the first few days. You can expect to feel tired, so ask family and friends for help with household chores and children for at least the first few weeks. Your health care provider may tell you to avoid tub baths, douches, driving, climbing, or lifting heavy things for several weeks. If you have to drive or need to carry small children, ask for suggestions about how and when you can do these tasks safely.

Full recovery generally takes four to six weeks, but some women feel tired for as long as six months or even a year after surgery. Most medical practitioners also recommend waiting six to eight weeks before resuming sex and/or active sports, but some women return to them earlier. Start with light exercise, such as walking, and gradually build up to your old routines.

Emotional Reactions

Some women feel only relief following hysterectomy, especially when the operation eliminates a serious health problem or chronic, disabling pain. But even if you were prepared for it and did not expect to feel depressed, you might cry frequently and unexpectedly during the first few days or weeks after surgery. This may be due to sudden hormonal changes. Many of us are also upset by losing any part of ourselves, especially a part that is so uniquely female. Acknowledging feelings of anger and grief after losing a part of yourself or some of your sexual responsiveness is an important part of the recovery process.

Some gynecologists recommend psychiatric help and prescribe antidepressants or tranquilizers (or other habit-forming drugs) while ignoring treatment of underlying physical or sexual conditions caused by the surgery. Often, talk therapy alone—or conversations with friends and family—enables us to cope with any posthysterectomy depression. Some women have started their own postsurgery support groups by networking in their community. Visit HERS Foundation (hersfoundation.org) for more resources.

VULVA

VULVITIS

Vulvitis, or inflammation of the vulva, may be caused by one of several medical conditions, medicated creams, or external irritants. It can also be caused by an injury; oral sex; a bacterial, viral, or fungal infection; sitting in a hot tub; allergies to common commercial products such as body soaps, powders, and deodorants; or irritation from sanitary napkins, synthetic underwear, or panty hose. Vulvitis often accompanies vaginal infections. Stress, inadequate diet, and poor hygiene can increase the likelihood of vaginal infections. Women with diabetes may develop vulvitis because the sugar content of their cells is higher, increasing susceptibility to infection. Postmenopausal women often develop vulvitis because as hormone levels drop, the vulvar tissues become thinner, drier, and less elastic and therefore more prone to irritation and infection.

Symptoms of vulvitis include itching, redness, swelling, burning, and pain. Sometimes fluid-filled blisters form that break open, ooze, and crust over (these could also be herpes). Scratching can cause further irritation, pus formation, and scaling, as well as secondary infection. Sometimes, as a result of scratching, the skin whitens and thickens.

Women with this problem tend to overclean the vulva, contributing to further irritation. Wash once a day with warm water only.

Medical Treatments for Vulvitis
The first step in treating vulvitis medically is to make a diagnosis. Depending on the cause, your health care provider may prescribe antifungal creams or antibacterial treatment. Cortisone cream or other soothing lotions can relieve severe itching. (Low-dose cortisone creams are good for a short time; fluorinated ones can cause thinning and atrophy of the skin if used for a long time, though these may be required for some conditions.) Postmenopausal women may be given a form of local estrogen. If you have a vaginal infection or herpes, treating these problems will usually clear up the vulvitis as well.

If the vulvitis persists or worsens, you may need a vulvar biopsy to rule out the possibility of cancer or chronic vulvar conditions such as lichen sclerosus, a skin disease that can produce itching, bruising, pain, and scarring. This biopsy can be done in the practitioner's office with local anesthetic.

Self-Help
Discontinue using any substances that might be a cause of vulvitis. All commercial preparations may be irritating, including antifungal agents and lubricants containing propylene glycol. Keep your vulva clean, cool, and dry—and remember to wipe from front to back. Hot boric acid compresses and hot sitz baths with comfrey tea are soothing. Use unscented white toilet paper (as perfumes and dyes may be aggravat-

ing) and soft cotton or linen towels, and wear cotton underwear to prevent chafing. Aveeno colloidal oatmeal bath and cold compresses made of plain, unsweetened, live-culture yogurt or cottage cheese also help relieve itching and soothe irritation. Calamine lotion can be used to address itching. Use a sterile, nonirritating lubricant such as K-Y jelly or Astroglide during intercourse and other genital sex.

VULVODYNIA

Vulvodynia is the term developed in 1976 by the International Society for the Study of Vulvovaginal Disease to describe chronic vulvar pain. Women with vulvodynia experience severe burning, pain, itching, stinging, and/or irritation in the vulva (external genitals).

Vulvar pain can be related to a known disorder such as a bad yeast infection or a herpes outbreak. Recently clinicians have learned that pelvic floor muscle spasm or tightness (caused by a variety of conditions) is a major source of vulvar pain.

Vulvar pain in the absence of relevant visible finding or clinically identifiable disease is called vulvodynia. There are two kinds of vulvodynia. In generalized vulvodynia, symptoms occur in different areas of the vulva, at various times and sometimes even when the vulva is not being touched. In localized vulvodynia (formerly called vestibulodynia, vulvar vestibulitis, or localized vulvar dysesthesia), women feel pain mainly in an area just around the vaginal opening (the vestibule), usually when that area is touched or pressed. (For more information about the anatomy of the vulva, see Chapter 1, "Our Female Bodies.")

Diagnosis

As many as 3 to 15 percent of women have chronic vulvar pain.[21] Even so, it can be hard to get a proper diagnosis for it, let alone successful treatment. If your vulva hurts, it is essential to find a health care provider who is familiar with vulvodynia. To rule out vulvovaginal conditions that are known causes of pain, she or he should do a full history, pelvic exam and pH examination of vaginal secretions (wet mount), and vaginal cultures if indicated. During a pelvic exam, the practitioner evaluates the architecture and appearance of your vulva. Then she or he will lightly touch areas on your vulva with a cotton swab (Q-tip) to see where it's sensitive. This may be painful; feel free to bring a close friend or partner with you into the exam room.

It started within the first few times I ever had sexual intercourse. Here I was with this wonderful partner, but the sex hurt so much it made us both cry—me from the physical pain, him because I hurt so much. Once it started, the pain would come back whenever something touched my vulva: a tampon, a finger, a speculum (that was the worst). I saw several nurses and doctors; the first doc told me I was just "tight" and needed to relax. Did she have any idea how insulting, demoralizing, and belittling that was? Finally, I found a physician who respected me, recognized that my pain was real, and was able to give it the label of vulvodynia. Even having a name for it helped. I've since tried many treatments, some more successful than others. Three years later, I'm thrilled to report that my wonderful partner and I are able to have pain-free sexual intercourse (as well as continue to share other kinds of physical intimacy)—my [vulvodynia] isn't totally gone, but it's on its way out!

Medical Treaments for Vulvodynia

Because the causes of vulvodynia remain uncertain, there is no standard treatment. You and your clinician will first attempt to identify and treat possible pain triggers, including:

- Irritants applied to the vulva or activities that have an impact on the vulva
- Inflammatory problem such as *Candida* or inflammatory vaginitis (an uncommon vaginitis)
- Viral infections such as herpes
- Vulvar skin problems
- Interstitial cystitis (causing urinary and bladder pain)
- Blocked Bartholin duct (a Bartholin gland cyst occurs when a pea-sized organ under the skin on either side of the labia gets blocked and fluid fills up in the gland)
- Pelvic floor muscle spasms

If pain persists, treatment may include:

- Application of estrogen cream in the vagina, especially if there is atrophy in the vaginal walls.
- Low-dose tricyclic antidepressant, such as amitriptyline, to reduce central nervous pain; some clinicians think there is a connection between pain and the abundance of nerves in the vulva area in some women.
- Physical therapy to evaluate and treat the back and/or pelvic floor; even if there are no apparent muscle spasms, pelvic floor exercises have been found to strengthen pelvic muscles and reduce vulva pain caused by touch.
- Topical anesthetic ointment applied prior to or after intercourse.
- Exploring possible relationship issues or past sexual experiences that could contribute to painful sex; referral to a sex therapist or counselor if needed.

Experts agree that it is a combination of treatments, not any one modality, that is usually successful. If other treatments fail, some experts offer surgery such as vestibulectomy, which is the surgical removal of the vestibule and the hymen. Others feel that the studies showing success of surgery are flawed because of lack of clear definitions of pain and a lack of clear criteria for selecting the women. Other experimental treatments include Botox, which some small studies have found helpful.

Find a supportive practitioner who is knowledgeable about the vulva and has the time and knowledge to explore treatment options with you. If you have a partner, it is important to educate him or her about vulvodynia and, together, explore options for physical intimacy (see Chapter 8, "Sexual Challenges"). Also consider connecting with a support group to share stories and successes.

The National Vulvodynia Association (nva .org) offers more information on pain management and treatment, including helpful lists of potential irritants, and can help you find referrals to clinicians and support groups in your area.

VULVAR CANCER

Vulvar cancer is relatively rare. Women who have had HPV infections seem to be at greater risk, and some experts believe that vulvar cancer rates will rise sharply in the future because of increased rates of HPV infections. There is no screening test for vulvar cancer, however, and many women are treated for other conditions before realizing a biopsy should be done.

Be aware of changes in your vulvar area such as persistent itching or irritation, and especially growths. Don't be afraid to look. Request a biopsy if you find a suspicious lump or lesion. Because vulvar cancer typically grows slowly, early detection can mean the difference between minor surgery and the more emotionally and physically devastating experience of losing one's genitals. More extensive surgery is also more likely to lead to complications such as problems with sexual functioning. If lymph glands are removed, fluid buildup in the thighs can cause swelling, making mobility difficult.

THE VAGINA

All women secrete moisture and mucus from the membranes that line the vagina and cervix. This discharge is clear or slightly milky and may be somewhat slippery or clumpy. When dry, it may be yellowish. When a woman is sexually aroused, under stress, or at midcycle, this secretion increases. It normally causes no irritation or inflammation of the vagina or vulva. If you want to examine your own discharge, collect a sample from inside your vagina—with a washed finger—and smear it on clear glass (such as a glass slide).

Many bacteria normally grow in the vagina of a healthy woman. Some of them, especially lactobacilli, help to keep the vagina healthy, maintaining an acid pH (less than 4.5), and control overgrowth of potentially bad bacteria.

VAGINAL INFECTIONS

When vaginal infections occur, you may have abnormal discharge, mild or severe itching and burning of the vulva, chafing of the thighs, and (in some cases) frequent urination. Chronic vaginal (and vulvar) symptoms sometimes result from skin conditions of the vulva and vagina, such as eczema or psoriasis.

Vaginal infections may be due to lowered resistance (from stress, lack of sleep, poor diet, other infections in our bodies); douching or use of scented sprays; pregnancy; taking birth control pills, other hormones, or antibiotics; diabetes or a prediabetic condition; cuts, abrasions, and other irritations in the vagina (from childbirth, intercourse without enough lubrication, tampons, or using an instrument in the vagina medically or for masturbation). Infections

are also transmitted during sex with an infected partner (see Chapter 11, "Sexually Transmitted Infections"). Chronic vaginal infections are infrequently a sign of serious medical problems such as HIV infection and diabetes.

Medical and Alternative Treatments

The usual treatment for vaginitis is some form of antibiotic—which can also disturb the delicate balance of bacteria in the vagina and may actually encourage other infections (such as yeast) by altering the vagina's normal acid/alkaline balance (pH). Some antibiotics also have unpleasant or even dangerous side effects.

As an alternative to antibiotics for vaginitis, some women find that natural and herbal remedies can help restore the normal vaginal flora and promote healing, though there are no studies showing how effective most of them are. Some women have tried soothing herb poultices or sitz baths (sitting in the tub with just enough water to immerse your thighs, buttocks, and hips). You should not rely on these remedies if you have an infection that involves your uterus, fallopian tubes, or ovaries.

Below is information about yeast (candida) infections and bacterial vaginosis. Trichomoniasis ("trich"), another common vaginal infection, is almost always transmitted sexually and thus is discussed in Chapter 11, "Sexually Transmitted Infections."

YEAST INFECTIONS

Candida albicans, a yeast fungus often called simply candida, grows in the rectum and vagina. It grows best in a mildly acidic environment. The pH in the vagina is normally more than mildly acidic. When we menstruate, take birth control pills or some antibiotics, are pregnant, or have diabetes, the pH becomes more alkaline. In a healthy vagina, the presence of some yeast may not be a problem. When our system is out of balance, yeastlike organisms can grow profusely and cause a thick white discharge that may look like cottage cheese and smell like baking bread. Sometimes this causes intense itching, while at other times it just causes intermittent burning or a sense of irritation.

One study about the risk of recurring yeast infections found that sexual behaviors, rather than the presence of candida fungus on the male partner, were associated with recurrences. Women who had not had candida infections in the vulvovaginal area during the previous year were able to masturbate with saliva without increasing their risk of a candida infection, whereas women with a recent history of such infection in the vulvovaginal area increased the likelihood of a recurrent infection if they masturbated with saliva.[22]

Diagnosis

The only way to be sure that an infection is caused by candida and not something else is to have vaginal secretions analyzed under a microscope. In some cases, it helps to get a lab culture done. Other conditions causing vaginal irritation may respond temporarily to treatment for candida and then recur a short time later, so accurate diagnosis is important. Self-diagnosis is inaccurate more than half the time, so hold off from self-treatment until diagnosis by a health care provider.

Medical Treatments for Yeast Infections

Treatment usually consists of some form of vaginal suppository or cream or an oral antifungal. The former is available over the counter, while pills require a prescription. Antifungal external creams such as clotrimazole may reduce or even eliminate the symptoms, sometimes without actually curing the infection. A small percent of woman have recurrent or chronic yeast infections. Prolonged oral treatment is sometimes required but should be based on a yeast culture.

Suppositories and creams have fewer side effects than oral medications, and they can be used during pregnancy. If a woman has a yeast infection when she gives birth, the baby will be likely to get yeast in its throat or digestive tract. This is called thrush and is treated orally with nystatin drops.

Other treatments for candida infection involve boric acid capsules or painting the vagina, cervix, and vulva with gentian violet. The latter is bright purple and stains, so a sanitary pad must be worn. This procedure can help, but in occasional cases, women have a severe reaction to gentian violet. Side effects are rare with boric acid, but it may cause vaginal burning and itching. Do not use boric acid near any cuts or abrasions, as it can enter the bloodstream and may cause nausea, vomiting, diarrhea, dermatitis, and kidney damage. Boric acid is never taken orally and is typically used only after other FDA-approved treatments have failed.

Self-Help

Some of us have had success with the following remedies: acidifying the system by drinking eight ounces of unsweetened cranberry juice every day, or taking cranberry concentrate supplements; inserting plain, unsweetened, live-culture yogurt in the vagina; inserting garlic suppositories (to prevent irritation, peel but don't nick a clove of garlic, then wrap in gauze before inserting). An effective and inexpensive treatment for candida infection is potassium sorbate, commonly used as a preservative in home brewing of beer. Dip a cotton tampon in a 3 percent solution (15 grams of dry potassium sorbate in 1 pint of water), then insert into the vagina at night and remove in the morning.

Also try to boost your immune system by reducing sugar in your diet and getting more rest. Avoid douches and don't use tampons for your period when you have an infection. If you have a male sex partner, have him apply antifungal cream to his penis twice a day for two weeks, especially if he's not circumcised.

For a long time I felt as though I were on a merry-go-round. I would get a yeast infection, take Mycostatin for three weeks, clear up the infection, and then find two weeks later that the itching and the thick, white discharge were back. Finally, I discovered that reducing my sugar intake and drinking unsweetened cranberry juice would help prevent repeat infections.

BACTERIAL VAGINOSIS

Bacterial vaginosis (BV) is a disturbance of the ecology of the vagina, with an overgrowth of certain microorganisms (possibly including mycoplasmas, gardnerella, and anaerobic bacteria). Many women with BV are unaware that they have it. Some practitioners believe it can be caused by routine douching; it may also be triggered by infections, including STIs. The symptoms can be confused with those of trich, though the discharge tends to be creamy white or grayish and is especially foul-smelling (some call it "fishy"), especially after intercourse. It sometimes comes and goes, getting better after a period and worse again as a woman's cycle progresses.

Medical Treatments for BV

Medication treatment is usually either metronidazole or clindamycin, taken orally or vaginally for five to seven days. Single-dose oral metronidazole may also be effective but less so (cure rates range from 40 to 60 percent). Metronidazole is sometimes used first, because it spares the lactobacilli in your vagina and is less likely to trigger a yeast infection. Vaginal treatment avoids systemic side effects but is more expensive than the five-to-seven-day pill regimens.

Some women will have another BV outbreak within nine months of initial treatment. Long-term condom use may help to prevent recurrent infection. Women with BV have more frequent infections following gynecologic surgery, and some studies suggest that BV increases the risk of giving birth prematurely if you have it during pregnancy.

Self-Help

Self-help treatments include general vaginitis prevention measures and taking extra vitamins B and C. You can help prevent recurrences by minimizing the use of tampons, avoiding douching, and using condoms (to offset the alkaline effect of semen). Alternative treatments may provide temporary relief but not an actual cure. Vaginal and oral use of yogurt doesn't help with BV.

THE BLADDER

The urinary bladder is an expandable muscular organ that stores our liquid waste (urine) so we can excrete it intermittently. This organ is obviously not exclusively female, but because it sits so close to the other organs that are unique to women, gender-specific issues exist.

URINARY TRACT INFECTIONS

Urinary tract infections (UTIs) are so common that most of us get at least one at some point in our lives. They are usually caused by bacteria, such as E. coli, that get into the urethra and bladder (and occasionally the kidneys) from the gastrointestinal system. Trichomoniasis, chlamydia, and viruses can also cause UTIs. Low resistance, poor diet, stress, and trauma to the urethra from childbirth, surgery, and catheterization can predispose you to getting them. A sudden increase in sexual activity can be a trigger (hence the term "honeymoon cystitis").

Pregnant women are especially susceptible, as pressure from the growing fetus keeps some urine in the bladder and ureters (the tubes carrying urine from the kidneys to the bladder), allowing bacteria to grow.

Postmenopausal women are also susceptible because of the effect of hormonal changes on the bladder and urethra. Occasionally, UTIs are caused by a congenital anatomical abnormality or, mostly in older women or women who have had many children, a prolapsed (fallen) urethra or bladder.

Cystitis (inflammation or infection of the bladder) is by far the most common UTI in women. While the symptoms can be frightening, cystitis in itself is not usually serious. If you suddenly have to urinate every few minutes and it burns like crazy even though almost nothing comes out, you probably have cystitis. There may also be blood and/or pus in the urine. You may have pain just above your pubic bone, and sometimes there is a peculiar, heavy odor when you first urinate in the morning.

It's also possible to get mild temporary symptoms (such as peeing frequently) without actually having an infection, simply because of drinking too much coffee or tea (both are diuretics), premenstrual difficulties, food allergies, vaginitis, anxiety, or irritation to the area from bubble baths, soaps, or douches. As long as you are in good health and not pregnant, you can usually treat mild symptoms yourself for twenty-four hours before consulting a practitioner.

Cystitis often disappears without treatment. If symptoms persist beyond forty-eight hours, recur frequently, or are accompanied by chills, fever, vomiting, and/or pain in the kidneys (near the middle of the back), see a doctor. These symptoms suggest that infection has spread to the kidneys, resulting in pyelonephritis, a serious problem that requires medical treatment. Also see your provider if you have blood or pus

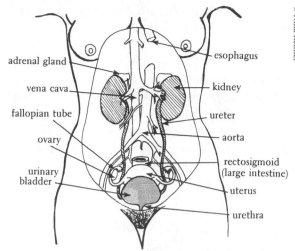

© Nina Reimer

in the urine, pain on urination during pregnancy, diabetes or chronic illness, or a history of kidney infection or diseases or abnormalities of the urinary tract. Untreated chronic infections can lead to serious complications, such as high blood pressure or premature births (if occurring during pregnancy).

Diagnosis

When cystitis does not respond to self-help treatments within twenty-four hours, or it recurs frequently, get a urine test. Make sure your provider asks for a clean voided specimen[23] and does a pelvic exam to rule out other infections. Your urine should be examined for evidence of blood and pus, then cultured. Sometimes, even when you have symptoms, the culture may come back negative (not show any infection). False-negative cultures may be due to mishandling or too-dilute urine; you may also get a false-negative report if your cystitis is caused by something other than bacterial infection. White blood cells in the urine plus a negative culture (acute urethral syndrome) may indicate a chlamydia infection (see p. 290). Some women have bacteria in the urine without symptoms; especially in pregnant women, this should be treated

PREVENTING UTIs AND AVOIDING REINFECTION

Drink lots of fluids every day. Try to drink a glass of water every two or three hours. For an active infection, drink enough so you can pour out a good stream of urine every hour.

Urinate frequently and try to empty your bladder completely each time. Never try to hold your urine once your bladder feels full.

Keep yourself clean. Wipe from front to back after urinating or having a bowel movement to keep the bacteria in your bowels and anus away from your urethra. Wash your genitals from front to back with plain water or very mild soap at least once a day.

Wash before sex. Wash your hands and genitals before sex and after contact with the anal area (especially before touching the vagina or urethra). That goes for your partner(s), too.

Prevent irritation. Any sexual activity that irritates the urethra, puts pressure on the bladder, or spreads bacteria from the anus to the vagina or urethra can contribute to cystitis. To prevent irritation, avoid pressure on the urethral area or prolonged direct clitoral stimulation during sex or masturbation. Make sure your vagina is well lubricated before penetration of any kind. Rear-entry positions and prolonged vigorous intercourse tend to put additional stress on the urethra and bladder. Emptying your bladder before and immediately after sex is a good idea. If you tend to get cystitis after sex despite these precautions, you may want to ask your medical practitioner for preventive drugs (sulfa, ampicillin, nitro-furantoin); a single tablet after sex can prevent infections and usually doesn't have the same negative effects as taking antibiotics for a longer time.

Try changing your birth control. Women taking oral contraceptives have a higher rate of cystitis than those who don't take them. Some diaphragm users find that the rim pressing against the urethra can contribute to infection. (A different-size diaphragm or one with a different rim may solve this problem.) Contraceptive foams or vaginal suppositories may irritate the urethra. Condoms that are not lubricated may put pressure on the urethra, or the dyes or lubricants may cause irritation.

Change menstrual pads often. The blood on the pad provides a bridge for bacteria from your anus to your urethra. Wash your genitals twice a day during your period. Some women also find that tampons or sponges put pressure on the urethra.

Wear loose clothing. Tight jeans may cause trauma to the urethra, as may some physical activities such as bicycling or horseback riding.

Avoid or reduce caffeine and alcohol. Both can irritate the bladder. If you drink either, be sure to drink enough water to dilute them.

Acidify your urine. Some women find that unsweetened cranberry juice, a cranberry concentrate supplement, or vitamin C every day makes urine more acidic and helps prevent UTIs. The hippuric acid in cranberry juice may help prevent bacteria from sticking to the bladder lining (mucosa). If you have an infection, try combining 500 mg of vitamin C with cranberry juice four times a day, or eat half a cup of fresh cranberries in plain, live-culture yogurt instead. Whole grains, meats, nuts, and many fruits also help to acidify the urine. Avoid strong spices such as curry, cayenne, chili, and black pepper.

Avoid refined (white) sugars and starches. White flour, white rice, and ordinary pasta may facilitate urinary tract infections by feeding bacteria.

Try certain vitamins or herbal remedies. Vitamin B$_6$ and magnesium/calcium supplements may help to relieve spasm of the urethra that can predispose you to cystitis. Drinking teas made of uva ursi, horsetail or shavegrass, barberry, echinacea, cornsilk, cleavers, lemon balm, or goldenseal may be beneficial to the bladder. Consult an herbalist to learn more about their specific properties and the correct doses.

Keep up your resistance. Eat well, get more rest, and find ways to reduce stress as much as possible.

---

with antibiotics to prevent kidney infection and other complications.

Medical Treatments for UTIs

For symptoms that are severe or indicate a kidney infection, medications are usually started immediately. For milder infections, many health care providers prefer to wait for culture results before prescribing a drug. Most UTIs respond rapidly to a variety of antibiotics. Drugs commonly used include ampicillin, nitrofurantoin, tetracycline, ciprofloxacin, a sulfamethoxazole and trimethoprim combination (Bactrim/Septra), and sulfonamides (Gantrisin). (Women who have a deficiency of glucose-6-phosphate dehydrogenase should not take sulfonamides.) You may get a single large dose or several doses spread out over three to ten days.

If symptoms persist longer than two days after you start taking drugs, contact your health care provider again. The organisms may be resistant to the antibiotics you are using. Eating plain, unsweetened live-culture yogurt or taking acidophilus in capsule, liquid, or granule form may help to prevent diarrhea or yeast infection by replacing the normal bacteria in your intestines that can be destroyed by the drugs.

Acetaminophen may relieve pain from UTIs. Some practitioners recommend a drug called Pyridium, an anesthetic that relieves pain but does not treat the infection itself. (Pyridium dyes the urine a bright orange, which will permanently stain clothing. It also can cause nausea, dizziness, and possibly allergic reactions.)

Surgical treatment for UTIs should be limited to specific situations in which a woman's anatomy is clearly causative. Pelvic exercises known as Kegels (see p. 643) can forestall the need for this operation and help prevent future infections.

Even with drugs and/or surgery, many women continue to have recurrent urinary tract infections. Sometimes it helps to treat chronic infections with long-term, low-dose medications.

URINARY INCONTINENCE

Urinary incontinence is a condition where women lose urine unintentionally. It often first appears during pregnancy as a result of pressure from the growing fetus on the bladder. Damage related to birth traumas may cause ongoing urinary incontinence, as can pelvic surgery. Some women will develop incontinence with advanced age, even without any specific traumas. If the condition is mild, simply using menstrual pads to collect leaking urine may be an adequate solution. A thorough evaluation can help determine what treatment approaches might be most effective. These include bladder training, pelvic flow exercises, medication, and surgery.

PAINFUL BLADDER SYNDROME/ INTERSTITIAL CYSTITIS (PBS/IC)

Painful bladder syndrome/interstitial cystitis (PBS/IC) was for many years thought to be an inflammatory condition of the bladder wall, but recently it has been recognized as poorly understood chronic pain syndromes that develop for multiple reasons. A clinical diagnosis is based primarily on symptoms of urgency/frequency of urinating and pain in the bladder and/or pelvis.[24] Standard treatments of many decades are no longer routinely considered effective. One large urological study from 2000 concluded that "no current treatments have a significant impact on symptoms with time."[25]

PBS/IC is at least five times more common in women than men, affecting close to 500,000 females in the United States, with an average age of onset of about forty years; 25 percent of those affected are under age thirty.

PBS/IC has symptoms similar to those of the common urinary tract infection known as cystitis. However, with PBS/IC, routine urine cultures are negative, and there is usually no response to antibiotics. You may feel pelvic pain and pressure and an urgent need to urinate, sometimes as often as sixty to eighty times a day. You may also have vaginal and rectal pain. Pain during sexual intercourse is common. The symptoms can vary from mild to severe.

HOW TO DO KEGEL EXERCISES

Kegel exercises are a particular set of exercises that strengthen the pelvic muscles involved in urination. Doing them can help women who have urinary incontinence and may be helpful for women who have vulvovaginal pain conditions.

The pelvic floor muscles, also called the pubococcygeus (PC) muscles, surround our three openings (bladder, vagina, and rectum). An easy way to find the pelvic floor muscles is to clench your muscles by pretending you're holding in pee. Or you can put your finger halfway inside your vagina and try to squeeze your finger with your vagina. Think of pulling muscles up and in, and try to relax your abdominal muscles and buttocks. It's easy to involve them in these exercises, but if you use your abdomen, you're not exercising the pelvic floor. Try squeezing up and in for ten seconds and then relaxing for ten seconds. Repeat for a few minutes. You also may experiment with quick flicks or squeezes in and out, to get the feel for the muscle. Kegels are most effective when held for five seconds and done in sets of five or ten throughout the day.

Diagnosis

PBS/IC may be incorrectly diagnosed as urethral syndrome or trigonitis, or you may be told there's nothing wrong and that you have a "sensitive bladder." A complete battery of urologic tests typically produces negative results. Conditions that have similar symptoms include

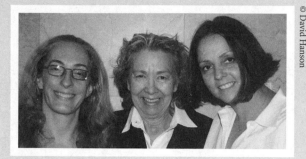

From left to right: Dr. Elizabeth Kavaler, Kay Zakariasen, and Dr. Jennifer Hill

"I WANTED TO KNOW WHAT OTHER PATIENTS HAD EXPERIENCED"

KAY ZAKARIASEN

My struggle to learn about the nature, benefit, harm, and alternatives to standard urological treatments for painful bladder syndrome/interstitial cystitis syndrome (PBS/IC).*

My own experience with urological treatment for PBS/IC led me to the New York Academy of Medicine to find out why, after standard treatment, chronic and unbearable symptoms had begun. What I found in the medical literature about dilation, hydrodistention, instillations of chemicals, and many more treatments stunned me.

I had one bladder infection, cleared up with one antibiotic, and then had no symptoms. Unfortunately, a gynecologist's referral to a urologist and two more opinions convinced me that my urethra was "too narrow" and would have to be dilated for the rest of my life. I was told, "You'll be fine."

I had ten dilations, one about every six months for five years. Then I suddenly had the feeling that I had to urinate—desperately—but no infection was detected. I also experienced severe intestinal pain after eating. Several doctors later, I began to conclude that the treatment I had was the cause of my problem. Three decades later I finally found help and told my story in a National Women's Health Network newsletter article.[26]

Since then, I have been sharing my story and medical findings. The urological literature emphasized the importance of widening urethras, but there were urologists who disagreed with this approach, calling dilation a "failure" and a "quality of care problem in urology." One urologist I interviewed on film called it "voodoo" and suggested that it was the economic mainstay of many private practices.

I wanted to know what other patients had experienced. With the help of several doctors supportive of my efforts, I developed a questionnaire (cystitispatientsurvey.com); 750 responses were analyzed by Dr. Elizabeth Kavaler, M.D., and several other doctors. Jennifer Hill,

---

* I want to thank the many doctors (including Dr. Virginia Sharpe), many volunteers (including Elena M. Paul, executive director of Volunteer Lawyers for the Arts), and the patients who completed our survey, as well as thirty who provided medical information and personal stories in interviews. More information can be found at Kitchener-Waterloo Interstitial Cystitis Support (skatecrooked.com/kwics/).

M.D., authored the article publishing their findings.[27] Only 25 percent of patients reported some improvement in symptoms, not enough to justify surgeries.*

Surgical interventions include dilation, hydrodistention, and instillations of caustic chemicals. To justify such treatments, doctors need to demonstrate that these techniques provide more benefit than harm and that they are reasonably safe and effective. I now realize that this is a field with minimal evidence of effectiveness for the surgeries that are routinely performed. Research currently under way will, I hope, offer better solutions for women with PBS/IC. In the meantime, I believe that less-invasive approaches offer a far wiser course.

* See ourbodiesourselves.org for patient experiences with this disease and which treatments they found to be either harmful or helpful.

bladder infections, kidney problems, vaginal infections, endometriosis, and sexually transmitted infections (STIs).

Medical Treatment for PBS/IC

There is no consistently effective treatment or cure for PBS/IC. However, the most commonly recommended approaches are:

- **Medication,** including nonsteroidal anti-inflammatory drugs, antispasmodics, and antihistamines. Pentosan polysulfate sodium (Elmiron), an oral medication, may protect the bladder from irritants in the urine.
- **Low-dose antidepressants,** which appear to have antipain properties
- **Diet changes,** eliminating caffeinated beverages, alcohol, artificial sweeteners, spicy foods, citrus fruits, and tomatoes
- **Transcutaneous electrical nerve stimulation (TENS)** to block pain, using a small portable unit worn on the body

The following approaches all involve surgery, the benefits of which are sometimes unproved, and all of which pose significant risks:

- **Bladder distention (hydrodistention)** stretches the bladder by filling it with water while you are under regional or general anesthesia.
- **Dimethyl sulfoxide (DMSO, Rimso-50),** an anti-inflammatory medication, is placed directly into the bladder.
- **Oxychlorosene sodium (Clorpactin)** is placed directly into the bladder; regional or general anesthesia may be necessary for this.
- **Major surgery** (partial or complete removal of the bladder, or of certain nerves leading to the bladder) is often followed by severe complications and should be done only as a last resort.

Developing effective IC therapies is a major challenge facing all researchers in this field. The American Urological Association is planning to publish the first guidelines regarding methodology for diagnosis and treatment during 2011. In 2010, a large multicenter NIH-funded study reported on findings that myofascial physical therapy (specialized stretching of the thin tissue that covers all the organs of the body) was shown to be effective when compared with conventional massage techniques.[28]

OTHER PELVIC CONDITIONS

OBSTETRIC FISTULA

Obstetric fistula is a childbirth injury that typically affects girls and women living in acute poverty throughout Africa and South Asia. Fistula is caused by prolonged and obstructed labor when the constant pressure of the baby's head against the soft tissues of the vagina creates a hole between the bladder and the vagina, and sometimes between the rectum and the vagina. This leaves girls and women leaking urine and/or feces continuously from the vagina. It may also cause serious nerve damage to the legs, making it difficult or impossible to walk. Girls and women with fistula are often isolated and highly stigmatized. In most cases, the cost of an operation and the distance to a medical facility providing fistula services make surgical repair impossible. Fistula is entirely preventable, and it rarely or never occurs in the developed world. Women with this condition who immigrate to the United States or Canada may encounter health care providers who have never seen it before. For more information, see "Obstetric Fistula" at ourbodiesourselves.org.

FEMALE GENITAL CUTTING

Female genital cutting (FGC)—also called female genital mutilation or female circumcision—is a traditional cultural practice in some African countries as well as in several countries in Asia and the Middle East. It involves cutting parts of the external genitals of girls or young women as a rite of passage into womanhood and to curb sexuality. FGC may consist of removing the hood of the clitoris, part or all of the clitoris and/or labia minora (inner lips), and, in some cultures, part or all of the external genitalia. The vaginal opening may also be narrowed or stitched (infibulation). Pricking, piercing, burning, scraping, slashing, and corroding the female genitals are also considered to be FGC by the World Health Organization (WHO). As a result of an influx of refugees and immigrants, thousands of women in the United States are living with the results of these practices.

Short-term health complications of FGC include excessive bleeding, infection, and shock, mostly due to unsanitary conditions, failed procedures by inexperienced circumcisers, or inadequate medical services once a problem occurs. Long-term health complications are abscess formation, scar neuromas, dermoid cysts, keloids, recurrent urinary tract infections, painful sexual intercourse, and vulval adhesions that block the vagina. In women who are infibulated, obstruction of the urethra and vagina by scar tissue may result in urine retention and urethral and bladder stones, irregular or prolonged menstrual flow, chronic urinary tract infections, and chronic pelvic infection, which often leads to scarring of the fallopian tubes and infertility. Sexual and psychological issues are likely to emerge over time. In 2006, a major World Health Organization study provided strong evidence that FGC increases the risk of complications during childbirth and can lead to one to two additional perinatal deaths per one hundred births. For more information, see "Female Genital Cutting," p. 793.

Many circumcised women seek treatment for problems or issues related to FGC but may not always acknowledge or understand the connection. It is critical for health care providers to be sensitive to women in both discussing this issue and treating its negative consequences.

PELVIC RELAXATION AND UTERINE PROLAPSE

Pelvic relaxation is a condition in which the muscles of the pelvic floor become slack and no longer support the pelvic organs properly. In severe cases, the ligaments and tissues that hold the uterus in place may weaken enough to allow the uterus to fall (prolapse) into the vagina. Women sometimes experience pelvic relaxation and/or uterine prolapse after one or more very difficult births, but the tendency can also be inherited. Uterine prolapse is often accompanied by a falling of the bladder (a condition known as cystocele) and rectum (rectocele).

The first sign of pelvic relaxation is often a tendency to leak urine when you cough, sneeze, or laugh suddenly. If your uterus has fallen into the vagina, you may have a dull, heavy sensation in your vagina or feel as if something is falling out. You may have constipation, difficulty accomplishing a bowel movement, or an inability to control your bowels. These symptoms are usually worse after you have been standing for a long time.

Medical Treatments for Pelvic Relaxation and Uterine Prolapse

Medical intervention is usually not necessary for pelvic relaxation or even mild uterine prolapse. If the prolapse is severe enough to cause discomfort, you can ask your doctor to insert a pessary—a rubber device that fits around the cervix and helps to prop up the uterus. Disadvantages include difficulty in obtaining a proper fit, possible irritation or infection, and the need to remove and clean the pessary frequently. A surgical procedure called a suspension operation can lift and reattach a descended uterus, and often a fallen bladder or rectum as well. Many medical practitioners recommend hysterectomy for prolapsed uterus, but it is usually unnecessary and should be done only as a last resort in appropriate cases. It's best to consult a surgeon who has expertise in this area and keeps up with new research. Urologists have special training in this kind of pelvic surgery.

Prevention and Self-Help

The best way to prevent pelvic relaxation and uterine prolapse is to do regular Kegel exercises and leg lifts, which strengthen the muscles of the pelvic floor and lower abdomen (see "How to Do Kegel Exercises," p. 643). Check whether your pelvic muscles are in good shape by trying to start and stop the flow of urine while sitting on the toilet. If you can't stop the flow, you need to do more Kegels. Some health care providers recommend doing them up to a hundred times a day, especially during pregnancy, when the pelvic muscles are under particular stress. You may also strengthen a slightly prolapsed uterus by relaxing in the knee-chest position (kneeling with your chest on the floor and your bottom in the air) several times a day. Some women find that certain yoga positions, such as the shoulder stand and headstand, relieve the discomfort of a prolapsed uterus.

POLYCYSTIC OVARIAN SYNDROME (PCOS)[29]

Polycystic ovary syndrome (also called anovulatory androgen excess, polycystic ovarian disease, or Stein-Leventhal syndrome) is the most common hormonal and reproductive problem that affects women of childbearing age. It is a medical condition that may include a variety of ailments, making it difficult to diagnose. PCOS usually starts around the time of puberty but may become noticeable when a woman is in her twenties or thirties. Between approximately 5 and 8 percent of women experience this disorder.

PCOS is defined by the presence of any two of the following characteristics:

- Irregular menstrual cycles or lack of ovulation (release of an egg) for an extended period of time
- Elevated levels of androgens (male hormones) in the blood, or evidence for elevated

androgens such as acne or excess unwanted hair growth (and head hair loss)
- Many small follicles (benign fluid-filled sacs) on the ovaries (resulting from not releasing eggs)

PCOS is diagnosed in large part by excluding other possible conditions that can cause similar signs and symptoms. Your health care provider will first administer blood tests or other exams to see if your body is making high doses of steroids, or if there are pituitary, adrenal, or ovarian tumors.

What Causes PCOS?

The exact cause of PCOS is unclear, although risk increases in women who are overweight. PCOS is more common in certain families. There is evidence for a genetic cause, but the exact gene(s) responsible have yet to be identified.

PCOS results from a combination of several related factors. Many women with PCOS have insulin resistance, in which the body cannot use insulin efficiently. This leads to high blood levels of insulin, called hyperinsulinemia. It is believed that hyperinsulinemia is related to increased androgen levels, as well as to obesity and type 2 diabetes. In turn, obesity can also cause insulin resistance and increase the risk for or worsen PCOS.

Large amounts of androgens can block egg growth and ovulation. Because they are male sex hormones, they can also cause women to develop male secondary sex characteristics such as facial hair or hair thinning at the front of the head.

How Does PCOS Affect Ovulation?

When a woman has an ovulatory problem, her reproductive system does not produce the necessary amounts of hormones to develop, mature, and release a healthy egg. In this case, the ovaries become enlarged and develop many small fol-

licles. These follicles produce androgens, which further interfere with ovulation. Some researchers believe that the cysts contain eggs that didn't mature and didn't get released during ovulation. Others disagree. Studies have shown that not every woman with PCOS has these numerous follicles. Nor does every woman with these numerous follicles have PCOS. Some women with polycystic ovaries have regular menstrual cycles.

PCOS Symptoms

The signs and symptoms of PCOS are related to hormonal imbalance (excess male hormones), lack of ovulation, and insulin resistance and may include:

- Irregular, infrequent, or absent menstrual periods
- Hirsutism—excessive growth of body and facial hair including hair on the chest, stomach, and back
- Acne or oily skin
- Enlarged and/or polycystic ovaries
- Problems with fertility
- Being overweight or obese, especially around the waist (central obesity)
- Male-pattern baldness or thinning hair
- Skin tags—small pieces of skin on the neck or armpits
- Acanthosis nigricans—darkened skin areas on the back of the neck, in the armpits, and under the breasts

In addition, women with PCOS may be at increased risk for developing certain health problems, including:

- Type 2 diabetes
- Elevated cholesterol levels. Triglycerides—fatty acids in the bloodstream—may be higher than normal in some women with PCOS, whereas HDL, the "good cholesterol," may be lower than normal. This could raise

the risk of heart attacks because arteries and other blood vessels are more likely to be narrowed or clogged over time.

- High blood pressure
- Elevated blood clotting factors
- Missed periods followed by prolonged and heavy bleeding
- Endometrial cancer. Lack of ovulation for an extended period of time may cause excessive thickening of the endometrium (the lining of the uterus). Abnormal cells may build up in the lining of the uterus when it is not shed regularly during a menstrual period. Eventually, some of these abnormal cells may turn cancerous.
- Some studies show a relationship between PCOS and breast cancer.

The symptoms of PCOS may resemble other conditions or medical problems. Always consult your physician for a diagnosis.

Diagnosis

In addition to a complete medical history, a physical examination, including a pelvic exam, can be used initially to diagnose PCOS.

A variety of tests can also be used to detect PCOS. Blood tests are used to detect increased levels of androgens and other hormones. Other blood tests can measure blood sugar, cholesterol, and triglyceride levels.

Physicians sometimes use an ultrasound (also called a sonogram)—a diagnostic technique that uses high-frequency sound waves and a computer to create images of blood vessels, tissues, and organs. Ultrasounds are used to view internal organs as they function and to assess blood flow through various vessels. Ultrasound can determine if a woman's ovaries are enlarged and if cysts or follicles are present, and also evaluate the thickness of the endometrium.

Sometimes it can be difficult to diagnose PCOS with certainty because of how it varies,

both from woman to woman and even over time in the same woman.

Medical and Self-Help Treatments for PCOS

Specific treatment for PCOS will be determined by your clinician based on your age, overall health, and medical history. In addition, your health care provider will take into account the extent of the disorder and expectations for improvement; your tolerance for specific medications, procedures, and therapies; and your preferences. Treatment also depends on whether or not you want to become pregnant.

For women who do not want to become pregnant, treatment is focused on treating the symptoms and preventing long-term consequences of the condition. Treatment may include the following.

Weight reduction: A healthy diet and increased physical activity allow more efficient use of insulin and decrease blood glucose levels, and also lower risk of heart disease and diabetes. Some women with PCOS who lose weight will start having regular periods.

Oral contraceptives: Birth control pills may be prescribed to regulate menstrual cycles, decrease androgen levels, control acne, prevent balding or hair thinning, and decrease facial hair.

Cyclic progesterone: Can be prescribed intermittently to ensure women don't go too long without a period.

Spironolactone: A less common but often helpful treatment that can minimize excess hair growth. Other procedures such as bleaching, electrolysis, and laser hair removal may also be used to decrease facial hair.

Diabetes medication: Metformin, a medication used in the treatment of type 2 diabetes, is often used to decrease insulin resistance in PCOS. Some preliminary studies of women with PCOS who are insulin resistant show that such drugs may also help reduce androgen levels, hair growth, acne, balding, and body weight and may help a woman ovulate more regularly. No long-term studies of this form of treatment are available. Some studies have shown a reduction in the risk of miscarriage in pregnant PCOS patients taking metformin, while others have not. Your clinicians will discuss this with you if you become pregnant.

For women who want to become pregnant, treatment is focused on weight reduction and promoting ovulation and may include the following.

Weight reduction: A healthy diet and increased physical activity allow more efficient use of in-sulin and decrease blood glucose levels and may help a woman ovulate more regularly.

Ovulation induction medications such as Clomid: These medications stimulate the ovary to make one or more follicles (sacs that contain eggs) and release the egg for fertilization. Metformin is sometimes used for this purpose as well.

Surgery: In cases of infertility where drugs don't work, surgical techniques that make small holes in one or both ovaries may be suggested. This surgery often restores ovulation, though not always permanently. Adhesions—scar tissue that can twist the ovaries or make them cling to other organs—are a potential drawback. Because of these concerns, this procedure is rarely performed today.

CHAPTER 23

The United States does not ensure access to health care and related services. While the federal health care reform law passed in 2010 will make substantive and important improvements, many of us will struggle to get the health care that we need.

Access alone, however, does not guarantee the care we receive will be medically and culturally appropriate or even effective. In order to increase the quality of care, we need to learn how to navigate the health care system maze. This complex task is somewhat easier when we understand medical insurance and health care options, have access to care providers we trust, and know how to find accurate and up-to-date health information.

This chapter addresses some of the social, political, and economic factors that affect our health and the quality of the care we receive and focuses on what we can do as individuals to get good reproductive and sexual health care. For additional information on the broader factors that affect our health, see Chapter 26, "The Politics of Women's Health."

DETERMINING WHEN WE NEED HEALTH CARE

We regularly make decisions that affect our health: every day we make choices like whether to fasten a seatbelt, use a condom, or have a cigarette. These self-care decisions, including what we eat and how we manage stress, can have profound effects on our well-being and need for medical care.

No matter what choices we make, almost all of us will at some point turn to health care providers for advice, testing, or treatment. Sometimes a team of professionals is needed to manage different aspects of care and coordinate different services and treatment plans.

When it comes to reproductive and sexual health, determining when we need care can sometimes be difficult because most aspects of reproductive health and sexuality are not diseases or disorders. Medical care can sometimes lead to medicalization—meaning that normal body processes such as menstruation, childbirth, and menopause come to be defined as diseases that need close monitoring and medical intervention. Medicalization can chip away at our confidence in our bodies and expose us to risks and costs from unnecessary medical tests and treatments.

On the other hand, there are many times when health care providers are needed to sort out whether a troubling symptom is normal or a sign of a problem. And we rely on the expertise of health care providers when we experience illness, chronic pain, or injury. Underuse of health care in these situations may lead to poor health outcomes or drive up the eventual cost of our care.

MAKING HEALTH CARE DECISIONS

Making good health care decisions can be challenging. A good decision involves gathering and evaluating information, weighing what's important to you, finding the resources needed to maximize the quality of care you receive, and dealing with the associated costs. All tests and medical treatments have potential positive and negative effects, and each of us values these potential effects differently.

Benefits of a test or treatment may include:

- Gaining important information about your health
- Avoiding or terminating an unwanted pregnancy
- Achieving a wanted pregnancy
- Getting welcome relief from symptoms
- Improving your ability to function in your job or recreational activities
- Acquiring information that will allow you to make better choices regarding your health and health care
- Increasing your chance of living longer

We must balance the likelihood of these benefits with possible negative effects, which may include:

- The possibility that the test or treatment will be ineffective
- The possibility that the test may give unreliable information that may require more

costly or risky tests to confirm, or lead to unnecessary treatment

- Impact on the ability to conceive and carry a healthy pregnancy or to breastfeed a child in the future
- Impact on sexuality or body image
- Increased chance of health problems in the future, such as cancer risk from radiation or certain hormone treatments
- Impact on family and community support systems
- Financial costs
- Effect on ability to work
- Pain and discomfort
- Emotional effects

For some tests and treatments, especially those that are newer, long-term effects are uncertain. Even when research is available, it is more likely to address physical effects than emotional well-being, effects on family or work, or financial costs. As a result, we must often make health care choices without complete information.

Our choices matter because getting too little, too much, or the wrong health care can have serious negative consequences. In addition, the right care may not be the same for all women. Many of the challenges to getting the right care in a timely manner may not be under your individual control. You may lack the time or money needed to follow up on appointments or treatments; there may be errors in your medical record that lead to delays; or your care providers may not tell you about the full range of options because of financial conflicts of interest or simply because they are too busy. We need to advocate for changes in the system, while recognizing the system's limitations and making the best choices we can with the resources available.

I went to my doctor because I was having an awful, burning pain during sex. She did a test to see if cell changes in my vagina could be leading to dryness. The result came back showing a bacterial infection and cell changes consistent with inflammation, which she said was most likely caused by the infection. She prescribed an antibiotic and I was pain-free within a week. Later, my doctor insisted that we do Pap tests every three months just in case the cell changes were from abnormal cells that "fell off of my cervix." I had done a lot of research on my symptoms and infection and asked a few friends who had medical backgrounds, and we all agreed that such frequent Paps were overkill, especially since I was low risk (I was monogamous with my partner). I got reminders by phone and even a certified letter from the doctor's office reminding me that I "needed" the Pap tests. I know they were just covering themselves in case I had cervical cancer and sued them. But I know I made the right decision, and I've had normal Paps and no pain for nearly a decade since then.

HOW THE NEW HEALTH CARE REFORM LAW AFFECTS WOMEN'S ACCESS TO HEALTH CARE AND HEALTH INSURANCE

In early 2010, national comprehensive health care reform became law. While far from perfect, this law takes critically important steps to remedy some of the many challenges that women face dealing with the current health care system. Under the health reform law, which will be phased in over several years, millions of people will have greater access to more affordable and comprehensive health care and insurance. Unfortunately, health care reform includes burdensome restrictions on insurance coverage of abortion care and unacceptable limits on access to coverage for certain immigrant women. For a more detailed discussion, see "Health Care Reform and the Politics of Women's Health," p. 770.

HELP FINDING HEALTH INSURANCE

The website healthcare.gov explains how health care reform affects individuals, families, children, and employers. By answering a few simple questions, you'll learn about the different insurance plans available and where you might be able to find low-cost health care if you are currently uninsured. Starting in 2014, insurance "exchanges" will be available to individuals who do not have access to other coverage through their employers and to small businesses.

COVERAGE OF IMPORTANT HEALTH CARE SERVICES

Under the law, health plans must cover a broad range of health services that are particularly important for women, including certain preventive care and screenings, such as mammograms and Pap tests, without any cost-sharing (such as a co-payment). Starting in 2014, insurance plans must include coverage of "essential benefits," which will include maternity care, prescription drugs (which should include contraceptive drugs and devices),* and mental health care.

ADDITIONAL PROVISIONS AFFECTING WOMEN

The new reform law has many components, only some of which have received media atten-

---

* A panel appointed by the Institute of Medicine is set to recommend whether to include prescription contraceptives as a preventive service, in which case they would be covered without charge beginning in 2012.

tion. Here are a few other provisions that are important to women:

- Women will have direct access to obstetrical and gynecological care, meaning you won't have to obtain prior approval from your health plan when seeking care from these providers.
- Pregnant women will gain insurance coverage of additional options for labor and birth:
  - Medicaid will now cover births at freestanding birth centers.
  - Nurse-midwives will receive more equitable reimbursement under Medicare.
- Young people—who are more likely to be uninsured than any other age group—will be able to remain on their parents' health insurance policy until age twenty-six.
- Older women on Medicare will benefit from a provision that will eliminate the Medicare "donut hole"—a gap in prescription drug coverage that requires seniors to spend a considerable amount out of pocket. (For more information, see "Medicare Basics," p. 569.)

RESTRICTIONS ON IMMIGRANT WOMEN AND WOMEN SEEKING ABORTIONS

There are a number of troubling restrictions that many women's health care advocates are seeking to remedy:

- Immigrants must wait five years before being eligible for Medicaid; however, once eligible, immigrants are eligible for sliding scale insurance subsidies.
- Immigrants who lack documentation of their legal status will be ineligible to buy insurance through the exchanges or to enroll in Medicaid.

Several groups offer information and advocacy about the reform law and track its implementation with respect to women, including:

- National Women's Law Center (nwlc.org)
- EQUAL Health Network (equalhealth.info)
- Raising Women's Voices (raisingwomens voices.net)

- Insurance coverage of abortion is treated differently from any other health care service. Anyone who purchases a subsidized health plan with abortion coverage through an exchange is required to make two separate payments for this health insurance: one for abortion coverage and another for the remainder of the premium. This unfair and burdensome requirement could deter women from purchasing plans that cover abortion and deter health plans from offering it.

SOURCES OF HEALTH INFORMATION

Accurate information about your health and about the full range of health care options available to you is needed to make good health care decisions. To begin with, it is important to listen to and trust what your body tells you. Knowing your symptoms, understanding prior or ongo-

TRACKING YOUR OWN HEALTH

It can be helpful to keep a log of symptoms, triggers, or behaviors relevant to your health condition and to track the effectiveness and side effects of treatments. Bringing this information with you is one way to get the most out of visits to a health care provider.

There are many ways to monitor your health. Tracking your menstrual cycle and signs of ovulation can help you manage problems related to menstruation, achieve a wanted pregnancy, or avoid an unwanted pregnancy. (For more information, see "Charting Your Menstrual Cycles," p. 26.) A pain diary can help you notice what triggers your pain or makes it better or worse. If you have started a new medication, keeping a journal of your symptoms and side effects can help you determine if the treatment is working and identify possible adverse effects. Tracking your nutritional habits or physical activity may make it easier to succeed at making long-term changes.

A simple paper or online journal often works fine. There are also many mobile phone applications and online health sites designed specifically for this purpose.

One benefit of online health management tools is that people with similar health concerns can track their data together and support one another in finding and sticking to the best treatment plans. Websites like FertilityFriend (fertilityfriend.com) allow you to chart your ovulation cycle and, if you want, share charts with friends, your care provider, or online contacts. Sites such as PatientsLikeMe (patientslikeme.com) and CureTogether (curetogether.com) allow registered users to track their symptoms and treatments and pool the data from multiple users so that people can see what worked and what didn't for others with the same symptoms or diseases. Several sites sell health data (without personal identifying information) to pharmaceutical companies, who typically use the data to track drug safety and look for new uses for drugs. Carefully review each privacy policy to make sure your personal health information is secure.

I could not take the excruciating burn in my vulva (vulvodynia) a single moment more. It not only completely inhibited my sex life, it eventually took over my life when I could barely walk. As traditional health care and medicine failed (often making the pain even worse), I found an abundance of information online and people at CureTogether and other communities with my same unlikely condition. Tracking every symptom out of desperation and using the sites to compare my symptoms and triggers with other women's, I was finally able to uncover underlying hormonal causes and find treatments that worked.

Some sites run ads for medications or other health products and many accept funding from drug and device companies. When websites accept funding from pharmaceutical or medical device companies, it can influence the content available on the site or make it more difficult to identify reliable information. For more information, see "Evaluating Health Information in the Media," p. 664.

ing health problems, knowing the health status of your sexual and household partner(s), and learning and recording as much information as possible about your family history can help you to more fully understand your current health and improve communication with health care providers.

INFORMATION FROM HEALTH CARE PROVIDERS

Discussing medical problems with a health care provider can be enormously satisfying or frustrating, or somewhere in between. When your health care provider has looked thoroughly at your health history and current symptoms and discussed with you your values, priorities, and concerns, she or he can engage with you in shared decision making and help you make the best choice for *you*.

When we couldn't find the heartbeat at my ten-week prenatal appointment, I had an ultrasound and found out that I had miscarried. My doctor offered me medication or a D&C to complete the miscarriage, and also told me that I could wait and see if my body would do it on its own. I asked for a day or two to think about it and she told me to take my time. I read up on the pros and cons of each option and talked to my friend who was a midwife. I had had my son at home naturally and I really felt that I wanted to complete this pregnancy naturally, too, so I decided to wait. But after two more weeks, still nothing had happened. By then the risks seemed to be increasing and I was having a difficult time emotionally being in this state of limbo. I decided on the D&C at that point. I think it would have been the wrong choice for me right after I found out I miscarried, but in the end it was the right one.

While there is much they can provide, doctors and other health care providers may be constrained by such factors as:

- Financial incentives built into the system that reward the use of procedures and prescriptions over talk time and preventive care
- Pressures or more subtle influence from drug company representatives to recommend certain medications or devices over others that may be more appropriate
- "Standards of care" that have been shown to be the most effective for the most people but still may not be appropriate or desirable for certain individuals
- Lack of time to keep up with all of the latest research or the skills necessary to evaluate research and tailor treatment to individual patient situations

- Inability to recommend certain testing or preventive care if insurance won't cover it
- Fear of a lawsuit resulting from a missed diagnosis or a bad outcome, which can drive hospitals and providers to overuse tests and treatments
- A mistrust of patients' abilities to understand or make good use of complex information
- Sexism, racism, homophobia, and class bias as a result of their training or upbringing
- Lack of knowledge or negative attitudes toward prevention, self-care, less invasive procedures, nonmedical alternatives, and complementary and alternative medicine

It is common to want to trust doctors or other health care providers completely and always accept their advice. While this can feel reassuring, you may ultimately receive better care by becoming more informed, asking more questions, and treating the relationship as a partnership with shared decision making. Changing our relationships to care can require courage in the face of uncertainty and may not always be welcomed by providers, but it is a good step in obtaining the care that is most appropriate for each of us.

My son was only seven weeks old and breastfeeding heartily when I developed what I thought was just a really bad clogged duct. After two days of intense pain, my ob-gyn performed an ultrasound and found an abscess. She very sympathetically told me I needed surgery and would have to stop breastfeeding immediately. She prescribed medication to dry up my milk supply and scheduled the surgery for the next day.

I was devastated by the idea of stopping breastfeeding. I called my friend, a pediatric nurse practitioner and lactation consultant, for sympathy, and she mentioned that she had heard of instances where a woman continued breastfeeding during and after the surgery. When

THE TIME CRUNCH

In most settings, the typical office visit for a gynecology exam or prenatal visit is just ten to fifteen minutes. The complexity of care options, the proportion of women with chronic medical problems, and the average number of medications a patient takes have all increased over recent years, but the length of office visits has not. Obstetrician-gynecologists, who provide much of the health care for women's reproductive and sexual health needs, face high malpractice insurance and other overhead costs and recoup those costs by seeing more patients or doing more reimbursable procedures. This takes away from their ability to schedule longer appointments.

You can make the most of your medical appointments by being organized and proactive (see "Making the Most of Your Health Care Visit" p. 676), but we also need to advocate for better access to care models that allow deeper interaction with care providers and better coordination of care. Alternative models of care include the following.

Group medical appointments: In Centering Pregnancy group prenatal care, visits are ninety minutes with no waiting room time and incorporate health assessment, support, and education. The successful model is now being adapted to other areas of health care. For more information, visit centeringhealthcare.org.

Woman and family-centered medical home: The WFCMH concept is new but is likely to expand in coming years. In this model, each woman has a personal physician or other care provider who knows her and her history and coordinates all care and referrals. The medical home concept also encompasses patient-centered features such as online scheduling and expanded office hours and uses new technologies to measure outcomes and enhance patient education and communication.

Midwives, nurse-practitioners, and physicians' assistants: These types of care providers may have lower overhead costs and therefore sometimes offer longer appointments. They also may have more education in preventive care and patient education. However, if you have complex health needs, some of the care you need may be outside the scope of practice of these providers, and you may be referred to specialists.

---

my ob-gyn called that night to check in, I asked if this was possible. She told me that it's rarely done, because the risk of the incision becoming infected is high, but she listened when I expressed how important it was to me to continue nursing. In the end we agreed to try, because I felt willing to take the risk.

The recovery was pretty intense—in order for the milk not to cause an infection, the incision had to heal from the deepest part outward. A home nurse came twice a day to clean out and repack the wound to keep it from closing up, and each time she did so, milk would spray out from deep inside my breast! But my breast healed relatively quickly—and two years later my son is still happily nursing.

SUPPORT, SELF-CARE, AND SELF-HELP GROUPS

There are many kinds of groups that you can join to learn about and discuss health topics and treatments. Participating in a group provides the opportunity to talk with other people in our situation, to trade ideas, to feel less alone, to motivate one another, and sometimes to learn new self-care skills. Self-help groups are based on the belief that we are capable of understanding medical information, that our health information rightfully belongs to us, and that we can learn more collectively than we can individually. When these groups are independent of health care institutions and professionals, we can freely question, challenge, and evaluate accepted medical treatments and explore nonmedical therapies and providers.

Some physicians, medical centers, and hospitals offer groups or classes on a wide variety of health topics. These groups often emphasize self-care and activities that we can do to manage our care in conjunction with our providers. Local support groups are also offered by nonprofit organizations such as the American Cancer Society, La Leche League, or the Endometriosis Association. If the kind of group you seek does not already exist in your area, consider starting one of your own.

Increasingly, women are tapping into existing support groups online. New technologies vastly expand the number of people we can potentially connect with for support and information sharing. If you have a rare condition that doesn't affect many people or if you have decreased mobility, the Internet may be your best source of support from people with similar health issues:

During my long four months of bed rest, because of my online community I always had someone to chat with who could understand my pain—other moms going through the same experience. We
no longer felt alone. It was also a source of hope as we would see the "bed rest graduates" and understand that there was indeed a light at the end of the tunnel. We just had to hang in there and support one another.

Tips for finding a good support group online include:

- Look for websites that have information on the condition or topic you are seeking, and see if any groups are mentioned there.
- If you find an online group, look through previous discussions (if publicly available) to see how active the group is. When was the most recent post? How many people are involved? Does one person dominate all of the discussion? Are the participants supportive of each other?
- Before participating, take some time to listen to what people are talking about. Evaluate whether or not you feel that this is a safe space for you to share your questions, concerns, and knowledge.
- If you do find groups that meet your needs, remember that there are a wide range of opinions on any given topic and it's okay for people to disagree. Ideally, however, the conversation remains respectful.
- Verify information. Remember, people posting don't necessarily have medical knowledge or experience. Bring new information to your health care provider or verify it with another trustworthy source.
- Check the moderation policy to make sure that comments aren't explicitly censored if they don't support a certain point of view.
- Always bear in mind that once you post information, you cannot control where it goes or who reads it.

DIRECT-TO-CONSUMER ADVERTISING OF DRUGS

My doctor told me I was at high risk of invasive breast cancer. I told him I wanted to reduce that risk.
—Ad for an osteoporosis drug

The only birth control proven to treat premenstrual dysphoric disorder.
—Ad for YAZ

I'm proud of him because be asked about Viagra . . . I love him because he did it for us.
—Ad for Viagra

Ads for prescription and over-the-counter drugs are everywhere—on the Internet and on TV, on billboards and in magazines. Some of these ads promise not only to solve our medical problems but to bring us happiness, contentment, and the good life.

Other ads appeal to our fears about our health. Their underlying message is this: You appear to be healthy, but a deadly heart attack, a hip fracture, or some other medical catastrophe could occur at any time. Therefore, you should take a prescription drug to prevent such problems.

Drug companies claim that direct-to-consumer (DTC) advertising is good because the ads educate the public and encourage people to be more involved in their medical choices. But drug companies have a serious conflict of interest when it comes to educating the public: They have a vested interest in convincing people to take their drugs. The more peo-ple use their products, the larger the drug companies' profits. In 2005 the pharmaceutical industry spent $4.2 billion advertising drugs directly to consumers.[1]

Ads aimed at healthy people who can be persuaded to take a drug daily for the rest of their lives clearly target the industry's most desirable customer base. The overselling of postmenopausal hormones, supported by the depiction of natural menopause as a "hormone deficiency disease" that needed "hormone replacement therapy," was the forerunner to this type of sales pitch, which now permeates the media. Aging, social anxiety disorder, heartburn, restless leg syndrome, and overactive bladder are all examples of symptoms or normal physiological events that are now presented to consumers as being in need of long-term drug treatment.

We need to recognize misleading pharmaceutical marketing practices and base drug treatment decisions on scientifically accurate evidence. Be particularly skeptical of heavily advertised drugs and those that come with coupons or free samples. They are the newest, most expensive drugs with the shortest track records of safety. The Food and Drug Administration (FDA) does not require new drugs to be proved better than competing, often cheaper drugs already on the market. In addition, drug trials typically last no more than a few months and long-term safety studies are almost never done, so problems with long-term use may not show up until years after FDA approval.

The FDA's website (fda.gov) offers extensive information about medicines, including safety alerts about the latest recalls and warnings for specific drugs. The international nonprofit group Healthy Skepticism (healthyskepticism.org) counters misleading drug promotion and maintains a regular "AdWatch" section on its website. Be cautious when looking for information on other websites, as many are substantially sponsored by pharmaceutical companies. Being skeptical about drug ads and promotions is smart: it can protect both our health and our wallets.

HEALTH INFORMATION ONLINE

While the amount of material available on the Internet is vast, the quality of the information varies greatly. Some sites push dubious medicine, both conventional and alternative; some are concerned only with selling you their products; and some sites are biased by the drug companies, professional societies, and other advertisers who support them.

Below are some questions to ask to help evaluate the quality of online health information:

Who is responsible for the content on the site? Any good site should make it easy for you to learn who is responsible for the site and its content. Look for a link that says "Who We Are" or "About Us." It is also useful to understand whether the information is created by a health care provider, a person dealing with a medical condition, or a professional spokesperson, for example, so you can better judge the content. If there is no information available about who owns the site or develops the content, be wary.

Who/what pays for the site? It is important to consider how sources of funding for a site or its content provider may affect the content. Does the site sell advertising? Does it sell products or services? Is it sponsored by a drug company? Is it funded through industry grants or donations? (Nonprofit organizations are often funded this way.) The source of funding can affect what content is presented, and how. For example, drug-company-sponsored information tends to downgrade or ignore nonmedical or nonpharmacological approaches (which are often more effective) and is slow to present innovative alternatives or preventive treatments. Try to figure out if the author(s) and site owner(s) have a financial interest in, or anything else to gain from, proposing one particular point of view over another.

Is there research to support the information on the site? Many health-oriented websites do not provide references to support the statements made. This may be because the site is written by a patient speaking from personal experience, because a statement is generally accepted to be true, or for other, less trustworthy reasons. The presence of references to medical and scientific literature can be a positive aspect of a site, as it allows readers to track down the source material and verify the author's statements. However, a list of scientific sources does not mean a site is automatically trustworthy. For example, an organization with a political agenda (such as anti–abortion rights groups) may present references that—upon closer inspection—do not actually support the claims being made.

When was the material written or compiled? It is important to have a sense of whether the content is frequently updated or has been updated recently. It is not always possible to determine this, and copyright dates are not a reliable measure of when individual pieces of content were last updated. Medical research can easily become outdated; what may have been accepted in the recent past (such as routine hormone replacement therapy for postmenopausal women) may not be the current standard of medical care. **Does the site allow anyone to alter or update content?** Sites like Wikipedia allow anyone with Internet access to edit, revise, or update content according to voluntary community standards. Based on the success and popularity of Wikipedia, several organizations and companies have begun to offer health-related wiki tools. While these resources can sometimes provide balanced and up-to-date content, remember that people who offer edits and revisions may be those most motivated to share their insights—because of either very positive or very negative experiences. Company representatives or paid consultants may also alter content and may not be identifiable.

Does the information sound too good to be true? Be wary of "cures" for incurable diseases or treatments that seem too good to be true. Question sites that credit themselves as the sole source of information on a topic as well as sites that disparage other sources of knowledge. Also be aware that terms like bioidentical, herbal, or natural do not have regulated meanings and do not guarantee either safety or good outcomes.

Does the site ask you for personal information? If so, read its privacy statement to find out if your information will be shared by others without your permission. When choosing to participate in discussion forums or other online communities where you share personal information, think about whether there are any potential consequences of the information being publicly available (such as job discrimination or insurance claim denials).

What About Websites Run by Patients?

Sometimes, someone who has learned a lot about her or his own health condition or worked hard to find the most up-to-date research about treatment options will "pay it forward" by making this information more easily available to others.

These sites, usually free of financial conflicts of interest, can sometimes provide excellent, up-to-date information from a consumer perspective—a perspective too often missing from other sources of information. However, the content developers may not be skilled at understanding medical information and research literature or keeping the site updated. And they may not have exactly the same medical condition or symptoms as you, or the same values, preferences, and priorities that you bring to your health care decisions.

Also, beware of sites or social media pages that look as if they are from individual patients but are actually slick advertising campaigns created by corporate interests such as pharmaceutical companies or hospitals. In some cases, the "patient" is fabricated altogether, but pharmaceutical and device companies may also recruit real patients to tell their stories online, selecting those patients who have treatment success stories and who didn't experience or are willing to downplay negative side effects. Even on sites that purport to be patients' personal web pages, look for an "About" link or any ads or company logos, clues that the content is sponsored and potentially biased. Federal regulations now require bloggers to disclose when they receive advertising revenue, free product samples, or anything else of value, so also look for disclosure statements.

Finally, you should be aware that your online privacy could be violated by individuals who run websites or by individuals with access to your computer. For example, when you comment on a blog, the blog's administrators may be able to detect where you are located or where you work (if you post your comment using a computer at work) by looking at the IP address attached to your comment. It may also be pos-

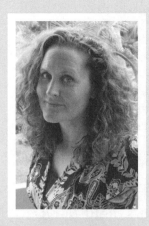

"THE REACH OF THE BLOG HAS BEEN MIND-BOGGLING."

JILL ARNOLD
THEUNNECESAREAN.COM

In 2005, when I was almost thirty-eight weeks pregnant, my midwife informed me that she suspected macrosomia (a too big baby) based on ultrasound results and told me I needed a cesarean section to prevent injury to my baby. I didn't think that major surgery was necessary because all of the babies born into my family are big. But I didn't want to put my baby at risk, either. I began frantically searching the Internet for information to support this recommendation. I found journal articles and websites with the statistics that I needed to make an informed decision to refuse the cesarean, but the process was arduous and stressful. Based on what I found, I waited until labor began spontaneously, refused the cesarean at the hospital, and had a healthy 10-pound baby vaginally. I went on to have another baby at a freestanding birth center who weighed over 11 pounds.

I launched TheUnnecesarean.com in 2008 with the hope of reaching other women who found themselves hungry for the same information for which I searched high and low three years prior. My hope was not that the site would constitute an authoritative source of advice on cesareans; rather, I envisioned a starting place for consumers to begin their own research, read peer-level commentary, and meet other people who might help direct them to whatever missing piece of information they need to feel secure in their decision-making process.

Now the blog has several contributors who all bring different perspectives but share the philosophy of trusting women to make decisions about their bodies and their births and a commitment to offering a safe space for women to explore the full range of birth choices. The reach of the blog has been mind-boggling. We reached nearly half a million readers in the past year and some of our blog posts have influenced mass media coverage of birth issues. The blog was even referenced at the National Institutes of Health Consensus Development Conference on Vaginal Birth After Cesarean. I started the site with the mind-set that if I could help prevent just one family from going through what we did, it would be worth it. The fact that it has been helpful to so many people makes me very happy.

sible for someone in your household to monitor your Internet activity using certain tools and techniques.

EVALUATING HEALTH INFORMATION IN THE MEDIA

"Tequila Plant May Help Fight Bone Loss"
"U.S.-Developed Vaccine 'Could Eliminate' Breast Cancer"
"Extract May Help Treat Bladder Infection"
"Abortion Pill Might Help Battle Breast Cancer"

What do these recent headlines from major U.S. news outlets have in common? They report on studies that were conducted in mice, not humans.

Overzealous or oversimplified headlines are only one problem in mass media health reporting. In a 2009 survey of health journalists commissioned by the Kaiser Family Foundation, journalists overwhelmingly said that budget constraints have seriously hurt the quality of health coverage and that pressure to be the first to break a story leads to fewer opportunities to conduct thorough research before filing a story. Respondents felt this leads to more "quick hit" stories about new treatments or technological breakthroughs rather than in-depth coverage of health care policy and complex health issues. Nearly half (44 percent) of staff journalists participating in the survey said that their organizations sometimes or frequently based stories on press releases without substantial additional reporting. And perhaps most shockingly, 11 percent of staff journalists said that their organizations sometimes or frequently allowed advertisers, the sales staff, or sponsors to influence story selection or content.[2]

HealthNewsReview.org is a website provided by the Foundation for Informed Medical Decision Making, an independent organization that evaluates the quality of the reporting on health stories by examining whether and how a story answers these ten questions:

1. What's the total cost?
2. How often do benefits occur?
3. How often do harms occur?
4. How strong is the evidence?
5. Is this condition exaggerated?
6. Are there alternative options?
7. Is this really a new approach?
8. Is it available to me?
9. Who's promoting this?
10. Do they have a conflict of interest?

For more information on HealthNewsReview.org's rating criteria and to see the ratings on more than one thousand health stories in major news outlets, visit healthnewsreview.org.

UNDERSTANDING RESEARCH LITERATURE

New research is published constantly, and even the most diligent health care providers have difficulty staying on top of every new study that may affect their area of practice. When your own health is at stake, you may be more motivated than your care providers to seek out and find the most current research about your specific needs.

Finding Research Studies

Nearly all research published in peer-reviewed health journals can be found by searching MEDLINE, a database available through PubMed (ncbi.nlm.nih.gov/pubmed). PubMed provides study abstracts (structured summaries providing key information about the design and main results of the research) at no charge. There may be a fee, however, for access to a full article.

Another excellent source of research is the Cochrane Database of Reviews (www2.cochrane.org/reviews). The Cochrane Collaboration creates systematic reviews of the best research about the safety and effectiveness of health and medical interventions. Abstracts of the reviews and plain-language summaries are available online for free.

Increasingly, people can obtain access to research studies and other professional publications such as clinical guidelines through open access journals, through public access articles, or by requesting articles from a library. One benefit of using the library is that a trained librarian may be able to search for you or show you how to make the best use of databases. Some hospitals or treatment centers have libraries and services to help patients learn more about their condition. State universities with medical schools are often required to make their medical libraries open to the public, and the medical librarians at these institutions can offer expert assistance. You might also be able to ask a friend at an academic institution (with free access to medical journals) to help you retrieve specific articles.

Reading a Research Study

Reading research can be daunting at first, and understanding it takes practice. Once you read a few studies you will notice that they are organized predictably into several sections.

- A research paper begins with an **abstract** that summarizes the study's methods and results and the researchers' conclusions.
- The full article begins with an **introduction** that frames the research problem and reviews the existing research in the area.
- The researchers should then include a **methods section** that explains exactly how they conducted their study, including how they recruited participants, what intervention or procedure was tested, and how data were collected and processed.

- This is followed by a **results section,** which often includes tables, charts, or graphs. If the study is comparing two or more groups, the researchers will state whether differences in outcomes among those groups are statistically significant, meaning they are unlikely to have occurred by chance and are therefore likely to be associated with the intervention or behavior being studied.
- The article will end with a **discussion section** that reviews the major findings, discusses the strengths and limitations of the study, and makes recommendations for further research or changes in practice. It is important in reading a study to focus on the

DO THESE RESULTS APPLY TO ME?

One of the most important questions to ask yourself when you are looking at a research paper is, "Do these results apply to me?" To answer this question, you actually have to ask two related questions, "Am I similar to the women in the study?" and "Will the test or treatment be the same for me as it was in the study?"

You are most likely to experience the same benefits and harms of an intervention that are reported in a study if you share characteristics with the people who participated in the study. You may (or may not) be similar to the study participants in terms of your sex, age, diagnosis, previous health history, current health, pregnancy status, and other characteristics. For instance, a study of the safety of labor induction conducted among women who had given birth al-

ready cannot be applied to women who are giving birth for the first time. Similarly, a new STI prevention strategy may be more or less effective depending on whether the study is conducted on college students in the United States or women visiting a family planning clinic in Africa. The study participants will usually be described in the methods section of the paper, although some information about the participants may also be listed in the results section.

Even if the women studied are similar to you, the context in which the care was provided might be different. The dose of the drug, the timing of the test or treatment, the skill of the practitioner, and the other care given along with the intervention may influence how effective or safe a procedure is. If your situation is different, you may not be able to expect the same results. A good research paper will describe these issues in detail, usually in the methods section of the paper.

CAN WE BELIEVE THE EVIDENCE IN EVIDENCE-BASED MEDICINE?[3]

When we and our providers seek solutions to our health problems, we depend on medical research to explain which treatments work best, the likelihood that a particular treatment will help, and the risks involved. We expect this evidence-based medicine, as it is called, to identify the best possible care.

Sources that health professionals turn to include research published in respected medical journals, continuing education courses presented by experts, and clinical practice guidelines established by expert review committees that evaluate medical research to define standards of good care.

What few people realize is that medical research has undergone a quiet but radical transformation. Before 1970, the vast majority of clinical research was funded by government sources.[4] By 2009, 85 percent of clinical trials were commercially funded.[5] In 1991, 70 percent of clinical research was commercially funded, but about 80 percent of this research was still being done in universities, where academic checks and balances supported the independence of researchers. By 2004, however, only 26 percent of this research was conducted in academic medical centers. The rest was conducted by for-profit research companies, a trend that continues today.[6]

When drug and medical device companies fund research directly through private contracts, they are able to influence the study design and the published results. For starters, drug companies can select the characteristics of the people included in a study to highlight the benefits of the drug and minimize the risks—including studying the product on healthy, younger people who take few other medications and are therefore less likely to have adverse effects, even though the drug is more likely to be taken by older people taking multiple medications. The drug companies are not required to compare their products with other known treatments, and they can end studies if the results don't appear favorable. Though they still must report results of most studies to the FDA, drug companies don't have to publish studies that don't come out the way they had hoped. And many of the authors of the research articles published in even the most respected medical journals have access only to data the drug companies choose to make available to them.

Because of these limitations, medical literature often gives an unbalanced picture of drug risks, benefits, and alternatives. Two studies published in 2003, one in the *Journal of the American Medical Association* (*JAMA*) and the other in the *British Medical Journal,* found that commercially funded studies were 3.6 to 4 times more likely than noncommercially funded studies to show positive results for the sponsor's product.[7] Another *JAMA* study that looked only at highest-quality studies found even stronger bias: The odds that commercially funded research found the sponsor's product the treatment of choice were 5.3 times greater than for studies funded by non-profits.[8] And yet another study found that when clinical studies are commercially funded and authors have financial ties to the sponsor (sometimes as paid speakers or consultants), the odds are 8.4 times higher that the results of the study will support use of the sponsor's drug.[9]

Another problem with commercially funded studies is that the articles published are sometimes "ghostwritten" by companies hired by pharmaceutical companies. In 2010, thousands of court documents stemming from a civil lawsuit over the safety of hormone therapy (HT) were made public. Analysis of these documents revealed that Wyeth pharmaceutical company, maker of the popular hormone drugs Premarin and Prempro, paid ghostwriters to produce twenty-six scientific papers promoting the benefits and downplaying the risks of HT and then found academic physicians willing to put their names on them and submit them to peer-reviewed journals.[10] In addition to downplaying the perceived risks of breast cancer and promoting cardiovascular benefits of hormone therapy, the articles promoted off-label, unproven uses, such as the prevention of dementia and Parkinson's disease—both of which were later debunked by the Women's Health Initiative study.

Unfortunately, the agencies we count on to protect the interests of health consumers are increasingly compromised. More than half of the funding for the Center for Drug Evaluation and Research, the division of the U.S. Food and Drug Administration that approves new drugs and oversees drug safety, comes from user fees paid by drug companies. Medical journals, trusted to evaluate articles independently, themselves depend on money from pharmaceutical advertising and from selling reprints of commercially favorable published articles to corporate sponsors, whose drug reps then distribute them to physicians. So-called expert committees that produce the clinical practice guidelines that inform and direct health care professionals are often dominated by researchers with active financial ties to one or more companies that make the drugs under consideration. And about 70 percent of continuing medical education courses for doctors are paid for by drug companies and other medical industries. Since doctors must participate in continuing medical education to maintain their medical licenses, it becomes increasingly difficult to avoid exposure to industry-sponsored messages.

The fundamental reason that companies create and distribute this information is to fulfill their primary fiduciary responsibilities to their shareholders and investors. Increasing product sales increases corporate bottom lines. Our health is relegated, at best, to a secondary consideration.

We need to demand complete transparency so we'll know when medical experts quoted by the media are receiving research funding or advising/consulting/speaking fees from drug and biomedical companies. We need to advocate for stricter standards in both the regulatory agencies and the medical journals that evaluate and publish research results. And we must insist that clinical guidelines that inform our doctors' decisions be free of commercial interest. The commercial takeover of our medical knowledge is, at its core, not a scientific problem but a political one. Reorienting our health care system to the service of public rather than private interests will occur only when an engaged and active citizenry creates a political force that stands at least equal to the political power of the drug industry.

Some change is already under way. Harvard Medical School instituted new rules in 2010 prohibiting professors from getting paid by drug companies to deliver educational talks and from accepting personal gifts, travel, or meals from drug companies. The new rules also restrict the amount of money professors can earn from consulting to drug companies or serving as board members. Some medical journal editors are requiring drug companies to register studies in advance, before rather than after the results are known, so that negative results are easier to track. And following the lead of Minnesota, more states are requiring drug companies to disclose payments to doctors. Some drug companies have begun posting doctors' names and compensation online. ProPublica compiled these disclosures into one database—projects.propublica.org/docdollars—that allows patients to search for their doctor. As ProPublica notes, "Receiving payments isn't necessarily wrong, but it does raise ethical issues."

methods and results sections, as the abstract and discussion section often focus on the authors' interpretations or opinions rather than on the actual findings. In some cases, the authors' statements in these sections may not be supported by the information in the methods and results sections.

OUR RIGHTS TO INFORMED CONSENT AND REFUSAL

Informed consent is a process of communication between you and your health care providers during which you learn all of the necessary information to choose whether you want to undergo a test or treatment. The concept of informed consent is founded on two fundamental propositions:

- It is your body, and you should be able to decide what is done to it.

- You are likely to make a better decision about your care if you have and can understand information on which to base a rational decision.

No one can treat or even touch you until you make an informed decision to accept or reject treatment. When you and your health care providers take informed consent seriously, you can have a true partnership with your caregivers, with shared authority, decision making, and responsibility.

In order to make an informed choice, you need to understand:

- Your specific health and illness situation
- The recommended treatment or procedure
- The risks and benefits of the recommended treatment or procedure, with a special emphasis on the risk of death or serious disability
- Medically reasonable alternative treatments and procedures, together with the risks and benefits of each

- Likely results if you refuse any treatment
- Probability of success, and what the health care provider means by "success" (for example, will the treatment cure the condition, or will it only alleviate symptoms?)
- Major problems anticipated in recuperation, including how long it will be until you can resume your normal activities
- What equipment or personal support you may require during your recovery
- The cost of the treatment or procedure, and how much of the cost your health plan will cover

Informed consent is a process, not just a written sheet to be signed. For consent to be informed, you must understand all that is being explained. It is not enough for a physician or another practitioner to catalog the risks and benefits in a hasty or complicated manner, to do so when you are under the effects of medication, to speak to you in a language you do not understand well, or to rely on a child or another family member to translate rather than a professional interpreter.

The consent form itself can be used as evidence of consent, so do not sign it if you do not understand and agree with what is written. You may cross out, reword, or otherwise amend a prepared form. Consent forms may sometimes be too technical in their language or be provided at a time when you are not prepared to review them thoroughly and discuss their implications. Hold on to the form until you feel you have all the information you need in order to add your signature.

You also have a right to know if a medication is being used for a purpose not approved by the U.S. Food and Drug Administration—otherwise known as "off-label" use. Ask your health care provider or a pharmacist for this information. You can also check drug reference books found in local libraries, online sources such as the FDA's website, or the medication's package insert for the approved purposes. Physicians and other providers are legally allowed to use medications for any purpose, even if the FDA has not reviewed evidence for that purpose. Because many routinely used obstetric drugs, many hormonal preparations, and some psychiatric drugs are given for purposes not specifically approved by the FDA, it is especially important for women to understand and ask about such off-label use.

CLINICAL TRIALS

Informed consent is particularly important when the treatment offered is part of a clinical trial or research program. In research settings, where you may be given an unproven or experimental drug or other therapy, practitioners must follow federal regulations that govern such research. The researcher must give you a copy of any informed consent form that you sign, as well as the name of a person who can provide you with additional information, and should review any potential harms from participation. You are never obligated to participate in research. Even if you decide to, you can change your mind at any time.

If the research project that you are asked to participate in includes treatments or diagnostic tests, it is important to ask whether the institution conducting the study will provide and pay for treatment, including treatment for conditions that may be found by the tests. You can learn more about the protections for patients involved in clinical trials at clinicaltrials.gov.

THE RIGHT TO REFUSE TREATMENT

You have a legal right to refuse any medical treatment at any time, even if you agreed to it previously. This right applies to all competent adults and mature minors—those who can understand and appreciate the information necessary to give informed consent. Simply disagreeing with your provider's recommendation does not mean that you are incompetent. In life-or-death matters involving decisions for others who are unable to decide for themselves, individual providers and hospitals may try to resist your choice to refuse treatment on behalf of them. All states have passed laws that allow people to authorize the withholding or withdrawal of medical treatment, even though such an order may lead to their death. Accepting one part of a treatment plan does not mean that you must accept the whole thing. You always have the right to leave the hospital if your wishes are not respected (with the exception, in some cases, of a psychiatric facility). Enlisting the support of a family member or some other advocate may be particularly helpful in such situations. For more information about refusing treatment, see *The Rights of Patients: The Basic ACLU Guide to Patient Rights* by George Annas (see Recommended Resources).

The right to refuse treatment is of particular importance to women regarding our reproductive autonomy. While it is generally recognized that people have a right to bodily integrity and informed consent, both legal decisions and political actions have dictated that women sometimes lose these rights upon becoming pregnant. Examples of such actions include court orders forcing women to undergo cesarean sections and medical tests performed without consent. In several cases, pregnant women who have refused a recommended cesarean section or who have used drugs have been arrested and charged with endangering fetal health.

National Advocates for Pregnant Women (NAPW) (advocatesforpregnantwomen.org) is a national nonprofit organization that advocates on behalf of all women, especially those who are most marginalized and most likely to be targeted for these punitive actions: women

of color, low-income women, and women who use drugs. NAPW uses a variety of strategies, from litigation and public education to organizing on the local and national level, to ensure that women do not lose their constitutional and human rights as a result of pregnancy or under the guise of "fetal rights," children's rights, or family protection. For more information about NAPW, see p. 815.)

ACCESSING HEALTH CARE

One of the first health care choices we make is choosing a health care provider. You can get reproductive and sexual health care from many kinds of care providers including family medicine physicians, obstetrician-gynecologists (ob-gyns), midwives, and nurse-practitioners. For information on kinds of maternity care providers, see "Choosing a Practitioner and a Place for Your Birth," p. 362.

While most insurance plans require members to choose a primary care provider to coordinate care and make referrals to specialists, obstetrician-gynecologists and nurse-midwives can usually be contacted directly without a referral and in some cases can act as your primary care provider, making necessary referrals for other health concerns. The recently adopted national health reform law will expand the number of health insurance plans that must allow direct access to an ob-gyn without a referral.

Good health care providers will work to create a relationship with you based on mutual trust and respect. They will provide accurate, unbiased information and address your questions and concerns. They will ask detailed questions about your health history and sexual history using safe, nonjudgmental language. To find a good health care provider, learn as much as you can about the practitioners in your area by

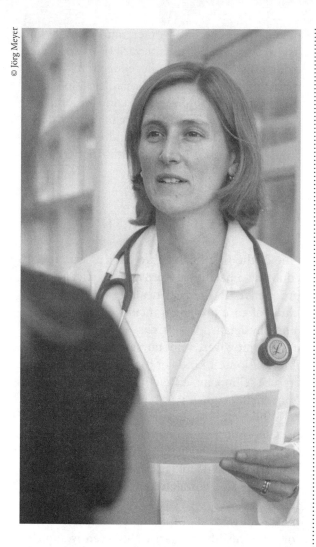

asking health care providers you respect whom they recommend. Also talk to friends and check consumer reviews and feedback online.

CHOOSING A HEALTH CARE PROVIDER

Here are some questions to consider when choosing a health care provider:

- If you have insurance coverage, does it cover the provider you are considering?

- What is his or her training and experience? Is she or he board certified in her/his specialty?
- Is the provider licensed in your state? State licensure databases will often provide the educational background of, any specialty certifications of, and any disciplinary actions taken against the provider.
- Is the provider female or male, and is that important to you?
- Is she or he familiar with any special health problems or concerns you have?
- Does the provider participate in a database that tracks and reports clinical outcomes or is she or he willing to discuss these data?
- How long will you have to wait for an appointment? Are evening or weekend appointments available for routine visits? How easy is it get to get an appointment for an urgent medical visit?
- If you have an urgent medical need and your chosen provider is not available, who else in the practice would see you, and are you comfortable with your provider's colleagues?
- How long is a typical appointment slot? Will the provider take the time to explain health issues to you?
- Is the provider willing to communicate with you on the phone or through email?
- What is the provider's relationship with industry? (For example, is a conflict of interest policy in place with regard to the pharmaceutical industry?)
- Is the provider attentive to needs related to your culture, race, gender identity, age, disability, or sexual orientation?
- Does she or he speak your language or provide a medical interpreter?
- Will she or he support your use of complementary, alternative, and traditional medicine?
- Is the office accessible for your disability or size?
- Is the office in a convenient location?

A Female or Male Provider?

Many of us hope, and often believe, that female physicians will be different from their male colleagues—perhaps by listening better and being more understanding or caring. Unfortunately, female physicians emerge from the same stressful and sometimes dehumanizing medical training process that affects all doctors. Once in practice, female physicians face the same financial and time constraints as male physicians and thus may disappoint us in similar ways.

At the medical plan I belong to, I chose one of the two women doctors because I believed a woman would be less likely to push drugs and surgery and would look with me first for the less invasive nonmedical alternatives. In the first visit, she suggested not only thyroid medication but also a routine X-ray; she talked crisply, rapidly, coolly, with many complicated medical terms. I felt as if I were sitting across from a medical school curriculum.

Although you cannot assume that a female physician will be better than a male physician, there may be some relevant differences. Studies have found that female physicians spend more of the visit on preventive care and counseling than male physicians and patients of female physicians report higher satisfaction with their care.[11] In addition, women who go to female doctors are more likely to be up-to-date on screening tests including Paps.[12]

At present, most nurse-practitioners and nearly all midwives are women. While they often learn in a hierarchical learning model similar to that for physicians and face some of the same constraints as physicians, their training often emphasizes woman-centered and holistic care, and they sometimes have more flexibility and time to provide care. Typically nurse-practitioner and midwifery education places a strong emphasis on prevention and wellness as well as the assessment of common health problems.

In the end, the sex of your provider matters less than his or her style, approach to health care, and ability to provide you with the kind of care and communication you need. Take the time to interview and ask your provider about her or his attitudes toward care and common practices. Don't be afraid to change providers if you do not feel that you have a good match.

THE IMBALANCE OF POWER IN THE DOCTOR/PATIENT RELATIONSHIP

The doctor-patient relationship is often one of inequality, an exaggeration of the power imbalances inherent in many client-professional relationships in our society. While some doctors take a more participatory and egalitarian approach to care, many still work within a paternalistic mind-set and make assumptions about patients who don't "cooperate" easily. If we forget to mention a detail about a prior symptom or diagnosis, we are "bad historians." If we choose not to take a drug prescribed or can't afford to finish a treatment plan we are "noncompliant." If we seek a second opinion, do our own research or suggest a test, diagnosis, or treatment, we are "difficult patients." And if the doctor cannot figure out the cause of the condition, it must be "all in our heads."

When these attitudes exist, you may feel intimidated and fail to ask questions or request a clearer explanation. However, it is important that you have the opportunity to both understand and question your own care.

If necessary, bring along an advocate who can ensure your questions are answered and help assess your care and treatment (see "Making the Most of Your Health Care Visit," p. 676).

If you consistently feel that your concerns aren't heard or your participation in your own

COMPLEMENTARY AND ALTERNATIVE THERAPIES

Women have long used massage, herbal medicine, and other methods to heal ourselves, soothe members of our families, assist birth, and tend the ill. Many women continue to use traditional healing methods, which range from ginger tea for a cold to entire medical systems—such as traditional Chinese medicine and ayurvedic medicine—that have their own diagnostic techniques and treatments. These healing methods are diverse, yet most are rooted in the following principles:

- Health is not merely the absence of disease but a state of well-being in which the body, mind, and spirit are balanced.
- Disease and treatment affect the whole body, not just one part.
- Human energy flow (variously called chi or qi, prana, life force, or vital energy) can be affected by disease or treatment.
- Each person has a great capacity for self-healing.

In North America, these diverse health care practices are sometimes called complementary and alternative medicine, often referred to as CAM. CAM health practices include both practitioner-administered therapies such as acupuncture, chiropractic, and massage, and self-care practices such as meditation and visualization. Integrative medicine is the practice of combining both Western and CAM approaches to care.

People may explore alternative therapies because they seem safer than conventional medical or surgical approaches, appeal to the desire to use natural methods to manage health, align with cultural values, or counteract side effects of other treatments.

Until recently, there was little scientific evidence about the safety and effectiveness of many complementary health practices. In recent years this has begun to change, and agencies such as the U.S. National Institutes of Health's National Center for Complementary and Alternative Medicine (nccam.nih.gov) now provide research-based information on treatments such as acupuncture, yoga, herbs, and dietary supplements. As more and better research is done, we will have a clearer idea of what complementary therapies are helpful and safe to use. In the meantime, it is important to remember that a therapy described as "natural" or "herbal" is not necessarily safe or effective, and may have adverse effects or interactions with medications or other treatments.

Complementary health practitioners work in a range of settings, including clinics, private offices, health spas, and homes. To find a practitioner, ask for referrals from a health care provider, friends, or family, or seek local referrals from national organizations.

Alternative modes of healing may seem to promise a richer way of practicing health care than the standard drugs and surgery used in conventional Western medicine. However, holistic practices and practitioners can have some of the same weaknesses, as well as additional problems of their own.

The tips below can help you choose and evaluate a provider or treatment.

Check your state department of health website for licensure information: Many states require licenses for practitioners of acupuncture, chiropractic, massage, reflexology, or other therapies. While a license does not guarantee safety or efficacy, it is a good first step in evaluating a provider.

Competence matters: National certification exams exist for some complementary therapies; however, no piece of paper guarantees a person's ability to heal (nor does the lack of a recognized credential mean that a person isn't skillful or knowledgeable). Expect practitioners to be able to describe their training and experience in relation to the treatment they provide and ask about their experience in cases similar to yours. Be wary of practitioners who have no indicators of their qualifications.

Seek practitioners who listen carefully and are willing to try different approaches and teach you skills to improve your health. Ask for personal referrals, interview several practitioners, and trust your intuition. If you are not comfortable with a practitioner for any reason, or a practitioner is willing to consider only one specific kind of treatment, go to someone else.

Look for practitioners who are willing to be part of a team of providers: Avoid those who insist that any other therapy will undermine treatment.

Clarify how many appointments you will need: Be wary of providers who try to get you to commit to a long series of treatments before you begin.

If a treatment isn't helping after a reasonable time, do not continue it: Most CAM methods should lead to benefits within a month or two, or after three or four treatments.

Avoid practitioners who ask you to purchase expensive equipment or remedies, especially if they sell these from their office.

Beware of miracle cures: Don't trust sweeping claims about curing cancer, AIDS, or other serious diseases.

Ask about the cost of treatment: If you have health insurance, check to see whether the treatment is covered. If you are unable to pay the full rate, ask the provider if she or he will accept a reduced payment.

Beware of alternative diagnostics: This includes iridology (which claims to diagnose disease through examination of the iris), muscle testing, and machines that purport to detect energy fields. Alternative laboratory tests are almost always a waste of money and generally are not regulated by the federal government.

Explore the politics of the method you want to use: Ask yourself, "Who profits from this mode of healing?" Complementary and alternative healers can also be profiteers or use shamanic, Native American, and other traditional practices in exploitive ways, for example to add a veneer of mysticism to what they do.

Avoid practitioners who seem to blame you for your health problems: Trust-health care isn't respected, find a new health care provider, if possible. If the problem is really significant, you may want to submit a formal complaint (see "Voicing Our Complaints," p. 685).

MAKING THE MOST OF YOUR HEALTH CARE VISIT

Find out how the practice or clinic works: Know the hours of operation, evening and weekend coverage, what to do in an emergency, and numbers to call for appointments, prescriptions, and referrals. Ask what hospitals the practice uses and who will care for you if you need to be in the hospital.

Bring someone you trust with you: It is often helpful to have another pair of eyes and ears to "record" what happens at appointments. (See "Patient Advocates," p. 677). If you do not have a friend or relative to accompany you, ask your doctor if you can record the visit so that you can review important conversations and instructions when these are needed.

Track your health information, and bring it with you to visits: Practitioners often do not recall the details of your specific case, so they will benefit from this important information about your previous experience. Keeping a journal of symptoms and other issues related to your condition can help your provider better understand what you are experiencing (see "Tracking Your Own Health" p. 655). If possible, research relevant issues before your visit, and discuss your findings with your health care provider.

List all your questions and make sure that they are addressed: Take into account that providers typically spend only relatively short amounts of time with each patient, so it helps to be prepared before your visit.

Bring any medicines, herbal preparations, or over-the-counter preparations you are taking to avoid receiving duplicate medications or medications that interact poorly: If needed, ask your provider for detailed instructions for taking new medications or making changes in your existing medications.

Ask your provider for an explanation of anything you do not understand: If necessary, ask for images or diagrams that explain your condition or materials in your language or at your literacy level. Ask for a written statement of the treatment plan in order to monitor your care or in case you choose to seek a second opinion later. When no medical emergency exists, take as much time as you need to think about any decisions.

Confirm how the practice uses email or digital communication tools: Can you submit questions about treatment or routine matters such as scheduling and prescription renewal via email or online? Can you sign up to get a text message reminding you when your next appointment is?

If you need more time for the visit, ask for another appointment: You can also ask to schedule longer visits, though this is not always possible.

If you have tests, make sure you get test results, an explanation of any abnormal findings, and recommendations for follow-up. Request a printed or electronic copy of the results, since it may show additional helpful information. Find out exactly when you can expect the results and who will contact you. If notification occurs only when there is a problem with the results, ask to be contacted regardless.

PATIENT ADVOCATES

The more complicated your symptoms or diagnosis, the more you will want to bring someone to your health care appointments who can help you keep track of the details and advocate on your behalf.

Doctors, nurses, and other health care professionals are required, according to the federal law called the Health Insurance Portability and Accountability Act of 1996 (HIPAA), to keep your information private. You'll want to have a conversation with your advocate, regardless of whether that person is related to you, about keeping your information private, too. You'll also want to make sure her or his presence doesn't prevent you from bringing up important but sensitive topics such as domestic abuse or sexual history. Choose someone whose presence does not prevent you from being completely honest about these issues, or ask your advocate to leave the room for part of your visit when you discuss those issues with your provider.

Before your visit, discuss with your advocate what you want and expect to happen. Make sure you both understand the kinds of diag-

RIGHTS REGARDING MEDICAL RECORDS

You have a legal right to view, obtain, or even correct your hospital and medical records. Since 2003, this right has been backed by federal law, the Health Insurance Portability and Accountability Act (HIPAA) legislation and regulations. A written statement of your rights is provided when you see a health care provider or are admitted to the hospital. These rights include all hospital and individual provider records about you, except, in some cases, psychotherapy notes.

The time frame for making records available to you varies by state, and providers are allowed to charge per printed page. If you request your records at each appointment, test, or hospital visit, those charges may be waived, since their purpose is to cover the cost of records re-

trieval. If you obtain health care through the Department of Veterans Affairs (VA) you can download certain health data directly from the VA website (myhealth.va .gov) by clicking the "download my data" blue button, a feature that Medicare beneficiaries may soon be able to access as well.

Regulations and standards affecting patient access to medical records are very likely to change as the federal government offers incentives for hospitals and health care providers to increase their use of electronic medical records. A robust advocacy movement is also afoot to remove barriers to patient medical record access. For up-to-date information about your rights under HIPAA and state laws, visit the Center on Medical Record Rights and Privacy at Georgetown University (medicalrecordrights.georgetown .edu).

nostic tests, treatments, or surgical procedures proposed. Ask your advocate to keep a record of events that occur. Anticipate situations that may make you feel powerless or inadequately informed and make a list of your questions. No good hospital (or individual provider) should object to patients having an advocate, and many actively encourage it.

Large hospitals and health plans may employ patient advocates or representatives who can help cut through red tape. Yet because they represent the hospital, these people may not be free to represent your interests if they conflict with the interests of the hospital or provider. Even so, many patient advocates do an excellent job.

RECOGNIZING AND OVERCOMING BARRIERS TO GETTING GOOD HEALTH CARE

FINANCIAL BARRIERS

The high cost of health care creates particular hardships for women because, on average, women use health care services, especially reproductive health care services, more than men. We typically have more provider visits, fill more prescriptions, purchase more over-the-counter medications, and make greater use of complementary and alternative medicine. As a result, even those of us who have health care insurance often find that we cannot afford the health care that we need.

The up-front cost of insurance premiums represents only one part of our actual health care expenses. In order to use our health care insurance, we typically have to pay a co-pay (a fixed sum per visit, procedure, or medication) or coinsurance (a percentage of the visit or procedure). In addition, many insurance plans require an annual deductible of anywhere from several hundreds to several thousands paid out-of-

pocket before the insurance kicks in—making insurance essentially unusable for people who lack sufficient funds to cover this initial payout. Annual deductibles are particularly problematic for pregnant women, who are likely to carry a pregnancy over two different years and thus would need to reach the annual deductible twice before insurance pays for their maternity care.

These considerations make choosing an insurance policy a complicated task even when competing plans are clearly presented. It's tempting to choose what looks to be a less expensive insurance plan (that is, a plan with lower up-front premiums). However, those plans often have higher co-pays, coinsurance, and annual deductibles that can quickly add up to more money than the difference between a lower and a higher premium. As a result, those of us who opt for what looks to be a cheaper plan may find that we end up actually spending more on our health care.

It's impossible to predict future medical needs, so choosing an insurance plan is always a matter of guesswork. However, try to make the best possible guess by drawing up a comprehensive list of all of the health care services and products that you are likely to use and then checking whether they are completely or partially covered on a variety of lower-premium and higher-premium plans. This information should be available through your employer's human resources department and through the state insurance exchanges. It is particularly important to find out whether any medication you use regularly is covered, whether alternative and complementary methods you use are covered (fully, partially, or not at all), and whether you need to go through your primary care provider (which means a co-pay or coinsurance) in order to see a specialist. Once you have made your list—being sure to add in one or two unexpected health problems—you can try to calculate how much you actually would have to pay out-of-pocket on various plans.

Here are some additional ways to control the cost of health care.

Finding Low-Cost Options

Negotiate for the lowest price: Hospitals and health care providers (including labs) often quote higher fees to uninsured patients than the insurance companies have negotiated. You can call the billing department of the institution or provider and ask what its best rate is. Then (in a separate conversation) tell the person billing you that you are willing to pay only that rate. Or, offer cash, on the spot, for an amount that is half what the billing cost is.

Don't be afraid to ask if there are less expensive options available: Lower-cost treatments or tests are often just as effective as, and sometimes more effective than, the option your care provider recommends.

Go to a Planned Parenthood clinic: Planned Parenthood offers low-cost or free reproductive health care to uninsured women in many communities throughout the United States. Services include family planning, breast and cervical cancer screening, mammograms, and sexually transmitted infection testing, counseling, and treatment. To find a Planned Parenthood clinic near you, go to plannedparenthood.org and enter your zip code under "Find a Health Center."

Go to a community health center (CHC): There are CHCs in all fifty states. These centers are federally funded and provide care to all individuals; fees are set on a sliding-scale basis. Search for the nearest center at the Health Resources and Services Administration website (findahealth center.hrsa.gov). CHCs do not provide abortion care, owing to federal funding restrictions. Other low-cost options may include city/county public health clinics, community clinics, or clinics provided through medical, nursing, or dental schools.

Consult your care provider by phone or email: You may be able to get prescription refills, orders for lab tests, or referrals to specialists without having a visit with your primary care provider.

Find out if your care provider works in more than one facility: Costs may be lower at another location.

See a nurse-practitioner, physician assistant, or nurse-midwife: In some settings, these professionals may provide the same services as a doctor but at a lower cost.

Keep copies of your test results: You may be able to avoid repeating blood and other laboratory tests if there is a record showing they have been done recently.

If you are hospitalized, ask to see a social worker: A social worker can help you navigate the system and discuss options for paying the hospital bill and the cost of follow-up care or rehabilitation.

Look into the cost of obtaining care in another country: Some people find that it is more economical to travel abroad to receive health care. Unfortunately, it may be more difficult to assess the safety of overseas health care options, and you may not have recourse (e.g., the ability to sue or file a formal complaint) if you are harmed as a result of services you receive in another country.

Extending Medicaid Coverage

Medicaid is a government program that provides health insurance to people with low incomes.

Eligibility for Medicaid depends primarily on your income but also on other factors, such as whether you are pregnant. There are also other special situations that may extend your Medicaid coverage.

Contact your caseworker or congressperson if you are about to lose public assistance because you have become employed: If you are receiving Medicaid or other public assistance (financial assistance from a government program) and get a job, you may no longer qualify for these benefits, but in some cases your eligibility can be extended.

If you are pregnant, find out if you qualify for Medicaid at a higher income level than if you weren't pregnant: The Kaiser Family Foundation offers a table showing eligibility by state: statehealthfacts.org/comparemapreport.jsp?rep=43&cat=17.

If you need family planning services, find out if your state has special Medicaid eligibility that will provide coverage: In many states, family planning services are available through Medicaid for women (and sometimes men) at the same income level as pregnant women. The Guttmacher Institute offers a list of family planning eligibility by state (guttmacher.org/statecenter/spibs/spib_SMFPE.pdf).

Obtaining Drugs as Cheaply as Possible

Find out if the company that makes your medication has a patient assistance program: These programs distribute a limited amount of free and discounted medication to patients who cannot afford the drugs or do not have insurance. The downside is that the application may be too complex and jargon-filled. In many communities, charitable organizations (such as Catholic Charities) employ someone to help people fill out and submit this kind of application. Hospital case or social workers may also be able to help.

Call around to pharmacies before filling your prescription: The cost to fill a prescription may vary among pharmacies, especially when you are paying out of pocket. Some pharmacies have a list of specific drugs that they provide at very low cost as a way to attract patients.

Ask your health care provider or pharmacist about economical ways to manage your medication: In some cases medicine can be ordered at a higher dose for the same cost and the pills can be cut in half to provide the desired dose. This is a much better alternative than taking partial doses or skipping days or weeks, which can be more dangerous than not taking the medication at all.

Ask your provider if a generic or over-the-counter drug may be a cheaper but equally effective alternative to a brand-name prescription drug. There's no reason to pay more, assuming the options are equally safe and effective.

Look into options for obtaining prescription drugs more cheaply. Some medications can be ordered online from other countries, such as Canada. Be aware, however, that drug regulations vary from country to country, and some websites that sell drugs are not reliable.

HEALTH CARE DISPARITIES

Access to health care is far from equal. Women of color are less likely than white women to receive regular mammograms, and they are more likely than white women to report not having had a Pap test in the past three years.[13] Black and Latina women are more likely than white women to receive no prenatal care or to receive care later in their pregnancy.[14]

Women of color are less likely to get prompt, adequate follow-up for abnormal cancer screening tests such as mammograms. This may contribute to the higher rates of death from breast cancer among black women compared with white women. Similarly, even though women of color are more likely than white women to report being in fair or poor health, they are less likely to have a regular health care provider, less likely to have health care insurance, and less likely to see a health care provider when ill.[15] (For more detailed information and discussion, see "Disparities in Women's Health," p. 761).

Low-income women are more likely to receive care from medical and nursing students and residents (physicians training in a particular area of medicine), who are learning and refining their skills. The same treatment options that may be available to women with insurance and/or higher incomes may not be discussed, and instead, more emphasis may be placed on disease management.

The recently adopted national health care reform law takes steps to increase access by offering continuing education support for providers who work in underserved communities and grants to increase retention and representation of minority faculty members and health professionals.

BIAS AGAINST SUBSTANCE ABUSERS

Women who have current drug and alcohol problems and women who have histories of such problems also sometimes experience discrimination. For example, women who are believed to be drug users may be denied pain medication during labor or in the course of painful illnesses, because of misinformation and prejudice about drug use, or experience hostile comments from medical staff members. Some women have been turned over to the police rather than offered appropriate medical care. Despite laws prohibiting discrimination, drug-using women often face extensive barriers to accessing appropriate drug treatment:[16]

I can't go into a doctor's office and say, "Look, I'm a heroin addict," to tell them everything that I need to tell them about what I've done to my body and health. I don't think there is a doctor in this city that I can go to and be comfortable with and they can be comfortable with me and treat me totally equal as anybody else, you know?[17]

Sometimes health care providers set up narcotics contracts with former or current substance abusers if they are in true pain or recovering from surgery. The contract usually requires regular check-ins and a very limited supply of the medication. Ask your doctor about such a contract so you can obtain the pain-relief or other medications you need.

LANGUAGE AND CULTURE

Many providers do not understand the beliefs and practices of each specific culture, including issues such as women's physical and sexual modesty around male health care providers. This puts some of us, especially immigrants, at a disadvantage. Even though Title VI of the Civil Rights Act of 1964 states that individuals cannot be discriminated against based on language, and every individual with limited English skills is entitled to care in her language, an interpreter may not always be available. It is helpful to request an interpreter in advance, when you make an appointment, if it is not an emergency visit. Sometimes an interpreter can be scheduled to be available by phone.

Most states offer health assessments to refugees soon after arrival, but the assessment sites vary in the type of services available and the quality of care, and time frames vary among states. Refugees are eligible for Refugee Medical Assistance, a federally funded, state-administered program with benefits similar to Medicaid, for their first eight months in the United States. Families with minor children are eligible for Medicaid. After eight months, refugees are subject to the same access limitations to health care as U.S. citizens. Finding or maintaining employment is a priority for refugees, but the employment available may not carry health benefits and may also lead to loss of eligibility for Medicaid benefits. Mental health and reproductive health services are increasingly recognized as essential to refugees, but traditionally, there has been an emphasis on screening refugees only for infectious diseases such as tuber-culosis.

DISABILITY ISSUES

Those of us with chronic illnesses and/or physical and developmental disabilities often experience barriers to receiving comprehensive health care, including lack of accessible transportation, limited income and insurance coverage, and inaccessible practitioners' offices and/or equipment such as examination tables that do not adjust. The recently adopted national health care reform law begins to address this problem by establishing standards for medical diagnostic equipment so people with disabilities can access vital preventive care.

Providers are not always knowledgeable about particular disabilities or conditions, so the responsibility is on us to provide medical information and educate them about our disability or illness and appropriate care. It is often difficult to be a teacher while also being an advocate for ourselves at a time when we need medical care. Another problem is dealing with providers who see only the disability and fail to address our reproductive and sexual health needs.

Some hospitals and health care systems have patient advocates who can provide help (see "Patient Advocates," p. 677).

To find providers who are capable and sensitive, contact a national advocacy organization for your specific disability or illness. Many keep lists of recommended providers or can direct you to a local organization for referrals. For more information and resources, check out the links section at the Center for Research on Women with Disabilities at Baylor College of Medicine (bcm.edu/crowd). There are also sections on reproductive health, sexuality, and access to health care.

HOMOPHOBIA, TRANSPHOBIA, AND HETEROSEXISM

Many lesbian, gay, bisexual, and/or transgender people experience financial, personal, and cultural barriers to getting appropriate health care.[18] Obstacles can include the following.

Lower income and lack of health insurance: According to the Lesbian Health & Research Center, lesbians generally have lower incomes than women who partner with men and are less likely to have health insurance coverage from a partner or themselves. Trans people often have a difficult time finding work and so have little income despite many expenses, especially if they are using sex hormones. Lower income and lack of health insurance make paying for screening and preventive health services (and treatment when it is necessary) more difficult. (See p. 80, "Transsexual Health Issues" for a discussion of the health insurance tangle for gender-variant people.)

Homophobic attitudes and inadequate training among health care providers: Some health care providers exhibit homophobic attitudes or have inadequate training for cultural competency in treating lesbians and bisexual women. Markers that can make us feel excluded include the intake forms, the pamphlets lining the wall, and the language used by the provider and intake staff.

Many health care providers (except for my local Planned Parenthood) have intake forms that ask marital status. I always change it to relationship status and handwrite whatever is true for me at the time. I hope they get it.

Providers may assume we have sex with men and make health care recommendations based on that assumption.

Last time a doctor asked me what birth control I was using (which, she admitted, was completely irrelevant to the reason for my visit), I said that I didn't need to use any at the moment. She wrote "not sexually active" on my form, and I left the room furious, not only at her but at myself for not challenging her.

On the flip side, some health care providers do not ask lesbians about safer sex practices, because providers assume wrongly that women who have sex with women aren't at risk for sexually transmitted infections.

Attitudes and training have improved significantly, especially in larger cities, but many health care settings continue practices that make LGBT people either less likely to seek care or less likely to be open with providers about sexual orientation, sexual practices, and health care needs. All this can affect long-term health.

I bounced around from one provider to another, looking for someone I could feel comfortable disclosing to about being sexually active with women and men, as well as being a sex worker. The reactions I encountered were very negative and judgmental. Eventually I stopped disclosing. I am happy to say that I finally found a good place to go here in New York. It is a health clinic especially for LGBTQ people. The doctors there are nonjudgmental. I have a provider now who knows all about me, and I always feel comfortable talking to her.*

The ability to be out to a health care provider can improve the quality of the care we receive. When we can be fully honest about our lives, our concerns, and our health risks and behaviors, our providers are in a better position to

---

* For more information about the Callen-Lorde Community Health Center, see callen-lorde.org.

care for us, in part because we are more comfortable asking questions, discussing sensitive information that may be critical for diagnosis of a problem, and seeking help when we need it.

For many of us, coming out to a new provider is the first order of business, so we can determine right away if she or he is a good fit for us.

Even if we are not ready to come out to a provider, it is essential that providers know our risk behaviors, so they can consider all of the information in order to properly care for us:

I practice in advance how to maintain my privacy and still get the care I need—ways of refusing to answer offensive or unnecessary inquiries and of asking direct, specific questions about what I need to know.

How can you increase your chances of finding a provider who is sensitive to your concerns? The Human Rights Campaign offers these tips.[19]

Ask for referrals: Ask friends or local LGBT centers for the names of LGBT-friendly health care providers. You can find the centers closest to you by searching the Community of LGBT Centers (lgbtcenters.org.) Also check out the Gay and Lesbian Medical Association's health care provider directory ("Find a Provider") (glma.org.)

Inquire by phone: When you call to make an appointment, ask if the practice has any LGBT patients. If you're nervous about asking, remember you don't have to give your name during that initial call.

Bring a friend: If you're uneasy about being open with your health care provider, consider asking a trusted friend to come with you.

Bring it up when you feel most comfortable: Ask your doctor for a few minutes to chat while you're still fully clothed—maybe even before you're in the exam room.

Know what to ask: Learn about the specific health care issues facing LGBT people.

You have the right to be spoken to in the way that you identify your gender, sexual orientation, and/or relationship status. Some staff members or health care providers who do not regularly work with LGBT communities may default to a heterosexual or gender-normative script (meaning they assume all women are attracted to men and, if you have a vagina, then you identify as a woman). If that happens, remind them of who you are and what issues are relevant to and appropriate for you.

Health history forms may include a space to identify a nickname or other name you prefer to be called. For those of us who are transgender, this is a good place to write in your gender and preferred pronoun. You can reiterate this as you complete questions asking about gender (which you may need to adapt/expand) and also verbally remind the receptionist that you would like the staff to address you by your identified gender and pronoun.

Gender identity is protected under privacy guidelines, so disclosing it in the process of receiving health care does not mean it will be released or shared elsewhere. Intake forms don't often have a line for sexual orientation, but you can go ahead and write it in to help keep assumptions from being made.

You also have the option not to disclose your orientation or gender identity during your exam. It is difficult for the health care staff to do their best job without all pertinent information. But do what feels right for you at the time. Remember, it's your right to get the care that you need.

For more information about particular health issues for LGBT people, see Chapter 4, "Gender Identity and Sexual Orientation."

MULTIPLE BARRIERS FOR INCARCERATED WOMEN

Women who are incarcerated face particularly difficult barriers navigating the health care system and accessing appropriate medical services. Incarcerated women typically are in poorer health than other women, even before they enter prison, and they are more likely to have experienced sexual abuse and other violence; to live with mental health challenges and with addictions; and to suffer from a variety of physical ailments including hepatitis C, arthritis, asthma, STIs, and post-traumatic stress disorder (PTSD). The complexities of PTSD, mental illness, and addiction, plus physical illnesses, make it difficult to arrange and coordinate proper care in an underfunded system.

When women are sent to prison they lose the care they may have been receiving. This means that if they were in therapy, it is interrupted, treatment protocols are stopped, diagnoses are not followed up, and relationships with health care providers are disrupted. Within the prison system, requests to see a health care provider or therapist are first made to prison guards, who function as gatekeepers to medical care.

The medical care offered in prison is limited in scope and often privatized. Because of the need to limit expenses, prison health care administrators may be reluctant to send women to see a specialist outside the prison. Pregnant women often encounter inadequate prenatal health care and a lack of nutritious food. They are often forced to give birth in front of guards or in shackles. (Only nine states explicitly prohibit the shackling of women during labor and birth and even in these states, there have been reports of shackling.) Often their babies are taken from them immediately after the birth while they themselves receive no or little postpartum care.

Upon leaving prison women need to reapply

for Medicaid and must wait for an appointment to see a health care provider. Treatment protocols that they may have received in prison are disrupted. Criminalized women both in prison and outside often find that their health complaints are not taken seriously but rather are assumed to be "drug seeking" behavior. They are labeled as "manipulative" when they try to advocate for themselves.

While there are no immediate systemic solutions to these problems, there are a number of steps women prisoners can take to try to minimize the negative impact of incarceration on health care. If you are a woman prisoner, try to:

- Keep copies of your prescriptions so that you can show them to your various medical providers inside and outside prison. While prison health care providers often will not take your word for your medication needs, they may be more willing to honor a written prescription.
- Ask for and hold on to copies of your medical records so that whoever is treating you will know about your other health issues. This is particularly important in order to avoid being given medications that have negative interactions with other conditions or medications.
- When you are approximately one month from your prison discharge date, ask to meet with a nurse, social worker, or chaplain to help you contact a health care provider on the outside so that your care will be disrupted as little as possible.
- Ask the prison health care provider if you can be given one month's supply of your medications when you are discharged from prison. This is particularly important for psychiatric medications, some of which are associated with severe withdrawal symptoms if you stop taking them.

- Remember that as a prisoner you have a right to receive medical attention. Practice being your own advocate by calmly and persistently asking to see a medical professional. There may be a prisoners' advocacy organization in your area that can help you. For more information, see "Women's Anti-prison Activism" on the Our Bodies Ourselves website, ourbodiesourselves.org.

ENFORCING OUR RIGHTS

Our rights as patients mean little if they cannot be enforced effectively. The method of enforcement we use will depend on state laws and the rights involved. Some of the most common ways to exercise and enforce our rights are listed below. You can obtain further information and possible assistance by contacting women's health groups, consumer groups, or legal services organizations (see Recommended Resources).

VOICING OUR COMPLAINTS

When we are sick or in pain, we may be reluctant to complain about our treatment out of fear of alienating our health care providers. However, many of us find that giving voice to our concerns not only improves the care we receive, but also contributes to our own sense of well-being.

It is sometimes useful to discuss your intentions with your practitioner before actually lodging any complaints against her or him, since this may provide the incentive necessary to improve the situation. This can sometimes be the basis for positive and lasting relationships between a woman and her care provider, as conscientious providers want to be told if there is a problem and want a chance to remedy or address it.

Complaints are important because they alert

health care providers to potential problems that, if corrected, can improve care for everyone. If you are unhappy with the results of a medical encounter or experience any inappropriate behavior on the part of the provider, do not hesitate to report the problem. Write down the events as soon as they occur and draft a letter that clearly states what happened and when. If friends or family members have firsthand knowledge of what happened, ask them to record their thoughts and observations right away. Make certain that all your medical records and supporting materials are together before you lodge a complaint, as your care provider may become defensive or try to manipulate the information included in your record after that point. To arrange to obtain your records or have them transferred to another provider you do not need to speak to the previous provider or justify your decision; you can simply ask the office staff to send your records. You will be asked to sign a release and sometimes there may be a small fee for copying papers.

Assess how serious your complaint is. For example, if the doctor consistently runs late and you're spending too much time in the waiting room, that's a complaint that needs to be discussed with the doctor or practice manager first. If the doctor is disrespecting you, then you do much better to politely (at first) call attention to that, ask that he or she show the proper respect, and try to improve the relationship. If you can't—find a new doctor!

On the other hand, if a health care provider is physically, emotionally, or sexually abusive or violates your privacy or safety, then a more formal complaint process should be undertaken. To make a formal complaint, you will need to know where to send it.

- If your complaint is lodged against a licensed health professional, send it to the appropriate licensing board and send a copy to the rel-

evant county and state professional societies. You can also contact a local women's health group for assistance and encouragement. Especially in the case of sexually inappropriate behavior, consider discussing your experience with a reliable lawyer or women's law group.
- To file a complaint against a state-licensed facility (hospital, nursing home, clinic, etc.), contact the appropriate licensing agency as well as the consumer protection division of the state attorney general's office.

Consider sending a copy of your complaint letter to the following people or organizations, depending on their relevance to your care: the individual provider involved; the provider who referred you; the administrator or director of the clinic, hospital, or managed care organization; the hospital's patient affairs or other patient satisfaction office; the organization that will pay for your visit or treatment, if different from the organization providing care (such as your union, insurance plan, or Medicare); the local health department; your neighborhood health council or community board; community agencies; local women's groups and women's centers.

WORKING TOWARD TRANSPARENCY

As consumers of health care services, we should be able to determine for ourselves if the treatments we are receiving are safe and effective, what our care will cost, whether our care providers are competent, and whether the settings in which we receive care adhere to best practices and reliably protect patient safety. Transparency exists when the information we need to make these determinations is easy to access and understand.

Hospitals and insurers collect and report extraordinary amounts of data about the costs, processes, and outcomes of care. For instance, hospitals track their cesarean section rates, rates of various complications of hysterectomy and other gynecological surgeries, incidence of infections, and costs of services. Unfortunately, few hospitals report these data to the public. Recent health care reform legislation has mandated even more data collection, and future widespread adoption of electronic health records will enable collection and analysis.

Increasingly, the federal government is reporting hospital quality and cost data in ways that are useful and meaningful to consumers. Medicare's online "Hospital Compare" tool (hospital compare.hhs.gov), for example, allows patients to compare some quality of care and patient sat-isfaction measures for nearby hospitals, but most of the data reported come from Medicare payments, so data pertaining to many reproductive and sexual health issues such as family planning, cancers that affect younger women, and pregnancy and birth remain inaccessible, since Medicare plays a minor role in funding these services. Until federal or state governments prioritize the public reporting of costs and outcomes of all types of health care, consumer advocates are filling in the gap by tracking down data themselves or using Freedom of Information Act requests to obtain the data, then making them available to other consumers.

Major Forces Affecting Women's Sexuality and Reproductive Health

Violence against women is pervasive in the United States and around the world. Often the violence comes from those closest to us. Almost one in every four women in the United States has been raped and/or physically assaulted by a current or former spouse, live-in partner, boyfriend, or date; young women, low-income women, women of color, immigrant and elderly women, and women with disabilities are disproportionately affected.[1] On average, more than three women are murdered by husbands or boyfriends every day in the United States.[2] Even greater numbers of women experience verbal and emotional abuse—from partners, family members, or caregivers, for example—that may inflict less immediate physical harm but nonetheless leaves lasting scars.

The World Health Organization recognizes sexual violence, intimate-partner violence, and other abuse of women and children as public health problems of epidemic proportions.[3] The United Nations has repeatedly called for the "elimination of all forms of violence against women." The International Criminal Court in The Hague has recognized rape used in war as a war crime. And in the United States and many other countries, law enforcement agencies increasingly provide specialized training for officers dealing with abuse situations. Yet violence against women is so woven into the fabric of acceptable behavior that many of us who experience violence feel that we are at fault or have no right to complain about violent treatment.

The vast majority of violence against both men and women is inflicted by men.[4] They may feel justified by strong societal messages that say rape, battering, sexual harassment, child abuse, and other forms of violence are acceptable, or at least understandable. Every day we see images of male violence against women in the news and in advertising, and in all forms of entertainment media. The prevalence of these images makes it appear that violence against women is simply an accepted fact of life.

There were eight of us girls pre-partying at a friend's house in our early twenties. I'm not sure how we got to this point in the discussion, but someone asked, "How many of us here have been a part of sexual abuse or violence?" To my surprise, seven of the eight girls raised their hands. I don't know why I was surprised, since I was one of the seven, but this moment is forever burned in my mind.

In the broadest sense, violence against women is any assault on a woman's body, physical integrity, or freedom of movement inflicted by an individual or through societal oppression. It includes physical, verbal, and emotional and also abuse, rape, sexual assault, murder by a partner or spouse, "honor" killings by a family member (for sexual activity or identity that "dishonors" the family), forced sterilization, female genital cutting, stalking, sexual coercion in the workplace, preparing women and girls for prostitution through rape and psychological manipulation, and trafficking of women and girls.

Every form of violence limits our ability to make choices about our lives. Sexual violence is particularly insidious because sexual acts are ordinarily and rightly a source of pleasure and loving human contact. Persistent cultural images linking sex with violence have caused violence itself sometimes to be seen as sexual or erotic.

Historically, violence against women and children has been hidden under a cloak of silence and tolerance. Four decades of feminist activism and the rise of a movement against domestic violence have resulted in greater awareness. The health care and justice professions are more likely to acknowledge the problem and to respond more effectively but they still have a long way to go. We must continue to be outspoken about the ongoing need to address the violence in women's lives.

UNDERSTANDING VIOLENCE AGAINST WOMEN

One man's act of violence against a woman may seem to result from individual psychological problems, or from sexual frustration, childhood abuse, unbearable life pressures, or drug or alcohol abuse. All these factors may contribute to the dynamic of violence. But these reasons, often given to explain or even justify violent actions, oversimplify a complex reality.

Violence against women is about power and coercive control exerted over another person in the context of a relationship, culture, or social and institutional system (for example, inti-

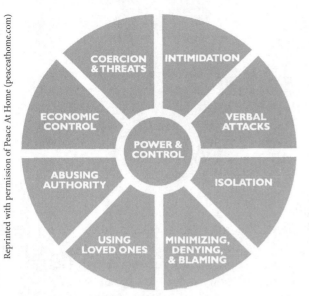

The Power and Control Wheel, developed by the Domestic Abuse Intervention Project of Duluth, Minnesota, is one model for understanding the dynamics of violence and abuse.

mate partner, parent/child, employer/employee, teacher/student). The power to exert such coercive control is rooted in the power imbalances that exist between men and women. The U.S. culture—like most other cultures in the world—assigns a superior position to men and an inferior or dependent position to women. Most people have been taught to relate to the world in terms of dominance and control, and men in particular have been taught that violence is an acceptable method of maintaining control, resolving conflicts, and expressing anger.

When rapists select their victims or bosses sexually harass employees, they act out of a wish to control or punish. When images in the media present women only in terms of bodies and sexuality, this hypersexualizing can be understood as a means of limiting and controlling women through presenting and valuing them only as sexual objects. When a batterer uses beatings or the threat of harm to coerce a partner, confine her to the home, prevent her from seeing friends and family, and/or keep her from pursuing outside work, the abuser is exerting dominance and coercive control.

Little by little, he isolated me from my friends, he convinced me to quit working, he complained about how I kept the house, he kept track of the mileage on the car to make sure that I wasn't going anywhere. Eventually, when the beatings were regular and severe, I had no one to turn to.

A young woman who was tackled by a boy at her high school describes her experience:

He pinned me down, and then sat on me in such a way that his genitalia were rubbing against my face and called me a bitch while the people watching laughed. I reported the incident about a month ago, and the school has yet to do anything about it, probably due to the fact that he is very well liked amongst staff and other students.

On the surface, it may seem that men benefit from male dominance, control, and violence. On a deeper level, men's violence against women harms men, too, not only because it harms the women and girls in their lives but also because it keeps men from having positive and loving relationships with their partners, daughters, mothers, and sisters. Growing numbers of men are recognizing this and working with women to stop the violence.

MARGINALIZED IDENTITY AND VIOLENCE AGAINST WOMEN

While violence is often targeted toward us simply because we are women, some factors put particular women at greater risk. Women of color; older women; young women; women without legal immigration status; refugees; lesbians;

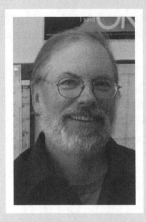

THE "WHITE RIBBON CAMPAIGN" TO ENGAGE AND MOBILIZE MEN

CRAIG NORBERG-BOHM
MEN'S INITIATIVE FOR JANE DOE INC.

In 1991, on the second anniversary of one man's massacre of fourteen women in Montreal, Canadian men created the White Ribbon Campaign to urge men everywhere to speak out against violence against women. Today, this is a worldwide campaign in sixty countries that has collected more than 5 million signatures to the pledge, "I promise to never commit, condone, or remain silent about violence against women."

While violence affects us all, men have a particular relationship to violence against women and the means to help stop it. This campaign asks men to eliminate the social values among males that support and foster violence against women. Although not all men are violent, each man has a role and responsibility to play in ending this violence. That starts by changing long-accepted and deeply rooted beliefs about male authority.

The White Ribbon campaign focuses not on individual acts of violence but rather on broader social frameworks that encourage unhealthy behaviors. It fosters a deep mutual accountability among men to one another and to women. We seek to uphold our commitments as fathers, partners, friends, colleagues, brothers, and sons of women and girls and to broaden definitions of masculinity to include men and boys who support, nurture, and foster authentic and respectful relationships.

At local White Ribbon Days around the United States and the world, this campaign celebrates nonviolence as a demonstration of our manhood and holds this value as an example for our children and other men. To find out more about White Ribbon Day Massachusetts, visit janedoe.org/whiteribbonday. For more about White Ribbon Day Worldwide, visit white ribbonday.com.

poor women; women who are transsexual, are transgender, or otherwise identify as gender nonconforming; and women with disabilities are especially likely to encounter violence. Violence against women may occur alongside other hate-based violence aimed at a particular race, nationality, or religion.

Violence against women and racism are pro-

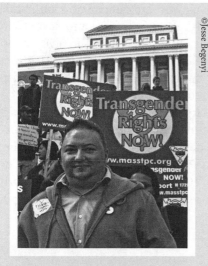

©Jesse Begenyi

HOW VIOLENCE AGAINST TRANSGENDER PEOPLE IS RELATED TO VIOLENCE AGAINST WOMEN

GUNNER SCOTT
MASSACHUSETTS TRANSGENDER POLITICAL COALITION

I was born female and now live and identify as male. For the first half of my life I lived as a woman and I was the target of men's violence through harassment, intimidation, domestic violence, and demeaning of my feminine gender expression.

Violence against trans people represents a form of "gender terrorism" whose underlying motivation is to maintain the social system in which men dominate women through the use of emotional, verbal, and physical acts of force, and in which the line between the genders must be rigidly maintained to support the social construct of a world that privileges masculinity over femininity.* In fact, antitransgender violence is a form of violence against women, because this violence targets gender whether that transgender person is a transgender woman or a transgender man. For someone who is female-to-male like myself, the message is that I will never be a "real man" and for male-to-females they will never be "real women." Many transgender people are past, present, and future women.

The above remarks are adapted from Gunner Scott's speech at the Jane Doe organization's White Ribbon Day rally in March 2010.
* This concept was adapted from the study "Conflicting Identities and TransGender Violence," by Tarynn M. Witten and A. Evan Eyler, 1999.

foundly connected. Rape, for example, has been used as a means of dominating other races and a tool of cultural genocide in wars, military and colonial occupations, and throughout the history of slavery.

Samhita Mukhopadhyay, executive editor of Feministing.com, writes that while "it is illegal to rape a black woman, since rape is officially illegal," many things "make it difficult for black women to prove they have been raped." These include stereotypes of women of color as hypersexual, the rape of enslaved African-American women over three centuries of U.S. history, and continuing racial and class inequity. No wonder, she writes, "the rape of a woman of color rarely makes the front page of any national newspaper."[5]

Women of color who call the police for protection against violence may ask themselves, "Will I be treated fairly by a police officer of another race or culture?" or "Will I be accused of betraying our 'people'?"

The man who raped me was white, and the cops here are all white. I didn't report it. I just told a few people I trusted. It helped, but I still feel scared knowing he's out there and that nobody would do anything about it.

Those of us who are gender nonconfirming also face high rates of physical and sexual violence, and may often hesitate to involve the police for fear that they will mock our identities, dismiss our complaints, and/or become violent toward us themselves.

Other marginalized women also face high levels of assault and abuse. For more information, see "Violence Against Immigrant Women," p. 699, and "Violence Against Women with Disabilities," p. 710. For more on the abuse concerns of older women, see "Elder Abuse and Neglect," p. 575.

VIOLENCE AGAINST NATIVE WOMEN

It has been a little-known fact to all but Native communities that American Indian and Alaska Native women experience by far the highest rates of rape and sexual assault in the United States. The U.S. Department of Justice estimates they are 2.5 times more likely than women in general to be sexually assaulted and nearly 1 in 3 will be raped in her lifetime. Most victims who do report their assaults describe their attackers as non-Native.

Why are sexual crimes against indigenous women so frequent? In 2007, Amnesty International released "Maze of Injustice: The Failure to Protect Indigenous Women from Sexual Violence in the USA," a groundbreaking report that outlined the various barriers to justice that Native women face.[6] The report discusses chronic underresourcing of law enforcement and health services, both in tribal lands and in surrounding areas;

confusion over jurisdiction (tribal police are not allowed to arrest non-Natives and must report crimes by non-Natives to the federal justice system, which rarely takes action); erosion of tribal authority (tribal courts are not allowed to give sentences long enough to fit violent crimes like rape and sexual assault); discrimination in law and practice; and indifference to the suffering of Native women.

In sum: "The United States government has created a complex maze of tribal, state and federal jurisdictions that often allows perpetrators to rape with impunity—and in some cases effectively creates jurisdictional vacuums that encourage assaults." Sarah Deer, a member of the Muscogee (Creek) Nation and a tribal law specialist, names history as a further factor, specifically the rape of Native women and children as a tool of colonization.[7]

Amnesty International issued a follow-up report in 2008 citing some promising initiatives but also identifying many crucial areas where change still needs to occur. In a statement to Congress urging more funding for the Bureau of Indian Affairs (BIA) and the Indian Health Service (IHS), Deer termed these epidemic levels of sexual violence "violations of our human rights on many levels," adding that they are "but one example of the significant disparities that exist for American Indian and Alaska Native peoples in accessing health services and justice in the United States." Among her recommendations is the recognition of the right of tribal authorities to prosecute crimes committed on tribal land, regardless of whether a suspect is Native or non-Native.[8]

The federal government has taken some steps to improve ties with tribal communities and increase protections for women. In 2010, President Obama signed the Tribal Law and Order Act, which strengthens tribal law enforcement authority and requires the Justice Department to disclose data on cases in Indian Country that it declines to prosecute. Tribal and BIA officers will have greater access to improved criminal databases. The bill also aims to reduce domestic violence and other crimes through enhanced programs to combat alcohol and drug abuse and to help at-risk youths. Amnesty International welcomed the legislation.

In early 2011, the Justice Department announced the formation of the Violence Against Women Federal and Tribal Prosecution Task Force. One of the task force's objectives is to produce a trial practice manual on the federal prosecution of acts of violence against women in Indian Country. It will also explore concerns raised by experts and recommend best practices in prosecution strategies involving domestic violence, sexual assault, and stalking.

Still, much work remains to be done at the tribal, state, and federal levels to reduce the rate of violence against Native women. Deer says opportunity must also be provided for Native women to speak and be heard. "Our issues," she notes, "have been invisible for too long."

"Native women have been resisting rape in North America for over five hundred years. It has been an invisible problem to the larger dominant culture because of myths and misconceptions about Native people. We are an extremely marginalized population but Native women are strong and capable. We have always been leaders in our communities."

COMMON REACTIONS TO EXPERIENCING VIOLENCE

We usually experience violence as a private crisis. Many survivors feel isolated because of a lack of support, and because of the shame that surrounds sexuality and victimization in our culture. Isolation is one of the tools used by child abusers and abusive intimate partners. This creates a difficult set of reactions that may be experienced by women who have been raped, battered, sexually harassed, abused as children, robbed violently, or hurt by other forms of violence. Such reactions are common to many people who have experienced trauma, including soldiers in wartime.

It helps some of us to recognize the commonality in our experiences. The mental health professions have classified some of the common reactions listed below as post-traumatic stress disorder (PTSD). This term is used to describe the reexperiencing of trauma and the recurrent, intrusive, and distressing recollection of the event in images, thoughts, or perceptions. It can include flashbacks, hallucinations, nightmares, dissociation (feeling of detachment from one's body or surroundings), an intense negative response to reminders of the trauma, troubled sleep, irritability or outbursts of anger, difficulty concentrating, and hypervigilance.

Some common reactions to experiencing violence include:

- Self-blame and feelings of shame and guilt
- Fear, terror, and feeling unsafe
- Anger and rage
- Anger turned inward, depression, and suicidal feelings
- Substance abuse
- Eating disorders
- Physical symptoms
- Self-harm
- Grief and loss
- Loss of control, powerlessness
- Changes in sexuality and intimacy

Although these are common reactions, they may vary greatly from one person to another. Four women speak about the impact of sexual violence on their lives:

I was in a sexually abusive relationship in my early twenties, and that has had an impact on my physical health as I have a very difficult time with internal exams. I had cervical cancer at 22, so I know how important my annual exam is but I have to summon my strength every time.

How do you come to love your own body after sexual abuse? There was a point in my life that

I hated my body. I hated myself. I had no self-confidence, and I hid under a green oversized Columbia jacket, one that could fit my father, while I was barely one hundred pounds. I would wear it in every season, summer through winter, indoors or outdoors. It was my protection. I didn't fit that saucy Latina image; I was a lost bird that wore oversized clothing.

If a person I am with gets angry or has a behavior that seems aggressive, even if they are playing around, I get very nervous and can have panic attacks. I consider myself to be a very strong person, but when something triggers me I can feel so small and insecure again, regardless of how far I have come.

In a relationship, I have trouble giving up control. Sexually, I cannot let go enough to really enjoy myself, and I am therefore content to abstain from sex.

As we move through the healing process, different reactions may increase or decrease in intensity.

REGAINING OUR LIVES

Recovery is a gradual process. Reflecting on the following points can help us move through the healing process:

The violence was not your fault. Myths about violence against women get expressed in destructive ways: "It must have been her behavior, she must have provoked him somehow, it must have been what she was wearing, where she was . . ." These things have nothing to do with responsibility for the assault. You did not ask to be hurt and violated, and you did not deserve it.

You made the best choices you could. Whatever dicisions you made before, during, and after the assault were limited by the situation.

There is no right way to feel or heal. Your reactions and healing process are connected to who you are as an individual. Culture, economic background, and prior traumatic experiences can influence the healing process in both positive and negative ways. We all take different paths to healing, and we must respect the choices each survivor makes.

Healing takes time, and there may be setbacks. Even when you have healed significantly, an event such as learning about a similar victimization or being in the environment where the violence occurred can temporarily trigger trauma

Recommended Reading: For a candid discussion among several women about sexual violence—how it has affected their relationships and what has helped them heal—see p. 132 in Chapter 5, "Relationships."

symptoms. This does not mean you have lost all the healing that has occurred. Some of us experience real doubt about whether we will ever fully feel comfortable again in our own bodies:

I don't know for sure if the feeling of guilt and disgust will all totally vanish. There are times

VIOLENCE AGAINST IMMIGRANT WOMEN

Immigrants and refugees in the United States experience high rates of violence and sexual abuse. Many immigrant women crossing the U.S.-Mexico border will make birth control provisions in advance, since sexual assault is so prevalent.[9] Some immigrant women and girls are trafficked into the United States and forced into sex work as payment for their travel expenses. Others are brought to the United States by international matchmaking agencies that market women as "mail-order brides."

Immigrant women are particularly vulnerable to sexual assault.[10] School-aged immigrant girls are almost twice as likely as their nonimmigrant peers to have experienced recurring incidents of sexual assault.[11] Further, Latina college students experience the highest incidence of attempted rape compared with white, African-American, and Asian women college students.[12] This increased vulnerability may stem from increased isolation[13] or from younger immigrant girls being actively targeted by sexual assault perpetrators who see them as legally and socially vulnerable.[14]

Women with undocumented or temporary immigration status often fear that reporting crimes will lead to deportation[15] or that disclosure about sexual activity may affect relationships in their cultural community or with family members.[16] This is especially true for women who are dependent on a spouse, parent, adult child, or employer to attain legal immigration status, or who lack access to accurate legal information.

With the passage of the Violence Against Women Act (VAWA) in 1994 and more recent legislation, access to protection and legal services has been greatly expanded. Immigrants who experience domestic violence can receive custody, child support awards, and protective orders from family courts. For example, immigrant parents whose partners are abusive generally are awarded child custody even when the abuser is a U.S. citizen. A full range of services is available, including shelters, transitional housing programs, and other services necessary to protect the health and safety of women and children. Some community and migrant health clinics provide health care regardless of immigration status.

Despite these legal remedies, immigrant women often encounter a system that is not knowledgeable about their legal rights, is insensitive to their needs, and, in the worst cases, is discriminatory. Few advocates, attorneys, and justice system personnel understand the lethal danger of immigration-related abuse.[17] For example, threats of deportation against an immigrant spouse or intimate partner almost always exist when physical or sexual abuse is also present.[18] Immigration-related abuse in relationships that do not yet include physical or sexual abuse can be a predictor of future violence.[19]

To locate an advocate or lawyer with expertise in immigrant victims' issues, consult the state-by-state directory provided by Legal Momentum, iwp .legalmomentum.org/reference/service -providers-directory. The Immigrant Women Program at Legal Momentum also offers technical assistance to legal professionals. Information is also available at the National Women's Health Information Center (womenshealth.gov/ violence).

when I can't stand myself, when anxiety takes over, but these feelings have been lessening as the years have passed.

You deserve support. Connecting with people who believe you and who can provide support and comfort can help you heal.

Rape crisis centers and domestic violence organizations are available and often will help without regard to immigration status. A family member, friend, clergy member, or counselor may also be able to help, particularly if she or he has a real understanding of the dynamics of violence. For many, connecting with survivors online is a huge help. You may decide to try other kinds of healing based on art, music, writing, physical activity, or meditation.

RAPE

Rape, one of the most common forms of sexual assault, is defined slightly differently in each state. Most state laws define rape as penetration with the use of force and without the person's consent.* Penetration in the vagina, anus, or

* The term statutory rape is a legal term that describes sexual activity where one participant is below the age required to legally consent to sex. In most states, the age of consent for sex is between sixteen and eighteen. Even if a child or teen says yes to having sex, the law considers the act to be rape.

mouth can be committed with a body part or instruments such as bottles or sticks.

The National Violence Against Women Survey reported that almost 18 percent of women said they have experienced a completed or attempted rape at some point in their lifetime, and most of these women were raped by someone they knew.[20] Rape can be committed against us at any age, but girls and young women are at particular risk. In this same survey, which interviewed only women over eighteen, almost 22 percent reported that they were younger than age twelve when they were raped, and over half were under age eighteen.[21]

During rape, as in any sexual assault, survival is the primary instinct, and we protect ourselves as best we can. Some women choose to fight back; others do not. Choosing not to fight back is also a survival strategy.

Women are often blamed for rape and attempted rape. The media, and even family and friends, may look for what we did to encourage it.

Because we live in a culture that blames women for sexual violence and downplays the actions of perpetrators, and because so few of us get comprehensive sex education that would teach us about rape, we may not realize that we have been sexually assaulted until sometime after the incident(s).

No one had a frank discussion with me about how abuse happens. I had no idea what to do when I found myself in an abusive situation and could not even identify what was happening as abusive because I foolishly believed that you can only be abused if you are weak or stupid, and I saw myself as intelligent and strong.

This does not mean that the assault was not real, but simply that cultural messages are difficult to unlearn.

" 'Rape' is only four letters, one small syllable," writes Latoya Peterson, a hip-hop feminist

SEXUAL ASSAULT

Sexual assault is any kind of sexual activity committed against another person without that person's consent—for example, vaginal, oral, or anal penetration, inappropriate touching, forced kissing, child sexual abuse, sexual harassment, or exhibitionism. Force or threat of force may be used to gain the person's compliance, but this is not always the case. What is legally considered sexual assault varies by the laws that are in effect where the assault takes place. Because rape is one of the most common forms of sexual assault, many people use the terms rape and sexual assault interchangeably.

and editor of Racialicious (racialicious.com), "and yet it is one of the hardest words to coax from your lips when you need it most."[22]

Having been taught as teens that rape involved attack by a stranger, she and her friends experienced many assaults that they did not recognize as sexual assault: "Being pressured into losing your virginity in a swimming pool pump room to keep your older boyfriend happy; waking up in the night to find a trusted family friend in bed with you; having your mother's boyfriend ask you for sexual favors; feeling the same group of boys grope you between classes, day after day after day." Peterson and her friends told no adults about these assaults. "After all, who could we tell? This wasn't rape—it didn't fit the definitions. This was not-rape. We should have known better."[23]

One woman who was repeatedly assaulted by her long-term boyfriend before she finally ended the relationship experienced a similar sense of disconnect:

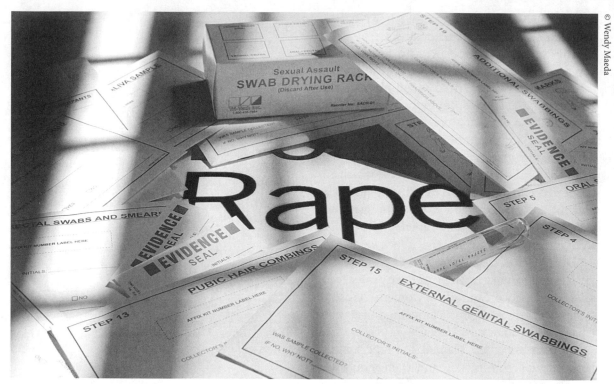

Rape kit, courtesy of the Boston Area Rape Crisis Center

At that time I knew that rape and physical assault were inexcusable acts of violence generally committed against women. I just didn't realize that what was being done to me was rape. For that reason, it took me years to realize why I felt so traumatized.[24]

When rape happens in a long-term relationship, it is a form of domestic abuse (see "Intimate Partner Violence," p. 709), and support can be particularly difficult to find.

CAMPUS RAPE

Rape is the most common violent crime on college campuses today.[25] The National Institute of Justice estimates there are an estimated 35 rapes per 1,000 female college students per year,[26] yet only 5 percent of the attempted or completed rapes are ever reported to law enforcement officials.[27]

Colleges and universities are required by federal law (the 1990 Clery Act) to have a policy in place that addresses rape and sexual assault on campus. This policy must include a disciplinary procedure against the perpetrator that is separate from what happens if the crime is reported to the police.[28]

Students who choose to report a rape or sexual assault to campus police personnel or a campus official do not have to decide at that moment whether to file a criminal complaint.

Many college administrations underreport or play down sexual assault incidents so as not to harm the school's reputation or finances. If the school's sexual assault counselors are administrators rather than service providers for sexual assault survivors, their priority may be the interests of the school, not access to justice. If you feel your college is not responding to your concerns, or that you are being dismissed, contact one of the organizations listed above.

Most of the rapes that happen on campuses occur between people who know each other. Schools are required to let students change dormitories and to grant a stay-away order against the attacker.

One college student who was raped after drinking at a party eventually decided that she wanted to confront the rapist. Because he was a fellow student, she knew how to contact him:

I saw a counselor a few months later and finally after seven months of not going out, had a mutual friend help me get my rapist into the counselor's office for a session. I confronted him and told him how I felt about what happened, the results of what he did (nightmares, sexual fear in certain positions), and that next time he wanted to have sex with a drunk person, to just get her a cup of water and tuck her into bed instead, waiting until she was sober to make advances.

"AN ACTIVE YES": REFLECTIONS ON RAPE AND CONSENT

In the book *Yes Means Yes!* contributors write about "visions of female sexual power and a world without rape." Below are excerpts from two essays.

Let's be clear. By "rape," I mean a sexual encounter without consent. Consent is saying yes. Yes, YES! "No" is useful, undoubtedly, but it is at best incomplete. How can we hope to provide the tools for ending rape without simultaneously providing the tools for positive sexuality?
　—Lee Jacobs Riggs, "A Love Letter from an Anti-Rape Activist to Her Feminist Sex Toy Store"

By making absolutely sure your partner wants to be involved in what you're doing sexually, you are not only on the right side of the law but are going to have a hotter time in bed.

Consent is a basic part of the sexual equation. If there's any uncertainty, or if you find that you're using some power to coax someone into sex when they clearly aren't that into it, you need to rethink what you're doing and why you're doing it.

The burden is not on the woman to say no, but on the person pursuing a sexual act to get an active yes.
　—Rachel Kramer Bussel, "Beyond Yes or No: Consent as Sexual Process"

WAS I RAPED?

I did not physically resist. Is that rape?

Just because you didn't resist physically doesn't mean it wasn't rape. In fact, many victims make the good judgment that physical resistance would cause the attacker to become more violent.

I knew the person. Is that rape?

Rape can occur when the offender and the victim have a preexisting relationship (sometimes called "date rape" or "acquaintance rape"), or even when the offender is the victim's spouse. It does not matter whether the other person is an ex-boyfriend or a complete stranger, and it doesn't matter if you've had sex in the past. If it is nonconsensual this time, it is rape.

Adapted from material developed by the Rape, Abuse & Incest National Network (RAINN). Special thanks to RAINN for permission.

I don't remember the assault. Was I raped?

Just because you don't remember being assaulted doesn't necessarily mean it didn't happen and that it wasn't rape. Memory loss can result from excessive alcohol consumption or the ingestion of GHB or other so-called rape drugs. That said, without clear memories or physical evidence, it may not be possible to pursue prosecution. Talk to your local crisis center or local police for guidance.

We were all drinking. Was I raped?

Alcohol and drugs are not an excuse—or an alibi. The key question is still: Did you consent? Regardless of whether you were drunk or sober, if the sex is nonconsensual, it is rape. If you were so drunk or drugged that you passed out and were unable to consent, it was rape. Both people must be conscious and willing participants.

"GRAY RAPE"

Anti-rape activists have worked for years to make date (or acquaintance) rape understood as the crime that it is. Then in 2007, a *Cosmopolitan* article by Laura Sessions Stepp, "A New Kind of Date Rape," stirred the waters by asserting that "gray rape" "falls somewhere between consent and denial" and happens owing to "casual sex, hookups, missed signals, alcohol."[29] By implying that certain rapes happen because of miscommunication or because of what a woman does, the idea of gray rape influenced many people and gave victim blamers fresh fodder. The term gray rape masks the reality that any nonconsensual sexual activity is sexual violence, period. It makes it easier for us to blame ourselves (and for others to blame us) for all but the most obvious sexual assault. Gray rape is really date or acquaintance rape with a misleading name.

Sometimes we don't want to think of unwanted sexual activity as rape, because we don't want to see ourselves as victims. Yet by not seeing nonconsensual sex for what it is—sexual assault—we risk feeling the effects for a long time, and we also risk not knowing what wanted, consensual sex can feel like.

SEXUAL ASSAULT BY A WOMAN

Although the majority of rapes are committed by men, women do rape. Rape by a woman can happen to any woman, regardless of her sexual orientation. Because of widespread ignorance and denial surrounding sexual assault of women by women, a woman may feel that no one will believe her if she reports what happened.

I kept it to myself because it was an embarrassing thing: I was bigger than she was. When people hear about rape, they think of a man raping a woman. It's hard to envision one woman raping another.

One woman lived in an off-campus group house where friends of friends passing through town often stayed over:

I set up the sofa bed for [my housemate's guests] and retired to my own bed in another room. I

Recommended Resources: Woman-on-Woman Assault

National Coalition of Anti-Violence Programs: avp.org/ncavp.htm
The NCAVP, a program of the New York City Anti-Violence Project (AVP), is a coalition of more than forty LGBT victim advocacy and documentation programs. The AVP hotline is available twenty-four hours a day in both English and Spanish and provides emotional and practical support to victims of violence (212-714-1141).
The Network/La Red: thenetworklared.org
The Network/La Red offers confidential support, information, and referrals in English and Spanish to LGBT partner abuse survivors (617-742-4911).

---

awoke to find one of the girls on top of me having sex, my body responding and feeling horrified, violated, betrayed by my own body and knowing I would be the only person in the world who would see this as I experienced it, rape.

Fear of not being believed—and, for those of us who are lesbian or bi and/or trans, experiences of homophobia and transphobia—may make many of us reluctant to call a crisis line, go to an emergency room, call the police, or tell our friends. If you are not lesbian or bisexual, you may fear that people will assume you are. Everyone deserves respectful assistance. Woman-to-woman sexual assault must be acknowledged so that all women can get the support and assistance they deserve and need.

MEDICAL CONSIDERATIONS REGARDING RAPE

If you have been raped, it is critical to obtain medical attention as soon as possible, even if you have no obvious injuries. It is understandable to want to take a shower and try to forget what happened, but bathing may wash away evidence that could be crucial if charges are filed (see sidebar on rape kits, p. 706). Even if you do not think you want to go to the police right now it is important to gather evidence in case you change your mind. Note that statutes of limitations—laws that set the maximum amount of time that can pass after a crime is committed before legal action is taken—vary by state; check the Rape, Abuse & Incest National Network (rainn.org) for specifics in your state. Since rape perpetrators seldom rape only once, your evidence may also provide critical information that can help others.

Hospital Exam

A friend or advocate can help you through the step-by-step examination process. Trained rape

RAPE KITS AND THE GOVERNMENT BACKLOG

A rape kit (also known as a sexual assault evidence collection kit, or SAFE kit) is designed specifically for collecting physical evidence of sexual assault. A specially trained health care provider collects and stores in sterile envelopes anything the rapist might have left on or in a woman's body—including hairs, blood, and semen—as well as photographs of bruises, scratches, and injuries. The collection process can take about four hours and can be done only with consent. This medical evidence will be made available to police or others only with your written permission. DNA testing of the materials in the kit can provide forensic evidence to support the prosecution in a case against the rape suspect, if legal action is pursued.

The DNA testing is usually performed by a local law enforcement agency and can cost the agency up to $1,000. Owing to lack of funds and, in some cases, not taking sexual assault seriously enough, many municipalities have a large backlog of untested rape kits. Many choose to test only those kits for which there is an identified suspect as well as a promising legal case. An estimated 180,000 rape kits a year remain untested, leaving on the shelves potential evidence that could prove a woman's claims, identify an attacker, or exonerate a suspect.

The backlog in rape kit testing is a serious public health and safety issue. The long delay creates extra stress for sexual assault survivors, adding to feelings of isolation, helplessness, and abandonment. Advocates have testified repeatedly before Congress, pressing for legislation that would require quicker testing and provide more funds. (The federal government helps cities and states foot the bill through grants to local law enforcement agencies.) New York City has achieved dramatic success in eliminating rape kit backlog. It can be done.[31]

---

crisis advocates are available through the organizations listed in the resources box on p. 703.

Clothing you wore during an assault may have evidence on it, so bring it with you if you changed before going to the hospital, or ask a friend to bring a change of clothing to the hospital so you can leave your clothes there if needed.

If possible, request a trained sexual assault nurse examiner in the emergency room. Some hospitals have specialized programs staffed by nurses or doctors who have received extensive training in the medical, legal, and emotional issues associated with sexual assault.[30] The programs are designed to provide sensitive medical exams and collect the best evidence possible for prosecution. Under the Violence Against Women Reauthorization Act of 2005, there is no charge for a rape exam; the physical samples and information gathered are considered criminal evidence.

Rape can cause physical injuries to any part of the body. You should request a thorough examination that includes and/or results in the following.

A verbal history of the sexual assault and related medical concerns: You will be asked to give a detailed description of the assault, which will be written down. Although it may be difficult to talk about these details, it is important for the medical provider to know where to check for injuries and what evidence to document for possible prosecution. Do not answer irrelevant questions about your sexual history, past drug use, or mental health counseling; should you go to trial, the perpetrator's defense might try to gain access to your records.

A pelvic or rectal exam: You will have a pelvic exam if you were raped vaginally and a rectal exam if you were raped anally. (For more information on these exams see Chapter 2, "Intro to Sexual Health.") You or your advocate should check the clinician's written record for accuracy and objectivity as soon as possible after the exam. Try to do this while the clinician is still present.

Checking for external injuries: The practitioner will examine and treat you for any external injuries and may photograph bruises or other marks to document the assault. Take pictures of any bruises that emerge after the exam and call the examiner so the information can be added to your record.

Prevention of sexually transmitted infections (STIs): You should be offered antibiotic injections as a preventive measure against STIs that are treatable by antibiotics. Medications are available to decrease the risk of some other STIs, including HIV. (For more information, see "Decreasing Risk *After* Exposure," p. 286.) If you are offered testing for HIV, be aware that immediately after the assault is too soon for HIV antibodies to show up. Also, the test results could become part of your medical and legal record. Because some STIs are not detectable until six weeks have passed, you should get tested again for STIs six weeks after the rape.

Prevention of pregnancy: If it is possible that you will become pregnant as a result of the rape, the practitioner may offer you emergency contraception (EC), sometimes called "the morning-after pill." Catholic hospitals may not offer EC. If you are seventeen or older, you can buy emergency contraception at pharmacies without a prescription. (For more information, see "Emergency Contraception," p. 251.) A pregnancy resulting from rape cannot be detected until several weeks later.

Follow-up exam: Although you may feel physically recovered shortly after the rape, a follow-up visit that includes tests and treatment for STIs and a pregnancy test, if indicated, is an important part of taking care of yourself.

WHAT TO DO IF SOMEONE YOU CARE ABOUT HAS BEEN SEXUALLY ASSAULTED

If a friend or family member has been sexually assaulted, you might not know what to say. Just being there and listening is helpful. If she feels ashamed or guilty, reassure her that the rape was not her fault and that her feelings are normal. Even if you feel you might have reacted differently, remember that her reactions are uniquely hers. Help her to think about what changes, if any, she would like to make that will help her feel safer, whether related to her physical surroundings or her interactions with people at home or at work. Resist pressuring her to do things she is not yet ready to do. When in doubt about what to do or say, ask what she wants or needs from you. For more ideas on how you can be supportive, see "What to Do If Someone You Care About Has Been Raped" at ourbodies ourselves.org.

LEGAL CONSIDERATIONS REGARDING RAPE

Although improvements have been made in the legal system, prosecution of a rapist can still be a drawn-out and painful process. Most communities have rape crisis centers that provide advocates to help women navigate the legal system. Many local district attorney offices offer victim/witness advocates who can provide information and support. In some states, sexual assault can be reported anonymously.

Even if you do not intend to report the assault now, write down everything you can remember so if you decide to file a criminal complaint later, your statement will be accurate. This statement can be useful should you decide to pursue a sexual assault protection order or other civil law remedies. For guidance, contact the Victim Rights Law Center (victimrights.org.), which focuses on legal services for victims of sexual assault.

Many anti-violence activists focus on making the existing criminal justice system work better for those who experience sexual assault and domestic violence. Hard work by feminist activ-

PROTECTING OURSELVES AND EACH OTHER FROM SEXUAL ASSAULT

The responsibility to prevent rape should be on the people who rape—not on the potential victims. Rape is never our fault, but in a society where sexual assault is so prevalent, it is wise to try to take steps, when possible, that may reduce our risk.

Safety in social situations: Pay attention to how you feel, and trust your instincts. If you want to end a date or leave a party, say so, even if you are afraid or embarrassed. If you have a drink, keep an eye on it, as blackout-inducing drugs can be slipped into drinks. If a friend is drinking heavily, make sure she gets home safely and is not left alone. If you see a situation in which another woman is possibly being subjected to unwanted sexual advances, you may be able to interrupt the situation safely by asking her to accompany you in finding a women's washroom. This can give her a break from the pressure and a chance to reassess the situation.

Safety in intimate relationships: Learn to recognize potentially abusive relationships. An abusive or unhealthy relationship involves disrespect, fear, jealousy, possessiveness, and controlling behavior.

Safety at home: Make sure entrances are well lit and windows and doors are securely locked. Identify alternative ways out of your home besides doors. Use only your last name on your mailbox. Find out who is at your door before opening it for anyone.

Safety in your neighborhood: Arrange to walk home with people you trust. Get to know the people who live in your apartment building or on your street.

Safety on the street: Be aware of what is going on around you. Walk at a steady pace and look as if you know where you are going. If possible, walk in the middle of the street, avoiding dark places. Carry a whistle and keep it where you can easily reach it. If you drive, always check the backseat of your car before getting in, and keep the car doors locked while driving. When taking public transportation, try to find a seat near other people, and avoid subway cars occupied by groups of men.

Calling for help on the highway: Dial 911 for emergency services. Some highways may indicate another number for state police; this will vary by state. If you are summoned to pull over by an unmarked vehicle, especially at night or in a secluded area, you do not have to stop immediately. Slow down, turn on your emergency flashers, and drive to a well-lit, populated place before stopping. Keep your doors locked and roll down the window only an inch. Ask to see a badge and photo ID. If you have a cell phone, use it to contact a police dispatcher to check the person's authenticity.

These tactics can help, but they are not foolproof. Practice tactics for dealing with situations that make you feel most at risk and least powerful. Try to remain calm and act as confident and strong as possible.

---

ists in the late twentieth century, for example, achieved better handling of domestic violence cases, through improved federal and state laws and more informed awareness in many police departments. Some activists cite deep flaws in the criminal justice system. In the anthology *Yes Means Yes!* former rape-crisis worker Lee Jacobs Riggs writes, "I felt drained and frustrated (not to mention flat-out dirty) operating within a framework that positioned the criminal legal system as the primary remedy for sexual violence."[32] In cases when prosecution of a rapist is successful, the verdict and who gets convicted too often reflect the inequities present in the U.S. legal system, which imprisons people of color and poor people at a higher rate than white and/ or middle-class perpetrators of similar crimes.

INTIMATE PARTNER VIOLENCE

Intimate partner violence and battering, also known as domestic violence, are among the most common yet least reported crimes in the world. All couples at times disagree, argue, and have feelings of anger; not all aggressive behavior between partners constitutes domestic violence.

While a single act of physical or psychological violence between intimate partners is an act of domestic violence, most domestic violence involves a pattern of behavior that causes fear and intimidation in which one person in the relationship exerts coercive control over the other person. Within that pattern, acts of physical or psychological violence may occur frequently or rarely, but the threat is always present and serves to shore up the abuser's coercive control.

I was living with my then-girlfriend, and everything was okay for a while. Then she started to . . . force me into doing things that I didn't want to do. She wouldn't take no for an answer to anything. If she wanted it, she would get it.

A young homeless woman who moved in with an older man says of her experience:

It started with him ensuring that all ties with friends and family were broken . . . he would ask me to make unreasonable demands from

VIOLENCE AGAINST WOMEN WITH DISABILITIES

Women with disabilities are at higher risk for violence and abuse. The abuse is often more intense, longer lasting, and perpetrated by a greater number of abusers.[33] If help with daily care is needed, a woman may be physically dependent on her abuser. Assistants and relatives may withold medication or refuse access to mobility aids until money, sex, or other favors are given.[34]

The stereotypes of women with disabilities may increase vulnerability to sexual assault. Women with developmental disabilities are often stereotyped as innocent and childlike or as hypersexual. In either case, complaints of sexual assault may not be taken seriously.

Communication barriers, including hearing or speech impairments, may make reporting an assault more difficult. Fear of nursing homes or women's shelters not set up to accommodate disabilities may also discourage reporting. Finding appropriate help and alternative living arrangements can be exceedingly difficult.

There has been progress. The historic 1994 Violence Against Women Act was amended in 2000 to include language addressing the needs of women with disabilities, including providing funding for expanded protection, services, and education. Increasingly, the domestic violence service community is addressing the needs of clients with disabilities. Constructing barrier-free shelters, renovating existing shelters to be fully accessible to all abused women and children, and having the option to house or provide caretakers are important parts of the effort to respond comprehensively to violence against women.

For additional information, visit the National Women's Health Information Center (womenshealth.gov/violence) and the Center for Research on Women with Disabilities (bcm.edu/crowd).

---

them, such as borrowing money, and when they refused, he managed to convince me that they didn't care about me at all. Within a year, he had me convinced that he was the only person that cared for me. Once I got pregnant, he became very abusive. There was a lot of yelling and name-calling. He had me feeling completely worthless. I couldn't make a decision without asking him. I justified it to myself saying that he wasn't really abusive because he never hit me, which I now understand is absurd.

Intimate partner violence can be expressed by an array of threatening and harmful behaviors intended to reinforce coercive demands and to assert power and control. It may include physical violence, threatening with weapons, sexual assault, verbal and emotional abuse, control of finances or physical freedom, destruction of objects, and threats of harm or actual harm to loved ones including children or pets.

When I first dated my husband, I explained my childhood sexual abuse history and expressed my need for clear consent. But, a few years later, when I was pregnant with our first child, he stopped paying attention to my sexual boundaries and while I slept he anally raped me. I awoke, hit him, pushed him away, and said no. A year or two later, he sexually assaulted me in my sleep again. Many of the things he chose to do were things I said I was not okay with when awake. My husband has since admitted that he knew it was wrong, that he knew I wouldn't like it, and that he did it anyway.

Intimate partner abuse often follows a pattern. Over time, the abuser sets the stage by doing things that will make the partner increasingly susceptible to coercion. These can include:

- Exploiting vulnerabilities such as immigration status, childbirth, financial debt, or illness
- Wearing down resistance through emotional abuse or isolation from family and friends
- Increasing emotional dependency, for example, by inflicting injuries and then caring for those injuries

The abuser then introduces coercion by communicating a demand—for sex, perhaps, or not to leave the house without permission. The abuser makes a credible threat of meaningful negative consequences if the partner does not comply, like a threat of physical or sexual violence. When the abuser delivers the threatened negative consequences, this increases the likelihood that the abused person will comply with future demands and threats.[35] After that, the abuser can often get what he or she wants with just a hint of negative consequences, a particular scowl, or a quick "You know what you're supposed to do."

Intimate partner abusers are often skilled manipulators and use tactics designed to cause a woman and/or her family members, her employer, or the legal system to believe that she is mentally incompetent, unfit to parent, or otherwise unqualified to retain her constitutional rights. Abusers use such tactics to coercively

control the women in their lives, including wives, mothers, and grandmothers.

When the battered partner attempts to leave or does leave the relationship, the abuser may stalk her in an attempt to regain control. (See "Stalking," p. 717.) If intimate partner violence is not adequately addressed in its early stages, it can escalate in magnitude and severity and ultimately end in murder. For information on civil protection orders and other safety measures, see "Legal Considerations for Intimate Partner Violence," p. 716.

Women who obtain assistance from advocacy programs and legal services attorneys increase the likelihood that they will be able to obtain and enforce protection orders. They can

RECOGNIZING ABUSIVE BEHAVIOR

The following list identifies a continuum of abusive behaviors that come from the batterer's desire for coercive control. The more behaviors that apply to the relationship, the more dangerous the situation may be.

Overprotective and jealous behavior:
Abuse occurs with an escalation of behaviors that begins with actions that may not be overtly seen as abusive. Often, overprotective behavior is seen as "He/she cares so much about me" or "He/she really loves me" or "He/she doesn't like it when I wear revealing clothing—that is so sweet." While these actions do not always predict abusive behavior down the road, they can indicate overprotection as a form of control or reveal jealous motives that can lead to abuse. These actions can be confusing; they can seem to indicate special attention or loving concern, especially since popular culture often portrays such behavior as romantic, but they may escalate to increasing levels of coercive control, emotional and economic abuse, and/or physical violence.

Emotional and economic abuse:

- Destructive criticism/verbal attacks/blaming/disrespect/insults
- Intimidation/pressure tactics
- Immigration-related abuse/threats of deportation and/or threat to withdraw or not file immigration papers on your behalf

- Lying
- Minimizing/denying the abusive or controlling behavior
- Threatening suicide or self-harm as a method of control or manipulation
- Isolating you from friends and family, supportive persons, and important activities
- Depriving you of access to needed assistive devices such as eyeglasses, hearing aids, or walkers, or access to needed services such as transportation, medical or dental care, counseling, or home health aide assistance
- Threats or unwarranted actions to remove children from your custody, turn your family against you, have you declared mentally ill or incompetent, throw you out of your home, place you in an institution, or have you deported or arrested
- Threats of harm to you, your children, family members, or pets
- Surveillance, stalking
- Controlling all the money or withholding necessary resources
- Preventing you from getting or keeping a job
- Taking away something you desire if you don't do what the abuser demands

Acts of violence: These may be directed against you, your children, your family members, or other beloved people or pets.

- Making angry gestures
- Destroying objects
- Sexual violence

improve their safety by combining protection orders with safety planning. To locate advocates in your community, see "If You Are Being Abused" on p. 711.

THE IMPACT OF INTIMATE PARTNER VIOLENCE ON CHILDREN

Growing up in an atmosphere of intimate partner violence can be devastating to children. They may live in constant fear and can be torn physically and emotionally between their adult caretakers. They may develop severe physical and emotional responses to the violence, including symptoms of post-traumatic stress disorder. Children who grow up with intimate partner violence may come to believe that violence is an appropriate way to resolve conflicts. They arc morc likcly to be abused later on, and more likely to abuse others. Indeed, many adult perpetrators of violence were exposed to intimate partner violence or were themselves abused as children. Many came of age in families where male dominance and abuse were never questioned and where physical punishment "in the name of love" was accepted. When our families teach us to accept male dominance, manipulation, and violence as a way to relate to others, this "education" is difficult to defy:

I was raped and beaten by my father. By the time I . . . started dating, I had lost my voice. I didn't think that I had the right to say, "No, you can't do this to me."

There are innovative programs working to teach nonviolence and conflict resolution skills to teenagers, schoolchildren, and community members. These efforts aim to teach girls and young women that they have a right to be free from violence and terror, and to teach boys and young men a better way to relate to girls, women, and the world. One group that works to do this—by addressing teen dating violence—is the nonprofit organization Break the Cycle (breakthecycle.org).

IF YOU ARE EXPERIENCING INTIMATE PARTNER ABUSE

If you are in a dangerous relationship right now, there are things you can do that may help you to be safer, ensure the safety of your children, and work toward ending the relationship, if that is what you want to do. No one answer is right for everyone. Assess the suggestions below in light of your own situation. In some cases, it may be important to be extra cautious about leaving a trail (on the computer, for example, or in notes kept in an insecure place), as you may be exposed to further risk if your partner learns what you are doing. Overall, your safety can increase as you become more aware, inform others, find support, and implement a safety plan.

WHY DO WOMEN STAY?

A common question asked is "Why does she stay?" This question takes the focus off the real issue: "Why does the partner beat, coerce, and threaten her?"

There are many reasons why someone stays with an abusive partner. We may feel trapped and unable to leave, either because we still feel love for our partner and hope the abuse will end, because we are physically prevented from leaving, or because we feel so beaten down that leaving no longer feels like an option. Abuse often escalates at the point of separation, and we may feel safer staying. If we have children, we may think that we will not be able to support them and ourselves if we leave. People to whom we turn for support—clergy, police, friends, family—may not take the situation seriously or may not know how to intervene or provide help. A woman whose husband raped her while she slept said:

When I told my family doctor, she made a ton of excuses for him.

We may know about the existence of women's shelters but feel that moving to a shelter will cause too much upheaval for us and/or our children. We may know that we can obtain a protection order that allows us to stay in our home with our children and have the abuser removed and ordered to stay away, but we may be afraid of involving the police and ashamed that others will learn of our situation. We may be afraid to leave if we believe our immigration status is dependent on the "goodwill" of the abuser. If we have been living with abuse for a long time, we may be so worn down physically and emotionally that we cannot see a way out or imagine a future without pain and fear.

Call the National Domestic Violence Hotline (1-800-799-SAFE). Hotline advocates are available 24/7 to provide crisis intervention, safety planning, and information on and referrals to local domestic violence agencies in all fifty states and U.S. jurisdictions. Translators are available for many languages.

Build a support network. Get connected with your local women's service for abused women, join a support group, and develop a network of friends who understand domestic violence.

Teach your children how to call 911 for emergency assistance. It's important that they know what to do in case of emergency, especially if you cannot call yourself.

Look online for additional resources. See the sidebar on p. 711 for sites that offer trustworthy information and help.

Learn computer safety. It is quite easy for others to track websites you have visited, so consider using a trusted friend's computer or one at your local library. Email and instant messaging are not safe or confidential ways to talk to someone about the danger or abuse in your life. Tips on Internet and computer safety are available from the National Network to End Domestic Violence: nnedv.org/internetsafety.html.

Prepare a safety plan (see the sidebar on p. 715). Write it down if you can keep it in a place the abuser cannot find. Let others you trust know your plans when appropriate.

Study the abuser's patterns. Are there times

MAKING A SAFETY PLAN

Making a safety plan while you are dealing with a violent partner can give you hope in what so often feels like a hopeless situation. It can also bring you closer to leaving a dangerous situation in a safer and more organized way. In many communities, advocacy organizations can help you develop a plan to increase your safety and that of your children. To find a domestic violence victim advocate in your community, call your state domestic violence hotline for a referral. For national organizations to contact, see the sidebar on p. 711.

Carry important phone numbers for yourself and your children. Keep these numbers in a place that the abuser cannot find. Do not use your computer to store this information unless you are sure it cannot be accessed. Make sure your cellphone does not have any tracking software.

Find someone to tell about the abuse and develop a signal for distress. Ask neighbors to call the police if they hear sounds indicating that violence is occurring.

Think of one or two places where you can go and not be tracked down if you have to leave in a hurry.

If possible, open a bank account or a credit card just in your own name. Keep this information where your abuser does not have access to it.

Pack a bag with essentials in case you decide to leave in an emergency or unexpectedly. Keep this bag where you can get easy access to it, but not where your abuser can find it. Often, this bag is best left with a trusted friend or family member. Items to include: money, checkbook, bank cards, credit cards; copies of your identification, driver's license, and car registration along with extra car keys; important phone numbers; copies of birth certificates, Social Security and health insurance cards, welfare identification, copies of passport or immigration card and immigration papers, work permit; divorce or other court papers and child custody orders; school and medical records; prescriptions and needed medications; house deed, mortgage; insurance papers and policies; information on past abuse, such as photos and police reports including restraining orders or orders of protection.

Rehearse an escape route.

Periodically review and update your safety plan.

Increasing Safety After You Leave

Withdraw as much money as you can from a joint account and deposit it into a personal account.

Use different routes as you go home, to work, or about your daily tasks.

Avoid the places that you know your abuser goes to often.

Tell your child care provider who has permission to pick up your kids. Warn the provider's staff if you think the abuser may attempt to kidnap your children. Tell them to call the police if he/she appears for any reason.

Get a protection order, if it is right for you. Know what it includes and what will happen if the abuser violates it. Keep it with you at all times.

when the abuser is calmer and less volatile? For example, after an incident of violent abuse, there may be a brief period of "making up" or apology. Although you may most want to leave when the abuser is explosively angry and violent, it may be safer to leave during a time of relative calm.

LEGAL CONSIDERATIONS FOR INTIMATE PARTNER VIOLENCE

There is no single right way to handle abusive intimate partners. Each woman must decide what is best for herself and her family. Abusers can be prosecuted for crimes such as rape, assault, and battery. In addition, special laws protect battered women in all fifty states and all U.S. jurisdictions. These laws are quite similar from one state to another. Immigrant women are included in many protections.

The laws enable you to go to a local court and obtain an immediate protection order against the batterer. Orders of protection—often called civil protection orders, restraining orders, or protection-from-abuse orders—can provide different kinds of protection. They can order the abuser to leave the family home, to stay away from you and your children, and not to molest, assault, harass, stalk, threaten, or physically or sexually abuse you in the future. They can give you legal custody of your children. They can order the abuser to pay child support, medical bills, and the costs of car or house repairs, such as broken locks.[36] You can obtain protection orders even when you continue living with your abuser. Protection orders in all states except North Carolina offer protection to women in lesbian relationships.

Since the easy accessibility of firearms makes intimate partner violence particularly deadly, federal law specifies that people against whom a court has issued an intimate partner violence protection order cannot legally own or purchase firearms.

In addition to abuse prevention orders, all states have antistalking laws, though the legal definitions of "stalking" vary among them. Recognizing that women are often at greater risk right after leaving the batterer, these laws impose criminal sanctions against batterers who continue to harass or stalk. (For more information, see "Stalking," p. 717.)

Some abusers are intimidated enough by the legal system to be stopped by a court order. If this is the case, a protection order can provide safety and some reduction in the severity of the abuse. However, restraining orders don't work in all cases. Some batterers become violently enraged by what they see as betrayal. In these instances, going to court may actually make you and your children less safe. An advocate at your local domestic violence organization may be able to help you decide whether getting a civil protection order is best for you.

You may be able to improve your safety under a protection order by pursuing other legal remedies first, such as applying for and securing welfare benefits. If possible, immigrant women should consider initiating a case for victim-related immigration benefits and filing for a protection order only after receiving information confirming that the Department of Homeland Security believes that they have filed a valid case.

If you have had to defend yourself against a violent attack and have been charged with a crime, seek legal representation with an attorney who has experience defending battered women and who understands the dynamics of violence against women. The National Clearinghouse for the Defense of Battered Women (ncdbw.org or call 1-800-903-0111, ext. 3) or your statewide domestic violence or rape crisis coalition can inform you about legal resources and connect you with someone familiar with your state's self-defense laws. The Battered Women's Justice Project (bwjp.org) also provides resources and information.

MEDICAL CONSIDERATIONS FOR INTIMATE PARTNER ABUSE

Ideally, all hospitals would be required to train the staff about violence against women. Some hospitals do but some do not, and in some the training is inadequate. As one Boston-area activist commented, "In Massachusetts, hospitals seem to universally include three or four questions related to safety in the forms that folks complete, but I suspect that many hospital staff would not know what to do if someone disclosed violence in responding to these questions." If you find that the hospital where you are being treated has no one to advocate for you as a victim, ask someone to call the local domestic violence shelter and request an advocate.

Since the person taking you to the hospital may be your abuser, the hospital staff should separate you so you can talk freely about your experience and injuries. The hospital staff should also assist you in getting help from the social services department.

ENDING INTIMATE PARTNER VIOLENCE

There are alternatives to enduring intimate partner violence. More and more women are leaving violent partners and making new lives free of violence. Women everywhere have been organizing to help battered women leave abusive situations, provide shelter, and demand a more responsive legal system. Efforts have been developed in every state to establish collaborative, community-based responses to intimate partner violence. These task forces bring together advocates, attorneys, health care professionals, police, judges, prosecutors, and relevant women's organizations in the community to identify and resolve problems that battered women face when seeking help. To get involved in curbing partner abuse in your community, contact your state or local domestic violence program or coalition.

STALKING

After ending the relationship, I was stalked for more than six months. Despite the fact that the relationship had ended, my ex continued to call me fifty or more times a day, show up at my apartment with bloodied wrists, paste my old emails together, and send himself love notes in my name, and reported to the college that I was making death threats to him.

Recommended Resources: For more information on stalking, visit the National Center for Victims of Crime, Stalking Resource Center (ncvc.org/src).

IN TRANSLATION: UPENDING THE NOTION OF VIOLENCE AS "NORMAL"

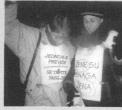

NAŠA TELA, MI

knjiga koju su pisale žene za žene

original je izdao
Bostonski kolektiv knjige o ženskom zdravlju

The Serbian adaptation of *Our Bodies, Ourselves.*

Group: Women's Health Promotion Center

Country: Serbia

Resource: *Naša Tela, Mi,* a Serbian adaptation of *Our Bodies, Ourselves*

Website: centarzdravljezena.org.rs

Domestic violence against women is a widespread problem in Serbia, due to conflict, poverty, and unemployment across the country.

Our Bodies Ourselves' Serbian partner, Women's Health Promotion Center, notes that reporting of violence against women remains pathetically low. This is mainly because gender-based violence is perceived as "normal," and there is a corresponding lack of political and social will to increase awareness and track crimes against women and girls. In addition, women are often unaware of their rights and understandably lack confidence in institutions charged with protecting their well-being.

Since the early 1990s, the center has helped draw public and government attention to women's health and make it a central part of social and health policy. Some examples: a manual and screening questionnaire on domestic violence—the first of its kind in Serbia—which is now part of routine medical evaluations in public and private health care settings; an action plan on promoting women's health that has been incorporated into the country's national response on gender equality; and special guidelines on protecting and assisting women exposed to violence that are now used by the Ministry of Health.

A key player in Serbia's social movement, Women's Health Promotion Center notes that its Serbian adaptation of *Our Bodies, Ourselves* has been pivotal to the movement's success. The book has helped highlight violence in the community, put women's health on the political agenda, and brought meaningful—and lasting—change to the lives of women and girls.

While legal definitions of stalking vary from one place to another, a good working definition of stalking is "intentional behavior directed at a specific person that would cause a reasonable person to feel fear." A more complete definition identifies stalking as "a course of conduct directed at a specific person that involves repeated (two or more occasions) visual or physical proximity, nonconsensual communication, or verbal, written, or implied threats, or a combination thereof, that would cause a reasonable person fear."[37] Stalking is serious, is often violent, and can escalate over time.[38]

According to the U.S. Department of Justice, both men and women are victims of stalking, but women are three times more likely to be stalked. Three in four victims know their stalkers, and 30 percent of stalking cases involve a current or former intimate partners who may monitor a partner's behavior, follow her, go to her place of work, or track her down if she has gone into hiding. Current or former intimate partner stalkers are more likely to reoffend and to approach the victim with a weapon.[40] In many jurisdictions, batterers who continue to stalk after a protection order are subject to arrest.

Many women who experience stalking feel forced to move residences, change jobs, or alter daily habits. Stalking can also involve damaged property and strains on personal relationships.[41]

CYBERSTALKING AND ONLINE SAFETY

According to data from the 2009 National Crime Victimization Survey,[39] approximately one in four people who experience being stalked reported some form of stalking online, such as via email (83 percent) or instant messaging (35 percent). Cyberstalking is often conducted as a form of surveillance and harassment by an abusive partner, but people report cyberstalking by acquaintances and strangers as well.

Though it is most often thought of as sending or posting obscene, hateful, or threatening messages and images, cyberstalking can also involve identity theft, posting false accusations, monitoring a person's online activities, and using personal data to empty bank accounts or ruin someone's credit score. Stalking via social media sites such as Facebook may involve adding strangers as friends to get information about someone or leaving vulgar or harassing comments on someone's public profile page.

Stalking and harassment in digital spaces should be taken just as seriously as stalking and harassment in person and should be reported to the authorities. In 2005, Congress extended the federal Violence Against Women Reauthorization Act to include cyberstalking.

The National Network to End Domestic Violence offers numerous resources to help victims and agencies respond effectively to the ways that technology affects victims of domestic and dating violence, sexual violence, and stalking. For online privacy and safety tips, visit nnedv.org/resources/safetynetdocs. Also check out the Electronic Privacy Information Center (epic.org) for tips and tools to protect online privacy.

Sometimes stalkers not only stalk the woman, but also follow partners, children, or other family members to "get" at the woman being stalked.

Although stalking is considered a crime in all U.S. states, prosecution presents challenges in many places. In thirteen states, the initial offense is considered a misdemeanor, and it is not until there is a repeat offense that stalking is considered a felony. Many actions such as persistent calling, sending gifts, emailing, or waiting at the victim's place of work or home are not crimes and are, in fact, considered—in different circumstances—positive actions. For this reason, stalking can be difficult to prove. For many of us who seek help from law enforcement agencies, the only course of action is to charge offenders with nonstalking crimes, such as burglary, vandalism, sexual assault, and violation of a protection order. Many law enforcement personnel lack the proper training to handle stalking cases.[42] According to a Network for Surviving Stalking survey, police often do not take stalking seriously, with half of the participants reporting they were told they were being paranoid; 17 percent were told by police officials that they were lucky to receive such attention.[43]

Stalking is unpredictable and dangerous. Here are some tips on how to proceed if you are being stalked:

- Change your patterns—vary your actions and your travel routes.
- Keep a log of all encounters with the stalker and a record of all attempts to reach you.
- Don't communicate with the stalker or respond to attempts to contact you.
- Make a safety plan. (See "Making a Safety Plan" on p. 715.)
- Let your friends, family, and neighbors know you are being stalked. Circulate a picture and physical description of the stalker.
- Protect your personal information (bank account information, private records) by using a safe for documents and a shredder for discarded documents.
- Install dead bolt locks (ask your local locksmith for recommendations) and hide all keys. Nonpickable locks and restricted locks are expensive, but if you have the money, it may be worth the investment. If you have the funds, install an alarm/security system.

SEXUAL ABUSE OF CHILDREN AND ADOLESCENTS

When I was sleeping over at my grandparents', I awoke in the middle of the night and noticed my cousin touching my private parts. He told me to shush and that everything was fine. He explained to me that this is what cousins do and that it was okay, but it should still remain our little secret. Since he was ten years older than me I listened to him. He did it whenever he came over, and I never knew what he was doing was wrong until two years later when my best friend moved back to her grandmother's without her mom. She had to come back because her stepfather had raped her, and it had started out with just the touching. It wasn't until this moment that I knew what my cousin had told me was a lie. I became very scared to tell everyone. I didn't want my mom to get mad at me and I didn't want to be taken away from my family. I decided to keep it a secret.

Sexual abuse of a child occurs when an older or more knowledgeable child or adult forces, tricks, threatens, or pressures a child into sexual awareness or activity. Sexual abuse is an abuse of power over a child and a violation of a child's right to normal, healthy, trusting relationships.

Although the common image is of a male abusing a female child or teen, women also commit sexual abuse, and boys are also victims.

Trusted adults who abuse children and teenagers include parents, uncles, aunts, siblings, cousins, stepparents, grandparents, coaches, babysitters, teachers, clergy, and day care operators. The abuse is called incest when the abuser is functioning in the role of a family member, whether or not he or she is biologically related to the child. (In some states, however, foster parents are not included.)

The extent of incest and childhood sexual abuse is hard to measure because of lack of reporting and uniform definitions and the limits of memory. Also, partly because children rarely receive education that would help them recognize sexual abuse, children frequently do not know that they are experiencing sexual abuse at the time, or cannot give a name to it, even though many later do. A conservative estimate is that one in five girls and one in thirteen boys in the United States have been sexually abused as children. Other sources cite figures of about one out of six boys and one out of four girls. In 2004, the U.S. Department of Justice reported that 15 percent of all sexual assault and rape victims were under age twelve, and 29 percent were between age twelve and seventeen.[44]

Incest and sexual abuse of children take many forms, including different kinds of body contact (for example, sexual kissing, sexual touching and fondling, and oral, anal, or vaginal sex). Sometimes the abuser uses sexually suggestive language, or shows private parts, or exposes children to adult sexual activity like pornographic movies. Abuse may also include verbal pressure for sex, and having children pose for pornography. The abuse often begins gradually and increases over time.

The use of physical force is rarely necessary to engage a child in sexual activity because children are trusting and dependent and are taught not to question adult authority. Because of this, children may have no physical signs of harm. Sexual offenders often use the child's trust and dependence to initiate sexual contact and to ensure continued sexual access to the child.

Sexual abuse in childhood has lifelong consequences. Some children and teens run away from home to escape abuse; experience depression; or use drugs, alcohol, food, or sex to dull the emotional pain. Victims of sexual abuse who act out may do so by abusing others. Often survivors of childhood sexual abuse blame themselves long after the abuse has ended—for not saying no, not fighting back, telling or not telling, having dressed or acted a certain way, or trusting the abuser. The young woman whose cousin molested her continues:

Today I am in college and this secret has turned me off toward men. I get very jumpy when a man tries to touch me or kiss me and that is why I have not had sex with a man. I just can't do it. And it makes me mad because I would love to have a husband and a family but I just can't bring myself to let a man hold me.

It can help to remember that what happened was not your fault. Those of us who have been sexually assaulted in any way are not to blame.

Healing from the trauma of incest or early sexual abuse can be helped by talking about it with people who can understand and empathize. Try to find someone who will listen to your individual experience rather than decide in advance what you should be feeling or what effect the abuse has had on you. Talking with others in counseling or in support groups may break the silence, help us gain perspective, and end the isolation. Some of us find it helpful to confront family members who abused us. Survivors must be prepared for the possibility that the abuser will deny the assaults and fail to provide an appropriate response when confronted. As with any decision about healing, we must make our own decisions about the steps we want to take.

SEXUAL HARASSMENT

Sexual harassment is unwanted sexual attention. It includes leering, touching, repeated comments, subtle suggestions of a sexual nature, pornography in the workplace, and pressure for dates. Sexual harassment is not limited to the workplace or school. It can include doctors with patients, welfare workers with clients, and police officers with the public, and occur during any interaction involving an abuse of power. In addition to men harassing women, women can harass other women, and men can be harassed by other men or by women. Sexual harassment can escalate, and people who are being sexually harassed are at increased risk of being physically abused or raped.

In the workplace, we may experience a direct or implied threat, such as, "Have sex with me or you will be fired." A hostile work environment can interfere with the ability to do our job, whether the harasser is an employer, a supervisor, a coworker, a client, or a customer.

Socializing at work often includes flirting or joking about sex. While this is sometimes a pleasant relief from routine or a way to communicate with someone, this banter can turn insulting or demeaning. It becomes sexual harassment when it creates a hostile, intimidating, or uncomfortable working environment. Refusal to comply with the harasser's demands may lead to reprisals, which can include escalation of harassment; poor work assignments; sabotaging of projects; denial of raises, benefits, or promotion; and sometimes the loss of a job. Harassment can drive women out of a job or the workplace altogether. Poor women, immigrant women, older women, and teenagers are especially vulnerable to sexual harassment because they often have less power in the workplace and greater difficulties finding other employment.

When sexual harassment happens in a school setting, it can have devastating effects on a young person's life. One sixteen-year-old girl describes her experience:

It came to the point where I was skipping almost all of my classes, therefore getting me kicked out of the honors program. I dreaded school each morning, I started to wear clothes that wouldn't flatter my figure, and I kept to myself. I'd cry every night when I got home, and I thought I was a loser. . . . Sometimes the teachers were right there when it was going on. They did nothing.[45]

A college student looks back:

My coach sexually harassed me for the majority of my senior year in high school. I was heavily involved in the activity, and we had a close relationship—one I had always assumed was strictly platonic. I turned 18 early senior year, and after my birthday things began to get strange. I didn't really think anything of it, but his actions got progressively more blatant. After talking to older girls that had already graduated, I learned he was well practiced in his harassment—he never did anything physically obvious, but the things he said, asked, and implied made me so uncomfortable I couldn't go near him. I stopped participating in the activity I had dedicated my high school career to. Even now that I have moved across the country and stopped all communication, thinking about the activity, him, or anything related makes me nauseous. My male adviser in college makes me uncomfortable, even though he has been nothing but polite and professional. I blame myself for not noticing, for running away instead of standing up to him. I used to see myself as a strong, take-no-shit woman. I'm afraid I'll never be the same.

Because there is a strong taboo against identifying sexual harassment, when we first experience it, we may be aware only of feeling stressed.

We may develop headaches, anxieties, or resistance to going to the setting in which it occurs. It may take us a while to realize that these symptoms come from being sexually harassed. We may blame ourselves and wonder if we did something to provoke the harassment. We may also be afraid to say no or to speak out because of possible retaliation. But when we take the risk and talk with other women, we often find others who are being or have been harassed and have responses similar to ours.

I experienced a graduate school sexual harassment scenario with an adviser and trusted colleague. It got ugly, then it got uglier, and we have managed to bring reconciliation (through a long arduous process and a restoration of power) to ourselves and to the department. Facing that situation, challenging the behavior, defining my own boundaries, reclaiming power, and then, eventually, opening up to reconciliation, forgiveness, and dialogue, was one of the most empowering experiences of my life.

SEX WORK AND VIOLENCE AGAINST WOMEN

Sex work is an umbrella term that refers to a variety of jobs within the sex industry, including prostitution, exotic dancing, phone sex, and work in the pornography industry. The majority of women involved in sex work in the United States do so involuntarily, out of economic desperation. Women involved in prostitution are often recruited when they are young, frequently by boyfriends, family members, or other people they know. Some have run away from home as teens—sometimes to avoid sexual abuse or physical violence, or to escape antigay or antitrans hostility—before being coerced into sex work with promises of money and security.

I ran away from home, and I met a woman who brought me to her boyfriend, who I later found out was a pimp, and that guy raped me, over and over. . . . He then brought me to his friend, another pimp, and sold me to him, and from the age of 12 years old until I was 35 and too drugged out to work, I was a prostitute.

Poverty and the lack of economic alternatives are what drive most people into sex work. The majority of sex workers worldwide are women of color, and/or very poor. Women (and children) at the bottom of the sex work ladder end up having to work in higher-risk settings and perform the unsafe acts demanded by some clients, like sex without a condom. They are often trafficked across state lines or from other countries. (For more information, see "Sexual Exploitation of Women and Sex Trafficking," p. 789.)

A smaller number of women who work in the sex industry actively choose to do so for various reasons, including money (for those in control of earnings); a sense of power and independence; or as a way of working out personal issues. Activists among voluntary sex workers affirm that sex work, when chosen, is a valid and not shameful occupation and that good working conditions, decent health care, control of one's earnings, and protection from harm are crucial. They advocate for resources and services that will provide sex workers with medical testing and treatment, condoms, and help with negotiating safer sex. One such activist group is the Sex Workers Project in New York (sexworkers project.org), which uses "human rights and harm reduction approaches" to protect and promote "the rights of individuals who engage in sex work, regardless of whether they do so by choice, circumstance, or coercion."

All sex workers are at risk of violence—from pimps, from clients, from bosses in the porn industry, and from the police.

When I turned 18, I worked as an exotic dancer. There were several cases of women, myself included, getting attacked by clients after our shifts or if we went outside to have a cigarette. In my case, it was a client that we saw quite regularly and knew by name. The boss found out when I showed up for work with bruises, and he told me that if I reported the client to the police not only would I lose my job, but that the police wouldn't care because I was just a stripper. He then gave me three nights off with minimal pay so my bruises could heal enough to be covered with special body makeup. He was more concerned about losing money from clients than he was about the safety of his employees.

Sex workers who are prostitutes (especially those who are not free to insist on condom use) risk contracting sexually transmitted infections, including HIV and hepatitis. Most health studies so far have focused on sex workers as vectors of disease rather than as disease victims.

Sex workers, especially those who are transgender, have little or no protection from police harassment and lack police protection when victimized by crimes such as robbery, battery, and rape. The criminal justice system currently prosecutes sex workers, while the johns (those who hire sex workers) most often go free.

Activists have organized to fight the exploitation and violence many sex workers face and to change public perceptions so that police come to view prostitutes as victims instead of criminals. Some activists work in the streets to protect and to free women who are caught in sex work. They seek to create better economic opportunities for women, and campaign to eliminate the sex industry entirely. One example of such activism is the Minneapolis group called Breaking Free (breakingfree.net). An excellent film about this kind of work in Chicago is *Turning a Corner* (see Recommended Resources). See also "The Sex Trade and Feminism," an interview with DePaul University professor Ann Russo, and other articles available on womenandprison .org/sexuality.

Could legalization or decriminalization of prostitution reduce the levels of violence and health risk faced by some sex workers? In some countries and places in the United States, such as Nevada, prostitution has been legalized. This puts sex work under state regulation and thus hypothetically ensures better working conditions. However, legalization creates a two-tiered system, in which only U.S. citizens get to register, get tested for STIs, receive safer sex materials, and work in marginally safer environments. Sex workers who are not citizens (some immigrants, for example, and those who have been trafficked) would not necessarily be covered by even these minimal state protections.

Sex workers have organized in the United States and Europe to advocate for decriminalization, the abolition of all laws that punish sex workers. In what is known as the Swedish model, some decriminalization groups seek laws that would make it illegal to be a customer of a sex worker or to engage in sex trafficking, pimping, or owning brothels. Such laws, which aim to reduce the demand side of prostitution, would put the johns, rather than the sex workers, at risk of being arrested and fined. Others believe that only complete decriminalization of all parties involved in sex work could create safer working environments. As of 2011, only a handful of U.S. states have ended the practice of prosecuting minors under age eighteen on prostitution offenses and instead focus on offering them protection and access to services.

DEFENDING OURSELVES

The most important step in ending violence against women is to stop people from using violence to get their way. For some women, learning self-defense boosts physical and emotional self-confidence. The actual use of these skills when we are in danger is a choice made at a particular moment. We each make the best decision we can based on our resources and knowledge at the time.

The study of self-defense includes many activities: assertiveness training, exercise, and boxing and other sports that promote self-confidence, self-knowledge, and self-reliance. Self-defense is not simply responding to violence with violence. Self-defense classes may help us think clearly if we are under attack, so that we can mobilize our thoughts, assess the situation, judge the level of danger, and then carry out the response we have chosen.

I have experienced such profound changes in my self-image and in the way that I see the world

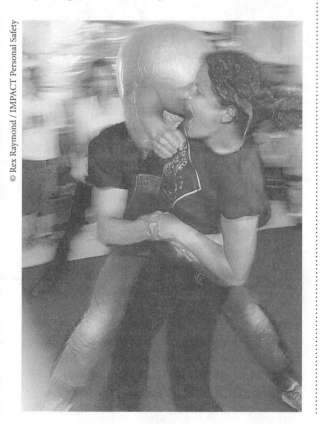

© Rex Raymond / IMPACT Personal Safety

and relate to people that I really can't separate my study of self-defense from the rest of my life.

Myths can prevent us from defending ourselves effectively against a physical assault. These include the belief that we do not know how to defend ourselves, or that the assailant is invulnerable. Women have defended themselves against attacks through both resourcefulness and force.

Street techniques, which depend upon surprise and causing damage, do not work as well against repeated assault by people with whom we live. Other skills developed in the practice of self-defense may be useful. As we develop abilities to think quickly and clearly, and to find sources of help, we will be able to consider how we might resist or minimize the abuse or how we might eventually leave the abuser and the violence behind us.

ENDING VIOLENCE AGAINST WOMEN

Over the past forty years, women have focused much effort on the problem of violence against women and have made great progress.

We have talked openly about our experiences, built rape crisis centers and shelters, advocated for changes in laws, been joined in our efforts by men, and become recognized as part of the international public health and human rights movements. We have also influenced other survivor movements, such as the one working on abuse by clergy. For more information about the history of the movement to end violence against women, see "Ending Violence Against Women: A Brief History" at ourbodiesourselves.org.

There is still much to be done. We need to:

- Recognize that violence against women is a risk throughout the life span, and advocate to

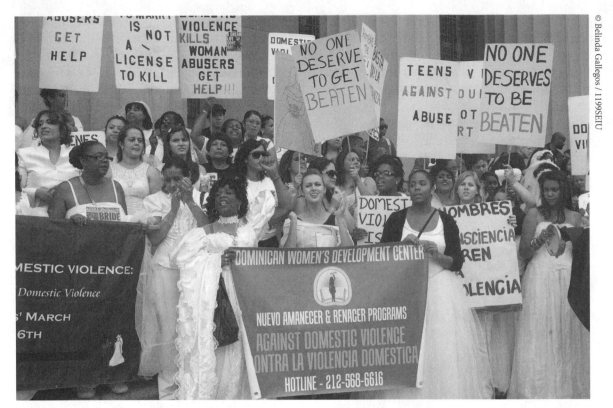

Women take part in the Brides March Against Domestic Violence in New York City in 2010. The march was started ten years earlier in remembrance of Gladys Ricart, who was murdered by an abusive former boyfriend on the day she was to marry her fiancé.

make necessary services available to women of all ages, abilities, and backgrounds.

- Speak out against the messages in our society that glorify and encourage violence, domination, and exploitation.
- Teach and model nonviolence.
- Intervene whenever we see the seeds or expression of violence against women, realizing that our silence helps to perpetuate it.
- Strengthen family, community, and neighborhood sanctions against violence as opposed to relying exclusively on the criminal justice system.
- Work to maintain a strong network of services for all of us who are at risk of and who have survived violence.

- Insist that our government officials take violence against women seriously and make it a key part of their agendas.

We must pursue our vision of a violence-free world loudly and clearly. Noeleen Heyzer, the former executive director of what is now known as the United Nations Development Fund for Women, describes that vision:

Imagine a world free from gender-based violence: where homes are not broken into fragments; where tears are no longer shed for daughters raped in war, and in peace; where shame and silences break into new melodies; where women and men gain power and courage to live to their full potential.[46]

■ ■CHAPTER 25

Every day I see research linking chemicals that pollute our environment with adverse effects on women's reproductive health, from infertility to birth [impairments] to early puberty in girls. . . . I am convinced that countries that do not protect the Earth will not protect their women, and countries that do not protect their women will never protect the Earth. The time has come for the U.S. to enact policies that do both.

—Alison Ojanen-Goldsmith, in "Young Feminists—Poison Earth, Poison Woman: Making the Connection."[1]

Where and how we live and work have a direct impact on our health. We absorb chemicals, toxics, and other manufactured hazards found in the home, workplace, and environment through the air we breathe, the products we apply to our skin, the substances we come into contact with, and the food we consume.

Occupational health and environmental health are sometimes considered separate fields of study, and different government agencies deal with each: The Occupational Safety and Health Administration (OSHA) focuses on workplace health and safety, while the Environmental Protection Agency (EPA) works to protect the environment at large. Yet many of the problems in both arenas are similar and overlap. For example, chemicals that put workers at risk in a manufacturing plant are likely also to contaminate water supplies and threaten air quality. So decreasing the use of toxic substances in the workplace protects not only workers, but also people who live nearby, as well as consumers who purchase products made at the plant.

Occupational and environmental hazards affect many aspects of our health, resulting in a myriad of cancers, neurological disorders, allergies, and behavioral changes. In 2010, the President's Cancer Panel (PCP) stated, "The true burden of environmentally induced cancer has been grossly underestimated. With nearly 80,000 chemicals on the market in the United States, many of which are used by millions of Americans in their daily lives and are un- or under-studied and largely unregulated, exposure to potential environmental carcinogens is widespread."[2]

An increasing body of scientific evidence points to the connection between the health of our environment and our reproductive health and the health of our children, including elevated rates of cancer in reproductive organs, premature births, miscarriages, and birth impairments. In keeping with the focus of this edition of *Our Bodies, Ourselves*, this chapter focuses on the impact of environmental pollution on women's reproductive and sexual health.

IMPACTS ON FETAL, INFANT, AND CHILD DEVELOPMENT: WHY THE YOUNGEST ARE MOST VULNERABLE

Children often experience worse effects than adults exposed to the same damaging substances. Children are smaller and have more vulnerable immune systems, and their metabolism, physiology, and biochemistry are different from adults', so these contaminants can cause greater damage to the nervous system, brain, reproductive organs, and endocrine (hormonal) system. Fetuses and babies are much less able to metabolize and inactivate dangerous contaminants. Many sensitive and important chemical and hormonal processes take place from conception through adolescence and can be interrupted or affected by harmful exposures. Perversely, some of the worst chemicals and contaminants in use today are present in children's products, toys, and foods. As the number and concentration of chemicals have increased, so has the number of childhood illnesses: Leukemia, brain cancer, and other cancers linked to environmental car-

Environment refers to where we live, work, and play, as well as to the broader ecology. Because we live in a highly industrialized world, all of our bodies contain measurable amounts of chemicals, pesticides, and other toxic materials that we are exposed to through the air, soil, food, water, workplace, and home.

Acute: Resulting from short-term, high-level exposure. Often used to denote an illness that comes on quickly and severely.

Bioaccumulation: The uptake of toxics at higher rates than those found in the natural environment and leading to a higher concentration in bodily tissues over time. Through bioaccumulation, toxics move up the food chain, with animals (humans) at the top of the food chain absorbing the highest amounts. This process is especially hazardous for our reproductive health, as toxics the mother has absorbed over time can be passed on to her children, especially through breast-feeding.

Body burden: The cumulative amount of natural and synthetic chemicals that are present in the human body at a given point in time.

Carcinogens: Chemicals that cause cancer.

Chronic: Resulting from long-term exposure. Often used to denote a disease that progresses slowly and over a long duration.

Endocrine disrupting chemicals (EDCs): Chemicals that interfere with normal hormone function.

Endocrine system: A system of glands, each of which secretes a type of hormone into the bloodstream. The endocrine system regulates body functioning, with hormones affecting mood, growth and development, tissue function, metabolism, sexual function, and reproductive processes.

Estrogen: The primary female sex hormone. Estrogen is essential for the formation of breasts and reproductive organs, regulating the menstrual cycle, and helping to maintain a healthy heart and bones. Many synthetic and natural compounds affect estrogen production, which is a concern, since women with higher lifetime estrogen levels are more likely to develop breast cancer.

Polychlorinated biphenyls (PCBs): Exposure to PCBs, organic compounds widely used in manufactured products, has been linked to skin conditions; reproductive disorders such as reduced growth rates, developmental disabilities, and neurological effects; a compromised immune system; and an increased risk of certain cancers. Although banned from manufacture in the United States in 1977, PCBs are slow to break down.

Persistent organic pollutants (POPs): Organic compounds that do not easily degrade in the natural environment, meaning that a variety of toxics can still be found in nature years after they have been banned and/or disused. They thus pose a significant threat to environmental and human health.

cinogens have increased more than 20 percent since 1975.[3]

Most children in the United States are exposed to potentially hazardous chemicals before they are even born. A father's sperm or mother's eggs, if damaged through pesticide, chemical, or other exposure, could potentially affect an embryo's development. According to the 2010 report of the President's Cancer Panel (PCP), studies have found a total of three hundred chemicals present in the umbilical cords of newborns, prompting the authors to assert, "To a disturbing extent, babies are born 'pre-polluted.'"[4] Exposure to potential contaminants while in the womb may irreversibly and negatively affect important development, predisposing babies to illnesses and susceptibilities throughout their lives. Because of this, the PCP urges those considering having a child to "avoid endocrine disrupting chemicals and known or suspected carcinogens prior to a child's conception and throughout pregnancy and early in life, when damage is greatest."[5] (See "Key Terms to Know," p. 729, for a definition of endocrine disrupting chemicals and other key words in this chapter.)

BREAST MILK CONTAMINATION

Once a child is born, exposure can continue through breastfeeding. Toxics are easily stored in a woman's fat through the process of bioaccumulation, and mothers pass them to newborns through their milk. Even so, breast milk is still considered the healthiest form of infant feeding in all but rare cases, because the many benefits are so significant for both mothers and babies.

Many chemicals considered hazardous to babies' health, especially when they are consumed in breast milk, have been banned in the United States, yet traces of these banned chemicals are still found in women's breast milk.[6] Some women and babies are at especially high risk because of diet or environmental exposures; for example, among indigenous people in the high Arctic, babies take in seven times more PCBs than the typical infant in Canada or the United States.[7]

Breast milk offers tremendous protective qualities and benefits that outweigh the risks of low-level exposure to toxics in most cases. Babies who are formula-fed are more likely than babies who are breastfed to develop ear infections, diarrhea, asthma, diabetes, lower respiratory tract infections, and eczema. Both sudden infant death syndrome (SIDS) and childhood leukemia, while rare, are more common in babies who are formula-fed.[8]

Women can make individual adaptations to limit the toxics in breast milk. For example, women at Akwesasne (see sidebar, p. 745) adjusted their fish intake during their reproductive and nursing years to reduce exposure to PCBs and other contaminants. Equally important at Akwesasne and other communities, people are mobilizing to challenge polluters, holding them accountable for environmental degradation, and demanding adequate remedies.

WHO'S RESPONSIBLE FOR THE PROTECTION OF OUR HEALTH?

Too often, individuals rather than government institutions or companies are expected to take primary responsibility for health and safety. For example, employers may require employees to wear personal protective equipment (which may be ill-fitting and cumbersome) instead of changing a risky practice or substituting a less hazardous substance. Or we are told that our behavior is what makes us get sick or stay well. But we can't avoid being exposed to toxic substances or dangerous conditions that we cannot control. Furthermore, our personal "choices" are limited by economic constraints, access to information, family obligations, workplace rights, and available alternatives.

Many environmental health hazards are caused by industrial practices and pollution that expose individuals and communities to chemicals, often without the people affected being given any information about potentially harmful effects. We may know little, for example, about pesticides sprayed on the foods we eat and chemicals used in our homes and workplaces.

It's the responsibility of industry and government to ensure that information is properly disseminated and regulations are properly enforced, and to fund scientific studies that analyze the potential impact of different hazards, as well as respond to communities most affected. There are state and federal right-to-know laws that provide some access to critical information about exposure and potential effects, but these laws will make a difference only if communities insist on their implementation.

THE PRECAUTIONARY PRINCIPLE OF PUBLIC HEALTH

Meanwhile, in a world of constant exposure to chemical contaminants, and after decades of public health nightmares like DDT and asbestos, we can no longer assume that products are safe. Only a few hundred of the tens of thousands of chemicals in use are adequately tested; many substances suspected to cause cancer or reproductive health problems are not regulated at all.[9]

Community activists, researchers, and advocates from the fields of science and health are calling for the increased use of a new kind of risk paradigm that encourages anticipatory action in the absence of scientific certainty. This Precautionary Principle states, "When an activity raises threats of harm to human health or the environment, precautionary measures should be taken even if some cause and effect relationships are not fully established scientifically."[10]

Jennifer Coleman of the Oregon Environmental Council explains: "Today, tens of thousands of synthetic chemicals are 'innocent until proven guilty'—that is, they are not thoroughly tested for hazards to health or the environment before they are used to make consumer goods. We need a chemical policy that ensures the safety of all consumer products before they reach the shelves. Until that occurs, we must work on banning or restricting the use of potentially harmful chemicals one at a time."[11]

The Precautionary Principle requires taking action in the face of uncertainty, shifting the burden of proof to those who create risks, and analyzing alternatives to potentially harmful activities. For more information, visit the Science & Environmental Health Network, which has numerous articles, statements, and government positions concerning the Precautionary Principle: sehn.org/precaution.html.

ADVOCATING FOR OURSELVES AND OUR COMMUNITY

Advocacy is another important part of protection and remedial action. Women are pushing for more research on risks that are poorly understood, launching community-based health projects, calling for enforcement of regulations to keep our environment safe, and insisting that communities that are most vulnerable are protected against and compensated for unnecessary health burdens.

More work and advocacy are being done through national and international networks, often linking researchers and health-care providers to women working for change in their communities. One key organization is the Collaborative on Health and the Environment (CHE) (healthandenvironment.org), an international partnership that pays special attention to reproductive and cross-generational impacts. Elise Miller, the director of CHE, explains why activism on this issue is desperately needed:

Only recently has research focused on how certain chemicals may disrupt women's reproductive health. With the leadership of scientists, health professionals, and patient advocates, these concerns are now starting to be prioritized. Our great hope is that future generations of women and their partners will not have to struggle with the rampant incidence of infertility, endometriosis, and other reproductive health disorders we see today.[12]

TYPES OF HAZARDS: CONTAMINANTS AFFECTING OUR HEALTH TODAY

LEAD

Everyone is exposed to trace amounts of lead through air, food, water, dust, and various products. Lead occurs naturally in the environment and has many industrial and commercial uses (it is used in plumbing pipes and car batteries, for example). Lead is a neurotoxic, meaning it affects our nerve cells. Even small amounts can be dangerous, since the substance accumulates in tissue and bone over time. Sickness from lead is often referred to as "lead poisoning." Acute exposure can result in vomiting, diarrhea, seizures, coma, and death. Chronic exposure can result in brittle bones; anemia (iron deficiency); damage to the brain, nervous system, liver, kidney, and blood system; and general weakness.

Children and pregnant women are most susceptible to serious health effects of lead. Dr. Louis W. Sullivan, former Secretary of the Department of Health and Human Services, called lead the "number-one environment threat to the health of children in the United States."[13] Lead crosses the placenta in a mother's womb to reach her developing fetus,[14] and occupational health studies show increased miscarriages and stillbirths among women who work with the substance. Long-term exposure can also reduce male fertility. Even limited prenatal and/or childhood contact can affect children's intellectual development, behavior, growth, and hearing, and may result in early puberty for girls. Those under the age of six are most vulnerable. Children who eat a diet rich in iron and calcium absorb less lead, since calcium prevents absorption. (Pregnant women also need to ensure their calcium intake is high.) Dairy products, red meat, dark leafy greens, tofu, and beans, can help to increase iron and calcium levels.

Historically lead was an ingredient in both paint and gasoline; while those uses have mostly been discontinued, there is a persistent concern about lead paint in housing, especially in older homes and in poorer neighborhoods where remediation has been lax.

The EPA estimates that lead paint poisoning affects more than 1 million American children. Owing to a lack of adequate nutrition and an abundance of substandard housing, children from low-income families are eight times more likely to experience lead poisoning than those from higher-income families. African-American children are five times more likely to be poisoned than white children. In New York

Contact your state health department for tips on having your home tested and treated for lead. For general information on lead and its impacts, contact the National Lead Information Center Hotline at 1-800-424-LEAD. For information about lead in drinking water, call the EPA's Safe Drinking Water Hotline at 1-800-426-4791.

City, as of 2009, more than 80 percent of the children poisoned by lead are children of color.[15]

Lead exposure in the home can occur through lead pipes and lead-based paint, particularly in older buildings. The EPA considers lead-based paint to be in good condition if it's not chipping. Chipped or otherwise degraded paint should always be removed by a trained worker; never sand or burn off paint that may contain lead, as dry chips, fine particles, and vapor are easily inhaled.

Airborne lead emissions also raises concerns.

In 2011, the U.S. and Illinois Environmental Protection agencies launched a joint investigation after lead levels at an elementary school in Chicago's Pilsen neighborhood were found to be at or above federal limits. "Lead pollution exceeded health standards during a fifth of the days monitored and, on one day in December, spiked more than 10 times higher—findings that alarm even veteran investigators," reported the *Chicago Tribune*.[16] The school is near several industrial polluters, including a coal-fired power plant, and community activists have long asserted that the neighborhood is disproportionately affected by air pollution.

Occupational exposure is the most common source of lead poisoning for adults. Under the state and federal lead standard laws, employers are legally required to limit employee exposure. If extensive exposure does occur, employers must institute a medical surveillance program, including blood testing; lead-specific medical exams and treatment, if necessary; and relocation if a worker's health is at risk. Workers should contact the Occupational Safety and Health Administration (osha.gov, 202-219-8151) or the

RADIATION EXPOSURE

Radiation exposure is a possible reproductive health risk. More research is needed to determine if nonionizing radiation—the radiation we're exposed to from microwaves, electronics, and voltage lines—can damage reproductive health. Ionizing radiation, which we're exposed to through medical technologies, nuclear power plant emissions, uranium mining, and weapons testing, can pose very serious risks to our reproductive systems.

According to the Breast Cancer Fund, "Exposure to ionizing radiation is the best- and longest-established environmental cause of human breast cancer in both men and women."[17]

The Navajo Nation and other indigenous and rural communities located near uranium mines face higher risks of ionizing radiation. Employees in laboratories using radioactive materials are also at risk. For more information about these complex risks, visit Toxipedia (toxipedia .org), and the Indigenous Environmental Network (ienearth.org).

National Institute for Occupational Safety and Health (cdc.gov/niosh, 1-800-CDC-INFO) for more information.

Symptoms of lead poisoning may occur right after exposure, or months or years later. Therefore, it is important for anyone concerned about lead exposure to be tested. The CDC recommends that each state provide testing for children who are potentially exposed, including all children who live in or regularly visit a house built before 1950 or renovated before 1978, and those whose parents work with lead. The CDC also recommends that children who are receiving Medicaid or whose families receive federal or state assistance be tested free of charge.

MERCURY

Mercury is used in some thermometers, thermostats, auto parts, scientific instruments, batteries, dental fillings, eye makeup (as thimersol, a mercury-based preservative), over-the-counter drugs, chlorine production, and lighting, including tanning beds. Release into the environment stems primarily from coal-fired power plants; metal production, primarily gold production; cement production; waste disposal, specifically biomass burning; and iron and steel production. The last mercury mine in the United States closed in 1992.

The FDA has banned the use of mercury compounds in all cosmetics except those used around the eyes, where levels are very limited. Still, some cosmetics, including skin-lightening creams, have been found to contain mercury (see "What's in Our Cosmetics," p. 742.). A small number of states have banned other consumer products containing mercury (such as toys and jewelry) or products containing more than a low level of mercury.

Mercury can damage the central nervous system, the endocrine system (which regulates

WHAT IS BODY BURDEN?

Many of our day-to-day exposures to toxics are small and limited, with chemicals and other materials entering our body through the food we eat, products we use, and home and work environments. But while each contact may be small, it's the accumulation of toxics over time—our total "body burden"—that matters.

Scientists estimate that each person carries approximately seven hundred chemicals in her or his body at any given time.[18] While some chemicals leave the body relatively quickly, others stay in the fat, bones, and muscle. A woman's total body burden is especially worrisome during pregnancy and lactation, as chemicals pass from her to the fetus through the placenta and to her baby through breast-feeding.

hormonal activity), the heart, the lungs, the immune system, and the kidneys. Exposure is linked to numerous problems, including but not limited to sensory impairment, lack of coordination, seizures, pneumonia, decreased pulmonary function, depression, memory loss, brain damage, and—at very high doses—sudden death.

Mercury is especially harmful to pregnant women and fetuses, infants, and children, who may experience neurological disorders as well as decreased brain function, delayed onset of walking, and permanent kidney damage. Additionally, boys may experience decreased sperm count.

Symptoms of mercury poisoning include itching, burning, or pain; skin discoloration;

shedding of skin; muscle weakness; red face; loss of teeth, hair, and nails; and increased sensitivity to light. Mercury poisoning may manifest itself up to several months after initial exposure.

PESTICIDES

Pesticides are some of the most commonly and heavily utilized synthetic products. Based on most recent data, the EPA estimates that more than 1.2 billion pounds of pesticides are used annually in the United States alone—with 5 billion pounds used worldwide[19]—primarily for pest control and mostly in agriculture, in industry, and in and around people's homes. Seventy-five percent of U.S. households use at least one indoor pesticide.[20] Owing to widespread agricultural use, pesticide exposure also occurs through residue on foods and exposed water sources.

Pesticide exposure has been linked to many developmental problems and effects on the reproductive system, including: impact on placenta cells; delayed neurodevelopment; abnormal ovary and menstrual function; decreased sperm count; early puberty; delayed testis, prostate, and penis development; infertility; miscarriage; stillbirth; lowered birth rate; endocrine disruption; premature birth; and increased risk of cervical, vaginal, testicular, and childhood brain cancers. Exposure to some agricultural

REDUCING YOUR COMMUNITY'S PESTICIDE EXPOSURE

- When possible, avoid using pesticides in homes and on lawns and gardens. Instead, use inexpensive, nontoxic products such as vinegar, baking soda, boric acid, insecticidal soaps, and pest control products made from essential oils. You can also use beneficial predators and parasites (like ladybugs and nematodes). When it comes to pets, skip the chemicals and use pesticide-free flea-prevention applications.
- If you do use pesticides, wear protective clothing. Wearing a long-sleeved shirt, long pants, nonabsorbent gloves and shoes, goggles, and a respirator mask helps minimize risk. Wash exposed skin, gloves, clothing, shoes, or boots immediately after exposure. Wash clothes soiled with pesticides separately from other laundry in hot water and detergent.

- Never smoke, eat, or drink while handling pesticides—doing so offers the chemicals a pathway into your body.
- Do not apply pesticides right before a heavy rain or in places where they might wash into sewers or directly into bodies of water. Use pesticides when the wind is no more than a light breeze and the temperature is cool, such as early morning or evening, to reduce the air travel to nearby areas.
- Follow disposal directions on the pesticide label for leftover substances and empty containers. Never pour pesticides down the sink, toilet, or sewer drain or onto the ground. Never reuse a pesticide container.

To learn more, check out the "Reducing Pesticide Exposure" page on the New York State Department of Health website (health.state.ny.us/environmental/pests/reduce.htm), and Vassar College's Environmental Risks and Breast Cancer project (erbc.vassar.edu).

---

pesticides among women during pregnancy may be associated with autism in their children. Many people are sensitive to pesticides and experience skin, lung, respiratory, and eye irritation when exposed.

In addition to affecting fetal development, pesticide exposure prior to conception and during the prenatal and postnatal phases can affect a child's long-term health. The *Journal of Agromedicine* reported in 2007 that "every chemical class of pesticides has at least one agent capable of affecting a reproductive or developmental endpoint in laboratory animals or people."[21] An article in a 2006 issue of *Environmental Health Perspectives* stated: "Every child conceived today in the Northern Hemisphere is exposed to pesticides from conception throughout gestation and lactation regardless of where it is born."[22]

Pesticide exposure is especially common in farm communities. A study looking at Mexican farmworkers in 2000–2001 found that mothers exposed to pesticides through agricultural work had a fivefold increased chance of their fetus developing anencephaly, a neural tube defect that results in a partial or complete absense of the brain and skull. Fathers exposed through farmwork faced twice the risk.[23]

People who live near farms that use pesti-

PERSISTENT ORGANIC POLLUTANTS

According to the United Nations Environment Programme, Persistant Organic Pollutants (POPs) "are chemical substances that persist in the environment, bioaccumulate through the food web, and pose a risk of causing adverse effects to human health and the environment."[24] POPs are extremely resistant to the natural breakdown process experienced by other substances and thus remain in the environment up to decades after initial production. POPs are also stored in animal and human fats, which makes them of particular concern for breastfeeding, as mother's milk acts as a route of exposure, bringing toxics from the mother's fat to her baby. Exposure has been linked with wildlife and human diseases, disorders, and birth impairments.[25]

The control of POPs is addressed through the 2001 Stockholm Convention on Persistent Organic Pollutants, of which the United States is a signatory. The convention notes the presence of POPs in areas far from their original use, including the Arctic, indicating that communities far from agricultural, industrial, and other areas with high chemical use could still be affected by them. Twelve chemicals known as the "Dirty Dozen" are listed for "priority action" by the Stockholm Convention. These include pesticides like aldrin and DDT and the industrial chemicals PCBs. For a full list and description of sources of POPs, go to uspopswatch.org/global/dirty-dozen.htm.

PESTICIDES ON YOUR FOOD: FROM SAFEST TO WORST OFFENDERS

The best way to avoid exposure to pesticides through your food is to purchase and eat certified organic food and food from farmers you know do not use pesticides on their crops (many farmers are not officially certified but make great efforts to farm responsibly).

Keep in mind that not all crops are treated equally. The Environmental Working Group maintains a Shopper's Guide to Pesticides (foodnews.org) that identifies forty-nine fruits and vegetables and ranks them from most safe to least safe in terms of pesticide residue. This list can be helpful if you're wondering which foods to prioritize buying organic.

The clean fifteen: The fifteen least sprayed vegetables and fruits are onions (best), avocados, sweet corn (frozen), pineapple, mango, sweet peas (frozen), asparagus, kiwi, cabbage, eggplant, cantaloupe (domestic), watermelon, grapefruit, sweet potato, and honeydew melon.

The Dirty Dozen: The twelve most sprayed vegetables and fruits are celery (worst), peaches, strawberries, apples, blueberries (domestic), nectarines, bell peppers, spinach, kale, cherries, potatoes, and imported grapes.

cides are also at increased risk of experiencing negative health effects. A 2007 study of women in California found that the rate of autism was six times higher among children of women living within 500 meters of farms that use certain pesticides than among women who lived farther from such farms.[26]

In addition to being affected in the womb, infants and children experience more negative effects from pesticides than adults, owing to their size and biology. According to the Pesticide Action Network (panna.org), "Pound for pound, [children] drink 2.5 times more water, eat 3–4 times more food, and breathe 2 times more air. They therefore absorb a higher concentration of pesticides than do adults."[27]

While many pesticides have been banned or their use has been reduced, they continue to affect human and environmental health for decades. Several pesticides are considered persistent organic pollutants (POPs), meaning that they can stay in the environment and humans for years if not decades. Many of us have com-

pounded exposures rather than one-time exposure (see "What Is Body Burden?" p. 734).

ENDOCRINE DISRUPTING CHEMICALS

Endocrine disrupting chemicals, or EDCs, are industrial and pharmaceutical chemicals that mimic naturally occurring hormones. EDCs can block or interfere with the complex hormonal messages that affect many of the body's functions, including thyroid function, sexual development and behavior, metabolism, and nervous and immune system function. Research on EDCs reveals occupational and environmental threats to women's general and reproductive health.[29]

While there is still much debate as to the full effect of EDCs on human health, scientists have become increasingly concerned, particularly in the past two decades. Low-level exposure still needs to be better understood, but the dangers of high-level exposure have been proved to affect

DDT: THE MOST POPULAR EDC

According to the EPA, "DDT [dichloro-diphenyltrichloroethane] is likely one of the most famous and controversial pesticides ever made," with more than 4 billion pounds being produced and applied since its first production in 1940.[28] DDT has been used most prominently on agricultural crops and as pest control, especially in tropical areas where malaria is rampant. It is still used for malaria control in many parts of the world.

In humans, DDT is linked to reproductive disorders, including decreased fertility. While DDT use was banned in

the United States in 1973, its status as a persistant organic pollutant (POP) means that it can stay in the environment for decades. A 2005 study by the CDC found the chemical present in the blood of many of those tested,[30] and trace amounts of the chemical have made their way to remote regions of the Himalayas, hundreds of miles from where it was initially used.[31] It can also enter U.S. households through products imported from countries where DDT regulations are more lax and where the pesticide is sprayed in order to stem malaria infection, such as those in Asia and Africa.

reproductive health. The most famous, diethyl-stilbestrol, or DES—a synthetic estrogen—was found to cause long-term health problems for the children of pregnant women who were prescribed DES in the 1950s and 1960s to prevent miscarriages during pregnancy. The effects included higher rates of vaginal cancers among the teenage daughters. DES was banned in the 1970s,[32] long before it was determined to be an EDC.

EDCs are present in our food supply and in air and water, as well as in industrial municipal waste and in many synthetic household and personal-care products. They may be associated with increased risk of breast cancer and other cancers in women; breast milk contamination; and other reproductive problems including endometriosis, miscarriage, tubal pregnancy, and reduced fertility. Most scientists agree that breast cancer risk is affected by how much estrogen we have in our bodies and for how long over our lifetime. If the body's estrogen levels are changed by chemicals that act like estrogens, our risk of breast cancer may increase.

EDCs affect fetal, infant, and children's health, often much more than they do adult health, because of children's developing and highly sensitive endocrine systems. Because many important and complex processes take place during fetal development and infancy, EDCs could have life-long effects.

WHERE DO WE FIND EDCS?

According to TEDX—the Endocrine Disruption Exchange—EDCs include any chemical or substance that affects development and function. This broad category includes pesticides; materials used in plastics such as bisphenol A (BPA); flame retardants; some cosmetics; glues and sealants; and some cleaning products. Some EDCs are persistent organic pollutants (POPs), which means they stay in the environment for years. Others leave the environment relatively

quickly. With hundreds of thousands of products and processes containing or using EDCs, we experience low-level exposure daily.

Diet is a main source: as with other chemicals, EDCs that are fat-soluble (as many are) make their way up the food chain, meaning that they accumulate in the fat of animals and animal products over a period of years, finally being consumed by humans at higher levels than are found in the natural environment. Women are more vulnerable to chemical exposure than men, in part because of their bodies' fat content.

Research suggests that indoor air quality also heavily affects our exposure. The presence of dust and chips of wood that has been sprayed with EDCs such as glues, sealants, and wood polish, combined with the use of chemicals and other substances in the home, may rival diet as a primary route of exposure.

DIOXINS

Dioxins are a by-product of industrial processes that use or burn chlorine. They are notorious for causing harmful human exposure at Love Canal, a neighborhood in Niagara Falls, New York, where dioxin-contaminated toxic waste was buried by Hooker Chemical (it later became a Superfund site); and at Times Beach, Missouri, a small town outside St. Louis that was evacuated in 1983 following the largest civilian dioxin exposure in the United States. Dioxins were also present in Agent Orange, an herbicide used during the Vietnam War that resulted in serious birth impairments in the children of some of those exposed.

Major sources include municipal waste facilities, hospital incinerators, chemical and pesticide manufacturing plants, backyard burn barrels, and pulp and paper bleaching plants. Dioxins are one of the most common chemicals affecting Americans today. According to the EPA, the average level of dioxin found in the population is at or near levels linked to adverse health effects observed in animals and people.[33] Any additional exposure above such levels could therefore damage our health. Dioxin exposure occurs primarily through eating contaminated food, particularly fish, meat, and dairy products. Dioxin can cause cancer and reproductive disorders.[34]

BPA

Bisphenol A, or BPA, is an organic compound widely used in hard plastic products, including reusable food containers, baby bottles, sippy cups, and the lining of baby formula containers and canned food. It is also present in a wide range of household items, from children's toys to dental sealant. The chemical industry produces 7 billion pounds of BPA in the United States each year. Exposure occurs when the chemical contaminates food and drink.

The compound is considered an endocrine disrupting chemical (EDC), and more than two hundred studies have produced a long list of serious chronic disorders associated with it— cancers, infertility, heart disease, liver abnormalities, genital abnormalities in male babies, early puberty in girls, cognitive and behavioral impairments, reproductive and cardiovascular system abnormalities, diabetes, asthma, obesity, attention deficit disorder, and attention deficit hyperactivity disorder.[35] According to a 2007 study by the CDC, 93 percent of the U.S. population age six and up have been exposed to BPA.[36] The Environmental Working Group (EWG) found BPA in more than half of ninety-seven cans of brand name fruit, vegetables, soda, and other common canned goods.[37] Of particular concern is its use in toys and plastic containers aimed at young children, who are more vulnerable to side effects than adults, owing to natural differences in metabolism and size. Fetuses are also affected in utero and at the earliest stages of development. According to the Oregon Environmental Council, premature babies are exposed to levels of BPA ten times greater than the general population.[38]

In 2011, China and Malaysia set bans on BPA, joining Canada and all of the European Union. Some U.S. cities and states have banned baby bottles containing BPA, yet proposed federal legislation banning BPA in all baby products remains stalled.

While BPA-free products are becoming more available across the country, they are often more expensive than products containing the compound, potentially putting lower-income groups at higher risk. Indeed, minority children in the United States may face higher rates of BPA exposure: the presence of BPA was recently found in the umbilical cords of nine out of ten African-American, Asian, and Hispanic women tested by the EWG.[39]

TIPS TO AVOID BPA EXPOSURE

- Watch for the numeral 7 on the bottom of plastic containers. That often means they contain BPA.
- Don't microwave plastic food containers made with BPA (better to use glass or porcelain), and discard old or damaged bottles (scratches can promote leaching).
- Choose glass, stainless steel, or BPA-free polypropylene (PP #5) bottles. Visit Safe Mama (safemama.com) for an updated list of BPA-free products.
- Minimize the use of canned foods and canned drinks.
- Ask your dentist for BPA-free sealants and composite fillings.

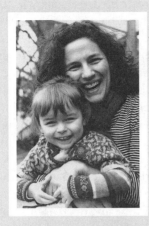

© Andy Utz

WHY I WORK TO IMPROVE ENVIRONMENTAL HEALTH

LISA FRACK
SOCIAL MEDIA MANAGER, ENVIRONMENTAL WORKING GROUP

When I was pregnant with my second child, I read Sandra Steingraber's book *Having Faith*, about the amazing—and quite terrifying—interconnectedness of pregnancy and the environment. I had, of course, heard about the serious downsides of alcohol, smoking, and drugs on a baby's development—and had chosen to avoid them all while pregnant. I'd even had a blood lead-level test because we were remodeling an old house.

But what I hadn't chosen to avoid—because I didn't know about them—were the thousands of other chemicals that my baby and I were exposed to every day: chemicals in my cleaning supplies, the house paint, the creams and shampoos I'd received as gifts for my new baby, and my nail polish, to name but a few.

What took me from this new knowledge and some product changes to a career in environmental health was one chemical: bisphenol A (BPA). As a working mother, I pumped breast milk at work for my partner and day care providers to feed my baby. Turns out, the feeding bottles we used contained the toxic hormone disruptor BPA, and to make matters worse, they were hand-me-downs, which are more likely to leach chemicals.

Well, that did it! I stopped using our toxic baby bottles once I knew about BPA, but plenty of others were still using them, and safer alternatives weren't easy to identify or buy. So I decided to shift my focus from just protecting my own family to working for the Washington, DC-based organization Environmental Work Group (EWG), to protect other caregivers and their children. EWG informs people about the chemicals that affect our health and offers practical, effective tips on how to avoid them. We also advocate for stronger laws—at both the national and the state level—since current laws are notoriously outdated and weak. It has to be easier for a parent to assess the toxicity of all the products out there!

Environmental health science continues to show that exposure to toxic chemicals during pregnancy and early childhood can have long-term adverse health effects. One of my most important responsibilities is my children's health. Fighting for their environmental health is one way I can fulfill that responsibility—for all children.

POLYCHLORINATED BIPHENYLS (PCBS)

Polychlorinated biphenyls, or PCBs, are one of the most toxic and hazardous chemicals used in modern manufacturing. Historically, they have been used extensively throughout industry, specifically in transformers, capacitors, and coolants. Concerns about health and environmental effects led to a ban on PCBs for most uses in the United States in 1979. But some uses are still allowed, and PCBs are persistent contaminants (POPs) that can stay in our bodies and environment for decades. Health problems resulting from PCB exposure include thyroid disorders, breast cancer, endometriosis, low birth weight, menstrual disorders, and possibly early puberty, as well as miscarriage and hormonal changes.

Some areas are considered PCB "hot spots." Along New York's Hudson River, into which the General Electric company released thousands of pounds of PCBs, strict fish advisories remain for women of child-bearing age to help minimize their exposure to PCBs. Two hundred miles of the river, some of which runs through New York City, is considered a Superfund site.[40] Lake Erie and Lake Ontario are two other bodies of water marked as potentially hazardous.

PHTHALATES

Phthalates are chemicals that make plastic more pliable. They can be found in many common products, including pills, wallpaper, adhesives, food containers, vinyl, shower curtains, building materials, cosmetics, medical devices, toys and other children's items, packaging, water bottles and soda cans, paints, textiles, polyvinyl chloride (PVC, commonly used in flooring), pesticides, insecticides, and food. Phthalate use is slowly being phased out in the United States: its use in children's products is in some cases banned and is often restricted, especially in toys and products meant for a baby's mouth, such as pacifiers.[41]

According to the CDC, nearly all Americans have phthalates in their urine. Eating is the main way the substance enters our bodies, either through leaching from food containers into food and liquids or from the food products themselves.[42] Phthalates are easily released into the air when plastics age and break down.

Phthalate exposure is associated with asthma and allergies (especially in children), autism, endocrine disruption, obesity, decreased sperm count, low birth weight, premature birth, and ADHD. The EPA rates phthalates as "probable human carcinogens."[43]

WHAT'S IN OUR COSMETICS?

Most women in the United States use multiple cosmetic and personal care products—including lotions, toothpaste, and makeup—every day. We apply these products directly to some of the most vulnerable parts of our bodies. Our skin is permeable; our eyes and mouths offer an entry

BAD REACTION TO COSMETICS? TELL THE FDA

In 2011, the FDA launched tools for the public to report rashes, hair loss, infections, or other problems after using a product, even if product directions were not followed. The FDA also wants to know if a product has a bad smell or unusual color—which could signal contamination—or if the item's label is incomplete or inaccurate. For more information, go to fda.gov/ForConsumers.

to the rest of the body, particularly the bloodstream; our lungs inhale hundreds of potential contaminants. Many of the chemicals commonly used in cosmetics are associated with allergies, multiple chemical sensitivity (MCS), asthma, shortness of breath, changes in hormone function, different cancers, brain development, reproductive disorders, skin diseases, and birth impairments. According to the EWG, one in five personal care products contains chemicals linked to cancer. Even chemicals that have been banned from other products owing to their adverse health effects, like lead and mercury, still make their way into common cosmetics such as lipstick and mascara.[44]

Babies are also heavily exposed to personal care products, from baby wipes to powders. Fetuses can be exposed in the womb: A 2009 study by the EWG, for example, found chemicals from cologne present in the umbilical cords of newborns.

Cosmetics and household products contain some of the highest rates of synthetic chemicals, yet their regulation is minimal. While food and drug additives must be tested before they are sold, cosmetic products don't face the same requirements. Many suspected reproductive toxics are used in everyday cosmetics. The European Union has banned the use of more than 1,100 chemicals in personal care products, according to the Campaign for Safe Cosmetics. The United States has banned or restricts only 11.[45]

For more information on cosmetics and health, see "More Products, Less Regulation," p. 50, as well as the Campaign for Safe Cosmetics (safecosmetics.org), which also features a video on "The Story of Cosmetics," and the EWG's Cosmetic Safety Database (cosmeticdatabase.org), where you can search products and ingredients.

COMBINATION EXPOSURE: WHY A LITTLE HERE AND THERE MATTERS

The risks associated with chemicals in cosmetics are often downplayed, as usually there is only a small amount present in any product. But most of us use a multitude of products in our daily lives, many of which have dozens of chemical ingredients. This combined exposure warrants

EARLY PUBERTY MAY INCREASE THE RISK OF BREAST CANCER

According to Vassar College's Environmental Risks and Breast Cancer project (erbc.vassar.edu), personal care products may be associated with premenopausal breast cancer in young African-American women. When the use of personal care products such as hair relaxers was discontinued among individual girls with signs of premature puberty, those signs receded, suggesting a link between chemicals in certain products and early puberty.[46] And early puberty increases the risk of breast cancer.[47]

Early puberty is of concern for all girls. According to the Breast Cancer Fund, a significant portion of U.S. girls start breast development before the age of 8. In addition to breast cancer, early puberty is linked to polycystic ovary syndrome, depression, and anxiety.[48] While the causes of early puberty are still being investigated, endocrine-disrupting chemicals—including those that mimic estrogen—are a possible culprit.[49]

standard, cosmetic manufacturers in particular are able to claim that their products are safe when in fact they may pose serious health threats.[51] These low standards are upheld because of industry's close ties to government, their heavy lobbying, and the many loopholes in our laws.

Lack of knowledge about what chemicals are doing to our health goes far beyond just the cosmetic sector. During a special CNN report in 2010 on toxic chemicals in the womb, Phil Landrigan, a pediatrician and director of the Children's Environmental Health Center at Mount Sinai School of Medicine, said, "For eighty percent of the common chemicals in everyday use in this country we know almost nothing about whether or not they can damage the brains of children, the immune system, the reproductive system, and the other developing organs. . . . It's really a terrible mess we've gotten ourselves into."[52]

To protect consumers, the federal government must require industry to test for combination exposures. Until we understand more about the effects of multiple chemicals, it is important to do what you can to reduce your total exposure.

that chemicals be tested in combination rather than in isolation.

Many chemicals are simply tested for their obvious effects, such as short-term allergic reactions, rather than their longer-term or combined effects. In addition, many chemicals are not even listed on some products. The EWG found that the average perfume includes fourteen ingredients not included on the label, most of which the FDA had not assessed; the fragrance industry has tested only 34 percent.[50]

According to the Campaign for Safe Cosmetics, in the absence of a U.S. governmental safety

SHARED RISKS, UNEQUAL BURDENS

While everyone is affected by environmental conditions, gender, race, ethnicity, and class intersect with workplace and environmental conditions so that health hazards are borne unequally by people with low incomes and people of color. The movement to right such wrongs is called the environmental justice movement.

Economic and social power determines how much we are able to protect ourselves from environmental and occupational health hazards. Some people can afford to buy bottled water or food without additives, to get better health care,

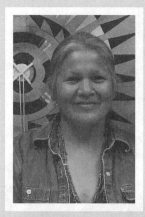

© Nancy Ackerman

THE AKWESASNE MOTHER'S MILK PROJECT

Katsi Cook, a guiding midwife and educator in the Mohawk community in Akwesasne, New York, initiated the award-winning Akwesasne Mother's Milk project in 1984. She wanted to help answer Mohawk women's questions about toxic chemicals' effects on breast milk quality and reproductive health. The community's high levels of exposure to PCBs and other contaminants puts its women at increased risks for reproductive health effects. The project continues, setting the model for community-based research at Akwesasne and other communities.

"The waters of the earth and the waters of our bodies are the same water," Cook said. "Breastfeeding is an inherent human right and a critical element of our Mohawk subsistence lifestyle that is protective of the health of the generations."[53]

Cook's organization, First Environment Collaborative of Running Strong for American Indian Youth (Indianyouth.org/women.html), is currently working with Akwesasne's health departments and clinical services to implement the Centering Pregnancy empowerment model of prenatal care. This woman-centered model of care provides physical assessment, peer support, and community building and education that support and nourish women as they become mothers.

or even to move to a less-polluted neighborhood. Others cannot. People of color are more likely to work in more dangerous workplaces, and to live in inadequate housing, closer to environmental hazards.

Research done by the Commission for Racial Justice (United Church of Christ) helped launch the environmental justice movement in the 1980s. The Commission's work pointed out that three of the five largest commercial hazardous-waste landfills in the United States are located in mostly black or Latino communities; three out of five blacks and Latinos live in communities with uncontrolled toxic-waste sites; and about half of all Asians/Pacific Islanders and Native Americans live near uncontrolled waste sites.[54]

The work continues on through many networks, with the Environmental Justice Resource Center at Clark Atlanta University (ejrc.cau.edu) being one of the best sources of information and inspiration.

EFFECTS OF PESTICIDES AT HOME AND ABROAD

Of the 3 million farmworkers in the United States, most are migrants, usually Latinos, and about one in four are women. Female farm-

ENVIRONMENTAL AND REPRODUCTIVE INJUSTICES

Those of us who work for reproductive justice must pay serious attention to environmental injustices that affect our ability to become pregnant, have a healthy pregnancy, and give birth to and raise a healthy child. Instead, individual women are blamed for these problems, [and are] often told to avoid dangerous jobs, move out of contaminated areas, improve our educational status or eliminate language barriers.

Moreover, women of color often work in industries that pose severe risks to our health. Farmworkers are exposed to many dangerous chemicals that cause spontaneous miscarriages and create lifelong physical damage. . . . These preventable risks are not individual problems for women to deal with but instead require that we create a society based on human rights in which it is unacceptable to profit from chemicals that harm us.[55]

—*Loretta Ross**
*National Coordinator, SisterSong
(sistersong.net) and organizer for reproductive justice and environmental justice*

*Read more about Loretta Ross's work in "Organizing for Change: Reproductive Health and Justice," p. 813.

workers' health issues are often neglected, with their occupational health exposure monitored less than that of men. According to the Committee on Women, Population and the Environment (cwpe.org), farmworker studies disproportionately focus on men's health exposure, with few being done on women. When women are considered, they are often classified as farmers' wives, a designation which excludes them from large studies considering pesticide-induced cancer. Without proper research, appropriate interventions for women have not been designed and implemented. The committee also notes that women face more of a burden than their male counterparts because of gender prescribed roles, such as washing dirty, pesticide-ridden clothes of a farmworking partner.

One of the most serious hazards facing Inuit women in northern Canada is the damage to the food supply from the atmospheric movement of contaminants from the United States and globally. This puts women at high risk for reproductive damage to themselves and their children, particularly breastfed children. Women there have needed to adjust their diet so that they are not as exposed to top-of-the-food-chain sources of food.

Pesticides, drugs, industrial chemicals, and processes banned in the United States are often exported to developing countries where regulations are nonexistent or ill-enforced. Poorer countries often have weaker environmental regulations in order to attract industrial business interests from abroad. Many U.S. companies, for example, work in countries with little or no workplace or toxic regulations, producing chemicals and products that could not be so easily and cheaply produced at home, risking the health and lives of workers in those countries. Some international agreements, such as the North American Free Trade Agreement (NAFTA), weaken countries' abilities to enforce regulations because of industries' dominance over their politics and economies.

IN TRANSLATION: CONSTRUCTING TOILETS AND PLANTING TREES

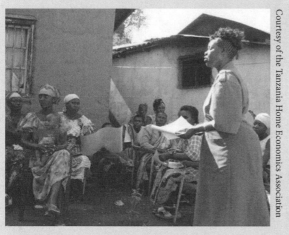

A nurse-midwife in Tanzania facilitating a community health workshop.

Group: Tanzania Home Economics Association

Country: Tanzania

Resource: Kiswahili materials adapted from *Our Bodies, Ourselves* for East Africa

Website: ourbodiesourselves.org /programs/network

Tanzania, located in East Africa, has a population that is almost 80 percent rural and quite poor. While the population's exposure to manufactured chemicals and toxins differs from that of populations in industrialized nations, the majority of Tanzanians face other environmental challenges, such as little or no access to clean water and food, crowded living spaces, and inadequate waste disposal and sanitation. This increases their risk for diseases such as diarrhea, hepatitis A, typhoid, cholera, and malaria. Many of these are serious public health issues in their own right. However, some chemicals commonly used to contain the spread of disease can also affect the health and well-being of entire communities. DDT, for example, a chemical used to control malaria in parts of Asia and Africa, is linked to a range of reproductive disorders, including decreased fertility.

Tanzania Home Economics Association (TAHEA), Our Bodies Ourselves' partner in Tanzania, has adopted a comprehensive approach to the problem, one that looks at the relationship between both individual and collective health and the environment. As TAHEA uses its Kiswahili materials based on *Our Bodies, Ourselves* to increase awareness about reproductive and sexual health, the group also educates the community on practices that foster the growth of germs and transmit disease, and works in partnership with local health, water, sewage, medical, and academic departments to identify sustainable solutions.

This collaborative effort has already helped train more than 450 women in different villages on the importance of sanitation. Thirty of these women are now peer educators, reaching out to even more communities with information on general hygiene, human waste containment, water sources protection, and environmental effects on reproductive health, as well as overall community health and economic development.

(continued)

ACTION STRATEGIES: IN THE WORKPLACE

Women have a long history of collective action for health at work. The millworkers of Lowell, Massachusetts, struggled against hazardous conditions in the 1840s. In 1909, thousands of women in New York City's garment industry went on strike to protest sweatshop working conditions and low wages. In 1943, two hundred African-American women "sat down" at their machines in a North Carolina tobacco plant when a coworker died on the job after years of exposure to excessive heat, dust, and noise. In 1979, women led a strike to improve health and safety conditions at a poultry farm in Mississippi. Nurses often speak out about the hazards of understaffing and mandatory overtime that affect both nurses and patients. With plenty of experience behind us, we continue to take action.

In protecting women's reproductive health and justice, a strong coalition has fought against "fetal protection policies." These policies target women on the job (particularly women of reproductive age), excluding them from hazardous jobs in the name of protecting an actual or potential fetus. This so-called protection leaves the workplace just as hazardous, puts men's reproductive health at risk, and "protects" women right out of a job. A coalition of labor, environmental, women's rights, and reproductive health organizations fought these policies all the way to the Supreme Court. In 1991, in the famous case of *United Auto Workers (UAW) v. Johnson Controls* (battery manufacturers), the Court ruled that the exclusion of fertile women, regardless of childbearing intentions, from jobs because of potential fetal injury is illegal discrimination based on sex. The American Civil Liberties Union, which supported the UAW, argued that women should be the ones to make decisions about their reproductive and economic roles. The coalition emphasized that the workplace needs to be cleaned up for everyone's sake—for women, men, and future generations.

PRECAUTIONS FOR PREGNANT WOMEN

If you are pregnant and work with hazardous substances, you may have certain rights to a job transfer or to paid or unpaid leave. Under an amendment to the U.S. Civil Rights Act, women "disabled by pregnancy" must be treated the same as other temporarily disabled workers, like those who have had heart attacks or accidents. (Disabled, in this instance, is a legal term meaning unable to do specific tasks.) Some states also have pregnancy disability acts.

Before starting a new job, ask whether the company has a specific reproductive health policy, what it is, and whether it applies to both men and women. Some companies ask employees to sign waivers stating that they are aware of the job's possible reproductive hazards and will not hold the employer liable. Some lawyers think these waivers can be challenged in court. If your employer has a policy that seems unclear or unfair on fertility, pregnancy, childbirth, or any other issue related to reproductive health, contact your nearest committee coalition on occupational safety and health (COSH) (look under "local groups" on the national council website: coshnetwork.org) or other workplace health advocacy groups or occupational/environmental health clinics for support (see Recommended Resources).

HOW TO CREATE CHANGE IN THE WORKPLACE

If you are thinking about taking action in your workplace, consider the possible consequences. Although the law says that you cannot be fired for raising health and safety issues, the reality may be different. In the United States, you have the right to call an OSHA inspector to check health and safety conditions in your workplace. You can remain anonymous when you file an OSHA complaint. However, this does not ensure that your employer will not figure out who submitted the request, especially in small workplaces or when you have already been vocal about a potential problem.

Action on a particular health and safety problem often starts informally. Be sure to understand the difference between risk factors (hazards in the environment or workplace that may endanger health) and health outcomes (actual injury or sickness) and the consequences of focusing on one or the other. Try to show the connections. Show how a problem affects everyone.

Whenever possible, try to form an ongoing workers' health and safety committee. Instead of responding just to emergencies, a committee can work preventively to uncover potential problems before anyone gets hurt and approach management about them. Members of a group may be less likely to be singled out as "troublemakers" and subjected to special harassment or dismissal than individuals working alone.

Know your group's strengths, weaknesses, barriers, and opportunities. You may find support in unexpected places. Ask what other workers in your shop or community can contribute to your efforts. For example, female workers battling unhealthy indoor environmental conditions might enlist male maintenance or security workers who can help with ventilation, furniture, machines, or safety issues. Small acts of solidarity on the part of many women from all racial and socioeconomic classes can lead to substantial gains.

Susan McQuade, health and safety specialist at the New York Committee for Occupational Safety and Health (nycosh.org), talks about the committee's work:

We educate women entering the construction trades on reproductive hazards that can be encountered on the job. New York Committee for Occupational Safety and Health (NYCOSH) trainers use the UAW v. Johnson Controls case to demonstrate how unions have fought to better protect their members from exposure to reproductive hazards. This is particularly important for new workers who may feel pressured to accept less-than-adequate protections when exposed to hazards that can affect their reproductive health. But, while women face some unique health and safety issues, the vast majority of hazards on any construction site affect both men and women. Increased knowledge, coupled with activities organized to address health and safety concerns, are the best tools for reducing exposure to reproductive and other workplace hazards.

Here are some suggestions for improving workplace safety.

Substitute safer alternatives: Research and press your employer to research whether a safer substance or equipment (chemical or process) can be used. For example, encourage the employer to replace solvents with water-based products and to use natural, biodegradable cleaning products.

Isolate or enclose the process: Can the hazardous job be moved to a different time or area when/where fewer people or even none will be exposed to danger? Can the worker be isolated from the operation, or can the process be completely enclosed? Ventilating hoods or fans can keep workers from breathing fumes.

Improve housekeeping: Keep toxic materials from being reintroduced into the air by cleaning up. Keep dust levels down to protect workers' lungs. Move obstacles out of work areas and exits to prevent accidents. Wear masks and gloves, and use safety equipment.

Improve maintenance: Is equipment regularly serviced and repaired?

Accept personal protective equipment as a last resort: It is the employer's responsibility to ensure that workers are adequately protected; workers should not have to adapt to the workplace. Personal protective equipment (PPE) is particularly burdensome for women when they are pregnant. Other protections should be implemented first for all workers. Some groups, like occupational health and safety clinics and COSH groups, can help you think through whether the PPE strategy is effective and fair.

Secure protections: Under the Americans with Disabilities Act, which includes pregnancy, women may be able to successfully secure certain protections in the workplace, such as relocation or altered work processes. To effectively activate such protection requires good strategy with other workers, advocacy groups, and unions. But don't let them "protect you" out of a job.

Create committees: Organized groups can gather information, educate coworkers, help set priorities, and provide leadership and per-

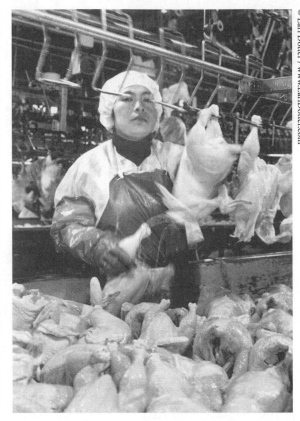

A "guest worker" from Central America handles chickens that are about to be processed.

sistence to create change. A health and safety committee is most effective as part of a union. In the United States, a unionized company is required by law to negotiate health and safety issues with the union. For nonunionized workplaces, there may be legal guarantees providing for health and safety committees, depending on where you live. For example, in Washington State, workplaces with more than ten employees must have such a committee. Check with the national COSH network or similar networks in other countries to learn about committees in your area.

Negotiate contracts: Contract negotiations offer the opportunity to address hours, wages,

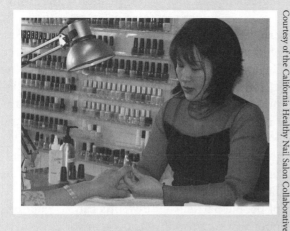

ORGANIZING FOR WORKERS RIGHTS

ANUJA MENDIRATTA AND JULIA LIOU
MEMBERS OF THE CALIFORNIA HEALTHY NAIL
SALON COLLABORATIVE
CAHEALTHYNAILSALONS.ORG

"You can't imagine how many chemicals are being used by workers in nail salons every day," says Connie Nguyen, a former cosmetologist who developed respiratory problems. "Most do not have any knowledge about the health hazards of the product that they're using."

In the United States, the beauty industry is booming and nail salons offering "mani/pedis" are all the rage. Yet little attention has been paid to the impact of occupational exposures on the health of women working in salons. Daily, for long hours, nail salon technicians, most of whom are of reproductive age, handle polishes and other products containing a variety of un-regulated chemicals known or suspected to cause cancer, allergies, respiratory problems, and neurological and reproductive harm. The California Healthy Nail Salon Collaborative is working to raise the profile of this issue, build the capacity of salon workers to advocate for their rights, and advocate for safer salon products, additional research, and greater regulatory protection for the salon sector.

---

and working conditions. If you belong to a union, discuss mobilizing around health issues with your union representative or organizer.

When there is no other recourse, workers may want to consider striking or other job actions organized by a labor union. Class action lawsuits are difficult to win and are usually filed only against large companies that can afford to pay damages, rather than small companies, where many women of color and low-income women work. Unions, COSH groups, and other advocacy groups (see Recommended Resources) can help you decide whether class action is a good strategy for your situation.

ACTION STRATEGIES: IN OUR HOMES AND COMMUNITIES

Protecting our communities starts at home. Many products that we use in our households on a daily basis pose a threat to our health and the health of our neighbors. Scientists are continually presenting new data about harmful health effects stemming from the use of cleaning products, plastics, storage containers, pest control, and other household products. The best way to protect ourselves is to stay informed.

Regardless of what products are on the "most wanted" list from year to year, you can always take precautions by reducing the number of synthetic products you use, by replacing them with homemade cleaners (such as vinegar and baking soda, which are safer and less expensive to use), or by buying brands that are known to be environmentally sensitive and use few synthetic materials. Simply reducing the number and amount of products used in your house can be the greatest step toward reducing exposure.

Some important questions to ask yourself are:

- What are we buying, using, and storing, and how are we disposing of these things?
- What is in our furniture and carpets?
- Is there lead paint on our walls or asbestos wrapping on our hot water pipes?
- How can we test the water, and who is responsible for the local water supply?
- How can we tell if our food is safe, and how can we buy food that is the safest?
- What's in the personal-care products, pesticides, and cleaning supplies that we use?
- How can we get a landlord to clean up a building?

But environmental health goes far beyond the home, and we shouldn't have to fight harmful side effects on our own. Luckily, we don't have to. Thousands of grassroots groups across the country are increasingly concerned about environmental conditions—from polluted water to toxic landfills—and many people are working together to ensure a safer environment. Experienced activists agree on some basic ways to take effective action in our homes and communities.

Be a careful consumer: Read labels. It is important to have access to full disclosure of all ingredients in your food, including the use of growth hormones in dairy products, genetically engineered organisms in fruits and vegetables, and pesticide use on produce and feed given to livestock. However, some of this information is difficult to come by, with companies slipping through loopholes of government regulations. Find out where pollutants come from and what products they're used in, and refuse to buy them. Visit GoodGuide.com to search for products that are healthy and socially responsible. Boycotts are especially effective when networks of people participate. Boycotts can also address poor working conditions of farmworkers.

Investigate environmental conditions: Get information under worker and community right-to-know legislation, and use the online scorecard (scorecard.goodguide.com). Contact groups listed in the Recommended Resources section to learn about workplace and community monitoring and campaigning for preventive measures.

Find out who paid for a study when you obtain or your group obtains information. The answer should help you evaluate the data. Insist that information be presented in terms you can understand, not in scientific jargon. Join with local organizations battling poor environmental and occupational health to learn about what's happening in your community. Share what you learn on Facebook, Twitter, and other social networks.

Talk to your neighbors: Develop labor-neighbor alliances between neighbors and unions around toxic exposure from factories, landfills, and waste shipment. Monitor health concerns, symptoms, and suspected exposure in the community. Conduct a community and workplace health survey. Pay attention to reproductive patterns in your area, such as the number of miscarriages and rate of birth impairments, and to the incidence of cancers. Consider using the research and organizing being done by your local health department and local advocacy groups to connect your observations with the community at large. Contact other groups doing similar work.

Document your health: Keep a log of exposures, symptoms, and diagnoses that you and other family members or housemates have received. The health care providers you see should (but may not) keep an accurate medical and occupational/environmental history. If they don't, ask them to, and ask to see these records every time you visit the doctor. Discuss possible patterns and health concerns stemming from the environment and work.

Work in coalition. Join with other organizations and movements. Don't limit your protest to "not in my backyard"—your efforts will be more effective, just, and inspiring if they don't develop at the expense of others whose resources and power are more limited than yours. Organizations such as the Center for Health, Environment & Justice (chej.org); the Environmental Justice Resource Center at Clark Atlanta University (erjc.cau.edu); the Collaboration on Health and the Environment (healthandenvironment.org); Physicians for Social Responsibility (psr.org); the Toxics Use Reduction Institute (turi.org); and the National Council for Occupational Safety and Health (coshnetwork.org) can advise U.S. grassroots groups about filing legal challenges, conducting surveys, building relationships with sympathetic scientists, getting a company to accept a "neighbors' inspection," and using national data systems and community right-to-know provisions.

The CHEJ also provides workshops for women leaders. Coalitions of environmental, labor, and other social justice groups are pushing beyond right-to-know (the basic right of access to certain information about on-site toxics) and promoting right-to-act (the right to refuse work, change production activity, or enforce an emergency shutdown).

For one of the best collections of ideas, resources, and strategies visit the Women's Health and the Environment website (womenshealthandenvironment.org), a project of Women's Voices for the Earth. Its tool kit has sections on "What We Know: New Science Linking Our Health and the Environment," "What You Can Do: Everyday Actions to Protect Your Health," and "What We Can Do: Community Efforts to Protect Our Health."

WOMEN CHANGING THE WORLD, PROTECTING THE ENVIRONMENT

Taking action is often complicated—there are bureaucracies to fight, chemistry to learn, and the power of polluters to deal with—but it is definitely not impossible. Consider the efforts of these women who exposed environmental health hazards and worked to eliminate them. Each one has left a lasting impact on the world.

Alice Hamilton, who lived from 1869 until 1970, is one of the most significant grandmothers of today's environmental movement. One of the first women physicians, Hamilton is considered the founder of the field of occupational health. She made a home at Jane Addams's Hull House in Chicago, working with immigrant workers facing severe job hazards. Her book *Exploring the Dangerous Trades* revealed how lead affected workers and their children. She helped create workers' compensation, industrial medicine, and justice for workers.

Rachel Carson, whose book *Silent Spring* (1962) exposed the widespread use and dangers of pesticides in our environment. Her research brought this to public attention, led to the U.S. ban on DDT, and helped launch the American environmental movement. Carson's efforts live on through organizations such as the Silent Spring Institute (silentspring.org), an excellent resource for news and studies on environmental health issues and links between the environment and breast cancer.

Lois Gibbs organized the Love Canal Homeowners Association in 1978, forcing New York State to recognize that toxic waste had contaminated the Niagara Falls community. Members did health surveys, signed petitions, confronted officials, picketed, blocked buses, and testified in Washington until the government evacuated one thousand families, bought their homes, and established a safety plan and a health fund to cover future problems. Gibbs now leads the Center for Health, Environment & Justice (chej.org), organized the BE SAFE Campaign for Precautionary Action in support of communities, and frequently testifies before Congress on environmental protection issues.

Hazel Johnson, often called the mother of the environmental justice movement, founded People for Community Recovery (peopleforcommunityrecovery.org) in 1979, when she learned about Southeast Chicago's high cancer rate among African-American women. She documented health problems by going door to door, testified in Congress, and helped to educate and empower her community. Johnson died in early 2011, after many years of leading "toxic tours" of Chicago neighborhoods.

Peggy Shepard, a former journalist, cofounded West Harlem Environmental Action, now WE ACT for Environmental Justice (weact.org), a coalition of young feminists and older neighborhood women, in 1988, to challenge the location of a sewage treatment plant. The group won a sizable settlement and the right to oversee plant remediation. This victory also established a community's right to seek redress of a grievance. She later served as the first female chair of the National Environmental Justice Advisory Council to the U.S. Environmental Protection Agency, and is cochair of the Northeast Environmental Justice Network. Shepard and WE ACT are still doing community-based action,

research, and public education linking health care to environmental justice. She partners with Columbia University's Columbia Center for Children's Environmental Health on its pregnancy and environment project.

Patty Martin was mayor of a small town in Washington state in 1992 when she, along with farmers and neighbors, discovered that hazardous waste was being blended into fertilizers, causing crop failure, environmental damage, and health risks. In 2000, after being targeted by agribusiness and losing her campaign for reelection, Martin founded Safe Food and Fertilizer (safefoodandfertilizer.org); in the fall of 2003, she took the fight to the federal courts. She continues to support the health of farming communities and the food supply.

Sandra Steingraber (steingraber.com) has been an inspiring leader in bringing attention to environmental conditions that impair reproductive health. An ecologist, cancer survivor, and mother, Steingraber wrote a powerful book—*Living Downstream: An Ecologist's Personal Investigation of Cancer and the Environment*—that has been transformed into a film. *Having Faith: An Ecologist's Journey to Motherhood* explores how mothers can care for their children in a toxic world. Her report *The Falling Age of Puberty in U.S. Girls,* written for the Breast Cancer Fund, is another major contribution. In 2006 she was honored with a Hero Award from the Breast Cancer Fund for leadership in preventing environmental causes of breast cancer.

Theo Colborn is influencing the way we look at reproductive health. She has transformed what we know about endocrine disrupting chemicals (EDCs), chemicals that subtly affect our hormonal chemistry and development. Her 1997 book *Our Stolen Future: Are We Threatening Our Fertility, Intelligence, and Survival? A Scientific Detective Story,* cowritten with Dianne Dumanoski and John Peter Meyers, brought this issue to public attention; it has since been translated into eighteen languages. She founded TEDX—the Endocrine Disruption Exchange (endocrinedisruption.com)—where health providers and the general public can learn about the impacts of toxics on reproductive health, pregnancy, and early childhood.

Combating the environmental and health risks in our workplaces, homes, and neighborhoods, as well as trying to make sense of all the un-knowns, is not easy. But more and more of us are building knowledge, working across differences, pushing for answers, and fighting for prevention and for precautionary measures. Women like Loretta Ross, Theo Colborn, and Katsi Cook are urging us to join them in their daily battles. We have nothing to lose and everything to gain—for ourselves, our families, and our communities—by joining them.

TWO ENVIRONMENTAL CRISES THAT INSPIRED ACTION

Looking at past environmental and oc-cupational health disasters helps us to understand the community trauma and dedication that have shaped efforts today to protect public health across the world. Here are brief profiles of two of the most troubling and inspiring lessons.

Love Canal

The story of Love Canal, a neighborhood in Niagara Falls, New York, is one of the most famous instances of environmental contamination in U.S. history, brought to light thanks to the dedication of com-munity activists, principled scientists, and investigative journalists.

Over the early decades of the twenti-eth century, a dried-up canal in Niagara Falls was turned into a municipal and in-dustrial dump site, with more than 21,000 tons of toxic waste buried at the 16-acre site. Desperate for land to serve an ex-panding population, the city bought the plot from Hooker Chemical, the polluter, in 1953 for one dollar. A school was soon built on the property, and by 1957, the city had constructed low-income and single-family residences next to the site. By the 1970s, health problems emerged, with residents reporting birth impairments and high rates of cancer.

Local activism was led by Love Canal resident Lois Gibbs, whose son developed epilepsy, asthma, urinary tract infections, and a low white blood cell count. When she asked for her son to be removed from the school, the city refused. Gibbs's or-ganization, the Love Canal Homeowners Association, conducted a survey of neigh-borhood children and found evidence of elevated rates of birth impairments.[56]

Despite the efforts of activists and concerned parents, Hooker Chemical and the local health department contin-ued to claim that the health concerns were unconnected to the buried waste. After years of continued complaints, the EPA and New York State Department of Health began to take action, with the department finding evidence of an abnor-mal incidence of miscarriage in the area. Pregnant women and children were en-couraged to leave; a state of emergency was declared in 1978.

Tests would later show evidence of 248 separate chemicals, 11 of them suspected carcinogens, in the neighborhood. Dioxin was of particular concern. While usually measured in parts per trillion, at Love Canal, water samples had dioxin levels in parts per billion—a much higher concentration.

Eckardt Beck, an EPA administrator in the 1970s, recalls a visit to the area: "Corroding waste-disposal drums could be seen breaking up through the ground of backyards. Puddles of noxious substances were pointed out to me by the residents. Some of these puddles were in their yards, some were in their basements, others yet were on the school grounds. Everywhere the air had a faint, choking smell. Children returned from play with burns on their hands and faces."[57]

The EPA calls Love Canal "one of the most appalling environmental tragedies in American history." President Carter declared the site a federal health emergency, and this triggered the creation of the federal Superfund legislation, which provides some protections that we didn't have before. It was the women of deep conviction and courage at Love Canal who helped shape the modern struggle for environmental protection and justice in the United States.

Bhopal

In December 1984, the world's worst industrial catastrophe occurred when a pesticide plant owned by U.S.-based Union Carbide Corporation (UCC) and located in the city of Bhopal, India, accidentally leaked methyl isocyanate (MIC) gas and other toxics, exposing more than 500,000 people, including more than 200,000 children. MIC is used to produce the pesticide carbaryl, used primarily as an insecticide. Those exposed immediately experienced coughing, burning eyes, foaming at the mouth, and vomiting, with some suffocating to death as a result of their bronchial passages constricting in reaction to chemical exposure. Long-term effects included chronic respiratory infections, cancers, and reproductive and birth impairments. It is estimated that more than 16,000 people died from gas exposure, either immediately after the disaster or in the years following, with 120,000 to 150,000 becoming chronically ill.[58]

About 3,000 pregnant women were exposed to the gas leak. The Pesticide Action Network UK (pan-uk.org) states, "Among women who were pregnant at the time of the disaster, 43 percent aborted [miscarried]. In the years that followed, the spontaneous abortion rate remained four to ten times worse than the national Indian average. Only 50 percent of prepubescent girls who were exposed to the gas had normal menstrual cycles."

A 2009 study reports that babies in their mother's wombs at the time of exposure exhibited hyperresponsive immune systems.[59] Pregnant women also experienced increased rates of stillbirth and increased infant mortality. Other reproductive health concerns associated with the disaster include early menopause, pelvic inflammatory disease (PID), excessive menstrual bleeding, and suppression of lactation. Children of exposed mothers were born with harelips, cleft palates, cerebral palsy, and misformed limbs, hands, and feet. According to PAN UK, "In spite of persistent demands of women survivor organizations, [the] reproductive health of gas-exposed women continues to be a neglected area in terms of official surveillance, research and therapeutic intervention."[60]

Union Carbide, now owned by Dow Chemical, has evaded responsibility for this tragedy for more than twenty-five years. But an international network of concerned scientists and advocates continue to press for accountability. Dedicated community activists in Bhopal in connection with international groups such as Health Care without Harm (noharm.org) have created the Sambhavna Clinic, using traditional and Western medical approaches to support the recovery of health in the community. People worldwide look to the Bhopal activists for leadership and inspiration in how to take on polluters and how to sustain multigenerational health.

For more information on the Bhopal Medical Appeal, visit bhopal.org. For more information on international coalition and legal strategy, see bhopal.net. To see how UC/Dow tells its story of the disaster, see bhopal.com.

CHAPTER 26 ■ ■ ■ ■ ■ ■ ■ ■ ■ ■ ■ ■ ■ ■ ■ ■ ■ ■

Women are healthier in places where policies promote equal access to health care and education; clean, safe neighborhoods and workplaces; fair and livable incomes; and the power to participate democratically in decisions that affect our lives. In fact, these markers of social and economic equality have significant influence over our health and longevity.[1, 2]

This chapter provides an overview of economic and political trends that shape women's health. The first half looks at the health status of women in the United States, focusing on indicators of sexual and reproductive health. It also addresses U.S. health care reform and the brewing political storms over reproductive health and justice. The second half discusses the status of women's health from a global perspective and looks at how U.S. policy affects women's reproductive and sexual health in developing countries.

WOMEN'S HEALTH IN THE UNITED STATES

By many measures, the health of women in the United States has improved dramatically since the women's health movement began in the late 1960s. Many of the issues that the early women's health movement advocated for have become policy. Abortion is legal, and more research is directed toward women's health issues. Women are now more often health care professionals (accounting for 49 percent of medical school graduates in 2007, compared with 9 percent in 1970) and assertive patients.[3] Women's participation in late-phase clinical trials of new drugs has improved; approximately 50 percent of enrollees are now women, and sex-based data analysis has also improved. We are living longer and enjoying higher incomes, more equal access to resources, and greater independence than earlier generations.

But our lives are still unevenly restricted by race, ethnicity, and class, as well as by gender, sexual orientation, and age. The global economic downturn has fallen most heavily on women, and the problem is compounded by the increasingly uneven distribution of wealth.

Although the United States spends more on health care per person than any other country, it has some of the worst statistics among developed countries for infant mortality, maternal health, unintended pregnancy, and sexually transmitted infections. Acts of harassment, including violence, increasingly obstruct access to family planning and abortion care. Americans are more likely to lack coverage for health care and are in worse health by several measures than citizens of other developed nations.

The Patient Protection and Affordable Care Act (PPACA)—the health care reform bill signed

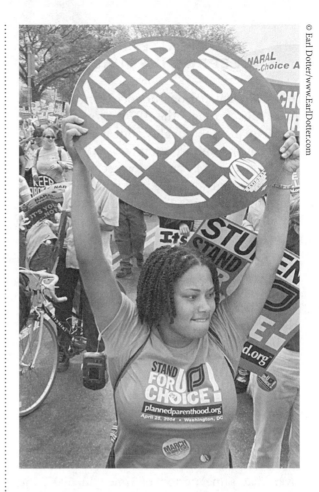

© Earl Dotter/www.EarlDotter.com

into law in 2010—begins to address some of the problems of inadequate coverage and a fragmented health care delivery system. However, the law limits immigrants' rights, and it places new restrictions on our rights to reproductive health care. These setbacks came as a rude shock to many who expected greater support from Democrats when they controlled Congress between 2008 and 2010. Conservative political campaigns continue to use reproductive health care as a divisive wedge issue, waging formidable and concerted attacks on access to family planning, including abortion and contraception.

POLITICAL ECONOMY DEEPENS INEQUALITY

The turbulent periods of social activism from the 1930s through the 1970s won important gains in income equality. But beginning with the Reagan administration in the 1980s, the divide between rich and poor became a chasm. Economic and social policies swung in favor of deregulating corporate practices, cutting public funding for social programs such as education and public health, and draining public reserves with tax breaks for the wealthy and spending on wars.

Between 1947 and 1973, income growth was distributed roughly equally across income classes, with the poorest 20 percent of families seeing income growth at least as fast as the richest 20 percent. But between 1979 and 2005, the trend reversed. Households at the bottom fifth of the income scale saw income growth of just $200 over the entire twenty-six-year period (adjusted for inflation). In contrast, household income grew by almost $6 million for a small number of households in the top 0.1 percent over that same period of time.[4] In 2009, the bottom 20 percent of the population received only 3.4 percent of the aggregate income in the country, while the top 20 percent received a full 50.3 percent of the nation's income.[5]

The administration of George W. Bush manipulated concerns about national security to deflect attention from the virtual abandonment of government oversight and accountability. The global economic crash and the collapse of the U.S. financial sector followed in 2008, resulting in persistent high unemployment, record rates of home foreclosures and personal bankruptcies, and rising health care costs

The election of President Barack Obama in 2008 and the early days of the Obama administration in 2009 brought hope for the restoration of policies based on science and evidence and a new emphasis on equity in shaping economic and social policies that affect women's health. Congress passed the Lilly Ledbetter Fair Pay Act, and the administration's economic stimulus package promised some relief from the cratering economy. But the recession proved difficult to reverse.

ECONOMIC RECESSION DISADVANTAGES WOMEN

Women traditionally have had less financial security than men. Our economic insecurity contributes to worse access to health care and worse health. The sharp economic downturn of 2008 compounded the damage as women lost jobs, income, and health care coverage. Women working full-time in 2009 were paid only 77 cents for every dollar paid to their male counterparts, earning a median salary of $36,278 versus $47,127 for men.[6] Some of this disparity can be attributed to the disproportionate share of economically valuable but unpaid home tasks and child care carried out by women also working outside the home; however, sex discrimination in the workplace and fewer employment options also play critical roles, as does the fact that women on the whole receive lower rates of pay than men for the same work.

The poverty rate among women rose to 14 percent in 2009, the highest rate in fifteen years, versus 10.5 percent for men.[7] The poverty rate is higher among women of color: 25 percent of African-American women were living below the poverty line in 2009, as were 24 percent of Hispanic women.

The recession has been marked by the greatest decline in the number and percent of full-time jobs since 1969. From 2007 to 2010, the number of working women with earnings decreased by 1.3 million (from 74.3 million to 73.0 million). The number of working men with earnings decreased by 2.5 million (from 84.5 million to 81.9 million).

A third of working mothers are the sole family wage earners either because they are single parents or because their spouse is unemployed or out of the labor force. In August 2010, unemployment among single women who head families was 13.4 percent—the highest in more than twenty-five years.

Households headed by single women are particularly vulnerable to poverty: Nearly four in ten single mothers (38.5 percent) lived in poverty in 2009. It is not surprising, therefore, that an increasing number of children are also now living in poverty. In 2009, 1.4 million children fell below the poverty line, bringing the number of poor children in the United States to 15.4 million. Over half of poor children lived with single mothers in 2009, and children now represent 35 percent of all those living in poverty in the United States.

There was one positive development during this period: The poverty rate declined for older Americans, including women sixty-five and older living alone. Poverty among older women living alone dropped to 17 percent in 2009 from 18.9 percent in 2008. This is where Social Security truly acted as a safety net: Without Social Security benefits, an additional 14 million older Americans would have fallen into poverty in 2009.[8, 9]

DISPARITIES IN WOMEN'S HEALTH

There are differences in health status by race and ethnicity that cannot be explained based only on physical or genetic characteristics. These differences are influenced primarily by social and economic inequities and policies, including increased exposures to environmental toxins, lack of access to health care and to education, and residential segregation. Different treatment by health care providers can also play a role. These differences are referred to as disparities.

Health, United States (cdc.gov/nchs/hus .htm) is the federal government's annual report on the population's health, including life expectancy, rates of illness, and major causes of death. It identifies numerous significant differences in health status by race and ethnicity. In most cases, women of color experience worse health than white women, though some aspects of cultures and communities may protect health (Latinas have a lower rate of low birth weight infants than whites, for example).[10] A third of women self-identify as a member of a racial or ethnic minority group, and this share is estimated to increase to more than half by 2045.[11]

Some glaring health disparities based on race or ethnicity include:

- Life expectancy at birth increased for the population as a whole from 1970 to 2007. Life expectancy for black women increased more than that for white women but still consistently lags behind. White women's life expectancy was 80.8 years, up from 75.6, while black women's life expectancy was 76.8 years, up from 68.3.
- The infant death rate among African Americans is more than double that of whites; heart disease death rates are more than 40 percent higher; and the death rate for all cancers is 30 percent higher. African-American women have a higher death rate from breast cancer, despite having a mammography screening rate that is nearly the same as the rate for white women. The rate of new AIDS cases among black women is 55.7 per 100,000, compared with 3.8 for white women.[12]
- Hispanics living in the United States are almost twice as likely to die from diabetes as are non-Hispanic whites, and to have higher

CONFLICTS OF INTEREST

Individuals and institutions with clear conflicts of interest often distort the public debate and media coverage of controversial issues in women's health. One example is the mammography screening controversy in late 2009, when the findings and recommendations of the U.S. Preventive Services Task Force were distorted by the American College of Radiology and the American Cancer Society. For more information, see "Debate Around Breast Cancer Screening Guidelines," p. 591.

A second example is the vehement opposition of the American Congress of Obstetricians and Gynecologists (ACOG) to any state-level proposals that certified professional midwives (CPMs)—who are trained to attend women only in out-of-hospital settings such as the home or freestanding birth centers—be licensed and regulated in order to further increase the safety of planned home birth.

Our Bodies Ourselves and hundreds of experts in the maternity care field have supported such regulation over the past decade and often have collaborated to challenge misleading representations of home birth safety data in both the mainstream press and medical literature. Visit ourbodiesourselves.org/cpm for more information.

A third example is the opposition of many anesthesiologists to the reintroduction of nitrous oxide (N_2O) as a safe and versatile alternative to epidurals for women coping with pain during labor in the hospital setting. All the evidence gathered from both recent and earlier studies points to the extraordinary advantages that N_2O offers, and women in all other advanced industrialized countries are provided with N_2O as an option. Advocates and researchers in the United States are hopeful that current efforts will expand N_2O access beyond the few hospitals that offered it in 2010. For more information, see "Nitrous Oxide," p. 415.

rates of high blood pressure, obesity, and tuberculosis. There are a number of differences among Hispanic populations. For example, the rate of low-birth-weight infants is lower for all Hispanics than for whites, but for Puerto Ricans the low-birth-weight rate is 50 percent higher than the rate for whites.

- The infant death rate among Native Americans and Alaska Natives is almost double and the rate of diabetes is more than twice that for whites. The Pima of Arizona have one of the highest rates of diabetes in the world. Native Americans and Alaska Natives also have disproportionately high death rates from unintentional injuries and suicide.

- Health indicators suggest that Asians and Pacific Islanders, on average, are the healthiest population groups in the United States, although new cases of hepatitis and tuberculosis are higher in these groups than in whites. There is also great diversity within this population group, and health disparities for some specific segments are quite marked. Women of Vietnamese origin, for example, suffer from cervical cancer at nearly five times the rate of white women.

- Tobacco use during pregnancy has declined steadily since 1989 to 10.4 percent in 2007 but varies by race. The rate was highest among Native American/Alaska Native women (24.4 percent) and lowest among Asian/Pacific Islander women (1.5 percent).[13]

There are also health disparities between women and men. For example, women are more likely than men to experience mental health problems, including depression, anxiety, phobias, and post-traumatic stress disorder. In 2008, 40 percent of Native American/Alaska Native women and women of multiple races reported ever having had depression, followed by 36.5 percent of white women.[14]

WOMEN IN THE MILITARY

The proportion of military veterans who are female has increased by more than 25 percent in recent years. More than 1.8 million women were veterans as of 2008, and women are expected to account for 9 percent of the veteran population by 2013. This has raised new issues about women's rights and health status. There has been a high rate of reported sexual assaults on women within the military. At the same time, military health care services are prohibited by law from providing abortions. The majority of new female veterans are of childbearing age and are more likely than female veterans of previous eras to obtain their health care from Department of Veterans Affairs (VA) facilities. Women are expected to account for one in seven enrollees in health programs sponsored by the VA over the next ten years.[15]

DISPARITIES IN MATERNAL AND INFANT HEALTH

MATERNAL HEALTH CARE CRISIS

Far too often, the care women receive during pregnancy and birth is not based on the most reliable research about what is safe and effective. Unnecessary medical and surgical interventions that don't improve outcomes are overused, particularly elective labor inductions and cesarean sections, and practices known to improve maternal and child outcomes and maternal satisfaction are underused. (For more information, see Chapter 15, "Pregnancy and Preparing for Birth.")

According to Amnesty International, the United States spends $86 billion a year on hospital charges related to pregnancy and childbirth, the highest of any single area of medicine. Yet the United States ranks behind forty other countries in a woman's lifetime risk of dying from pregnancy-related complications.[16] In 2007, 548 women died in childbirth in the United States,[17] but complications and near misses push the consequences much higher. According to an Amnesty International report on maternal health:

[The] likelihood of a woman dying in childbirth in the USA is five times greater than in Greece, four times greater than in Germany, and three times greater than in Spain. More than two women die every day in the USA from pregnancy-related causes. Maternal deaths are only the tip of the iceberg. Severe complications that result in a woman nearly dying, known as a "near miss," increased by 25 percent between 1998 and 2005. During 2004 and 2005, 68,433 women nearly died in childbirth in the USA. More than a third of all women who give birth in the USA—1.7 million women each year—experience some type of complication that has an adverse effect on their health.[18]

A combination of lack of affordable, accessible health insurance, lack of comprehensive coverage in some health insurance policies, gaps in access to Medicaid and related programs, and social and economic conditions and citizenship status all contribute to high rates of maternal complications. African-American women are nearly four times more likely to die from pregnancy-related complications than white women; these rates and disparities have not improved in twenty years. According to Amnesty International:

In high-risk pregnancies, the disparities are even greater, with African-American women 5.6 times more likely to die than white women. Among women diagnosed with pregnancy-induced hypertension (eclampsia and pre-eclampsia), African-American and Latina women were 9.9 and 7.9 times more likely to die than white women with the same complications.

Discrimination profoundly affects a woman's chances of being healthy in the first place. Women of color are less likely to begin their pregnancies in good health for a range of reasons including lack of access to primary health care services. They are also less likely to have access to adequate maternal health care services. Compared with white women, Native American and Alaska Native women are 3.6 times, African-American women 2.6 times, and Latina women 2.5 times as likely to receive late or no prenatal care. They are also more likely to experience poorer quality of care, discrimination, or culturally inappropriate treatment.[19]

Melissa Gilliam, an ob-gyn and former chair of the board of the Guttmacher Institute, adds to these factors too few educational and professional opportunities for minority women; unequal access to safe, clean neighborhoods; and, for some African Americans, a lingering mistrust of the medical community.[20]

INFANT MORTALITY

Preterm birth, birth before thirty-seven weeks gestation, is the leading cause of newborn death, and very premature babies (before thirty-two weeks) who survive may suffer lifelong consequences, including cerebral palsy, blindness, and other chronic conditions.[21] The rate of preterm births in the United States improved slightly in 2008, declining to about 12.3 percent, or 523,033 infants.[22]

Preterm birth rates were highest for black infants (18.4 percent), followed by Native Americans (14.2 percent), Hispanics (12.2 percent), whites (11.6 percent), and Asians (10.8 percent).

The causes of preterm births appear to be multifaceted and resist direct or routine medical interventions. According to the March of Dimes, about half of premature births result from spontaneous preterm labor, the causes of which are unknown. One-third of premature births can be attributed to an infection in a woman's uterus, which may not have presented any symptoms. Research is being done to determine if there's a genetic link—if women who were born prematurely may be more likely to deliver early themselves.[23]

Research by physician Michael Lu and others links intergenerational poverty, racism, and social isolation to chronic stress that triggers changes in women's immune and vascular systems, making them more vulnerable to having a preterm birth.[24] Organizations such as HealthConnect One (healthconnectone.org) in Chicago are working to reduce disparities by training and providing assistance to frontline community organizations. HealthConnect One's community-based doula program, for example, focuses on connecting underserved women to women in their community who are specially trained to provide support during pregnancy, birth, and the early months of parenting. Also encouraging is the Centering Pregnancy program in Connecticut, part of the Centering Healthcare Institute (centeringhealthcare.org), which promotes a model of group care that integrates health assessment, education, and support. Both of these peer-to-peer programs are exemplars for improving and promoting women's health.

POLITICIZING REPRODUCTIVE HEALTH

TEEN PREGNANCIES AND SEX EDUCATION

Owing in part to the politicization of reproductive health care, the rates of unintended pregnancies and sexually transmitted infections are also higher in the United States than in virtually every other country with comparable economic and social indicators.

The teen pregnancy rate in the United States dropped 41 percent between 1990 and 2005 (from 116 pregnancies per 1,000 women age fifteen to nineteen to 69.5 per 1,000)—the result of more and better contraceptive use among sexually active teens. Teen birth and abortion rates also declined, with births dropping 35 percent between 1991 and 2005 and teen abortion declining 56 percent between its peak in 1988 and 2005.[25]

Political efforts to limit access to contraceptive methods during the two terms of President George W. Bush led to temporary reversals in these trends. There was heavy investment in sex education programs aimed exclusively at promoting abstinence and prohibited by law from discussing the benefits of contraception. Teens' use of contraceptives declined.[26] In 2006, there was a rise in teen pregnancies (ages fifteen to nineteen) to 71.5 pregnancies per 1,000 women. These trends included sharp reversals in declining teen pregnancy rates among African-

American teens, Latina teens, and non-Hispanic whites.

As a result of the rise in teenage birth rates, many states began to reconsider abstinence-only curricula. In 2007, for example, after receiving nearly $9 million in federal funds for abstinence-only programs, Ohio embraced more comprehensive sex education, becoming the eighth state to reject federal funding dedicated to abstinence-only programs. A congressional investigation found that much of the federally approved abstinence-only curricula included false, misleading, or distorted information about reproductive health.[27]

Teen births declined again in 2009, perhaps in response to new policies and to the recession.[28] However, the new majority in the U.S. House of Representatives of 2011 has announced its intention to revert to the Bush policies.

Another severe example of politics trumping science during the Bush administration was the FDA's refusal to approve over-the-counter (OTC) sale of the emergency contraceptive Plan B, despite encouragement from medical advisory experts. Two FDA officials resigned in protest in 2005 after the FDA announced it would postpone the approval of OTC Plan B indefinitely. One year later, the FDA ruled that Plan B could be sold without a prescription, but only for women over age eighteen. In 2010, the U.S. District Court for the Eastern District of New York ruled that the FDA must lower the OTC cutoff to seventeen and urged the FDA to do away with age restrictions entirely. The government opted not to appeal the decision, thus allowing the cutoff age to be reduced to seventeen in 2011.

Starting in 2010, the U.S. Department of Health and Human Services, under a new administration, divided a five-year, $375 million grant among twenty-eight programs that have been proved to lower pregnancy rates. While some programs are involved in condom dis-

Related Reading: See the chapters on "Un-expected Pregnancy," "Sexually Transmitted Infections," and "Safer Sex."

tribution, others aim to boost teens' scholastic performance and increase their involvement in extracurricular and community activities.

SEXUALLY TRANSMITTED INFECTIONS

Sexually transmitted infections among teens and young adults in the United States are at epidemic proportions. Young people age fifteen to twenty-four account for nearly half of the 19 million new cases of all STIs in the United States each year.[29, 30] Most STIs disproportionately affect women, especially young women, and the burden is most severe among young women of color.

Researchers have found that women in low-income, racially segregated communities with high incarceration rates and limited health care access are most at risk, even when they participate in low-risk sexual activities[31] (see "Who Gets Infected?" on p. 282 for further discussion). Chlamydia, the most commonly reported infectious disease in the United States,[32] is also one of the most underdiagnosed and can lead to pelvic inflammatory disease and infertility. Expanded screening and treatment for this STI would benefit many women.

Human papillomavirus (HPV) infections are the most commonly spread infections. While most HPV infections clear up on their own, some types of the virus can lead to cervical cancer. Pap tests are a highly effective method for early detection of precancer and cervical cancer, but lower-income women have worse access to this common screening test. According to the CDC, in 2008, 69 percent of women defined as poor by federal standards had a Pap test within the previous three years, compared with 79 percent of women whose income was at least twice the poverty level.

New vaccines can prevent infection by the most common types of HPV if girls obtain the shots before they are sexually active. The District of Columbia and dozens of states—many of which have been lobbied by vaccine makers to expand vaccination requirements—have introduced legislation to require, fund, or educate the public about the HPV vaccine.[33] However, since 30 percent of infections are now caused by virus types for which the HPV vaccines do not provide protection, universal access to Pap tests remains critically important. Unfortunately, many girls in underserved communities (where HPV infection rates are often high) have less access to both the Pap test and the HPV vaccine.

For example, as of September 2009, when the CDC released its first state-level statistics for the HPV vaccine Gardasil, only 15.8 percent of girls in the relatively poor state of Mississippi had received the vaccine, compared with 54.7 percent of girls in the relatively wealthy state of Rhode Island. Partly because of greater access to Pap testing, the cervical cancer mortality rate in Rhode Island was already 50 percent lower than in Mississippi—which means the girls in Rhode Island are at much lower risk of contracting HPV to start with.[34]

HIV Infection Rate

African Americans face the most severe burden of HIV in the United States. From 2005 to 2008, the rate of HIV diagnoses among blacks increased from 68 in 100,000 persons to 74 in 100,000—the largest increase in rates of HIV diagnoses during that time of any race or ethnicity.[35] Women account for more than one in four new cases of HIV infection in the United States.

Of these newly infected women, about two out of three are African American.[36]

Approximately one in sixteen black men and one in thirty black women will be diagnosed with HIV at some point in their lives. The HIV prevalence rate for black women (1,122.4 per 100,000) is nearly four times higher than the rate for Hispanic/Latina women (263 per 100,000) and nearly eighteen times higher than the rate for white women (62.7 per 100,000).[37] AIDS is now the leading cause of death for African-American women ages 25 to 34.[38] And as with complications of pregnancy, lack of early detection and lack of access to treatment lead to a rate of death from AIDS-related illnesses among African-American women that is twenty-one times the rate among non-Hispanic white women.

Unprotected sex with an infected partner is the leading cause of HIV infection in women. The CDC cites lack of awareness of HIV status as one issue leading to ineffective efforts at prevention. The CDC and others also underscore that the "socioeconomic issues associated with poverty, including limited access to quality health care, housing, and HIV prevention education, directly and indirectly increase the risk for HIV infection and affect the health of people living with HIV."[39]

U.S. HEALTH CARE SYSTEM

To understand why the economic downturn has greatly reduced women's access to health care, it helps to understand the structure of the U.S. health care system.

The best way to be sure there is enough money to afford care for everyone is to cover everyone. Since everyone needs health care at some point, it is most affordable if everyone chips in, including those who are still healthy. Most other developed countries accomplish this, usually through systems of public and private coverage. They also use the negotiating power of the government to moderate health care prices, such as prices for drugs and for hospital care. They ensure a large supply of primary care services, to lessen the need for expensive specialty care. But the United States has historically done none of these.

The United States spends more than any country on health care, about 16 percent of gross domestic product in 2008. Despite this, it is the only industrialized country where not all residents are automatically covered for health care services. In 2010, close to 51 million Americans did not have health insurance coverage for some time during the year.[40] In 2007, 45 percent of women, compared with 39 percent of men, had been underinsured or uninsured for a time in the past year.[41] Even women with health insurance report problems affording health care. Unaffordable cost-sharing requirements and annual or lifetime limits on covered services have a disproportionate impact on women. More than half (52 percent) of working-age women report problems accessing health care because of costs, compared with 39 percent of men.[42]

Public programs guarantee coverage for some people. The federal Medicare program covers most people age sixty-five and older and people with certain disabilities, and the federal/state Medicaid program covers some of the very poor and disabled. Two public health services that pay for and provide care are the Indian Health Service and the Department of Veterans Affairs (VA). About 44 percent of personal health expenditures are covered by public programs, 36 percent by private insurance, and 16 percent by out-of-pocket payments.

Most people under age sixty-five who have private health insurance receive it through an employer. But there is no law requiring employers to provide coverage. Increasingly, workplace-based health care benefits have become a privilege enjoyed by those in the largest workplaces with the highest-paid employees. Private insurance companies can make money on large groups, where expenses are somewhat predictable, and even more on large groups of healthy people.

But private insurers are reluctant to cover individuals and small groups, because it is difficult to predict who will have an expensive accident or illness. Without a large group of healthy people paying premiums, the insurer can lose out. And insurance companies calculate that if individuals don't have to buy insurance, only people who are already sick will do so. For these reasons, individuals and small employers have the hardest time finding a private insurance company that will agree to cover them, much less one that is affordable and pays claims reliably. In addition, insurance companies spend a lot of money trying to avoid paying claims and to exclude people who already need care—known in insurance-speak as those having a preexisting condition—or who might get sick.

As a result of this dysfunctional system, insurance premiums have risen, and employers have increasingly stopped offering coverage. Widespread job losses have led to equally widespread losses of employer-based health care for those who were fortunate enough to be covered in the first place.

Women are less likely than men to have jobs that offer employment-based private health insurance. This means, for example, that middle-age women who are single, divorced, or widowed and not yet old enough for Medicare are often uninsured. And even under Medicare, the long-term care that many women require is not covered. Women are more likely to be covered by Medicaid than men, owing to rules on eligibility during pregnancy, but the coverage frequently does not continue after the birth of the child. And in states where Medicaid payments are low, many providers do not accept Medicaid patients.

The spiraling cost of health care is attributable in part to administrative costs, which account for 25 percent of private insurance costs, compared with 3 percent in the federal Medicare program. Public systems like Medicare are much more efficient because they cover everyone over age sixty-five, even though older people generally need more health care as they age. Because they are public, they do not make profits. In addition, U.S. drug companies, hospitals, and other providers increase charges annually.[43] Other countries use the power of the government to negotiate with these providers and hold down prices. In the United States, private insurance companies haven't done the job.

AN ECONOMIC CRISIS BECOMES A HEALTH CARE CRISIS

With the economy in decline, funding for many safety net programs, including local nonprofit food and housing programs, has been cut. And as unemployment insurance benefits run out, many of the unemployed have been unable to keep up health insurance payments on their own.

The situation is often worst for those workers who never had employer-based care to begin with. They often cannot even find an insurance plan that will take them, especially if plans detect preexisting conditions, which can include pregnancy and past medical treatment for domestic violence. They usually cannot afford the higher self-paid premiums. Poverty and poor health go hand in hand: An employment crisis becomes a health care crisis, while a health care crisis can drive a family into poverty.

People of color and people with low incomes are the least likely to have stable health insurance coverage. Black women age eighteen to sixty-four are nearly twice as likely to be uninsured as white women, while Hispanic women

WOMEN HEALTH CARE WORKERS

Women account for approximately 80 percent of the health care workforce, an employment sector that includes nurses, nurses' aides, home health care workers, physicians, dental hygienists and assistants, medical assistants, medical secretaries, cleaners, nutritionists, phlebotomists, cafeteria workers, and more. With a few exceptions (such as physicians), most of these jobs are poorly paid.

Minority and immigrant women make up a significant number of those in lower-paying positions. For example, In 2008, African Americans and Hispanics made up 34.5 percent and 13.1 percent, respectively, of nursing, psychiatric, and home health aides.[44] In that year, home health aides earned an average income of $20,850,[45] a salary that is under the poverty line for a family of four.[46]

Occupational hazards shared by women in health care include back injuries due to heavy lifting, exposure to infectious diseases and hazardous chemicals, long hours and shift work, abuse from disturbed or disgruntled patients, and chronic disrespect from higher-up administrative and clinical staff members. In fact, nurses' aides have the highest rate of workplace injuries and illnesses in the country.[49]

In addition to concern for occupation health and hazards, women health care workers must think about their own health care. Nearly 30 percent of all direct-care health workers in the United States lack health coverage themselves.[50] Historically, direct-care health workers have faced enormous struggles obtaining the right to unionize. Some women have found it helpful to contact organizations such as the Service Employees International Union (seiu.org), Jobs with Justice (jwj.org), or National Nurses United (nationalnursesunited.org) for support organizing for better working conditions, salaries, and access to medical coverage.

are almost three times as likely not to have insurance.[47] More than a third of low-income women age eighteen to sixty-four lack health insurance, compared with 18 percent of women overall.

Insurance access—or lack thereof—has a very real impact on health and quality of life. Low-income women are twice as likely as higher-income women to report problems getting health care, such as not filling a prescription, not seeing a specialist when needed, or skipping a recommended medical test, treatment, or follow-up visit.[48] Other women who are more likely to lack health insurance include women who are divorced; who work in service jobs such as waitressing; who work part-time or as temps; or who provide full-time care for children, aging parents, or ill family members.

CONSEQUENCES FOR REPRODUCTIVE HEALTH

The economic decline and loss of health insurance coverage have had negative consequences for reproductive health care. The Guttmacher Institute found that the rate of uninsured women of reproductive age rose faster—and was significantly higher—than the rate for the U.S. population overall.[51] The share of women age fifteen to forty-four who were covered by private (mostly employer-based) insurance fell 4 percentage points between 2008 and 2009, from nearly 39 million to only 36.7 million. In 2009, 22.3 percent of all women of reproductive age were uninsured and 14.8 percent were covered by Medicaid, compared with 20.1 percent and 13.2 percent, respectively, in 2008. The analysis further noted:

[These] bleak new data confirm previous Guttmacher research on the severe impact of the recession. In 2009, we documented that because of economic hardship, nearly half of low- and middle-income women wanted to delay pregnancy or limit the number of children they have, but that many had to skimp on their contraceptive use—or forgo it entirely—to save money. We also found that publicly funded family planning providers were struggling to meet a growing need for subsidized contraceptive care, even as they had to make do with fewer resources.

Taken together, Guttmacher concludes, "the evidence paints a grim picture of fast-growing numbers of women struggling to afford contraceptives at a time when many say they can least afford to have a child (or an additional child)."

Yet while these data all underscore the critical importance of publicly funded family planning clinics as a crucial safety net for women who cannot otherwise afford the services and supplies they need to prevent an unintended pregnancy, those very services have become increasingly politicized.

HEALTH CARE REFORM AND THE POLITICS OF WOMEN'S HEALTH

In March 2010, President Obama signed the Patient Protection and Affordable Care Act

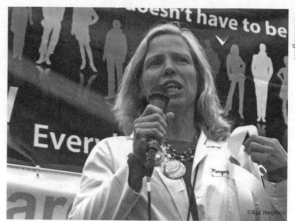

Dr. Margaret Flowers speaks at a 2009 rally sponsored by the "Mad-as-Hell Doctors," in Washington, D.C. Dr. Flowers is the Congressional Fellow of Physicians for a National Health Program, where she works on single-payer health care reform.

(PPACA) into law. The act aims to expand health care coverage to 32 million uninsured Americans, mostly those who are locked out of the private insurance market because they are not part of a large group, already have a health condition, or can't afford coverage. They will be eligible either for the public Medicaid program or for new, private insurance options.

The PPACA proposes to make insurance affordable through a combination of cost controls, subsidies, and mandates. It is estimated to cost $848 billion over a ten-year period, but the cost would be fully offset by new taxes and revenues and was projected on signing to actually reduce

Related Reading: For more discussion on how health care reform affects women and how to obtain the care you need, see Chapter 23, "Navigating the Health Care System."

the U.S. budget deficit by $131 billion over the same period. It also has separate provisions intended to stabilize and improve the federal Medicare program for seniors and people with disabilities. Some of the provisions are of particular importance to women. The program is being challenged by the Republican majority in the House of Representatives and in the courts. The following describes the law as enacted.

EXPANSION OF COVERAGE

Three provisions on coverage went into effect immediately in 2010: Small employers can get tax credits for providing insurance to their employees; young adults can remain covered on their parents' plans until age twenty-six if they are not covered through their own jobs; and new, temporary "high risk pool" plans, called the Pre-Existing Condition Insurance Plan (PCIP), became available for people who have been uninsured for at least six months owing to a preexisting condition (this plan will close when the health insurance exchanges open in 2014). Other provisions are outlined below.

Insurance exchanges for individuals and small employers: Beginning in 2014, new state-run health insurance exchanges will be available to individuals and employees of small businesses. (People already covered by Medicare or other insurance will not be affected.) The exchanges will offer choices of insurance plans with regulated benefits and premiums. Most uninsured individuals and some businesses will be mandated to pay into the exchanges; people earning up to 400 percent of the poverty limit will get subsidies. Members of Congress and their staffs will be required to obtain their insurance through the exchanges.

Medicaid and the Children's Health Insurance Program: The act maintains current funding levels for the Children's Health Insurance

Program (CHIP) through fiscal year 2015. It also expands eligibility for Medicaid to include everyone with an income below 133 percent of the federal poverty level and increases assistance to states to help cover the costs of adding people under Medicaid, as of 2014. The majority (69 percent) of adult beneficiaries of Medicaid are female.

This expansion removes two present barriers to Medicaid eligibility: First, some states cover only people with much lower incomes, such as by cutting off eligibility at 50 percent of the federal poverty level. Second, some states require "categorical eligibility," meaning that in addition to having low income, people must fall into certain categories of need—have young children, for example, or certain serious health conditions.

Medicaid is the largest source of public funding for family planning services for low-income women, as well as the largest funder of maternity services. Twelve percent of women of reproductive age rely on Medicaid for their care; the percentage ranges from 6 percent of women in Nevada and New Hampshire to 24 percent of women in Maine.[52] Expansion of Medicaid services means an expansion of critical family planning and contraceptive services for women, one reason that increased access to health care helps reduce the number of unintended and un-

> **Recommended Resources:** For excellent summaries and expert analysis on health care reform visit these organizations:
>
> - EQUAL Health Network: equalhealth.info
> - Raising Women's Voices: raisingwomensvoices.net
> - National Women's Law Center: nwlc.org
> - Kaiser Family Foundation: kff.org

wanted pregnancies. Expanding access to these services and to community health centers generally will also dramatically increase access to testing and treatment for sexually transmitted infections.

CONSUMER PROTECTIONS

Preexisting conditions: The act prohibits insurance companies from denying coverage to people because of preexisting conditions. The prohibition applied immediately to children; adults will be protected starting in 2014.

Elimination of annual and lifetime limits: A key cause of bankruptcy by individuals even though they have insurance is the annual and lifetime limits some plans imposed on how much insurers would pay. The lifetime limits were eliminated in 2010; annual limits will be eliminated in 2014.

Elimination of gender rating: Many individual and small group insurance plans charge women more for insurance coverage than men of the same age and health status. The act eliminates this practice for plans offered through the exchanges.[53]

Limits on age rating: Plans in the exchanges will be able to charge older people only three times more than younger ones; there is currently no limit, and many individual plans charge older enrollees up to seven times more. This does not apply to Medicare, which does not use age rating.

No referrals for ob-gyn and midwifery care: Plans can no longer require preauthorization or referrals for ob-gyn care.

QUALITY IMPROVEMENTS AND LOWER COSTS

To improve quality and lower costs, the law mandates the following:

Free preventive care: The act requires new private plans and Medicare to cover preventive services with no co-payments or deductibles. This dramatically expands women's access to screening for cervical and breast cancer and other forms of preventive reproductive and sexual health care.

Increased funding for community health centers and primary health care: The act increases funding by $11 billion over five years to these partly publicly supported neighborhood clinics in underserved areas, known to offer high-quality primary care and often dental and other services. This will allow for nearly double the number of patient visits over the next five years. This funding went into effect in fiscal year 2010 and is an essential aspect of health care, particularly for low-income women and their families.

Improvements to Medicare, long-term care: The law creates a number of programs critical for older women. Several initiatives will explore and evaluate programs to improve the quality of care through Medicare. One goal is to ensure that health care professionals and systems will have the evidence about the best medical treatments and incentives to practice accordingly.

The law also expands community-based options for long-term care. These programs are especially important for women, as they live longer than men. There are also improvements to the prescription drug program (Medicare Part D), including phasing out of the gap in coverage known as the "donut hole." For more information, see "Medicare Basics," p. 569.

Time for mothers to express breast milk: The act amended the Fair Labor Standards Act (FLSA), giving breastfeeding mothers in all fifty states the right to pump at work. The act requires that employers provide a reasonable—though unpaid—break time for an employee to express breast milk for her nursing child for up to one year after the child's birth, whenever the employee has need to express milk.

WHERE THE ACT FALLS SHORT

The law is under attack from the U.S. Chamber of Commerce and parts of the insurance industry that oppose expanding population-wide benefits and oppose almost all forms of government involvement and oversight. Congress is proposing to reverse or at least chip away at elements of the reform.

In addition, there are concerns about whether the combination of regulations and delivery system reforms will effectively control costs. State and federal regulators have some new powers to control health insurance premiums. The law did not adopt popular proposals to offer a public option through the insurance exchanges. Our Bodies Ourselves has long supported proposals for publicly financed systems such as H.R. 3000, sponsored by U.S. Representative Barbara Lee (D-Calif.), which would provide affordable care to every resident and could effectively use the public sector's bargaining power to control health care prices. (See the sidebar on single-payer proposals, p. 778.)

Two explicit exclusions are additionally significant for women: the exclusion of some immigrants, and restrictions on abortion and contraceptives.

Coverage for immigrant women: According to the National Latina Institute for Reproductive Health (NLIRH), the Patient Protection and Affordable Care Act "will cover an estimated 9 million uninsured Latinos and increase funding for community health centers, which is a lifeline for many in our neighborhoods. In addition, 4.4 million Americans in Puerto Rico and territories will receive $6.3 billion in new Medicaid funding, increased flexibility in how to use fed-eral funding, access to the Exchange and $1 billion in subsidies for low-income residents." [54]

At the same time, immigrant women, a highly vulnerable population, will continue to face high barriers to accessing basic health care. The act bars undocumented immigrants from receiving Medicaid or from enrolling in health insurance exchanges. About half of the nation's 12 million immigrants would be excluded. This is a human rights violation and bad public health policy.

The bill also imposes a five-year waiting period on permanent, legal residents before they are eligible for assistance such as Medicaid or subsidies for purchasing insurance through the exchange.

Threats to abortion and contraception care: The law took several significant swipes at reproductive health care. Advocates are exploring options to ameliorate the impact of each provision, while opponents seek to tighten these limits. The main provisions, which concern limits on access to abortion and prescription contraceptive services, are covered in more detail below.

THE POLITICS OF REPRODUCTIVE RIGHTS

Owing to the combination of well-funded and sometimes violent opposition and a diffuse political defense, the issue of abortion has become increasingly stigmatized over the past several decades. As a result, women's health in general—an issue relevant to more than half the population—has become a hot-button issue.

During the 1980s, conservatives focused their efforts on a crusade to limit and ultimately strip women of their rights to sexual and reproductive health services both at home and abroad. This agenda has been used to win support for conservative, pro-corporate political candidates, whose economic and financial interests otherwise have little in common with many of the voters who elect them. President Reagan (who, as governor of California, approved a law in 1967 liberalizing access to abortion[55]) instituted the so-called global gag rule, which mandates that no U.S. family planning assistance can be provided to nongovernmental organizations that use funding from other sources to perform abortions in cases other than when a pregnancy poses a threat to the woman's life or is a result of rape or incest; or that use other funding to provide counseling and referral for abortion; or that lobby to make abortion legal or more available in their country. (See p. 785 for more on the global gag rule.)

This battle continued during the 1990s, with court challenges and local and state initiatives. However, the Clinton administration did not support restraints on reproductive health and promptly overturned the global gag rule. Then came the administration of George W. Bush, which cooperated with strategies of the far right to support candidates at the local, state, and national levels representing extreme anti–abortion rights agendas. Antichoice advocates aimed to control the public dialogue around sex and reproduction through aggressive messaging strategies based on the spread of misinformation while continuing efforts through the executive branch, federal and state legislatures, and the courts to hinder gains in reproductive and sexual health policies and programs.

One legislative legacy that has had far-reaching implications is the Hyde Amendment. First adopted in 1976, it prohibits using U.S. federal funds to pay for abortions in programs administered through the Departments of Labor and Health and Human Services, including Medicaid. Exceptions are granted in cases of rape or incest, or a threat to the woman's life. The Hyde Amendment is not permanent law; it is an amendment to a federal appropriations bill specific to those two federal departments, and

it must be reintroduced for consideration during every two-year session of Congress. Yet over the years, the Hyde Amendment's restrictions have been included in an ever-wider range of programs—for instance, abortions are no longer covered for any federal employee or members of the military. This is exceptional treatment of a legal and common medical procedure.

U.S. POLICY IN THE OBAMA YEARS: FROM RELIEF TO RETRENCHMENT

The ongoing debate over the health care reform law underscores the formidable political obstacles to women's health and equality in the United States. In 2009, President Obama and the Democratic-controlled Congress increased funding for evidence-based teen pregnancy prevention programs. They also revived a long-stalled authorization for the State Children's Health Insurance Program. The Justice Department awarded $127 million to Native American and Alaskan Native communities, in part to enhance law enforcement and better serve women who have been sexually assaulted. Benefits were extended to same-sex partners of federal employees, and restrictions were lifted on federal funding for embryonic stem cell research. And President Obama overturned the global gag rule, yet again. The pro–reproductive rights public was optimistic that its champions had regained legitimacy.

But the far right engaged in a sustained and angry assault on Democrats generally—and the president in particular—throughout efforts to pass health care reform, extend unemployment benefits, and bolster the economy. These attacks escalated the war on women at both the state and the federal levels, posing the greatest threats to our reproductive and sexual rights since before the Supreme Court decision on *Roe v. Wade* legalized abortion in 1973.

What stunned advocates was not just the

losses, but the perception that abortion had been expendable from the beginning of negotiations on the law. Women could not rely on a vigorous defense from any power bloc. It seemed that reproductive rights and justice had been "thrown under the bus"—leading the Women's Media Center to respond with an online health care campaign called Not Under the Bus.

In part, this was the culmination of years in which advocates and elected officials generally refrained from a full-court defense of reproductive rights. Whether afraid to speak out or bowing to pragmatism, Democrats routinely failed to present a united front in countering attacks on abortion, and they abandoned attempts to win the argument. Instead, they opted for so-called common ground strategies, seeking to prevail by accommodating anti–abortion rights positions and candidates.

As a result, the Patient Protection and Affordable Care Act includes a series of explicit limits on coverage for abortion and contraception including the following.

Limits on federal funding for abortions through the exchanges: The act requires every enrollee—female or male—in a health plan offered through the new exchanges that include abortion coverage to make two payments. One of these payments would go to pay the bulk of the premium; the other would go to pay the share of the premium that would ostensibly cover abortion care. The basis for this provision is to ensure that women who receive federal subsidies to help pay for the premium cannot use federal funds for an abortion.

This language was included at the insistence of a bloc of Democratic members of Congress, led by Sen. Ben Nelson of Nebraska, whose votes were needed for passage, since Republicans vowed uniformly to oppose the act. Analysts are concerned that the law will jeopardize coverage for abortion care—even for policies paid for with private dollars—because the administrative complexities for insurance companies may discourage them from offering abortion coverage.

This provision was underscored by President Obama when he signed an executive order on March 24, 2010, after the act was passed, emphasizing that no federal dollars would be used to pay for abortion through the newly created health insurance exchanges or through community health centers, except in the case of rape, incest, or a threat to the life of the mother. This order codifies in statute the limitations on using federal funds to pay for abortions imposed by the Hyde Amendment, described above, and includes the same exceptions. However, the executive order will outlast any two-year renewal of the Hyde Amendment.

Limits on coverage for abortion through new temporary health insurance programs, known as the Pre-Existing Condition Insurance Plan (PCIP): The act created the temporary Pre-Existing Condition Insurance Plan (PCIP), which will provide insurance to high-risk pools of citizens. PCIP is a federally authorized, state-administered health insurance plan that must accept any individual who has been uninsured for at least six months and who has a preexisting health condition. Enrollees, who would pay a premium, are usually low income and would benefit from immediate care. Since the women entering PCIP have experienced serious enough medical conditions that insurers have been unwilling to sell them insurance, they're at a heightened risk for needing an abortion for health reasons should they become pregnant. PCIP is set to be disbanded in 2014, when the insurance exchanges become operational.

On July 14, 2010, the Department of Health and Human Services issued an interim final rule stating that abortion would not be covered by PCIP except in the cases of rape or incest, or where the life of the woman would be endangered. This order again codifies in statute the limitations on using federal funds to pay for abortions that are imposed by the Hyde Amendment—and it went beyond any expected restrictions on coverage in PCIP. The act itself didn't mandate such restrictions for PCIP, and the Nelson Amendment, described above, applied only to the new health insurance exchanges, which start in 2014.

It was "a whoosh moment" for reproductive rights advocates, said Jill Adams, director of Law Students for Reproductive Justice. The reality sank in that reproductive rights had become truly politically precarious. EQUAL Health Network fellow Keely Monroe and codirector Ellen Shaffer argued that the provisions should be reversed, noting that the administration's decision "would create new restrictions on abortion not already mandated by federal law, and elevate its status as a policy." [56]

Shaffer also noted, "We wrote off earlier compromises as part of the price for health care reform, to be fixed down the road. The road has come to our door. A procedure experienced by at least a third of women during our lives, abortion has become stigmatized, a toxic issue. It is not enough to appoint and elect many fine, smart, progressive women—and pro-choice men—to government. They and we need militant mobilized advocacy for reproductive choice and justice." [57]

Prescription contraceptives not covered under preventive health services: The act calls for preventive services to be covered at no cost to the patient, but the list of covered services is determined by the U.S. Preventive Services Task Force. Bowing to political pressure from the U.S. Conference of Catholic Bishops and others, the Obama administration called for a panel appointed by the Institute of Medicine to determine whether contraceptives are indeed preventive and related to health. Should the panel so decide, women will be able to use the benefit starting in 2012.

In addition, the law includes conscience-clause language that protects only individuals or entities that refuse to pay for or provide coverage for an abortion, or even refer for abortion, removing earlier language that provided balanced nondiscrimination language for those who provide a full range of choices to women in need.

Women's groups saw this as a major loss, and advocates seek to reverse all of these provisions.

ONGOING THREATS

After the Republican gains in the 2010 midterm elections, the 112th Congress opened in 2011 with more than forty-five additional anti–abortion rights legislators in the U.S. House of Representatives and five in the Senate. They immediately introduced legislation to further restrict access to and funding for abortion and family planning services, and efforts are likely to include reinstating (and making permanent) the global gag rule. [58]

Meanwhile, women are facing an increased number of restrictions at the state level. In a 2010 report detailing major trends in anti-abortion legislation and abortion restrictions enacted at the state level, the Center for Reproductive Rights noted that five states had already passed bans on insurance coverage of abortion care, even with premiums paid with private money. [59]

Other states are considering a similar ban. As of early 2011, thirty-two states have enacted laws subjecting women to mandatory delays and/or biased counseling. Such counseling requires that abortion providers give their patients materials developed by the state, including pictures of fetal development and information about alternatives to abortion. These materials may contain medically inaccurate and misleading information about health risks.

"For women who have unwanted pregnan-

Related Reading: For more information on restrictive state and federal legislation and obstacles to access, see "History of Abortion in the United States," p. 337; and "Organizing for Change: Reproductive Health and Justice," p. 813.

cies or who have been victims of rape, incest, or abuse, these requirements can also result in unnecessary emotional suffering," Amie Newman wrote at RH Reality Check. "These bills also interfere with the doctor/patient relationship, forcing physicians to give each woman 'one size fits all' treatment, instead of allowing the physician to treat each patient individually according to his or her professional judgment."[60]

Another among the numerous trends to limit access to abortion—as well as contraception—is the effort to confer "personhood" on fertilized eggs. Ballot initiatives have been attempted in Colorado, Montana, and Nevada, and while they have been defeated, proponents of these laws, who state unequivocally that they aim to ban contraception as well as abortion, continue to push for such measures. As the Center for Reproductive Rights notes, these initiatives to define personhood from the moment of conception would in fact ban many forms of contraception and some reproductive technologies such as in vitro fertilization.

THE FUTURE OF HEALTH CARE REFORM

By 2014, when the most sweeping health insurance reforms will take effect, there will be an unprecedented expansion of Medicaid and a new federal tax credit to make health insurance more affordable for low- and moderate-income fami-

lies. The Congressional Budget Office estimates that by 2019, 32 million people will have secured health insurance coverage under the new law, as long as Congress continues to support and fund health care reform.

As women's health advocates have noted, the PPACA is not a single-payer system and does not even include a public option. However, it opens the door to states that seek to experiment with single-payer plans; broadens policy space to move further toward universal coverage; and takes steps in the right direction by expanding public sector programs such as Medicaid and aiming to reduce administrative waste.[61]

The Obama administration, elected on a wave of voter mobilization, succeeded in enacting a historic health care reform law, as well as numerous other achievements. But it has yet to generate the momentum for a comprehensive economic and political movement to transform access to and equality of health care and other social services. We must continue to advocate for policies that take into account the needs of all women.

WOMEN'S HEALTH AROUND THE GLOBE

ECONOMICS, EDUCATION, AND WOMEN'S HEALTH

Gender relations of power constitute the root causes of gender inequality and are among the most influential of the social determinants of health.

> —Gita Sen, Piroska Östlin, Asha George, Women and Gender Equity Knowledge Network

Women's health is no less contested in other regions of the world than in the United States, but the politics surrounding women's health in the United States, especially related to sexual and re-

WHY OUR BODIES OURSELVES ENDORSES SINGLE-PAYER HEALTH CARE

Single-payer models build on systems like Medicare. They are publicly financed, instead of being administered through private insurance plans, and cover everyone. One single payer—the government—replaces the many private insurance plans that now waste billions on administration. Even more important, it gives the government the authority to negotiate prices with drug companies, hospitals, and other health care providers, the key to controlling costs while protecting care.

Our Bodies Ourselves has supported single-payer proposals since they were first introduced in Congress in the 1970s, including H.R. 3000, sponsored by Representative Barbara Lee (D-Calif.). It remains the only plan that explicitly includes women's reproductive health services, including abortion.

We believe these plans would best address women's needs and improve our health. Coverage would be completely independent from employment and from marriage. The plans would better allocate resources and reduce payment incentives that have been obstacles to investing in training more primary care professionals and that lead to overuse and misuse of drugs and medical procedures.

Other specific advantages of a single-payer system include the following.

It would encourage better care for chronic illnesses: Women use chronic care services far more than men. Because caring for people with chronic disease now accounts for more than 75 percent of all health care spending, women will benefit substantially from more efficient and effective ways to deal with severe chronic illnesses.

It would eliminate substandard tiers of care: Women who are unemployed and have functional limitations that exclude them from the private health insurance market would receive health and medical care on a par with women in general.

It would address the cost issues that send women into debt and bankruptcy: Medical debt is an enormous concern for many women. A 2009 Commonwealth Fund study found that 45 percent of women accrued medical debt or reported problems with medical bills in 2007 compared with 36 percent of men.[62]

It would reduce the incidence of medical malpractice: Assuring people they would not have to worry about paying for medical care if they experienced bad medical outcomes would relieve the pressure on medical malpractice premiums.

A single-payer system would enhance the working environment for health care professionals: There would be less need to spend hours on pointless documentation in order to justify billing for services.

For more information, visit ourbodies ourselves.org/singlepayer.

productive health and rights, have an impact on women beyond our national boundaries. This section discusses some of the major challenges to women's health and rights internationally, focusing particularly on sexual and reproductive health in developing countries.

LIFE EXPECTANCY AND SOCIAL DETERMINANTS

Women's health status varies greatly depending on socioeconomic status, class, race, ethnicity, and education. The same, of course, can be said of men. However, the intersection of gender inequality with social determinants and race has a profound effect on women's physical and mental health, as well as the health practices women are exposed to and the care they are able to access. Together, these social factors may play a far greater role in a woman's health and life expectancy than innate physical well-being.

In many societies, women are less likely to have educational opportunities and to be literate than men. They often lack decision-making power within the household, as well as in the community. The extent to which women have freedom of mobility and can make autonomous decisions has a great impact on their ability to seek health care and on their sexual and reproductive health.[63]

A woman's life expectancy at birth averages eighty-six years in Japan, eighty-three years in western and southern Europe and Canada, eighty in the United States, seventy-five in Saudi Arabia, seventy-two in Southeast Asia, fifty-three in sub-Saharan Africa, and forty-four in Afghanistan.[64, 65] While this great variation is influenced by a country's income and wealth and how evenly that wealth is distributed, life expectancy, especially for women, is also powerfully influenced by sexual and reproductive health and the accessibility of health care services.

For example, a woman in sub-Saharan Africa has a 1 in 22 chance of dying of causes related to pregnancy and childbirth over the course of her reproductive life, compared with a 1 in 5,900 lifetime risk for a woman in the developed world.[66] In Africa, after years of slow improvement, life expectancy for women in eleven countries has fallen below fifty years, largely owing to the impact of HIV/AIDS. Although women have longer life expectancy than men in most of the world, when diseases related to sexual and reproductive health are considered, women are 2.2 times more likely to experience disability-adjusted life years lost (DALYs) than men.[67]

Life expectancy is also related to whether economic resources have been used to provide basic public health services, such as safe drinking water and sanitation; basic or primary-level health care, including immunizations, antenatal care, and well-child programs; and education at least through the primary level to ensure literacy.

CONNECTION BETWEEN EDUCATION AND FAMILY PLANNING

Access to education has a powerful effect on a woman's ability to exert more control over personal choices, including whether and when to have children. Better-educated women are more likely to delay childbearing, and literate mothers are better able to care for their children. Policies that promote the education of girls and women therefore lead to reductions in the birth and infant mortality rates, as well as improved health for women and for the community as a whole. Women with more education will generally have fewer children than women with less education, regardless of economic status. Education alone, however, does not guarantee a woman's autonomy to make decisions, even regarding her own health and that of her children. An oppressive fundamentalist regime, for example, can make educational gains irrelevant for women, curtailing mobility, access to contraception, and safe abortion and increasing her vulnerability to gender-based violence. War and sustained civil conflicts can destroy any opportunity for economic advancement. In other words, knowledge is power only when we have the opportunity to use it.

THE EFFECTS OF THE GLOBAL ECONOMY

As economies become more integrated and with the rise of capitalist economic development, women's education levels are rising, and more women are joining the ranks of the formal labor force. These processes are enabling women to live longer, but they are also changing the health risks that women face on a global level. Breast cancer is by far the most common form of cancer in the world, with an estimated 1.3 million new cases in 2008, and it is the second leading cause of cancer deaths, topped only by lung cancer.[68] Cancer was once thought of as primarily a disease of the wealthy, but the majority of cancer cases now occur in developing countries.

Changes in lifestyles, such as eating more overall and eating more processed foods, often come along with the other changes brought about by globalization, and these factors are contributing to increases in obesity, diabetes, and heart disease among women. Women in most countries tend to smoke less than men, but women are increasingly being targeted by transnational tobacco companies as a potential growth market.[69]

In the past, businesses anchored in particular countries perceived a benefit in providing financial support for education, public health, and roads and other infrastructure. As businesses circle the globe seeking the lowest wages and the least restrictive governments, this social contract is under fire, as are public funding and public accountability for services.

Global trade agreements increasingly play a role in determining critical national policies that affect health—from sustainable economic development to the prices and availability of pharmaceuticals and health care and the rights of public health authorities to regulate the safety of food and to reduce harm from tobacco and alcohol products. Campaigns are focusing on expanding the availability of generic drugs, which cost less than patented brand-name drugs, and to involve health concerns directly in trade policy and negotiations.[70]

RECOMMENDED RESOURCES: GLOBAL GENDER NEWS

- **Interagency Gender Working Group** (igwg.org) and its listserv provide near-daily updates of gender news, publications, and events. The IGWG promotes gender equity within population, health, and nutrition programs with the goal of improving reproductive health/HIV/AIDS outcomes and fostering sustainable development.
- **Women Watch** (un.org/womenwatch), a joint United Nations project, provides UN system-wide news and resources on gender equality issues.

MATERNAL HEALTH AND WELL-BEING

BIRTH RATES AROUND THE GLOBE

As more women have secured access to contraception to avoid unwanted pregnancies, fertility has fallen to an average of 2.5 lifetime births per woman. However, this global birth rate average

THE MILLENNIUM DEVELOPMENT GOALS AND THE POLITICS OF WOMEN'S HEALTH

In 2000, 189 countries agreed to a set of eight Millennium Development Goals (MDGs; un.org/millenniumgoals) aiming to reduce poverty and hunger and improve health, gender equity, and environmental sustainability. The MDGs were an important global milestone not only because of their near universal buy-in, but because they are evidence based and provided specific targets to be reached within a fifteen-year timeframe, and are being carefully monitored. Millennium Development Goal 5 specifically calls for a 75 percent reduction of 1990 maternal mortality levels by 2015.

While only a few countries are on track to reach this goal, recent estimates show that the maternal mortality rate has declined in a number of countries after years of stagnation, and the focus of the MDGs on maternal health has served as a rallying cry in the past decade for activists and policy makers to secure long-overdue global attention to an underfunded challenge.

However, conservative political forces in the United States and abroad were still able to limit women's reproductive rights through initially excluding universal access to reproductive health care from the framework of the Millennium Development Goals. This occurred despite preexisting international agreements in support of reproductive health and rights from the 1994 International Conference on Population and Development and the 1995 World Conference on Women, a reminder that decisions made about women's health in the United States have far-reaching consequences for women's access to health care around the globe. Only through tenacious advocacy was a new target for reproductive health added to MDG 5 for maternal health in 2007. Target 5b, as it is known, aims to achieve universal access to reproductive health care including family planning by 2015.[72]

---

masks stark disparities. In the United States, where 79 percent of married women use contraception, women give birth to an average of two children. (Differences by race, ethnicity, and religion are fairly small; white women have an average of 1.8 children, compared with 2.1 children for black women and Asian/Pacific Islanders, and a high of 3.1 children for Latinas.) Women in Africa have the most children, 4.6, while women in Europe have the least, 1.5.[71]

In sub-Saharan Africa as a whole, fewer than one-fourth of married women use contraception. The average woman gives birth to 5.2 children, with large variations within and between countries. For example, in Niger, only 11 percent of women use a method of contraception, and women have on average more than seven births each.

In Europe, where 70 percent of married women use contraception, birth rates have fallen below replacement level (2.1 births per woman) in all but a few countries.[73] A number of European countries now offer financial incentives to encourage women and families to have more children and supportive workplace policies aim to make childbearing more compatible with remaining in the workforce. Women in the United Kingdom take thirty-nine weeks of maternity leave, of which ten weeks are paid, while Estonia provides twenty-nine weeks of paid leave. Iceland and Sweden each provide more than ten weeks of paid paternity leave. Conversely, neither the United States nor Australia provides paid maternity leave.[74]

Some of these policies are paying off, as evidenced by slower declines in the birth rate or even small increases, as seen in Norway, France, and Sweden. However, experts do not expect that these pronatalist policies will cause the birth rate to rise above replacement level.[75] Still, such policies have made an impact on gender equality in wages and labor force participation.[76]

MATERNAL MORTALITY

In 2008, an estimated 358,000 maternal deaths occurred around the world, a 34 percent decline from 1990 levels. Although significant, this decline is not sufficiently rapid to reach the target of a three-quarters reduction within the time frames of the Millennium Development Goals.[77] While in developed countries such as Sweden, as few as 5 women die per 100,000 live births (the rate is 11 per 100,000 in the United States), in some sub-Saharan African countries, as well as in Afghanistan, nearly 1,400 women die per 100,000 live births. Six countries account for more than 50 percent of all maternal deaths: India, Nigeria, Pakistan, Afghanistan, Ethiopia, and the Democratic Republic of the Congo. Overall, 99 percent of all maternal deaths occur in developing countries, and this differential is the largest single public health disparity between low- and high-income countries.[78]

The leading causes of maternal death include hemorrhage, hypertensive disorders such as eclampsia, infections, and unsafe abortions, but there are geographic variations. For example, hemorrhage is most common in Africa and Asia, while hypertensive disorders and unsafe abortion are leading causes in Latin America and the Caribbean.[79] Most maternal deaths result from preventable causes and could be averted if societies placed a higher value on women's lives, enabled women to avoid unwanted pregnancies, and provided more and better-quality prenatal and maternity care, including emergency obstetric care as well as postnatal care, including access to family planning.

Skilled attendance at birth is a critical step to protecting women's lives—trained professionals can manage complications and identify when women in labor or postpartum require higher levels of care—but access to skilled birth attendants is extremely unequal in many developing countries.[80] Only 6 percent of all births in Ethiopia are attended by a trained professional, yet that number disguises wide disparities according to wealth: 30 percent of births to wealthy women are attended by a professional, as compared with only 1 percent of births among the poorest women.[81]

Often unacknowledged in the focus on reducing maternal deaths is the extent of illness and disability that can result from obstetric complications. Severe complications, such as those requiring admission to an intensive care unit, may occur in anywhere from almost 1 percent to more than 8 percent of births.[82] In some cases, women with obstructed labor who do not receive adequate care may develop a fistula—a tear in the wall between a woman's vagina and the bladder and/or rectum that can cause chronic incontinence. The consequences of obstetric fistulas can be devastating to affected women, who may be abandoned by their families and shunned by their communities. Treatment of an obstetric fistula requires surgical reconstruction, and prevention through access to emergency obstetric care is critical.

Because young adolescent mothers are more likely to have obstructed labor and to develop

ROLE OF MEN IN FAMILIES

The United Nations Programme on the Family in early 2011 released a new publication, "Men in Families and Family Policy in a Changing World," covering trends and issues among governments as well as in the private sector. The report addresses the evolving roles of men in families and the corresponding need to develop social policies paying attention to the rights and responsibilities of all family members. To learn more or to download the report, visit un.org/en/development/desa.

obstetric fistulas, efforts to combat child marriage and delay the first birth are essential strategies. (For more information, visit endfistula.org.)

Eight million children per year die before the age of five, representing, in some developing countries, as many as one child in ten. The leading causes of child deaths are neonatal factors, pneumonia, diarrhea, and malaria. Children are more likely to die if they were born less than twenty-four months after a previous birth.[83] Women who have frequent or closely spaced births have higher rates of anemia and other nutritional deficiencies and suffer more frequent complications of pregnancy and childbirth, including death. Women in developing countries generally would prefer not to have their births so closely spaced.[84] However, in communities where having a large family is a woman's only way to improve her social status and where being childless or not having sons is grounds for divorce or abandonment, women may feel pressured to have many closely spaced children. Improving life expectancy and reduc-

ing maternal and child mortality require a sufficient investment in the accessibility and quality of health care—both primary health care and emergency obstetric care, family planning and safe abortion services, and basic health education, including the health benefits of birth spacing.

The reasons for unmet need are varied and

FAMILY PLANNING AND GLOBAL FUNDING POLICIES

The ability to plan one's family is essential to a woman's health, autonomy, and empowerment. In the 1960s, only 9 percent of all married women used modern methods of contraception, as compared with about 55 percent of married women in 2010. Africa has the lowest rates of contraceptive use—only 23 percent of married women use a modern method of contraception—while in developed regions, about 70 percent of women or more use contraception.[85, 86]

Owing to increased demand for family planning, as well as a large increase in the number of women of reproductive age due to past high fertility, more than 137 million women globally have an unmet need for family planning—they do not want to become pregnant within two years, but are not using a method of contraception, either modern or traditional, to prevent this.[87] Traditional methods include periodic abstinence and withdrawal. Most women with unmet need live in developing countries, particularly in sub-Saharan Africa, where as many as 45 percent of women want to prevent or delay a pregnancy but are not using contraception.

IN TRANSLATION: BARRIERS TO CONTRACEPTION AND ABORTION

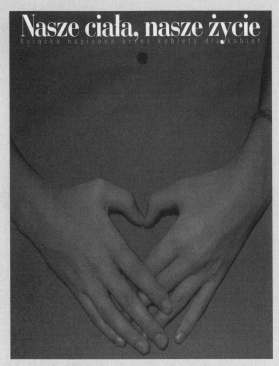

The Polish adaptation of *Our Bodies, Ourselves*

Group: Network of East-West Women

Country: Poland

Resource: *Nasze Ciała, Nasze Życie* (*Our Bodies, Our Life*), a Polish adaptation of *Our Bodies, Ourselves*

Website: neww.org.pl

Poland's postcommunist transformation to a market economy has resulted in a massive overhaul of its health sector. Network of East-West Women, OBOS's partner in Poland, reports that traditional gender attitudes, along with laws that en-able doctors to deny care they consider morally objectionable, and exorbitant health care fees levied by powerful pharmaceutical companies and private clinics, are serious barriers for girls and women seeking contraceptives and accurate information on sexual and reproductive health.

The entrenched influence of the Catholic Church, conservative media, and political groups has made the situation particularly difficult for women, who feel constant pressure to carry pregnancies to term and are continually denied access to information about their health and their rights.

Polish law is extremely restrictive of abortion, and a growing number of policy makers assume an anti-abortion rights stance that disregards the needs of pregnant women. There is widespread use of abortion pills bought online, and thousands of women have turned to illegal and expensive private clinics or have traveled abroad for abortion procedures. Given these social, political, and economic constraints, Network of East-West Women is committed to ensuring women become decision makers in their own care.

To this end, the Polish adaptation of *Our Bodies, Ourselves* is invaluable. In its preface, the authors state that "it is of vital importance for Polish women to know where and how to get help in case they are sick, what questions they should ask when talking to a physician, what rights they have as patients."

The book, which has been distributed throughout the country, is empowering women as health consumers by explicitly explaining that they have the right to de-

include lack of access to modern methods at reasonable or no cost; fear of contraceptive side effects; misperceptions about the risk of becoming pregnant; and opposition (real or perceived) from husbands, mothers-in-law, or religious groups. The availability of a good range of short- and long-acting methods to meet the varied needs of women—as well as good-quality and respectful service delivery—has been shown to increase contraceptive use.[88]

The United States is the leading international donor for family planning assistance, though funding has been a political football for many years. International family planning funds have been tied to the global gag rule policy, which disqualifies foreign nongovernmental organizations from receiving U.S. funds if they provide legal abortion services or counseling and referral for abortion (even if legal) or lobby to make abortion legal or to expand access in their country. This policy (discussed more on p. 774) was rescinded again by President Obama in January 2008, in what was considered a major victory for reproductive rights globally. The gag rule is an example of how the political battles over abortion in the United States harm the lives and health of women around the world.

The U.S. contribution to the United Nations Fund for Population Activities, UNFPA, has also been a subject of controversy in recent years, owing primarily to its work in China. China's one-child policy is used by anti–reproductive rights politicians as a false rationale for blocking appropriations to UNFPA, despite evidence that UNFPA's presence supports women's rights and in no way provides "assistance for abortion,

abortion services, or abortion-related equipment and supplies as a method of family planning."[89]

What gets lost in these debates is that while development assistance for some health problems expanded rapidly, international family planning assistance declined over the past decades. In fiscal year 2010, the U.S. government appropriated $648.5 million for family planning (including a $55 million contribution to UNFPA), a moderate 15 percent increase over fiscal year 2009. Stagnating funding for family planning, despite growing demand, reflected the limited support for sexual and reproductive health during President George W. Bush's administration. Funds for maternal and child health were also limited to $549 million, while funds earmarked for global HIV/AIDS programming reached $5.7 billion, a sign of the political support rallied against the HIV/AIDS epidemic after over a decade of advocacy.[90] The increase in funding for HIV/AIDS and other infectious diseases in the U.S. foreign assistance budget shows that funding follows political will.

Declining support for international family planning is not unique to the United States, although it is perhaps more acute because of the substantial role that U.S. funding has played. In addition to reducing maternal and child mortality, the Millennium Development Goals include a target to achieve universal access to reproductive health services, including family planning, by 2015.[91] The United Nations estimates that $24.6 billion annually is needed between 2011 and 2015 to reach these goals—a little more than double the current global spending on family planning and maternal and newborn services.

IN TRANSLATION: ABORTION IN LATIN AMERICA AND THE CARIBBEAN

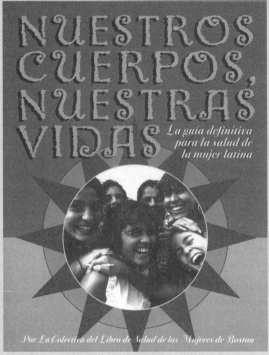

A Spanish adaptation of *Our Bodies, Ourselves* for the Americas and Caribbean

Group: A collaboration of nineteen women's organizations in the Americas and Caribbean

Country: Coordinated in the United States

Resource: *Nuestros Cuerpos, Nuestras Vidas (Our Bodies, Our Lives)*, a Spanish adaptation of *Our Bodies, Ourselves*, and peer health educator training materials for the Americas and Caribbean

Website: ourbodiesourselves.org/publications/ncnv.asp

Latin America and the Caribbean have some of the most restrictive abortion policies in the world. El Salvador, Chile, and Nicaragua, for example, do not allow abortions under any circumstance. Women seeking care after a miscarriage may be interrogated first for possible prosecution for suspected abortion, and some states in Mexico have begun such prosecutions. Providers in Costa Rica can be sent to prison.

While most other countries make allowances in certain situations (to save a woman's life or health, or in cases where pregnancy is the result of rape), the ideology and power of the Catholic Church hierarchy, as well as legal, judicial, and medical obstacles, make it nearly impossible to talk about abortion or to seek care. Despite these restrictions, these regions have some of the highest rates of abortion worldwide. Most of the abortions are unsafe, according to the nonprofit organization Ipas, and account for about one out of nine maternal deaths.[92]

The authors of *Nuestros Cuerpos, Nuestras Vidas,* the Spanish-language cultural adaptation of *Our Bodies, Ourselves*, chose to speak directly to the ethical and spiritual dimensions of abortion decisions in ways that would address Catholic women's concerns. They drew on the work of Catholics for Choice, which courageously challenges church doctrine by placing a woman's decision on abortion within the context of her sacred responsibility for life—emphasizing a woman's right and moral agency to make these difficult decisions, while recognizing that many women throughout the world would rather risk their lives than bear a child they cannot care for. The book also draws heavily from the rich bonds that Latin American women have with their families and communities, voicing the culturally harmonious relational message "If you don't care for yourself, you can't take care of others."

Nineteen women's organizations representing twelve countries worked together to promote personal health while mobilizing for social change and to create a resource that inspires and guides Latinas throughout the Americas. The translation and topics, including abortion and HIV/AIDS, reflect enormous differences in social and economic realities and access to care across Latin America.

To reach Latina women and girls in the Caribbean, Central and South America, as well as those living *entre mundos*–between worlds–in the United States, *Nuestros Cuerpos, Nuestras Vidas* emphasizes engagement in a critical analysis of social, economic, political, and religious issues affecting women and girls every day. Additionally, it contextualizes women's ability to access timely, safe, and legal abortion care within other areas of economic, educational, and social life that leave them vulnerable to exploitation. It offers a window into the stories and social movements of women and girls throughout this region and the world, as they strive for–and achieve–equality and wellness.

A simultaneous investment in family planning and maternal and newborn health would ultimately cost less than investing in maternal and newborn services alone, because it would prevent unintended pregnancies and avert maternal and infant deaths.[93]

The Obama administration is addressing women's health from a more comprehensive perspective than in the past in its Global Health Initiative—a $63 billion effort over six years to help partner countries improve health outcomes and strengthen health systems.[94] The initiative will focus on improving the health of women, newborns, and children, but the specific actions to be taken are still under development.

RESTRICTIONS ON ABORTION WORLDWIDE

Legal restrictions on abortion do not affect its incidence. The countries where abortion is the most accessible, in fact, have the lowest rates of abortion. Legal restrictions do, however, influence the safety of the procedure.[95] Where abortion is legal and permitted on broad grounds, it is generally safe, and where it is legally restricted, it is often performed unsafely or in unsafe conditions. In South Africa, the incidence of infection resulting from abortion decreased by 52 percent and the number of deaths decreased by 90 percent after the abortion law was liberalized in 1996.[96]

Eighteen countries, Australia, Benin, Bhutan, Cambodia, Chad, Colombia, Ethiopia, Guinea, Iran, Mali, Nepal, Niger, Portugal, St. Lucia, Swaziland, Switzerland, Thailand, and Togo, as well as Mexico City, liberalized their laws to increase access to safe abortion between 1997 and 2010. Three countries, El Salvador, Nicaragua, and Poland, tightened restrictions on abortion.

Lack of access to safe, legal abortion has a dramatic impact on women's health.[97]

- There are 19 million unsafe abortions each year.
- An estimated 5 million women are hospitalized each year for treatment of abortion-related complications, such as hemorrhage and sepsis.
- Complications due to unsafe abortion procedures account for an estimated 13 percent of maternal deaths worldwide, or 50,000 per year based on new WHO estimates of maternal deaths.
- Almost all abortion-related deaths occur in developing countries. They are highest in Africa, where there were an estimated 650 deaths per 100,000 abortions in 2003, compared with 10 per 100,000 abortions in developed regions.[98]

VIOLENCE AGAINST WOMEN

Violence against women takes many forms around the world and can occur at any stage in the life of a female from infanticide to abuse of widows.[99] Among women ages fifteen to forty-four, acts of violence cause more death and disability than cancer, malaria, traffic accidents, and war combined.[100] Violence against women destroys lives, fractures communities, and inhibits development.

Women's rights advocates and the UN system—including the newly formed UN Women (unwomen.org), which acts as a focal point for women's issues within the UN—have succeeded in raising awareness globally about the problem of gender-based violence. The 16 Days of Activism Against Gender Violence Campaign launched by the Center for Women's Global Leadership at Rutgers University is one example. Since 1999, this campaign has symbolically linked November 25, the International Day for the Elimination of Violence Against Women, to December 10, International Human Rights Day.

This campaign is now marked in all regions of the globe (see: 16dayscwgl.rutgers.edu). However, awareness-raising alone cannot address the problem; we also must ensure that resources are in place to protect women and address social norms that foster violence.

INTIMATE PARTNER VIOLENCE

In many societies, patriarchal values and traditional ideals of masculinity condone violence against women as a means of asserting authority. Men may perceive that they have the right to dominate their wives and partners physically and sexually, and the cultural and legal environment supports that perception. Intimate partner violence is often underreported because of assumptions that it is merely common practice, or because of perceptions of stigma on the part of women who are victimized. Globally, an estimated one-third of all women have experienced physical, sexual, or emotional intimate partner violence at some point in their lives.[101] Intimate partner violence is a leading cause of femicide—the murder of women because they are women. In South Africa, a woman is killed every six hours by an intimate partner.[102] In India, there are twenty-two dowry-related murders each day.[103] And in Guatemala, an average of two women are murdered each day.[104]

In many settings, there is very little recourse for women experiencing domestic violence—no legal action, no safe houses, and no option for divorce—and in countries where these protections exist, they are in insufficient supply. In some societies, women are blamed, punished, or even killed for being victims of sexual violence. Without the economic means and the cultural support to live independently of men, women cannot leave abusive situations.

Increasingly, intimate partner violence is recognized as a pervasive public health problem demanding attention and action. Spurred by the WHO study, research on gender-based violence has increased substantially. Today, more than three hundred studies in ninety countries have documented the extent of intimate partner violence and some have illuminated its consequences for the health and well-being of women,[105] including the recent International Men and Gender Equality Survey, IMAGES, conducted among 8,000 men and 3,500 women in six countries.[106] Numerous recent publications document promising interventions,[107] and several global organizations are raising awareness and involving men in fighting gender-based violence. The White Ribbon Campaign (whiteribbon.ca), an effort by men to end violence against women, began in Canada in 1991 and is now in place in sixty countries. Men Engage (menengage.org), begun in 2004, is a global network of four hundred nongovernmental organizations and a number of UN agencies working to engage boys and men to achieve gender equality, promote health, and reduce violence.

IMPACT OF POLITICAL AND MILITARY CONFLICTS

War disrupts the social and health care services that women need and can make travel to clinics or hospitals dangerous or impossible. Poor obstetrical care during wartime can lead to high rates of maternal and infant mortality, while access to contraception and abortion may be restricted as women's fertility is recruited in the national mission of producing future soldiers. Long-term wars can inure men to violence. Indeed, studies suggest that intimate partner violence increases during and immediately after wartime.[108]

Violence targeted at women in association with political or military conflicts seems to be growing, especially in so-called ethnic or civil wars. Rape of women as a weapon of war has been documented in countries such as Rwanda, the Democratic Republic of Congo (DRC), Sierra Leone, Zimbabwe, Sudan, Liberia, Uganda, Bangladesh, Vietnam, and Bosnia. Between 250,000 and 500,000 women and girls, for example, were raped during the 1994 Rwandan genocide alone.[109] And in the DRC, at least 200,000 cases of sexual violence, mostly involving women and girls, have been documented since 1996, though the actual numbers are considered to be much higher.[110] In some circumstances, sexual violence is condoned by the government.

When women survive wartime rape, they still must deal with forced pregnancies or dangerous abortions, sexually transmitted infections (including HIV), and the social stigma of having been "spoiled" for marriage. In 2002, the International Criminal Court in The Hague defined sexual offenses during war as a crime against humanity.[111] For more information, visit Say No—UNITE (saynotoviolence.org) and V-Day (vday.org).

SEXUAL EXPLOITATION OF WOMEN AND SEX TRAFFICKING

In developing countries, poor women and women with little or no formal education have few means of support. Economic need drives some women to become commercial sex workers. Other women, particularly undocumented immigrants in developing and industrialized nations, are forced into the sex trade. All of these women are at an elevated risk of a host of STIs, including syphilis, gonorrhea, hepatitis, chlamydia, and HIV/AIDS, as well as violence perpetrated by clients and others who market and profit from the women's sexual services.

Policy responses to commercial sex have generally fallen into one of two camps. A harm reduction approach focuses on protecting the sex worker and her clients from STIs and treating any infections she acquires. Although such practices may protect the health and safety of

sex workers and clients, they ignore the circumstances that lead women into commercial
sex—poverty, marginalization, addiction, and
limited education and employment opportunities. The clients of commercial sex workers
may prefer that society place emphasis on reducing the transmission of infections and stop
there.

Rehabilitation approaches focus on creating alternative employment opportunities for
women in sex work. While some of these approaches open new doors for women, many do
not provide sufficient income for women to be
able to leave sex work.[113] Further, staged raids
on commercial sex establishments to rescue sex
workers, common to some rehabilitation programs, are generally more disempowering to
women who have been "rescued" than effective
as a means for women to leave commercial sex
work.[114]

Decriminalizing sex work and ensuring that
sex workers are protected from violence and
abuse are essential for fulfilling all women's
human rights. Some advocates believe the most

sensible solution is to formally recognize sex
work as an occupation, so sex workers can access labor rights and benefits workers in other
industries receive.[115] This would entail removing
laws and policies that prevent sex workers from
finding safe places to live and work. By bringing the sex industry out of the underground
economy, sex workers could obtain greater
protection and access needed health and social
services. At the same time, steps are needed to
ensure that women have feasible options for
leaving the sex industry.

Child prostitution is a particularly heinous
aspect of the commercial sex industry. UNICEF
estimates that approximately 1 million children
(mainly girls) enter the multibillion-dollar commercial sex trade every year. Parental abuse and
neglect cause children to run away from home;
homeless children may be sold to commercial
sex organizations; the trade might seem to offer
a chance for a lot of money; and in an environment of armed conflict, children who become
separated from their parents may seek protection from the military in return for sex.

HUMAN TRAFFICKING

Human trafficking—the illegal buying and selling of human beings—is the fastest-growing
criminal industry in the world.[116] Because this
trade is underground, accurate statistics are elusive, but the 2010 *Trafficking in Persons Report*
estimates that 12.3 million people are enslaved
in forced labor, bonded labor, and forced sex
work around the world. Women and girls make
up 80 percent of all people trafficked annually,[117]
with the majority of women (79 percent) trafficked for sexual exploitation.[118]

Many trafficked people are targeted for various forms of exploitation in the sex industry,
including sex work, pornography, stripping,
live-sex shows, and sex tourism. However, people may be trafficked for other forms of labor

IN TRANSLATION: HELPING WOMEN FIND SAFETY IN SOUTH ASIA

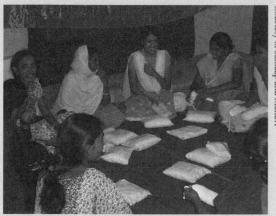

Courtesy of Sanlaap and Manavi

Community session on menstrual health in West Bengal.

Groups: Sanlaap and Manavi

Country: India

Resource: "Aamaar Shaastha, Aamaar Sattaa" ("My Health, My Self"), a Bengali booklet based on *Our Bodies, Ourselves*

Website: sanlaapindia.org and manavi.org

In South Asia, nearly 150,000 girls and women are trafficked every year, with India and Pakistan as the main destinations for children under sixteen years of age.[119] Prostitution and trafficking provide money that can sustain families who have no other viable means of support. As a result, in a country as poor as India—where practices such as female infanticide, sex-selective abortion, nutritional and educational neglect of girls, and dowry deaths are common—family members and relatives play a significant role in the trafficking process.

Our Bodies Ourselves' partners in South Asia, Sanlaap (established in 1987 in Kolkata) and the New Jersey-based Manavi, work to change the conditions that lead to human trafficking. Sanlaap provides education, health care, vocational training, legal aid, and safe-respite locations in the red-light districts of Kolkata in the eastern state of West Bengal. Kolkata is an important transit point for traffickers in Mumbai, on the western coast of India, and Pakistan. Sanlaap also works with vulnerable children of sex workers to prevent them from entering the industry. It promotes safe migration, sensitizes law enforcement and the judiciary, and uses a successful psychosocial intervention model that has been replicated by government and international agencies.

Sanlaap and Manavi have published a Bangla adaptation of sections from *Our Bodies, Ourselves* on sexual health and taking care of ourselves. This resource is used in Sanlaap's work on trafficking and the health care of survivors. It is also important to Manavi's work in the United States on domestic violence in South Asian communities. Manavi was one of the first groups to recognize the physical, emotional, and economic abuses South Asian women—particularly young brides—are sometimes subjected to in the United States by their spouses and their extended families.

Since the mid-1980s, Manavi has introduced innovative domestic violence intervention methods that combine Western-style counseling with culturally appropriate traditional techniques. Manavi has drawn attention to factors that promote and sustain inequality and encourage violence as an acceptable form of human interaction. It has helped immigrant women to overcome the many barriers—cultural, social, linguistic, legal, and political—that encourage their silence.

exploitation, such as sweatshop labor, domestic servitude and maid service at motels and hotels, and agricultural work.

What distinguishes trafficking is the use of force, coercion, and lies to recruit, transport, and exploit people as forced labor or slaves. False enticements include the promise of a good job or false marriage proposals that turn into bondage situations. Some young women and girls are sold by their own families who can no longer afford to feed and shelter them. The growth of websites promoting sex tourism fuels the rapid growth of the trafficking industry.

A twenty-two-year-old sex worker in Calcutta recalls how she was trafficked from her native Bangladesh at age seventeen:

I didn't come of my own wish; I was sold. They picked me up from the street over there and brought me. . . . For the first two or three days, I was very stubborn about not joining this line [of work]. They starved me for those two or three days and never even gave me water to drink.

The tactics used to instill fear in victims and to keep them enslaved—whether in a field, a factory, a brothel, or a war zone—include rape, beatings, starvation, forced drug use, confinement, and isolation.[120] Traffickers also trap victims into cycles of debt, control victims' money, confiscate passports and other identifying documents, threaten falsely that victims will be imprisoned or deported for immigration violations if they contact authorities, and threaten to injure or kill family members back home if they resist.

In 2000, the United Nations negotiated international standards against human trafficking and began tracking the situation in every country. That same year, the U.S. Trafficking Victims Protection Act (TVPA) made human trafficking a federal crime. It was enacted to prevent human trafficking overseas; to protect victims (including U.S. citizens) and help them rebuild their lives in the United States; and to prosecute traffickers of humans under federal penalties. The TVPA created the T visa, a special temporary immigration visa for human trafficking victims that allows victims to sue their traffickers in federal district court and provides access to a range of social services, legal assistance, and

Recommended Resources: The National Human Trafficking Resource Center has a 24/7 hotline (1-888-3737-888) for crisis calls from victims and to receive tips about trafficking situations. The federal government's Campaign to Rescue & Restore Victims of Human Trafficking (acf.hhs .gov/trafficking) also provides resources and information.

Visit the Polaris Project (polarisproject .org) and Free the Slaves (freetheslaves .net) to learn more and to join advocacy efforts against trafficking.

public benefits. Many organizations, including Amnesty International (amnesty.org), are working to end human trafficking and to improve the conditions that lead to trafficking.

FEMALE GENITAL CUTTING

Between 100 and 140 million girls and women in the world have experienced female genital cutting (FGC), also known as female genital mutilation (FGM), a traditional cultural practice that is also an extreme violation of human rights, including the right to bodily integrity. More than 3 million girls each year on the African continent alone are subject to the practice, which usually involves excising the clitoris and may include partial or total removal of the labia and suturing the vagina, leaving a small opening for menstrual flow. While FGC/M is viewed in practicing cultures as a rite of passage to prepare girls for womanhood or for other sociocultural reasons, its fundamental purpose is the control of female sexuality. The practice can have serious health consequences, including hemorrhage, shock, pain, infection, difficulties during childbirth, and psychological and sexual problems.[121]

FGC is practiced in at least twenty-eight countries in sub-Saharan and northeastern Africa, as well as a few countries in Asia and the Middle East. It is generally performed on preadolescent and adolescent girls, but in some countries, such as Mali, it is often performed on girls between the ages of one and five. While FGC is practiced by people from all educational levels and social classes, among urban and rural residents, and among many different religious and ethnic groups, increasing recognition of FGC as a human rights issue has led to it becoming less common among urban and more educated residents in most countries for which survey data are available.[122]

The prevalence of FGC in a number of practicing countries is nearly universal: 85 percent or more of women ages fifteen to forty-nine in Egypt, Eritrea, Guinea, Mali, Sierra Leone, and Somalia are circumcised. In Burkina Faso, Central African Republic, Côte d'Ivoire, Egypt, Eritrea, Kenya, and Tanzania, a decline in the percentage of younger women who have been circumcised suggests that the practice is declining. For example, in Kenya, where circumcision usually occurs before age fourteen, less than 15 percent of girls ages fifteen to nineteen are circumcised, compared with 35 percent of women ages thirty-five to thirty-nine. On the other hand, in the Gambia, Mali, and Somalia, the prevalence among young women is virtually unchanged from that of older women.

Through a joint program, the UNFPA and UNICEF have brought together governments, NGOs, religious leaders, and small community groups to substantially reduce the practice within seventeen participating countries by 2012. Opportunities for nondirective dialogues among women and men of all ages have demonstrated promise as vehicles for the necessary social change and altered power dynamics, which will help to eliminate this harmful practice.

Egypt and Eritrea are among the numerous countries that have passed legislation prohibiting FGC. While these laws may discourage the practice, they appear to spur the "medicalization" of FGC.

Parents are also increasingly turning to the medical profession rather than to traditional circumcisers to perform the procedure. For example, nearly a third of circumcisions in Egypt are now medically performed. The medicalization of FGC is controversial, considered to be both unethical and in some countries outlawed, while at the same time likely to be safer than a procedure performed in the bush by a traditional circumciser. Greater success has been achieved through recognizing the cultural significance of the practice and the fact that parents view the procedure as an obligation. Alternative rite-of-passage programs and ceremonies help girls and their families acknowledge the transition to adulthood without the "cut."[123]

In several countries, women have been recognized as refugees under the 1951 UN Convention Relating to the Status of Refugees (Geneva Refugee Convention) on the grounds that they would be at risk of FGC if they returned to their country. However, there are still only a tiny number of such cases. In the United States, the Citizenship and Immigration Services and international laws and treaties recognize gender-based violence as a human rights violation. Still, women are often denied asylum in the United States because the definition of a refugee entitled to protection is too narrow.

SELECTED MEDICAL CONCERNS

CERVICAL CANCER: A NEGLECTED HEALTH CHALLENGE

Cervical cancer kills 275,000 women each year, with the majority of those deaths occurring in developing countries.[124] It is the leading cause of cancer death among adult women in the developing world and the second most common cancer among women worldwide. The largest number of cervical cancer cases and subsequent deaths occur in South and Southeast Asia, but women in Africa are most likely to die of the disease compared with other regions of the globe.[125]

Cervical cancer is caused by several types of the human papillomavirus (HPV), with two specific types causing about 70 percent of all cervical cancers.[126] HPV is associated with other cancers as well. Cervical cancer is both preventable and treatable, making the disparities in the likelihood of dying of the disease a matter of social justice. Several effective screening methods exist to identify precancerous lesions and early stages of the disease, including Pap tests, visual inspection methods, and, more recently, HPV DNA testing.[127] However, Pap tests require trained cytologists plus laboratory facilities to read tests accurately, and many countries with weak health care systems lack the resources to ensure access. In other countries, where Pap tests are more widely available, they are provided on an opportunistic basis, with poor women least likely to receive the test and wealthier women potentially being tested more than medically necessary.[128]

HPV DNA testing as a newer technology remains prohibitively expensive for many health care systems, although more affordable technologies are being researched. Visual inspection of the cervix by a trained health care provider remains a feasible option for low-resource settings when provided in tandem with on-site treatment methods such as cryotherapy.[129]

HPV Vaccines

Two HPV vaccines have been available since 2006 to prevent infection from the types of HPV responsible for the majority of cervical cancer cases—Gardasil, made by Merck, and Cervarix, by GlaxoSmithKline. Both vaccines have been found to be at least 95 percent effective in preventing the types of HPV responsible for most cancers when given to girls before they become sexually active, or to women without prior infection with these HPV types. These vaccines are licensed in more than one hundred countries.[130] However, they remain widely unavailable in many low- and middle-income countries owing to a combination of financial and organizational challenges that signal a lack of commitment to addressing this disease.

As recently developed vaccines, Gardasil and Cervarix remain under patent and are prohibitively expensive for many health care systems. Donation programs have enabled vaccine demonstration programs in some settings, but these will not be sustainable. Moreover, viable financing programs will require that the manufacturers offer reasonable pricing. The Global Alliance for Vaccines and Immunisation (GAVI), a global mechanism to finance immunization programs, is currently working on plans to support subsidized purchases for low-resource settings.[131]

The World Health Organization recommends that the vaccine be targeted to young adolescent girls, who must receive three doses of the vaccine for it to be fully effective, but adolescent girls tend to have extremely limited contact with health services. Demonstration programs have found that school-based programs may be an effective mechanism to reach young girls, but they will miss girls who leave school prior to adolescence.[132]

Messaging around the vaccine is also critical to address low awareness about cervical cancer and HPV, as well as to prevent misconceptions about the rationale for targeting young girls.[133] Without a concerted and coordinated global effort to ensure access to the vaccine to prevent future cases in tandem with screen-and-treat programs to address the current burden of cervical cancer, the gross disparities between women in rich and poor countries will persist.

HIV/AIDS EPIDEMIC

Perhaps no other worldwide catastrophe has so poignantly revealed the vulnerability of women in society as the AIDS epidemic. The ability of the international community to secure broad-based access to the HPV vaccine is being watched closely by HIV activists, since a future vaccine for HIV/AIDS, one of the great hopes of the medical world, is likely to face similar struggles.[134]

As of 2010, an estimated 33.3 million people are living with HIV/AIDS worldwide,[135] nearly half of them (15.9 million) women. Two out of three people infected with HIV (22.5 million)

live in sub-Saharan Africa. In this region, thirteen women are infected for every ten men, and three-quarters of HIV-positive young people are female. Most women contract HIV during unprotected heterosexual sex. Gender power imbalances, transactional sex driven by poverty, and greater biological vulnerability put women at higher risk of HIV than men.

The pandemic of HIV/AIDS has led to the deaths of more than 25 million people worldwide in the last thirty years. Families, communities, societies, and whole countries have been ravaged by this ultimately preventable disease. The impact of the HIV epidemic also falls more heavily on women, who assume the bulk of caregiving when their male partners, children, and parents fall ill.

Women with HIV and women whose partners die of AIDS often suffer discrimination and abandonment. In a study in India, almost 90 percent of the HIV-positive women interviewed were infected by their husbands. Despite being monogamous, they were often blamed for their husbands' illnesses. In some contexts, women's lower status in the family and community make it less likely that they have access to health care, including antiretroviral treatment.[136] In many places, a woman will be expelled from her home and her family when it is learned that she is infected, even though she has remained faithful.

As the epidemic has progressed, it has become increasingly feminized, especially among youth. Young women age fifteen to twenty-four are 2.5 times more likely to be infected than young men, too often as a result of gender-based violence and coerced sex. Studies have consistently found that women subject to violence by a sexual partner are more likely to be infected with HIV.[137] These findings contribute to a growing global recognition of the need for women-centered prevention efforts that focus on addressing harmful gender norms, gender-based violence, and the economic vulnerability of women.[138]

Stepping Stones is a widely acclaimed community-based HIV prevention program that engages young and older men and women in critical reflection and cross-generational dialogue about harmful gender norms, including gender-based violence, and how they increase the risk of HIV. Thousands of participants have been introduced to the Stepping Stones curricula in a number of African countries. In a recent evaluation conducted in South Africa, home to the greatest number of people living with HIV in the world (5.5 million), Stepping Stones training was associated with a significant reduction in intimate partner violence perpetrated by young men. After two years of follow-up, those who had participated in the Stepping Stones program reported a 38 percent reduction in intimate partner violence as well as a one-third reduction in the incidence of genital herpes (HSV-2) infections in comparison with a control group.[139]

The President's Emergency Plan for AIDS Relief (PEPFAR)

A significant accomplishment of the George W. Bush administration was the creation of the President's Emergency Plan for AIDS Relief (PEPFAR; pepfar.gov), initiated in 2003. At a cost of $15 billion over five years, it massively increased the resources available to treat and fight HIV. The plan was reviewed and expanded in 2008 as the United States Global Leadership Against HIV/AIDS, Tuberculosis, and Malaria Act, authorizing up to $48 billion for prevention, care, and treatment of these diseases in low-resource settings.

While PEPFAR had some shortcomings—including a focus on abstinence-only programs as a primary prevention strategy despite a lack of scientific evidence to support the effectiveness of such programs—PEPFAR funding enabled 2 million people to access lifesaving antiretroviral treatment and provided care and support to millions more.

In low- and middle-income countries, 5.2 million people now receive treatment, a 30 percent increase over 2008, but still only 36 percent of total need. Nearly 10 million people in poor countries who are in immediate need of these lifesaving drugs are not receiving them.[140] The new plan includes funding to continue the treatment for those currently receiving it and a pledge to provide treatment to 2 million more people over the next five years.[141] These shortfalls suggest that demand for antiretroviral drugs (ARVs) will continually outpace supply until more attention is devoted to prevention.

HIV and Pregnancy

The continuing rate of new HIV infections and the unlikelihood of donors and countries fully meeting the growing demand for lifelong treatment have led to a greater emphasis on prevention, including prevention of mother-to-child transmission of HIV. Of the 2.5 million children under the age of fifteen living with HIV worldwide, the great majority have become infected through the birthing process or through breast milk.[142]

The risk of transmission during birth can be substantially reduced by administering ARVs to the mother, beginning early in pregnancy, and to the infant during delivery and for four to six weeks afterward. If formula feeding is not

Recommended Reading: For an analysis of PEPFAR and where and how its money is spent, visit AVERT, the international HIV and AIDS charity based in the UK (avert.org/pepfar.htm).

IN TRANSLATION: HIV ACTIVISTS TRAVEL ON FOOT AND BY CANOE TO RAISE AWARENESS

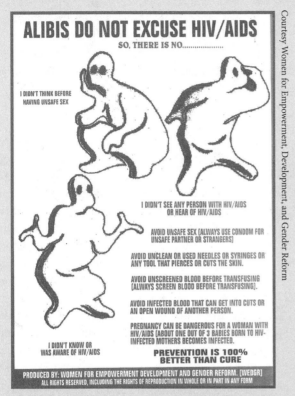

WEDGR created this poster with culturally relevant information for distribution in rural Nigeria.

Group: Women for Empowerment, Development, and Gender Reform

Country: Nigeria

Resource: Print and nonprint materials based on *Our Bodies, Ourselves* in pidgin English and Yoruba

Website: ourbodiesourselves.org/ programs/network

Nigeria's growing AIDS epidemic is attributed to a number of factors, including limited access to sexual health information; a failing health system unable to provide testing and care to large segments of the population; and cultural practices such as polygamy and early marriage that leave women and girls disproportionately vulnerable to infection.

Though HIV prevalence is even higher in South Africa and Zambia, Nigeria's ethnic and political structure has hampered effective wide-scale intervention. This has made grassroots groups—such as Women for Empowerment, Development, and Gender Reform (WEDGR), Our Bodies Ourselves' partner in Nigeria—critical to the global fight on HIV transmission, prevention, and care.

WEDGR is adapting content from *Our Bodies, Ourselves* into local dialects—Yoruba and pidgin English—and using creative ways to bring information to those who most need it. The organization is raising awareness in communities with the highest numbers of HIV-positive women in the country through outreach on the local canoe system that ferries passengers from remote farms to markets; peer educator training for village hairdressers; an outreach walk to cover a wide network of villages; and a groundbreaking effort to sensitize and include men as partners in change.

Successes, however, have been hard won, with challenges ranging from rising fuel costs to reluctant male participation. Stigma attached to the virus has also generated anger against WEDGR, resulting in a brutal and fatal attack on outreach workers in 2009. This was followed by a deliberate fire that destroyed the organization's office. More recently, members of the project team were kidnapped and released after a month in exchange for ransom paid by family, friends, and community chiefs.

In the aftermath of these terrifying incidents, WEDGR remains steadfast in its commitment to building conciliatory bridges and raising consciousness about HIV. Nonetheless, the experience is a disheartening reminder of the danger human rights defenders face as they take on the most urgent social and health issues. WEDGR hopes its story will mobilize the global community to rise in defense of activists around the world.

feasible or safe (owing to cost, lack of access to clean water, or social stigma), a breastfed infant has the best chance of avoiding infection if the mother receives a triple-ARV regimen for at least the last third of her pregnancy and continuing throughout the breastfeeding period.

In the last decade, programs to test pregnant women for HIV and to treat those who are infected have greatly expanded, many supported by PEPFAR funds. Despite the progress, less than half of HIV-positive pregnant women receive treatment to prevent transmission of the virus to their infants during pregnancy, during labor and birth, and while breastfeeding. As a result, 370,000 infants became infected with HIV in 2009.[143] Some women refuse the drug because of the stigma still associated with HIV. As noted above, HIV-positive women fear social ostracism, divorce, expulsion from the household, and financial destitution.

These programs have helped reduce the number of infants born with HIV in developing countries, but there is still a long way to go. Mothers are often not able to access ongoing antiretroviral treatment for themselves, with the result that they may not survive to raise their children. Follow-up efforts during and after pregnancy are critical to ensure that women who are eligible are actually enrolled in treatment programs.

Regardless of their HIV status, many women will want to or will face societal pressure to bear children, but health workers may assume that women with HIV should not have children. Activists in Namibia and South Africa have documented several cases of forced sterilization of HIV-positive women.[144] In other settings, health workers may refuse to perform abortions for women with HIV based on their misperceptions of infection risk.[145] Women living with HIV have the same rights to safe and affordable contraceptive and abortion services as HIV-negative women. Women with HIV also require support to be able to conceive safely if they wish to have a child and to bring that pregnancy safely to term.[146]

Testing New Drugs

Pharmaceutical companies are increasingly testing new drugs in poor and developing countries. African and Asian women, in particular, have been recruited for HIV/AIDS medication trials—especially medications aimed at preventing vertical transmission from mothers to babies—and contraceptive treatments. While clinical trials are an important stage in the process of developing better medical treatments, it is crucial to ensure that women recruited for clinical trials are adequately informed and protected.

Human rights activists are concerned that drugs deemed too risky for testing in America are increasingly "outsourced" to India or Africa, where more lax government oversight and greater economic deprivation can lead to abuse. For these reasons, human rights activists call for greater transparency regarding the use of human subjects, increased international regulation of drug testing, better enforcement of human rights treaties (especially the Convention on the Elimination of All Forms of Discrimination Against Women), and assurances that pharmaceutical products will be made available at affordable prices for women in developing countries once the clinical trials have ended.

HIV Prevention Methods

Male Circumcision

Globally, adult male circumcision has emerged in recent years as a promising means of protection against HIV infection. Recent evidence indicates that circumcision can reduce a man's risk of getting HIV by as much as 60 percent.[147] The extent to which male circumcision also reduces the risk of sexually transmitting HIV infection to female partners remains under investigation. Several African countries have introduced male circumcision policies and programs as a new component of their existing HIV prevention strategies.[148] In addition, more STI prevention approaches are actively involving men, focusing on gender and men's attitudes and practices.

Condoms

Male condoms remain the mainstay of HIV prevention programs, since they are affordable and effective at preventing transmission of HIV and other sexually transmitted infections. However, the global supply of male condoms is low and in many developing countries is largely financed by donations from international entities such as the U.S. Agency for International Development (USAID). The United Nations Population Fund (UNFPA) estimated that at least 13.1 billion condoms were needed in 2005 to significantly reduce the spread of HIV, and another 4.4 billion were required for family planning purposes. In actuality, 10.4 billion male condoms were estimated to have been used globally in 2005—around 4.4 billion condoms for family planning and 6 billion condoms for HIV prevention. Only 2.3 billion condoms were donated in 2005—representing less than 15 percent of the need.[149] Thus, only four condoms were available in 2008 for every adult male of reproductive age in sub-Saharan Africa.[150]

Although international funding for HIV treatment has grown exponentially in the past decade, funding for HIV prevention has not kept pace, in part owing to policy debates and confusion over the direction that prevention programs should take. The necessity of ensuring a sustainable supply of condoms has often been overshadowed within these debates. Meanwhile, commodity supply specialists estimate that owing to increases in the number of contraceptive users and growing demand for condoms for HIV prevention, by 2020, an estimated $424 million will be required in commodity support to satisfy the demand for contraceptives, including condoms, in donor-dependent countries. Even if donor funding were to remain at or near current levels, the shortfall would be almost $200 million annually.[151]

Female condoms provide another practical and effective method of HIV prevention, but they remain a neglected tool in the arsenal of HIV prevention programs. Although the female condom is available in more than a hundred countries, its use is widespread in only a small number of them, including South Africa and Zimbabwe, where concerted efforts have been made to market and promote the device.[152] A recent review found that female condoms were generally considered to be acceptable by users; however, the international donors responsible for purchasing the bulk of female condoms from the Female Health Company, the sole manufacturer of the device, uniformly cite its high price, approximately 75 cents per condom, as a key barrier to broader availability.[153]

In response, FHC developed the FC2 female condom at a cost reduction of at least 30 percent. Given the substantial price reductions for FC2, as well as in patented antiretroviral therapies over the past decade, the price argument is specious and suggests a failure of collective action on the part of governments and international agencies to ensure that an effective method of HIV prevention is able to get into the hands of women who wish to use this method.

Microbicides and PrEP

Female-controlled methods to reduce the transmission of STIs and HIV have long been sought as a means to help bring the pandemic of AIDS under control. The empowerment of women to control infection transmission is an essential tool in cultures where negotiating safer sex practices may be difficult, dangerous, or even impossible.

Two forms of female-controlled protection are preexposure prophylaxis (PrEP) and genital microbicides. PrEP involves taking certain antiretroviral medication (the drugs that people living with HIV use to manage the virus in their bodies) on a consistent basis as a means of protecting oneself against infection. A recent U.S. study of at-risk gay men found that those taking emtricitabine/tenofovir were far less likely to contract HIV. Worldwide, further studies are under way to explore the effectiveness of this method in other risk groups and using other antiretroviral medications.[154]

Microbicides, substances that when inserted in the vagina or rectum could substantially reduce the risk of getting or transmitting STIs, including HIV, have been under study for many years, often with disappointing results. More recent work with topical antiretrovirals used in gel form has shown promise in reducing the risk of viral transmission.

In July 2010, South African scientists who led the CAPRISA 004 trial announced that 1 percent tenofovir gel reduced women's risk of acquiring HIV from their male partners by 39 percent.[155] The researchers found that women who used the gel 80 percent or more of the times they had sex had reduced their HIV risk by 54 percent. Women who used the gel less than half the times, however, reduced their HIV risk by only 28 percent, indicating, not surprisingly, that the more consistently the microbicide gel was used, the less likely its user was to become HIV positive. What was surprising, however, was that tenofovir gel also showed 51 percent effectiveness against herpes (HSV-2) infection; this was important in itself—and also because people infected with herpes are more likely to acquire and transmit HIV.

Still, it will probably be three to four years before tenofovir gel becomes publicly available, as more studies are needed to confirm its effectiveness and safety. Another large study involving tenofovir gel is under way, with results expected in 2012 or 2013, and smaller key studies are being readied for rapid start-up. Confirmation from these studies that the gel has a protective effect would be likely to expedite efforts to bring it to market. Several other potential microbicides are also in clinical trials, with a larger number in development.

This new antiretroviral-based class of candidates may be more potent and offer greater protection against HIV infection than any of those tested to date. Like any drug, they will raise different kinds of questions. Antiretroviral-based microbicides are likely to be available only by prescription (at least initially, until more is known about them) and may raise questions of drug resistance. They may not protect against other STIs, since they target HIV specifically. Still, tenofovir's activity against herpes was a fine surprise, and some ARV-based candidates may lend themselves to combination with other anti-infectives, contraceptives, and new delivery systems.

Owing to the many years of work by advocates around the world, millions of people have now heard about microbicides and agree on the need for them. Now it is up to us as advocates to ensure that funding is available and public demand for microbicides is maintained so that these candidates continue to move through the product pipeline as efficiently and as rapidly as possible.

EMERGING ISSUES: BIOPOLITICS, WOMEN'S HEALTH, AND SOCIAL JUSTICE

We are well into what some have termed the biotech century, and a range of new reproductive and genetic technologies and practices are under development and being brought to market. Many offer significant benefits, including advanced tools for biomedical research, improved medical treatments, and new options for forming families. But many also pose unique safety challenges and raise questions about their social consequences and ethical meanings.

Assisted reproductive technologies are an obvious area of interest for those concerned with women's health (see "The Ethics of Fertility Treatments," p. 498). Other issues raised by human biotechnologies and related technologies include the patenting of human genes; the appropriate use of genetic testing; the questionable marketing of direct-to-consumer tests to determine your (or your children's) genetic makeup; the civil liberties and racial justice implications of forensic DNA databases; the use of synthetic biology techniques to create novel forms of life; and the prospect of extreme practices such as creating cloned or genetically redesigned human beings.

Advocates for women's health are among the growing number of civil society leaders, scholars, and policy experts who are concerned about the societal implications of these technologies and who want to ensure that their introduction will be grounded in values of social justice, human rights, ecological integrity, and the common good.

An informal network of organizations and individuals concerned about new reproductive and genetic technologies gathered in summer 2010 for the first of three planned annual meetings, now collectively known as the Tarrytown Meetings. The Center for Genetics and Society is the lead organization, and Our Bodies Ourselves is proud to be centrally involved in planning and implementation. These meetings focus on the policies, practices, and other societal changes needed to ensure responsible use and accountable governance of these technologies, both nationally and globally, and to promote a fuller awareness of their benefits and risks among the public, opinion leaders, policy makers, and others. For more information, see geneticsandsociety.org.

EMBRYONIC STEM CELL RESEARCH

Since human embryonic stem cells were first isolated in 1998, some scientists, biotechnology companies, and research advocates have made dramatic claims about their medical potential, promising treatments and cures for a wide range of chronic, degenerative, and acute diseases—including diabetes, Parkinson's disease, cancer, and Alzheimer's disease.

Their predictions have won impassioned support from many patient advocacy groups and stirred hopes in all who want to alleviate the suffering that these diseases inflict. Although some of these claims have been exaggerated, and although no treatments based on embryonic stem cells have been produced so far, many researchers believe that significant breakthroughs may be close at hand.

In addition to building excitement, embryonic stem cell research has also generated heated controversy. The critical voices most often heard during debates are those with strong moral objections to *all* embryonic stem cell work, on the grounds that it uses and then destroys human embryos for the sole purpose of harvesting stem cells. Yet a number of reproductive rights advocates have concerns, too—specifically about a type of stem cell research known as research cloning.

Objections to Research Cloning

The crucial distinction between embryonic stem cell research and research cloning is often blurred in the public debate. Embryonic stem cell research uses embryos initially produced in fertility clinics to help women become pregnant. So long as those embryos are donated with informed consent, which some people wish to do when they no longer need them for reproductive purposes, most women's health advocates have no objections to their use in research.

Research cloning—also called somatic cell nuclear transfer, embryo cloning, and therapeutic cloning—requires young women to undergo invasive and risky egg extraction procedures solely for the purpose of research. If it were to be perfected, research cloning would open a gateway not just to therapeutic applications but to efforts to clone a human being or to engineer the traits of future children (see "Genetic Modification of Future Generations" on p. 806). Unlike dozens of countries around the world, the United States has not yet established a federal prohibition on reproductive cloning, making it more likely that unethical researchers would use cloned embryos to attempt to produce a cloned baby.

Still, some reproductive rights advocates have hesitated to speak out against research cloning out of apprehension that their concerns will be used by anti–abortion rights activists to elevate the legal and moral status of embryos in efforts to deny access to abortion.

With new developments such as induced pluripotent stem cells (iPS cells)—specially treated cells that can be processed to behave somewhat like embryonic stem cells—research cloning may not even be necessary for generating patient-specific and disease-specific stem cell lines that could be used for medical therapies.

Concerns About Egg Extraction

Many feminists and social justice activists are concerned about research cloning and the egg extraction required for it. The envisioned treatments could require many thousands of donated eggs, requiring thousands of women to undergo the substantial risks of multiple egg extraction, which uses high doses of potent drugs. Although women already undergo these procedures in infertility clinics, the risks—even as inadequately defined as they are—may be justified because there is a demonstrated possibility that a baby will result. It is unwarranted to ask women to undergo these risks solely for research cloning. Not only are the benefits unclear, but there are not yet sufficient data on health risks to make true informed consent possible.

In addition, many women's health advocates are concerned about the creation of a larger market in human eggs. Women providing eggs for other people's fertility treatments generally receive reimbursements that range from $5,000 to $10,000, and some ads on college campuses have offered as much as $50,000 to $100,000 for eggs from women with desired traits (so-called Ivy League eggs).

It is unlikely that many women would provide eggs for research without reimbursement, and economically disadvantaged and young women would be most vulnerable to such incentives. Whether eggs are for research or helping others to have a baby, all women have the right to be informed about the potential risks. For this reason, advocacy groups are now calling for a national registry that would track the long-term effects of these procedures on women who donate eggs.

ASSISTED REPRODUCTIVE TECHNOLOGIES AND FERTILITY TOURISM

New developments in assisted reproductive technologies (ART) have enabled many people to have biologically related children who previously could not. At the same time, these technologies continue to raise complicated ethical questions that are often difficult for individuals and society to resolve.

Drawing the line with ARTs is both an individual and a social concern. In countries such as Canada, the United Kingdom, South Korea, and Australia, public policies have already been established to ensure greater safety for everyone involved with fertility procedures—parents, children, women who donate eggs, and gestational, or surrogate, mothers. These countries have prioritized the need for public discourse to ensure that these technologies—powerful enough to create human life outside a woman's body and to alter the species—are used in ways that society deems ethically acceptable.

Procedures that enable women to have a gestational—but not genetic—tie to a child, or that result in children with several sets of parents, pose new social and logistical dilemmas. Other procedures that test the genes of fetuses or embryos for genetic conditions open the way to further stigmatize people with disabilities; every day, more conditions are classified as diseases requiring intervention. A small but vocal group of scientists and others envision a future in which parents routinely choose their offspring's sex, physical traits, and even intelligence, prospects that would alter family and social relationships in disturbing ways.

As assisted reproduction technologies have mushroomed into a multibillion-dollar fertility industry, ethical and social challenges multiply. And as people seek to avoid policies in one country by traveling to another country to seek the services of a gestational mother, or to obtain embryos or donated eggs not available in their own countries, a rapidly growing phenomenon of cross-border reproductive tourism—also called fertility tourism—has magnified these problems.

For example, because the services of gestational mothers are less expensive in India than in the United States, India has become the leading go-to source of such services. Women with few other economic options are becoming gestational mothers with little assurance that contracts specifying particular payments will be honored, and with little protection for their own well-being and autonomy. These women are sometimes required to leave their own children for part or all of the duration of the pregnancy, live in dormitories attached to fertility clinics, and deliver by C-section even when that is not medically indicated.

The remarkable and exponential growth of infertility services across the globe, as well as the increasing use of ARTs that have not been adequately assessed for safety, requires new and more effective alliances among feminists, public health advocates, ethicists, and others who recognize the serious threats to women's health and human rights—especially for more vulnerable women enticed by misleading advertising and prospects of income.

One group that has taken the lead in such movement building is SAMA: Resource Group for Women and Health, located in New Delhi. In 2010, SAMA brought together scholars, activists, and researchers from around the world to develop strategies that will address these issues and also call for more efforts to identify and remove the environmental causes of infertility. "Unraveling the Fertility Industry," a report from the conference, is available at samawomenshealth.org.

PATENTING OF HUMAN GENES AND WOMEN'S HEALTH: WHO OWNS OUR GENES?

Since 1980, the U.S. Patent and Trademark Office (USPTO) has issued patents on the genes of living organisms, despite the widespread objection that genes are products of nature and not human-made inventions. The controversy has intensified with the patenting of human genes in the early 1990s.

In 2007, Rep. Xavier Becerra (D-Calif.) introduced the Genomic Research and Accessibility Act (H.R. 977) to prohibit the patenting of human genes and human genetic information. This act cited many justifications, from the points of view of both researchers and patients. Numerous researchers have been concerned that the patenting of and monopoly on a particular human gene reduce information sharing, innovation, quality control, and competition. For health consumers, patenting reduces availability of tests, increases cost, limits alternatives, and prevents second opinions.

The American Civil Liberties Union (ACLU), the Public Patent Foundation, and twenty co-plaintiffs filed a lawsuit in 2009 against the USPTO, Myriad Genetics, and the University of Utah Research Foundation, charging that patents on two human genes associated with breast and ovarian cancer are unconstitutional and invalid. The suit focused on the BRCA1 and BRCA2 genes, mutations of which are related to increased risk of breast and/or ovarian cancers, and for which Myriad Genetics controls the patents—effectively controlling the available testing for important mutations.

Breast Cancer Action and Our Bodies Ourselves—the only two women's health groups that are co-plaintiffs—believe that when one company controls all the testing, less information and fewer resources are available to both patients and researchers. Some doctors and researchers involved with the lawsuit contend that this monopoly has long held up not only competing, cheaper tests but also important gene-based research.

In 2010, a U.S. federal district court judge's ruling in the case invalidated the patents, arguing that the company deserved praise for what is "unquestionably a valuable scientific achievement," but not a patent, because the "claimed isolated DNA is not markedly different from native DNA as it exists in nature."[156] Essentially, the relevant genes are found in nature and thus, like other products of nature, are not patentable.

The judge did not address the question of whether the USPTO had violated the Constitution. After the decision, the U.S. Department of Justice withdrew its support for human gene patents, agreeing that genes themselves are not patentable. The ruling has the potential to make the study of and testing for important genetic variations cheaper and more readily accessible. This court decision was appealed in 2010 to a federal appellate court. For updates on the case, visit aclu.org/brca.

GENETIC MODIFICATION OF FUTURE GENERATIONS

Inheritable genetic modification (IGM, also called germline engineering) means changing the genes passed on to future generations. The genetic changes would be made during in vitro fertilization (IVF)—a process by which egg cells are fertilized by sperm outside the body—in eggs, sperm, or early embryos. The modified genes would appear not only in the person who developed from that gamete or embryo, but also in all succeeding generations. It would be by far the most consequential type of genetic modification, as it would open the door to irreversibly altering the human species—and these permanent changes could include unintended consequences.

Genetically modified plants and animals are now relatively common, but IGM has not been tried in humans. The production of cloned or genetically modified animals requires repeated attempts, the vast majority of which result in nonviable fetuses or in animals that die shortly after birth or have reduced life spans. Because cloning or IGM in humans would likewise result in large numbers of failed attempts, any research program would represent unethical experimentation on humans.

Some advocates of IGM say it can be used for medical purposes—such as to avoid the birth of children with genetic impairments or diseases. Even if this were possible, safe, and desirable, the same end can almost always be achieved using the embryo selection technique called preimplantation genetic diagnosis (see p. 488). Disability rights advocates point out that even embryo selection exerts pressures on women to produce the "perfect baby" and can create new forms of discrimination and prejudice based on genetics.

A disturbing number of influential scientists and biotechnology entrepreneurs are openly promoting the idea of using IGM in efforts to produce children with so-called genetic enhancements, referring to better looks, talents, and intelligence. Whether used for purposes of therapy or enhancement, inheritable genetic modification would be likely to entail harmful effects that are impossible to predict, regardless of how much previous research is conducted.

Many early discussions of inheritable genetic modification proposed drawing a line between its use for the treatment of disease and its use for enhancement of traits, such as height, eye color, strength, coordination, and intelligence. However, people often disagree about what constitutes an enhancement and what constitutes a necessary medical intervention. Many procedures that were introduced for medical purposes—such as plastic surgery—became commercialized for clearly nonmedical use soon after their introduction. In addition, some potential modifications would fall somewhere between treatment and enhancement—strengthening the immune system, for example, or increasing general alertness. It is increasingly clear that our society has not found effective ways to distinguish between what is an enhancement and what is a necessary medical intervention.

Some proponents of human genetic enhancement say they look forward to the day when parents can quite literally assemble their children from genes listed in a catalog. Fortunately, there is growing public debate—fostered by prominent ethicists and public health advocates—pointing to inherent dangers with such scenarios.

Princeton University biologist Lee Silver envisions the possibility that inheritable genetic modification will eventually lead to the emergence of genetic castes and human subspecies. "The GenRich class and the Natural class will become . . . entirely separate species," he has written, "with no ability to cross-breed, and with as much romantic interest in each other as a current human would have for a chimpanzee."[157]

As George Annas, chair of the Department of Health Law, Bioethics & Human Rights at Boston University School of Public Health, has noted, to the extent such visions are at all realistic, such a division of the human species is a sufficient argument against pursuing human inheritable genetic modification.[158] The profound social impacts of inheritable genetic modifications, as well as their potential impact on the entire species, mean that no individual scientist, corporation, or country has the moral authority to make the decision to use such technology.

Some advocates of IGM (and of reproductive cloning and sex selection) are attempting to appropriate the language of the reproductive rights movement, claiming that these high-tech procedures are extensions of individual choice and privacy rights. This claim blurs the difference between the right for which women have fought for so many years—the right to terminate an unwanted or unsustainable pregnancy—and a very different thing: the right of individuals (parents) to manipulate the biological traits of a future child. Women's health advocates need to challenge this co-optation of language in the public debate on biotechnology issues.

Given the far-reaching consequences of these technologies, we owe it to ourselves, our children, and future generations to think carefully about which ones we can responsibly and beneficially use as a society. The key question is where and how we would draw the line. Our Bodies Ourselves believes that the United States should join the emerging international consensus and pass laws against human reproductive cloning and inheritable genetic modification.

CHAPTER 27 ■ ■ ■ ■ ■ ■ ■ ■ ■ ■ ■ ■ ■

On May 31, 2009, anti-abortion rights activist Scott Roeder shot and killed Dr. George Tiller during Sunday morning services at Tiller's church in Wichita, Kansas. The target of constant protests, Tiller had survived a clinic bombing, previous shooting, and multiple legal challenges to close his practice, Women's Health Care Services—one of only three clinics in the country that performed abortions after twenty-one weeks.

Within days of Tiller's death, Steph Herold, a twenty-one-year-old recent college grad who was working as an abortion counselor in Pennsylvania, created the website I Am Dr. Tiller (IAmDrTiller.com). She sent the link to feminist blogs and women's clinics, asking for stories from individuals working to make abortion safe, legal, and accessible. Submissions came in

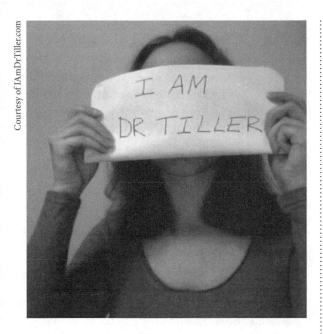

Courtesy of IAmDrTiller.com

from nurses, medical students, escorts, volunteers at abortion funds, and abortion doctors themselves—all of whom held up a sheet of paper or sign proclaiming "I Am Dr. Tiller." Criticism by Fox News host Bill O'Reilly only increased the site's popularity.

Herold also created a Twitter account—@iamdrtiller—to promote the stories and, later, to continue sharing facts and information around reproductive rights and justice and to connect with other pro-choice activists. She also founded a blog run by a group of young feminist activists (read her story on p. 816).

Using new media tools and technologies, it's easier for us to find and build community and make our voices heard. Today, anyone with a mobile phone or Internet connection can share information, create awareness, and attract the attention of policy makers or other stakeholders. While traditional forms of activism—such as street protests, boycotts, and well-crafted media campaigns—are still necessary and effective ways of gaining support and attention for some causes, the Internet and social media have trans-formed not only how we organize but also our ideas about what organizing or activism means.

There has never been a greater likelihood that one voice can make a difference. In fact, a far-reaching campaign is often started by just one person taking action—and today it might begin with blogging or raising awareness on Facebook, or tweeting about an injustice happening this very second. What may start as a small group of voices united by a common goal or grievance can develop into an organized and sustainable movement.

One group using the latest technological tools to effect change, the crowd-sourced initiative Hollaback! (ihollaback.org), formed to counter the street harassment frequently encountered by women and LGBTQ individuals. The movement encourages people to share their stories and to report instances of street harassment, from unwanted verbal attention to acts of touching or groping, using mobile technology such as the Hollaback! iPhone app. From its founding in New York City in 2005, Hollaback! has grown into an international movement.

We also have access to more information and viewpoints than ever before. Politicians, activist groups, and media sources keep us informed via email, text messages, and social networks. Racialicious (racialicious.com), Colorlines (colorlines.com), Feministing (feministing.com), Pam's House Blend (pamshouseblend.com), Feministe (feministe.us/blog), Pandagon (pandagon.net), INCITE! Women of Color Against Violence (inciteblog.wordpress.com), Shakesville (shakespearessister.blogspot.com), and The F Word (thefword.org.uk) are more than sites to visit for daily news and activism; they're feminist communities where readers share, commiserate, and challenge one another. The do-it-yourself dynamic of blogs enables a wide variety of voices to reach a larger audience and become part of the dialogue.

Through social media, more teens and young

women are speaking out and taking a stand. Julie Zeilinger was a fifteen-year-old high school student in Pepper Pike, Ohio, when she launched fbomb (thefbomb.org) in 2008 with the goal of creating a community and dialogue for teenage girls "who care about their rights as women and want to be heard." Within two years, Zeilinger's site had published submissions from all over the world.[1]

In this new era, traditional gatekeepers have been replaced by a decentralized assembly of digitally empowered citizen journalists. Organizing takes place independent of geographical boundaries, and stories have the potential to reach large audiences quickly. On the flip side, communities have never been more diffuse, and standing out among so many voices can be difficult. Online petitions and other forms of viral protest are sometimes dismissed as ineffective slacktivism. And access to new technology isn't universal; a digital divide exists between the digitally adept and those without access to digital tools and/or those who lack the knowledge and skills to be media creators as well as consumers. Spending a few hours a week in a school computer lab isn't the same as having a laptop or iPad in your backpack.

While social networking and digital media have certainly become important catalysts for change, providing new and effective forms of expression, we need to work to increase access so all of us have the tools and the means to tell our own stories.

MAKING OUR VOICES HEARD

STRENGTH IN NUMBERS

This impulse toward activism usually begins when something affects us or someone we know. We may be motivated by a health problem or by injustices in our neighborhoods and schools. A friend or family member may alert us to issues we care deeply about and want to work to improve.

Organizing does not take experts or a lot of money. What it does take is a committed group of individuals willing to invest time and energy to work together toward a common goal. The Internet and mobile technology (which has even higher use among African Americans and Latinos than among whites)[2] have made it easier for more people from diverse backgrounds to share information and get involved in causes that matter most to them.

Creating change on a larger level takes many voices. After we have taken a few steps on our own, we may want to get involved with groups working on an issue or start a group of our own. Here are some questions for groups to consider in the early stages of organizing:

- Can we clearly define our issue?
- What do we already know about the issue? What don't we know? What research has already been done, and by whom?
- What will be the scope of our work? Do we have enough people to manage the work we want to do?
- Which online/offline communications tools will we use to spread our message? Which communication tools are used by the people most affected by this issue?
- Are there organizations or individuals already working on the problem? If so, how can we work together?
- How many women are affected? Are the women most affected involved in efforts to create solutions?
- Who are the opposition? How are they supported/funded?
- What approaches to the problem are we considering? What resources are needed to accomplish them? Where will we find the needed resources?

• How will our group be organized? What will be our group norms on inclusiveness, diversity, decision making, and logistics?

The answers to these questions will help you to create a supportive group infrastructure and work toward formulating an action plan. Think of specific objectives and consider what tools and resources you need to realize each goal. Remember to focus on telling people's stories, which helps to personalize the issue.

Don't assume that everyone will know about an event if you post it on Facebook. Think about whom you're trying to reach and adapt your message—and your medium—accordingly.

In our group, very few women had experience speaking publicly to or before the media. So we set aside some meetings to role-play, to practice speaking before a group, and to learn how to say the most important things in the least amount of time. We also practiced saying the things we wanted people to hear, even if they were not related to the interviewer's question. Doing all this is a great way to break through shyness and stage fright.

GET YOUR MESSAGE OUT

Need help making your voice heard? These groups work with individuals and organizations, helping them to tell their own stories and develop media expertise.

• **The OpEd Project** (opedproject.org) trains female experts in all fields to write for the op-ed pages of major print and online forums of public discourse. The OpEd Project works with universities, nonprofits, corporations, women's organizations, and community leaders and offers seminars open to the public in major cities across the nation. Scholarships are available.

• **The Women's Media Center** (womensme diacenter.org) aims to make women visible

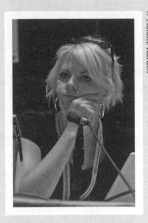

© Natalie Kardos

YOUR PRESENCE IS REQUIRED

Deanna Zandt (deannazandt.com), a media technologist and the author of Share This! How You Will Change the World with Social Networking, *would like to see more women sharing stories on Twitter, editing entries on Wikipedia, and dismantling the dominant paradigm everywhere.*

We all know that we can get the word out about the things we care about—but social media is so much more than a tool to broadcast to the masses. It's where people and organizations are increasingly coming together to *listen* to one another—a fairly transformational act in the age of information overload.

What we see when we participate on social networks are tiny acts of radical storytelling that, when compiled over time, paint a picture of a person's life. Through that portrait, we can influence the power structures that surround us: the cultural norms by which we act; the laws that govern us; the expectations we experience based on our gender, race, class, sexuality, abilities, and more.

When we share and listen, a magical thing happens in our brains: We start to trust one another more. And once we start trusting one another, we start empathizing with one another more. Empathy is critical to any kind of social change movement; it is the opposite of apathy.

The trust we create with one another on social networks is what fuels the empathetic response we have, to one another, even if we don't know one another that well. That trust-created empathy is what will lead us away from the isolation that we've experienced as a culture in the last century's focus on mass communications and market demographics—siloing people and separating them. These technologies are all about connecting, engaging, sharing.

Your presence is required in this work: We need you here in the online social space. Change won't happen on its own. It requires you to show up, and to participate. Tech will not solve our problems—*we* will solve our problems, working together.

and powerful in the media. In addition to offering media training workshops to the public, women can apply for the Progressive Women's Voices Project, an all-expenses paid program that trains women to position themselves as thought leaders/experts in their fields; craft strong media messages and newsworthy pitches; and prepare for both friendly and hostile broadcast interviews.

- **Barefoot Workshops** (barefootworkshops .org) is a New York City–based nonprofit organization that teaches individuals and organizations how to use digital video, new media, and the arts to transform their communities and themselves.

- **"Get Noticed! How to Publicize Your Book or Film"** (aidandabet.org/resources/get-noticed) is your DIY guide to promoting a project. Written by Jen Angel, Matt Dineen, and Justine Johnson, this fifty-plus-page booklet covers everything from writing press materials to using social media and pitching stories to reporters at independent and mainstream media outlets.

ORGANIZING FOR CHANGE: REPRODUCTIVE HEALTH AND JUSTICE

In recent years, women of color and their allies have organized a reproductive justice movement that examines how issues of race and class affect women's abilities to exercise their reproductive rights. This dynamic movement is growing, and today many organizations and networks are taking part. The largest among them is SisterSong, a network of eighty local, regional, and national organizations (and many other affiliate organizations) representing five primary ethnic populations/indigenous nations in the United States: African American, Arab American/Middle Eastern, Asian/Pacific Islander, Latina, and Native American/Indigenous.

The reproductive justice movement promotes a broader understanding of women's rights and health, placing abortion within a larger framework that includes maternal and infant health, economic justice, racial equality, and ending violence against women. There are three main frameworks for addressing reproductive oppression: reproductive rights (legal structures), reproductive health (service delivery), and reproductive justice (movement building).

Organizations and individuals are working to strengthen each of these pillars and, by doing so, they are improving access for all women.

SISTERSONG WOMEN OF COLOR REPRODUCTIVE JUSTICE COLLECTIVE

Website: sistersong.net

In 2010, the Georgia state legislature took up a bill that aimed to limit access to reproductive services. The new twist: The bill falsely proclaimed that women of color were being targeted by abortion providers. So-called "pro-life freedom rides" in the summer of 2010 co-opted important civil rights legacies in order to try to deny women of color access to reproductive choice. This followed on the heels of a controversial anti–abortion rights billboard campaign that called black children "an endangered species."

"You cannot save black babies by discriminating against black women," said Loretta Ross, national coordinator of SisterSong. "Civil rights

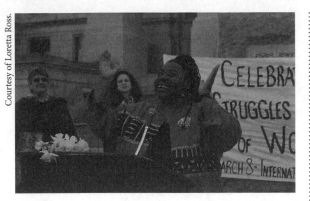

Loretta Ross, a founder and the National Coordinator of the SisterSong Women of Color Reproductive Health Collective, speaks at a Georgia rally for immigration rights in March 2011.

has always been about expanding freedoms for black people, not rolling back the clock to the nineteenth century like these anti-abortionists want. Should black women again become breeders for their cause?"

True freedom, she added, ensures human rights for all people, including reproductive rights and reproductive health care options for women.

When anti–abortion rights activists arrived by bus in Atlanta on July 24, SisterSong, along with SPARK Reproductive Justice NOW (sparkrj.org) and SisterLove (sisterlove.org) were waiting, their voices ready. This is Ross's story from the counterrally:

More than fifty supporters came from Project South, Advocates for Youth, Feminist Women's Health Center, the Malcolm X Movement, and of course, SPARK, SisterSong, and SisterLove. The folks were mostly African American, but a number of Latinas and some white activists came in solidarity. It was a decidedly young group, with only a few elders like me sitting back and watching them lead. We had a spirited rally for about an hour, with speeches and statements of

solidarity, like from the Religious Coalition for Reproductive Choice.

Then the anti-abortionists' bus and cars pulled up in front of the King Center. Staying on our side of the street as they disembarked, we started chanting. "Trust Black Women" as loudly as we could, holding up signs that read "You Can't Steal Civil Rights" and "Women's Rights are Human Rights." Paris Hatcher and Tonya Williams from SPARK, and Heidi Williamson of SisterSong, led the rally with spirit and energy that really excited our side and kept everyone engaged and having fun.

We were quite surprised when the antis piled off the bus—all but four of whom were white as far as we could tell! For a campaign organized by the African-American outreach director for Priests for Life, Alveda King, it was surreal seeing all these white folks carrying signs that said "Abortion Is the #1 Killer of Black America." Can you imagine the optics of the scene? Here's a group of white folks claiming to save black babies being protested by mostly African-American women and men who are shouting "Trust Black Women!" Once we saw their signs, Paris instantly created a new chant: "Racism Is the #1 Killer of Black America, Not Black Women!" The ironies of the day seemed endless—when was the last time black folks protested at a white folks' rally at the center named after Dr. Martin Luther King?

After marching in front of the tombs and reassembling on the sidewalk until they were told to move on, the antis left their side of the street and walked around the back of our demonstration to hold their prayer service on the grass behind the amphitheater where we were, possibly upon orders by the park police. Suddenly, there were no barriers, no police, nothing between the two groups. At first, everyone kept their distance—we shouted, they sang; we held up signs, they held up their hands. Then things got interesting when they decided to cross the invisible barrier and start praying over us. The park police providentially appeared and kept both sides apart.

It seemed a bit ridiculous when they started singing "We Shall Overcome" to counter our singing "Lift Ev'ry Voice." Eventually, the heat of the day wore everyone out. They moved across the street again (not in front of the King Center) in order to finish their praying. We climbed to the top of the amphitheater to look down on them to continue our chant, "Trust Black Women!" I think we frustrated them because I'm sure many of these white folks assumed the black community of Atlanta would welcome them as saviors of the black race. It was obvious they were more than a little uncomfortable at being shouted down by black women. After about an hour and a half of this back and forth, they boarded their bus and left and so did we, but not without singing, "Nah, nah, nah, nah, nah, nah. Hey-hey-hey. Good-bye."

NATIONAL ADVOCATES FOR PREGNANT WOMEN

Website: advocatesforpregnantwomen.org
In October 2010, Colorado voters rejected a ballot measure seeking to classify "preborns" as "legal persons with protection under the law." With implications that went far beyond attempting to restrict abortion, this measure would have granted fetuses, embryos, and even fertilized eggs legal status separate from the women who carry them. The National Advocates for Pregnant Women (NAPW), an advocacy group working on behalf of all pregnant women, published a commentary criticizing the Colorado measure's sponsor Personhood USA's "radical fetal-separatist agenda" and helped defeat the ballot measure. Other states, including Montana and Nevada, have attempted without success to pass similar laws.

Lynn M. Paltrow, founder and executive director of NAPW, wrote, "Pregnant women could be sued, subject to child welfare interventions, or even arrested if they engaged in activities at work and at home that might be thought to create a risk to the life of the 'preborn.' Legally separating the 'preborn' from the pregnant women who sustain them will ensure that in jobs, education, and civic life, pregnant women will, once again, be unequal to men."[3]

Speaking out against laws that undermine the rights of women, the NAPW formed to expand the reproductive rights movement to all parenting and pregnant women, including those who plan to continue their pregnancies to term. Through a wide array of advocacy work—including local and national organizing, litigation, public policy development, and public education—the organization works to secure reproductive rights for all women, especially underrepresented and at-risk groups such as women of color, low-income women, and women addicted to drugs or alcohol. In addition to safe and legal abortion, the organization lobbies for access to adequate prenatal health care, alternative birthing practices, support for vaginal birth after cesarean (VBAC), and nonpunitive drug treatment services for pregnant women.

NAPW's legal advocates vocally oppose the shackling of inmates during labor and the criminalization of drug addiction in pregnancy and have provided litigation support in a variety of related cases across the country. Relying on a network of more than two thousand local and national activists, the group has challenged the arrests of pregnant women charged with child endangerment for drinking alcohol and has formed alliances with other organizations to file amicus (friend of the court) briefs explaining how so-called fetal rights laws dehumanize and criminalize pregnant women.

STEPH HEROLD: ONLINE ACTIVIST

Websites: abortiongang.org and
iamdrtiller.com

Steph Herold is a reproductive justice activist
who has worked in direct service abortion care
and reproductive health advocacy.

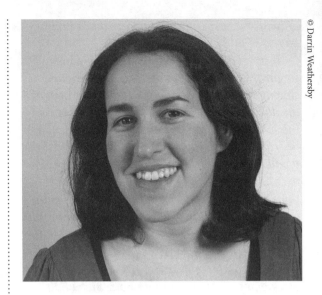

© Darrin Weathersby

*In 2010, I created the Abortion Gang blog as
a space specifically for young people in the
reproductive justice movement, with the goal of
raising our visibility and highlighting our activism.*

*There were a number of articles in the
mainstream media that year claiming that young
people weren't pro-choice enough or were not
engaged in meaningful activist work. I wanted to
counteract those attitudes with tangible evidence.
The next time someone wondered what young
people were doing, I could point to numerous
activities documented on the blog.*

*The name "Abortion Gang" came out of the
seemingly endless health care reform debates.
Then-representative Bart Stupak was accused
of having an "abortion gang"—a group of
congressmen who were committed to voting no
on the bill unless Stupak's antichoice abortion
language was included. My first reaction was:
Why does this antichoice, antiwoman politician
get to have an abortion gang? He doesn't know
the first thing about abortion, women's health,
and reproductive justice, to say the least. If there's
anyone who could disqualify from being in an
abortion gang, it's Bart Stupak. So I decided to
start the real abortion gang, one composed of
people fully committed to abortion rights.*

*When the blog first appeared, we received
some criticism from within the feminist
community, asking why we focus specifically on
abortion. I explained that calling ourselves an
abortion gang means that we are committed to
destigmatizing not only abortion care work but
also reproductive justice activism. We support
all aspects of reproductive justice work and do*

*not shy away from controversy and complexity.
We embrace and analyze it in order to better
understand why we do what we do, and to
explore the power of justice and compassion.*

*In the past year and a half, I've launched the
Abortion Gang blog, the I Am Dr. Tiller project,
and both Twitter accounts associated with these
initiatives. The success of each of these campaigns
speaks volumes to the power of social media and
the Internet as organizing tools.*

*A case study of just how powerful online
campaigns can be is the Twitter hashtag I started
in the fall of 2010, #IHadAnAbortion. I asked
women to tweet their abortion stories as a way to
counteract the stigma associated with abortion. I
had no idea what to expect, if there was going to
be any response at all. What happened in the next
twenty-four hours amazed me: Women shared
their stories, women who had previously been
completely absent from the pro-choice activist
community. It didn't take long for the media to
catch on, and soon enough, CNN, PBS, and a
variety of mainstream media, online and off,
were talking about this phenomenon. Did they
understand it? Usually not. But their coverage
showed that this campaign struck a nerve, and*

this exposure led more women to speak out and find a new community of people who support them and their reproductive choices.

That isn't to say the world of social media advocacy isn't without its complexities and problems. If you looked at the hashtag a few weeks later, it's dominated by antichoice cruelty and misinformation. That is the reality of online organizing: when you open up a conversation, everyone has access to it.

SEXUALIZATION OF YOUNG GIRLS AND WOMEN

WHEN SEXUALITY EQUALS POWER

A clever advertising tactic is to manipulate the message that many feminists have tried to promote: Girls have the power to be anything and to do anything they want. It's not surprising that in what author and activist Ariel Levy calls "raunch culture," advertisers and other media have reinterpreted this idea. In a male-centered culture, where female athletes gain praise and recognition when they pose in *Playboy* and pop stars focus first and foremost on how sexy and attractive they are, this girl power gets translated into a distorted message that tells girls they can wear anything they want and no one can tell them otherwise.

In this interpretation, power has nothing to do with character or achievement but instead equates to the power of sexual attraction. For tweens and teens navigating this landscape, the pressure and expectation to be pretty, thin, *and* sexy can become an all-consuming task.

Levy aptly observes: "Adolescent girls in particular—who are blitzed with cultural pressure to be hot, to seem sexy—have a very difficult time learning to recognize their own sexual desire, which would seem a critical component of feeling sexy."[4] The notion that performance of sexuality equals power and control is particularly perilous for girls navigating their way to adulthood.

APA TASK FORCE ON THE SEXUALIZATION OF GIRLS

The APA Task Force on the Sexualization of Girls, formed by the American Psychological Association, issued a report in 2007 (updated in 2010)[5] addressing the omnipresence and damaging effects of sexualized images of girls and young women in every media format studied, including advertising, television, movies, music videos, music lyrics, magazines, sports media, video games, and online.

As expected, the images and depictions of women presented reflect a narrow—and unrealistic—standard of beauty that serves to undermine women. And, according to the report, sexualization has a host of negative psychological consequences for girls and young women—it affects their "cognitive functioning, physical and mental health, sexuality, and attitudes and beliefs" and harms "girls' self-image and healthy development." (See Chapter 3, "Body Image," for more discussion.)

The report also took an important step in identifying the components of sexualization, noting that it occurs when:

- a person's value comes only from his or her sexual appeal or behavior, to the exclusion of other characteristics
- a person is held to a standard that equates physical attractiveness (narrowly defined) with being sexy
- a person is sexually objectified—that is, made into a thing for others' sexual use, rather than seen as a person with the capacity for independent action and decision making
- sexuality is inappropriately imposed upon a person

RAISING VOICES, SHARING STORIES

In response to this widespread problem, feminist and youth groups are promoting their own positive messages about sexuality tied to thinking critically about media representations of girls and women. New Moon Girls (newmoon.com) is both a magazine and a moderated online community for girls ages eight and older. Designed to help girls develop healthy body image, the site features articles on girls changing the world, stories about arts and culture from around the world, and a safe and moderated chat room where girls can express themselves and share ideas. Girls can also create and share their own artwork, poetry, and videos through the site.

Dedicated to the health and well-being of girls and young women, Hardy Girls Healthy Women (hghw.org) is a nonprofit that works to give girls opportunities to explore new interests and build alliances with other girls. The organization trains adults who work with girls in second to twelfth grade and develops programs that encourage girls to think critically about media depictions of women and recognize and address unfairness. On the website, a program participant named Beth says: "When I see an ad that is selling women instead of the product, I recognize it. When I hear a sexist comment, I recognize it. And when I feel the need to speak my mind, I do, and without feeling out of line."[6]

Geared toward an older demographic, Name It, Change It (nameitchangeit.org) is a nonpartisan organization that works to end sexist and misogynistic coverage of women candidates in the media. The site has exposed sexist comments by radio hosts, pundits, bloggers, and journalists that undermine women candidates and leaders.

Finally, if you're tired of stories that misrepresent girls and women—or leave us out of the picture entirely—visit Women, Action & the Media (womenactionmedia.org), also known as WAM! This organization aims to change the narrative by connecting and supporting media makers, activists, academics, and funders working to advance women's media participation, ownership, and representation. Among its many offerings is an active and informative Listserv that welcomes students as well as professionals.

SPARK SUMMIT SPARKS ACTION

In October 2010, Hunter College—in partnership with the Women's Media Center, Hardy Girls Healthy Women, Ms. Foundation, and numerous other educators and organizations—held the first-ever SPARK Summit (sparksummit.com) to counter the increasing sexualization of girls in the media.

SPARK in this instance stands for Sexualization Protest: Action, Resistance, Knowledge. Speakers tackled a wide variety of issues, including the marketing of padded bras and thong underwear to little girls, the passive or hypersexualized roles of girls and women in TV and films, and the link between self-sexualization and low self-esteem in teens. More than three hundred people attended the summit, with hundreds more participating online.

At the Women Media Center's action station—dubbed "Changing the Conversation/Amplifying Your Voice"—girls created their own video journalism, submitted posts to WMC's blog, and reported on incidents of sexism through the WMC's Sexism Watch campaign. Some girls went on to be featured on NPR and CBS, in The Huffington Post, in *El Diario,* and in other media outlets.

As one speaker at the summit explained, the focus wasn't antisex but, rather, antiexploitation. Women and girls need to think critically about the messages they're receiving and "take sexy back"—in other words, reclaim their sexuality in a healthy and positive way.

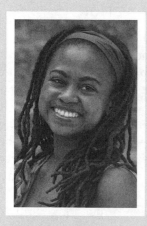

JAMIA WILSON

Named one of the Real Hot 100 by the Younger Women's Task Force (ywtf.org)—an award that celebrates achievements—activist Jamia Wilson, vice president of programs at the Women's Media Center, explains why media literacy is fundamental to empowering girls and young women.

Girls deserve access to media literacy education and information about how to create their own positive media, so they can better understand the choices they have—and the impact that billions of dollars in advertising has on the *lack* of choices they're presented with daily.

With six media conglomerates controlling the vast majority of media content, we're seeing a dramatic decrease in alternative and positive representations of girls in entertainment and news media. Studies show that the more TV a girl watches, the fewer options she believes she has in life. The media and marketers tell us from the time we are very little that this is what we have to look, dress, and act like if we want to fit in. We're asking for alternatives that do not render our bodies as expendable objects.

The messages are becoming more limiting with the emergence of pole-dancing kits for little girls, padded bikini tops for toddlers, highly sexualized costumes for all ages, and thongs and lingerie for tweens. We have the Powered by Girl "Library of Really!?!" on the SPARK website, featuring some of the current sexualized media messages and products.

Our sexuality is not a commodity for marketers to sell or co-opt. We must tell our stories on our own terms.

CHALLENGING MAINSTREAM SCIENCE AND INDUSTRY

According to the Natural Resources Defense Council, more than 80,000 chemicals in use in the United States have never been fully tested for their potential adverse impact on humans or the environment. While the European Union has banned 1,100 dangerous chemicals from use in personal care products, the FDA has banned or restricted only 11. (For more information on toxics and chemicals and their effect on our health, see Chapter 25, "Environmental and Occupational Health.")

Consider the case of bisphenol A (BPA), a chemical used to make plastics more durable. Despite overwhelming scientific evidence that BPA disrupts the endocrine system and has been shown to cause cancer as well as developmental and reproductive problems, the product is still used in water bottles, baby bottles, the lining of aluminum cans, and other food and drink packaging. Seven states and a few cities have passed laws prohibiting the sale of baby bottles containing BPA, but the federal government has yet to pass a nationwide ban on the chemical's use in food and drink containers. (Notably, the European Union and Canada have already banned the use of BPA in baby bottles.)

For years, activist groups have taken up the slack, delving into critical issues about the safety of our food, water, and air and carrying out their own research into the effects of chemicals in the environment. The Silent Spring Institute, for example, works to identify and cast light on the links between environmental issues and women's health, particularly breast cancer. Formed in 1994 to investigate the higher rates of breast cancer on Cape Cod, the organization took its name from Rachel Carson's landmark 1962 book *Silent Spring*, which helped launch the environmental movement. The coalition of scientists, physicians, and public health activists at the institute has undertaken research into, among other issues, the environmental causes of breast cancer, rates of household exposure to endocrine disrupters, and the presence of hormone-disrupting chemicals in septic systems.

In an open letter on the organization's website (silentspring.org), Silent Spring Institute executive director Julia G. Brody details the important questions we should be asking about the link between environmental issues and breast cancer and other diseases: "In the past decade, the very personal question, 'Why did I get breast cancer?' has been transformed. New voices ask, 'Why do we have breast cancer rates higher than generations before and among the highest in the world? What can we do as a community of women and men to change the legacy for our daughters?' "

BREAST CANCER ACTION

Website: bcaction.org

In the past two decades, the fight against breast cancer has become a popular cause. Walks, runs, and fund-raisers exist in every major city in the United States. Breast Cancer Action (BCA) has used this growing public interest to challenge the cancer industry—that is, hospitals, pharmaceutical companies, research institutes, and other organizations—and insist on increased focus on prevention.

BCA's Think Before You Pink initiative (thinkbeforeyoupink.org) has challenged a number of misguided breast cancer awareness campaigns that trivialize or sexualize breast cancer—for example, taking to task one manufacturer for selling pink ribbon thongs imprinted with the slogan "I've lost my boobies, but not my sex appeal."

BCA also targets pinkwashers, or companies profiting from pink-cause marketing that make or sell products that could increase the risk of breast cancer. One such pinkwashing campaign was KFC's "Buckets for the Cure,"[7] an attempt by the fried chicken franchise to raise breast cancer awareness in partnership with Susan G. Komen for the Cure. BCA exposed the hypocrisy of linking fast food—and franchises disproportionately located in low-income neighborhoods with limited access to fresh, healthful food options—to efforts to reduce the rate of breast cancer.

In an interview on NPR, Barbara Brenner, former executive director of BCA, countered the assumption that all the marketing and awareness around the disease have solved the problem, saying that "if shopping could cure breast cancer, it would be cured by now." She continued, "Awareness we have, the question is, what are we doing about it? And when companies can just slap a pink ribbon on any product, then

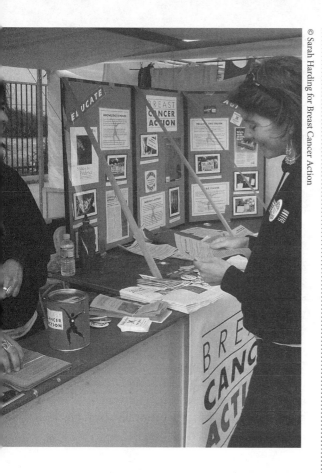

we're in trouble, because many of those products don't do anything for breast cancer. And many of them are actually harmful to our health."[8]

In 2008, Think Before You Pink took on the mainstream dairy industry. Yoplait was selling pink-lidded yogurt to raise money for breast cancer. Yoplait's yogurt, however, was made from milk containing recombinant bovine growth hormone (rBGH), an artificial hormone injected into cows to make them produce more milk; rBGH may be associated with increased rates of breast, prostate, colon, and other cancers. BCA started an online campaign to raise awareness about the issue and helped activists get their message directly to the CEO of Yoplait's par-

ent company, General Mills. As a result of the campaign, Yoplait changed to rBGH-free milk. Shortly after, the second-largest dairy product manufacturer, Dannon, followed suit.

The backlash against pinkwashing is gaining momentum and more people—and media—are questioning if the focus on awareness is helping women. In the article "The Downside of Awareness Campaigns," the *Los Angeles Times* reported this troubling statistic: "The stark reality is that in the 26 years since the campaign [National Breast Cancer Awareness Month] began, deaths from breast cancer have dropped only slightly—about 2 percent per year, starting in 1990." Certain breast cancer–related issues, such as overdiagnosis and overtreatment, the article continues, don't make it into the mainstream literature or most large-scale advocacy compaigns.[9]

When buying pink products or donating to breast cancer causes, find out about the company's environmental practices (to learn whether the company contributes to the problem) and how much of the money raised actually goes to support breast cancer research or treatment.

Many women with breast cancer are inspired to ask questions and get involved in efforts to find the answers. One woman recalls how meeting and working with other women transformed her experience:

I was first diagnosed with breast cancer in September of 1991 at the age of forty-two. I was angry, depressed, and hopelessly paralyzed. I was certain that I would die—never to see my children grow up. Within two months, I found a small group of women who were meeting at a coffee shop in my neighborhood. What began as a support group turned into a call to action. I recall bringing homemade petitions to the group and asking people to sign letters to senators, representatives, and even the president of the United States asking for more money for research. We found women in other support groups who were also wanting to mobilize—to channel our anger and our energy. We started to talk about things like environmental exposures and prevention. . . . As I think back to those first years, I remember clearly the faces of the women in those groups. Some are still alive, many are not. Now it is clear to me how much becoming active in a movement was a vital piece of my getting through treatment and getting well again. For this I am eternally grateful.

GLOBAL ACTIVISM

STORIES FROM AROUND THE WORLD

In our increasingly plugged-in and interconnected world, it's never been easier to read stories and view videos created by women working to secure sexual and reproductive health rights around the world. You don't have to look any farther than Facebook, Flickr, or YouTube to be awed by the range of actions held during the 16 Days of Activism Against Gender Violence (16dayscwgl.rutgers.edu), the international campaign that runs from November 25 (International Day Against Violence Against Women) to December 10 (International Human Rights Day), or to connect deeply with one girl's story about how she is creating change in her community.

In recent years, more attention has been paid to the idea that to overcome poverty in developing countries, more must be done to invest in the health, education, and empowerment of girls (see, for example, Half the Sky Movement [halftheskymovement.org] and The Girl Effect [thegirleffect.org]), reinforcing the strategies that a number of women's organizations have been supporting for decades.

The Global Fund for Women (globalfundforwomen.org), for instance, advances human rights by channeling resources into women-run organizations worldwide working toward women's economic security, health, education, and leadership. It trusts local activists to come up with solutions that best address the needs of their own communities and countries. Since 1988, it has awarded grants to more than 4,200 women's groups in 171 countries—from helping the multicultural feminist organization The Fiji Women's Rights Movement (fwrm.org.fj) address inequalities in Fiji's legal system to supporting the work of Labrys (labrys.kg), a group advocating for lesbian, gay, bisexual, and transgender rights in Kyrgyzstan.

In Mexico, Semillas (semillas.org.mx) does similar work, awarding grants to organizations that work in four primary areas: human rights, women and work, sexual and reproductive rights, and gender violence. Learn about other women's funds around the world at the International Network of Women's Funds (inwf.org) and the Women's Funding Network (wfnet.org), both of which act as umbrella organizations, linking women's funds together.

INTERNATIONAL WOMEN'S HEALTH COALITION

Website: iwhc.org

In September 2009, the Indonesian government passed a new health law that expanded reproductive health services for women. Prior to its passage, abortion was essentially illegal. The new law allows access to abortion in cases of rape or when the life of the woman is threatened. While far from perfect, it's an encouraging start in a country lacking comprehensive reproductive health care for women.

One primary advocate of the new law was the Jakarta-based Yayasan Kesehatan Perempuan (YKP), or Women's Health Foundation, which works with health workers and the Indonesian government to promote women's rights. Funding from the International Women's Health Coalition (IWHC) helped YKP get its message across to policy makers and community leaders and influence the government's decision to pass the law. The IWHC is also helping YKP promote other reproductive health issues, including increasing access to emergency obstetric care by trained midwives or birth attendants to reduce the maternal mortality rate.

Since 1984, the IWHC has distributed more than $16.5 million in grants to organizations advocating women's rights and health in Africa, Asia, and Latin America. The organization aims to have both a local and a global impact by focusing on two areas that are occasionally at odds: local activism and international policy. In addition to working closely with community and regional organizations and networks in Africa, Asia and the Middle East, and Latin America, the IWHC has collaborated with other global women's health and rights organizations to influence United Nations deliberations. It also has served as an intermediary between UN agencies and local and grassroots advocates on key issues regarding reproductive and sexual health. The IWHC's collaborations with the World Health Organization focus on access to safe abortion services, sexuality and sexual health, and reproductive health and rights.

The IWHC also runs an informative blog, Akimbo (blog.iwhc.org), that provides coverage of global news and policies related to women's health and rights. On the anniversary of *Roe v. Wade* in 2011, one of Akimbo's contributors posted a video about a dangerous abortion procedure that cost a woman her life in rural India. The video stressed that, even in places where abortion is nominally legal, it is not necessarily safe or accessible. The video and post underscored the importance of continuing to advocate for better access to safe abortion procedures and reproductive health care for women worldwide.

MOVING FORWARD

Social networks and new technologies have made information incredibly accessible, and the participation of a multitude of voices has made generating awareness and support for women's issues a more organic and dynamic process. At the same time, the challenges facing the women's health movement are formidable, and the political atmosphere in the United States has seldom been this volatile.

Regardless of the ever-changing ways we organize and communicate, and despite the nature and complexity of our present challenges, we can find our strength where we have always found it—in community. Together we stand a greater chance of addressing immediate issues while also taking on entrenched stereotypes and power structures.

When we—with our endless variety of backgrounds and experiences—are willing to cross boundaries to listen and learn from one another, anything is possible.

IN TRANSLATION: WOMEN'S RIGHTS ARE HUMAN RIGHTS

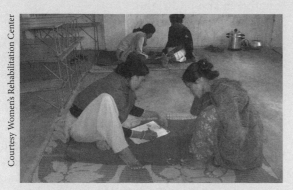

A WOREC community health provider in session.

Group: Women's Rehabilitation Centre (WOREC)

Country: Nepal

Resource: *Hamro Sharir, Hamro Ho (Our Body, Ourselves)*, a set of five Nepali booklets based on *Our Bodies, Ourselves*

Website: worecnepal.org

Since 1991, Our Bodies Ourselves' partner in Nepal, the Women's Rehabilitation Center (WOREC), has been central to the country's civic progress and political transition from a monarchy to a fledgling democracy. WOREC fights against many forms of gender violence, including early marriage and sexual trafficking, and promotes the health rights of women at both the community and the national level.

In 2007, WOREC was part of a coalition responsible for the inclusion of reproductive health rights in Nepal's interim constitution, and it is now working to ensure that the same rights are included in the country's final constitution. The group also worked with government officials on a national health strategy focused on women. More recently, WOREC collaborated with partners and policy makers on gender and violence training for twelve district governments and nonprofit organizations across the country.

The organization has published five booklets based on *Our Bodies, Ourselves*, adapted to the needs of women and girls in Nepal. Prior to publication, WOREC used the information in a nationwide outreach at health fairs, clinics, and health centers to educate women and girls about their bodies and the influence of cultural and social factors on their well-being.

Challenging the status quo in a deeply patriarchal society has often placed the organization's members in danger. The group has advocated on behalf of rape survivors to bring perpetrators to justice and educated Dalits (a socially and economically disadvantaged group) on their right to fair wages.

Attacks on WOREC have included physical and sexual intimidation, verbal abuse, and death threats. With little support from law enforcement authorities, WOREC continues to put itself on the front line to bring health information to thousands of women and girls across the country.

The nature of WOREC's work, coupled with ongoing intimidation and limited support, has often left members demoralized and isolated in their activism. This is sobering, and it demands renewed commitment to holding perpetrators accountable, so activists who defend women's rights can do so with dignity and safety.

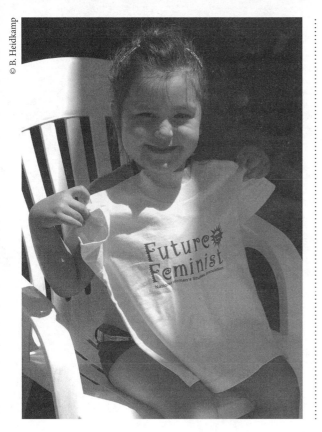

© B. Heidkamp

It wasn't until I went to a social justice conference that I fully grasped the longevity of the struggle of which I am only the latest small part. I knew that many women had come before me, of course, but to see the generations interacting at this conference was a revelation to me. We have to keep listening and challenging and supporting each other. It's a long road. But I get goose bumpy thinking of going forward with so many amazing women, of all ages and backgrounds, and I'm grateful that they are my friends and allies.

RECOMMENDED RESOURCES

For additional recommended resources, visit the Our Bodies Ourselves website, ourbodiesourselves .org/book/library.asp.

CHAPTER 1:
OUR FEMALE BODIES

Accord Alliance: AccordAlliance.org. Promotes the health and well-being of people and families affected by disorders of sex development (DSD). Has replaced the Intersex Society of North America, which closed in 2008.

Bobel, Chris. *New Blood: Third-Wave Feminism and the Politics of Menstruation.* New Brunswick: Rutgers University Press, 2010.

Centre for Menstrual Cycle and Ovulation Research: Cemcor.ubc.ca.

Loulan, JoAnn, and Bonnie Worthen. *Period.: A Girl's Guide.* Minnetonka, MN: Book Peddlers, 2001.

MRKH Organization: information and support to those with Mayer-Rokitansky-Küster-Hauser syndrome, mrkh.org.

Nalebuff, Rachel Kauder. *My Little Red Book.* New York: Twelve, 2009.

re: Cycling: blog of the Society for Menstrual Cycle Research: menstruationresearch.org/blog.

Reis, Elizabeth. *Bodies in Doubt: An American History of Intersex.* Baltimore: Johns Hopkins University Press, 2009.

Singer, Katie. *The Garden of Fertility: A Guide to Charting Your Fertility Signals to Prevent or Achieve Pregnancy—Naturally—and to Gauge Your Reproductive Health.* New York: Harper, 2001.

Wechsler, Toni. *Taking Charge of Your Fertility, 10th Anniversary Edition: The Definitive Guide to Natural Birth Control, Pregnancy Achievement, and Reproductive Health.* New York: Harper, 2006.

CHAPTER 2:
INTRO TO SEXUAL HEALTH

Center for Young Women's Health: youngwomenshealth.org.

Coalition for Positive Sexuality: positive.org.

Feminist Women's Health Center: fwhc.org.

National Women's Health Network: nwhn.org.

North Carolina Office on Disability and Health: fpg.unc
.edu/~ncodh/publications.cfm. Provides booklets and
other information on women's health, including reproductive health care.

Planned Parenthood Info for Teens—Going to the Doctor:
plannedparenthood.org/info-for-teens/our-bodies/going
-doctor-33816.htm.

Scarleteen: Find-a-Doc: scarleteen.com/find_a_doc.

Stewart, Elizabeth G., and Paula Spencer. *The V Book: A
Doctor's Guide to Complete Vulvovaginal Health*. New York:
Bantam, 2002.

VaginaPagina: vaginapagina.com.

Vaginaverite: vaginaverite.com.

CHAPTER 3:
BODY IMAGE

Brown, Harriet, ed. *Feed Me! Writers Dish About Food, Eating, Weight, and Body Image*. New York: Ballantine Books,
2009.

Byrd, Ayana D., and Lori L. Tharps. *Hair Story: Untangling
the Roots of Black Hair in America*. New York: St. Martin's
Press, 2002.

Disability Studies, Temple U.: disstud.blogspot.com. Covers disability news and history and provides a portal to the
disability blog world.

Douglas, Susan J. *Enlightened Sexism: The Seductive Message That Feminism's Work Is Done*. New York: Times
Books, 2010.

Fat Nutritionist: fatnutritionist.com. Michelle Allison is an
online nutritionist who writes about health and body acceptance; the site includes numerous articles and blog links.

Levin, Diane E., and Jean Kilbourne. *So Sexy So Soon: The
New Sexualized Childhood and What Parents Can Do to
Protect Their Kids*. New York: Ballantine, 2008.

Maine, Margo, and Joe Kelly. *The Body Myth: Adult Women
and the Pressure to Be Perfect*. New York: Wiley, 2005.

Martin, Courtney. *Perfect Girls, Starving Daughters: How
the Quest for Perfection Is Harming Young Women*. New
York: Berkley, 2008.

Redd, Nancy Amanda. *Body Drama: Real Girls, Real Bodies,
Real Issues, Real Answers*. New York: Gotham Books, 2007.

Steiner-Adair, Catherine, and Lisa Sjostrom. *Full of Ourselves: A Wellness Program to Advance Girl Power, Health,
and Leadership*. New York: Teachers College Press, 2006.

Weitz, Rose, ed. *The Politics of Women's Bodies: Sexuality,
Appearance, and Behavior*. 3rd ed. New York: Oxford University Press, 2009.

CHAPTER 4:
GENDER IDENTITY AND SEXUAL ORIENTATION

Baumgardner, Jennifer. *Look Both Ways: Bisexual Politics*.
New York: Farrar, Straus and Giroux, 2007.

Bernstein Sycamore, Matti, ed. *Nobody Passes: Rejecting the
Rules of Gender and Conformity*. Berkeley: Seal Press, 2006.

Bornstein, Kate, and S. Bear Bergman, eds. *Gender Out-
laws: The Next Generation*. Berkeley: Seal Press, 2010.

Carbado, Devon W., Dwight A. McBride, and Donald
Weise, eds. *Black Like Us: A Century of Lesbian, Gay and
Bisexual African American Fiction*. San Francisco: Cleis,
2002.

Clare, Eli. *Exile and Pride: Disability, Queerness and Liberation*. Boston: South End Press, 2009.

Conway, Lynn. ai.eecs.umich.edu/people/conway/conway
.html. Website by a University of Michigan professor
emerita, including photo gallery of Transsexual Women's
Successes.

Diamond, Lisa M. *Sexual Fluidity: Understanding Women's
Love and Desire*. Cambridge, MA: Harvard University
Press, 2008.

Hermann, Joanne. *Transgender Explained for Those Who
Are Not*. Bloomington: AuthorHouse, 2009.

Makadon, Harvey J., Kenneth H. Mayer, Jennifer Potter,
and Hilary Goldhammer. *Fenway Guide to Lesbian, Gay,
Bisexual, and Transgender Health*. Philadelphia: American
College of Physicians, 2008. See fenwayhealth.org for more
on LGTB health.

Serano, Julia. *Whipping Girl: A Transsexual Woman on Sexism and the Scapegoating of Femininity*. Berkeley: Seal
Press, 2007.

CHAPTER 5:
RELATIONSHIPS

Black, Claudia. *Deceived: Facing Sexual Betrayal, Lies, and
Secrets*. Center City, MN: Hazelden, 2009.

Clunis, Merilee, and G. Dorsey Green. *Lesbian Couples: A Guide to Creating Healthy Relationships.* 4th ed. Berkeley: Seal Press, 2004.

Coontz, Stephanie. *Marriage, a History: How Love Conquered Marriage.* New York: Penguin, 2006.

DePaulo, Bella. *Single with Attitude: Not Your Typical Take on Health and Happiness, Love and Money, Marriage and Friendship.* CreateSpace Publishing, 2009.

Eason, Dossie, and Janet W. Hardy. *The Ethical Slut: A Practical Guide to Polyamory, Open Relationships and Other Adventures.* 2nd ed. Berkeley: Celestial Arts, 2009.

Hernández, Daisy, and Bushra Rehman, eds. *Colonize This! Young Women of Color on Today's Feminism.* Berkeley: Seal Press, 2002.

Lerner, Harriet. *The Dance of Anger: A Woman's Guide to Changing the Patterns of Intimate Relationships.* New York: Harper, 2005.

Richardson, Brenda Lane, and Brenda Wade. *What Mama Couldn't Tell Us About Love: Healing the Emotional Legacy of Racism by Celebrating Our Light.* New York: Harper, 1999.

Walker, Rebecca. *One Big Happy Family: 18 Writers Talk About Polyamory, Open Adoption, Mixed Marriage, House-husbandry, Single Motherhood, and Other Realities of Truly Modern Love.* New York: Riverhead, 2009.

CHAPTER 6:
SOCIAL INFLUENCES
ON SEXUALITY

Abbott, Elizabeth. *A History of Celibacy.* New York: Scribner, 2000.

Carpenter, Laura, and John DeLamater, eds. *Sexuality Across the Lifecourse.* New York: New York University Press, 2011.

Fields, Jessica. *Risky Lessons: Sex Education and Social Inequality.* Piscataway, NJ: Rutgers University Press, 2008.

Fowles, Stacey May, and Megan Griffith Greene, eds. *She's Shameless: Women Write About Growing Up, Rocking Out and Fighting Back.* Toronto: Tightrope Books, 2009.

Luadzers, Darcy. *Virgin Sex for Girls: A No-regrets Guide to Safe and Healthy Sex.* New York: Hatherleigh Press, 2006.

Roberts, Tara, ed. *What Your Mama Never Told You: True Stories About Sex & Love.* Boston: Houghton Mifflin, 2007.

Ruttenberg, Danya, ed. *The Passionate Torah: Sex and Judaism.* New York: NYU Press, 2009.

Tanenbaum, Leora. *Slut! Growing Up Female with a Bad Reputation.* New York: Harper, 2000.

Valenti, Jessica. *The Purity Myth: How America's Obsession with Virginity Is Hurting Young Women.* Berkeley: Seal Press, 2009.

Wade, Jenny. *Transcendent Sex: When Lovemaking Opens the Veil.* New York: Pocket Books, 2004.

CHAPTER 7:
SEXUAL PLEASURE AND
ENTHUSIASTIC CONSENT

Corinna, Heather. *S.E.X.: The All-You-Need-to-Know Progressive Sexuality Guide to Get You Through High School and College.* New York: Marlowe, 2007.

Friedman, Jaclyn, and Jessica Valenti, eds. *Yes Means Yes! Visions of Female Sexual Power and a World Without Rape.* Berkeley: Seal Press, 2008.

Herbenick, Debby. *Because It Feels Good: A Woman's Guide to Sexual Pleasure and Satisfaction.* New York: Rodale Books, 2009.

Hutcherson, Hilda. *Pleasure: A Woman's Guide to Getting the Sex You Want, Need, and Deserve.* New York: Putnam, 2006.

Kerner, Ian. *She Comes First: A Thinking Man's Guide to Pleasuring a Woman.* New York: Harper, 2004.

Nelson, Tammy. *Getting the Sex You Want: Shed Your Inhibitions and Reach New Heights of Passion Together.* Beverly, MA: Quiver, 2008.

Newman, Felice. *The Whole Lesbian Sex Book: A Passionate Guide for All of Us.* 2nd ed. San Francisco: Cleis, 2004.

Ogden, Gina. *The Return of Desire: A Guide to Recovering Your Sexual Passion.* Boston: Trumpeter Books, 2008. (Also see Gina Ogden's other books: *The Heart and Soul of Sex: Making the ISIS Connection,* and *Women Who Love Sex: Ordinary Women Describe Their Paths to Pleasure, Intimacy, and Ecstasy.*)

Price, Joan. *Better Than I Ever Expected: Straight Talk About Sex After Sixty.* Berkeley: Seal, 2006.

Schell, Jude. *Lesbian Sex: 101 Lovemaking Positions.* Berkeley: Celestial Arts, 2008.

CHAPTER 8:
SEXUAL CHALLENGES

Brownworth, Victoria A., and Susan Raffo, eds. *Restricted Access: Lesbians on Disability*. Berkeley: Seal Press, 1999.

Center for Research on Women with Disabilities, Baylor College of Medicine: bcm.edu/crowd.

ChronicBabe.com: chronicbabe.com. Articles, community forums, and resources for women with chronic illness.

Clare, Eli. *Exile and Pride: Disability, Queerness and Liberation*. Cambridge, MA: South End Press, 2009.

FWD (feminists with disabilities): a blogroll of disability blogs, disabledfeminists.com/blogroll.

Kaufman, Miriam, Cory Silverberg, and Fran Odette. *The Ultimate Guide to Sex and Disability: For All of Us Who Live with Disabilities, Chronic Pain and Illness*. 2nd ed. San Francisco: Cleis, 2007.

Kroll, Ken, and Erica Levy Klein. *Enabling Romance: A Guide to Love, Sex and Relationships for People with Disabilities (and the People Who Care About Them)*. Horsham, PA: No Limits Communications, 2001.

National Vulvodynia Association: nva.org. Resources, support services, and educational booklets for women and their partners.

Stewart, Elizabeth G., and Paula Spencer. *The V Book: A Doctor's Guide to Complete Vulvovaginal Health*. New York: Bantam, 2002.

CHAPTER 9:
BIRTH CONTROL

Gordon, Linda. *The Moral Property of Women: A History of Birth Control Politics in America*. Champaign: University of Illinois Press, 2007.

Guttmacher Institute: information about contraceptive use and policies in the United States, guttmacher.org/sections/contraception.php?scope=U.S.%20specific.

Hatcher, Robert A., James Trussell, Anita L. Nelson, Felicia H. Stewart, and Deborah Kowal. *Contraceptive Technology*. 19th edition. New York: Ardent Media, 2008.

Nationwide Emergency Contraception Hotline: (888) NOT-2-LATE, 24/7 in English and Spanish. Not-2-Late .com has information in English, Spanish, French, and Arabic.

National Women's Law Center Family Planning Report Card for States: hrc.nwlc.org/states.

Planned Parenthood: plannedparenthood.org/health-topics/birth-control-4211.htm.

Singer, Katie. *The Garden of Fertility: A Guide to Charting Your Fertility Signals to Prevent or Achieve Pregnancy—Naturally—and to Gauge Your Reproductive Health*. New York: Avery Publishing Group, 2004.

"U.S. Medical Eligibility Criteria for Contraceptive Use, 2010": cdc.gov/mmwr/PDF/rr/rr5904.pdf.

Weschler, Toni. *Taking Charge of Your Fertility: The Definitive Guide to Natural Birth Control, Pregnancy Achivement, and Reproductive Health*. New York: Harper, 2001.

CHAPTER 10:
SAFER SEX

American Sexual Health Association: ashastd.org.

Foley, Sallie, Sally A. Kope, and Dennis P. Sugrue. *Sex Matters for Women: A Complete Guide to Taking Care of Your Sexual Self*. New York: Guilford Press, 2002.

Fulbright, Yvonne K. *The Hot Guide to Safer Sex*. Alameda, CA: Hunter House, 2003.

Go Ask Alice! goaskalice.columbia.edu/Cat7.html.

HIV InSite: Safer Sex, hivinsite.ucsf.edu.

Planned Parenthood Safer Sex: plannedparenthood.org/health-topics.

San Francisco Sex Information: sfsi.org, 415-989-7374. Free, anonymous, nonjudgmental sex info via web, phone, email.

Scarleteen: scarleteen.com/article/sexuality/safe_sound _sexy_a_safer_sex_how_to.

Pleasure Project: thepleasureproject.org.

Winks, Cathy, and Anne Semans. *The Good Vibrations Guide to Sex: The Most Complete Sex Manual Ever Written*. 3rd ed. San Francisco: Cleis, 2002.

CHAPTER 11:
SEXUALLY TRANSMITTED INFECTIONS

American Social Health Association (ASHA): ashastd.org.

The Body: HIV/AIDS Resource Center for Women, the body.com/content/art44411.html.

Centers for Disease Control: Sexually Transmitted Diseases, cdc.gov/STD.

Centers for Disease Control: *2010 STD Treatment Guidelines,* cdc.gov/std/treatment/2010.

Guttmacher Institute: HIV/AIDS and STIs, guttmacher.org/sections/sti.php.

Krishnan, Shobha S. *The HPV Vaccine Controversy: Sex, Cancer, God, and Politics. A Guide for Parents, Women, Men, and Teenagers.* Westport, CT: Praeger, 2008.

Nack, Adina. *Damaged Goods? Women Living with Incurable Sexually Transmitted Diseases.* Philadelphia: Temple University Press, 2008.

Sexuality Information and Education Council of the United States (SIECUS): siecus.org.

Warren, Terri. *The Good News About the Bad News: Herpes—Everything You Need to Know.* Oakland, CA: New Harbinger Publications, 2009.

CHAPTER 12:
UNEXPECTED PREGNANCY

Abortion Care Networks. "Mom, Dad, I'm Pregnant:" momdadimpregnant.com

Austin-Small, Ophelia. *Surprise Motherhood: A Guide to Unexpected Adult Pregnancy.* Self-published, 2007.

Davis, Deborah. *You Look Too Young to Be a Mom: Teen Moms Speak Out on Love, Learning, and Success.* New York: Perigee Books, 2004.

Guttmacher Institute. "*Facts on American Teens' Sexual and Reproductive Health,*" guttmacher.org/pubs/FB-ATSRH.html.

National Abortion Federation. "Unsure About Your Pregnancy? A Guide to Making the Right Decision for You," prochoice.org/pubs_research/publications/downloads/index.html#pregnant.

Planned Parenthood. "Thinking About Parenting," plannedparenthood.org/health-topics/pregnancy/parenting-21521.htm.

Williams-Wheeler, Dorrie. *The Unplanned Pregnancy Book for Teens and College Students.* Virginia Beach, VA: Sparkledoll Productions, 2004.

CHAPTER 13:
ABORTION

Abortion Conversation Project: abortionconversation.com.

Baumgardner, Jennifer. *Abortion & Life.* New York: Akashic Books, 2008.

Frankfort, Ellen, and Frances Kissling. *Rosie: The Investigation of a Wrongful Death.* New York: Doubleday, 1979.

Freedman, Lori. *Willing and Unable: Doctors' Constraints in Abortion Care.* Nashville, TN: Vanderbilt University Press, 2010.

Guttmacher Institute: guttmacher.org.

Joffe, Carole. *Dispatches from the Abortion Wars: The Costs of Fanaticism to Doctors, Patients, and the Rest of Us.* Boston: Beacon Press, 2009.

National Abortion Federation (NAF): prochoice.org.

Paul, M., et al., eds. *Management of Unintended and Abnormal Pregnancy: Comprehensive Abortion Care.* West Sussex, U.K.: Blackwell Publishing, 2009.

Planned Parenthood: plannedparenthood.org, 800-230-PLAN.

Religious Coalition for Reproductive Choice: rcrc.org.

CHAPTER 14:
CONSIDERING PARENTING

Bynoe, Yvonne, ed. *Who's You Mama? The Unsung Voices of Women and Mothers.* Berkeley, CA: Soft Skull Press, 2009.

Casey, Terri. *Pride and Joy: The Lives and Passions of Women Without Children.* New York: Atria Books/Beyond Words, 2007.

Child Welfare Information Gateway. "Adoption." childwelfare.gov/adoption.

Kruger, Pamela, and Jill Smolowe. *A Love like No Other.* New York: Riverhead Hardcover, 2005.

Leibovich, Lori. *Maybe Baby: 28 Writers Tell the Truth About Skepticism, Infertility, Baby Lust, Childlessness, Ambivalence, and How They Made the Biggest Decision of Their Lives.* New York: HarperCollins, 2006.

Peri, Camille, and Kate Moses. *Mothers Who Think: Tales of Real-Life Parenthood.* New York: Washington Square Press, 2000.

Ratner, Rochelle, ed. *Bearing Life: Women's Writing on Childlessness.* New York: Feminist Press, 2001.

Register, Cheri. *Beyond Good Intentions: A Mother Reflects on Raising Internationally Adopted Children.* St. Paul, MN: Yeong & Yeong Book Company, 2005.

Roberts, Dorothy. *Shattered Bonds: The Color of Child Welfare.* New York: Basic Books, 2003.

Single Mothers by Choice: singlemothersbychoice.com.

Vissing, Yvonne Marie. *Women Without Children: Nurturing Lives.* New Brunswick, NJ: Rutgers University Press, 2002.

CHAPTERS 15 AND 16: PREGNANCY AND PREPARING FOR BIRTH; LABOR AND BIRTH

Block, Jennifer. *Pushed: The Painful Truth About Childbirth and Modern Maternity Care.* Cambridge, MA: Da Capo Press, 2007.

Boston Women's Health Book Collective. *Our Bodies, Ourselves: Pregnancy and Birth.* New York: Simon & Schuster, 2008.

Childbirth Connection. "What Every Pregnant Woman Needs to Know About Cesarean Birth," rev. ed. 2006, childbirthconnection.org/article.asp?ck=10164.

Childbirth.org. "Birth Stories," childbirth.org/articles/stories/birth.html.

Coalition for Improving Maternity Services: motherfriendly.org.

Davis, Elizabeth, and Debra Pascali-Bonaro. *Orgasmic Birth: Your Guide to a Safe, Satisfying, and Pleasurable Birth Experience.* Emmaus, PA: Rodale, 2010.

Gaskin, Ina May. *Ina May's Guide to Childbirth.* New York: Bantam Books, 2003.

Goer, Henci. *The Thinking Woman's Guide to a Better Birth.* New York: Perigee Books, 1999.

Greenfield, Marjorie. *The Working Woman's Pregnancy Book.* New Haven, CT: Yale University Press, 2008.

Lothian, Judith, and Charlotte DeVries. *The Official Lamaze Guide: Giving Birth with Confidence.* Minnetonka, MN: Meadowbrook Press, 2010.

March of Dimes. "Pregnancy," marchofdimes.com/pregnancy.

Mysko, Claire, and M. Amadeï. *Does This Pregnancy Make Me Look Fat? The Essential Guide to Loving Your Body Before and After Baby.* Deerfield Beach, FL: HCI, 2009.

Rogers, Judith. *The Disabled Woman's Guide to Pregnancy and Birth.* New York: Demos Medical Publishing, 2006.

Science & Sensibility: A Research Blog About Healthy Pregnancy, Birth & Beyond, scienceandsensibility.org.

Simkin, Penny, and P. Klaus. *When Survivors Give Birth: Understanding and Healing the Effects of Early Sexual Abuse on Childbearing Women.* Seattle, WA: Classic Day Publishing, 2004.

Simkin, Penny, et al. *Pregnancy, Childbirth and the Newborn, Revised and Updated: The Complete Guide.* Minnetonka, MN.: Meadowbrook Press, 2010.

TheUnnecesarean.com: Pulling Back the Curtain on the Unnecessary Cesarean Epidemic, theunnecesarean.com.

van der Ziel, Cornelia. *Big, Beautiful, and Pregnant: Expert Advice and Comforting Wisdom for the Expecting Plus-Size Woman.* New York: Da Capo Press, 2006.

The Well-Rounded Mama: wellroundedmama.blogspot.com.

CHAPTER 17: THE EARLY MONTHS OF PARENTING

Hale, Thomas W. *Medications and Mothers' Milk.* 14th ed. Amarillo, TX.: Hale Publishing, 2010.

Huggins, Kathleen. *The Nursing Mother's Companion.* 6th ed. Boston: Harvard Common Press, 2010.

Kabat-Zinn, Myla and Jon. *Everyday Blessings: The Inner Work of Mindful Parenting.* New York: Hyperion, 1997.

Kendall-Tackett, Kathleen. *The Hidden Feelings of Motherhood: Coping with Stress, Depression, and Burnout.* 2nd ed. Amarillo, TX: Pharmasoft Publishing, 2005.

La Leche League International: llli.org.

Lim, Robin. *After the Baby's Birth: A Woman's Way to Wellness: A Complete Guide for Postpartum Women.* Rev. ed. Berkeley: Celestial Arts, 2004.

MomsRising.org: momsrising.org.

Placksin, Sally. *Mothering the New Mother: Women's Feelings and Needs After Childbirth, A Support and Resource Guide.* 2nd ed. New York: Newmarket Press, 2000.

Postpartum Support International: postpartum.net.

Smith, Linda. *Impact of Birth Practices on Breastfeeding.* 2nd ed. Boston: Jones & Bartlett Publishers, 2009.

CHAPTER 18:
MISCARRIAGE, STILLBIRTH, AND OTHER LOSSES

Douglas, Ann. *Trying Again: A Guide to Pregnancy After Miscarriage, Stillbirth, and Infant Loss.* Dallas: Taylor Trade Publishing, 2000.

Gross, Jessica Berger. *About What Was Lost: Twenty Writers on Miscarriage, Healing, and Hope.* New York: Plume, 2006.

Kohn, Ingrid, and Perry-Lynn Moffitt with Isabelle A. Wilkins. *A Silent Sorrow: Pregnancy Loss Guidance and Support for You and Your Family.* 2nd ed. New York: Routledge, 2000.

Layne, Linda. "Designing a Woman-Centered Health Care Approach to Pregnancy Loss: Lessons from Feminist Models of Childbirth." In *Reproductive Disruptions: Gender, Technology, and Biopolitics in the New Millennium,* ed. Marcia Inhorn. Oxford: Berghahn Books, 2007, pp. 79–97.

———. "Making Memories: Trauma, Choice, and Consumer Culture in the Case of Pregnancy Loss." In *Consuming Motherhood,* eds. Janelle Taylor, Linda Layne, and Danielle Wozniak. New Brunswick, NJ: Rutgers University Press, 2003.

———. *Motherhood Lost: A Feminist Account of Pregnancy Loss in America.* New York: Routledge, 2003.

McCracken, Elizabeth. *An Exact Replica of a Figment of My Imagination: A Memoir.* New York: Little, Brown, 2008.

CHAPTER 19:
INFERTILITY AND ASSISTED REPRODUCTIVE TECHNOLOGIES

The Broken Brown Egg: African American Infertility & Reproductive Health Awareness, thebrokenbrownegg.org.

Crockin, Susan L., and Howard W. Jones, Jr. *Legal Conceptions: The Evolving Law and Policy of Assisted Reproductive Technologies.* Baltimore: Johns Hopkins University Press, 2009.

Eggsploitation: eggsploitation.com.

Ehrensaft, Diane. *Mommies, Daddies, Donors, Surrogates: Answering Tough Questions and Building Strong Families.* New York: Guilford Press, 2005.

Ford, Melissa. *Navigating the Land of IF: Understanding Infertility and Exploring Your Options.* Berkeley, CA: Seal Press, 2009.

The InterNational Council on Infertility Information Dissemination: inciid.org.

Orenstein, Peggy. *Waiting for Daisy: A Tale of Two Continents, Three Religions, Five Infertility Doctors, an Oscar, an Atomic Bomb, a Romantic Night, and One Woman's Quest to Become a Mother.* New York: Bloomsbury, 2007.

Spar, Debora L. *The Baby Business: How Money, Science, and Politics Drive the Commerce of Conception.* Boston: Harvard Business School Press, 2006.

Sterling, Evelina Weidman, and Ellen Sarasohn Glazer. *Having Your Baby Through Egg Donation.* Indianapolis: Perspective Press, 2005.

Tsigdinos, Pamela Mahoney. *Silent Sorority: A Barren Woman Gets Busy, Angry, Lost and Found.* BookSurge Publishing, 2009.

Vercollone, Carol Frost, Heidi Moss, and Robert Moss. *Helping the Stork: The Choices and Challenges of Donor Insemination.* New York: Wiley, 1997.

CHAPTER 20:
PERIMENOPAUSE AND MENOPAUSE

Baxter, Susan, and Jerilynn C. Prior. *Estrogen Errors: Why Progesterone Is Better for Women's Health.* Westport, CT: Praeger, 2009.

Boston Women's Health Book Collective. *Our Bodies, Ourselves: Menopause.* New York: Simon & Schuster, 2006.

Edelman, Julia Schlam. *Menopause Matters.* Baltimore: Johns Hopkins University Press, 2009.

Kagan, Leslee, Herbert Benson, and Bruce Kessel. *Mind Over Menopause: The Complete Mind/Body Approach to Menopause.* New York: Free Press, 2004.

Manson, JoAnn E., and S. Shari Bassuk. *Hot Flashes, Hormones and Your Health: Breakthrough Findings to Help You Sail Through Menopause.* Ohio: McGraw Hill, 2008.

Nelson, Miriam, and Sarah Wernick. *Strong Women, Strong Bones*. New York: Perigee, 2006.

Porter, Gayle K., and Marilyn Gaston. *Prime Time: The African American Woman's Complete Guide to Midlife Health and Wellness*. New York: Random House Ballantine, 2001.

Prior, Jerilynn. *Estrogen's Storm Season: Stories of Perimenopause*. Vancouver, BC: Centre for Menstrual Cycle and Ovulation Research, 2005.

Seaman, Barbara. *The No-Nonsense Guide to Menopause*. New York: Simon & Schuster, 2008.

Sterling, Evelina W., and Angie Best-Boss. *Before Your Time: The Early Menopause Survival Guide*. New York: Fireside, 2010.

CHAPTER 21:
OUR LATER YEARS

Bateson, Mary Catherine. *Composing a Fuller Life: The Age of Active Wisdom*. New York: Knopf, 2010.

Butler, Robert N. *The Longevity Revolution: The Benefits and Challenges of Living a Longer Life*. New York: Public Affairs, 2008.

Cruikshank, Margaret. *Learning to Be Old: Gender, Culture, and Aging*. Lanham, MD: Rowman & Littlefield Publishers, 2009.

Foley, Sallyie. *Sex and Love for Grown-ups: A No-nonsense Guide to a Life of Passion*. New York: Sterling Publishing, 2005.

Goldman, Connie. *Who Am I . . . Now That I'm Not Who I Was?* Minneapolis: Nodin Press, 2009.

Guillette, Margaret Morganroth. *Agewise: Fighting the New Ageism in America*. Chicago: University of Chicago Press, 2010.

Horn, Janet, and Robin H. Miller. *The Smart Woman's Guide to Midlife and Beyond*. Oakland, CA: New Harbinger Publications, 2008.

Kliger, Leah, and Deborah Nedelman. *Still Sexy After All These Years? The 9 Unspoken Truths About Women's Desire Beyond 50*. New York: Penguin, 2006.

Movement Advancement Project (MAP) and Services and Advocacy for Gay, Lesbian, Bisexual & Transgender Elders (SAGE). "Improving the Lives of LGBT Older Adults," March 2010, lgbtmap.org/improving-the-lives-of-lgbt-older-adults-at-national-aging-in-america-conference.

Roszak, Theodore. *The Making of an Elder Culture: Reflections on the Future of America's Most Audacious Generation*. Gabriola Island, BC, Canada: New Society Publishers, 2009.

CHAPTER 22:
SELECTED MEDICAL PROBLEMS

Ballweg, Mary Lou. *Endometriosis: The Complete Reference to Taking Charge of Your Health*. New York: McGraw-Hill, 2003.

Breast Cancer Action: bcaction.org.

Carlson, Karen J., et al. *The New Harvard Guide to Women's Health*. Cambridge: Harvard University Press, 2004.

Cooper, Raymond, and Fredi Kronenberg, eds. *Botanical Medicine: From Bench to Bedside*. New Rochelle, NY: Mary Ann Liebert Publications, 2009.

Love, Susan M., and Karen Lindsey. *Dr. Susan Love's Breast Book*. 5th ed. New York: Da Capo Lifelong Books, 2010.

The National Women's Health Information Center, U.S. Dept of Health and Human Services: womenshealth.gov.

National Women's Health Network: nwhn.org.

Parker, William H. *A Gynecologist's Second Opinion: The Questions and Answers You Need to Take Charge of Your Health*. New York: Penguin/Plume, 2002.

Stewart, Elizabeth G., and Paula Spence. *The V Book: A Doctor's Guide to Complete Vulvovaginal Health*. New York: Bantam, 2002.

CHAPTER 23:
NAVIGATING THE
HEALTH CARE SYSTEM

Abramson, John. *Overdosed America: The Broken Promise of American Medicine*. New York: HarperCollins, 2008.

Agency for Healthcare Research and Quality: Improve Your Healthcare, ahrq.gov/questionsaretheanswer.

Annas, George J. *The Rights of Patients: The Basic ACLU Guide to Patient Rights*. Carbondale: Southern Illinois University Press, 2004.

Center on Medical Rights and Privacy at Georgetown University Health Policy Institute: medicalrecordrightsgeorgetown.edu/records.html.

Greenhalgh, Trisha. *How to Read a Paper: The Basics of Evidence-Based Medicine.* 4th ed. West Sussex, UK: BMJ Books, June 2010.

HealthCare.gov: information about health reform and finding health insurance and health care.

Institute of Medicine. *Health Literacy—A Prescription to End Confusion.* Washington, D.C.: National Academies Press, 2004.

Sered, Susan, and Rushika Fernandopulle. *Uninsured in America: Life and Death in the Land of Opportunity.* Berkeley: University of California Press, 2005.

Torrey, Trisha. *You Bet Your Life: The 10 Mistakes Every Patient Makes.* Minneapolis: Langdon Street Press, 2010.

Woloshin, Steven, Lisa M. Schwartz, and H. Gilbert Welch. *Know Your Chances: Understanding Health Statistics.* Berkeley: University of California Press, 2008.

CHAPTER 24:
VIOLENCE AGAINST WOMEN

Bass, Ellen. *The Courage to Heal: A Guide for Women Survivors of Child Sexual Abuse.* 20th anniversary edition (revised, expanded). New York: Harper Paperbacks, 2008.

Chain of Change (chainofchange.net), a project of Beyondmedia Education (beyondmedia.com) in Chicago, organizes youth activists to strategize how to end violence by exposing its roots through the creation of media.

Ensler, Eve. *The Vagina Monologues.* New York: Villard, 2008.

Friedman, Jaclyn, and Jessica Valenti, eds. *Yes Means Yes! Visons of Female Sexual Power and a World Without Rape.* Berkeley: Seal Press, 2009.

Herman, Judith. *Trauma and Recovery: The Aftermath of Violence—from Domestic Abuse to Political Terrorism.* New York: Basic Books, 1997.

Lehman, Carolyn. *Strong at the Heart: How It Feels to Recover from Sexual Abuse.* New York: Farrar, Straus and Giroux, 2005.

Lloyd, Rachel. *Girls Like Us: Fighting for a World Where Girls Are Not for Sale, an Activist Finds Her Calling and Heals Herself.* New York: Harper, 2011.

"No!" 2004. Documentary by Aishah Shahidah about rape in African-American communities, notherapedocumentary.org.

Orloff, Leslye, ed. *Empowering Survivors: Legal Rights of Immigrant Victims of Sexual Assault for Advocates Working with Immigrant Victims of Sexual Assault.* Washington, DC: Legal Momentum, 2010.

Potter, Hillary. *Battle Cries: Black Women and Intimate Partner Abuse.* New York: NYU Press, 2008.

Renzetti, Claire, Jeffrey Edleson, and Raquel Kennedy Bergen, eds. *Sourcebook on Violence Against Women.* Rev. ed. Thousand Oaks, CA: Sage Publications, 2010.

Turning a Corner. 2008. This film tells the stories of people involved in the sex trade and their efforts to raise public awareness of systematic injustice and to promote needed reforms. Available through womenandprison.org/store, and beyondmedia.com/catalog.

CHAPTER 25:
ENVIRONMENTAL AND
OCCUPATIONAL HEALTH

Association of Occupational and Environmental Health Clinics: aoec.org. National network providing information and resources on patient care.

Association of Reproductive Health Professionals: arhp.org. Resources for health care providers and patients regarding toxic exposures and reproductive outcomes.

Beyond Pesticides: beyondpesticides.org. Resources and strategies on pesticide impacts and alternatives.

The Campaign for Safe Cosmetics: SafeCosmetics.org. Provides information on detrimental health effects associated with cosmetics.

Center for Health, Environment and Justice: chej.org. Community and national strategies and resources.

The Centers for Disease Control, Agency for Toxic Substances and Disease Registry: atsdr.cdc.gov. Toxic profiles, public health programs, community assessments, and links to national resources.

The Collaborative on Health and the Environment: healthandenvironment.org. Fact sheets, working groups, and updated data on environment and reproductive health.

Committees on Occupational Safety and Health (COSH): nycosh.org (includes national listing of all COSH groups). Committees are located across the United States, focusing on occupational health education and advocacy, and can provide information and services for grievanced workers.

The Endocrine Disruption Exchange: endocrinedisruption .com. Resources for health practioners and communities, including information on critical windows of development.

Environmental Defense Fund: scorecard.org. Community database (search by zip code), with detailed information on chemicals, health effects, and actions to take.

Environmental Working Group: ewg.org. Fact sheets and reports, with a focus on advocacy. See also the EWG Skin Deep project, cosmeticsdatabase.com.

CHAPTER 26:
THE POLITICS OF WOMEN'S HEALTH

Black Women's Health Imperative: blackwomenshealth.org. Takes action to eliminate health disparities for black women.

Center for Policy Analysis on Trade and Health: cpath.org. Conducts research and adds a public health voice to the debate on trade and sustainable development.

Equal Health Network: equalhealth.info. Brings together partners from public health, women's health, and the public to advocate for equitable, quality, universal, affordable—EQUAL—health care.

Levy, Barry S., and Victor W. Sidel. *War and Public Health.* New York: Oxford University Press, 2007.

National Women's Health Network: nwhn.org. Improves the health of all women by providing a critical analysis of health issues in order to affect policy and support consumer decision making.

National Women's Law Center: nwlc.org. Champions laws and policies that work for women and families, including health care and reproductive rights, poverty and income support, education and Title IX, and more.

Population Reference Bureau, *The World's Women and Girls 2011 Data Sheet:* prb.org/Publications/Datasheets/2011/worlds-women-and-girls.aspx. Produced with support from the U.S. Agency for International Development through the IDEA project. Includes data for 181 countries on a variety of reproductive health and gender equality indicators. Copies are available to download at prb.org. To request free print copies, contact idea@prb.org.

Shepard, Bonnie. *Running the Obstacle Course to Sexual and Reproductive Health: Lessons from Latin America.* Westport, CT: Greenwood Publishing Co., 2006.

Turshen, Meredeth. *Women's Health Movements: A Global Force for Change.* New York: Palgrave Macmillan, 2007.

United Nations Entity for Gender Equality and the Empowerment of Women: unwomen.org. A clearinghouse for United Nations initiatives.

CHAPTER 27:
ACTIVISM IN THE
TWENTY-FIRST CENTURY

Applied Research Center: arc.org. This racial justice think tank and home for media and activism also publishes Colorlines (colorlines.com), a daily news site offering award-winning reporting, analysis, and solutions to today's racial justice issues.

Baumgardner, Jennifer, Amy Richards, and Winona LaDuke. *Grassroots: A Field Guide for Feminist Activism.* New York: Farrar, Straus and Giroux, 2005.

Electronic Frontier Foundation: eff.org. Works to protect freedom in the networked world and provides information on privacy, transparency, fair use, and free speech.

Martin, Courtney E. *Do It Anyway: The New Generation of Activists.* Boston: Beacon Press, 2010.

Morgan, Robin. *Fighting Words: A Toolkit for Combating the Religious Right.* New York: Nation Books/Avalon Publishing, 2006.

Murray, Anne Firth. *From Outrage to Courage: Women Taking Action for Health and Justice.* Monroe, ME: Common Courage Press, 2007.

Shirky, Clay. *Here Comes Everybody: The Power of Organizing Without Organizations.* New York: Penguin Press, 2008.

Trigg, Mary K., ed. *Leading the Way: Young Women's Activism for Social Change.* Piscataway, NJ: Rutgers University Press, 2010.

Turshen, Meredeth. *Women's Health Movements: A Global Force for Change.* New York: Palgrave Macmillan, 2007.

CHAPTER 1:
OUR FEMALE BODIES

1. David Landes, "Swedish Group Renames Hymen 'Vaginal Corona,' " The Local, the local.se/23720/20091208.

2. Angela Moreno, "In Amerika They Call Us Hermaphrodites," in *Intersex in the Age of Ethics*, ed. A. D. Dreger (Hagerstown, MD: University Publishing Group, 1999), p. 137.

3. G. C. Windham et al., "Age at Menarche in Relation to Maternal Use of Tobacco, Alcohol, Coffee, and Tea During Pregnancy," *American Journal of Epidemiology* 159 (2004): 862–71. Also: W. C. Chumlea et al., "Age at Menarche and Racial Comparisons in U.S. Girls," *Pediatrics* 111 (2003): 110–13.

4. Sandra Steingraber, "The Falling Age of Puberty in U.S. Girls," Breast Cancer Fund, 2007, breastcancerfund.org/media/publications/falling-age-of-puberty.

5. Ani DiFranco, "Blood in the Boardroom," © 1993 by Ani DiFranco/Righteous Babe Music.

6. Andrew Adam Newman, "Rebelling Against the Commonly Evasive Feminine Care Ad," *New York Times*, March 15, 2010.

7. Simone N. Vigod, Lori E. Ross, and Meir Steiner, "Understanding and Treating Premenstrual Dysphoric Disorder," *Obstetrics & Gynecology Clinics of North America* 36 (2009): 916.

8. K. J. Sales and H. N. Jabbour, "Cyclooxygenase Enzymes and Prostaglandins in Pathology of the Endometrium," *Reproduction* 126 (2003): 559–67.

9. For more information on the misleading Yaz ads, see nytimes.com/2009/02/11/business/11pill.html.

10. European Medicines Agency, Committee for Proprietary Medicinal Products, "Summary Information on Referral Opinion Following Arbitration Pursuant to Article 30 of Council Directive 2001/83/EC for Prozac and Associated Names,"

emea.europa.eu/docs/en_GB/document_library/referrals_prozac_30/wc50000.9147.pdf.

11. Cathleen Morrow and Elizabeth H. Naumburg, "Dysmenorrhea," *Primary Care: Clinics in Office Practice* 36 (2009): 19–32.

CHAPTER 3:
BODY IMAGE

1. Randi Hutter Epstein, "When Eating Disorders Strike in Midlife," *New York Times*, July 13, 2009, nytimes.com/ref/health/healthguide/esn-eating-disorders-ess.html.

2. Timothy A. Judge and Daniel M. Cable, "When It Comes to Pay, Do the Thin Win? The Effect of Weight on Pay for Men and Women," *Journal of Applied Psychology* 96, no. 1 (2010): 95–112, timothy-judge.com/Judge%20and%20Cable%20%28JAP%202010%29.pdf.

3. R. Gonzalez Rey and M. Parra, "The Beauty Advantage," *Newsweek*, July 19, 2010, newsweek.com/feature/2010/the-beauty-advantage.html.

4. Amanda Lenhart, "Teens and Sexting," Pew Internet and American Life Project, December 15, 2009, pewinternet.org/Reports/2009/Teens-and-Sexting.aspx.

5. "Lucy," "Transgender Women and Body Image," *Lovely Lucy: My Life as a Transgender Woman in Academia*, lucyinacademia.blogspot.com/2010/04/transgender-women-and-body-image.html.

6. Kathy Peiss, *Hope in a Jar: The Making of America's Beauty Culture* (New York: Henry Holt, 1998), pp. 41–42.

7. Dr. S. Allen Counter, "Whitening Skin Can Be Deadly," *Boston Globe*, December 16, 2003, p. C12.

8. Ellen Gabler and Sam Roe, "Some Skin-Whitening Creams Contain Toxic Mercury, Testing Finds," *Chicago Tribune*, May 18, 2010, chicagotribune.com/health/ct-met-mercury-skin-creams-20100518,0,4522094.story.

9. Ellen Gabler and Sam Roe, "Mercury Content of Skin-lightening Creams," *Chicago Tribune*, May 25, 2010, media.apps.chicagotribune.com/tables/skincreams.html.

10. AFP, "Vaseline Launches Skin-Whitening Facebook India App," July 13, 2010, google.com/hostednews/afp/article/ALeqM5g0O0kuPQsHSvuTd2t-YTrq1Rxaew.

11. Jorge Rivas, "ELLE Cover Lightens the Most Beautiful Woman in the World," *Colorlines*, January 12, 2011, colorlines.com/archives/2011/01/elle_cover_lightens_the_most_beautiful_woman_in_the_world.html.

12. Gil Kaufman, "L'Oréal Denies Altering Beyoncé's Skin Color in Ad," MTV.com, August 8, 2008, mtv.com/news/articles/1592434/loreal-denies-altering-beyonces-skin-color-ad.jhtml.

13. R. Ritchie, "Black Women Say They Have Had Enough, They Are Going Natural," WPTV.com, November 27, 2010, wptv.com/dpp/news/local_news/special_reports/Special-Report%3A-Going-Natural.

14. Geoffrey Jones, *Beauty Imagined: A History of the Global Beauty Industry* (New York: Oxford University Press, 2010), p. 301.

15. Hillary Chura, "On Cosmetics: Marketing Rules All," *New York Times*, November 18, 2006.

16. Vanessa Williams, "Dark and Lovely, Michelle," The Root.com, January 13, 2009, theroot.com/views/dark-and-lovely-michelle.

17. Mark Clothier. "P&G's Consumer Changes to He from She with Men's Line." Bloomberg Businessweek, June 4, 2010. Accessed at businessweek.com/2010-06-04/p-g-s-consumer-changes-to-he-from-she-with-men-s-line-update2-.html.

18. Marco Roso and Katerina Llanes, "The W4W Buzz," *Dis* magazine, October, 2010, dismagazine.com/dysmorphia/beauty/10144/the-w4w-buzz/.

19. Lisa Wade, "Revisioning Aspirational Hair," *Sociological Images*, November 18, 2010, thesocietypages.org/socimages/2010/11/18/revisioning-aspirational-hair/.

20. PR Newswire, "Toxic Chemicals in Cosmetics: New Bill Reforms Personal Care Products Law," July 21, 2010, prnewswire.com/news-releases/toxic-chemicals-in-cosmetics-new-bill-reforms-personal-care-products-law-98936514.html.

21. Susan Salisbury, "Safety of Chemical-Laden Grooming Items Uncertain," *Palm Beach Post News*, July 30, 2010, palmbeachpost.com/money/safety-of-chemical-laden-grooming-items-uncertain-832902.html.

22. Ibid.

23. Brian Walsh, "Cracking Down on Toxic Makeup," *Time*, July 21, 2010, ecocentric.blogs.time.com/2010/07/21/cracking-down-on-toxic-makeup/.

24. D. Lazovich et al., "Indoor Tanning and Risk of Melanoma: A Case-Control Study in a Highly Exposed Population," *Cancer Epidemiology, Biomarkers & Prevention*, May 26, 2010.

25. C. Mosher and S. Danoff-Burg, "Addiction to Indoor Tanning," *Archives of Dermatology* 146, no. 4 (2010): 412–17.

26. My New Pink Button, 2010, mynewpinkbutton.com.

27. American Society of Plastic Surgeons, "Report of the 2010 Plastic Surgery Statistics," plasticsurgery.org/Documents/Media/2010-Statistics/ASPS_2010_Plastic_Surgery_Statistics_20711.pdf.

28. Ibid.

29. Ibid.

30. Food and Drug Administration, FDA Approved Labeling Text—Botox, 2010, fda.gov/downloads/Drugs/DrugSafety/UCM176360.pdf.

31. Catherine Saint Louis, "This Teenage Girl Uses Botox. No, She's Not Alone," *New York Times*, August 11, 2010, nytimes.com/2010/08/12/fashion/12SKIN.html.

32. Natasha Singer, "Is the Mom Job Really Necessary?" *New York Times*, October 4, 2007, nytimes.com/2007/10/04/fashion/04skin.html?_r=4&oref=slogin&pagewanted=all.

33. Ed Diener, Brian Wolsic, and Frank Fujita, "Physical Attractiveness and Subjective Well-Being," *Journal of Personality and Social Psychology* 69, no. 11 (July 1995): 120–29.

34. D. Zuckerman, "Reasonably Safe?" *Reproductive Health Matters* 18, no. 35 (2010): 94–102.

35. Ruth Brandon, *Ugly Beauty: Helena Rubinstein, L'Oréal, and the Blemished History of Looking Good* (New York: HarperCollins, 2011), p. 229.

36. Ibid., 377–78.

37. M. Milkie, "Social Comparisons, Reflected Appraisals, and Mass Media: The Impact of Pervasive Beauty Images on Black and White Girls' Self-Concepts," *Social Psychology Quarterly* 62 (1999): 190–210.

38. Vanessa R. Shick, Brandi N. Rima, and Sarah K. Calabrese, "Evulvalution: The Portrayal of Women's External Genitalia and Physique Across Time and the Current Barbie Doll Ideals," *Journal of Sex Research*, November 11, 2009.

39. J. Gohmann, "The Vagina Dialogues," *Bust* magazine, June/July 2009, bust.com/component/option,com_zine/id,2/view,article/.

40. Angela Bonavoglia, "Cosmetic Vaginal Surgeons Clueless," Women's Media Center, February 24, 2010, womensmediacenter.com/blog/2010/02/cosmetic-vaginal-surgeons-clueless/.

41. V. Braun, "In Search of (Better) Sexual Pleasure: Female Genital 'Cosmetic' Surgery," *Sexualities* 8 (2005): 407–24.

42. Bonavoglia, "Cosmetic Vaginal Surgeons Clueless."

43. L. Liao, L. Michala, and S. Creighton, "Labial Surgery for Well Women: A Review of the Literature," *BJOG: An International Journal of Obstetrics & Gynaecology* 117 (2010): 20–25.

44. "Vaginal 'Rejuvenation' and Cosmetic Vaginal Procedures," *Obstetrics & Gynecology* 110 (2007): 737–38.

45. S. Kobrin, "More Women Seek Vaginal Plastic Surgery," *Women eNews*, November 14, 2004, womensenews.org/story/health/041114/more-women-seek-vaginal-plastic-surgery.

46. "ACOG Advises Against Cosmetic Vaginal Procedures Due to Lack of Safety and Efficacy Data," press release of the American College of Obstetricians and Gynecologists, September 1, 2007, acog.org/from_home/publications/press_releases/nr09-01-07-1.cfm.

47. Working Group on a New View of Women's Sexual Problems, "Challenging the Medicalization of Sex," New View Campaign, 2000, newviewcampaign.org/manifesto1.asp.

48. Laura Fitzpatrick, "Plastic Surgery Below the Belt," *Time*, November 19, 2008, time.com/time/health/article/0,8599,1859937,00.html#ixzz1DXjtKMz0.

49. Carrie Melago, "Ralph Lauren Model Filippa Hamilton: I Was Fired Because I Was Too Fat!" *New York Daily News*, October 14, 2009, nydailynews.com/lifestyle/fashion/2009/10/14/2009-10-14_model_fired_for_being_too_fat.html.

50. A. Doherty and G. Dines, "Living in a Porn Culture" New Left Project, April 15, 2010, newleftproject.org/index.php/site/article_comments/living_in_a_porn_culture/.

51. R. Weitz, "Changing the Scripts: Midlife Women's Sexuality in Contemporary U.S. Films," *Sexuality & Culture* 14, no. 1 (2009): 17–32.

52. Ibid.; M. M. Lauren and D. M. Dozier, "Maintaining the Double Standard: Portrayals of Age and Gender in Popular Films," *Sex Roles* 52 (2005): 437–46.

53. L. Wade, "How and Why People of Color Are Included in Advertising," The Society Pages, December 6, 2008, thesocietypages.org/socimages/2008/12/06/how-and-why-people-of-color-are-included-in-advertising-6th-in-a-series/.

54. D. Stewart, " 'Young Hollywood' Is White, Thin," Jezebel, jezebel.com/#!5461571/young-hollywood-is-white-thin.

55. Michelle Diament, "Can Disability Be Sexy?" *disabilityscoop*, May 14, 2010, disabilityscoop.com/2010/05/14/can-disability-be-sexy/8048/.

56. Ibid.

57. Ischmeiser, "Screenshot: Lose the Biggest Loser Already," *Bitch* magazine, bitchmagazine.org/post/screenshot-lose-the-biggest-loser-already.

58. Maura Kelly, "Should 'Fatties' Get a Room? (Even on TV?)," *Marie Claire*, October 25, 2010, marieclaire.com/sex-love/dating-blog/overweight-couples-on-television.

59. C. Leive, "On the C.L.: The Picture You Can't Stop Talking About: Meet 'the Woman on p. 194,' " *Glamour*, August 17, 2009, glamour.com/health-fitness/blogs/vitamin-g/2009/08/on-the-cl-the-picture-you-cant.html.

60. C. Strawn, "*Glamour* Honors Plus-Size Models in Its November Issue," *The Frisky*, October 2, 2009, the frisky.com/post/246-glamour-honors-plus-size-models-in-its-november-issue/.

61. S. Marikar, "Lizzie Miller Fuels Debate About Plus-Size Acceptance," ABC News, September 2, 2009, abcnews.go.com/Entertainment/BeautySecrets/story?id=8463526.

62. The latest in the series is Jean Kilbourne, *Killing Us Softly 4: Advertising's Image of Women* (Northampton, MA: Media Education Foundation, 2010).

63. Newscore, "ABC Slams Lane Bryant: We Never Rejected Plus-Size Lingerie Ad," FoxNews.com, April 22, 2010, foxnews.com/entertainment/2010/04/22/abc-slams-lane-bryant-rejected-plus-size-lingerie-ad/.

64. G. Bellafante, "Plus-Size Wars," *New York Times*, July 28, 2010, nytimes.com/2010/08/01/magazine/01plussize-t.html?_r=2&pagewanted=all.

65. Mimi Nichter and Nancy Vuckovic, "Fat Talk: Body Image Among Adolescent Girls," in Nicole Sault, ed., *Many Mirrors: Body Image and Social Relations* (Piscataway, NJ: Rutgers University Press, 1994), p. 7.

66. N. Hellmich, "Do Thin Models Warp Girls' Body Images?" *USA Today*, September 26, 2006, usatoday.com/news/health/2006-09-25-thin-models_x.htm.

67. C. Stewart, "Disney Provokes Girls' Body Image-Image Anxiety?" *Orange County Register*, June 16, 2010, ocregister.com/articles/provokes-253659-anxiety-women.html.

68. Disney, Inc., "Consumer Products," disneyconsumerproducts.com/Home/display.jsp?contentId=dcp_home_ourfranchises_disney_princess_us&forPrint=false&langauge=en&preview=false&imageShow=0&pressRoom=US&translationOf=null&region=0.

69. P. Bronson, "Do Disney Princesses Make Young Girls Obsessed with Thinness?" *Newsweek*, December 1, 2009, newsweek.com/blogs/nurture-shock/2009/12/01/do-disney-princesses-make-young-girls-obsessed-with-thinness.html.

70. "Dove Reveals Results of Second Global Study," Dove Self-Esteem Fund media release, April 2007, campaignforrealbeauty.com.au/dove-self-esteem-fund/pdfs/Dove_Global_Study_2007.pdf.

71. Peggy Orenstein, "Real-Life Disney Princess Exposed the Danger Line," *Women's News* (February 13, 2011), womensenews.org/story/parenting/110212/real-life-disney-princess-exposed-the-danger-line.

72. CNN, "Kiss My Fat Ass, Says Meghan McCain," CNN.com, March 17, 2009, politicalticker.blogs.cnn.com/2009/03/17/kiss-my-fat-ass-says-meghan-mccain.

73. J. Rao, "It's the Year of the Value Diet" CNBC, June 18, 2010, cnbc.com/id/37492840/It_s_The_Year_ofThe_Value_Diet.

74. T. Mann et al., "Medicare's Search for Effective Obesity Treatments: Diets Are Not the Answer," *American Psychologist* 62, no. 3 (2007): 220–33.

75. U. Ghitza et al., "Peptide YY3-36 Decreases Reinstatement of High-Fat Food Seeking During Dieting in a Rat Relapse Model," *Journal of Neuroscience* 27, no. 3 (2007): 11522–32.

76. A. Field et al., "Relation Between Dieting and Weight Change Among Preadolescents and Adolescents," *Pediatrics* 112, no. 4 (2003): 900–90.

77. K. Gapinski, K. Brownell, and M. LaFrance, "Body Objectification and Fat Talk: Effects on Emotion, Motivation, and Cognitive Performance," *Sex Roles* 48 (2003): 378–79.

78. Y. May Chao et al., "Ethnic Differences in Weight Control Practices Among U.S. Adolescents from 1995 to 2005," *International Journal of Eating Disorders* 41, issue 2 (2008): 124–33.

79. Denise Brodey, "Blacks Join the Eating Disorder Mainstream," *New York Times*, September 20, 2005, nytimes.com/2005/09/20/health/psychology/20eat.html?pagewanted=all.

80. Catherine Steiner-Adair and Lisa Sjostrom, *Full of Ourselves: A Wellness Program to Advance Girl Power, Health, and Leadership* (New York: Teachers College Press, 2006).

81. T. Andreyeva et al., "Changes in Perceived Weight Discrimination Among Americans, 1995–1996 Through 2004–2006," *Obesity* 16, no. 5 (2008): 1129–34.

82. Laura Fraser, *Losing It: False Hopes and Fat Profits in the Diet Industry* (New York: Penguin, 1998), p. 53.

83. Centers for Disease Control and Prevention, *Obesity and Overweight*, cdc.gov/nchs/fastats/overwt.htm.

84. M. Magowan, "Congresswomen Urge Healthy Media for Youth" *San Francisco Chronicle*, April 15, 2010, sfgate.com/cgi-bin/blogs/mmagowan/detail?entry_id=61396.

85. American Psychological Association, report of the Task Force on the Sexualization of Girls, apa.org/pi/women/programs/girls/report-full.pdf.

86. Rose Weitz, *Rapunzel's Daughters: What Women's Hair Tells Us About Women's Lives* (New York: Farrar, Straus, 2005), p. 225.

CHAPTER 4:
GENDER IDENTITY
AND SEXUAL ORIENTATION

1. Julia Serano, *Whipping Girl: A Transsexual Woman on Sexism and the Scapegoating of Femininity* (Berkeley: Seal Press, 2007), p. 27.

2. Joanne Herman, *Transgender Explained for Those Who Are Not* (Bloomington, IN: Author House, 2009), p. 51.

3. Ibid., p. 28.

4. Henk Asscheman et al., "A Long-Term Follow-up Study of Mortality in Transsexuals Receiving Treatment with Cross-Sex Hormones," *European Journal of Endocrinology* (January 25, 2011): D01: 10.153/EJ-10-1095. See also Louis J. Gooren, E. J. Giltay, and M. C. Bunck, "Long-Term Treatment of Transsexuals with Cross-Sex Hormones: Extensive Personal Experience," *Journal of Clinical Endocrinology and Metabolism* 93 (2008): 19–25.

5. Wylie C. Hembree et al., "Endocrine Treatment of Transsexual Persons: An Endocrine Society Clinical Practice Guideline," *Journal of Clinical Endocrinology and Metabolism* 94, no. 9 (2009): 3132–54, endo-society .org/guidelines/final/upload/Endocrine-Treatment-of -Transsexual-Persons.pdf.

6. Dr. Louis Gooren, personal correspondence, December 2010.

7. See also Louis J. Gooren and E. J. Giltay, "Review of Studies of Androgen Treatment of Female-to-Male Transsexuals: Effects and Risks of Administration of Androgens to Females," *Journal of Sexual Medicine* 5, issue 4 (2008): 765–76.

8. Hembree et al., "Endocrine Treatment of Transsexual Persons," table 11.

9. Ibid.

10. H. Makadon et al., *Fenway Guide to Lesbian, Gay, Bisexual, and Transgender Health* (Philadelphia: American College of Physicians, 2008), p. 381.

11. The World Professional Association for Transgender Health, "Medical Necessity Statement," 2008, wpath .org/medical_necessity_statement.cfm.

12. Norman Spack, "Transgenderism," *Medical Ethics* 12, issue 3 (Fall 2005).

13. M. Potter, "Tips for Providing Paps to Trans Men," Sherbourne Health Center, checkitoutguys.ca/sites/ default/files/Tips_Paps_TransMen_0.pdf.

14. Mautner Project, National Lesbian Health Organization, "Transgender Health," at mautnerproject.org/health_ info/transgender_health.cfm.

15. Makadon et al., *Fenway Guide*, p. 381.

16. Ibid., p. 347.

17. Norman Spack, "Key to Successful Treatment of Transgender Patients May Involve Delay of Puberty," April 24, 2010, media.aace.com/article_display.cfm? article_id=4975.

18. Saber's Story, Minnesota Transgender Health Coalition, mntranshealth.org. Type "Saber's Story" into "Search." Used with permission.

19. Makadon et al., *Fenway Guide*, pp. 169, 170, 140.

20. Ibid., p. 148.

21. Ibid., p. 147.

22. Ibid., p. 168.

23. Ibid., p. 238.

24. Ibid., p. 227.

25. Ibid. For a survey-based study suggesting that older lesbians may have an increased risk for breast, ovarian, and endometrial cancer but a decreased risk for cervical cancer, see E. Zaritsky and S. L. Dibble, "Risk Factors for Reproductive and Breast Cancers Among Older Lesbians," *Journal of Womens Health* 19, no. 1 (2010): 125–31.

26. Petra Doan, "The Tyranny of Gendered Spaces: Reflections from Beyond the Gender Dichotomy," *Gender, Place, and Culture*, Special Issue on Transgendered Geography, 2010.

27. H.R. 3017, Employment Non-Discrimination Act of 2009, 111th Cong., at govtrack.us/congress/bill.xpd? bill=h111-3017.

28. Pat Parker, *Movement in Black,* expanded ed. (Ithaca, NY: Firebrand Books, 1999). Thanks to Rev. Irene Monroe for this reference.

29. C. Whitney, "Intersections in Identity-Identity Development Among Queer Women with Disabilities," *Sexuality and Disability* 24, no. 1 (2006): 39–52.

30. *Black Lesbians Matter*, Zuna Institute, 2010, zunainstitute.org/index.php?option=com_content&task=view &id=113&Itemid=148.

31. For an essay that offers an analysis of racism and classism among white lesbian feminist activists and white transgender activists, see Emi Koyama, "Whose Feminism Is It Anyway? The Unspoken Racism of the Trans Inclusion Debate," in *The Transgender Studies Reader*, ed. Susan Stryker and Stephen Whittle (New York: Routledge, 2006), pp. 698–705.

CHAPTER 5:
RELATIONSHIPS

1. Single in America Study, funded by Match.com and conducted by MarketTools in association with biological anthropologist Dr. Helen Fisher, social historian Stephanie Coontz, evolutionary biologist Justin Garcia, and the Institute for Evolutionary Studies at Binghamton University. The study is based on the attitudes and behaviors of a representative sample of 5,200 U.S. single people ages 21 to 65-plus. Results are available at blog.match.com/singles-study.
2. U.S. Census Bureau, "American Community Survey," 2005–2009, census.gov/acs/ww.
3. U.S. Census Bureau, "America's Families and Living Arrangements," 2000–2007.
4. "American Community Survey."
5. Ibid.
6. "Support for Same-Sex Marriage Edges Upward: Majority Continues to Favor Gays Serving Openly in the Military," October 6, 2010, The Pew Research Center for the People & the Press, pewresearch.org/pubs/1755/poll-gay-marriage-gains-acceptance-gays-in-the-military.
7. Freedom to Marry, "States," freedomtomarry.org/states/.
8. Jeffrey S. Passel, Wendy Wang, and Paul Taylor, *Marrying Out: One-in-Seven New U.S. Marriages Is Interracial or Interethnic*, Pew Research Center, June 4, 2010, pewsocialtrends.org/files/2010/10/755-marrying-out.pdf.

CHAPTER 6:
SOCIAL INFLUENCES
ON SEXUALITY

1. From *Sister Outsider* (Freedom, CA: Crossing Press, 1984), pp. 53–59.
2. Cara Kulwicki, personal correspondence.
3. Carol Roye, "What Exactly Is a Hymen?" Our Bodies Ourselves website, ourbodiesourselves.org/book/companion.asp?id=13&compID=130.
4. J. Friedman and J. Valenti, eds., *Yes Means Yes! Visions of Female Power and a World Without Rape* (Berkeley: Seal Press, 2008), pp. 77–91.
5. Ibid., pp. 74–75.
6. Thank you to psychologist Judy Leavitt for this concept.
7. Asra Q. Nomani, originally published in *Living Islam Out Loud: American Muslim Women Speak*, ed. Saleemah Abdul-Ghafur (Boston: Beacon Press, 2005), pp. 155–156.

8. A. F. Bogaert, "Asexuality: Prevalence and Associated Factors in a National Probability Sample," *Journal of Sex Research* 41, no. 3 (2004): 279–87.
9. Susan Scherrer, "Coming to an Asexual Identity: Negotiating Identity, Negotiating Desire" *Sexualities* 11, no. 5 (2008): 621–41, ncbi.nlm.nih.gov/pmc/articles/PMC2893352/.

CHAPTER 7:
SEXUAL PLEASURE
AND ENTHUSIASTIC CONSENT

1. Recent research by Beverly Whipple, Barry Komisaruk, and their team has demonstrated that there are at least four nerve pathways that respond to stimulation of the genital regions: the pudendal, the pelvic, the hypogastric, and the vagus nerves. Stimulation of different nerves in the clitoris, vagina, and cervix produces different responses. Whipple and Komisaruk have documented the areas of the brain that are activated with different forms of stimulation and from imagery or thinking alone by conducting fMRIs of the brain during orgasm. A review of their research can be found in *The Science of Orgasm* and in *The Orgasm Answer Guide*.
2. Persistent genital arousal disorder causes a woman to sustain unwanted, persistent, and intense genital arousal, unaccompanied by sexual desire, which is only temporarily relieved by orgasm. The condition can be extremely distressing and may be caused by medications such as the antidepressant trazodone, or a combination of physical, psychological, or emotional factors. See, for example, L. A. Brotto et al., "Women's Sexual Desire and Arousal Disorders," *Journal of Sexual Medicine* (January 2010): 586–614.
3. Shere Hite, *The Hite Report: A National Study of Female Sexuality* (New York: Seven Stories Press, 2004).
4. Gina Ogden, *The Heart and Soul of Sex: Making the ISIS Connection* (Boston: Trumpeter, 2006), and *The Return of Desire: A Guide to Rediscovering Your Sexual Passion* (Boston: Trumpeter, 2008).
5. Helen Singer Kaplan, *Disorders of Sexual Desire* (New York: Brunner/Mazel, 1979); B. Zilbergeld and C. R. Ellison, "Desire Discrepancies and Arousal Problems in Sex Therapy," in S. R. Leiblum and L. A. Pervin, eds., *Principles and Practice of Sex Therapy* (New York: Guilford, 1980), pp. 65–104.
6. B. Whipple and K. Brash-McGreer, "Management of Female Sexual Dysfunction," in M. L. Sipski and C. J. Alexander, eds., *Sexual Function in People with*

Disability and Chronic Illness: A Health Professional's Guide (Gaithersburg, MD: Aspen Publishers, 1997), pp. 509–34.

7. R. Basson, "Female Sexual Response: The Role of Drugs in the Management of Sexual Dysfunction," *Obstetrics & Gynecology* 98 (2001): 350–53.

8. B. Whipple, G. Ogden, and B. R. Komisaruk, "Physiological Correlates of Imagery-Induced Orgasm in Women," *Archives of Sexual Behavior* 21, no. 2 (1992): 121–33.

9. The G-spot was named by the sex researchers Dr. John Perry and Dr. Beverly Whipple. See A. Ladas, B. Whipple, and J. Perry, *The G Spot: And Other Discoveries About Human Sexuality* (New York: Holt, 2005).

10. E. A. Jannini et al., "Who's Afraid of the G-spot?" *Journal of Sexual Medicine* (January 2010): 25–34; and D. Rabinerson and E. Horowitz, "G-spot and Female Ejaculation: Fiction or Reality?" *Harefuah* 146, no. 2 (2007): 145–47 (in Hebrew).

11. J. B. Korda, S. W. Goldstein, and F. Sommer, "The History of Female Ejaculation," *Journal of Sexual Medicine* 7, no. 5 (2010): 1965–75.

12. F. Cabello, "Female Ejaculation: Myth and Reality," in J. J. Baras-Vass and M. Perez-Conchillo, eds., *Sexuality and Human Rights: Proceedings of the XIIIth World Congress of Sexology*, pp. 325–33 (Valencia, Spain: Nan Libres, 1997).

13. Friedman and Valenti, *Yes Means Yes!* pp. 43–51.

14. Ibid., pp. 20–21.

15. Ibid., pp. 309–310.

16. Joanna L. Grossman, "Courts Divide Over the Constitutionality of Sex Toy Bans," FindLaw.com, November 10, 2009, writ.news.findlaw.com/grossman/20091110.html.

17. Stacey May Fowles, "The Fantasy of Acceptable Non-Consent," in *Yes Means Yes!* p. 120.

CHAPTER 8: SEXUAL CHALLENGES

1. D. M. Ferguson, B. Hosmane, and J. R. Heiman, "Randomized, Placebo-Controlled, Double-Blind, Parallel Design Trial of the Efficacy and Safety of Zestra in Women with Mixed Desire/Interest/Arousal/Orgasm Disorders," *Journal of Sex and Marital Therapy* 36, no. 1 (2010): 66–86. Abstract: "Over 256 women, age 21 to 65, with acquired mixed female sexual disorders participated in a 16-week randomized, placebo-controlled, double-blind study of Zestra, a topical botanical preparation. Routine outcome instruments measured efficacy and safety. Zestra was well tolerated. The only significant safety finding was mild-to-moderate genital burning seen only in Zestra-treated subjects (14.6%). Zestra provided significant desire, arousal, and treatment satisfaction benefits for a broadly generalized group of women with sexual difficulties" (ncbi.nlm.nih.gov/pubmed/20063238).

2. Food and Drug Administration, "Briefing Information for the June 18, 2010, Meeting of the Advisory Committee for Reproductive Health Drugs," fda.gov/AdvisoryCommittees/CommitteesMeetingMaterials/Drugs/ReproductiveHealthDrugsAdvisoryCommittee/ucm215436.htm.

3. D. Wilson, "Drug for Sexual Desire Opposed by Panel," *New York Times,* June 18, 2010, nytimes.com/2010/06/19/business/19sexpill.html.

4. Alessandra Graziottin, "Dyspareunia and Vaginismus: Review of the Literature and Treatment," *Current Sexual Health Reports* 5, no. 1, (2008): 43–50, springerlink.com/content/k6w1681521n14305/.

5. D. Herbenick, "Vaginismus: 6 Facts You Should Know," 2009, mysexprofessor.com/womens-sexuality/vaginismus-6-facts-you-should-know/.

6. B. Whipple and B. R. Komisaruk, "Elevation of Pain Thresholds by Vaginal Stimulation in Women," *Pain* 21 (1985): 357–67; B. Whipple and B. R. Komisaruk, "Analgesia Produced in Women by Genital Self-Stimulation," *Journal of Sex Research* 24 (1988): 130–40; Barry R. Komisaruk and Beverly Whipple, "The Suppression of Pain by Genital Stimulation in Females," *Annual Review of Sex Research* 6 (1995): 151–86.

7. B. Whipple, C. A. Gerdes, and B. R. Komisaruk, "Sexual Response to Self-Stimulation in Women with Complete Spinal Cord Injury," *Journal of Sex Research* 33 no. 3 (1996): 231–40; B. R. Komisaruk and B. Whipple, "Functional MRI of the Brain During Orgasm in Women," *Annual Review of Sex Research* 16 (2005): 62–86; Marca L. Sipski, Craig J. Alexander, and Ray C. Rosen, "Orgasm in Women with Spinal Cord Injuries: A Laboratory-Based Assessment," *Archives of Physical Medicine and Rehabilitation* 76 (1995): 1097–1102.

8. K. Best, "Epilepsy Drugs May Reduce Method Effectiveness," *Network* 2, no. 19 (Winter 1999): 12.

9. Victoria Department of Human Services, Australia, "Traumatic Brain Injury and Sexual Issues," *Better Health Channel.*

10. Sexual Health Network, "Possible Effects of a Traumatic Brain Injury on a Person's Sexuality," sexualhealth.com/article.php?Action=read&article_id=336&channel=3&topic=12.

11. Society of Obstetricians and Gynaecologists of Canada, "Contraception, Disability and Illness, Female Contraceptive and Reproductive Issues: Epilepsy," 2006, games.sexualityandu.ca/professionals/illness-1-4.aspx.

12. J. Guan et al., "Sexual Dysfunction in Patients with Chronic Renal Failure," *Zhonghua Nan Ke Xue* 9, no. 6 (September 2003): 454–56, 461.

13. P. Enzlin et al., "Sexual Dysfunction in Women with Type 1 Diabetes: Long-Term Findings from the DCCT/EDIC Study Cohort," *Diabetes Care* 32, no. 5 (2009): 780–85.

14. A. Giraldi and E. Kristensen, "Sexual Dysfunction in Women with Diabetes Mellitus," *Journal of Sex Research* 47, issue 213 (2010): 199–211; L. P. Wallner, A. V. Sarma, and C. Kim, "Sexual Functioning Among Women with and Without Diabetes in the Boston Area Community Health Study," *Journal of Sexual Medicine* 7 (2010): 881–87.

15. M.T. Filocamo et al., "Sexual Dysfunction in Women During Dialysis and After Renal Transplantation," *Journal of Sexual Medicine* 6, no. 11 (2009): 3125–31.

16. J. Bringer et al., "Which Contraception to Choose for the Diabetic Woman?" *Diabetes & Metabolism* 27, no. 4 (2001): S35–41; S. Wysocki and S. Schnare, "Current Advances in Oral Contraceptives: OC Use in Patients with Common Medical Conditions," in *Preventing Unintended Pregnancy: Advances in Hormonal Contraception*, National Institute of Child Health and Human Development conference, 2001, npwh.org/Oral-Contraception/.

17. L. E. Duncan et al., "Does Hypertension and Its Pharmacotherapy Affect the Quality of Sexual Function in Women?" *American Journal of Hypertension* 13 (2000): 640–47.

18. A. Manolis and M. Doumas, "Sexual Dysfunction: The 'Prima Ballerina' of Hypertension-Related Quality-of-Life Complications," *Journal of Hypertension* 26, no. 11 (2005): 2074–84.

19. R. Basson and W. W. Schultz, "Sexual Sequelae of General Medical Disorders" *Lancet* 369 (2007): 409–24.

20. *Merck Manual of Geriatrics*, "Effects of Medical Disorders on Sexuality," merck.com/mrkshared/mm_geriatrics/sec14/ch114.jsp.

21. G. Jackson et al., "The Second Princeton Consensus on Sexual Dysfunction and Cardiac Risk: New Guidelines for Sexual Medicine," *Journal of Sexual Medicine* 3, no. 1 (2006): 28–36.

22. K. Perez, M. Gadgil, and D. S. Dizon, "Sexual Ramifications of Medical Illness," *Clinical Obstetrics and Gynecology* 52, no. 4 (2009): 6691–6701.

23. Manolis and Doumas, "Sexual Dysfunction."

24. S. C. Smeltzer and N. C. Sharts-Hopko, *A Provider's Guide for the Care of Women with Physical Disabilities and Chronic Medical Conditions* (Chapel Hill: North Carolina Office on Disability and Health, 2005), fpg.unc.edu/~ncodh/publications.cfm.

25. W. T. Van Berlo et al., "Sexual Functioning of People with Rheumatoid Arthritis: A Multicenter Study," *Clinical Rheumatology* 26 (2007): 30–38.

26. A. M. Abdel-Nasser and E. I. Ali, "Determinants of Sexual Disability and Dissatisfaction in Female Patients with Rheumatoid Arthritis," *Clinical Rheumatology* 25 (2006): 822–30.

27. Monika Ostensen, "New Insights into Sexual Functioning and Fertility in Rheumatic Diseases," *Best Practice & Research Clinical Rheumatology* 18 (April 2004): 219–32.

28. Society of Obstetricians and Gynaecologists of Canada. "Contraception, Disability and Illness, Female Contraceptive and Reproductive Issues: Rheumatoid Arthritis," 2009, games.sexualityandu.ca/professionals/illness-1-7.aspx.

29. Smeltzer and Sharts-Hopko, *A Provider's Guide for the Care of Women.*

30. Ostensen, "New Insights into Sexual Functioning and Fertility."

31. A. G. Tristano, "The Impact of Rheumatic Diseases on Sexual Function, *Rheumatology* 29 (2009): 853–60.

32. M. Petri et al., "Combined Oral Contraceptives in Women with Systemic Lupus Erythematosus," *New England Journal of Medicine* 353 (2000): 2550–58.

33. J. P. Buyon et al., "The Effect of Combined Estrogen and Progesterone Hormone Replacement Therapy on Disease Activity in Systemic Lupus Erythematosus: A Randomized Trial," *Annals of Internal Medicine* 142 (2005): 753–62.

34. A. J. McDougall and J. G. McLeod, "Autonomic Nervous System Function in Multiple Sclerosis," *Journal of Neurological Science* 215, no. 1–2, (2003): 79–85.

35. Smeltzer and Sharts-Hopko, *A Provider's Guide for the Care of Women.*

36. Society of Obstetricians and Gynaecologists of Canada, "Contraception, Disability and Illness, Female Contraceptive and Reproductive Issues: Multiple Sclerosis," games.sexualityandu.ca/professionals/illness-1-2.aspx.

37. A. Koivusalo et al., "Sexual Functions in Adulthood After Restorative Proctocolectomy for Pediatric Onset Ulcerative Colitis," *Pediatric Surgery International* 25, no. 10 (2009): 881–84.

38. K. Perez et al., "Sexual Ramifications of Medical Illness."

39. F. Biering-Sørensen et al., "Sexual Function in Patients with Spinal Cord Injuries," *UgesKrift for Laeger* 164, no. 41 (October 7, 2002): 4764–68 (in Danish).

40. B. R. Komisaruk et al., "Brain Activation During Vaginocervical Self-stimulation and Orgasm in Women with Complete Spinal Cord Injury," *Brain Research* 1024 (2004): 77–88.

41. P. Rees, C. Fowler, and K. Maas, "Sexual Dysfunction in Neurological Disorders," *Lancet* 369 (2006): 512–25.

42. L. Pereira, "Obstetric Management of the Patient with Spinal Cord Injury," *Obstetrical and Gynecological Survey* 58, no. 10 (October 2003): 678–87.

43. W. M. Helkowski et al., "Autonomic Dysreflexia: Incidence in Persons with Neurologically Complete and Incomplete Tetraplegia," *Journal of Spinal Cord Medicine* 26, no. 3 (Fall 2003): 244–47.

44. G. P. Earl, "Autonomic Dysreflexia," *American Journal of Maternal Child Nursing* 27, no. 2 (March April 2002): 93–97; Smeltzer and Sharts-Hopko, *A Provider's Guide for the Care of Women.*

45. International Planned Parenthood Federation, *IMAP Statement on Contraception for Women with Medical Disorders*, 1999, ippf.org/medical/imap/statements/eng/pdf/1999 06a.pdf.

46. G. Aydin et al., "Relationship Between Sexual Dysfunction and Psychiatric Status in Premenopausal Women with Fibromyalgia," *Urology* 67 (2006): 156–161.

47. Tristano, "The Impact of Rheumatic Diseases on Sexual Function."

48. Komisaruk and Whipple, "Suppression of Pain by Genital Stimulation in Females."

49. Manolis and Doumas, "Sexual Dysfunction"; S. H. Kennedy and S. Rizvi, "Sexual Dysfunction, Depression, and the Impact of Antidepressants," *Journal of Clinical Psychopharmacology* 29, no. 2 (2009): 157–164; A. Saval and A. E. Chiodo, "Sexual Dysfunction Associated with Intrathecal Baclofen Use: A Report of Two Cases," *Journal of Spinal Cord Medicine* 31 (2008): 103–05; C. L. Harden, "Sexuality in Men and Women with Epilepsy," *CNS Spectrums* 11, supp. 9 (2006): 13–18; E. R. Schwarz and J. Rodriguez, "Sex and the Heart," *International Journal of Impotence Research* 17, supp. 1: (2005): S4–6 (this article references male erectile problems primarily).

50. Smeltzer and Sharts-Hopko, *A Provider's Guide for the Care of Women.*

51. J. Hsia et al., "Estrogen Plus Progestin and the Risk of Peripheral Arterial Disease: The Women's Health Initiative," *Circulation* 109 (2004): 620–26.

52. D. M. Plourd and W. F. Rayburn, "New Contraceptive Methods," *Journal of Reproductive Medicine* 9 (2003): 665–71.

53. Ostensen, "New Insights into Sexual Functioning and Fertility in Rheumatic Diseases."

CHAPTER 9: BIRTH CONTROL

1. Elizabeth Miller et al., "Pregnancy Coercion, Intimate Partner Violence and Unintended Pregnancy," *Contraception* 81, issue 4 (April 2010): 316–22.

2. M. F. Gallo et al., "Nonlatex Versus Latex Male Condoms for Contraception," *Cochrane Database of Systematic Reviews* 1 (2006).

3. A. M. Minnis and N. S. Padian, "Effectiveness of Female Controlled Barrier Methods in Preventing Sexually Transmitted Infections and HIV: Current Evidence and Future Research Directions," *Sexually Transmitted Infections* 81 (2005): 193–200.

4. Physician labeling for the FemCap, contracept.org/docs/femcap-fda.pdf.

5. WHO/CONRAD, *Technical Consultation on Nonoxynol-9*, 2001, who.int/reproductivehealth/publications/rtis/RHR_03_8/en/index.html.

6. D. Wilkinson et al., "Nonoxynol-9 for Preventing Vaginal Acquisition of Sexually Transmitted Infections by Women from Men," *Cochrane Database of Systematic Reviews* 4 (2007).

7. A. Edelman et al., "Continuous Versus Cyclic Use of Combined Oral Contraceptives for Contraception: Systematic Cochrane Review of Randomized Controlled Trials," *Human Reproduction* 21, no. 3 (2006): 573–78.

8. Some researchers believe there may be unknown risks involved with extended use of contraceptive hormones to eliminate bleeding. See, for example, "Menstrual Suppression," position statement of the Society for Menstrual Cycle Research, menstruationresearch.org/position-statements/menstrual-supression-2007.

9. Food and Drug Administration, Center for Drug Evaluation and Research, "Guidance for Industry: Labeling for Combined Oral Contraceptives," March 2004, fda.gov/downloads/Drugs/GuidanceCompliance RegulatoryInformation/Guidances/ucm075075.pdf.

10. Robert A. Hatcher et al., *Contraceptive Technology*, 19th ed. (New York: Ardent Media, 2007), p. 243.

11. A. B. Berenson and M. Rahman, "Changes in Weight, Total Fat, Percent Body Fat, and Central-to-Peripheral Fat Ratio Associated with Injectable and Oral Contra-

ceptive Use," *American Journal of Obstetrics and Gynecology* 200, no. 3 (2009): 329.e1–e8.

12. L. M. Lopez et al., "Skin Patch and Vaginal Ring Versus Combined Oral Contraceptives for Contraception," *Cochrane Database of Systematic Reviews* 3 (2010).

13. Z. Harel et al., "Recovery of Bone Mineral Density in Adolescents Following the Use of Depot Medroxyprogesterone Acetate Contraceptive Injections," *Contraception* 81, no. 4 (2010): 281–91.

14. Berenson and Rahman, "Changes in Weight, Total Fat, Percent Body Fat, and Central-to-Peripheral Fat Ratio."

15. S. Wu et al., "Copper T380A Intrauterine Device for Emergency Contraception: A Prospective, Multicentre, Cohort Clinical Trial," *British Journal of Obstetrics and Gynaecology* 117, no. 10 (2010): 1205–10.

16. H. B. Peterson et al., "The Risk of Menstrual Abnormalities After Tubal Sterilization," *New England Journal of Medicine* 343, no. 23 (2000): 1681–87.

17. B. Xu and W. Huang, "No-Scalpel Vasectomy Outside China," *Asian Journal of Andrology* 2 (2000): 21–24.

18. P. J. Schwingl and H. A. Guess, "Safety and Effectiveness of Vasectomy," *Fertility and Sterility* 73, no. 5 (2000): 923–36.

19. W. D. Mosher and J. Jones, "Use of Contraception in the United States: 1982–2008," *Vital and Health Statistics* 23, no. 29 (2010).

20. M. J. Sneyd et al., "High Prevalence of Vasectomy in New Zealand," *Contraception* 64, no. 3 (2001): 155–59.

21. I. Schroeder-Printzen et al., "Vaso-Vasostomy," *Urologia Internationalis* 70 (2003): 101–07.

22. Y. Gu et al., "Multicenter Contraceptive Efficacy Trial of Injectable Testosterone Undecanoate in Chinese Men," *Journal of Clinical Endocrinology & Metabolism* 94 (2009): 1910–05.

23. K. Thompson and E. Lissner, "RISUG," malecontraceptives.org/methods/risug.php.

24. S. T. Truitt et al., "Combined Hormonal Versus Nonhormonal Versus Progestin-only Contraception in Lactation," *Cochrane Database of Systematic Reviews* 2 (2003).

25. H. von Hertzen et al., "Low Dose Mifepristone and Two Regimens of Levonorgestrel for Emergency Contraception: A WHO Multicentre Randomised Trial," *Lancet* 360 (2002): 1807.

26. Rachel K. Jones et al., "Better Than Nothing or Savvy Risk-Reduction Practice? The Importance of Withdrawal," *Contraception* 79 (2009) 407–10.

CHAPTER 10:
SAFER SEX

1. H. Weinstock et al., "Sexually Transmitted Diseases Among American Youth: Incidence and Prevalence Estimates, 2000," *Perspectives on Sexual and Reproductive Health* 36, no. 1 (2004): 6–10.

2. Sara E. Forhan et al., "Prevalence of Sexually Transmitted Infections Among Female Adolescents Aged 14 to 19 in the United States," *Pediatrics* 124, no. 6 (December 2009): 1505–12.

3. Center for Sexual Health Promotion, Indiana University School of Health, Physical Education and Recreation, "National Survey of Sexual Health and Behavior," *Journal of Sexual Medicine*, October 2010.

4. Minnis and Padian, "Effectiveness of Female Controlled Barrier Methods in Preventing Sexually Transmitted Infections and HIV."

5. H. Brückner and P. Bearman, "After the Promise: The STD Consequences of Adolescent Virginity Pledges," *Journal of Adolescent Health* 36 (2005): 271–78, jahonline.org/article/PIIS1054139X05000558/fulltext.

6. S. Blake et al., "Condom Availability Programs in Massachusetts High Schools: Relationships with Condom Use and Sexual Behavior," *American Journal of Public Health* 93, no. 6 (2003), ajph.aphapublications.org/cgi/content/full/93/6/955.

7. P. K. Kohler, L. E. Manhart, and W. E. Lafferty, "Abstinence-Only and Comprehensive Sex Education and the Initiation of Sexual Activity and Teen Pregnancy," *Journal of Adolescent Health* 42, no. 4 (2008): 344–51.

8. B. McKeon, "Effective Sex Education," Advocates for Youth, 2006, advocatesforyouth.org/storage/advfy/documents/fssexcur.pdf.

CHAPTER 11:
SEXUALLY TRANSMITTED
INFECTIONS

1. H. Weinstock, S. Berman, and W. Cates Jr., "Sexually Transmitted Diseases Among American Youth: Incidence and Prevalence Estimates, 2000," *Perspectives on Sexual and Reproductive Health* 36, no. 1 (2004): 6–10.

2. Forhan, "Prevalence of Sexually Transmitted Infections Among Female Adolescents."

3. Centers for Disease Control and Prevention, "Trends in Sexually Transmitted Diseases in the United States:

2009 National Data for Gonorrhea, Chlamydia and Syphilis," cdc.gov/std/stats09/trends.htm.

4. Centers for Disease Control and Prevention, "Sexually Transmitted Disease Surveillance 2009," cdc.gov/STD/stats09/default.htm.

5. CDC, "Trends in Sexually Transmitted Diseases in the United States: 2009," p. 9.

6. World Health Organization, "HIV/AIDS: Some Questions and Answers," p. 10, searo.who.int/en/Section10/Section18/Section2011.htm.

7. CDC, "Sexually Transmitted Disease Surveillance 2009."

8. Ibid.

9. Matthew Hogben and Jami S. Leichliter, "Social Determinants and Sexually Transmitted Disease Disparities," *Sexually Transmitted Diseases* 35, issue 12 (December 2008): S13–18.

10. Centers for Disease Control, "Sexually Transmitted Diseases Treatment Guidelines 2006. Special Populations: Women Who Have Sex with Women," cdc.gov/std/treatment/2006/specialpops.htm#specialpops5.

11. Margaret Brady, "Female Genital Mutilation: Complications and Risk of HIV Transmission," *AIDS Patient Care and STDs* 13, no. 12 (1999): 709–16.

12. Personal correspondence with Our Bodies Ourselves, November 19, 2010.

13. CDC, "Sexually Transmitted Disease Surveillance 2009."

14. Robert E. Fullilove, Adaora Adimora, and Peter Leone, "An Epidemic No One Wants to Talk About," *Washington Post*, March 21, 2008, washingtonpost.com/wp-dyn/content/article/2008/03/20/AR2008032003019_pf.html.

15. Ibid.

16. American Social Health Association, press release, January 13, 2009, ashastd.org/news/news_pressreleases_CDCsurveillancereport.cfm.

17. "HIV Infection Among Injection-Drug Users—34 States, 2004–2007," from CDC, in *Journal of the American Medical Association* 303, no. 2 (2010): 126–28.

18. For a review of forty-two studies on needle exchange, see David R. Gibson, Neil M. Flynn, and Daniel Perales, "Effectiveness of Syringe Exchange Programs in Reducing HIV Risk Behavior and HIV Seroconversion Among Injecting Drug Users," *AIDS* 15, issue 11 (2001): 1329–41.

19. ACE, *Breaking the Walls of Silence: AIDS and Women in a New York State Maximum-Security Prison* (New York: Overlook Press, 1998).

20. Donald Wright, "Progress Review: Sexually Transmitted Diseases," Department of Health and Human Services, Public Health Service, 2008.

21. CDC, "Sexually Transmitted Diseases Treatment Guidelines 2006," cdc.gov/std/treatment/2006/.

22. Ibid.

23. Ibid.

24. Ibid.

25. CDC, "Sexually Transmitted Disease Surveillance 2009," p. 34.

26. CDC, "Sexually Transmitted Diseases Treatment Guidelines 2006."

27. CDC, "Sexually Transmitted Disease Surveillance 2009."

28. Centers for Disease Control and Prevention, "STD Facts: Gonorrhea," cdc.gov/std/Gonorrhea/STDFact-gonorrhea.htm.

29. Ibid.

30. Centers for Disease Control and Prevention, "Trends in Sexually Transmitted Diseases in the United States: 2009 National Data for Gonorrhea, Chlamydia and Syphilis," p. 40, cdc.gov/std/stats09/trends.htm.

31. U.S. Preventive Services Task Force, Screening for Syphilis Infection: Recommendation Statement, July 2004, uspreventiveservicestaskforce.org/3rduspstf/syphilis/syphilrs.htm.

32. Centers for Disease Control and Prevention, "STD Facts: Trichomoniasis," cdc.gov/std/trichomonas/STDFact-Trichomoniasis.htm.

33. Centers for Disease Control and Prevention, "STD Facts: Human Papillomavirus," cdc.gov/std/HPV/STDFact-HPV.htm.

34. American Social Health Association, "Learn About HPV: Fast Facts," ashastd.org/hpv/hpv_learn_fastfacts.cfm.

35. American Association of Clinical Chemistry, "Lab Tests Online: HPV," labtestsonline.org/understanding/analytes/hpv/test.html.

36. Centers for Disease Control and Prevention, "Hepatitis B FAQs for Health Professionals," cdc.gov/hepatitis/HBV/HBVfaq.htm#overview.

37. Centers for Disease Control and Prevention, "Hepatitis B FAQs for the Public," cdc.gov/hepatitis/B/bFAQ.htm#overview.

38. Ibid.

39. Ibid.

40. H. I. Hall et al., "Estimation of HIV Incidence in the U.S.," *Journal of the American Medical Association* 300 (2008): 520–29.

41. Centers for Disease Control and Prevention, "Racial/Ethnic Disparities in Self-Rated Health Status Among Adults with and Without Disabilities—United States, 2004–2006," *Morbidity and Mortality Weekly Report* 57, no. 39 (October 3, 2008): 1069–73, cdc.gov/mmwr/PDF/wk/mm5739.pdf.

42. Ibid.

43. Centers for Disease Control and Prevention, "HIV Among African Americans," cdc.gov/hiv/topics/aa/index.htm.

44. D. J. Jamieson, "Cesarean Delivery for HIV-Infected Women: Recommendations and Controversies," *American Journal of Obstetrics & Gynecology* 173 (September 1973): S96–100.

45. Robert M. Grant et al., "Preexposure Chemoprophylaxis for HIV Prevention in Men Who Have Sex with Men," *New England Journal of Medicine* 363 (2010): 2587–99.

46. "Health Benefits of Breastfeeding in Children Born to HIV-Infected Mothers," in *HIV Transmission Through Breastfeeding: A Review of Available Evidence*, 2007 update, p. 21, whqlibdoc.who.int/publications/2008/9789241596596_eng.pdf.

47. K. Kayitenkore et al., "The Impact of ART on HIV Transmission Among HIV Serodiscordant Couples," program and abstracts of the XVI International AIDS Conference, 2006, Abstract MOKC101.

48. Department of Health and Human Services, AIDS Adult and Adolescent Treatment Guidelines, AIDS info.nih.gov/Guidelines.

49. R. Palmer, "Use of Complementary Therapies to Treat Patients with HIV/AIDS," *Nursing Standard* 22, no. 50 (2008): 35–41.

50. AIDS Care Project, part of Pathways to Wellness, is a public-health clinic for complementary therapies and HIV, pathwaysboston.org/specialty/aidscare.html.

51. M. Campsmith, P. Rhodes, and H. I Hall, "Estimated Prevalence of Undiagnosed HIV Infection: United States at the End of 2006," program and abstracts of the 16th Conference on Retroviruses and Opportunistic Infections, 2009, Abstract 1036.

CHAPTER 12:
UNEXPECTED PREGNANCY

1. The National Campaign to Prevent Teen and Unplanned Pregnancy, "Fast Facts: Unplanned Pregnancy: Key Data," May 2008, thenationalcampaign.org/resources/pdf/fast-facts-unplanned-key-data.pdf.

2. Lawrence B. Finer, "Unintended Pregnancy Among U.S. Adolescents: Accounting for Sexual Activity," *Journal of Adolescent Health* 47, no. 3 (2010): 312–14.

3. Guttmacher Institute, "An Overview of Abortions in the United States," January 2011, guttmacher.org/presentations/abort_slides.pdf.

4. National Women's Law Center, "When Girls Don't Graduate We All Fail: A Call to Improve High School Graduation Rates for Girls," 2007, accessed December 12, 2010.

5. Ibid.

6. U.S. Department of Health & Human Services Administration for Children & Families, Child Welfare Information Gateway, "Foster Care Statistics," childwelfare.gov/pubs/factsheets/foster.htm.

7. Ibid.

CHAPTER 13:
ABORTION

1. L. B. Finer et al., "Disparities in Rates of Unintended Pregnancy in the United States, 1994 and 2001," *Perspectives on Sexual and Reproductive Health* 33, no. 2 (2006): 90–96.

2. K. Pazol et al., "Abortion Surveillance—United States, 2006," *Morbidity and Mortality Weekly Report* 58, (November 27, 2009): 1–35, cdc.gov/mmwr/preview/mmwrhtml/ss5808a1.htm?s_cid=ss5808a1_e.

3. R. K. Jones and K. Kooistra, "Abortion Incidence and Access to Services in the United States, 2008," *Perspectives on Sexual and Reproductive Health* 43, no. 1 (2011): 41–50.

4. Ibid.

5. Rachel K. Jones, Lawrence B. Finer, and Susheela Singh, "Characteristics of U.S. Abortion Patients, 2008," May 2010, guttmacher.org/pubs/US-Abortion-Patients.pdf.

6. Lawrence B. Finer et al., "Reasons U.S. Women Have Abortions: Quantitative and Qualitative Perspectives," *Perspectives on Sexual and Reproductive Health* 37, no. 3 (2005): 110–18, guttmacher.org/pubs/psrhfull/3711005.pdf.

7. Jones and Kooistra, "Abortion Incidence and Access to Services in the United States, 2008."

8. Ibid.

9. National Cancer Institute, "Summary Report: Early Reproductive Events and Breast Cancer Workshop," March 4, 2003, cancer.gov/cancerinfor/ere-workshop-report.

10. G. E. Robinson et al., "Is There an 'Abortion Trauma Syndrome'? Critiquing the Evidence," *Harvard Review of Psychiatry* 17, no. 4 (2009): 268–90.

11. Brenda Major et al., "Psychological Responses of Women After First-Trimester Abortion," *Archives of General Psychiatry* 57 (2000): 777–84.

12. APA Task Force on Mental Health and Abortion, *Report of the APA Task Force on Mental Health and Abortion* (Washington, DC: American Psychological Association, 2008).

13. Guttmacher Institute, "State Policies in Brief: An Overview of Minors' Consent Law," guttmacher.org/statecenter/spibs/spib_OMCL.pdf.

14. S. K. Henshaw and K. Kost, "Parental Involvement in Minors' Abortion Decision," *Family Planning Perspectives*, 24, no. 5 (1992): 196–207, 213.

15. Picker Institute, *From the Patient's Perspective: Quality of Abortion Care* (Menlo Park, CA: Kaiser Family Foundation, 1999).

16. Pazol et al., "Abortion Surveillance—United States, 2006."

17. L. B. Finer and J. Wei, "Effect of Mifepristone on Abortion Access in the United States," *Obstetrics & Gynecology* 114, no. 3 (2009): 623–30.

18. Rachel K. Jones et al., "Abortion in the United States: Incidence and Access to Services, 2005," guttmacher.org/pubs/psrh/full/4000608.pdf.

19. Finer and Wei, "Effect of Mifepristone on Abortion Access in the United States."

20. E. Abdel-Aziz, I. M. Hassan, and H. Al-Taher, "Assessment of Women's Satisfaction with Medical Termination of Pregnancy," *Journal of Obstetrics and Gynaecology* 24, no. 4 (2004): 429–33; Christina Rørbye, Mogens Nørgaard, and Lisbeth Nilas, "Medical Versus Surgical Abortion: Comparing Satisfaction and Potential Confounders in a Partly Randomized Study," *Human Reproduction* 20, no. 3 (2005): 834–38.

21. S. K. Henshaw, "Unintended Pregnancy and Abortion: A Public Health Perspective," in *A Clinician's Guide to Medical and Surgical Abortion*, ed. M. Paul et al. (New York: Churchill Livingstone, 1999), pp. 11–22.

22. Ibid.

23. Pazol et al., "Abortion Surveillance—United States, 2006."

24. L. B. Finer et al., "Timing of Steps and Reasons for Delays in Obtaining Abortions in the United States," *Contraception* 74, no. 4 (2006): 334–44.

25. E. S. Lichtenberg and D. A. Grimes, "Surgical Complications: Prevention and Management," in *Management of Unintended and Abnormal Pregnancy: Comprehensive Abortion Care*, ed. M. Paul et al. (West Sussex, U.K.: Blackwell Publishing, 2009), pp. 224–51.

26. Leslie Reagan, *When Abortion Was a Crime: Women, Medicine and Law in the United States, 1897–1973* (Berkeley: University of California Press, 1997), pp. 11–12.

27. J. C. Mohr, *Abortion in America: The Origins and Evolution of National Policy, 1800–1900* (New York: Oxford University Press, 1978).

28. Carole E. Joffe, *Doctors of Conscience: The Struggle to Provide Abortion Before and After* Roe v. Wade (Boston: Beacon Press, 1996).

29. "Jane," "Just Call Jane," in *From Abortion to Reproductive Freedom: Transforming a Movement*, ed. Marlene Gerber Fried (Boston: South End Press, 1990), p. 100.

30. D. Kacanek et al., "Medicaid Funding for Abortion: Providers' Experiences with Cases Involving Rape, Incest and Life Endangerment," *Perspectives on Sexual and Reproductive Health* 42, no. 2 (2010): 79–86.

31. Adam Sonfield, Casey Alrich, and Rachel Benson Gold, "Public Funding for Family Planning, Sterilization and Abortion Services, FY 1980–2006," January 2008, guttmacher.org/pubs/2008/01/28/or38.pdf.

32. Shawn Towey, Stephanie Poggi, and Rachael Roth, "Abortion Funding: A Matter of Justice," National Network of Abortion Funds, ibisreproductivehealth.org/downloads/NNAF_Policy_Report.pdf.

33. NARAL Pro-Choice America Foundation, "Discriminatory Restrictions on Abortion Funding Threaten Women's Health," prochoiceamerica.org/assets/files/Abortion-Access-to-Abortion-Women-Government-Discriminatory-Restrictions.pdf.

34. National Abortion Federation, "Service Women Overseas Deserve Better Access to Safe and Legal Health Care," 2006, prochoice.org/policy/congress/women_military.html.

35. Theodore J. Joyce et al., "The Impact of State Mandatory Counseling and Waiting Period Laws on Abortion: A Literature Review," May 2009, guttmacher.org/pubs/MandatoryCounseling.pdf.

36. Guttmacher Institute, "Counseling and Waiting Periods for Abortion as of March 1, 2011," guttmacher.org/statecenter/spibs/spib_MWPA.pdf, accessed October 7, 2010.

37. National Cancer Institute, "Summary Report: Early Reproductive Events and Breast Cancer Workshop," cancer.gov/cancertopics/ere-workshop-report.

38. APA Task Force on Mental Health and Abortion, *Report of the APA Task Force on Mental Health and Abortion*.

39. Guttmacher Institute, "State Policies in Brief: An Overview of Minors' Consent Law," May 1, 2011, guttmacher.org/statecenter/spibs/spib_OMCL.pdf.

40. T. Joyce, R. Kaestner, and S. Colman, "Changes in Abortions and Births and the Texas Parental Notification Law," *New England Journal of Medicine* 354, no. 10 (2006): 1031–38.

41. Royal College of Obstetricians and Gynaecologists, "Fetal Awareness: Review of Research and Recommendations for Practice," March 2010, rcog.org.uk/files/rcog-corp/RCOGFetalAwarenessWPR0610.pdf.

CHAPTER 14:
CONSIDERING PARENTING

1. American Society for Reproductive Medicine, "Age and Fertility: A Guide for Patients," asrm.org/uploadedFiles/ASRM_Content/Resources/Patient_Resources/Fact_Sheets_and_Info_Booklets/agefertility.pdf.
2. Ibid.
3. Alison Taylor, "ABC of Subfertility: Extent of the Problem," *British Medical Journal* 327 (2003): 434–36.

CHAPTER 15:
PREGNANCY AND
PREPARING FOR BIRTH

1. Judith Dickson Luce, "Birthing Women and Midwife," in *Birth Control and Controlling Birth*, ed. Helen B. Holmes, Betty Hoskins, and Michael Gross (Clifton, NJ: Humana Press, 1980), p. 240.
2. M. Hatem et al., "Midwife-Led Versus Other Models of Care for Childbearing Women," Cochrane Database of Systematic Reviews, 2008, www2.cochrane.org/reviews/en/ab004667.html.
3. R. A. Rosenblatt "Interspecialty Differences in the Obstetric Care of Low-Risk Women," *American Journal of Public Health* 87, no. 3 (1997): 344–51.
4. K. C. Johnson, and B. A. Daviss, "Outcomes of Planned Home Births with Certified Professional Midwives: Large Prospective Study in North America," *British Medical Journal (Clinical Research Ed.)* 330, no. 7505 (2025): 1416; J. T. Fullerton et al., "Transfer Rates from Freestanding Birth Centers: A Comparison with the National Birth Center Study," *Journal of Nurse-Midwifery* 42, no. 1 (1997): 9–16.
5. A. de Jonge et al., "Perinatal Mortality and Morbidity in a Nationwide Cohort of 529,688 Low-Risk Planned Home and Hospital Births," *BJOG: An International Journal of Obstetrics and Gynaecology* 116, no. 9 (2009): 1177–84; E. K. Hutton, A. H. Reitsma, and K. Kaufman, "Outcomes Associated with Planned Home and Planned Hospital Births in Low-Risk Women Attended by Midwives in Ontario, Canada, 2003–2006: A Retrospective Cohort Study," *Birth* 36, no. 3 (2009): 180–89; P. A. Janssen et al., "Outcomes of Planned Home Birth with Registered Midwife Versus Planned Hospital Birth with Midwife or Physician," *Canadian Medical Association Journal* 181, nos. 6–7 (2009): 377–83.
6. Johnson and Daviss, "Outcomes of Planned Home Births."
7. Janssen et al., "Outcomes of Planned Home Birth."
8. J. R. Ickovics et al., "Group Prenatal Care and Perinatal Outcomes: A Randomized Controlled Trial," *Obstetrics & Gynecology* 110, no. 2 (2007): 330–39.
9. Eugene R. Declercq et al., "Listening to Mothers II: Report of the Second National U.S. Survey of Women's Childbearing Experiences," Childbirth Connection, October 2006, childbirthconnection.org/pdfs/LTMII_ExecutiveSum.pdf.
10. Ibid.
11. Ickovics et al., "Group Prenatal Care and Perinatal Outcomes."
12. "Obesity in Pregnancy," ACOG Committee Opinion, *Obstetrics & Gynecology* 106, no. 3 (September 2005): 671–75.
13. P. Simkin and P. Klaus, *When Survivors Give Birth: Understanding and Healing the Effects of Early Sexual Abuse on Childbearing Women* (Seattle, WA: Classic Day Publishing, 2004).
14. International Cesarean Awareness Network, "New Survey Shows Shrinking Options for Women with Prior Cesarean: Bans on Vaginal Birth Force Women into Unnecessary Surgery," February 20, 2009, ican-online.org/ican-in-the-news/trouble-repeat-cesareans.
15. National Institutes of Health, "NIH Consensus Development Conference: Vaginal Birth After Cesarean: New Insights," *Obstetrics and Gynecology* 115, no. 6 (June 2010): 1279–95.
16. American College of Obstetricians and Gynecologists, "ACOG Practice Bulletin No. 115: Vaginal Birth After Previous Cesarean Delivery," *Obstetrics & Gynecology* 116, no. 2, part 1 (2010): 450–63.
17. B. N. Gaynes et al., "Perinatal Depression: Prevalence, Screening Accuracy, and Screening Outcomes," February 2005, ahrq.gov/clinic/epcsums/peridepsum.htm. The full report is AHRQ Publication No. 05-EE006-2. This is a systematic review that reported a rate of 3 to 5 percent per trimester of pregnancy, with 7.5 percent of women experiencing an episode of major depression in pregnancy (i.e., depression that meets the criteria for a diagnosis).
18. O. Vesga-López et al., "Psychiatric Disorders in Pregnant and Postpartum Women in the United States," *Archives of General Psychiatry* 65, no. 7 (2008): 805–15. They found that 5.6 percent of pregnant women

versus 8.1 percent of nonpregnant women met diagnostic criteria for depression (but the difference was not significant).

19. "Depression During & After Pregnancy," December 2007, parents.berkeley.edu/advice/pregnancy/depression.html.

20. E. H. Turner et al., "Selective Publication of Antidepressant Trials and Its Influence on Apparent Efficacy," *New England Journal of Medicine* 358 (2008): 252–260; Irving Kirsch et al., "Initial Severity and Antidepressant Benefits: A Meta-Analysis of Data Submitted to the Food and Drug Administration," *PLoS Medicine*, 5, no. 3 (2008); H. Edmund Pigott et al., "Efficacy and Effectiveness of Antidepressants: Current Status of Research," *Psychotherapy and Psychosomatics* 79 (2010): 267–79.

21. S. Alwan et al., "Use of Selective Serotonin-Reuptake Inhibitors in Pregnancy and the Risk of Birth Defects," *New England Journal of Medicine* 356 (2007): 2684.

22. "Are Antidepressants Safe in Pregnancy? A Focus on SSRIs," *Therapeutics Letter* 76 (January–February 2010), ti.ubc.ca/letter 76.

23. L. S. Cohen et al., "Relapse of Major Depression During Pregnancy in Women Who Maintain or Discontinue Antidepressant Treatment," *Journal of the American Medical Association* 295, no. 5 (February 1, 2006): 499–507. This study was the subject of a *Wall Street Journal* exposé (July 11, 2006), because among the thirteen study authors there were sixty undisclosed conflicts of interest. There were also serious methodological problems with this study: (1) the study was not blinded or randomized and failed to report on key health outcomes; (2) women were considered to have discontinued if they were off antidepressants for one week or more in pregnancy, even if they took antidepressants the rest of the time, and any "recurrence" that occurred was linked or classified as being among "discontinuers" even if a woman had been on antidepressants for months before and after the recurrence occurred; (3) there was no protocol for gradual withdrawal from antidepressants, probably leading to some abrupt discontinuations that would increase the severity of withdrawal reactions; (4) the authors did not mention withdrawal reactions and failed to report a single withdrawal reaction; however, the timing of depression recurrences suggests that many were withdrawal reactions; (5) women were warned that if they withdrew from antidepressants, their depression might recur; (6) reporting of trial results was grossly inadequate—no serious or nonserious adverse reactions reported, no quality of life reported, no infant health outcomes reported. A factor making the results even harder to interpret is that the women in the study were warned ahead of time that if they stopped their antidepressants their depression might recur, but they were not warned about the possibility of drug withdrawal effects. This is likely to have led to some misdiagnoses.

24. E. D. Hodnett et al., "Continuous Support for Women During Childbirth," Cochrane Database of Systematic Reviews 3 (July 18, 2007), ncbi.nlm.nih/pubmed/17636733.

CHAPTER 16: LABOR AND BIRTH

1. Eugene R. Declercq et al., "Listening to Mothers II: Report of the Second National U.S. Survey of Women's Childbearing Experiences," Childbirth Connection, October 2006, childbirthconnection.org/pdfsLTMII_ExecutiveSum.pdf.

2. American College of Nurse-Midwives, "Position Statement: Prelabor Rupture of Membranes (PROM) at Term," October 2008, midwife.org/siteFiles/position/PROM_10_08.pdf.

3. ACOG Committee on Practice, "ACOG Practice Bulletin No. 80: Premature Rupture of Membranes. Clinical Management Guidelines for Obstetrician-Gynecologists," *Obstetrics & Gynecology* 109, no. 4 (2007): 1007–19.

4. Margareta Eriksson et al., "Warm Tub Bath During Labor. A Study of 1385 Women with Prelabor Rupture of the Membranes After 34 Weeks of Gestation," *Acta Obstetricia et Gynecologica Scandinavica* 75, no. 7 (1996): 642–44.

5. V. Berghella, J. K. Baxter, and S. P. Chauhan, "Evidence-Based Labor and Delivery Management," *American Journal of Obstetrics and Gynecology* 199, no. 5 (2008): 445–54.

6. J. L. Neal et al., "What Is the Slowest-Yet-Normal Cervical Dilation Rate Among Nulliparous Women with Spontaneous Labor Onset?" *Journal of Obstetric, Gynecologic, and Neonatal Nursing* 39, no. 4 (2010): 361–69.

7. R. M. Smyth, S. K. Alldred, and C. Markham, "Amniotomy for Shortening Spontaneous Labour," *Obstetrics and Gynecology* 11, no. 1 (January 2008): 204–5.

8. L. J. Mayberry, D. Clemmens, and A. De, "Epidural Analgesia Side Effects, Co-interventions, and Care of Women During Childbirth: A Systematic Review,"

American Journal of Obstetrics and Gynecology 186, no. 5 suppl. *Nature* (2002): S81–S93.

9. S. L. Clark et al., "Oxytocin: New Perspectives on an Old Drug," *American Journal of Obstetrics and Gynecology* 201, no. 3 (September 2009): 345–48.

10. Declercq et al., "Listening to Mothers II."

11. Z. Alfirevic, D. Devane, and G. M. Gyte, "Continuous Cardiotocography (CTG) as a Form of Electronic Fetal Monitoring (EFM) for Fetal Assessment During Labour," *Cochrane Database of Systematic Reviews*, July 9, 2006, www2.cochrane.org/reviews/en/ab0060 66.html.

12. Declercq et al., "Listening to Mothers II."

13. P. Simkin, and A. Bolding, "Update on Nonpharmacologic Approaches to Relieve Labor Pain and Prevent Suffering," *Journal of Midwifery & Women's Health* 49, no. 6 (2004): 489–504.

14. E. D. Hodnett, "Pain and Women's Satisfaction with the Experience of Childbirth: A Systematic Review," *American Journal of Obstetrics and Gynecology* 186, no. 5 suppl. *Nature* (2002): S160–S172.

15. Penny Simkin and Ruth S. Ancheta, *The Labor Progress Handbook*, 2nd ed. (Malden, MA: Blackwell Publishing, 2005).

16. Simkin and Bolding, "Update on Nonpharmacologic Approaches to Relieve Labor Pain and Prevent Suffering."

17. Ibid.

18. M. A. Rosen, "Nitrous Oxide for Relief of Labor Pain: A Systematic Review," *American Journal of Obstetrics and Gynecology* 186, no. 5 suppl. *Nature* (2002): S110–S126.

19. Ibid.

20. Declercq et al., "Listening to Mothers II."

21. S. Jordan et al., "The Impact of Intrapartum Analgesia on Infant Feeding," *BJOG: An International Journal of Obstetrics and Gynaecology* 112, no. 7 (2005): 927–34.

22. M. Anim-Somuah, R. Smyth, and C. Howell, "Epidural Versus Non-epidural or No Analgesia in Labour," *Cochrane Database of Systematic Reviews*, 2005, www2.cochrane.org/reviews/en/ab000331.htm.

23. Y. Beilin et al., "Effect of Labor Epidural Analgesia with and Without Fentanyl on Infant Breast-Feeding: A Prospective, Randomized, Double-Blind Study," *Anesthesiology* 103, no. 6 (2005): 1211–17.

24. J. Roberts, and L. Hanson, "Best Practices in Second Stage Labor Care: Maternal Bearing Down and Positioning," *Journal of Midwifery & Women's Health* 52, no. 3 (2007): 238–45.

25. K. R. Simpson and D. C. James, "Effects of Immediate Versus Delayed Pushing During Second-Stage Labor on Fetal Well-Being: A Randomized Clinical Trial," *Nursing Research* 54, no. 3 (2005): 149–57.

26. J. K. Gupta and G. J. Hofmeyr, "Position for Women During Second Stage of Labour," *Cochrane Database of Systematic Reviews*, 2004, ncbi.nlm.nih.gov/pub med/14973930.

27. L. L. Albers and N. Borders, "Minimizing Genital Tract Trauma and Related Pain Following Spontaneous Vaginal Birth," *Journal of Midwifery & Women's Health* 52, no. 3 (2007): 246–53.

28. J. S. Mercer et al., "Evidence-Based Practices for the Fetal to Newborn Transition," *Journal of Midwifery & Women's Health* 52, no. 3 (2007): 262–72.

29. Ibid.

30. Elizabeth Davis and Debra Pascali-Bonaro, *Orgasmic Birth: Your Guide to a Safe, Satisfying, and Pleasurable Birth Experience* (Emmaus, PA: Rodale, 2010).

CHAPTER 17:
THE EARLY MONTHS OF PARENTING

1. Eugene R. Declercq et al., "New Mothers Speak Out: National Survey Results Highlight Women's Postpartum Experiences," Childbirth Connection, child birthconnection.org/pdf.asp? PDFDownload=new -mothers-speak-out.

2. L. Righard, and M. O. Alade, "Effect of Delivery Room Routines on Success of First Breast-Feed," *Lancet* 336, no. 8723 (1990): 1105–7.

3. J. E. Swain et al., "Maternal Brain Response to Own Baby-Cry Is Affected by Cesarean Section Delivery," *Journal of Child Psychology and Psychiatry* 49, no. 10 (2008): 1042–52.

4. E. Moore, G. Anderson, and N. Bergman, "Early Skin-to-Skin Contact for Mothers and Their Healthy Newborn Infants," *Cochrane Database of Systematic Reviews*, 2007, www2.cochrane.org/reviews/en/ab00 3519.html.

5. D. Campbell et al., "Female Relatives or Friends Trained as Labor Doulas: Outcomes at 6 to 8 Weeks Postpartum," *Birth* 34, no. 3 (2007): 220–27.

6. Peter S. Blair, Peter J. Fleming, Iain J. Smith, Martin Ward Platt, Jeanine Young, et al., "Babies Sleeping with Parents: Case-Control Study of Factors Influencing the Risk of the Sudden Infant Death Syndrome," *British Medical Journal* 319 (December 1999): 1457–62; J. J. McKenna and T. McDade, "Why Babies Should

Never Sleep Alone: A Review of the Co-sleeping Controversy in Relation to SIDS, Bedsharing, and Breastfeeding," *Pediatric Respiratory Reviews* 6 (2005): 134–52.

7. McKenna and McDade, "Why Babies Should Never Sleep Alone: A Review of the Co-sleeping Controversy in Relation to SIDS, Bedsharing, and Breastfeeding." For more information on bedsharing, see policy statement, American Academy of Pediatrics, Task Force on Sudden Infant Death Syndrome, "The Changing Concept of Sudden Infant Death Syndrome: Diagnostic Coding Shifts, Controversies Regarding the Sleeping Environment, and New Variables to Consider in Reducing Risk," *Pediatrics* 116, no. 5 (2005): 1245–55; "Safe Co-Sleeping Habits," askdrsears.com/html/7/T070600.asp.

8. J. J. McKenna, "Scientific Studies of Mother-Infant Cosleeping with Breastfeeding: The Importance of the Mother-Infant Dyad and How and Why Things Can Go Wrong," Lamaze International Annual Conference, Phoenix, AZ, 2008.

9. S. Ip et al., *Breastfeeding and Maternal and Infant Health Outcomes in Developed Countries*, Agency for Healthcare Research and Quality, April 2007, ahrq.gov/downloads/pub/evidence/pdf/brfont/brfont.pdf.

10. L. M. Gartner et al., "Breastfeeding and the Use of Human Milk," *Pediatrics* 115, no. 2 (2005): 496–506.

11. Ip et al., *Breastfeeding and Maternal and Infant Health Outcomes.*

12. Ibid.

13. S. D. Colson et al., "Optimal Positions for the Release of Primitive Neonatal Reflexes Stimulating Breastfeeding," *Early Human Development* 87, no. 7 (2008): 441–49.

14. Jatinder Bhatia, Frank Greer, and the Committee on Nutrition, "Use of Soy Protein–Based Formulas in Infant Feeding," *Pediatrics* 121, no. 5 (May 2008): 1062–68.

15. S. E. Hoffbrand, L. Howard, and H. Crawley, "Antidepressant Treatment for Post-natal Depression," Cochrane Database of Systematic Reviews, 2001, www2.cochrane.org/reviews/en/ab002018.html.

CHAPTER 18:
MISCARRIAGE, STILLBIRTH, AND OTHER LOSSES

1. Anne-Marie Nybo Andersen et al., "Maternal Age and Fetal Loss: Population Based Register Linkage Study," *British Medical Journal* 320 (2000): 1708.

2. American College of Obstetricians and Gynecologists,
"Bleeding During Pregnancy," November 2008, acog.org/publications/patient_education/bp038.cfm.

3. J. Zhang et al., "A Comparison of Medical Management with Misoprostol and Surgical Management for Early Pregnancy Failure," *New England Journal of Medicine* 353 (2005): 761–69.

4. Nybo Andersen et al., "Maternal Age and Fetal Loss."

5. American College of Obstetricians and Gynecologists, "Early Pregnancy Loss: Miscarriage and Molar Pregnancy," May 2002, acog.org/publications/patient_education/bp090.cfm.

6. Pamela Prindle Fierro, "Vanishing Twin Syndrome," April 2006, od/twinpregnancyfaq/f/pregnancyfaq_e.htm.

7. Marian MacDorman and Sharon Kiremeyer, "Fetal and Perinatal Mortality, United States, 2005," National Vital Statistics Reports, January 2009, cdc.gov/nchs/data/nvsr/nvsr57/nvsr57_08.pdf.

8. Ibid.

9. Nybo Andersen et al., "Maternal Age and Fetal Loss."

10. March of Dimes, "Stillbirth," 2010, marchofdimes.com/Baby/loss_stillbirth.html.

11. MacDorman and Kiremeyer, "Fetal and Perinatal Mortality, United States, 2005."

12. CDC, "Recent Trends in Infant Mortality in the United States," October 2008, cdc.gov/nchs/data/databriefs/db09.htm.

13. U.S. Department of Health and Human Services, "Child Health USA 2008–2009: Very Low Birth Weight," mchb.hrsa.gov/chusa08/hstat/hsi/pages/203vlbw.html.

CHAPTER 19:
INFERTILITY AND ASSISTED REPRODUCTIVE TECHNOLOGIES

1. Centers for Disease Control and Prevention, "Fertility, Family Planning, and Reproductive Health of U.S. Women: Data from the 2002 National Survey of Family Growth," December 2005, cdc.gov/nchs/data/series/sr_23/_23_025.pdf.

2. CDC, Infertility FAQs, cdc.gov/reproductivehealth/infertility.index.htm.

3. Kaiser Family Foundation, Mandated Coverage of Infertility Treatment, January 2010, statehealthfacts.org/comparetable.jsp?ind=6868.cat=7.

4. CDC, "Assisted Reproductive Technology (ART)," cdc.gov/ART/index.htm.

5. CDC, American Society for Reproductive Medicine, and Society for Assisted Reproductive Technology,

2008 Assisted Reproductive Technology Success Rates: National Summary and Fertility Clinic Reports, December 2010, cdc.gov/ART/ART2008/PDF/ART_2008 _Full.pdf.

6. D. J. McLernon et al., "Clinical Effectiveness of Elective Single Versus Double Embryo Transfer: Meta-analysis of Individual Patient Data from Randomised Trials," *British Medical Journal* 341 (December 21, 2010): c6945.

7. Debora L. Spar, *The Baby Business: How Money, Science, and Politics Drive the Commerce of Conception* (Boston: Harvard Business School Press, 2006).

8. Jessica Arons, "Future Choices: Assisted Reproductive Technologies and the Law," Center for American Progress, December 17, 2007, americanprogress.org/ issues/2007/12/future_choices.html.

9. CDC, "Assisted Reproductive Technology Surveillance—United States, 2006," June 12, 2009, cdc .gov/mmwr/pdf/ss/ss5805.pdf.

10. Technology Marketing Corporation, "U.S. 'Baby Business' (Infertility Services) Worth $4 Billion," August 17, 2009, tmcnet.com/usubmit/2009/08/17/4326513 .htm.

CHAPTER 20:
PERIMENOPAUSE AND MENOPAUSE

1. "SWAN Highlights," April 25, 2003, swanstudy.org/ docs/SWAN_Highlights.pdf.

2. J. Prior, "Clearing Confusion About Perimenopause," *British Columbia Medical Journal* 47, no. 10 (2005): 534–38.

3. Dr. Jerilynn Prior, personal communication.

4. J. Prior and C. Hitchcock, "The Endocrinology of Perimenopause: Need for a Paradigm Shift," *Frontiers in Bioscience* 3 (January 1, 2011): 474–86. See also K. O'Connor et al., "Total and Unopposed Estrogen Exposure Across Stages of the Transition to Menopause," *Cancer Epidemiology, Biomarkers & Prevention* 18, no. 3 (March 2009): 828–36.

5. Dr. Jerilynn Prior, personal communication.

6. See, for example, a study from the University of California at San Francisco published in the July 12 *Archives of Internal Medicine*. Led by Deborah Grady, M.D., the study was ancillary to the Program to Reduce Incontinence by Diet and Exercise (PRIDE), a randomized, controlled trial, news.ucsf.edu/releases/ weight-loss-reduces-hot-flashes-in-overweight-and -obese-women.

7. Jerilynn Prior, "Progesterone Therapy for Symptom-

atic Perimenopause," cemcor.ubc.ca/files/uploads/ Progesterone_for_Symptomatic_Perimenopause.pdf.

8. Deborah Grady, "Management of Menopausal Symptoms," *New England Journal of Medicine* 355 (November 30, 2006): 2338–47, nejm.org/doi/full/10.1056/NEJ Mcp054015.

9. See, for example, D. R. Pachman, J. M. Jones, and C. L. Loprinzi, "Management of Menopause-Associated Vasomotor Symptoms: Current Treatment Options, Challenges and Future Directions," *International Journal of Women's Health* 2 (August 9, 2010): 123–35; D. R. Pachman et al., "Pilot Evaluation of a Stellate Ganglion Block for the Treatment of Hot Flashes," *Supportive Care in Cancer*, May 23, 2009; E. G. Lipov et al., "A Unifying Theory Linking the Prolonged Efficacy of the Stellate Ganglion Block for the Treatment of Chronic Regional Pain Syndrome (CRPS), Hot Flashes, and Posttraumatic Stress Disorder (PTSD)," *Medical Hypotheses* 72, no. 6 (June 2009): 647–61.

10. N. S. Gooneratne, "Complementary and Alternative Medicine for Sleep Disturbances in Older Adults," *Clinics in Geriatric Medicine* 24, vol. 1 (2009): 121–38.

11. P. Schüssler et al., "Progesterone Reduces Wakefulness in Sleep EEG and Has No Effect on Cognition in Healthy Postmenopausal Women," *Psychoneuroendocrinology* 33, no. 8 (September 2008): 1124–31, ncbi .nlm.nih.gov/pubmed/18676087.

12. See, for example, T. Hillard, "The Postmenopausal Bladder," *Menopause International* 16, no. 2 (June 2010): 74–80; A. A. Ewies and F. Alfhaily, "Topical Vaginal Estrogen Therapy in Managing Postmenopausal Urinary Symptoms: A Reality or a Gimmick?" *Climacteric* 13, no. 5 (October 2010): 405–18; I. Goldstein, "Recognizing and Treating Urogenital Atrophy in Postmenopausal Women," *Women's Health* 19, no. 3 (March 2010): 425–32.

13. Cynthia Gomey, "The Estrogen Dilemma," *New York Times Magazine*, April 14, 2010, nytimes.com/2010/ 04/18/magazine/18estrogen-t.html.

14. R. J. Rodabough et al., "Prevalence and 3-year Incidence of Abuse Among Postmenopausal Women," *American Journal of Public Health* 94, no. 4 (April 2004): 605–12.

15. Jerilynn Prior, "Ovarian Hormone Therapy for Women with Early Menopause," December 6, 2007, cemcor.ubc .ca/help_yourself/articles/oht_early_menopause.

16. Suzanne Oparil, "Hormone Therapy of Premature Ovarian Failure: The Case for "Natural" Estrogen," *Hypertension* 53 (2009): 745–46, hyper.ahajournals .org/cgi/content/full/53/5/745.

17. See, for example, C. Zhang et al., "Abdominal Obesity and the Risk of All-Cause, Cardiovascular, and Cancer Mortality: Sixteen Years of Follow-Up in US Women," *Circulation* 117, no. 13 (April 1, 2008): 1658–67; see also D. Canoy et al., "Body Fat Distribution and Risk of Coronary Heart Disease in Men and Women in the European Prospective Investigation into Cancer and Nutrition in Norfolk Cohort: A Population-Based Prospective Study," *Circulation* 116, no. 25 (December 18, 2007): 2933–43.

18. Mayo Clinic, "Osteoporosis: Risk Factors," November 20, 2010, mayoclinic.com/health/osteoporosis/DS00 128/DSECTION=risk-factors.

19. M. Audran and K. Briot, "Critical Reappraisal of Vitamin D Deficiency," *Joint Bone Spine* 77, no. 2 (2010): 115–19, ncbi.nlm.nih.gov/pubmed/20097593.

20. L. J. Dominguez, R. Scalisi, and M. Barbagallo, "Therapeutic Options in Osteoporosis," *Acta Bio Medica* 81, suppl. 1 (2010): 55–65, ncbi.nlm.nih.gov/pubmed/20518192; Byori Rinsho and N. Tsugawa, "Vitamin D and Osteoporosis: Current Topics from Epidemiological Studies," ncbi.nlm.nih.gov/pubmed? term=20408443; J. E. Isenor and M. H. Ensom, "Is There a Role for Therapeutic Drug Monitoring of Vitamin D Level as a Surrogate Marker for Fracture Risk?" *Pharmacotherapy* 30, no. 3 (2010): 254–64, ncbi .nlm.nih.gov/pubmed?term=20180609.

21. E. S. MacKinnon et al., "Supplementation with the Antioxidant Lycopene Significantly Decreases Oxidative Stress Parameters and the Bone Resorption Marker N-telopeptide of Type I Collagen in Postmenopausal Women," *Osteoporosis International* 22, no. 4 (2011): 1091–1101, ncbi.nlm.nih.gov/pubmed/20552330.

22. B. Mintzes, "For and Against: Direct to Consumer Advertising Is Medicalising Normal Human Experience: For," *British Medical Journal* 324, no. 7342 (2002): 908–9.

23. R. Wulffson, "Risk of Stopping Hormone Therapy: Hip Fractures," Examiner.com, October 28, 2010, examiner. com/women-s-health-in-los-angeles/risk-of-stopping -hormone-therapy-hip-fractures; and K. Kalvaitis, "Increased Incidence of Hip Fracture Reported After HT Discontinuation," *Endocrine Today,* October 11, 2010, at endocrinetoday.com/view.aspx?rid=76342.

24. V. Beral et al., "Endometrial Cancer and Hormone-Replacement Therapy in the Million Women Study," *Lancet* 365, no. 9470 (April 30, 2005): 1543–51, ncbi .nlm.nih.gov/pubmed/15866308.

25. P. Kenemans et al. for LIBERATE Study Group, "Safety and Efficacy of Tibolone in Breast-Cancer Patients with Vasomotor Symptoms: A Double-Blind, Randomized, Non-inferiority Trial," *Lancet Oncology* 10, no. 2 (February 2009): 135–46.

26. National Institutes of Health, "Dietary Supplement Fact Sheet: Black Cohosh," ods.od.nih.gov/factsheets/ blackcohosh.

27. National Center for Complementary and Alternative Medicine, "Menopausal Symptoms and CAM," January 2008, nccam.nih.gov/health/menopause/meno pausesymptoms.htm.

28. V. C. Wong et al., "Current Alternative and Complementary Therapies Used in Menopause," *Gynecological Endocrinology* 25, no. 3 (March 2009): 166–74.

29. National Center for Complementary and Alternative Medicine, "Menopausal Symptoms and CAM."

30. Prescribing practices are significantly different in Europe. See N. Carroll, "A Review of Transdermal Nonpatch Estrogen Therapy for the Management of Menopausal Symptoms," *Journal of Women's Health* 19, no. 1 (January 2010): 47–55, ncbi.nlm.nih.gov/ pubmed/20088658.

31. Women's Health Initiative, "What You Should Know About the HERS Study," October 1998, nhlbi.nih.gov/ whi/update_hers1998.pdf.

32. For example, a single randomized trial of oral contraceptive compared with a placebo showed that bleeding became irregular over three cycles before improving and that there was no benefit over a placebo in hot flashes and quality of life. See R. F. Casper, S. Dodin, and R. Reid, "The Effect of 20 mg Ethinyl Estradiol/1 mg Norethindrone Acetate (Minestrin™), a Low-Dose Oral Contraceptive, on Vaginal Bleeding Patterns, Hot Flashes and Quality of Life in Symptomatic Perimenopausal Women," *Menopause* 4, no. 3 (1997): 139–47.

33. L. Speroff, "Transdermal Hormone Therapy and the Risk of Stroke and Venous Thrombosis," *Climacteric* 13, no. 5 (October 2010): 439–42. From the abstract: "The case-control study by Renoux and colleagues is the first major analysis to compare transdermal and oral hormone therapy and conclude that, compared with an increased risk of stroke with oral therapy, there was no increased risk with transdermal treatment at a dose of 50 microg or less. This report is about as strong an observational study as can be achieved. Large numbers of cases (15 710) and controls (59 958) were available for analysis using the well-known UK GPRD. The use of this computerized database precludes selection bias by the investigators and recall bias by the women in the study. The results support the growing conventional wisdom that transdermal therapy at standard doses is free of the cardiovascular risks

associated with oral therapy." See also V. Olié, M. Canonico, and P. Y. Scarabin, "Risk of Venous Thrombosis with Oral Versus Transdermal Estrogen Therapy Among Postmenopausal Women," *Current Opinion in Hematology* 17, no. 5 (September 2010): 457–63.

34. A. Fournier, "Should Transdermal Rather Than Oral Estrogens Be Used in Menopausal Hormone Therapy? A Review," *Menopause International* 16 (2010): 23–32.

35. C. Campagnoli et al., "Differential Effects of Various Progestogens on Metabolic Risk Factors for Breast Cancer," *Gynecological Endocrinology* 23, suppl. 1 (October 2007): 22–31.

36. J. C. Prior and C. L. Hitchcock, "Progesterone for Vasomotor Symptoms: A 12-Week Randomized, Masked Placebo-Controlled Trial in Healthy, Normal-Weight Women 1–10 Years Since Final Menstrual Flow," *Endocrine Reviews* 31, no. 3, suppl. 1 (June 2010): S51.

37. H. B. Leonetti, S. Longo, and J. N. Anasti, "Transdermal Progesterone Cream for Vasomotor Symptoms and Postmenopausal Bone Loss," *Obstetrics & Gynecology* 94 (1999): 225–28; also B. G. Wren et al., "Transdermal Progesterone and Its Effect on Vasomotor Symptoms, Blood Lipid Levels, Bone Metabolic Markers, Moods, and Quality of Life for Postmenopausal Women," *Menopause* 10 (2003): 13.

38. National Institute on Aging, "Rates of Dementia Increase Among Older Women on Combination Hormone Therapy," May 27, 2003, nih.gov/news/pr/may2003/nia-27.htm.

39. Thanks to Karin Kolsky of the National Institute on Aging for adding to the information in this paragraph.

40. L. Rosenberg et al., "A Prospective Study of Female Hormone Use and Breast Cancer Among Black Women," *Archives of Internal Medicine* 166 (2006): 760–65.

41. S. Krishnan, L. Rosenberg, and J. R. Palmer, "Physical Activity and Television Watching in Relation to Risk of Type 2 Diabetes in the Black Women's Health Study," *American Journal of Epidemiology* 169, no. 4 (2009): 428–34.

42. Thanks to Julie Palmer, a BWHS researcher, for adding to the information in this paragraph.

CHAPTER 21:
OUR LATER YEARS

1. Ashton Applewhite, "Staying Vertical: Dispatches from the Old Old on Work and Happiness," November 11, 2009, stayingvertical.com/?q=node/227.

2. Gene Cohen, *The Creative Age: Awakening Human Potential in the Second Half of Life* (New York: Avon/HarperCollins, 2000); George Valliant, *Aging Well: Surprising Guideposts to a Happier Life* (Boston: Little, Brown, 2002); William Sadler and James Krefft, *Changing Course: Navigating Life After 50* (Centennial, CO: Center for Third Age Leadership Press, 2007); Sara Lawrence-Lightfoot, *The Third Chapter: Passion, Risk and Adventure in the 25 Years After 50* (New York: Farrar, Straus and Giroux, 2009).

3. National Center for Health Statistics, *Health, United States, 2009: With Special Feature on Medical Technology*, January 2010, cdc.gov/nchs/data/hus/hus09.pdf.

4. National Center for Health Statistics, *Health, United States, 2008, With Special Feature on the Health of Young Adults,* March 2009, p. 203, cdc.gov/nchs/data/hus/hus08.pdf#026.

5. Federal Interagency Forum on Aging-Related Statistics, *Older Americans 2010: Key Indicators of Well-Being.* July 2010, agingstats.gov/agingstatsdotnet/Main_Site/Data/2010_Documents/Docs/OA_2010.pdf.

6. Ibid.

7. Shirley Haynes, "Odds N Ends," *McKenzie River Reflections*, April 26, 2007, bit.ly/ecyDiH.

8. Pew Social Trends Staff, "Growing Old in America: Expectations vs. Reality," Pew Research Center, June 29, 2009, pewsocialtrends.org/pubs/736/getting-old-in-america.

9. Gretchen Livingston and Kim Parker, "Since Start of the Great Recession, More Children Raised by Grandparents," September 9, 2010, pewsocialtrends.org/pubs/764/more-children-being-raised-by-grandparents-great-recession.

10. Gary Gates, quoted in Jane Gross, "Aging and Gay, and Facing Prejudice in Twilight," *New York Times,* October 9, 2007, nytimes.com/2007/10/09/us/09aged.html.

11. Services and Advocacy for Gay, Lesbian, Bisexual & Transgender Elders (SAGE) and the LGBT Movement Advancement Project (MAP), "Improving the Lives of LGBT Older Adults," March 2010, sageusa.org/resources/resource_view.cfm?resource=183.

12. Gary Gates, quoted in Jane Gross, "Aging and Gay, and Facing Prejudice in Twilight."

13. Lisa Bennett and Gary J. Gates, "The Cost of Marriage Inequality to Gay, Lesbian and Bisexual Seniors," Human Rights Campaign Foundation, January 29, 2004, hrc.org/documents/cost_of_marriage.pdf.

14. Federal Interagency Forum on Aging-Related Statistics, "Older Americans 2010: Key Indicators of Well-Being."

15. Ibid.

16. R. S. Wilson et al., "Cognitive Activity and the Cognitive Morbidity of Alzheimer Disease," *Neurology* 75, no. 11 (September 14, 2010): 990–99, neurology.org/content/75/11/990.

17. Kirk R. Daffner, *Improving Memory: Understanding Age-Related Memory Loss* (Boston: Harvard Health Publications, 2010), pp. 9–11.

18. U.S. Preventive Services Task Force, "Screening for Breast Cancer," July 2010, uspreventiveservicestaskforce.org/uspstf/uspsbrca.htm.

19. American Congress of Obstetricians and Gynecologists, "First Cervical Cancer Screening Delayed Until Age 21; Less Frequent Pap Tests Recommended," November 20, 2009, acog.org/from_home/publications/press_releases/nr11-20-09.cfm.

20. National Gay and Lesbian Task Force Policy Institute, "Outing Age 2010: Public Policy Issues Affecting Lesbian, Gay, Bisexual and Transgender Elders," November 23, 2009, thetaskforce.org/reports_and_research/outing_age_2010.

21. Services and Advocacy for Gay, Lesbian, Bisexual & Transgender Elders (SAGE) and the LGBT Movement Advancement Project (MAP), "Improving the Lives of Lesbian, Gay, Bisexual and Transgender Older Adults."

22. Joan Price, *Better Than I Ever Expected: Straight Talk About Sex After 60* (Berkeley: Seal Press, 2005), p. 17.

23. Meika Loe, *Aging Our Way: Lessons for Living from 85 and Beyond* (New York: Oxford University Press, 2011).

24. Jan Leslie Shifren et al., *Sexuality in Midlife and Beyond* (Boston: Harvard Health Publications), p. 14.

25. Ibid., p. 5.

26. S. T. Lindau et al., "A Study of Sexuality and Health Among Older Adults in the United States," *New England Journal of Medicine* 357, no. 8 (2007): 762–74.

27. J. M. Wood, P. K. Mansfield, and P. B. Koch, "Negotiating Sexual Agency: Postmenopausal Women's Meaning and Experience of Sexual Desire," *Qualitative Health Research* 17, no. 2 (2007): 189–200.

28. AARP, "Sexuality at Midlife and Beyond: 2004 Update of Attitudes and Behaviors," assets.aarp.org/rgcenter/general/2004_sexuality.pdf

29. Barry R. Komisaruk et al., *The Orgasm Answer Guide* (Baltimore: Johns Hopkins University Press, 2010).

30. Ibid.

31. Price, *Better Than I Ever Expected,* p. 125.

32. Carol Rinkleib Ellison, *Women's Sexualities: Generations of Women Share Intimate Secrets of Sexual Self-Acceptance* (Oakland, CA: New Harbinger Publications, 2000).

33. "Manuscript in Preparation," Research Survey-Sexuality Profile of Older Women, Anita Hoffer, 2009.

34. Siobhan Benet, "HIV/AIDS in Mature Women Jumps 40 Percent," Women's eNews Inc., March 25, 2001, womensenews.org/story/hivaids/010325/hivaids-in-mature-women-jumps-40-percent.

35. P. J. Huffstutter, "Older But Wiser? Safe Sex After 50," *Los Angeles Times,* November 26, 2007, articles.latimes.com/2007/nov/26/nation/na-safesex26.

36. Federal Interagency Forum on Aging-Related Statistics, "Older Americans 2010: Key Indicators of Well-Being," table 14c, p. 94.

37. Institute of Medicine, *Retooling for an Aging America: Building the Health Care Workforce*, April 11, 2008, iom.edu/agingamerica.

38. Edward L. Schneider and Vito M. Campese, "Adverse Drug Responses: An Increasing Threat to the Well-being of Older Patients: Comment on 'Development and Validation of a Score to Assess Risk of Adverse Drug Reactions Among In-Hospital Patients 65 Years or Older,'" *Archives of Internal Medicine* 170, no. 13 (2010): 1148–49.

39. Jennifer W. Mack et al., "Racial Disparities in the Outcomes of Communication on Medical Care Received Near Death," *Archives of Internal Medicine* 170, no. 17 (2010): 1533–40, archinte.ama-assn.org/cgi/content/abstract/170/17/1533.

40. National Alliance for Caregiving and AARP, "Caregiving in the U.S. Executive Summary," November 2009, caregiving.org/data/CaregivingUSAllAgesExecSum.pdf.

41. AARP, "Valuing the Invaluable: The Economic Value of Family Caregiving, 2008 Update," November 2008, assets.aarp.org/rgcenter/il/i13_caregiving.pdf.

42. Margaret K. Nelson, "Listening to Anna," *Health Affairs* 26, no. 3 (2007): 836–40.

43. For more information, see National Center on Elder Abuse, "Domestic Violence: Older Women Can Be Victims Too," September 2005, ncea.aoa.gov/ncearoot/main_site/pdf/publication/OLDERWOMEN2-COLUMNFINAL10-11-05.pdf.

44. Administration on Aging, "World Elder Abuse Awareness Day," November 9, 2010, aoa.gov/aoaroot/aoa_programs/elder_rights/ea_prevention/weaad.aspx.

45. National Clearinghouse on Abuse in Later Life, "Frequently Asked Questions About Abuse in Later Life," 2006, ncall.us/docs/FAQs_DALL.pdf.

46. Ibid.

47. Gloria Steinem, "Transformative Thought," *Harvard Magazine,* May 28, 2010, harvardmagazine.com/commencement/2010-radcliffe.

48. Gene Cohen, "Research on Creativity and Aging: The Positive Experience of the Arts on Health and Illness," *Generations* 30, no. 1 (Spring 2006): 7–15, gwumc.edu/cahh/pdf/RESEARCH%20ON%20CREATIVITY%20AND%20AGING.pdf.

49. Pew Social Trends Staff, "Growing Old in America."

50. U.S. Census Bureau, "The Next Four Decades: The Older Population in the United States: 2010–2050. Population Estimates and Projections," May 2010, census.gov/prod/2010pubs/p25-1138.pdf.

CHAPTER 22:
SELECTED MEDICAL PROBLEMS

1. National Cancer Institute, *SEER Cancer Statistics Review 1975–2007*, table 4.6, Cancer of the Breast (Invasive), seer.cancer.gov/csr/1975_2007/results_single/sect_04_table.06.pdf.

2. W. A. Berg et al., "Combined Screening with Ultrasound and Mammography vs. Mammography Alone in Women at Elevated Risk of Breast Cancer," *Journal of the American Medical Association* 299, no. 18 (2008): 2151–63. See also K. M. Kelly et al., "Breast Cancer Detection Using Automated Whole Breast Ultrasound and Mammography in Radiographically Dense Breasts," *European Radiology* 20 (2010): 734–42.

3. Richard Knox, "In Mammogram Debate, Differences Aren't So Big," Southern California Public Radio, October 10, 2010. scpr.org/news/2010/10/10/in-mammogram-debate-differences-arent-so-big/.

4. D. J. Hunter et al., "Oral Contraceptive Use and Breast Cancer: A Prospective Study of Young Women," *Cancer Epidemiology Biomarkers & Prevention* 19, no. 10 (October 2010): 2496–2502.

5. Table from cancer.gov/cancertopics/pdq/screening/breast/HealthProfessional/page2.

6. Dr. Susan Love Research Foundation, "Screening and Diagnosis," dslrf.org/breastcancer/content.asp?CATID=31&L2=2&L3=8&L4=0&PID=&sid=132&cid=653.

7. See The Million Women Study, millionwomenstudy.org/introduction.

8. R. T. Chlebowski et al., "Estrogen Plus Progestin and Breast Cancer Incidence and Mortality in Postmenopausal Women," *Journal of the American Medical Association* 304, no. 15 (2010): 1684–92. See also Peter B. Bach, "Postmenopausal Hormone Therapy and Breast Cancer: An Uncertain Trade-off," *Journal of the American Medical Association* 304, no. 15 (2010): 1719–20.

9. Silent Spring Institute, "Breast Cancer and the Environment," silentspring.org/breast-cancer-and-environment.

10. See the U.S. Preventive Services Task Force guidelines on genetic screening for breast cancer, uspreventiveservicestaskforce.org/uspstf/uspsbrgen.htm.

11. Silent Spring Institute, "Breast Cancer and the Environment."

12. C. J. Allegra, D. R. Aberle, P. Ganschow, et al., "National Institutes of Health State-of-the-Science Conference Statement: Diagnosis and Management of Ductal Carcinoma in Situ," *Journal of the National Cancer Institute* 102 (2010): 161–69.

13. Diana Zuckerman, "Breast Implants After Mastectomy," Cancer Prevention and Treatment Fund, January 2010, stopcancerfund.org/posts/448.

14. Marcy Oppenheimer, "Safety and Benefits of Inamed Silicone Breast Implants," April 2005 FDA Analysis.

15. Based upon a fact sheet prepared by Marcie Richardson for Harvard Vanguard Medical Associates.

16. S. S. Coughlin et al., "Cervical Cancer Incidence in the United States in the US-Mexico Border Region, 1998–2003," *Cancer* 113 (2008): 2964–73.

17. J. V. Lacey et al., "Menopausal Hormone Therapy and Ovarian Cancer Risk in the NIH-AARP Diet and Health Study Cohort," *Journal of the National Cancer Institute* 98, no. 19 (2006): 1397–1405.

18. The incidence of PID is very low among lesbians.

19. Julie R. Palmer et al., "Prenatal Diethylstilbestrol Exposure and Risk of Breast Cancer," *Cancer Epidemiology, Biomarkers & Prevention* (August 2006): 15: 1509.

20. See William H. Parker et al., "Ovarian Conservation at the Time of Hysterectomy and Long-Term Health Outcomes in the Nurses' Health Study," *Obstetrics and Gynecology* 113, no. 5 (May 2009): 1027–37.

21. B. L. Harlow and E. G. Stewart, "A Population-based Assessment of Chronic Unexplained Vulvar Pain: Have We Underestimated the Prevalence of Vulvodynia?" *Journal of the American Medical Women's Association* 58 (2003): 82–88.

22. B. D. Reed et al., "Candida Transmission and Sexual Behaviors as Risks for a Repeat Episode of Candida Vulvovaginitis." *Journal of Women's Health* 12, no. 10 (December 2003): 979–89.

23. Wash the area carefully, urinate a little, then collect the rest of your urine in a sterile jar.

24. Philip Hanno, in *Campbell-Walsh Urology*, 9th ed. (Philadelphia, Saunders, 2007).

25. K. J. Propert et al., "A Prospective Study of Interstitial Cystitis: Results of Longitudinal Follow-up of the Interstitial Cystitis Data Base Cohort," *Journal of Urology* 163 (2000): 1434–39.

26. Kay Zakariasen and Jennifer R. Hill, "Treatment and Mistreatment of Chronic 'Urgency and Frequency'—

Gathering Women's Experiences About Interstitial Cystitis," *Women's Health Activist Newsletter*, March–April 2009.

27. Jennifer R. Hill et al., "Patient Perceived Outcomes of Treatments Used for Interstitial Cystitis," *Urology* 71 no. 1 (January 2008): 62–66.

28. Mary P. FitzGerald et al., "Randomized Multicenter Feasibility Trial of Myofascial Physical Therapy for the Treatment of Urological Chronic Pelvic Pain Syndrome," *Journal of Urology* 182 (August 2009): 570–80.

29. Based upon a patient information handout from Harvard Vanguard Medical Associates in Boston, MA.

CHAPTER 23:
NAVIGATING THE
HEALTH CARE SYSTEM

1. United States Government Accountability Office, "Prescription Drugs: Improvements Needed in FDA's Oversight of Direct-to-Consumer Advertising, gao.gov/new.items/d0754.pdf.

2. G. Schwitzer, *The State of Health Journalism in the United States* (Menlo Park, CA: The Kaiser Family Foundation, 2009), kff.org/entmedia/upload/7858.pdf.

3. This sidebar is based on the work of John Abramson, including the book *Overdosed America: The Broken Promise of American Medicine* (New York: HarperPerennial, 2008) and the article "The Effect of Conflict of Interest on Biomedical Research and Clinical Practice Guidelines: Can We Trust the Evidence in Evidence-Based Medicine?" *Journal of the American Board of Family Practice* 18 (2005): 414–18.

4. Thomas E. Andreoli, "The Undermining of Academic Medicine," *Academe* 85, no. 6 (November–December 1999): 32–37.

5. C. DeAngelis, "Conflicts of Interest—Facts and Friction," 26th Fae Golden Kass Lecture, Harvard Medical School, October 30, 2008.

6. R. Steinbrook, "Gag Clauses in Clinical Trial Agreements," *New England Journal of Medicine* 352 (2005): 2160–62.

7. Justin E. Bekelman, Yan Li, and Cary P. Gross, "Scope and Impact of Financial Conflicts of Interest in Biomedical Research: A Systematic Review," *Journal of the American Medical Association* 289 (January 2003): 454–65. See also Joel Lexchin, Lisa A Bero, Benjamin Djulbegovic, and Otavio Clark, "Pharmaceutical Industry Sponsorship and Research Outcome and Quality: Systematic Review," *British Medical Journal* 326 (May 2003): 1167–70.

8. B. Als-Nielsen, W. Chen, C. Gluud, and L. L. Kjaergard, "Association of Funding and Conclusions in Randomized Drug Trials: A Reflection of Treatment Effect or Adverse Events?" *Journal of the American Medical Association* 290 (2003): 921–28.

9. R. H. Perlis, C. S. Perlis, Y Wu, et al., "Industry Sponsorship and Financial Conflict of Interest in the Reporting of Clinical Trials in Psychiatry," *American Journal of Psychiatry* 162 (2005): 1957–60.

10. A. J. Fugh-Berman, "The Haunting of Medical Journals: How Ghostwriting Sold 'HRT,' " *PLoS Med* 7, no. 9 (2010), e1000335, doi:10.1371/journal.pmed.1000335, plosmedicine.org/article/info%3Adoi%2F10.1371%2Fjournal.pmed.1000335.

11. K. D. Bertakis, P. Franks, and R. Azari, "Effects of Physician Gender on Patient Satisfaction," *Journal of the American Medical Women's Association* 58, no. 2 (2003): 69–75.

12. S. A. Flocke, and V. Gilchrist, "Physician and Patient Gender Concordance and the Delivery of Comprehensive Clinical Preventive Services," *Medical Care* 43, no. 5 (2005): 486–92.

13. The Henry J. Kaiser Foundation, *Putting Women's Health Care Disparities on the Map: Examining Racial and Ethnic Disparities at the State Level*, 2009, kff.org/minorityhealth/upload/7886.pdf.

14. National Women's Law Center et al., *Making the Grade on Women's Health: A National and State-by-State Report Card*, 2007, hrc.nwlc.org.

15. The Henry J. Kaiser Foundation, *Putting Women's Health Care Disparities on the Map*.

16. Daniel Raymond, Harm Reduction Coalition, testimony to the New York City Council on the state of drug policy and addiction, February 2009, harmreduction.org/downloads/New%20York%20City%20Council%20Testimony,%20February%202009.doc.

17. Sheigla Murphy and Marsha Rosenbaum, interview from *Pregnant Women on Drugs: Combating Stereotypes and Stigma* (New Brunswick, NJ: Rutgers University Press, 1999). See also Wendy Choukin, "Cocaine and Pregnancy: Time to Look at the Evidence," *Journal of the American Medical Association* 285 (2001): 1626.

18. News Room, D.C., "New National Survey Shows Financial Concerns and Lack of Adequate Health Insurance Are Top Causes for Delay by Lesbians in Obtaining Health Care," newsroom.dc.gov/show.aspx/agency/lgbt/section/2/release/7561/year/2005.

19. The Human Rights Campaign, "Coming Out to Your Doctor," hrc.org/issues/3391.htm.

CHAPTER 24:
VIOLENCE AGAINST WOMEN

1. U.S. Department of Justice and the Centers for Disease Control, *National Violence Against Women Survey*, 1998, ojp.usdoj.gov/nij/pubs-sum/172837.htm. Though more than a decade old, these national statistics from 1998 are still considered the most comprehensive available.

2. Bureau of Justice Statistics, *Intimate Partner Violence, 1993–2001*, 2003, ojp.usdoj.gov/nij/topics/crime/intimate-partner-violence/measuring.htm.

3. World Health Organization, "Report on Violence and Health," October 2002, who.int/gender/violence/en/.

4. P. Tjaden and N. Thoennes, "Full Report of the Prevalence, Incidence, and Consequences of Violence Against Women—Findings from the National Violence Against Women Survey," National Institute of Justice, November 2000, ncjrs.org/pdffiles1/nij/183781.pdf.

5. Samhita Mukhopadhyay, "Trial by Media: Black Female Lasciviousness and the Question of Consent," in *Yes Means Yes!* ed. Jaclyn Friedman and Jessica Valenti (Berkeley: Seal Press, 2008), p. 154.

6. "Maze of Injustice: The Failure to Protect Indigenous Women from Sexual Violence in the USA," Amnesty International, 2007, amnestyusa.org/women/maze/report.pdf.

7. Interview with Sarah Deer, "Violence Against Native American and Alaska Native Women," Amnesty International, April 24, 2007, amnestyusa.org/askamnesty/live/display.php?topic=82.

8. Recommendations on Combating Sexual Violence Against American Indian and Alaska Native Women Through Fiscal Year 2010 Appropriations. Statement provided by Sarah Deer, amnestyusa.org/uploads/house_interior_testimony_deer.pdf.

9. Giselle Aguilar Hass, Nawal Ammar, and Leslye Orloff, "Battered Immigrants and U.S. Citizen Spouses," 2009, legalmomentum.org.

10. M. Decker, A. Raj, and J. Silverman, "Sexual Violence Against Adolescent Girls: Influences of Immigration and Acculturation," *Violence Against Women* 13, no. 5 (2007): 498 and 507. See also Jessica Mindlin, Leslye E. Orloff, Sameera Pochiraju, et al., "Dynamics of Sexual Assault and the Implications for Immigrant Women," and "Empowering Survivors: Legal Rights of Immigrant Victims of Sexual Assault for Advocates Working with Immigrant Victims of Sexual Assault" (Washington, DC: Legal Momentum, 2010).

11. Decker, Raj, and Silverman, "Sexual Violence Against Adolescent Girls," pp. 498, 503, 507.

12. L. Kalof, "Ethnic Differences in Female Sexual Victimization," *Sexuality and Culture* 4 (2000): 75–97.

13. S. M. Blake, R. Ledsky, C. Goodenow, and L. O'Donnell, "Recency of Immigration, Substance Abuse, and Sexual Behavior Among Massachusetts Adolescents," *American Journal of Public Health* 91 (2001): 794–98.

14. Decker, Raj, and Silverman, "Sexual Violence Against Adolescent Girls," pp. 498, 507.

15. Ibid.; see generally M. A. Dutton, G. A. Hass, and N. Ammar, "Battered Immigrant Women's Willingness to Call for Help and Police Response," *UCLA Women's Law Journal* (2003): 43, 89.

16. Decker, Raj, and Silverman, "Sexual Violence Against Adolescent Girls," pp. 498, 507.

17. Mary Ann Dutton et al., "Characteristics of Help-Seeking Behaviors, Resources and Service Needs of Battered Immigrant Latinas," *Georgetown Journal on Poverty Law and Policy* 7, no. 2 (2000): 245–306.

18. Giselle Aguilar Hass et al., "Lifetime Prevalence of Violence Against Latina Immigrants: Legal and Policy Implications," *Domestic Violence: Global Perspectives* (2000): 93–113.

19. Ibid., p. 109.

20. Tjaden and Thoennes, "Full Report of the Prevalence, Incidence, and Consequences of Violence Against Women," November 2000, ncjrs.org/pdffiles1/nij/183781.pdf.

21. Ibid.

22. L. Peterson, "The Not-Rape Epidemic," in *Yes Means Yes!* ed. Jaclyn Friedman and Jessica Valenti (Berkeley: Seal Press, 2009), p. 209.

23. Ibid.

24. Cara Kulwicki, "Real Sex Education," in *Yes Means Yes!* ed. Jaclyn Friedman and Jessica Valenti (Berkeley: Seal Press, 2009), p. 310.

25. R. Sampson, "The Problem of Acquaintance Rape of College Students," U.S. Department of Justice Office of Community Oriented Policing Services, Problem-Specific Guide Series #17, 2003.

26. Ibid., citing B. Fisher, F. T. Cullen, and M. Turner, *The Sexual Victimization of College Women* (Washington, D.C.: U.S. Department of Justice, 2000).

27. Ibid.

28. Jodi Gold and Susan Villari, eds., *Just Sex: Students Rewrite the Rules on Sex, Violence, Activism and Equality* (Lanham, MD: Rowan G. Littlefield Publishing, 2000).

29. Laura Sessions Stepp, "A New Kind of Date Rape," *Cos-*

mopolitan, September 2007, cosmopolitan.com/sex-love/tips-tips-moves/new-kind-of-date-rape.

30. Sexual Assault Resources Service and Sexual Assault Nurse Examiners Program, sane-sart.com.

31. D. Dwyer and L. Jones, "Rape Kit Testing Backlog Thwarts Justice for Victims: Lawmakers Seek Rules and Funds for Faster DNA Testing After Sexual Assault," 2010, abcnews.go.com/print?id=10701295.

32. Jaclyn Friedman and Jessica Valenti, eds., *Yes Means Yes! Visions of Female Sexual Power and a World Without Rape* (Berkeley: Seal Press, 2008), p. 107.

33. Center for Research on Women with Disabilities at Baylor College of Medicine, at womenshealth.gov/violence.

34. Margaret A. Nosek, Center for Research on Women with Disabilities, Baylor College of Medicine, bcm.edu/crowd/index.cfm?pmid=1410.

35. Mary Ann Dutton and Lisa A. Goodman, "Coercion in Intimate Partner Violence: Toward a New Conceptualization," *Sex Roles* 52, nos. 11/12 (June 2005): 746.

36. Leslye Orloff, ed., "Empowering Survivors: Legal Rights of Immigrant Victims of Sexual Assault for Advocates Working with Immigrant Victims of Sexual Assault" (Washington, DC: Legal Momentum, 2010); Kathleen Sullivan and Leslye Orloff, eds., "Breaking Barriers: A Complete Guide to Legal Rights and Resources for Battered Immigrants" (Washington, DC: Legal Momentum, 2004).

37. Patricia Tjaden and Nancy Thoennes, *Stalking in America: Findings from the National Violence Against Women Survey* (Washington, DC: U.S. Department of Justice, 1998), NCJ 169592. U.S.

38. The Stalking Resource Center and U.S. Department of Justice, "National Stalking Awareness Month 2011 Webinar," 2010, ncvc.org/src/main.aspx?dbID=DB_statistics195.

39. Bureau of Justice Statistics, "Stalking Victimization in the United States," 2009, bjs.ojp.usdoj.gov/content/pub/pdf/svus.pdf.

40. National Institute of Justice, "Stalking." ojp.usdoj.gov/nij/topics/crime/stalking/welcome.htm#tja.

41. M. P. Brewster, *Exploration of the Experiences and Needs of Former Intimate Stalking Victims, 1998*. Final report submitted to the National Institute of Justice. Grant No. 95-WT-NX-0002, NCJ 175475.

42. N. Miller, *Stalking Laws and Implementation Practices: A National Review for Policy Makers and Practitioners*, 2001. Final report submitted to the National Institute of Justice. Grant No. 97-WT-VX-0007, NCJ 197066.

43. Network for Surviving Stalking, University of Leicester, nss.org.uk.

44. U.S. Department of Justice, *The National Crime Victimization Survey*, Washington, DC: National Criminal Justice Reference Service (2004).

45. Nan Stein, "No Laughing Matter: Sexual Harassment in K–12 Schools," in *Transforming a Rape Culture*, ed. Emile Buchwald, Pamela Fletcher, and Martha Ross (Minneapolis: Milkweed Editions, 1993; rev. ed. 2004).

46. N. Heyzer, "Address to the Forty-Third Session of the U.N. Commission on the Status of Women," March 1, 1999.

CHAPTER 25: ENVIRONMENTAL AND OCCUPATIONAL HEALTH

1. Alison Ojanen-Goldsmith, "Young Feminists—Poison Earth, Poison Woman: Making the Connection," Women's Health Activist Newsletter, July/August 2009

2. President's Cancer Panel, "Reducing Environmental Cancer Risk: What We Can Do Now," 2010, deainfo.nci.nih.gov/advisory/pcp/annualReports/pcp08-09rpt/PCP_Report_08-09_508.pdf.

3. Ibid.

4. Ibid.

5. Ibid.

6. "Natural Resources Defense Council, Healthy Milk, Healthy Baby: Chemical Pollution and Mother's Milk," nrdc.org/breastmilk/chems.asp.

7. M. Nathaniel Mead, "Contaminants in Human Milk: Weighing the Risks Against the Benefits of Breastfeeding," *Environmental Health Perspectives* 116 (2008): A426–A34.

8. S. Ip et al., "Breastfeeding and Maternal and Infant Health Outcomes in Developed Countries," *Evidence Report/Technology Assessment* 153 (April 2007): 1–186.

9. President's Cancer Panel, "Reducing Environmental Cancer Risk: What We Can Do Now" (Washington, DC: U.S. Department of Health and Human Services, 2010), deainfo.nci.nih.gov/advisory/pcp/annualReports/pcp08-09rpt/PCP_Report_08-09_508.pdf.

10. "Precautionary Principle," Science and Environmental Health Network, sehnorg/winghtm.

11. Personal correspondence with author, January 2010.

12. Personal interview with author, January 2010.

13. United States Environmental Protection Agency, "An Introduction to Indoor Air Quality: Lead," epa.gov/iaq/lead.html.

14. Toxipedia, "Biological Properties of Lead," toxipedia .org/display/toxipedia/Biological+Properties+of+Lead.

15. New York City Department of Health and Mental Hygiene, "Lead Poisoning: Prevention, Identification, and Management," *City Health Information* 29, no. 5 (September 2010): 41–48, nyc.gov/html/doh/downloads/pdf/chi/chi29-5.pdf.

16. Michael Hawthorne, "High Levels of Toxic Lead Found in Air Outside Chicago School," *Chicago Tribune,* April 1, 2011.

17. Janet Gray, *State of the Evidence: The Connection Between Breast Cancer and the Environment*, 6th ed. (San Francisco: Breast Cancer Fund, 2010).

18. Coming Clean, "What Is Body Burden?" Chemical Body Burden website, chemicalbodyburden.org/whatisbb.htm.

19. Environmental Protection Agency, "2000–2001 Pesticide Market Estimate: Usage," epa.gov/pesticides/pestsales/01pestsales/usage2001.htm.

20. Environmental Protection Agency, "An Introduction to Indoor Air Quality," epa.gov/iaq/pesticid.html.

21. L. M. Frazier, "Reproductive Disorders Associated with Pesticide Exposure," *Journal of Agromedicine* 12, no. 1 (2007): 27–37.

22. Theo Colborn, "A Case for Revisiting the Safety of Pesticides: A Closer Look at Neurodevelopment," *Environmental Health Perspectives* 114 (2006): 10–17, doi:10.1289/ehp.7940, ehp03.niehs.nih.gov/article/fetchArticle.action?articleURI=info%3Adoi%2F10.1289%2Fehp.7940.

23. Graeme Stemp-Morlock, "Reproductive Health: Pesticides and Anencephaly," *Environmental Health Perspectives* 115, no. 2 (February 2007), ncbi.nlm.nih .gov/pmc/articles/PMC1817703/.

24. United Nations Environment Programme, "Persistant Organic Pollutants," chem.unep.ch/pops.

25. Francine Stephens, "Persistent Organic Pollutants: Chemicals That Won't Go Away and Hurt Us All," *Healthy Child, Healthy World,* June 21 2007, healthychild.org/blog/comments/persistent_organic_pollutants_chemicals_that_wont_go_away_and_hurt_us_all/.

26. Eric M. Roberts et al., "Maternal Residence Near Agriculture Pesticide Applications and Autism Spectrum Disorders Among Children in the California Central Valley," *Environmental Health Perspectives* 115, no. 10 (October 2007).

27. Pesticide Action Network, "Children," panna.org/your-health/children.

28. United States Environmental Projection Agency, "Persistent Organic Pollutants: A Global Issue, a Global Response," epa.gov/international/toxics/pop.html.

29. The Endocrine Disruption Exchange, "Endocrine Disruption Introduction," endocrinedisruption.com/endocrine.introduction.overview.php.

30. Centers for Disease Control and Prevention, "Third National Report on Human Exposure to Environmental Chemicals" (Atlanta, GA: Centers for Disease Control and Prevention, 2005), ehp03.niehs.nih.gov/article/fetchArticle.action?articleURI=info%3Adoi%2F10.1289%2Fehp.11748#b28-ehp-117-1359.

31. G. L. Daly and F. Wania, "Organic Contaminants in Mountains," *Environmental Science and Technology* 39, no. 2 (January 2005): 385–98.

32. Environment, Health and Safety Online, "Endocrine Disruptors and Human Health," July 31 2010, ehso .com/ehshome/endocrinedisrupters.htm.

33. United States Environmental Protection Agency, "Dioxins and Furans," epa.gov/pbt/pubs/dioxins.htm.

34. "Coming Clean, Case Study: Dioxin," Chemical Body Burden website, chemicalbodyburden.org/cs_dioxin .htm.

35. Mary Rothschild, "Study Says BPA Exposure, Risk Higher Than Assumed," *Food Safety News*, September 23, 2010, foodsafetynews.com/2010/09/study-says-bpa -exposure-worse-than-previous-estimates/.

36. A. M. Calafat et al., "Exposure of the U.S. Population to Bisphenol A and 4-tertiary-Octylphenol: 2003–2004," *Environmental Health Perspectives* 116 (2008): 39–44, doi:10.1289/ehp.10753, ehp03.niehs.nih.gov/article/info%3Adoi%2F10.1289%2Fehp.10753.

37. Environmental Working Group, "Bisphenol A: Toxic Plastics Chemical in Canned Foods," March 2007, ewg.org/reports/bisphenola.

38. Oregon Environmental Council, "SB 1032: BPA Legislative Fact Sheet," oeconline.org/our-work/smart -policy/2010-bpa-legislation-fact-sheet.

39. Environmental Working Group, "First BPA Detection in U.S. Infant Cord Blood," December 2, 2009, ewg .org/minoritycordblood/pressrelease.

40. Environmental Protection Agency, "Hudson River PCBs," epa.gov/Region2/superfund/npl/0202229c.pdf.

41. "Coming Clean, Case Study: Phthalates," Chemical Body Burden website, chemicalbodyburden.org/cs_ phthalate.htm.

42. Jane A. Hoppin et al., "Reproducibility of Urinary Phthalate Metabolites in First Morning Urine Samples," *Environmental Health Perspectives* 108, no. 10 (October 2000), mindfully.org/Pesticide/Phthalate -Metabolites-Urinary.htm.

43. United States Environmental Protection Agency, "Phthalates Action Plan Summary," epa.gov/opptintr/existingchemicals/pubs/actionplans/phthalates.html.

44. Campaign for Safe Cosmetics, "Unmasked: 10 Ugly Truths Behind the Myth of Cosmetic Safety," safecosmetics.org.

45. Campaign for Safe Cosmetics, "Laws and Regulations," safecosmetics.org/article.php?list=type&type=30.

46. Vassar College Environmental Risks and Breast Cancer project, erbc.vassar.edu/.

47. Ibid.

48. Breast Cancer Fund, "What We Know, What We Need to Know," breastcancerfund.org/assets/pdfs/publications/falling-age-of-puberty-adv-guide.pdf.

49. Ibid.

50. Campaign for Safe Cosmetics, "Not So Sexy: The Health Risks of Secret Chemicals in Fragrance," May 2010, p. 4, safecosmetics.org/article.php?id=644.

51. Ibid.

52. Stephanie Smith, "Toxic Chemicals Finding Their Way into the Womb," CNN, June 1 2010, articles.cnn.com/2010-06-01/health/backpack.cord.blood_1_toxic-chemicals-pregnant-women-cord-blood/2?_s=PM:HEALTH.

53. Katsi Cook, "Women Are the First Environment," *Indian Country*, December 23, 2003, p. 1.

54. Commission for Racial Justice, United Church of Christ, *Toxic Waste and Race in the United States* (New York: Public Data Access, 1987).

55. Loretta Ross, "Bridging the Environmental Justice and Reproductive Justice Movements," SisterSong Women of Color Reproductive Health Collective: Collective Voices (Summer 2009): 10–11.

56. Heroism Project, "Lois Gibbs: Environmental Activist," heroism.org/class/1970/gibbs.html.

57. Eckardt C. Beck, "The Love Canal Tragedy," *EPA Journal*, January 1979, epa.gov/history/topics/lovecanal/01.htm.

58. Centre for Science and the Environment, "25 Years After Bhopal Gas Disaster: A Selection of News," indiaenvironmentportal.org.in/files/Bhopal%20Gas%20Disaster%20-%2025%20years%20after.pdf.

59. Ibid.

60. Pesticide Action Network UK, "The Bhopal Aftermath—Generations of Women Affected," December 1999, pan-uk.org/pestnews/Issue/pn46/pn46p4.htm.

CHAPTER 26: THE POLITICS OF WOMEN'S HEALTH

1. World Health Organization, *Macroeconomics and Health: Investing in Health for Economic Development. Report of the Commission on Macroeconomics and Health* (Geneva: WHO, 2001).

2. *Unnatural Causes: Is Inequality Making Us Sick?* (California Newsreel, 2008). See unnaturalcauses.org.

3. Association of American Medical Colleges, *Women in U.S. Academic Medicine Statistics and Medical School Benchmarking, 2007–2008*, 2009, aamc.org/download/53434/data/wimstats_2008.pdf.

4. Economic Policy Institute, *State of Working America Preview: Income Inequality in Dollars and Cents*, November 3, 2010, epi.org/economic_snapshots/entry/swa_preview_income_inequality_in_dollars_and_cents.

5. Carmen DeNavas-Walt, Bernadette D. Proctor, and Jessica C. Smith, *Current Population Reports, P60-238, Income, Poverty, and Health Insurance Coverage in the United States: 2009* (Washington, DC: U.S. Government Printing Office, 2010), census.gov/prod/2010pubs/p60-238.pdf.

6. Ibid.

7. Ibid.

8. National Women's Law Center, "Analysis of New Census Data Shows Substantial Increase in Women's Poverty, Decline in Health Insurance Coverage, No Improvement in Wage Gap," September 16, 2010, nwlc.org/press-release/nwlc-analysis-new-census-data-shows-substantial-increase-womens-poverty-decline-health.

9. DeNavas-Walt, Proctor, and Smith, *Current Population Reports, P60-238, Income, Poverty, and Health Insurance Coverage in the United States: 2009*.

10. Centers for Disease Control and Prevention, "About Minority Health," cdc.gov/omhd/amh/amh.htm.

11. U.S. Census Bureau. *National Population Projections. Projections of the Population by Sex, Race, and Hispanic Origin for the United States: 2010 to 2050*, census.gov/population/www/projections/summarytables.html.

12. Centers for Disease Control and Prevention, "Subpopulation Estimates from the HIV Incidence Surveillance System—United States, 2006," *Morbidity and Mortality Weekly Report* 57, no. 3 (2008): 985–89.

13. U.S. Department of Health and Human Services, *Women's Health USA 2010*, 2010, mchb.hrsa.gov/whusa10/.

14. Ibid.

15. Ibid.

16. Amnesty International, "Deadly Delivery: The Maternal Health Care Crisis in the USA," 2010, amnestyusa.org/dignity/pdf/DeadlyDelivery.pdf.

17. U.S. Department of Health and Human Services, *Child Health USA 2010*, 2010, mchb.hrsa.gov/chusa10/hstat/hsi/pages/205mm.html.

18. Amnesty International, "Deadly Delivery."

19. Ibid.

20. Melissa Gilliam, "Health Care Inequality Is Key in Abortion Rates," *Philadelphia Inquirer,* August 10, 2008, guttmacher.org/media/resources/2008/08/10/Gilliam_op-ed.pdf.

21. National Center for Health Statistics, "Final Natality Data," 2011, marchofdimes.com/peristats/tlanding.aspx?reg=99&lev=0&top=3&slev=1&dv=qf.

22. March of Dimes, "Prematurity Campaign," 2010, marchofdimes.com/mission/prematurity_impact.html.

23. March of Dimes, "Prematurity Research," 2010, marchofdimes.com/research/prematurityresearch.html.

24. Michael C. Lu, "Racial and Ethnic Disparities in Birth Outcomes: A Life-Course Perspective," CIMS Mother-Friendly Childbirth Forum, March 2009.

25. J. Santelli et al., "Trends in Sexual Risk Behaviors, by Nonsexual Risk Behavior Involvement, U.S. High School Students, 1991–2007," *Journal of Adolescent Health* 44 (2009): 372–79, teenpregnancysc.org/documents/Santelli+et+al+2009+Trends+in+Sexual+and+Other+Risk+Behaviors.pdf.

26. Rebecca Ward, "Following Decade-Long Decline, U.S. Teen Pregnancy Rate Increases as Both Births and Abortions Rise," Guttmacher Institute, January 26, 2010, guttmacher.org/media/nr/2010/01/26/index.html.

27. Special Investigations Division, U.S. House of Representatives, Committee on Government Reform, *The Content of Federally Funded Abstinence-Only Education Programs* (Washington, DC: 2004).

28. Brady E. Hamilton, Joyce A. Martin, and Stephanie J. Ventura, "Births: Preliminary Data for 2009," *National Vital Statistics Report, 2010* 59, no. 3 (2010), cdc.gov/nchs/data/nvsr/nvsr59/nvsr59_03.pdf.

29. H. Weinstock, S. Berman, and W. Cates Jr., "Sexually Transmitted Diseases Among American Youth: Incidence and Prevalence Estimates, 2000," *Perspectives on Sexual and Reproductive Health* 36, no. 1 (2004): 6–10.

30. W. Cates Jr. et al. "Estimates of the Incidence and Prevalence of Sexually Transmitted Diseases in the United States," *Sexually Transmitted Diseases* 26 (1999): S2–S7.

31. Matthew Hogben and Jami Leichliter, "Social Determinants and Sexually Transmitted Disease Disparities: Sexually Transmitted Diseases," *Sexually Transmitted Disease* 35, no. 12 (December 2008): S13–S18.

32. Centers for Disease Control, "Sexually Transmitted Diseases in the United States, 2008: National Surveillance Data for Chlamydia, Gonorrhea, and Syphilis" (2009), cdc.gov/std/stats08/trends.htm.

33. National Council of State Legislatures, "HPV Vaccine," January 2010, ncsl.org/default.aspx?tabid=14381.

34. Peter B. Bach, "Gardasil: From Bench, to Bedside, to Blunder," *Lancet* 375 (March 20, 2010): 963–64.

35. Centers for Disease Control and Prevention, "HIV Among African Americans," September 9, 2010, cdc.gov/hiv/topics/aa/index.htm.

36. The National Women's Health Information Center, "Minority Women's Health," WomensHealth.gov (May 18, 2010), womenshealth.gov/minority/africanamerican/hiv.cfm.

37. "Racial/Ethnic Disparities in Self-Rated Health Status Among Adults with and Without Disabilities—United States, 2004–2006," *Morbidity and Mortality Weekly Report,* October 3, 2008.

38. The National Women's Health Information Center, "Minority Women's Health."

39. Centers for Disease Control and Prevention, "HIV Among African Americans," September 9, 2010, cdc.gov/hiv/topics/aa/index.htm.

40. "Census Bureau: Recession Fuels Record Number of Uninsured Americans," *Kaiser Health News*, September 17, 2010, smtp01.kaiserhealthnews.org/t/13983/384882/13463/0/.

41. Sheila D. Rustgi, Michelle M. Doty, and Sara R. Collins, "Women at Risk: Why Many Women Are Forgoing Needed Health Care," The Commonwealth Fund (2009), commonwealthfund.org/Content/Publications/Issue-Briefs/2009/May/Women-at-Risk.aspx.

42. S. D. Rustgi, M. M. Doty, and S. R. Collins, "Women at Risk: Why Many Women Are Forgoing Needed Health Care," *The Commonwealth Fund Issue Brief,* May 2009.

43. National Center for Health Statistics, "Highlights," *Health, United States, 2009,* cdc.gov/nchs/data/hus/hus09.pdf#highlights.

44. Bureau of Labor Statistics, "Employed Persons by Detailed Occupation, Sex, Race, and Hispanic or Latino Ethnicity," 2009, bls.gov/cps/cpsaat11.pdf.

45. Bureau of Labor Statistics, "May 2007 National Occupational Employment and Wage Estimates," 2007, bls.gov/oes/2007/may/oes_nat.htm#b31-0000.

46. U.S. Department of Health and Human Services, "The 2009 HHS Poverty Guidelines," aspe.hhs.gov/poverty/09poverty.shtml.

47. U.S. Census Bureau, "Annual Social and Economic Supplement," March 2008, census.gov/hhes/www/cpstc/cps_table_creator.html.

48. Rustgi, Doty, and Collins, "Women at Risk: Why Many Women are Forgoing Needed Health Care."

49. Carol Regan, "The Invisible Care Gap: Caregivers Without Health Coverage," Paraprofessional Healthcare Institute, May 2008, hchcw.org/wp-content/uploads/2008/05/phi-cps-report.pdf.

50. Ibid.

51. Guttmacher Institute, "Women of Reproductive Age Hit Hard by Recession, New Census Data Show," September 27, 2010, guttmacher.org/media/inthenews/2010/09/17/index.html.

52. "Medicaid's Role in Family Planning," *Guttmacher Institute,* October 2007, guttmacher.org/pubs/IB_medicaidFP.pdf.

53. National Women's Law Center, *Still Nowhere to Turn: Insurance Companies Treat Women Like a Pre-Existing Condition,* 2009, nwlc.org/our-resources/reports_toolkits/nowhere-to-turn.

54. National Latina Institute for Reproductive Health, "Our Issues: Access to Health Care," 2010, latinainstitute.org/issues/access-health-care.

55. Margaret Crosby, "A Contemporary Abortion Law for California," ACLU of Northern California, April 23, 2002, aclunc.org/news/opinions/a_contemporary_abortion_law_for_california.shtml.

56. Ellen R. Shaffer, "Abortion Rights at Risk," *Huffington Post,* July 20, 2010, huffingtonpost.com/ellen-r-shaffer/abortion-rights-at-risk_b_652922.html.

57. Ellen R. Shaffer, "New HHS Abortion Restriction Goes Beyond Current Law," Ellen Schaffer's Blog, July 20, 2010, ellenshaffer.blogspot.com/2010/07/new-hhs-abortion-restriction-goes.html.

58. Robert Pear, "Push for Stricter Abortion Limits Expected in House," *New York Times,* December 11, 2010, nytimes.com/2010/12/12/health/policy/12abortion.html.

59. Center for Reproductive Rights, "A First Look Back at the 2010 State Legislative Session," August 31, 2010, reproductiverights.org/en/feature/a-first-look-back-at-the-2010-state-legislative-session.

60. Amie Newman, "Report: States Pass Staggering Array of Anti-Choice Laws, Policies and Ballot Measures," RH Reality Check, September 3, 2010, rhrealitycheck.org/blog/2010/09/01/2010s-staggering-antichoice-legislation-policies-ballot-measures-states.

61. Ellen R. Shaffer and Judy Norsigian, "A Practical Guide Forward for Progressives on Healthcare," *Salon,* May 22, 2010, salon.com/news/opinion/feature/2010/05/22/progressives_practical_healthcare_guide.

62. Rustgi, Doty, and Collins, "Women at Risk: Why Many Women are Forgoing Needed Health Care."

63. Gita Sen and Piroska Östlin, "Unequal, Unfair, Ineffective and Inefficient. Gender Inequity in Health: Why It Exists and How We Can Change It," Final Report to the WHO Commission on Social Determinants of Health, WHO, 2007.

64. Population Reference Bureau, *2010 World Population Data Sheet* (Washington, DC: Population Reference Bureau, 2010).

65. United Nations, "World Population Prospects: 2008 Revision Population Database," 2008, esa.un.org/UNPP/index.asp?panel=2.

66. Susheela Singh, Jacqueline Darroch, Lori Ashford, and Michael Vlassoff, *Adding It Up: The Costs and Benefits of Investing in Family Planning and Maternal and Newborn Health* (New York: Guttmacher Institute and UNFPA, 2009).

67. Gita Sen and Piroska Östlin, "Unequal, Unfair, Ineffective and Inefficient."

68. International Agency for Research on Cancer, "GLOBOCAN 2008: Cancer Incidence and Mortality Worldwide in 2008," World Health Organization, 2009, globocan.iarc.fr/.

69. Centers for Disease Control and Prevention, "Differences by Sex in Tobacco Use and Awareness of Tobacco Marketing—Bangladesh, Thailand, and Uruguay, 2009," *Morbidity and Mortality Weekly Report* 59, no. 20 (May 28, 2010): 613–18.

70. Ellen R. Shaffer et al., "Global Trade and Public Health," *American Journal of Public Health* 95 (January 2005): 23–34.

71. Ibid.

72. Stan Bernstein with Charlotte Juul Hansen, *Public Choices, Private Decision: Sexual and Reproductive Health and the Millennium Development Goals* (New York: United Nations Millennium Project, 2006).

73. Population Reference Bureau, *2010 World Population Datasheet.*

74. Organisation for Economic Co-operation and Development, "Key Characteristics of Parental Leave Systems," January 7, 2010, oecd.org/dataoecd/45/26/37864482.pdf.

75. Anne H. Gautier, "The Impact of Family Policies on Fertility in Industrialized Countries: A Review of the Literature," *Population Research and Policy Review* 26, no. 3 (2007): 323–46, DOI: 10.1007/s11113-007-9033-x, rand.org/pubs/research_briefs/2005/RAND_RB9126.pdf.

76. Rebecca Ray, Janet C. Gornick, and John Schmitt, "Who Cares? Assessing Generosity and Gender Equality in Parental Leave Policy Designs in 21 Countries," *Journal of European Social Policy* 20, no. 3 (2010): 196.

77. WHO, "Trends in Maternal Mortality: 1990–2008,"

2010, whqlibdoc.who.int/publications/2010/9789241 500265_eng.pdf.

78. D. Jamison et al., eds., *Priorities in Health* (Washington, DC: World Bank, 2006).

79. K. S. Khan et al., "WHO Analysis of Causes of Maternal Death: A Systematic Review," *Lancet* 367, no. 9516 (April 1, 2006): 1066–74.

80. C. Ronsmans and W. J. Graham, "Lancet Maternal Survival Series Steering Group. Maternal Mortality: Who, When, Where, and Why," *Lancet* 368, no. 4542 (September 30, 2006): 1189–1200.

81. Demographic Health Surveys, "Measure DHS," stat compiler.com.

82. M. Minkauskiene et al., "Systematic Review on the Incidence and Prevalence of Severe Maternal Morbidity," *Medicina (Kaunas)* 40, no. 4 (2004): 299–309.

83. United Nations Interagency Group for Child Mortality Estimation, "Levels and Trends in Child Mortality" (New York: UNICEF, 2010).

84. John Ross and William Winfrey, "Contraceptive Use, Intention to Use and Unmet Need During the Extended Postpartum Period," *International Family Planning Perspectives* 27, no. 1:2 (March 27, 2001).

85. Susheela Singh et al., *Abortion Worldwide: A Decade of Uneven Progress* (New York: Guttmacher Institute, 2009), guttmacher.org/pubs/Abortion-Worldwide.pdf.

86. Population Reference Bureau, "World's Women and Girls 2011 Datasheet" (Washington, DC: PRB, 2011).

87. Singh, Darroch, Ashford, and Vlassoff, *Adding It Up.*

88. Ibid.

89. "Report of the China UNFPA Independent Assessment Team," U.S. Dept of State, 2002, state.gov/g/prm/rls/rpt/2002/12112.htm.

90. CHANGE: Center for Health and Gender Equity, "HIV/AIDS and Other STIs," 2010, genderhealth.org/the_issues/hiv_aids_and_other_stis.

91. Andrew Pavao and Miguel Ongil, "Euromapping 2010: Mapping European Development and Population Assistance," German Foundation for World Population and European Parliamentary Forum on Population and Development, 2010, euroresources.org/fileadmin/user_upload/Euromapping/EM2010/Euromapping2010_LoRes.pdf.

92. WHO, *Unsafe Abortion: Global and Regional Estimates of the Incidence of Unsafe Abortion and Associated Mortality in 2003* (Geneva: WHO, 2007).

93. Guttmacher, *Facts on Investing in Family Planning and Maternal and Newborn Health, in Brief* (New York: Guttmacher, 2010).

94. U.S. Department of Health and Human Services,

"President's Global Health Initiative," 2010, global health.gov/initiatives/index.html.

95. G. Sedgh et al., "Induced Abortion: Rates and Trends Worldwide," *Lancet* 370 (2007): 1338–45.

96. Singh, Darroch, Ashford, and Vlassoff, *Adding It Up.*

97. Ibid.

98. Ibid.

99. C. Watts and C. Zimmerman, "Violence Against Women: Global Scope and Magnitude," *Lancet* 359, no. 9313 (2002): 1232–37.

100. World Bank, *World Bank Study World Development Report: Investing in Health* (New York: Oxford University Press, 1993).

101. WHO, Multi-Country Study on Women's Health and Domestic Violence (Geneva: WHO, 2005).

102. S. Mathews, *Every Six Hours a Woman Is Killed by Her Intimate Partner: A National Study of Female Homicide in South Africa* (Cape Town: Medical Research Council, 2004).

103. National Crime Records Bureau, "Crime Against Women," chapter 5 in *Crime in India 2007* (New Delhi: Ministry of Home Affairs, 2008), p. 2.

104. Procurador de los Derechos Humanos, "Procurador de los Derechos Humanos Presente Informe Annual 2008" (Guatemala: Procurador de los Derechos Humanos, 2009).

105. C. Garcia-Moreno and C. Watts, "Violence Against Women: An Urgent Public Health Priority," *Bulletin of the World Health Organization* 89, no. 2-2 (2011).

106. G. Barker et al., *Evolving Men: Initial Results from the International Men and Gender Equality Survey (IMAGES)* (Washington, DC: International Center for Research on Women [ICRW] and Rio de Janeiro: Instituto Promundo, January 2010).

107. WHO, "Violence Prevention. The Evidence. A Series of Briefings (Geneva: WHO, 2009); WHO, "Preventing Intimate Partner and Sexual Violence Against Women" (Geneva; WHO, 2010); Family Violence Prevention Fund, endabuse.org.

108. Amy D. Marshall, Jillian Panuzio, and Casey T. Taft, "Intimate Partner Violence Among Military Veterans and Active Duty Servicemen," *Clinical Psychology Review* 25, no. 7 (2005): 862–76; Miranda Alison, "Wartime Sexual Violence: Women's Human Rights and Questions of Masculinity," *Review of International Studies* 33, no. 1 (2007): 75–90.

109. United Nations Special Rapporteur to the Commission on Human Rights, "Report on the Situation of Human Rights in Rwanda," E/CN.4/1996/68 (New York: United Nations, 2007), p. 7.

110. UNICEF Democratic Republic of Congo, cited in U.N. Security Council, *Report of the Secretary-General Pursuant to Security Council Resolution 1820, S/2009/362* (New York: United Nations, 2009), p. 5.

111. Watts and Zimmerman, "Violence Against Women."

112. Katy Robjant, Rita Hassan, and Cornelius Katona, "Mental Health Implications of Detaining Asylum Seekers: Systematic Review," *British Journal of Psychiatry* 194 (2009): 306–12.

113. Jayne Arnott and Anna-Louise Crago, "Rights Not Rescue: A Report on Female, Male, and Trans Sex Workers' Human Rights in Botswana, Namibia, and South Africa," Public Health Program, Open Society Institute, New York, 2009, soros.org/initiatives/health/focus/sharp/articles_publications/publications/rights_20090626/rightsnotrescue_20090706.pdf.

114. Laura Maria August, *Sex at the Margins: Migration, Labour Markets and the Rescue Industry* (London: Zed Books, 2007).

115. "Thematic Discussion Paper: Creating an Enabling Legal and Policy Environment for Increased Access to HIV & AIDS Services for Sex Workers." Product of discussions of the Thematic Task Team on Creating an Enabling Legal and Policy Environment in preparation for the First Asia and the Pacific Regional Consultation on HIV and Sex Work, October 2010, plri.org/sites/plri.org/files/Enabling%20Environment%20discussion%20paper.pdf.

116. Joy Ngozi Ezeilo, "Report Submitted by the Special Rapporteur on Trafficking in Persons, Especially Women and Children," United Nations General Assembly, May 2010, www2.ohchr.org/english/bodies/hrcouncil/docs/14session/A.HRC.14.32.pdf.

117. U.S. Department of State, *Trafficking in Persons Report* (Washington, DC: Office of Undersecretary for Democracy and Global Affairs and Bureau of Public Affairs, 2010), state.gov/g/tip/rls/tiprpt/2010.

118. United Nations Office on Drugs and Crime, *Global Report on Trafficking in Persons* (Vienna: UNODC, 2009), p. 11.

119. Jay G. Silverman et al., "HIV Prevalence and Predictors of Infection in Sex-Trafficked Nepalese Girls and Women," *Journal of the American Medical Association* 298, no. 5 (2007): 536–42.

120. U.S. Department of State. *Trafficking in Persons Report* (Washington, DC: Office of Undersecretary for Democracy and Global Affairs and Bureau of Public Affairs, 2010), state.gov/g/tip/rls/tiprpt/2010.

121. WHO, "Female Genital Mutilation," February 2010, who.int/mediacentre/factsheets/fs241/en/index.html.

122. C. Feldman-Jacobs and D. Clifton, "Female Genital Mutilation/Cutting: Data and Trends, Update 2010" (Washington, DC: Population Reference Bureau, 2010).

123. Rogaia Mustafa Abusharaf, ed., *Female Circumcision, Multicultural Perspectives* (Philadelphia: University of Pennsylvania Press, 2006).

124. International Agency for Research on Cancer, "Cervical Cancer Incidence and Mortality Worldwide in 2008," Globocan 2008, Lyon, 2010, globocan.iarc.fr/factsheets/cancers/cervix.asp.

125. Ibid.

126. WHO, "Cervical Cancer, Human Papillomavirus (HPV), and HPV Vaccines: Key Points for Policymakers and Health Professionals (Geneva: WHO, 2007), whqlibdoc.who.int/hq/2008/WHO_RHR_08.14_eng.pdf.

127. Cervical Cancer Action, "New Options for Cervical Cancer Screening and Treatment in Low-Resource Settings," 2010, cervicalcanceraction.org/pubs/CCA_cervical_cancer_screening_treatment.pdf.

128. S. Arrossi, M. Paolino, and R. Sankaranarayanan, "Challenges Faced by Cervical Cancer Prevention Programs in Developing Countries: A Situational Analysis of Program Organization in Argentina," *Revista Panamericana de Salud Publica* 28, no. 4 (October 2010): 249–57.

129. Cervical Cancer Action, "New Options for Cervical Cancer Screening and Treatment in Low-Resource Settings."

130. Cervical Cancer Action, "Strategies for HPV Vaccination in the Developing World," 2010, cervicalcanceraction.org/pubs/CCA_HPV_vaccination_strategies.pdf.

131. Ibid.

132. Ibid.

133. H. J. Larson et al., "The India HPV-Vaccine Suspension," *Lancet* 376, no. 9741 (August 2010): 572–3.

134. International AIDS Vaccine Initiative, *Current HPV Vaccines and Future AIDS Vaccines: Common Challenges and Unprecedented Opportunities* (New York: 2008).

135. UNAIDS, *Report on the Global Epidemic 2010* (Geneva; Joint United Nations Programme on HIV/AIDS, 2010), unaids.org/globalreport/Global_report.htm.

136. Niranjan Saggurti and Alankar Malviya, "HIV Transmission in Intimate Partner Relationships in India," UNAIDS, 2009, unaids.org.in/Publications_HIVTransmissionInIntimatePartnerRelationshipsInIndia.pdf.

137. WHO and UNAIDS, *Addressing Violence Against Women and HIV/AIDS: What Works?* (Geneva: WHO, 2010).

138. Ibid.

139. Ibid.

140. UNAIDS, *Report on the Global Epidemic 2010.*

141. The United State President's Emergency Plan for AIDS Relief, "About PEPFAR," pepfar.gov/about/index.htm.

142. WHO, "Paediatric HIV and Treatment of Children Living with HIV" (November 2010), who.int/hiv/topics/paediatric/en/index.html.

143. UNAIDS, *Report on the Global Epidemic 2010.*

144. International Community of Women Living with HIV/AIDS, "The Forced and Coerced Sterilization of HIV Positive Women in Namibia," 2009.

145. M. de Bruyn, "Safe Abortion for HIV-Positive Women with Unwanted Pregnancy: A Reproductive Right," *Reproductive Health Matters* 11, no. 22 (2003): 152–61.

146. S. Gruskin, "HIV and Pregnancy Intentions: Do Services Adequately Respond to Women's Needs?" *American Journal of Public Health* 98, no. 10 (October 2008): 1746–50. Epub August 13, 2008.

147. WHO, "New Data on Male Circumcision and HIV Prevention: Policy and Programme Implications" (Geneva: WHO, 2007).

148. WHO and UNAIDS, "Progress in Male Circumcision Scale-up: Country Implementation Update," July 2009, who.int/hiv/pub/malecircumcision/country_update_july09.pdf.

149. UNFPA, "Donor Support for Contraceptives and Condoms for STI/HIV Prevention 2007," 2008, unfpa.org/webdav/site/global/shared/documents/publications/2008/updated_donor_support_report.pdf.

150. UNAIDS, "Letter to Partners," 2010, data.unaids.org/pub/BaseDocument/2010/20100216_exd_lettertopartners_en.pdf.

151. Ibid.

152. The Female Health Company, "Female Health Company Quarterly Report of Financial Condition," May 2007, sec.edgar-online.com/female-health-co/10qsb-quarterly-report-of-financial-condition/2007/05/14/Section9.aspx._Avert.org; AVERT, "The Female Condom," 2010, avert.org/female-condom.htm.

153. A. Peters et al., "The Female Condom: The International Denial of a Strong Potential," *Reproductive Health Matters* 18, no. 35 (May 2010): 119–28.

154. Robert M. Grant et al., "Preexposure Chemoprophylaxis for HIV Prevention in Men Who Have Sex with Men," *New England Journal of Medicine* 363 (2010): 2587–99.

155. Family Health International, "Factsheet: Results of the CAPRISA 004 Trial on the Effectiveness of Tenofovir Gel for HIV Prevention," 2010, fhi.org/NR/rdonlyres/eh6buffl6gvlpwuspjystcj4jkfkqkblild6whxka2eljmt6lzzylm3xb2lbwyxhdf24hcvhqow2ap/CAPRISA004Effectiveness.pdf.

156. United States District Court, Southern District of New York. "Association for Molecular Pathology et al. v. United States Patent and Trademark Office et al.," (2010): 135, aclu.org/files/assets/2010-3-29-ampvuspto-opinion.pdf.

157. Lee Silver, *Remaking Eden: Cloning and Beyond in a Brave New World* (New York: Avon Books, 1997), pp. 4–7, 11.

158. George J. Annas, "Genetic Genocide," chapter 17 in *Worst Case Bioethics: Death, Disaster, and Public Health* (New York: Oxford University Press, 2010).

CHAPTER 27:
ACTIVISM IN THE
TWENTY-FIRST CENTURY

1. Sarah Crump, "Julie Zeilinger, Creator of thefbomb.org, Examines Teen Feminist Issues," *Cleveland Plain Dealer,* May 2, 2010, cleveland.com/arts/index.ssf/2010/05/julie_zeilinger_creator_of_the.html.

2. "Mobile Access 2010," *Pew Internet & American Life,* July 7, 2010, pewinternet.org/Reports/2010/Mobile-Access-2010.aspx.

3. Lynn M. Paltrow, "PersonhoodUSA: Promoting a Radical, Fetal-Separatist Agenda," *Huffington Post,* October 25, 2010.

4. Ariel Levy, *Female Chauvinist Pigs: Women and the Rise of Raunch Culture* (New York: Free Press, 2005).

5. American Psychological Association, *Report of the APA Task Force on the Sexualization of Girls,* apa.org/pi/women/programs/girls/report-full.pdf.

6. Image box on the Hardy Girls Healthy Women website, hghw.org/news/spark-summit-pushing-back-sexualization-girls.

7. Breast Cancer Action, "Buckets for the Cure," thinkbeforeyoupink.org/?page_id=1011.

8. Jacki Lyden, "Are Charities Doing Enough to Fight Breast Cancer?" NPR, October 25, 2010.

9. Christie Aschwanden, "The Downside of Awareness Campaigns," *Los Angeles Times,* October 4, 2011, articles/latimes.com/2010/oct/04/health/la-he-breast-awareness-month-20101004.

The Editorial Team

Senior Editor: Kiki Zeldes

Managing Editor: Christine Cupaiuolo

Contributing Editors: Judy Norsigian
Amy Romano
Wendy Sanford

OBOS Global Initiative
Coordinating Editor: Ayesha Chatterjee

Editorial Assistant: June Tsang

Additional Editors: Jackie Lapidus
Heather Stephenson

Book Interns: Natalie Chapman, Raquel Rios,
Meg Young

List of Contributors by Chapter

*1. Our Female Bodies: Sexual Anatomy,
Reproduction, and the Menstrual Cycle*
Revised by Marjorie Greenfield. Additional contributors: Chris Bobel, Hilary Gerber, Christine Hitchcock, Sheryl Kingsberg, Esther M. Leidolf, Marianne McPherson, Cathleen E. Morrow, Elizabeth Naumberg, Evelina Sterling, Trudy Van Houton, Toni Weschler, Meg Young.
Special thanks to: Jen Chapin-Smith, Joan Chrisler, and OBOS partners Women and Their Bodies (Israel) and Shokado Women's Bookstore (Japan).
Contributors to earlier editions: Marianne McPherson, Toni Weschler, Monica Casper, Cheryl Chase, Alice Dreger, Esther M. Leidolf, Chris Bobel, Esther Rome, Nancy Reame, Wendy Sanford, Abby Schwartz, Katherine Saldutti, Cindy Irvine, Nancy Woods, Leah Diskin, Nancy Miriam Hawley, Barbara Perkins, Roni Randall.

2. Intro to Sexual Health

Contributors: Heather Corinna, Marjorie Greenfield, Martha Ellen Katz, Evelina Sterling, Marcie Richardson, Elizabeth Stewart.

Special thanks to: Brittany Charlton, Karen Wolf, OBOS partner Mavi Kalem, Turkey.

3. Body Image

Revised by Jocelyn Sims. Additional contributors: Hanne Blank, Anita Hoffer, Jin In, Lisa Jervis, Jean Kilbourne, Courtney Martin, Nancy Redd, Rose Weitz, Courtney Young, Diana Zuckerman.

Special thanks to: Bridgit Brown, OBOS partner Groupe de Recherche sur les Femmes et les Lois au Senegal (GREFELS), Senegal.

Contributors to earlier editions: Sarai Walker, Lori Tharps, Demetria Iazzetto, Linda King, Jennifer Yanco, Allison Abner, Deborah Levine, Marsha Sexton, Judith Stein, Becky Thompson, Linda Villarosa, Kiki Zeldes, Wendy Sanford, the women of Boston Self Help Center, Frances Deloatch, Mary Fitzgerald, Jean Gillespie, Nancy Miriam Hawley, Janna Zwerner, Joan Lastovica, Oce, Rosemarie Ouilette, Jane Pincus, Esther Rome, Jill Wolhandler.

4. Gender Identity and Sexual Orientation

Revised by Wendy Sanford. Additional contributors: Rose Afriyic, Petra Doan, Cait Glasson, Ted Heck, Esther M. Leidolf, Elizabeth Sarah Lindsey, Irene Monroe, Su Penn, Norman P. Spack, Judy Anne Williams, Louis Gooren.

Special thanks to: Saber DeMare, Laura Edwards-Leeper, Gina Ogden, Devin Reynolds.

Contributors to earlier editions: Elizabeth Sarah Lindsey, Wendy Sanford, Loraine Hutchins, Rebecca Rabinowitz.

5. Relationships

With enormous thanks to the thirty-seven women who shared their stories.

6. Social Influences on Sexuality
7. Sexual Pleasure and Enthusiastic Consent
8. Sexual Challenges

Contributors: Saleemah Abdul-Ghafur, Rose Afriyie, Hanne Blank, Bella DePaulo, Stacey May Fowles, Jaclyn Friedman, Anita P. Hoffer, Cara Kulwicki, Elizabeth Sarah Lindsey, Gina Ogden, Jenni Prokopy, Tara Roberts, Kimberly Springer, Evelina Sterling, Beverly Whipple, Janna Zwerner (sexuality and disability).

Special thanks to: Melanie Davis; Janice Irvine; Rebecca G. Stephenson, PT, DPT, MS, coordinator of Wom-

en's Health Physical Therapy, Rehabilitation Services, Brigham and Women's Hospital; Leonore Tiefer.

Contributors to earlier editions: Lynn Rosenbaum, Janna Zwerner, Wendy Sanford, Nancy Miriam Hawley, Elizabeth McGee, Gina Ogden, Linda King, Judy Brewer, Denise Bergman, Eithne Johnson, Curdina Hill, Amy Alpern, Diana Chase, Francis Deloatch, Paula Doress-Worters, Bonnie Engelhardt, Mary Fitzgerald, Jean Gillespie, Ginger Goldner, Shere Hite, Janice Irvine, Nancy London, Jenny Mansbridge, Oce, Rosemarie Ouilette, Jane Pincus, Brenda Reeb, Marsha Saxton, Jean Lastovica.

9. Birth Control

Revised by Kirsten Thompson. Additional contributors: Kelly Blanchard, Heather Corinna, Marjorie Greenfield, Mary Ann Leeper, Lisa Perriera, Robin Wallace, Toni Weschler, Carolyn Westhoff, Susan Wysocki.

Special thanks to: Kate Curtis, Cynthia C. Harper, Polly Marchbanks, Michael Policar, Jill Schwartz, Naomi Tepper

Contributors to earlier editions: August Burns, Michelle Martelle, Maura Graff, Melanie Steeves, Emma Ottolenghi, Elaine Lissner, Kirsten Thompson, David Sokal, Toni Weschler, Susan Bell, Lauren Wise, Suzannah Cooper-Doyle, Judy Norsigian, Felice Apter, Charon Asetoyer, Sara Dickey, Anne Kelsey, Sophie Martin, Ava Moskin, Cindy Pearson, Linda Potter, Judith Richter, James Trussell, Kevin Whaley, Susan Wood, Ruth Bell, Pamela Berger, Jennifer S. Edwards, Charlotte Ellertson, Philip Hart, Nancy Miriam Hawley, Rachel Lanzerotti, Ken Legins, Pamela Morgan, Barbara Perkins, Susan Reverby, Wendy Sanford, Abby Schwarz, Felicia Stewart, Alice Steinhardt, James Trussell, Beverly Winikoff.

10. Safer Sex

Contributors: Susan Blank, Heather Corinna, Janet Dollin, Anna Forbes, Yvonne Piper, Gary Richwald, Laura Subramanian, Cosette Wheeler, Fred Wyand.

Special thanks to: Tonji Durant, Mary Ann Leeper (female condom), Ben Remsen of the AIDS Library of Philadelphia, Jill Schwartz.

Contributors to earlier editions: Laura Subramanian, Christie Burke, Amelia Glynn Hornick, Jennifer Block, Christie Burke, Sylvie Ratelle, Mary Crowe, Judy Norsigian, Katherine M. Stone of the Centers for Disease Control and Prevention, Catherine Liu of the American Social Health Association, Esther Rome, Fran Ansley, Hilde Armour, William McCormick, Michelle Topal, Pam White, Paul Wiesner, Michele Russell, Wendy Sanford, Maria Jobin-Leeds, Mary Ide, Wanda Allen, the Women of Color AIDS Council (especially Karen McManus, Malkia

Kendricks, and Charlotte, Colleen, Jackie, Shirley, and Yohani), Patricia O. Loftman, Peggy Lynch, Lucia Ortiz-Ortiz, Belynda Dunn, Anna Forbes, Sophie Godley, Mary Guinan, Laura Whitehorn, Amy Alpern, Marion Banzhaf, Laurie Cotter of ACT UP New York, Deborah Cotton, Risa Denenberg, Liz Galst, Jenny Keller, Vicky Legion, the Chicago Women's AIDS Project, Patricia O. Loftman, Janet L. Mitchell, Jamie Penney, Lindsey Rosen, Susan Rosenberg.

11. Sexually Transmitted Infections

Revised by Susan Blank and Gary Richwald. Additional contributors: Susan Clark Ball, Anna Forbes, Cynthia Gómez, Yvonne Piper, Rachel Walden, Cosette Wheeler, Fred Wyand.

Special thanks to: Tonji Durant, Esther Fine, Kimberley Warsett, Laura Whitehorn.

Contributors to earlier editions: Christie Burke, Sylvie Ratelle, Mary Crowe, Judy Norsigian, Katherine M. Stone of the Centers for Disease Control and Prevention, Catherine Liu of the American Social Health Association, Esther Rome, Fran Ansley, Hilde Armour, William McCormick, Michelle Topal, Pam White, Paul Wiesner.

12. Unexpected Pregnancy

Contributors: Alison Amoroso, Zobeida Bonilla, Meg Young.

Contributors to earlier editions: Judith Winkler, Alison Amoroso, Catherine Harris-Vincent, Jennifer Yanco, Linda King, Jane Pincus, Jill Wolhandler, Denise Bergman, Paula Harris-Vincent, Joyce Maguire Pavao, Carolyn Rudin, Kay Schlozman, Dianne Weiss.

13. Abortion

Contributors: Kelly Blanchard, Marlene Fried, Deborah Issokson, Carole Joffe, Laura Kaplan, Martha Katz, Sylvia Law, Lisa Perriera, Lauren Plante, Kirsten Thompson, Tracy Weitz, Beverly Winikoff, Susan Yanow.

Special thanks to: Dan Grossman, Erin Kate Ryan, Ellen Shaffer.

Contributors to earlier editions: Marlene Gerber Fried, Maureen Paul, Laureen Tews, Jill Wolhandler, Trude Bennett, Ruth Weber, Dana Gallagher, Centre de Santé des Femmes de Montréal, Carol Franzblau, Suzanne Hendrick, Luita Spangler, Laurie Williams, Vickie Alexander, Diane Balser, Pamela Berger, Sarah Buttenweiser, Helen Caulton, Concord Feminist Health Center, Terry Courtney, Debra Drassner, Carol Driscoll, Margie Fine, Marlene Gerber Fried, Linda Gordon, Nancy Miriam Hawley, Liz Hill, Debra Krassner, Elizabeth McGee, Judy Norsigian, Ana Ortiz, Jane Pincus, Stephanie Poggi, Loretta Ross, Wendy Sanford, Kira Sarpard, Meredith Tax, Susan Yanow.

14. Considering Parenting

Contributors: Alison Amoroso, Veronica Arreola, Onye Kachukwu C. Iloabachie Anaedozie, Jocelyn Sims, Sally Whelan.

Contributors to earlier editions: Merle Bombardieri, Meredith W. Michaels, Rachel Gaillard Smook, Merryl Pisha, Joan Ditzion, Mary Howell Raugust, Denise Bergman, Norma Swenson, Joan Rachlin, Joyce Maguire Pavao, Corinne Rayburn of the Center for Family Connections.

15. Pregnancy and Planning for Birth

Contributors: Jill Arnold, Zobeida Bonilla, Elizabeth Davis, Marjorie Greenfield, Katharine Hikel, Tekoa King, Christine Morton, De Nobleza, Debra Pascali-Bonaro, Miriam Zoila Pérez, Lauren Plante, Carol Sakala, Pamela Vireday, Claire Winstone.

Special thanks to: Henci Goer.

Contributors to earlier editions: Tekoa King, Maria Iorillo, Judith Bishop, Lisa Paine, Carol Sakala, Jane Pincus, Judy Luce, Audrey Levine, Robin J. Blatt, Linda Holmes, Marsha Saxton, Carol Sakala, Denise Bergman, Esther Entin, Ruth Bell, Robin Blatt, Jenny Fleming, Linda Holmes, Judy Luce, Mary (Bebe) Poor, Judi Rogers, Becky Sarah, Norma Swenson.

16. Labor and Birth

Contributors: Elizabeth Allemann, Jill Arnold, Zobeida Bonilla, Robyn Churchill, Elizabeth Davis, Henci Goer, Marjorie Greenfield, Katharine Hikel, Tekoa King, Christine Morton, Debra Pascali-Bonaro, Miriam Zoila Pérez, Lauren Plante, Carol Sakala, Pamela Vireday, Claire Winstone, Diony Young.

Special thanks to: Henci Goer.

Contributors to earlier editions: Tekoa King, Maria Iorillo, Judy Luce, Jane Pincus, Judith Bishop, Carol Sakala, Audrey Levine, Norma Swenson, Ruth Bell, Jenny Fleming, Nancy Miriam Hawley, Linda Holmes, Becky Sarah, Gail Sullivan.

17. The Early Months of Parenting

Contributors: Barbara Fildes, Alan Greene, Deborah Issokson, Alice LoCicero, Claire Mysko, Amie Newman, Beth Pimentel, Elizabeth Steiner, Annie Urban, Claire Winstone.

Contributors to earlier editions: Deborah Issokson, Alice LoCicero, Anne Merewood, Barbara L. Philipp, Tekoa King, Dennie Wolf, Mary Crowe, Laurie Williams, Helen Armstrong, Jane Honikman, Gail Levy, Veronica Miletsky, Carol Sakala, Dianne Weiss, Paula Doress-Worters, Esther Rome, Vilunya Diskin, Marty Reudi, Robbie Pfeufer Kahn.

18. Miscarriage, Stillbirth, and Other Losses

Contributors: Jen Dozer, Ruth Fretts, Arielle Greenberg, Linda Layne, Chukwuma Onyeije, Lauren Plante.

Contributors to earlier editions: Linda L. Layne, Wendy Garling, Catherine Romeo, Jane Pincus, Ellen Glazer.

19. Infertility and Assisted Reproductive Technologies

Revised by Evelina Sterling and Miriam Zoll. Additional contributors: Juaquita Callaway, Barbara Collura, Jen Dozer, Deborah Issokson, Maurizio Macaluso, Shree Mulay, Jeane Ungerleider.

Special thanks to: Tonji Durant and OBOS partner Women's Health Initiative in Bulgaria.

Contributors to earlier editions: Nancy King Reame, Rachel Gaillard Smook, Diane Clapp, Ruth Hubbard, Ami Jaeger, Wendy Sanford, Gena Corea, Ellen Glazer, Barbara Eck Menning, Marcie Richardson, Ester Shapiro, Lori Andrews, Geri Ferber, Nancy Reame, Barbara Katz Rothman, RESOLVE, Inc.

20. Perimenopause and Menopause

Revised by: Joan Ditzion and Marcie Richardson. Additional contributors: Ellen Bruce, Elaine Lissner, Jerilynn Prior, Evelina Sterling.

Special thanks to: Nancy Miller, Margaret Moloney, William (Bill) Parker, and the following OBOS partners: Sanlaap (India), Manavi (USA), Women for Empowerment, Development, and Gender Reform (Nigeria).

Contributors to earlier editions: Joan Ditzion, Nancy Fleming, Amy Alina, Diana Siegal, Lisa Begg, Loretta Finnegan, Jaqueline Lapidus, Paula Doress-Worters (formerly Paula Brown Doress), Norma Meras Swenson, Diana Laskin Siegal, Robin Cohen, Mickey Troub Friedman, Lois Harris, Kathleen MacPherson, Denise Bergman, Janine O'Leary Cobb, Linda King, Susan M. Love, Cindy Pearson of the National Women's Health Network, Jane Pincus, Lynn Rosenberg, Wendy Sanford, Stephanie Studentski, Mary Yeaton, Louise Corbett, Tish Anisimov, Lorraine Doherty, Ruth Hubbard, Audrey Michaud, Pamela Berger, Irene Davidson, Meg Hickey, Judy Norsigian, Josephine Polk-Matthews, Ruth Hubbard, Edith Fletcher, Barbara Krentzman, Lucile Longview Schuck, Anna Schenke, Anne Smith, Marian Saunders.

21. Our Later Years

Revised by Joan Ditzion. Additional contributors: Ellen Bruce, Leilani Doty, Margaret Morganroth Gullette, Jessica Haxton Retrum, Anita P. Hoffer, Jackie Lapidus, Alyson Martin, Ruth Palombo, Nushin Rashidian, Wendy Sanford.

Special thanks to: Kacey Bongarzone, Alice Fisher, Sadia Greenburg, Marjorie Harvey, Joanne LaPlante, Ginny Mazur, Charlotte Millman, Sarah Pearlman, Cynthia Phillips, Elaine Shapiro, Sarah Whitby, MSW, SHINE Program director.

Contributors to earlier editions: Joan Ditzion, Diana Siegal, Leilani Doty, Jacqueline Lapidus; see also list of contributors to earlier editions under Chapter 20, "Perimenopause and Menopause."

22. Selected Medical Problems

Revised by Marcie Richardson. Additional contributors: Paula Amato (PCOS), Mary Lou Ballweg (endometriosis), Kari Christianson (DES), Pat Cody (DES), Mary Costanza (breast cancer), Carol Drury (endometriosis), Judi Hirschfield-Bartek (breast cancer), Fran Howell (DES), Mitch Levine, William Parker, Elizabeth Steiner (breast cancer), Elizabeth Stewart (vulva), Kay Zakariasen (PBS/IC).

Special thanks to: Michelle Berlin, Mary Fillmore, Louise Gessel, Bonnie Hill, Elizabeth Kavaler, Kath Mazella, Diana Petitti, Gary Richwald, Gordon Schiff.

Contributors to earlier editions: Julia Brody, Barbara Brenner, Susan Troyan, Mary Lou Ballweg, Monica Casper, Adele E. Clarke, Martha Ellen Katz, Mitch Levine, Marcie Richardson, Kristina Graff, RAINBO, Marianne McPherson, Jaqueline Lapidus, Judy Norsigian, Susan Troyan, Cathie Ragovin, Judi Hirshfield-Bartek, Carmen Tamayo, Anne Kahn, Mimi Secor, Selma Mirsky, Lisa Whiteside, Kath Doyle, Nahid Toubia, Carol Englender, Endometriosis Association, Mary Crowe, Margaret Lee Braun, Pat Cody (DES Action), Dorothy Reider, Esther Rome, Debi Milligan, Women's Dignity Project.

23. Navigating the Health Care System

Contributors: John Abramson, Lisa Codispoti, Dave deBronkart, Barbara Fildes, Catherine Finn, Susan Sered, Gordon Schiff, Trisha Torrey, Rachel Walden, Karen Anne Wolf.

Special thanks to: Lois Aherns, Shannon Berning, Bridgette Courtot, Danielle Garret, Ellen Miller-Mack, Suede.

Contributors to earlier editions: Judy Ann Bigby, Susan Sered, George Annas, Shannon Berning, Laurie Rosenblum, Kiki Zeldes, Norma Meras Swenson, Wendy Sanford, Judy Norsigian.

24. Violence Against Women

Contributors: Heather Corinna, Cara Kulwicki, Margaret Lazarus, Judith Lennett, Craig Norberg-Bohm (sidebar on White Ribbon movement), Leslye Orloff, Miriam Zoila Pérez, Holly Ramsey-Klawsnik.

Special thanks to: Rev. Irene Monroe and OBOS partner Women's Health Promotion Center, Serbia.

Contributors to earlier editions: Margaret Lazarus, Laurie Rosenblum, Renner Wunderlich, Diane Rosenfield, Stacey Kabat, Marianne Winters, Dina Carbonell, Lois Glass, Suzanne Gosselin, Carol Mamber, Jill Stanzler, Alice Friedman, Lynn Rubinett, Lena Sorensen, Denise Wells, Nancy Wilbur, Terrie Antico, Wendy Sanford, Jackie Herskovitz, Judith Lennett, Laura Tandara, Gene Bishop, Andrea Fischgrund, Roxanne Hynek, Janet Jones, Freada Klein, Rachel Lanzerotti, Carol McEldowney, Judy Norsigian.

25. Environmental and Occupational Health

Revised by Mara Kardas-Nelson and Lin Nelson. Additional contributors: Katsi Cook, Carol Dansereau, Elise Miller, Loretta Ross, Marc Weisskopf.

Special thanks to: Namasha Schelling and OBOS partner Tanzania Home Economics Association.

Contributors to earlier editions: Lin Nelson, Barbara Sattler, Jaqueline Lapidus, Patricia Logan, Regina H. Kenen, MassCOSH Women's Committee: Letitia Davis, Marian Marbury, Laura Punnett, Margaret Quinn, Cathy Schwartz, Susan Woskie, Carol Dansereau, Maureen Gorman, Norma Grier, Elizabeth Gullette, Pat Hynes, Kristin Lacijan of NCAMP, Cheri Lucas-Jennings, Karen McDonell, Manju Mehta, Vernice Miller, Cydney Pullman, Dorothy Wigmore, Susan O'Brien, Ngazi Oleru, Judy Norsigian, the Shalan Foundation, Joan Bertin, Katsi Cook, Maureen Paul.

26. The Politics of Women's Health

Revised by Ellen Shaffer, with Rebecca Firestone and Karin Ringheim (global). Additional contributors: Susan Ball, Zobeida Bonilla, Lisa Codispoti, Marcy Darnovsky, Kezia Ellison, Anna Forbes, Polly F. Harrison, Jodi L. Jacobson, Susan Roll, Susan Sered, Susan F. Wood, Susan Yanow, Diana Zuckerman.

Special thanks to: Melissa Gilliam, Arden Handler, Mary Ann Leeper; OBOS collaborators on *Nuestros Cuerpos, Nuestas Vidas* in North, Central, and South America; OBOS partners Sanlaap (India) and Manavi (USA); Women for Empowerment, Development, and Gender Reform (Nigeria); Network of East-West Women—Polska (Poland).

Contributors to earlier editions: Ellen Shaffer, Gail Price-Wise, Marcy Darnovsky, Elizabeth J. Rourke, Sondra Crosby, Michael Grodin, Sharon Batt, Cindy Young, Christine Cupaiuolo, Norma Meras Swenson, Wendy Sanford, Judy Norsigian, Carol Sakala, Nalini Visvanathan, Vilunya Diskin, Hilary Salk, Judith Dickson Luce, Nancy Krieger, Anne Kasper, Steffi Woolhandler, Karen Kahn, Jacqueline Lapidus, Arnold Relman, Philip R. Lee, Roz Feldberg, Julie Friesen, Anne-Emmanuelle Birn, Nancy Worcester, Mariamne Whatley, Gabriela Canepa, Marilen Danguilan, Betsy Hartmann, Jennifer Yanco, Anita Anand, Asoka Bandarage, Elizabeth Coit, Jane Cottingham, H. Patricia Hynes, Marilee Karl, Una MacLean, Annie Street, Amy Alpern, David Banta, Gene Bishop, Robin Blatt, Lucy Candib, David Clarke, Mary Fillmore, Mary Howell, Sherry Leibowitz, Barbara Perkins, Joan Rachlin, Sheryl Ruzek, Kathy Simmonds, Mary Stern, Nancy Todd, Karen Wolf.

27. Activism in the Twenty-first Century

Revised by Heidi Moore. Additional contributors: Steph Herold, Hope Lewis, Susan Roll, Loretta Ross, Rachel Walden, Jamia Wilson, Deanna Zandt.

Special thanks to: OBOS partner Women's Rehabilitation Center, Nepal.

Contributors to earlier editions: Susan Roll, Victoria Passarella, Ellen Miller-Mack, Laurie Rosenblum, Eugenia Acuna, Judy Norsigian, Jane Pincus, Caty Laignel, Meizhu Lui, Suzanne Nam, Norma Meras Swenson, Rachel Lanzerotti.

General Thanks

Regina A., Onyeka Anaedozie, Polly Attwood, Natasha Beck, Barbara A. Beltrand CPA, Kali Blaze, Lucia Brea, Erin Callahan, Megan Carlson, Jen and Lexi Chapin-Smith, Caitlin Childs, Anna Cook, Juanita Crider, Nina J. Davidson, Jessica Devancy, Katie Emmet, Jasmine Galereave, Susan Galereave, Molly M. Ginty, Beth Grampetro, Consuela Green, Bernie Heldkamp, Amanda Huminski, Sarah Jackson, Jennifer Getting Jameslyn, Rebecca Kling, Carolyn Lejuste, Mags M., Ulises Martinez and the crew at Filter (Chicago), Mary Maxfield, Charlotte Mayerson, Hunter McCorkel, Alicia Merchant, Efia Miles, Nancy Miller, Jennifer Moon, Laurel O'Gorman, Lola Pellegrino, Cathryn Platine, Barbara Ray, S. E. Smith, Tasha Spencer, Jaime Taylor, Cierra Townsend, San Maday Travis, Sadie-Ryanne Vashti, Tara Vega, Jesse Zeldes.

Special Thanks To

Our Bodies Ourselves staff: Wendy Brovold, Anne Miller Sweeney, Sally Whelan, Nekose Wills.

OBOS interns and volunteers: Meredith Burns, Sarah Burton, Natalie Chapman, Morgan Clark, Katherine

Clavelle, Julie Eisen, Reed Ellis, Beth Katz, Sari Krumholz, Shannon O'Malley, Raquel Rios.

Photo and production assistance: Bernie Heidkamp.

Our Bodies, Ourselves **readers who submitted their photos for the cover, including:**

Lindsey Renée Bever; Lisa L. Boone; Marlies Bosch; Hillary Boucher; Margaret Park Bridges; Linda Burns; Candace C. Cabbil; Kim Comatas; Ciara J. Cooksey; Sarah Diehl; Tracy G. Eleazer; A'Llyn Ettien; Johanna Rincon Fernandez; Vanessa Shanti Fernando; Ruth L. Fischbach; Frances Ann Flint; Nancy Goldstein; Muriel Green; Emily Frost-Leaird; Noa Gutterman; Sarah Dove Heider; Debby Herbenick; Sandy Iredale; Tania Israel; Susan Jaszemski; Gamze Karadağ; Traci Lawson; Jennie Lee; Yasmeen Long; Nichole Lovett; Julia M.; Yaisa Mann; Katherine Marcovich; Lauren Martin; Katie O'Keefe McGuire; Jessica Meza; Kaamila Mohamed; Mary Gelb Park; Lesley Rafes; Molly Remer; Christine Ross; Alice Rothchild; Sally Rynne; Melissa Scholten-Gutierrez; Abby L. Schwarz; Simone Snyder; Jessica Lee Stovall; Malgorzata Tarasiewicz; June Tsang; Celeste Wang; Nekose Wills; Susan F. Wood.

The production crew at Simon & Schuster: Especially, Marcia Burch, Lisa Healy, Michelle Howry, Alex Preziosi.

Founders of the Boston Women's Health Book Collective: Ruth Bell Alexander, Pamela Berger, Vilunya Diskin, Joan Ditzion, Paula Doress-Worters, Nancy Miram Hawley, Elizabeth MacMahon-Herrera, Pamela Morgan (1949–2008), Judy Norsigian, Jane Pincus, Esther Rome (1945–1995), Wendy Sanford, Norma Swenson, Sally Whelan.

Current and recent Our Bodies Ourselves board members: Shahira Ahmed, MPH; Benjamin Albert, JD, MBA; Catherine Annas, JD; Barbara Anthony, MA, JD; Joanne Barker, MS; Bea Bezmalinovic, MBA, MPP; Anne Brewster, M.D.; Marcia Brown; Caroline Crosbie, MBA; Sally Deane, EdM, MPH; Nancy Forsyth; Kristin Guest, CMA, MBA; Jessica Halverson, MBA; Rachel Zack Ishikawa, MA, MPH; Myriam Hernandez Jennings, MA; Nancy Lyons, MPH; Julie Mottl-Santiago, CNM, MPH; Heather Nelson, PhD, MPH; Mary Poor, DVM, SM; Katie Reilly, RN, MPH; Penelope Riseborough; Patricia Roche, JD, MEd; Moises Russo, M.D., MBE; Bonnie Shepard, MPA, MEd; Amanda Buck Varella, JD; Rachel Wilson; Miriam Zoll.

Current and recent Our Bodies Ourselves advisory board members: Marjorie Agosin, PhD; Hortensia Amaro, PhD; Byllye Avery; Judy Bradford, PhD; Gloria Feldt; Teresa Heinz; Cathy Inglese; Paula Johnson, M.D.; Timothy Johnson, M.D.; Wanda Jones, PhD; Florence Ladd, PhD; Susan M. Love, M.D.; Meizhu Lui; Sally H. Lunt, EdD, JD; Ngina Lythcott, PhD; Evelyn Murphy, PhD; Cynthia Pearson; Vivian Pinn, M.D.; Mary Poor, DVM, SM; Ellen Poss, M.D.; Joan Rachlin, JD; Deborah Raptoulos, MEd, MSW; Gary A. Richwald, M.D., MPH; Moises Russo M.D., MBE; Isaac Schiff, M.D.; Gloria Steinem; Frederica Williams.

We thank the foundations that have supported OBOS in recent years, including Appleton Foundation; Archibald Foundation; Boston University School of Public Health; Brush Foundation; Common Benefits Trust; Conservation, Food and Health Foundation; Norton Cruz Family Foundation Fund; Fledgling Fund; Ford Foundation; Ipas; Kwitman Family Foundation; MacArthur Foundation; New Hampshire Charitable Foundation (donor directed grant); Seymour and Sylvia Rothchild Foundation; Sally and Terry Rynne Foundation; Schocken Foundation; Threshold Foundation; Tides Foundation (donor directed grant); Frederick and Margaret L. Weyerhaeuser Family Foundation; Mary Wohlford Foundation; the World Bank.

We thank the hundreds of individuals and organizations for their financial contribution to OBOS, including those who responded to our Word by Word campaign for this fortieth anniversary edition: Alison Amoroso; Sue Lindholm Barker; Diane Beeson; Barbara Berney; Gene Bishop; Connie Breece, CNM; Gillie Campbell; Vidal S. Clay; Carol Conway-Long; Barbara B. Crane; Elaine Dunbar; Mollie Glazer; Mary Godwyn; the Gordon Family; Helen Lingenfelter Gray; Kristin Guest; Nancy Holmstrom; Maya Honda; Lisa C. Ikemoto; Patricia J. Jenkyns, PT; Carole Joffe; Susan Jordan; Ziona K.; Ruth S. Kay; Miriam Atma Khalsa; Polly Russell Kornblith; Laura Lein; Elaine Lissner; Dr. Sally H. Lunt; Claudia Lux; Suzanne Marks; Erin Teare Martin; Karen J. Maschke; Jane Matthews; Joyce McFadden; Jenny Oberholtzer; Deborah Oyer; Joyce G. Perocchi; Susan Rose; Andee Rubin; Sally J. Rynne; Isaac Schiff, M.D., chief, Vincent Obstetrics and Gynecology Service, Massachusetts General Hospital; Jennifer P. Schneider; Sue Schwartz; Ellen R. Shaffer; Sara Shields, M.D.; Jan Stallmeyer; Lucy Stroock; Ruth Tuomala; Dr. Jan Werbinski; Hon. Ho-Tzu Chuang Yen; Sophia Yen, MD, MPH; Alliance for Humane Biotechnology; Harvard Vanguard Medical Associates; MIT Women's and Gender Studies Program; Ruth Kertzer Seidman and Aaron Seidman; Mark Munger and Katherine Bourne; Judy and Dave Archibald; Terri Rearick and Maria Rearick; Maria da Costa and Kai DaCosta; Hagop and Takouhy Mangerian and Armenhui Mangerian Jacobson; Craig and Anita McPherson; Amy Fine and Chester Hartman; Barbara Norton and Bradley Cruz; Kandace Olsen and Scott Peterson; Bill and Rachel Parker; Whitney Pinger, CNM, and WISDOM Midwifery; Mardge Cohen, M.D., and Gordon

Schiff, M.D.; Alice Rothchild and Dan Klein; Lee and Byron Stookey; UnCut/Voices Press, publishing against female genital mutilation, CEO Tobe Levin; WS103 students 1978–2009; Hannah J. Yanow and Lucy M. Yanow.

Donations in loving memory of: Rita Arditti (1934–2009), feminist activist for human rights and social and environmental justice—*abrazos* (Estelle Disch and everyone at OBOS); Elise Boulding (Gordon Fellman); Patricia Stocking Brown, a feminist scientist who worked to eliminate breast cancer (Bonnie Rose); Baby Chan Kenney (her parents); Dr. Charlotte Ellertson (Ibis Reproductive Health); Rachel Fruchter (Susan Reverby); Esther Gottesman, Ellen Ruth McAllister, Sheila Chatterjee, and Manasi Ray (Erik and Ayesha); Dr. Mary Raugust Howell (Yeou-Cheng Ma); Gracie James (Chris Bobel); Mary Martin Johnson (from her children Deborah, Cathy, Bruce, and Amy); Marjorie Carrère Lykes and Rita Arditti (Brinton Lykes); Roderick Mackenzie, 1934–2010 (Eila Kaarina Mackenzie); Esther R. Rome (Nathan Rome, Abby Schwarz); Esther Rome—passionate, joyful activist and OBOS founder—in apprecation of our "Menstruation Consciousness Raising" Workshops (Emily Culpepper); Amy Tavrow, beloved sister and daughter, who strongly supported women's health and rights (Paula Tavrow); Irving Kenneth Zola and Agnes Norsigian (Judy Norsigian).

Donations in honor of: Susan E. Bell (Susan Reverby); Gene Bishop (Evelyn Bishop); Janet Cook (Anna Cook and Hanna Clutterbuck); Carol Penney Guyer (Alisa Kenny-Guyer); Alexandra Esperanza Heidkamp-Pimentel and Oliva Violet Johnson Cupaiuolo (Christine Cupaiuolo); my daughter Alyson Isaac (Linda Oliver-Smith); Joan Israel (Nancy Reame); my daughter Kyra and colleague Norma Swenson (Judy Norsigian); our daughter Milla and other young women seeking peace and justice (Susan Bell and Philip Hart); Mom (Rachel Walden); the Musserians and Mangerians; the five founders and nearly 150 members of the National Women's Health Network's board of directors since 1975 (Cynthia Pearson, NWHN executive director); Judy Norsigian (Roz and Ross Feldberg, Yeou-Cheng Ma, Deborah and Vassilios Raptopoulos, Joan Rachlin and Seymour Small); the wonderful writers, editors, and researchers of Our Bodies Ourselves (Dr. Belisa); the board, staff, and founders at OBOS (Wendy Sanford and the board and staff of Public Responsibility in Medicine and Research—PRIM&R); my daughter Quinn and son Liam (Anne Miller Sweeney); Joan Rachlin (the Tiven-Gottesman family); Amy Romano (Fran Flanagan); Anne Shratter (Rosemarie Shratter); my mentors Marsha Saxton and the late Irving K. Zola (Janna Zwerner); Barbara Seaman (Alice Wolfson); Diana Laskin Siegal, for her contributions to many editions of *Our Bodies, Ourselves* (Paula Doress-Worters); daughters Naomi Siegal and Diane Benjamin, and granddaughter Anna Benjamin (Diana Laskin Siegal); Mrs. Norma Whelan, Dr. Raya Atlas Kane, Anya Whelan-Smith, and Jeff Smith (Sally Whelan); Dorothy Weber Sved, M.D. (Margery Sved); Takeia and Toya (Nekose Wills); Mrs. Norma Whelan and Leslie Whitaker (Virginia Raymond); the beautifully strong women in my family (June Tsang); forty more years! (our Armenian Feminist Gathering); Choices Women's Medical Center, founded by Merle Hoffman, also celebrating its fortieth anniversary.

ABOUT THE CONTRIBUTORS

EDITORIAL TEAM

Ayesha Chatterjee's leadership at Our Bodies Ourselves has resulted in resources based on *Our Bodies, Ourselves* in twelve languages. She serves on the board of directors of the Eastern Massachusetts Abortion Fund. Previously, she worked as a sexuality counselor in India and Central Asia.

Christine Cupaiuolo (christine2.com) covers women's health and public policy for Our Bodies Ourselves and Our Bodies, Our Blog. She also writes for other publications and edits articles and books on politics, culture, gender, and digital media.

Judy Norsigian, executive director of Our Bodies Ourselves, is a cofounder of the organization and has worked on all commercial editions of this book. She has been a women's health advocate and activist for forty years.

Amy Romano, MSN, CNM, is a nurse-midwife who has written extensively about evidence-based maternity care for books, online media, and professional journals. She has practiced full-scope midwifery in the home, birth center, and hospital settings and consulted for various maternity-related advocacy organizations.

Wendy Sanford has been a coauthor of *Our Bodies, Ourselves* since 1969. "What a privilege to work with women, men and genderqueers of many generations who are devoted to keeping *OBOS* useful. Happy fortieth, *OBOS*! Polly and Rory, I love you."

June Tsang attended Brandeis University, where she became passionate about women's health advocacy. She is grateful to Our Bodies Ourselves for following their tradition of educating young women and for granting her the opportunity to be involved in the process of this edition.

Kiki Zeldes has been part of the editorial team for the past four editions of *Our Bodies, Ourselves*. When not working on books, she develops content for and manages the Our Bodies Ourselves website.

CONTRIBUTORS

Saleemah Abdul-Ghafur is an occasional writer and an all-the-time activist. She compiled *Living Islam Out Loud: American Muslim Women Speak,* a seminal anthology of kick-ass women, because now, more than ever, the world needs to hear our voices.

John Abramson, M.D., MSc, a family physician, is the author of *Overdosed America: The Broken Promise of American Medicine* (overdosedamerica.com), is a lecturer in health policy at Harvard Medical School, and serves as an expert in litigation involving the pharmaceutical industry.

Rose Afriyie is a black feminist pursuing an MPP at the University of Michigan. Her policy areas of interest are gender and sexual health. She is currently writing a book about balancing economic security with passionate engagement in work and is a contributor to the website Feministing.

Elizabeth Allemann, M.D. (drallemann.com), is a family physician and acupuncturist in Missouri. She has attended births in hospitals, birth centers, and homes and believes it matters how we are born and how we give birth, and that maternity care must serve all mothers.

Paula Amato, M.D., is a reproductive endocrinologist and associate professor of obstetrics and gynecology at Oregon Health & Science University in Portland, Oregon.

Alison Amoroso, MEd, earned her master's degree at Harvard Graduate School of Education and her bachelor's at Duke. She recently authored *Unwanted Hair and Hirsutism: A Book for Women* published by Your Health Press. Alison is a longtime feminist activist and resides in Atlanta.

Onyekachukwu C. Iloabachie Anaedozie, MPH, CPH, is a Nigerian and New York City native who has made the decision to dedicate her career in public health to women's health. She currently works for the Department of Public Health in Philadelphia and lives with her husband, Obiora.

Jill Arnold is an activist and the founder of the childbirth advocacy blog TheUnnecesarean.com.

Veronica Arreola (vivalafeminista.com) is a professional feminist, a writer, and a mom who writes about feminism and motherhood.

Susan Ball, M.D., MPH, is an HIV specialist at New York–Presbyterian Hospital Weill Cornell Medical College.

Mary Lou Ballweg founded the Endometriosis Association (endometriosisassn.org) in 1980. The international organization's purpose is education, support, and research. She is the author of several books on the disease and many other published lay and scientific works.

Kelly Blanchard is president of Ibis Reproductive Health. Ibis's mission is to improve women's reproductive autonomy, choices, and health worldwide. Kelly's research focuses on improving access to and simplifying abortion, contraception, and HIV prevention products and services.

Hanne Blank (hanneblank.com) is the author of numerous books, including *Big Big Love: A Sourcebook on Sex for People of Size and Those Who Love Them* (Ten Speed Press) and *Virgin: The Untouched History* (Bloomsbury).

Susan Blank, M.D., MPH, is a medical officer with the Centers for Disease Control and Prevention's Division of Sexually Transmitted Disease Prevention, on assignment at the New York City Department of Health and Mental Hygiene.

Chris Bobel teaches women's studies at the University of Massachusetts Boston. She is the author of *The Paradox of Natural Mothering* and *New Blood: Third Wave Feminism and the Politics of Menstruation,* and coeditor of *Embodied Resistance: Breaking the Rules, Challenging the Norms.*

Zobeida Bonilla is an assistant professor in the Division of Epidemiology & Community Health at the University of Minnesota School of Public Health. She works with community health programs and coalitions that address the health needs of the Latino population throughout the country.

Ellen Bruce, J.D., is director of the Gerontology Institute in the John W. McCormack Graduate School of Policy and Global Studies at the University of Massachusetts Boston (geront.umb.edu). She teaches elder law and policy and has served on many nonprofit boards, including as president of the national board of the Older Women's League.

Juaquita D. Callaway, M.D. (holisticgynecology.com), is a holistic gynecologist in the metro Atlanta area. She blends conventional and natural treatment options to provide a comprehensive medical approach to women's health issues.

Kari Christianson is the DES Action USA program director (desaction.org) and a DES daughter. She advocates for all DES-exposed individuals on the National Cancer Institute DES Follow-up Study Steering Committee and the National Institute of Environmental Health Sciences Public Interest Partners.

Robyn Churchill, CNM, MSN (mamah.org), has been a midwife in greater Boston for more than ten years. She is the director of midwifery at Mount Auburn Hospital in Cambridge, Massachusetts. She has two teenagers and is an avid marathoner and rower in her spare time.

Lisa Codispoti is senior counsel at the National Women's Law Center (nwlc.org) with its Health and Reproductive Rights Team, where she helps lead the center's work on women and health reform, with a particular focus on ensuring low-income women's access to comprehensive health care.

Pat Cody was a pioneer in women's health. She founded DES Action, which brought mothers and the children affected together with doctors and researchers to make sure the effects of the drug were understood, and the children informed and cared for.

Barbara Collura has served as executive director of RESOLVE: The National Infertility Association since 2007. RESOLVE (resolve.org) is a nationwide advocacy and support organization for women and men diagnosed with infertility.

Katsi Cook (indianyouth.org) is an elder Mohawk midwife, a founding member of the National Aboriginal Council of Midwives of the Canadian Association of Midwives, and founding Aboriginal midwife of the Six Nations Birthing Centre at Six Nations, Ontario.

Heather Corinna is the director of Scarleteen (scarleteen.com) and CONNECT, and the author of *S.E.X.: The All-You-Need-to-Know Progressive Sexuality Guide to Get You Through High School and College,* and could not be more honored to have been part of this book.

Mary Costanza, M.D., professor of medicine at the University of Massachusetts Medical School, is a nationally known expert in breast cancer. After treating the disease for many years, she has focused her attention more recently on issues in screening and cancer control research.

Carol Dansereau is an environmental organizer/attorney who works with farmworkers in Washington State on pesticide issues. Before joining the staff of the Farm Worker Pesticide Project, she was director of the Washington Toxics Coalition and worked for other nonprofits.

Marcy Darnovsky, PhD, is associate executive director, Center for Genetics and Society (geneticsandsociety.org), a public affairs organization working to encourage responsible uses and effective societal governance of human biotechnologies, from a perspective grounded in social justice, human rights, and health equity.

Elizabeth Davis, BA, CPM (elizabethdavis.com), has been a midwife for more than thirty years and is cofounder of National Midwifery Institute, Inc. She is coauthor of *Orgasmic Birth: Your Guide to a Safe, Satisfying and Pleasurable Birth Experience* and the classic midwifery text *Heart & Hands.*

Dave deBronkart (epatientdave.com) almost died of Stage IV kidney cancer in 2007. He was saved by great medicine, started blogging and advocating for the e-patient movement (empowered, engaged, equipped, enabled) on epatients.net, and is patient cochair of the Society for Participatory Medicine.

Bella DePaulo, PhD (belladepaulo.com), earned her PhD at Harvard and is currently at UC Santa Barbara. She is the author of *Singled Out: How Singles Are Stereotyped, Stigmatized, and Ignored, and Still Live Happily Ever After* and the Living Single blog at the *Psychology Today* website.

Joan Ditzion is a founder of the Boston Women's Health Book Collective, coauthor of all editions of *Our Bodies, Ourselves,* and a geriatric social worker and educator. She appreciates the love and support of her husband, two sons and daughters-in-law, and new grandson.

Petra Doan, Ph.D., MRP (coss.fsu.edu/durp/people/petra-l-doan), teaches urban and regional planning for developing countries at Florida State University. As a transsexual woman, she also writes about the tyranny of gendered planning and its social and economic impact on sexual and gender minorities.

Janet Dollin, MDCM, FCFP, is a family physician and an associate professor at the University of Ottawa. She practices medicine, teaches, and mentors with a focus on women's health and leadership. She is a daughter, sister, wife, mother, aunt, and friend and lives in Ottawa, Ontario.

Leilani Doty, PhD, director, University of Florida Cognitive and Memory Disorder Clinics, works on elder/women's health, dementias, brain health, academic leadership, and communication. Google her name and topic words for articles; regarding brain health/exercise and dementia, try alzonline.net.

Jen Dozer is a writer, a registered nurse, and a mother after experiencing infertility.

Carol Ratliff Drury is the education program coordinator and associate director of the Endometriosis Association (endometriosisassn.org), a self-help organization founded in 1980 with international headquarters in Milwaukee, Wisconsin. She has a particular interest in conditions that often co-occur with endometriosis, especially candidiasis.

Kezia L. Ellison is a Pittsburgh native who has a master's in women's health from Suffolk University and a bachelor's in human biology from Brown University. She is the founder and president of Educating Teens about HIV/AIDS, Inc.

Barbara Fildes, MS, CNM, FACNM, is a certified nurse-midwife with more than thirty years of experience in a range of clinical settings. She is on the faculty of Dartmouth Medical School and is currently the manager of Regional Obstetrics Improvement, New England Alliance for Health at Dartmouth-Hitchcock Medical Center.

Catherine Finn, MSW, LCSW, is a health and medical writer. As a Senior Researcher at the Foundation for Informed Medical Decision in Boston, Cathy translates medical research to support the development of Shared Decision Making© programs in mental health, breast cancer, and palliative care.

Rebecca Firestone, ScD, MPH, is a researcher with Population Services International (psi.org), committed to policy advocacy and program evaluation in the field of sexual and reproductive health and rights.

Anna Forbes, MSS, an advocate, organizer, and writer, has worked in HIV/AIDS since 1985 and on women's health and rights since 1977. Now an independent consultant with an international client list, she has published numerous articles and eight childrens' books on HIV.

Stacey May Fowles (staceymayfowles.com) is an essayist, a journalist, and the author of two novels. Her writing has appeared in various magazines and journals. Most recently, she coedited the anthology *She's Shameless: Women Write About Growing Up, Rocking Out and Fighting Back.*

Ruth Fretts, M.D., is a practicing obstetrician and gynecologist who has been studying stillbirth for twenty-five years, an assistant professor at Harvard Medical School, and former chairperson of the Scientific Committee for the International Stillbirth Alliance. She lives with her husband and three children in Brookline.

Marlene Gerber Fried, PhD, is a longtime activist; founding president and board member, National Network of Abortion Funds; 2010–2011 acting president, professor, and faculty director, Civil Liberties and Public Program (CLPP), Hampshire College; and coauthor, *Undivided Rights: Women of Color Organize for Reproductive Justice.*

Jaclyn Friedman (jaclynfriedman.com) is the director of Women, Action & the Media and a charter member of CounterQuo, a coalition challenging how we respond to sexual violence. Her anthology *Yes Means Yes!* was one of *Publisher's Weekly*'s Top 100 Books of 2009.

Hilary Gerber is a medical student at Nova Southeastern University planning to be an obstetrician-gynecologist, a predoctoral research fellow who studied labor and delivery interventions, a former midwifery student, and a mother.

Cait Glasson (CaitieCat) is twice an immigrant: once coming home to Canada from the United Kingdom, once coming home to women's country. Both experiences have been happy, exciting, terrifying, and worth every moment. She blogs feministically at Shakesville (shakespearessister .blogspot.com).

Henci Goer (hencigoer.com) specializes in evidence-based maternity care. She is the author of *The Thinking Woman's Guide to a Better Birth* and *Obstetric Myths Versus Research Realities.* She is a resident expert on Lamaze International's website, where she moderates the "Ask Henci" forum.

Cynthia Gómez, PhD, is director of the Health Equity Institute at San Francisco State University (healthequity.sfsu .edu), linking science and practice in the pursuit of health equity for all. She is a leading HIV prevention scientist and formerly codirected the UCSF Center for AIDS Prevention Studies.

Arielle Greenberg (ariellegreenberg.net) is the author of two books of poetry and coeditor of several poetry anthologies. Her latest book is *Home/Birth: A Poemic,* written with Rachel Zucker. She is a birth activist and associate professor at Columbia College Chicago.

Alan Greene, M.D., is a Clinical Professor of Pediatrics at Stanford University School of Medicine, author of *Raising Baby Green and Feeding Baby Green,* founder and CEO of DrGreene.com, and founding president of the Society for Participatory Medicine. Follow Dr. Greene on Facebook and Twitter.

Marjorie Greenfield, M.D. (marjoriegreenfield.com), is a professor of ob-gyn at Case Western Reserve University School of Medicine and author of *The Working Woman's Pregnancy Book.* She dates her interest in women's health to the original 1973 edition of *Our Bodies, Ourselves.* Thanks, BWHBC!

Margaret Morganroth Gullette, PhD (brandeis.edu/centers/wsrc/scholars/profiles/Gullette.html), is the author of *Agewise: Fighting the New Ageism in America* and a scholar at the Women's Studies Research Center, Brandeis University. Her previous books include *Aged by Culture* and *Declining to Decline*.

Polly F. Harrison, PhD, an anthropologist, founded and directed the Alliance for Microbicide Development from 1998 through 2010. She previously led the Institute of Medicine's global health programs and worked in health research and policy analysis in Latin America. She is now senior adviser to AVAC.

Ted Heck, MCJ, works in HIV prevention at the Virginia Department of Health. Volunteer activities include antiviolence and advocacy work in LGBQ and especially T communities of Virginia. He lives as an out trans man with his partner and cats in Richmond.

Steph Herold is a reproductive justice activist who has worked in direct-service abortion care and reproductive health advocacy. She founded the website I Am Dr. Tiller and the blog Abortion Gang. She tweets from the handle @IAmDrTiller and lives in Brooklyn, New York.

Katharine (Trina) Hikel, M.D., was peer-trained in women's health at the Berkeley, California, Women's Health Collective and in conventional medicine at the University of Vermont College of Medicine. She lives in Vermont with her family and works as an activist in maternity care reform.

Judi Hirschfield-Bartek, RN, MS, OCN, has practiced as a clinical nurse specialist for more than thirty years and currently works at the Dana-Farber Cancer Institute. In 2010 she received the Silent Spring Institute's Rachel Carson Award for her breast cancer activism.

Christine Hitchcock, PhD, is research associate at the Centre for Menstrual Cycle and Ovulation Research (CeMCOR; cemcor.ubc.ca) at the University of British Columbia, Vancouver, BC, Canada. She studies menstruation and progesterone therapy for perimenopausal and menopausal hot flushes and night sweats.

Anita P. Hoffer, PhD, EdD, was formerly an associate professor (Harvard Medical School) and business specialist in women's health (Johnson & Johnson). Currently she educates women and their health care providers about sexuality throughout the life cycle, leads workshops, and does sex coaching.

Frances Howell is a DES daughter and executive director of DES Action USA (desaction.org), the national nonprofit organization for those exposed to the antimiscarriage drug diethylstilbestrol.

Jin In is Eastern born, Western bred with a global vision of empowering the world's poorest girls as a powerful lever to make our world better. She is the founding director and president of For Girls GLocal Leadership (4GGL.org).

Deborah Issokson, PsyD (reproheart.com), is a psychologist who specializes in perinatal mental health. She provides psychotherapy, training, supervision, and consultation to health care and mental health professionals. She maintains a private practice, Counseling for Reproductive Health & Healing, in Wellesley and Pembroke.

Jodi L. Jacobson is a longtime leader in the health and development community and an advocate with extensive experience in public health, gender equity, human rights, environment, and demographic issues. She is currently editor in chief of RH Reality Check (rhrealitycheck.org).

Lisa Jervis is the founding editor and publisher of *Bitch: Feminist Response to Pop Culture*. Her work has appeared in many magazines and anthologies, and she is the author of *Cook Food: A Manualfesto for Easy, Healthy, Local Eating* (cook-food.org).

Carole Joffe is a professor at the Bixby Center for Global Reproductive Health at UC San Francisco (ansirh.org). She is the author of *Dispatches from the Abortion Wars* and *Doctors of Conscience: The Struggle to Provide Abortion Before and After* Roe v. Wade.

Laura Kaplan is the author of *The Story of Jane: The Legendary Underground Feminist Abortion Service,* a former member of Jane, a board member of the National Women's Health Network, and a lifelong women's health advocate.

Mara Kardas-Nelson is a freelance journalist focusing on health and the environment. She is the assistant editor of *Equal Treatment*, the magazine of the Treatment Action Campaign, and has been published in the United States, Canada, and South Africa.

Martha Ellen Katz, M.D., has practiced medicine with a focus on women's health for thirty years. She works at the Harvard University Health Services, Cambridge, Massachusetts, and the Brigham and Women's Hospital, Boston, and teaches at the Harvard Medical School.

Jean Kilbourne (jeankilbourne.com), creator of the award-winning *Killing Us Softly* films and author of *Can't Buy My Love,* is internationally recognized for her pioneering work on the image of women in advertising and her critical studies of alcohol and tobacco advertising.

Tekoa King, CNM, MPH, is a clinical professor in the Department of Obstetrics, Gynecology and Reproductive

Health at UC San Francisco and a member of the faculty obstetrics clinical practice. She is also a deputy editor for the *Journal of Midwifery & Women's Health*.

Sheryl Kingsberg, PhD, is a clinical psychologist and professor in the Department of Reproductive Biology at Case Western Reserve University School of Medicine and is the chief of the Division of Behavioral Medicine in the Department of Obstetrics and Gynecology at Case Medical Center, University Hospitals of Cleveland.

Cara Kulwicki (thecurvature.com) is a feminist writer whose work centers on sexual assault and other forms of gender-based violence. She blogs at both the Curvature and Feministe.

Jacqueline Lapidus, MTS (jacquelinelapiduswords.net), is an editorial consultant experienced in the fields of health care, business, and travel and is also a poet, translator, and essayist. She has taught writing skills for medical decision making and women's health advocacy at Harvard and Suffolk.

Sylvia Law is a professor at New York University School of Law, and a scholar and activist on issues of health care and reproductive freedom. A founding board member of the Center for Reproductive Rights, she was a lawyer on many reproductive freedom cases.

Linda Layne, PhD (rpi.edu/~laynel), is the mother of two fine sons. Her work includes *Motherhood Lost: A Feminist Account of Pregnancy Loss in America,* the TV series *Motherhood Lost: Conversations,* collections on motherhood and consumption, and *Feminist Technology.* She is now studying single mothers by choice.

Margaret Lazarus (cambridgedocumentaryfilms.org) is an Academy Award–winning documentary filmmaker, author, women's rights and social justice activist, and university lecturer.

Mary Ann Leeper is a senior strategic adviser for Female Health Company, a leader in the development of pharmaceuticals and products that address global women's health issues. She is an authority on international public health issues.

Esther Morris Leidolf is a medical sociologist with a background in public health data management. She founded the MRKH Organization (mrkh.org) in 2000 and served as board secretary for the Intersex Society of North America. Her MRKH articles have been published internationally.

Judith Lennett is the founder and executive director of Northnode, Inc. (northnode.org), a nonprofit agency that works to secure the safety and well-being of frail elders, people with disabilities, and adults and children affected by intimate partner violence.

Mitch Levine, M.D., is a gynecologist committed to providing patients with a less invasive approach to women's health care, especially by avoiding unnecessary surgeries, including hysterectomies. He has been in practice at Women Care, in Cambridge, Massachusetts, since 1981.

Hope Lewis (northeastern.edu/law/academics/faculty/directory/lewis.html), professor of law, Northeastern University School of Law, has been an advocate for women's human rights for more than twenty years. She coauthored *Human Rights and the Global Marketplace.*

Elizabeth Sarah Lindsey is committed to equality, fighting poverty, and developing creative urban development solutions. She holds a master's in public affairs and urban planning from Princeton University. Elizabeth lives in Washington, DC, with her husband, Jonathan Rothwell.

Elaine Lissner is founder of the Male Contraception Information Project and, since 2005, director of Parsemus Foundation (parsemusfoundation.org), which focuses on contraceptive research, animal sterilization, and the impact of hormones on health.

Alice LoCicero, PhD, is a clinical psychologist with a long-standing interest in conventional and alternative approaches to women's health. She has a private practice in Cambridge, Massachusetts.

Maurizio Macaluso, MD, Dr PH, is an epidemiologist and is professor of pediatrics and director of the Division of Biostatistics and Epidemiology, Cincinnati Children's Hospital Medical Center. He was chief of the Women's Health and Fertility Branch at the CDC, where he led surveillance and research on infertility and assisted reproduction.

Alyson Martin is a freelance journalist living in New York City.

Courtney Martin (courtneyemartin.com) is the author of *Do It Anyway: The New Generation of Activists,* among other critically acclaimed books, an editor at Feministing, and a senior correspondent for *The American Prospect.*

Ginny Mazur, MA, LMHC, ATR, has served as community partnership director and in other jobs at Goddard House Skilled Nursing & Rehabilitation Center and Goddard House in Brookline Assisted Living (goddardhouse.org) for the past fifteen years.

Marianne McPherson, PhD, MS, is a mother and a public health researcher with a passion for young women's reproductive health, skiing, and tea. She's worked and studied at NICHQ, Our Bodies Ourselves, Ibis Reproductive Health, Harvard, and the Heller School.

Elise Miller, MEd, is the director of the Collaborative on Health and the Environment (healthandenvironment.org), an international partnership strengthening the scientific and public dialogue on environmental contributors to disease and disability and fostering initiatives to address these concerns.

Irene Monroe (irenemonroe.com) is a Huffington Post blogger and a queer religion columnist. A native of Brooklyn, Monroe is a graduate of Wellesley College and Union Theological Seminary, and served as a pastor before coming to Harvard Divinity School for her doctorate as a Ford Fellow.

Heidi Moore is a writer and editor in Chicago who focuses on culture, health, and environmental issues. Her writing has appeared in the *Chicago Tribune, Time Out Chicago*, and the Chicago guidebook, among other publications.

Cathleen E. Morrow, M.D., is associate professor in the Department of Community and Family Medicine at Dartmouth Medical School. Her clinical focus has been in women's health and obstetrics-gynecology throughout her career; she currently practices and teaches broad spectrum family medicine.

Christine Morton, PhD, is a medical sociologist whose research focuses on maternity care advocacy by doulas, childbirth educators, and, more recently, obstetric clinicians. She is the founder of ReproNetwork.org and is currently with California Maternal Quality Care Collaborative.

Shree Mulay (med.mun.ca/medicine/faculty/mulay,-shree .aspx) is the associate dean and professor in the Community Health and Humanities Division at Memorial University. She has worked for decades on issues related to unsafe contraceptives, assisted human reproduction, and reproductive tourism.

Claire Mysko (clairemysko.com) is a body image expert and the author of *You're Amazing!*—a self-esteem handbook for girls—and coauthor of *Does This Pregnancy Make Me Look Fat? The Essential Guide to Loving Your Body Before and After Baby.*

Elizabeth H. Naumburg, M.D., is currently an associate dean for advising and professor of family medicine at the University of Rochester. Her career has focused on women's health and the issues of gender and race in health care and medical education.

Lin Nelson teaches environment and community studies at Evergreen State College, Olympia, Washington. She works with organizations dealing with environment, workplace, women's lives, and reproductive rights. She's doing community-based research on how mining and metal smelting affect public health.

Amie Newman is a longtime womens' health advocate who has directed communications for a feminist health center, has served as submissions editor for *Our Truths, Nuestras Verdades,* and is currently managing editor for the award-winning reproductive health news publication RH Reality Check (rhrealitycheck.org).

Deanna Nobleza, M.D., is dual board certified in internal medicine and psychiatry and specializes in college mental health. Having previously worked at Princeton University, Dr. Nobleza is currently the director of student counseling at Thomas Jefferson University in Philadelphia.

Craig Norberg-Bohm cofounded in 1978 RAVEN (Rape and Violence End Now) in St. Louis, Missouri. Craig operates Massachusetts White Ribbon Day (jancdoc.org/white ribbonday), a men's campaign of Jane Doe Inc., the Massachusetts Coalition Against Sexual Assault and Domestic Violence.

Gina Ogden, PhD LMFT (ginaogden.com), is a sex therapist and workshop leader. She conducted a nationwide survey on sexuality and spirituality. Her latest books are *Women Who Love Sex, The Heart and Soul of Sex,* and *The Return of Desire.*

Chukwuma Onyeije, M.D. (chukwumaonyeije.com), is a board-certified maternal-fetal medicine specialist and clinical associate professor of obstetrics and gynecology at the Morehouse School of Medicine. His interests are technology, women's health, and patient empowerment through social media and participatory medicine.

Leslye Orloff is vice president and director of Legal Momentum's Immigrant Women Program and a cofounder and cochair of the National Network to End Violence Against Immigrant Women. She has written training curricula, manuals, and story collections bringing immigrant women's voices to national policy makers.

Margaret Owusu is an undergraduate at the University of Pennsylvania, where she is studying health and societies with a concentration in public health. After Penn, she will pursue a career in public health, focusing primarily on adolescent health.

Ruth Palombo, PhD, assistant secretary, Massachusetts Executive Office of Elder Affairs, designs programs that foster empowerment, independence, and well-being for older adults. She is a national leader in nutrition, aging, health promotion, chronic disease prevention, and end-of-life issues.

William Parker, M.D., is a clinical professor of obstetrics and gynecology at the UCLA School of Medicine and in private practice in Santa Monica, California. He is the author of the women's health care book *A Gynecologist's Second Opinion.*

Debra Pascali-Bonaro, LCCE, CD (DONA), is the director of the documentary *Orgasmic Birth: The Best-Kept Secret* (orgasmicbirth.com) and coauthor of *Orgasmic Birth: Your Guide to a Safe, Satisfying and Pleasurable Birth Experience.* Debra is chairperson of the International Mother-Baby Childbirth Initiative.

Su Penn (tapeflags.blogspot.com) was very happy to be asked to help with this edition of OBOS.

Miriam Zoila Pérez (miriamzperez.com) is a writer, blogger, and reproductive justice activist. She is an editor at Feministing and founder of Radical Doula. Pérez was presented with a 2010 Barbara Seaman Award for Activism in Women's Health.

Lisa Perriera, M.D., MPH, is an obstetrician-gynecologist who specializes in family planning. Her main areas of interest are the prevention of unintended pregnancy and contraceptive management of women with bleeding disorders and complicated medical conditions.

Elizabeth Pimentel, ND, trained as a naturopathic physician and midwife. She is committed to empowering women to take charge of their bodies and their health. She currently serves as associate dean of academics at the University of Bridgeport College of Naturopathic Medicine.

Yvonne Piper, MLIS, has worked in health and sex education since 1998. She attends UCSF School of Nursing and volunteers at San Francisco Sex Information and Women's Community Clinic. In addition to writing, she enjoys scuba diving, running, biking, reading, and gluten-free food.

Lauren Plante, M.D., MPH, is the director of maternal-fetal medicine at an academic medical center in Philadelphia, which probably would not like her to name it. She is board-certified in anesthesiology, critical care medicine, ob-gyn, and maternal-fetal medicine and still supports birth choices.

Diana Aquino Price is a fierce advocate for and scholar of feminist issues. She earned her BA from Barnard College in 2006 and is currently pursuing a graduate degree in Asian-American studies at University of California, Los Angeles.

Jerilynn Prior is a professor of endocrinology at the University of British Columbia, Vancouver, and scientific director of the Centre for Menstrual Cycle and Ovulation Research (CeMCOR; cemcor.ubc.ca). Her research has shown the importance of progesterone to women's health and that perimenopause is hormonally distinct from menopause.

Jenni Prokopy is founder and editrix of ChronicBabe.com, a resource for young women with chronic illness. An award-winning writer, speaker, and health expert, she shares her personal experience and rallies the expertise of others to help women live beyond illness.

Holly Ramsey-Klawsnik, PhD, Klawsnik & Klawsnik Associates, Canton, Massachusetts, is a licensed marriage and family therapist, licensed certified social worker, and researcher. Her research, clinical practice, teaching, and publications have focused on interpersonal violence, mental health issues, and self-care.

Nushin Rashidian is a freelance journalist living in New York City.

Nancy Redd (nancyredd.com) is a *New York Times* bestselling author of *Body Drama* and *Diet Drama* and a Harvard women's studies graduate. She is on a worldwide speaking tour designed to help all women love our bodies inside and out!

Jessica Haxton Retrum, PhD, LCSW, is a Postdoctoral Fellow in Public Health Systems and Service Research, CU Denver. She has eight years of clinical experience in health related social work and her doctoral research was related to social work in the field of gerontology.

Marcie Richardson, M.D., is an obstetrician-gynecologist who believes the only way that women can really be empowered is to understand and take charge of their bodies. To this end, she is privileged to have worked on multiple editions of *Our Bodies, Ourselves.*

Gary Richwald, M.D., MPH, is a communicable disease expert with training in internal medicine, epidemiology, and women's health. He teaches at UCLA and USC and is the medical adviser of the Los Angeles and Orange County HSV and HPV support groups.

Karin Ringheim, PhD, MPH, is an independent consultant in global health. She is a past adviser for the Population Reference Bureau and a past adviser for USAID and the World Health Organization. Publications include a book on homelessness and numerous articles on reproductive health and gender.

Susan Roll, PhD, is an assistant professor in the School of Social Work at the University of Maryland. Her research and teaching focus on urban poverty, community practice, and social welfare policy.

Loretta J. Ross is a cofounder and the national coordinator of the SisterSong Women of Color Reproductive Justice Collective (sistersong.net). She has a thirty-five-year-plus history in the feminist movement, from antirape organizing to reproductive justice activism.

Carol Sakala is director of programs at Childbirth Connection (childbirthconnection.org), a national not-for-profit organization that uses research, education, advocacy, and policy to improve the quality of maternity care and ensure that it meets the needs and interests of women, newborns, and families.

Gordon Schiff is a practicing internist, associate director of Brigham Center for Patient Safety Research and Practice, and associate professor of medicine at Harvard. He worked for more than three decades at Chicago's Cook County Hospital, where he directed the General Medicine Clinic.

Susan Sered, PhD, author of *Uninsured in America: Life and Death in the Land of Opportunity* and *Priestess, Mother, Sacred Sister: Religions Dominated by Women,* is on the faculty of Suffolk University. Her current research focuses on life challenges of criminalized women.

Ellen R. Shaffer, PhD, MPH, is codirector of the Center for Policy Analysis (centerforpolicyanalysis.org). The center sponsors the EQUAL Health Network, which campaigns for equitable, quality, universal, affordable health reform; and the Center for Policy Analysis on Trade and Health (CPATH), which explores the links between international trade agreements, vital human services, and health.

Grace Shih, M.D., MAS, is an assistant clinical professor in the Department of Family and Community Medicine at the University of California, San Francisco. When she's not seeing patients, you can find her cooking, hiking, or salsa dancing.

Jocelyn Sims is a Chicago area writer and editor. As an Asian-American woman, she has a particular interest in how Asian women are portrayed in television and film and researched the topic for her master's culminating project.

Norman Spack, M.D., is a pediatric endocrinologist and cofounder of Gender Management (GeMS) Service at Children's Hospital Boston/Harvard Medical School, which treats transgender youth and children with disorders of sex development (DSD).

Kimberly Springer (kimberlyspringer.com) is associate professor of women's studies specializing in mass media, social movements, and digital culture. Her books include *Living for the Revolution: Black Feminist Organizations, 1968–1980* and *Still Lifting, Still Climbing: Contemporary African American Women's Activism.*

Elizabeth Steiner, M.D., is a physician who specializes in family medicine: whole person, whole family, and whole community health. She teaches and does research to improve early detection of breast cancer.

Heather Stephenson was the managing editor of the 2005 edition of *Our Bodies, Ourselves,* editor of *Our Bodies, Ourselves: Menopause,* and executive editor of *Our Bodies, Ourselves: Pregnancy and Birth.* She is the publisher at the Appalachian Mountain Club.

Evelina Sterling, PhD, MPH, CHES, is a reproductive health researcher and educator as well as the author of several consumer health books focusing on women's health.

Elizabeth Stewart, M.D. (vbook.com), is the Director of the Vulvovaginal Service at Vanguard Medical Associates, Atrius Health, Boston. She has been caring for women with vulvovaginal problems and vulvodynia for over twenty years.

Kirsten Thompson, MPH (kirstenthompson.com), conducts reproductive health research and uses new media for public education at the University of California, San Francisco. She received her MPH from the Johns Hopkins Bloomberg School of Public Health and her BA from Bryn Mawr College.

Trisha Torrey is Every Patient's Advocate, an expert in patient empowerment and advocacy, and author of *You Bet Your Life! The 10 Mistakes Every Patient Makes.* Learn more about Trisha's work and expertise at everypatientsadvocate.com and on Twitter at @TrishaTorrey.

Jeane Ungerleider, LICSW, BCD, is Director of Counseling Services for Boston IVF, and cochairs the Ethics Committee at Boston IVF. She is a clinical social worker with particular expertise in women's health. She received her master's degree from Simmons College of Social Work.

Annie Urban is a social, political, and consumer advocate on issues of importance to parents, women, and children. She blogs regularly about the art and science of parenting at phdinparenting.com and can be found on Twitter at @phdinparenting.

Trudy Van Houton, PhD, is the director of the Clinical Applications of Anatomy course and codirector of the Human Body course at Harvard Medical School.

Pamela Vireday, BA, CCE, is a childbirth educator, size acceptance activist, and mother of four. She is the author of the website plus-size-pregnancy.org and the blog Well-Rounded Mama (wellroundedmama.blogspot.com).

Rachel Walden, MLIS, is a librarian at an academic medical center, where she connects people with medical resources and evidence. She blogs about women's health topics for Our Bodies, Our Blog (ourbodiesourblog.org) and at womenshealthnews.wordpress.com.

Robin Wallace, M.D., is a family doctor in the San Francisco Bay Area. She works with underserved and underinsured populations, with an emphasis on preventive and reproductive health care. Her contributions on family planning can also be found on Sex Really (sexreally.com).

Marc Weisskopf, PhD, ScD (hsph.harvard.edu/faculty/marc-weisskopf), is assistant professor of environmental and occupational epidemiology at the Harvard School of Public Health. He studies environmental influences on neurological disorders, plays hockey, and spends time with his wife, Cindy, and children Noah, Mira, and Micah.

Rose Weitz, PhD, is a professor at Arizona State University, the author or editor of numerous works on women's health and bodies, including the books *Rapunzel's Daughters: What Women's Hair Tells Us About Women's Lives* and *The Politics of Women's Bodies.*

Tracy Weitz, PhD, MPA, is an associate professor of obstetrics, gynecology, and reproductive sciences and director of the Advancing New Standards in Reproductive Health (ANSIRH) program of the Bixby Center for Global Reproductive Health (ansirh.org), both at the University of California, San Francisco.

Toni Weschler, MPH, is the author of the groundbreaking bestseller *Taking Charge of Your Fertility* (tcoyf.com) and a book on reproductive health for teens entitled *Cycle Savvy.* She is an internationally respected women's health educator with a master's degree in public health.

Carolyn Westhoff is a gynecologist and epidemiologist at Columbia University. She focuses her clinical practice and research on women's preventive services, contraception, and abortion.

Cosette Marie Wheeler, PhD, is a Regent's Professor of Pathology at the University of New Mexico (UNM) Health Sciences Center. She currently directs one of the nation's five NIH-funded cooperative research centers focused on sexually transmitted infections, the UNM Interdisciplinary HPV Prevention Center.

Sally Whelan is a cofounder of Our Bodies Ourselves. Sally has for the last ten years managed the organization's Global Initiative, where her leadership has resulted in the publication and in-country use of seventeen cultural adaptations of *Our Bodies, Ourselves* around the world.

Beverly Whipple, PhD, RN, FAAN, is professor emerita at Rutgers University and a certified sexuality educator, counselor, and researcher. She has coauthored seven books including the international best-seller *The G Spot and Other Discoveries About Human Sexuality.*

Judy Anne Williams, LICSW, is a clinical social worker, a Quaker, a youth worker, and a bisexual activist. Her work seeks to help us bring together our bodies, minds, hearts, and spirits into an integrated and blessed wholeness.

Jamia Wilson (jamiawilson.com) is vice president of programs at the Women's Media Center in New York. She serves on the leadership committee and cochairs the communications working group for SPARK Summit: Challenging the Sexualization of Girls.

Beverly Winikoff, M.D., MPH, is president of Gynuity Health Projects (gynuity.org) and a professor at Columbia University. At the Population Council, she developed the Ebert Program on Critical Issues in Reproductive Health. She graduated from Harvard University and earned her MD from New York University and MPH from Harvard.

Claire Winstone, PhD (speaking4baby.wordpress.com), is an infant mental health therapist treating early traumas and a prenatal/birth psychology educator who loves sharing with those who are passionate about mothers and babies her understanding of how birth and the prenatal period shape who we are.

Karen Anne Wolf, PhD, RN, NP, a nurse-practitioner and educator, has been an advocate for single-payer health care systems and care for underserved populations. She has contributed to publications and film projects on health care and writes for the website Nurse Together (nursetogether.com).

Susan Wood, PhD, is associate professor of health policy and director of the Jacobs Institute of Women's Health at the George Washington University School of Public Health and Health Services. Previously she was the assistant commissioner for women's health at the U.S. Food and Drug Administration until 2005, when she resigned on principle owing to the continuing delays of approval of over-the-counter emergency contraception by the FDA.

Fred Wyand is a sexual health educator and the editor of *HPV News,* published by the American Social Health Association (ASHA: ashastd.org). He is also director of ASHA's national resource centers for HPV and herpes.

Susan Wysocki, WHNP-BC, FAANP, is the president and CEO of the National Association of Nurse Practitioners in Women's Health (NPWH: npwh.org). She is a woman's health nurse-practitioner and a nationally recognized speaker, writer, and opinion leader in the field of women's health.

Susan Yanow, MSW, was the founding executive director of the Abortion Access Project. She currently consults for national and international organizations that support abortion as a fundamental human right and work to expand all women's access to abortion.

Courtney Young (thethirtymilewoman.wordpress.com) is a Manhattan-based popular culture writer. She has written for publications such as the *Nation,* the *Huffington Post,* and the *Daily Beast.* She is currently a staff writer for *Campus Progress.*

Diony Young has been editor of *Birth: Issues in Perinatal Care* since 1990. She authored the award-winning *Changing Childbirth: Family Birth in the Hospital* and many other publications. For more than thirty years she has advocated on numerous national and state maternal health advisory groups.

Meg Young is an undergraduate at Tufts University, where she hopes to study absolutely everything. During her gap year between high school and college she worked as an intern at Our Bodies Ourselves. She hails originally from Cornwall, Vermont.

Kay Zakariasen authored and ran an online patient survey (cystitispatientsurvey.com) with 1,800 respondents. She is also coauthor of an article in the journal *Urology* and coauthor of an article for the National Women's Health Network.

Deanna Zandt (deannazandt.com) is a media technologist and the author of *Share This! How You Will Change the World with Social Networking.* She is a consultant to key progressive media organizations and is a research fellow at the Center for Social Media at American University.

Miriam Zoll (miriamzoll.net) is a writer and communications strategist specializing in health and gender issues and the founding coproducer of the Ms. Foundation's Take Our Daughters to Work program. Her clients include UN agencies, USAID, and the Earth Institute, among others.

Diana Zuckerman, PhD, is president of the National Research Center for Women & Families (center4research .org), a nonprofit health organization. She previously worked in the U.S. Congress and at Vassar, Yale, and Harvard, has written five books, and is frequently quoted in national media.

Janna Zwerner, M.R.C., CRC, has been employed in the health and disability field for more than thirty years. She is currently the COO of the National Association of Chronic Disease Directors. She is particularly interested in sexuality and women with disabilities.

Page numbers in *italics* refer to illustrations.

Access Living, 191
Accord Alliance, 15
acne, 185, 225, 236, 238, 539, 631, 648
acquaintance rape, 704
active phase of labor, 403, 405–10, 412, 418
activism, twenty-first century, 808–25
    challenging mainstream science and industry, 819–22
    global, 822–23
    making our voices heard and, 810–13
    recommended resources for, 811, 823
    for reproductive health and justice, 813–17
    sexualization of young girls and women and, 817–19
Actonel, 532
Actonel with Calcium, 532
acupressure points, 25, 633
acupuncture, 305, 497, 613, 620
acute, defined, 729
acyclovir, 295
Adams, Jill, 776
Addams, Jane, 753
addiction:
    pregnancy and, 388
    to tanning, 52
    see also alcohol, abuse of; drug abuse
adenocarcinoma, 627
adenomyosis, 612, 613
adenosis, 628
ADHD, 177, 742
adhesions, 187, 650
Adiana, 242–45, 255
Administration on Aging, U.S., 558, 570, 575–76
adolescence, adolescents:
    abstinence in, 143, 271
    anovulation in, 26
    birth control and, 207, 208
    body image mentors for, 65
    breasts in, 15, *17*
    DES and, 739
    dieting of, 66
    grandparents and, 565
    marketing to, 64–65
    pregnancy in, *see* teen pregnancy
    sexualization of, 817
    statutory rape and, 700*n*
    STIs in, 258, 259, 271, 275, 276, 279, 280, 565, 766
    transsexual, medical intervention for, 83
    vaccination of, 277, 616, 617
    violence against, 701, 720–21
adoption, 127, 349, 434, 464, 475, 501, 525
    breastfeeding and, 444–45

depression after, 455
    as path to parenthood, 356–58
    unplanned pregnancy and, 313, 315
adrenals, 188, 189, *640*
advance directive forms, 571
advertising, 25, 817
    body image and, 45, 46, 47, 50, 59, 62–65, 70, 549–50
    breasts and, 13
    drugs, 660–61
    food, 68
    history of women in, 63
    menstrual flow and, 22
    osteoporosis and, 528, 531
Advil, 432, 443
advocacy, environmental health and, 731–32
Advocates for Youth, 272
Aetna, 489
Afghanistan, 779, 782
Africa, 48, 594, 646, 666, 738, 747, 798, 799, 823
    abortion in, 788
    birth rates in, 781
    cervical cancer in, 794
    family planning in, 783
    life expectancy in, 779
    sub-Saharan, 779, 781, 782, 783, 795
    see also specific countries
African Americans, 745, 810
    children, lead poisoning of, 732–33
    males, 60, 66, 117, 123, 126–27, 144, 301, 767
African American women, 96, 769
    abortion and, 813–15
    access to health care of, 680
    in aging studies, 542, 543, 545
    birth rates for, 781
    body image of, 47, *48*, 49, 50, 60, 66
    BPA and, 740
    breastfeeding of, 446
    cancer of, 543, 593–94, 616, 744, 754, 761
    colorism and, 50
    disparities in health of, 761, 764, 767
    fibroids in, 608, 630
    hysterectomy in, 630
    interracial marriage of, 125
    lesbians, 93
    life expectancy of, 761
    old age and, 549, 555
    perimenopause and menopause in, 509
    poverty of, 760
    pregnancy loss in, 469, 471
    queering of heterosexuality of, 145
    relationships and, 122–23, 125, 126–27

stereotypes of, 144, 695
    STIs in, 280, 282–83, 301, 766–67
    teen pregnancy of, 765
    as uninsured, 768
    violence against, 695–96, 699
    workpace activism of, 748
age:
    abortion and, 317
    birth control and, 209, 210, 226
    breast cancer screening and, 591–92
    feeling of, 578–79
    health insurance and, 569, 772
    infertility and, 476–77
    IVF and, 488
    marriage by, 114, 462
    at menopause, 17, 593
    at menstruation, 18, 26, 593, 594, 597
    for old age, 578
    Plan B and, 765
    pregnancy and, 385
    safer sex and, 259, 261
    stillbirth and, 469
    STIs and, 277, 279, 280, 299
Age4Action Network, 579
ageism, 508, 549
Agent Orange, 739
aging, 660
    feminized, 549
    fertility and, 351, 476–77
    medicalization of, 550
    miscarriage and, 351, 462, 477
    pregnancy loss and, 351, 462
    relationships and, 110, 137–38, 550–54
    research on, 542–43, 545
    single status and, 105
    vagina and, 187
    see also menopause; old age; perimenopause; postmenopausal women
Aging in Place Initiative, 570
Aging Our Way (Loe), 561
Aging with Dignity, 572
Aging with Options, 568
AGS Foundation for Health in Aging, 559
A Heartbreaking Choice, 335
AIDS, 241, 274, 276, 301–7, 761
    birth control as protection against, 201, 211, 218, 337
    birth control which fails to protect against, 224
    course of, 304
    death from, 283, 767
    global, 779, 785, 787, 789, 795–800
    reporting requirements and, 289
    safer sex and, 273
    see also HIV

North American Menopause Society (NAMS), 534, 543
North Carolina, 748
Norway, 627, 782
nose reshaping (rhinoplasty), 54
noses, 56, 517
notification laws, abortion and, 323, 343
Novarel, 484
NovaSure, 613
NOW, Love Your Body campaign of, 71
Nubain, 414
nucleic acid amplification DNA test (NAAT), 291, 293
nurse-midwives, 654, 679, *747*
nurse-practitioners, 286, 658, 673, 679
nurses, 366, 393, 412, 566, 748
   breastfeeding and, 440
   sexual assault, 706
Nursing Freedom, 454
nursing homes, 567, 569, 570, 572, 710
Nussbaum, Susan, 192
NuvaRing, 189, 197, 231, 251

Obama, Barack, 122, 697, 760, 770, 774–77, 785
Obama, Michelle, 50, 122
obesity, 648, 742, 762, 780
   cancer and, 593, 595, 610
   postmenopausal, 593
   pregnancy and, 385, 469
   risks of, 68
objects, objectification, 57, 141, 693, 817
obsessive-compulsive disorder, 67, 455, 456
obstetric fistula, 646, 782–83
obstetrician-gynecologists, 366, 519, 658
obstetricians, 363, 373, 384
occupational health, *see* environmental and occupational health
Occupational Safety and Health Administration, U.S. (OSHA), 728, 733
ochronosis, 47
Odette, Fran, 193
"Offensive Feminism" (Filipovic), 164
Office on Women's Health, U.S., 581
   Breastfeeding Helpline of, 438
Ogden, Gina, 155, 564
Ohio, sex education in, 765
oil-based lubricants, 177, 178, 213, 214, 268
   diaphragm and, 220
   female condom and, 215
Ojanen-Goldsmith, Alison, 727
old age, 547–83
   advocacy and, 581–83
   body image and, 549–50
   caregiving and, 572–77

common chronic diseases and, 556–57
decline of poverty in, 761
elder abuse and neglect in, 575–76, 693–94, 711
end-of-life care and, 571–72
going it alone in, 554
guidelines for sexual and reproductive health care in, 557–60
health and, 554–60
health and legal decisions and, 571
health information sources for, 559
household help and long-term care and, 570–71
housing and, 568, 570, 576
LGBT, 558
living fully in, 577–83
Medicare basics and, 569–70
navigating health care and, 566–68
new, 548–50
physical changes that affect sexuality in, 562–64
planning ahead in, 568–72
preventive measures and, 555–56
recommended reading for, 551, 564, 573, 577
relationships and, 550–54, 564
retirement and Social Security in, 568
sexuality and, 560–66
sexual pleasure in, 561, 565–66
Older Americans 2010 (U.S. government report), 566
Older Americans Act (1965), 579
Old Lesbians Organizing for Change, 550
oligomenorrhea, 26
omega-3 fatty acids, 25, 447
oncologists, 533, 600, 604
oophorectomy, 169, 506, 524, 529, 599, 621, 626, 630–32
   cysts and, 620
   long-term risks of, 631
   self-help and, 633–34
   sexuality and, 631–32
OpEd Project, 811
Operation Rescue, 340
opioids (narcotics), 414–16, 418
oral herpes, 263, 294, 295, 296
oral sex, 169, 173, 185, 215, 565, 721
   safer sex and, 263–64
   spermicides and, 222
   STIs and, 290, 292, 294, 296
Oregon Environmental Council, 740
O'Reilly, Bill, 809
Orenstein, Peggy, 64–65
Organic Birth (Davis and Pascali-Bonaro), 425

Organization of Teratology Information Specialists, 392
orgasm, 112, 113, 154–62, 168, 517, 631
   breastfeeding and, 450
   clitoris and, 5–6, 156–59, 177
   disabilities and, 157, 193
   effects of medications and hormones on, 188, 189
   fantasies and, 174
   intercourse and, 155, 159, 172
   lack of, 158–59
   male, 147
   masturbation and, 157, 158
   missing of, 157–58
   multiple, 158
   in old age, 562, 563, 564
   pornography and, 180
   power and, 147
   as sexual response, 154, 155
   simultaneous, 158
Orgasm Answer Guide, The (Komisaruk, Whipple, Nasserzadeh, and Beyer-Flores), 156
Orgasm Inc. (documentary), 183
Ortho Evra, 189, 229, 251
orthopedic surgeons, 567
Osher Lifelong Learning Institutes, 578
osmotic dilators, 333, 334
osteoarthritis, 543
osteopenia, 531, 538, 559
osteoporosis, 522, 523, 543, 556, 558–60, 596
   diet and, 527–30
   marketing of, 531
   prevention of, 528–32, 536
Osteoporosis International, 530
Ostlin, Piroska, 777
ostomy, 196
Our Bodies, Ourselves: Pregnancy and Birth, 382
Our Bodies, Ourselves, foreign adaptations of, 32, 48, *48,* 492, *492, 526, 527,* 718, 784–87, *784, 786, 791, 797, 797*
Our Bodies Ourselves, 805, 807
Our Bodies Ourselves Global Initiative, xii
ourbodiesourselves.org, resource section of, 158
Our Stolen Future (Colborn, Dumanoski, and Meyers), 754–55
"Outing Age 2010," 558
ovarian cancer, 225, 241, 559, 597–98, 599, 620–21, 805
   diagnosis of, 620–21
   medical treatment for, 621, 629, 630
   risk factors for, 620
   in trans men, 83

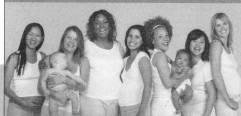
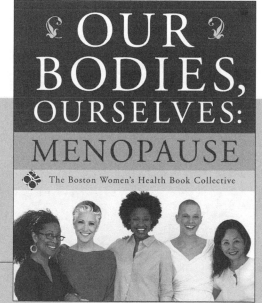
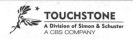